MDS	minimum data set (long-term care)
MET	basal metabolic equivalent
MI	myocardial infarction (heart attack)
MP	(see MCP)
MRI	magnetic resonance imaging
MRSA	methicillin-resistant *Staphylococcus aureus*
MS	multiple sclerosis
n	normal
NDT	neurodevelopmental treatment
NMES	neuromuscular electrical stimulation
NPO, npo	nothing by mouth (non per os)
NWB	non-weight bearing
OA	osteoarthritis
OBS	organic brain syndrome
ORIF	open reduction and internal fixation (i.e., of bones)
OSHA	Occupational Safety and Health Administration
OTAS	occupational therapy assistant student
OTR	registered occupational therapist
OTS	occupational therapy student (professional level)
P&A	percussion and auscultation
P-A, PA	posteroanterior; also for PA, physician assistant
p.c.	after meals (post cibum)
p/o	postoperative
PCA	patient-controlled administration (e.g., of medication)
PE	physical examination; also, pulmonary embolism
PET	positron emission tomography
PFM	peak flow meter
PFTs	pulmonary function tests
PH	past history
PI	previous illness
PIP	proximal interphalangeal
PLB	pursed lip breathing
PO, p.o.	by mouth (per os)
POV	power operated vehicle
PNF	proprioceptive neuromuscular facilitation
PNS	peripheral nervous system
PRN, prn	as required, as needed (pro re nata)
PROM	passive range of motion
PT	physical therapy, physical therapist
PTA	physical therapy assistant; also, post-traumatic amnesia
PTVS	post-traumatic vision syndrome
PVC	premature ventricular complex
PWB	partial weight bearing
q.	each, every
RA	rheumatoid arthritis
RAD	reactive airway disease
RAI	resident assessment instrument (long-term care)
RAP	resident assessment protocol (long-term care)
RCVA	right cerebrovascular accident (stroke)
RHD	rheumatic heart disease
R/O	rule out (as in diagnosis)
ROM	range of motion
RPE	rate of perceived exertion
RPP	rate pressure product
RSD	reflex sympathetic dystrophy
RSI	repetitive strain injury
RT	respiratory therapy
RVU	relative value unit
Rx	prescription
SICU	surgical intensive care unit
SCI	spinal cord injury
SLE	systemic lupus erythematosus
SNF	skilled nursing facility
SOB	shortness of breath
SROM	self range of motion
STSG	split-thickness (mesh of sheet) skin graft
TAM	total active range of motion
TBI	traumatic brain injury
TENS	transcutaneous electrical nerve stimulation
THR	total hip replacement
tid	three times a day
TIA	transient ischemic attack
TKA	total knee arthroplasty
TLC	tender loving care
TPM	total passive range of motion
TTWB	toe touch weight bearing
Tx	treatment
UE	upper extremity
US	ultrasound
VA	Veteran's Administration
VF	field of vision
WBAT	weight bearing at tolerance
WBC	white blood cell
W/C	wheelchair
WHO	wrist-hand orthosis

Physical Dysfunction Practice Skills for the Occupational Therapy Assistant

Physical Dysfunction Practice Skills for the Occupational Therapy Assistant

THIRD EDITION

Mary Beth Early, MS, OTR/L

Professor, Occupational Therapy Assistant Program
Department of Health Sciences
La Guardia Community College
City University of New York
Long Island City, New York

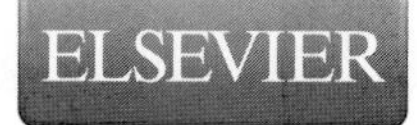

ELSEVIER
MOSBY

3251 Riverport Lane
St. Louis, Missouri 63043

EARLY: PHYSICAL DYSFUNCTION: PRACTICE SKILLS FOR THE OCCUPATIONAL THERAPY ASSISTANT

ISBN: 978-0-323-05909-1

Notices

Knowledge and best practice in this field are constantly changing. As new research and experience broaden our understanding, changes in research methods, professional practices, or medical treatment may become necessary.

Practitioners and researchers must always rely on their own experience and knowledge in evaluating and using any information, methods, compounds, or experiments described herein. In using such information or methods they should be mindful of their own safety and the safety of others, including parties for whom they have a professional responsibility.

With respect to any drug or pharmaceutical products identified, readers are advised to check the most current information provided (i) on procedures featured or (ii) by the manufacturer of each product to be administered, to verify the recommended dose or formula, the method and duration of administration, and contraindications. It is the responsibility of practitioners, relying on their own experience and knowledge of their patients, to make diagnoses, to determine dosages and the best treatment for each individual patient, and to take all appropriate safety precautions.

To the fullest extent of the law, neither the Publisher nor the authors, contributors, or editors, assume any liability for any injury and/or damage to persons or property as a matter of products liability, negligence or otherwise, or from any use or operation of any methods, products, instructions, or ideas contained in the material herein.

ISBN: 978-0-323-05909-1

Top left cover photo from Pendleton HM and Schultz-Krohn W: Pedretti's Occupational Therapy: Practice Skills for Physical Dysfunction, 6th ed, St Louis, 2006, Mosby.
Bottom left cover photo courtesy of Hank Morgan/Photo Researchers, Inc.

Vice President and Publisher: Linda Duncan
Content Strategist: Kathy Falk
Content Manager: Jolynn Grower
Publishing Services Manager: Julie Eddy/Hemamalini Rajendrababu
Project Manager: Kelly Milford/Prathibha Mehta
Designer: Karen Pauls

Printed in United States

Last digit is the print number: 9 8 7 6 5 4 3

To the students and graduates of the LaGuardia Community College Occupational Therapy Assistant Program, whose energy and enthusiasm have always inspired me to do my best to serve them, and who have enriched my life beyond measure.

I also dedicate this book to Hermine Plotnick and Naomi Greenberg. Hermine was on the committee that developed the LaGuardia program, and Naomi was its first director, remaining the director for decades. Both of these veteran occupational therapy educators embody the ideals of service, social justice, and inclusion that created and sustained two programs, as well as the articulation between them—an occupational therapy assistant program (at LaGuardia) and a professional occupational therapy program (at York College of the City University of New York, where Hermine was director).

CONTRIBUTORS

Carole Adler, BA, OTL
Rehab Case Manager, Spinal Cord Injury & Rehab Trauma Center
Patient Care Coordination
Santa Clara Valley Medical Center
San Jose, California

Denis Anson, MS, OTR
Director of Research and Development
Assistive Technology Research Institute
Misericordia University
Dallas, Pennsylvania

Serena M. Berger, MA, OT
Occupational Therapist
Westchester Rehabilitation Program
Visiting Nurse Service of New York
New York, New York

Ann Burkhardt, OTD, OTR/L, FAOTA
Adjunct Faculty
Occupational Therapy
Temple University
Philadelphia, Pennsylvania
Occupational Therapist
Therapy Resources Management
Fall River, Massachussetts

Estelle B. Breines, PhD, OTR, FAOTA
President
Geri-Rehab, Inc.
Lebanon, New Jersey

Sue Byers-Connon, MS, COTA/L, ROH
Former Instructor
OTA Program
Allied Health Division
Instructor, GED Program
Mt. Hood Community College
Gresham, Oregon

Patricia C. Coker-Bolt, PhD, OTR/L
Assistant Professor
College of Health Professions
Medical University of South Carolina
Charleston, South Carolina

Kerby Coulanges, MS, OTR/L
Occupational Therapy Supervisor
Department of Rehabilitation Services
Center for Nursing and Rehabilitation
Brooklyn, New York

Mariana D'Amico, EdD, OTR/L
Associate Professor
Department of Occupational Therapy
Georgia Health Sciences University
Augusta, Georgia

Beth Deverix, MBA/HCM, OTR/L
Clinical Specialist
Occupational Therapy
Genesis Rehabilitation Services
Andover, Massachusetts

Jessica Farman, MS, OTR/L
Director of Rehabilitation
Belmont Manor Nursing Center
Belmont, Massachusetts

Patricia Ann Gentile, DPS, OTR/L
Administrator
Certified Home Health Agency
Jamaica Hospital Medical Center
Jamaica, New York
Adjunct Instructor
Occupational Therapy Department
New York University
New York, New York

Glen Gillen, EdD, OTR/L, FAOTA
Associate Professor of Clinical Occupational Therapy
Department of Rehabilitation and Regenerative Medicine
Columbia University
New York, New York

Terri R. Gonzalez, EdD, OTR, LMT
Faculty
Allied Health Department
Laredo Community College
Laredo, Texas

Elza R. Guzman, MS OTR/L
Senior Occupational Therapist
Rehabilitation Medicine
New York Presbyterian Hospital-Weill Cornell
New York, New York

Pamela B. Harrell, OTR, CHT
Manager, Rehabilitation Services
Vanderbilt Orthopaedics Cool Springs
Vanderbilt University Medical Center
Nashville, Tennessee

Denise Haruko Ha, OTR/L, CBIS
Occupational Therapist II
Occupational Therapy Vocational Services
Adult Brain Injury Day Rehabilitation Center Rancho
Los Amigos National Rehabilitation Center
Downey, California

Emily Holzberg, MS, OTL, CHT
Occupational Therapist/ Certified Hand Therapist
Hand Rehabilitation Center
Dominican Hospital
Santa Cruz, California

Lynn E. Jaffe, ScD, OTR/L
Associate Professor
Occupational Therapy
Georgia Health Sciences University, Colleges of Allied Health and Graduate Studies
Augusta, Georgia

Jessica L. Koch, OTR/L
Occupational Therapy Alumni
Quinnipiac University
Hamden, Connecticut

Sonia Lawson, PhD, OTR/L
Associate Professor
Department of Occupational Therapy & Occupational Science
Towson University
Towson, Maryland

Cynthia J. Liska, BS, OTR
Instructor and Academic Fieldwork Coordinator
Department of Occupational Therapy
Navarro College
Corsicana, Texas

Michelle Mahone, OTR
Early Childhood Intervention of North Central Texas
MHMR of Tarrant County
Waxahachie, Texas

Maureen Michele Matthews, BSOT
Therapy Program Manager
Therapy Services Department
Santa Clara Valley Medical Center
San Jose, California

Michele D. Mills, MA, OTR
Assistant Professor
Division of Occupational Therapy
Long Island University
Brooklyn Campus
Brooklyn, New York

Miriam Watson Monahan, MS OTR/L, CDRS, CDI
Former Program Coordinator
Driver Rehabilitation Program
Fletcher Allen Health Care
Burlington, Vermont
Research Therapist
Institute for Mobility Activity and Participation
Public Health and Health Professions
University of Florida
Gainesville, Florida

Lynne F. Murphy, MS, OTR/L
Clinical Assistant Professor
Department of Occupational Therapy and Occupational Science
Towson University
Towson, Maryland

Jenny Nyblod, M Ed, OTR/L
Occupational Therapy Instructor
Occupational Therapy Program
Green River Community College
Auburn, Washington

Jane Clifford O'Brien, PhD, OTR
Program Director
Occupational Therapy Department
Westbrook College of Health Professions
University of New England
Portland, Maine

Eugenia Papadopoulos, MA, OTR/L, CHT
Clinical Specialist
Occupational Therapy—Rehabilitation Medicine
New York Presbyterian-Weill Cornell
New York, New York

Jill J. Page, OTR/L
Industrial Rehabilitation Consultant
Ergoscience, Inc.
Birmingham, Alabama

Steve Park, MS, OT
Associate Professor
School of Occupational Therapy
Pacific University
Forest Grove, Oregon

Michael Pizzi, PhD, OTR/L, FAOTA
Assistant Professor
Department of Occupational Therapy
Shenandoah University
Winchester, Virginia

Sally E. Poole, MA, OT, CHT
Clinical Assistant Professor
Department of Occupational Therapy
Steinhardt School of Culture, Education and Human Development
New York University
New York, New York
Co-owner
Hands-On Rehab
Valhalla, New York

Elizabeth A. Rivers, MA, OTR/L, RN
Clinical Instructor (Retired)
Department of Occupational Therapy
St. Catherine University
Burn Rehabilitation Clinical Specialist (Retired)
Burn Center, Physical Medicine and Rehabilitation
Regions Hospital
St. Paul, Minnesota

Regula H. Robnett, PhD, OTR/L
Professor
Department of Occupational Therapy
University of New England
Portland, Maine

Martha J. Sanders, PhD, MSOSH, OTR/L, CPE
Associate Professor
Occupational Therapy Department
Quinnipiac University
Hamden, Connecticut

Lori M. Shiffman, MS, OTR/L, BCPR
Owner and Occupational Therapist
Occupational Therapy Private Practice
Life Balance Rehabilitation
Midlothian, Virginia

Vicki Smith, EdD, MBA, OTR/L
Chair and Associate Professor
Department of Occupational Therapy
Keuka College
Keuka Park, New York

Jean W. Solomon, MHS, OTR/L
Occupational Therapist
Berkeley County School District
Moncks Corner, South Carolina

Christine M. Wietlisbach, OTD, MPA, CHT
Occupational Therapist, Hand Therapy/Employee Safety/Ergonomics
Eisenhower Medical Center
Rancho Mirage, California
Instructor, Occupational Therapy Sciences
School of Allied Health Professions
Loma Linda University
Loma Linda, California

PREFACE

The third edition of the *Physical Dysfunction Practice Skills for the Occupational Therapy Assistant* updates and expands this text designed specifically for the occupational therapy assistant (OTA) student. The authors embrace the notion that every person has a natural and compelling desire to function and participate in activities and occupations that he or she finds meaningful, productive, and interesting. Although the practice of occupational therapy has acquired many techniques and interventions over its history, the core of practice is the restoration of ability to participate in personally selected and valued occupations. Consequently, the present text focuses quite clearly on this core of practice, as is reflected in the organization of chapters and information within chapters. Throughout, the reader will see a pervasive emphasis on occupation, participation in occupation, and engagement in functional activities.

The text presents concepts and information needed for entry-level practice in physical disabilities and has been revised to conform to the American Occupational Therapy Association's (AOTA) *Occupational Therapy Practice Framework: Domain and Process, Second Edition (OTPF-2)* and to provide major content required by the Accreditation Council for Occupational Therapy Education's (ACOTE) *Standards for an Accredited Educational Program for the Occupational Therapy Assistant.* The text may also serve as a resource for occupational therapy practitioners at all levels seeking to understand the role of the OTA in physical dysfunction practice. Strict attention has been given to AOTA guidelines for practice, supervision, and service competency.

This edition continues to provide depth of content beyond entry level so that it may continue to serve as a resource to the OTA in the clinic. We have also recognized that individual schools and practitioners in different areas of the country may need specialized material to meet the needs of their local practice environment and have tried to include this information without compromising the parameters of technical level practice or unduly enlarging the book.

Certain assumptions were made when designing this book for the technical level student. First, the student should have completed basic anatomy and physiology and foundation occupational therapy courses. Second, the student should have completed or should be taking as a co-requisite a course in medical conditions or pathology. Third, the student must be willing to supplement this text with references, such as medical dictionaries and pathology texts, which will provide background information. We have made a sincere effort to write the book in such a way that it is understandable to an associate degree student, but it is not an elementary text.

The book is organized into seven sections. Part I covers theory and foundations for the role of the OTA in physical dysfunction practice. The history chapter included in previous editions has been deleted in response to suggestions from reviewers. The psychosocial chapter has been retitled and reworked to reflect recent understanding of the perspective of persons with disabilities, and to provide more direction for the reader in responding to patient concerns and behavior. Part II explains the occupational therapy process and documentation of service. Part III provides extensive information on evaluation and includes some evaluations that are beyond entry level but in which the OTA might reasonably be expected to achieve competency, at least in certain practice environments. Part IV introduces basic principles of intervention. Performance in areas of occupation is the focus of Part V, which includes chapters on activities of daily living, mobility, sexuality, work, technology, and leisure and social participation. Part VI opens with a chapter on the special needs of the older adult, but it also includes chapters on the major intervention modalities and techniques used for physical dysfunction. Part VII provides treatment applications for a variety of clinical conditions seen in physical disabilities practice, including cerebrovascular accident, traumatic brain injury, degenerative diseases, amputations, lower and upper extremity orthopedics, spinal cord injury, burns, oncology, HIV, cardiac dysfunction, and chronic obstructive pulmonary disease.

Special features include lists of key terms and objectives for each chapter, selected reading guide questions at the end of each chapter, text boxes highlighting special techniques, case studies and treatment plans, and a wealth of illustrations and photographs. A guide to selected acronyms has been included inside the back cover.

To make the best use of this text, we recommend that readers begin with the objectives, key terms, and reading guide questions for the targeted chapter. Then, making use of a medical dictionary as needed, the student should read the chapter or section completely, without taking notes and with an aim to understanding what is being read. During a separate session, the student should then do a second reading, make an outline or notes from the text, and attempt to answer the reading guide questions. This level of thoroughness and repetition is critical to mastery of the material.

Certain terms in this book have been used to describe both the occupational therapy service provider and the consumer. The consumer may be referred to as *patient, client, resident,* or *caregiver,* depending on the context of the intervention. The terms *practitioner* and *clinician* refer to providers of occupational therapy services at both levels of practice (i.e., both the occupational therapist and the OTA). The words *assistant,* OTA, and *occupational therapy assistant* are used to designate the technical-level practitioner. The terms *therapist* and *occupational therapist* indicate the professional-level practitioner. Occasionally the word *therapist* is used more generically to describe the provider of therapy but is intended to designate both levels of practitioners.

Mary Beth Early

ACKNOWLEDGMENTS

The first acknowledgment goes to the many contributors who provided the expertise and specialized information for the diverse chapters; this book would not exist but for their professional expertise and support. Jane O'Brien was especially helpful in finding contributors, as were Glen Gillen, Rebekah Walker, and Maureen Matthews. I am indebted to those who made contributions to the first and second editions. Again, special acknowledgment belongs to Lorraine Williams Pedretti and her contributors, whose pioneering efforts in their text, *Occupational Therapy: Practice Skills for Physical Dysfunction* (now in its seventh edition), inspired the first edition of this text.

I want to thank in particular Hermine Plotnick for her review of the history chapter, formerly Chapter 1, now deleted. Jan Froelich and Rosemary Early reviewed Chapter 2 and made helpful suggestions, much appreciated. Twenty-nine faculty members across the country responded to a publisher survey and provided detailed guidance; this was invaluable to me as I organized this project.

All of the editors and staff at Mosby have been supportive, professional, and endlessly helpful. I am grateful to Kathy Falk, Content Strategist, and Jolynn Gower, Content Manager, for their patient and reliable guidance and assistance. Jolynn demonstrated time and again great flexibility, ingenuity, and tact. I thank Sarah Vora, Editorial Assistant, for her management of details. Thanks are also due to Kelly Milford, Project Manager, for her careful scrutiny and stewardship of the production process.

CONTENTS

PART VII
Clinical Applications

PART I

Foundations

CHAPTER 1

Occupational Therapy and Physical Disabilities: Scope, Theory, and Approaches to Practice

MARY BETH EARLY

Key Terms

Occupation
Areas of occupation
Performance skills
Performance patterns
Context and environment
Activity demands
Client factors
Values, beliefs, and spirituality
Body functions
Body structures
Models
Practice model
Systems model
Volition
Habituation
Performance capacity
The lived body
Biomechanical approach
Kinetics
Statics
Sensorimotor approach
Neurophysiological
Reflex
Motor learning
Rehabilitation approach
Treatment continuum
Adjunctive methods
Enabling activities
Purposeful activity
Occupational roles
Evidence
Evidence-based practice

Chapter Objectives

After studying this chapter, the student or practitioner will be able to do the following:

1. Review the main concepts of the *Occupational Therapy Practice Framework: Domain and Process, 2nd edition (OTPF-2E).*
2. Apply the ideas of the *OTPF-2E* to the practice of physical disabilities.
3. Give examples in which impairment in body functions and structures impairs participation in occupation.
4. Discuss the importance of skills, habits, routines, rituals, and roles in performance of occupation.
5. Consider the effects of values, beliefs, and spirituality on occupational performance and on the rehabilitation process.
6. Illustrate ways in which different kinds of environments and contexts affect occupational performance.
7. Discuss why identifying client concerns is the recommended starting point for planning interventions.
8. Describe the model of human occupation and illustrate its application to a person with a physical disability.
9. Explain the principles of occupational therapy intervention that derive from the model of human occupation.
10. Describe the following approaches: biomechanical, sensorimotor/motor learning, and rehabilitation.
11. Differentiate these approaches from one another, and identify the practice situations in which each might be used.
12. Describe the *treatment continuum* and its four stages: adjunctive methods, enabling activities, purposeful activity, and occupational performance and occupational roles.
13. Discuss the role of evidence in selecting practice approaches and specific interventions.

This chapter reminds the reader of the scope and interests of occupational therapy (OT), as differentiated from other professions and scholarly disciplines. The authors expect that the material presented in the first part of this chapter is not entirely new to the reader. For many students, it will be a review. The latter part of this chapter discusses some of the theories and models used in OT practice in physical dysfunction.

In physical disabilities practice—where so many techniques and modalities address body functions and structures—clarifying the purposes and concerns of OT is essential. Students and new practitioners sometimes fall into the habit of medicalizing their thinking and their practice, perhaps sidetracked by the patient's symptoms, medical history, and test results or fascinated by mechanical devices (pulleys, weights, exercise machines) and modalities (hot packs, fluidotherapy, paraffin). In these new preoccupations, students and practitioners can easily lose sight of occupation and the occupational functioning in life roles that are important to the individual patient or client.

In its *Occupational Therapy Practice Framework: Domain and Process, 2nd Edition,*[2] henceforth referred to as *OTPF-2E,* the American Occupational Therapy Association (AOTA) outlines the unique focus of the profession and delineates the issues that OT should address. The purpose is to identify clearly the factors that the OT and occupational therapy assistant (OTA) should consider. In describing its unique focus, the OT profession lays claim to a certain territory within the broader areas of medicine and rehabilitation. By analogy, plumbers and electricians work within clearly marked territories. However, the territories of plumbers and electricians are necessarily shared with other professionals such as architects, engineers, and general contractors. This situation is also the case in our profession, where many aspects of practice overlap with those of other professions (e.g., physical therapists, physicians, social workers, psychologists). This overlap is all the more reason to be clear about the focus of OT.*

OT's domain of concern is occupation, and in particular "supporting health and participation in life through engagement in occupation."[2] No other profession has this focus. Occupation includes functional life activities (e.g., grooming, working, caring for children) and is classified by performance in eight areas of occupation (Figure 1-1). The main purpose of OT is to address performance issues that interfere with successful participation in occupation. For example, OT can help the person who has had a stroke and has weakness and impaired function of one side of the body to return to independence in dressing and self-care, working, and leisure activities.

Performance skills are the building blocks of performance in occupation. These skills (see Figure 1-1 and Table 1-1) apply flexibly and with many minute levels of precision to the entire range of human occupation, from caring for children to operating a forklift to designing web pages. The individual performing an occupation benefits from patterns such as habits, routines, rituals, and roles. Patterns help to make performance more automatic and thus less demanding of conscious attention. For example, the web page designer who knows HTML commands thoroughly may flow through the workday without having to think much about which command applies to a given task. Conversely, the student who is learning HTML must struggle more to find the right command for the desired effect.

The performance skills and patterns of the person who is engaged in an occupation are affected by the demands of an activity and the context or environment in which it is performed. Consider, for example, opening an envelope with a letter opener in an office or negotiating a racetrack on a videogame screen. The first activity (opening a letter) may be done differently at work (a social and cultural and physical context) than it would be at home (also a social, cultural, and physical context). The second activity (playing a videogame) is performed in a virtual context but may also have a social context if it is being played with someone else. A temporal context may also apply if racing against a clock.

The word context comes from the Latin word "contexere," meaning to weave together.[22] A context is the background into which something is interwoven. This word is used in many different ways. For example, a child who is having difficulty understanding a new word encountered in reading is told to "look for context clues" such as illustrations or other words that may help the child identify the mystery word. In another common use of the word context, after listening to a story or anecdote, someone who knows more about the situation may remark that "you've taken that out of context," suggesting that the speaker has failed to provide enough background information to give a fair idea of what actually happened. In both examples, we can see that context gives meaning. In the case of occupation, the context supplies the background and often the meaning of the activity—how and why it is performed. Contexts provide cues about what kind of occupational performance is expected and effective; the six categories of context and environment are shown in Figure 1-1.

Activities present their own demands (see Figure 1-1) somewhat independent of context. Activity demands take into account all of the parameters of a specific activity. A letter opener and a videogame controller must be operated with the hands. Objects such as these and the space and timing of activities may present challenges to persons with physical disabilities affecting body functions and body structures. Someone with the use of only one hand will have problems stabilizing objects that are manipulated with the other hand (e.g., opening a can with a can opener or taking the lid off a plastic food container) or performing personal hygiene and getting dressed in a "normal" timeframe. Body functions and body structures are part of the client factor aspect of OT's domain (see Figure 1-1).

Another element within client factors concerns the values and beliefs and spiritual aspects of an individual. These elements can strongly influence the rehabilitation process. For example, a person who has a strong belief in family and obligation to family may be upset over a new disability status,

*The reader should have access to a copy of the OTPF-2E to provide additional details on this subject.

Areas of occupation	*Client factors*	*Performance skills*	*Performance patterns*	*Context and environment*	*Activity demands*
Activities of daily living (ADL)* Instrumental activities of daily living (IADL) Rest and sleep Education Work Play Leisure Social participation *Also referred to as *basic activities of daily living (BADL)* or *personal activities of daily living (PADL).*	Values, beliefs, and spirituality Body functions Body structures	Sensory perceptual skills Motor and praxis skills Emotional regulation skills Cognitive skills Communication and social skills	Habits Routines Roles Rituals	Cultural Personal Physical Social Temporal Virtual	Objects used and their properties Space demands Social demands Sequencing and timing Required actions Required body functions Required body structures

Figure 1-1 Aspects of occupational therapy's domain. (From American Occupational Therapy Association: *Occupational therapy practice framework: domain and process,* ed 2, Bethesda, MD, 2008, the Association, p. 628).

Table 1-1 Performance Skill Categories and Examples

Category	Examples
Motor and praxis skills	Stabilizing, positioning, bending, reaching, transporting, lifting, gripping, pinching, manipulating
Sensory-perceptual skills	Positioning the body for action, locating keys by touch, timing one's movements
Emotional regulation skills	Responding to others, persisting in tasks, recovering from uncomfortable feelings without lashing out at others
Cognitive skills	Judging what is appropriate in a given situation, sequencing tasks, prioritizing, organizing, multitasking

Table 1-2 Client Factors and Examples

Client Factor	Examples
Values, beliefs, and spirituality	Honesty Each person has responsibility to others Search for meaning and purpose beyond self
Body functions	Mental Sensory Neuromusculoskeletal and movement-related Cardiovascular, hematologic, immunological, respiratory Voice and speech Digestive, metabolic, and endocrine Genitourinary and reproductive Skin and related structures
Body structures	Brain, CNS structures, spinal cord, peripheral and autonomic nervous systems Eye, ear Organs of voice and speech Heart, lungs, blood vessels, and immune system Digestive and metabolic organs Genitourinary and reproductive systems Bones, joints, muscles Skin and sensory receptors of skin and soft tissue

fearing that she will be unable to provide for her family. But this strong belief in the family may be helpful if family members can be involved in caregiving and even in therapy sessions. Spiritual beliefs may also influence rehabilitation outcomes; if the person believes that the accident or injury is "God's will" or punishment for sin, then the motivation to improve in therapy may be affected.

How Physical Dysfunction Affects Engagement in Occupation

Physical dysfunction is associated with changes in body functions and/or structures, classified in the OTPF-2E[2] as client factors (see Figure 1-1 and Table 1-2). Most changes that vary from the normal tend to disrupt performance of occupation. For example, a wrist fracture, with its necessary casting and period of immobilization, causes problems in dressing, bathing, handling money, driving a car, caring for a child, and so on. Some activities cannot be done independently while the cast is on (e.g., bathing an infant); others can be accomplished with modifications (e.g., donning a coat). Persons with physical disabilities cannot do the activities in the "normal," or customary, way because of impairments in underlying abilities needed to perform the activities. For example, a mother whose wrist is in a cast cannot bathe a squirming infant because she cannot hold the child with both hands; because of the cast, she lacks the necessary tactile sensitivity, strength, range of motion, and grasp.

The reader is now invited to practice applying these ideas to the case of Mrs. A (see p. 6). After reading the introductory history, we ask you to stop before reading the occupational analysis. Although the history provides little information, it is sufficient to give some idea of the body structures and functions affected, the likely impairments of performance skills, and the contexts that apply in Mrs. A.'s case. Cover the rest of the Case Study with a piece of paper, and write your own analysis of Mrs. A.'s case, focusing on how this patient's disability has affected her occupations and skills. When you are finished, check your work against the information in the box.

Were your ideas about Mrs. A. similar to those listed? You may have identified areas, performance skills, patterns, body structures and functions, and aspects of the context that were not discussed. If so, congratulate yourself. The point of this exercise has been to illustrate the complexities of occupation and the importance of considering the individual in context.

In the case of Mrs. A. the context would change dramatically if her injury had occurred 7 years earlier. Do you understand why? She would have been in the United States only 1 year; she would have had less time to develop her English skills; and most importantly in terms of her ability to cope with her injury, her daughters would be 4 and 2 years of age. They could not help her with the chores, and she would have the additional tasks of bathing and dressing them and perhaps also diapering the younger child. Other aspects of Dominican culture should be considered, and the reader is encouraged to consult the cited reference.[18]

Theories and Models

The rest of this chapter concerns models and approaches that OT practitioners use to structure their thinking about practice situations. Students beginning fieldwork typically are asked about their "frame of reference" or "theory" or "practice model." A supervisor may inquire, "Which frames of reference are you comfortable with?" or "Which theories did you learn in school?" A particular practice model may be named, and the student may be asked to tell what he or she knows about it. Students often suffer unduly as they struggle to answer. Our purpose is to show you that you *can* learn models and theories well enough to explain them to others. You will see that they are useful—and that *you* will find them useful. This discussion starts with a situation you might face someday.

Imagine that you are working in a skilled nursing facility. On Monday morning, your first day of fieldwork, you are assigned a new admission and go to visit the resident in his room, having first read the chart and learned the following facts:

- The resident is 87 years old, married, and of German-Jewish background.
- His diagnoses are congestive heart failure, multi-infarct dementia, and Parkinson's disease.
- He was admitted over the weekend after being discharged from a local hospital.

When you enter his room, you find him lying, fully clothed, on his back, in bed, with his knees drawn up. He seems to be staring into space and looks worried. You greet him by name, tell him your name, and ask him if he can sit up and talk with you. You assist him to sitting, although with difficulty because he seems stiff and almost uncooperative. Once up, he looks you in the eye and begins talking. You cannot make any sense of what he is saying, so you ask him to speak louder. Even understanding the words, you cannot tell what he is saying. After trying some simple questions ("How are you feeling today?" or "Would you like to come for a walk with me?"), you feel frustrated by incomprehensible responses. After helping the man to lie down again, you excuse yourself, promising to come back another time.

On returning to the chart area, you learn that his medical record from the hospital is now available. It is an inch and a half thick, and every page is filled with details. It is difficult to see where to start first. What is wrong with this man? How did he come to be in this situation? What can we do to help him? How should we do it? And where should we start?

It seems practical to start with the chart. But for what should you look? In a situation like this, a frame of reference or theoretical foundation is useful. It gives you a structure for organizing your thoughts. It identifies the most important areas in which to gather information. It provides concepts for analyzing the resident's problems and for developing broad goals. The next section of this chapter summarizes the Model of Human Occupation (MOHO), which has been used across all practice areas, from psychiatry to physical medicine, and with all age groups.

The model of human occupation gives a broad perspective for organizing the OT process. In physical disabilities, however, the main focus is at times much narrower, and in this case, practice approaches are useful. A practice approach allows the occupational therapist to focus on a selected area of the patient's problems, helps to define realistic goals, and helps in the selection of evaluation and treatment interventions that are likely to work. Practice approaches can be used in conjunction with a theoretical model. This chapter examines three approaches for OT: biomechanical, sensorimotor/motor learning, and rehabilitation. These approaches are compatible with the model of human occupation. Each focuses on one aspect of the larger picture of human occupation. The biomechanical and sensorimotor/motor learning approaches are specific to physical disabilities, but the rehabilitation approach is also used in other practice areas. Each approach is elaborated in later chapters.

Model versus Frame of Reference

Terminology can be confusing. Many scholarly authors, starting with Mosey,[21] have attempted to devise a structure to evaluate the theories and ideas that occupational therapists use to guide their practice. A frame of reference, as defined by Mosey, is based on a theory and contains specific elements, asking or answering specific questions about the patient. A frame of reference is theoretical, not necessarily practical. In other words, it may help us speculate on what is occurring with a patient. Ideally, it gives us a direction in which to look. However, it is not necessarily useful in our day-to-day interventions.

CASE STUDY

Mrs. A.

Mrs. A. is a 34-year-old seamstress who completed eleventh grade in the Dominican Republic. She moved to the United States 8 years ago with her two daughters, now ages 11 and 9, after separating from her husband. A devout Catholic, Mrs. A. has been an active member of her church, making handicrafts and participating in bazaars, potluck dinners, and other activities. She understands English fairly well but speaks haltingly and is embarrassed by her accent. She is right-handed and lives with her daughters in a small fourth-floor walk-up apartment in Red Hook, Brooklyn. She has a large extended family; a cousin lives in the neighborhood. As is common in the Dominican community, family relationships are important to Mrs. A., who has been sending money to her sister and other relatives in the Dominican Republic.

Two months ago she was injured at the factory where she has worked since coming to the United States. The right radial nerve was affected at elbow level, and the median nerve was damaged to a lesser extent. Partial to full recovery is expected within 10 months. Mrs. A. is able to support herself and her daughters with insurance compensation payments, but she is afraid that these will not last until she is able to recover completely. She is worried and depressed over this situation. She is concerned about the rumor that the factory may be closing and about the loss of income and her inability to send money to her family. The social worker reports that Mrs. A. has said repeatedly that her injury is God's will and punishment for wanting to divorce her husband now that he has taken up with another woman.[18]

Mrs. A. has been referred for OT for physical and functional restoration. She has weakness in the extensors of the wrist and the hand and the supinator muscle. Because the flexors and pronators are stronger than these affected muscles, her wrist drops into a flexed position, her fingers stay slightly curled, and she cannot turn her palm to face up.

Occupational Analysis of the Case of Mrs. A.

Areas of Occupation

Because of limitations in the right hand, Mrs. A. would have difficulty with grooming, oral hygiene, bathing, toilet hygiene, dressing, applying makeup, feeding and eating, and using the telephone. Mrs. A may have trouble sleeping through the night due to pain and worries. She is unable to work at her job as a seamstress. Her daughters are old enough to take care of their own dressing and bathing and may be able to help Mrs. A. with the housework, which would otherwise be difficult for her. If they are interested in learning to cook, they could be taught enough to relieve her of this responsibility until she is recovered. It is possible that her cousin might help with some chores and with the children.

Mrs. A. is worried about whether she will recover enough to return to her job. If her recovery is less than complete, her job should be analyzed to see if it can be adapted to allow her to perform it. Otherwise, given her low educational level, limited job skills, and relative lack of proficiency with English, Mrs. A. may have trouble finding another job.

Performance Skills

The motor skills of manipulating, reaching, and coordinating are disrupted. The abilities to move, transport, lift, calibrate, and grip are weakened or lost in the affected hand. Mrs. A. will likely tire easily because of the additional time demands of performing tasks one-handed. Skills related to handling and holding are challenged because the second hand cannot be used to stabilize. Disturbances in timing of tasks will result from one-handed performance. Mrs. A. must protect the injured hand from further injury that might result from sensory losses. Mrs. A. will need to rely on the assistance of others and will have to ask for help (communication and social skills). Her relationships with others will change because of her temporary dependent status.

Patterns

Habits, routines, rituals and roles may be altered. It will take longer to perform tasks. Some previous habits and routines may not be possible while the nerve is healing (e.g., keeping the kitchen spotless and washing the floor daily, keeping a regular schedule of housecleaning and laundry). Even the ritual of lighting the candles at Mrs. A.'s small home shrine to the Virgin of Altagracia[18] will be difficult because striking a match requires the use of both hands. Loss of the worker role and changes in the performance of parent and household maintainer roles may be psychologically devastating.

Body Structures and Functions

Sensory, neuromusculoskeletal, and movement-related functions are most obviously affected. Mrs. A. has limited strength in her right hand. Sensation is also likely to be affected. Whether range of motion is affected—and, if so, to what extent—is unclear. There is no reason to suspect any problems with cognitive functions. Based on Mrs. A.'s involvement with her church and her strong work history and family relationships, it appears she has good psychological and psychosocial skills. However, she is depressed over the injury, anxious about the future, fearful that she may have brought on the injury through sin, and embarrassed about her limited English-speaking ability. These factors may affect her experience of herself and her ability to cope with her situation.

Context and Environment

Mrs. A. is a young adult with two children in the middle years. Living on the fourth floor, Mrs. A. must carry groceries up the stairs, trash down the stairs, and laundry both down and up. Having only one useful hand is restrictive, although her daughters can help her. Coming from a Dominican background, with its strong emphasis on family solidarity, Mrs. A.'s daughters have been brought up to take on these responsibilities easily, and her cousin is likely to help as well. Besides Mrs. A.'s involvement with the church, it is not known if she has any relationships with neighbors or adults other than her cousin. Because she is no longer going to work every day, Mrs. A. is in some danger of becoming isolated. If Mrs. A. can call on her relationships with her cousin and with fellow church members, she should be able

CASE STUDY—cont'd

to manage her household adequately for at least a few months. With respect to returning to work, Mrs. A.'s employer most likely has replaced her already, because many skilled garment workers reside in the area. Because her injury occurred on the job, the employer will be required to rehire her, but doing so is probably not in his economic self-interest, especially if he must accommodate a residual disability. Nonetheless, Mrs. A. was a valued employee, with 8 years at the same job, and her work history may affect his feelings about accommodating her, which he is legally required to do.

A practice model (or approach), as defined by Reed,[25] has a practical focus. Its purpose is to guide the OT process to help us identify problems and technical solutions. Some practice models and approaches are derived from theories. Others have evolved from techniques that worked, even if the reason why they worked was unknown. The theories for these practice models were developed later to explain why these solutions or techniques were successful.

As an OTA, you will most likely be providing direct care to patients, performing evaluations and treatments, adapting equipment and environments, and working in a practical world—the world of people and their goals and problems. In the area of physical disabilities, most often you will be basing your work on one of the approaches in this book. These approaches focus on physical functions and on practical considerations of day-to-day life.

So, you might ask, why bother to learn a theoretical model if the practice approaches are more central to your work? The reason is that people are complicated and that their occupational functioning is complicated. Needs, desires, hopes, fears, personal histories, and family and cultural backgrounds affect a person's beliefs in the possibilities of therapy and willingness to try. It is not just a matter of a reflex here, some limitation in range there, or the need for a piece of adaptive equipment. Rather, the central question is how best to help each individual achieve the highest level of independent functioning possible in daily life activities. This question needs to be asked and answered from a broader perspective than any of the practice approaches can supply. In working with patients with physical disabilities, the patient's motivation, sense of hope, and drive to master the environment despite disability must be uppermost in the OTA's mind, even though the focus of day-to-day therapy may be on an isolated physical element such as the functioning of a muscle. For this reason, clinicians guide practice from theoretical models such as the model of human occupation.

The model of human occupation provides a clear, organized system for understanding occupational performance. The model of human occupation suggests how the various aspects of human occupation in the *OTPF-2E*[2] work together and how they are related. We can compare it to a building plan or blueprint.

Human Occupation

The core idea of the model of human occupation[14-17] is that humans have an inborn drive to explore and master their surroundings. The activity generated by this drive, of exploring and attempting to control the environment, is called *occupation.* The drive toward occupation can be nurtured and developed—or obstructed and crushed. In this model the individual and the environment are seen as interacting with and affecting one another.

The model of human occupation is a **systems model**. It is a holistic model (one that looks at the whole) rather than a reductionistic model (one that looks intensely at one part, such as muscular function). In this holistic model the human individual engaged in occupation is seen as a complex interaction of parts that cannot make sense viewed separately. In other words, therapists cannot look only at the right upper extremity or at the ability to sequence an activity without considering how this fits within the lives or occupation that individuals have shaped for themselves. Persons cannot be considered separately from their environments. Their families, communities, cultures, and the objects they use every day are forces that shape their nature as actors in the world.

Three Subsystems of Human Occupation

The model of human occupation seeks to explain complex interactions between the person, the activity or occupation, and the environment. Many reasons exist for difficulties in performing occupations. For example, a person may not be motivated. Or the person may keep repeating an ineffective action or sequence of actions, perhaps out of habit. Actions may be limited or ineffective because of inability to organize information into meaningful ideas or because of lack of strength or coordination. To organize these various aspects, the model of human occupation recognizes three interrelated components of human occupation: volition, habituation, and performance capacity (and the lived body) (Figure 1-2).

Volition

Another word for **volition** is *motivation.* Three key elements of volition are personal causation, values, and interests. *Personal causation* refers to the person's beliefs about personal effectiveness. Am I in control, or am I controlled by forces outside myself? Am I good at things? Can I succeed if I try?

Values are internalized images of "what is important and meaningful to do."[15] Values motivate behavior in many ways. For example, someone who is ill may make a special effort to get dressed and go to church. A father may neglect professional reading to spend more time helping his child with homework, because to him the child is more important.

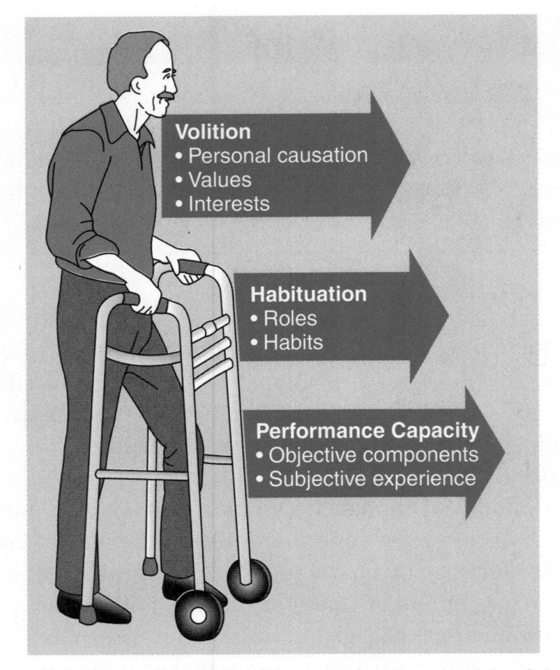

Figure 1-2 The interrelationships within the model of human occupation. (From Figure 2.6, page 22, Kielhofner G, editor: *A model of human occupation: theory and application,* ed 3, Baltimore, 2002, Lippincott Williams & Wilkins.)

Interests are "what one finds enjoyable or satisfying to do."[17] Interests are the things that attract people. When people are interested, they are energized, alive, and ready to attempt new things. Together and separately, personal causation, values, and interests supply motivation or volition to engage in occupation.

Habituation

Habituation refers to activities that have been performed enough times to become routine and customary. Two elements of habituation are habits and internalized roles. *Habits* are automatic routines or patterns of activity that a person seems to perform almost by reflex, without much conscious awareness. An example would be folding towels or locking a door when leaving. Habits help conserve energy; tasks are accomplished without too much effort or concentration, leaving more time and attention available for other things. Habits and habitat or environment are interdependent; the customary physical environment gives cues that are the same over time and that support regular performance of habits and role behaviors.[17]

Internalized roles are personalized occupational roles that consist of many different habits, routines, and skills. Some typical occupational roles are homemaker, student, and retiree. Although each role carries certain socially expected behaviors, these are internalized or personalized by the individual. For example, one homemaker may pay more attention to preparing food for family and guests, whereas another is more involved in keeping the house clean and organized. The internalized role of a particular student might reflect habits established in childhood, as when the adult student sets up to study at the kitchen table immediately on returning home, just as the person was taught to do in grade school 30 years ago. Also, it may reflect values and interests, as when the student organizes study time around a favorite television program.

Role change, or *role transition,* occurs as life moves forward and the person grows. Roles contract, expand, are modified, and sometimes are abandoned or replaced. Former roles are rediscovered and renewed. New ones are attempted. The grade school student becomes the high school student. The student becomes a worker. The worker becomes a student again. The worker changes to another field. Role change can be exciting or terrifying; occasionally it is both. Time for learning and adjustment is necessary before a new role becomes internalized.

Performance Capacity and the Lived Body

Performance capacity is "the ability for doing things."[16] Doing things depends on the body structures and functions already discussed and on the "subjective experience" of them. We live our lives through our bodies, giving each of us a subjective and personal experience. For example, stiffness of the fingers from arthritis may be experienced differently by a pianist or hairdresser than by someone whose work depends less on finger flexibility.

Kielhofner defines the lived body as "the experience of being and knowing the world through a particular body." [17] (The notion of the lived body is based on the work of Merleau-Ponty, a French phenomenological philosopher.[19]) By living through a particular body, we come to know the world—the experience of doing leads to knowing—and this is how we know and understand the world.

Performance capacity and performance skills are in many cases the primary focus of OT intervention for persons with physical disabilities. Performance skills depend on performance capacity. When the body is disabled, the sense of the lived body is different. For the person who is not disabled, there exists a seamless interaction of body and mind in which one does not notice one's body actions because these actions are effective expressions of mental intentions. Once the body is disabled, body actions become "a big deal." One has to notice, correct, and alter behavior because the body is not performing as previously experienced.

Complex Interactions and Interdependence

As noted, human occupation involves a complex relationship among volition, habituation, and performance capacity (as reflected in the lived body). Any of these three components will affect the others. Trends or patterns can develop. Successful completion of a goal can provide the energy and optimism to try more challenging tasks and the perseverance to keep trying despite minor setbacks. On the other hand, a perception that one has failed can reduce enthusiasm for new tasks and dampen willingness to try. The subjective experience of repeated successes, or of repeated failures, can set up and reinforce a persistent pattern. See Box 1-1 for definitions of terms used in the MOHO.[14-17]

Box 1-1

Model of Human Occupation: Definitions

Human occupation The act of doing work, play, activities of daily living, and other activities within the context of human life.
Environment Human and nonhuman object world in which human occupation is carried out.
Volition Motivation or the desire to act. Personal causation, values, and interests are aspects of volition.
Personal causation Individual's sense of own competence and effectiveness.
Values Internalized images of what is good, right, and important.
Interests Personal preferences in activities or people.
Habituation Patterns or routine behavior. Aspects of habituation include habits and internalized roles.
Habits Automatic routines. Actions carried out so regularly that they can be done without conscious effort.
Internalized roles Individual's personal interpretation and enactment of the (more general and less specific) occupational role.
Occupational roles Patterns for organizing productive activity, usually according to the product or service produced. Examples are grade-school student, homemaker, basketball player.
Role change/role transition Movement from one role to another, or movement within a role. Examples are going to work after finishing school and moving from full-time to part-time work.
Performance capacity The underlying capacities needed to do things, based on body structures and functions and on the subjective experience of them.

Model of Human Occupation's View of How Disability Affects Human Occupation

Now that you have a general understanding of the MOHO, consider what happens when a person encounters the challenge of a physical disability. Consider the case of a young, healthy, single woman who falls and fractures both wrists while rollerblading. She will probably experience this physical disability most immediately in performance capacity of the lived body because it takes away the functions of the hands. She will not be able to use her hands while they are in casts and will not be able to operate many switches, doorknobs, and faucet handles.

These changes also lead quickly to changed habits and roles because the necessary performance skills are not available and thus the habits cannot be carried out. She cannot bathe herself, prepare her own food, or perform her job. Ultimately, personal causation is affected, with the normal feedback of success from participating in accustomed roles reduced or eliminated. She is confined to her home and begins to feel isolated. She no longer enjoys the company of coworkers or the feeling of satisfaction from doing her job. Discouragement, helplessness, and apathy (lack of interest) may dominate her thinking. She begins to feel worthless, depressed, and self-pitying. She is forced into a new role, that of helpless patient, in which she receives more pleasant (less demanding and less frustrating) feedback from the environment. She sees herself as less capable, more dependent on others, and more needy of support. She watches television and sleeps all day. Although such dependence may be appropriate for a time, if prolonged it might undermine the volition subsystem and reduce motivation for independent living.

Box 1-2

Model of Human Occupation: Selected Concepts for Intervention

"Client change is the focus of therapy." (p. 296)
"Only clients can accomplish their own change." (p. 296)
"For doing to be therapeutic, it must involve an actual occupational form, not a contrived activity." (p. 297)
"For the client to achieve change through doing, what is done must have relevance and meaning for the client." (p. 297)
"Change in therapy involves simultaneous and interacting alterations in the person, the environment, and the relationship of the person to the environment." (p. 302)
"Change in therapy is part of a history of change in the person's life." (p. 302)
"The role of the therapist is to support and thereby enable clients to do what they need in order to change." (p. 310)

Compiled from Kielhofner G, editor: *A model of human occupation: theory and application,* ed 3, Baltimore, 2002, Lippincott Williams & Wilkins.

Few persons who sustain a physical disability react in this way. Many respond to the challenge with inventive solutions and creative and energetic changes in behavior. Environmental supports such as family or friends can ease the adjustment so that patients feel more in control. The disability is viewed as an inconvenience but not a serious obstacle to achieving life goals. Commonly, people dealing with a physical disability experience both optimism and despair alternately and with varying intensity. Important factors are the severity of the disability and whether it is temporary or permanent. The course of adjustment is usually not just one way or the other. Ups and downs are common.

General Principles of Occupational Therapy Intervention

The MOHO provides guidelines for designing and carrying out OT treatment. Some of these are discussed as follows and summarized in Box 1-2.[14-17]

Client change is the focus of therapy.[16] Even forms of therapy in which the practitioner provides equipment or devices still require the client to incorporate the devices and ways of using them.

Only clients can accomplish their own change.[16] Engagement and participation by the individual are required. Therapy cannot be done to someone. The person must be involved and active.

For doing to be therapeutic, it must involve an actual occupational form, not a contrived activity.[16] As discussed later in the chapter, contrived or enabling activities (e.g., stacking cones) are sometimes used as part of therapy, but these do not provide the opportunity to engage in occupation in ways that are "real" to the person or that engage the lived body in doing in the world. By participating in activities that match their needs, interests, and abilities, individuals can improve their ability to perform in daily life activities. The OT practitioner selects and designs activities to match the patient's characteristics and goals.

For the client to achieve change through doing, what is done must be relevant and meaningful to the client.[16] Therapy practitioners must start from the client's interests and history in selecting activities for therapy. Cleverness and creativity and careful gradation of the activity to the patient's capabilities will be necessary.

Change in therapy involves simultaneous and interacting alterations in the person, the environment, and the relationship of the person to the environment.[16] A dynamic among the person, task, and environment exists. In adjusting to a physical challenge, as well as learning new ways of doing things in the world, the person changes. But the environment also must change to accommodate the person—and how he or she experiences the self in relation to the environment changes as well.

Change in therapy is part of a history of change in the person's life.[16] As noted earlier, change in roles and occupations is ongoing. The change that occurs in therapy is just another episode of change, but how the change is experienced depends greatly on how the person sees the self. People have a sense of their own occupational nature, now challenged by physical disability. Therapy provides an opportunity for the person to modify the sense of self to accommodate the disability and the solutions that work for that person.

The role of the therapist is to support and thereby enable clients to do what they need in order to change.[16] The client needs support and information and guided experience in order to change, because change can be difficult and results discouraging. The therapist employs many strategies to assist the client in the process of changing. The therapist may do the following:

- Validate the client's experience
- Identify ways of managing tasks
- Provide feedback on performance
- Advise clients about alternatives
- Negotiate an intermediate step when a task seems too difficult
- Structure activities to provide meaningful challenges
- Coach performance by verbal cuing
- Offer words and gestures of encouragement
- Provide physical support and adaptations as needed.

These strategies represent only a selection of the many principles in the MOHO[16,17] (see Box 1-2).

Practice Approaches

We now examine the practice approaches most often used in physical disabilities practice: the biomechanical approach, the motor learning and sensorimotor approaches, and the rehabilitation approach. Each is described, and its relationship to the model of human occupation is discussed and illustrated.

Biomechanical Approach

The **biomechanical approach** to the treatment of physical dysfunction considers the human body as a living machine. Techniques in this approach derive from **kinetics**, the science of the motions of objects and the forces acting on them.[20] To some extent, the principles of **statics**, the study of the forces acting on objects at rest, are also used in this approach. The object here is the human body, which is studied at rest and in motion. Treatment methods employ principles of physics[30] related to forces, levers, and torque (Box 1-3).

Box 1-3

Biomechanical Approach: Definitions

Kinetics Study of the motions of objects and the forces acting on them.
Statics Study of the forces acting on objects at rest.
Force Measurable influence acting on a body.
Lever Rigid structure fixed at a point called the fulcrum and acted on at two other points by two forces, causing movement in relation to the fulcrum; a seesaw and a crowbar are examples.
Torque Rotary or twisting force.
Joint Point where two bones meet and around which motion occurs.
Range of motion Extent, measured in degrees of a circle, to which movement can occur at a joint.
Strength Work against resistance (including the force of gravity), measured in pounds.
Endurance Exertion or work sustained over time.

Typical evaluation and treatment techniques used in this approach are measurement of joint range of motion (ROM) and muscle strength, therapeutic exercise, and orthotics. Therapeutic activity for kinetic purposes, or the application of movement principles in the performance of activities, is also part of this approach. Sanding with a weighted sander to improve strength or weaving on an upright loom to increase shoulder ROM are examples. The goals of the biomechanical approach are to (1) evaluate specific physical limitations in ROM, strength, and endurance; (2) restore these functions; and (3) prevent or reduce deformity.

The biomechanical approach is most appropriate for patients whose central nervous system (CNS) is intact but who have lower motor neuron or orthopedic disorders. These patients can control isolated movements and specific movement patterns but may have weakness, low endurance, or joint limitation. Disabilities typically addressed with this approach include orthopedic conditions (e.g., rheumatoid arthritis, osteoarthritis, fractures, amputations, hand trauma), burns, lower motor neuron disorders (e.g., peripheral nerve injuries), Guillain-Barré syndrome, spinal cord injuries, and primary muscle diseases (e.g., muscular dystrophy). Biomechanical principles are also applied in ergonomics and work hardening, with an emphasis on proper positioning and the optimum fit between the biomechanics of the individual and the work environment.

The biomechanical approach targets the performance capacity level of the model of human occupation and focuses on physical skills (e.g., lifting the hand) and body structures and functions that support them (e.g., ROM, strength). Its principles can also be applied directly to occupations and to contexts (e.g., when the height of a chair and a desk are lowered to fit a person of less than standard height).

Sensorimotor and Motor Learning Approaches

When earlier generations of occupational therapists tried to apply biomechanical principles to patients with a damaged CNS, they were frustrated by their patients' inability to carry out the desired motions. These patients could not coordinate and regulate their movements because their muscles were not receiving normal directions from the CNS. Biomechanical treatment approaches, which demand controlled voluntary movement, clearly were inappropriate for patients who lacked such control.

Methods using the sensorimotor approach were developed for treatment of patients who have CNS dysfunction. The normal CNS functions to produce controlled, well-modulated (regular and adjusted) movement. The damaged CNS cannot coordinate and produce such movement smoothly or with ease.

Sensorimotor approaches to treatment use neurophysiological mechanisms to normalize muscle tone and elicit more normal motor responses.[28] They provide controlled input to the nervous system; this controlled input is meant to stimulate specific responses. Some approaches use reflex mechanisms, and the sequence of treatment may be based on the recapitulation of ontogenetic development.[28] In other words, these approaches might employ primitive reflexes such as those that infants display or those that humans share with other creatures such as fish. Therapy is directed at incorporating these reflexes into purposeful activity and at integrating them so that their power is reduced and movement becomes more controlled and voluntary. Chapter 21 describes the sensorimotor approaches. Box 1-4 lists definitions of terms related to sensori-motor approaches.

The sensorimotor approaches target the MOHO component of performance capacities. Sensorimotor approaches have been criticized when they do not include purposeful activity or the involvement of patients as creators and actors in their own occupational world. Sensorimotor approaches are used by other health practitioners including physical therapists, speech therapists, and physiatrists. They are not tools exclusively of OT. Although some approaches were developed by occupational therapists, others were designed or discovered by practitioners of these other disciplines.

The principles of the sensorimotor approaches can be used as an OT method when the practitioner applies them to purposeful activity. The AOTA advises that the techniques of an approach not associated with purposeful activity may be used "to prepare the client or patient for better performance and prevention of disability through self-participation in occupation."[6] These techniques should be a part of OT only when they are used to stimulate or condition the nervous system so that purposeful activity can be attempted, ideally during the same treatment session.

Motor learning is an approach associated with the sensorimotor approach that focuses on the acquisition of motor skills through practice and feedback.[24,27,29] Motor learning acknowledges the individual's involvement in the learning process and requires active practice and reflection from the patient. It uses motor training by therapists, with opportunities for patients to create their own movement solutions to challenges. The context or practice environment for movement activities is a major focus. Therapy practitioners attempt to design practice conditions that will challenge the person sufficiently to involve the thinking processes that guide motor behavior.[24] Motor control is discussed in Chapters 6 and 10.

The motor control approach addresses the volition and habituation and performance capacity components of the MOHO. The primary focus is the performance of motor functions. However, volition is involved as the person is engaged in solving movement problems. Habituation is involved through practice in a variety of situations and the generation of new movement patterns. The motor learning approach is based in learning theory.

Box 1-4

Sensorimotor Approach: Definitions

Central nervous system (CNS): The brain and spinal cord.
Neurophysiological: Pertaining to the study of the physical and chemical nature of the nervous system.
Muscle tone: Resistance of a muscle to being stretched by an external force.
Motor response: Movement or muscle action evoked by sensory input; may be voluntary or involuntary.
Reflex mechanism: Involuntary motor response to sensory input.
Recapitulation of ontogenetic development: Theory that the organism in its development goes through the same stages as did the species in its development from lower organisms; as applied to recovery from CNS damage, also implies that recovery must go through the same stages as individual human development (i.e., from infancy).

Rehabilitation Approach

The term *rehabilitation* means a restoration to a former state or to a proper state.[20] In medicine it means the return to the fullest physical, mental, social, vocational, and economic usefulness that is possible for the individual. It refers to the ability to live and work with remaining capabilities. Therefore the focus in the treatment program is on abilities rather than disabilities.

Rehabilitation is concerned with the intrinsic worth and dignity of the individual and with the restoration of a satisfying and purposeful life. The rehabilitation approach uses measures that enable a person to live as independently as possible despite residual disability. Its goal is to help the patient learn to work around or compensate for physical limitations.[25]

The rehabilitation approach assumes that the patient is an active, involved, contributing member of the rehabilitation team. The occupational therapist must identify the patient's capabilities and assets so that these can be engaged to overcome the effects of the disability on function. The therapist must consider the best research evidence and be aware of advances in methods and equipment (rehabilitation technology). Always, the therapist must place primary importance on the envisioned outcome of the individual functioning as he or she desires in his or her environments of choice.

Intervention methods of the rehabilitation approach include techniques and modalities such as the following:

- Self-care evaluation and training
- Acquisition and training in assistive devices
- Acquisition and training in use of adaptive clothing
- Homemaking and childcare
- Work simplification and energy conservation
- Work-related activities
- Leisure activities
- Prosthetic training
- Wheelchair management
- Home evaluation and adaptation
- Community transportation
- Architectural adaptations
- Acquisition and training in the use of communication aids and environmental control systems

In relation to occupation, the rehabilitation approach focuses on the occupations themselves and on performance skills rather than on body structures and functions. The aims of a rehabilitation program are to enable role performance and to minimize the effects of residual disability on role performance. The rehabilitation approach takes the influence of the environment into account and provides methods to adapt the environment to the individual.

The rehabilitation approach addresses most of the elements of the MOHO. Including the patient as a member of the rehabilitation team engages the volition subsystem. However, the patient's values, interests, and sense of personal causation are not addressed directly. Habituation is the main focus of intervention, and performance of occupation is emphasized. As mentioned, the environment and possible changes to the environment are also considered. The performance capacity level is emphasized less in this approach than in the biomechanical and sensorimotor approaches.

Therapists commonly use methods of the rehabilitation approach in combination with methods from the biomechanical or sensorimotor approaches. Biomechanical or sensorimotor principles can be applied *during* rehabilitation activities to reinforce the functioning of sensorimotor and cognitive functions. An example is the use of cross-diagonal patterns (a sensorimotor approach) to normalize muscle tone and coordination during dressing. This complements and enhances the success of rehabilitation. At the same time, it ties the sensorimotor technique to purposeful activity.

Limitations of These Practice Approaches

The three practice approaches just described have proved useful in evaluating and treating problems commonly encountered in physical disabilities practice. Used separately or together, however, they do not provide a complete view of the person. Di Joseph[11] urged occupational therapists to consider not only motor control but also motor behavior—that is, "a person acting purposefully within and upon his or her environment." She further stated that ignoring the emotive and cognitive aspects of motor behavior is a reductive approach that fails to consider all factors in the production of "purposeful action." Treatment goals for patients must be based on an evaluation of mind, body, and environment. These goals should be reached through activities compatible with the needs and values of the person and not necessarily with those of the therapist. Interaction between the person and the environment is essential to functional independence.[26] The person is mind and body, not just a motor system to be evaluated and "treated."[11] This approach is essential throughout the treatment continuum, discussed below.

Treatment Continuum in Physical Disabilities Practice

A *continuum* is a "continuous series of elements passing into each other."[22] A **treatment continuum** begins with the onset of injury or disability and ends with the restoration of the patient to maximal independence. It is not a series of steps but a gradual movement from disease and disability toward health and ability. The best prognosis for many conditions leaves the patient with some residual disability. For every patient the end point of the continuum is the maximal *possible* functional return.

Figure 1-3 is a model for the treatment continuum in physical disabilities practice. The stages in this treatment continuum overlap and can occur simultaneously. Although four stages are identified within it, the treatment continuum is not meant to illustrate a strict step-by-step progression. It takes the patient through a logical progression from dependence to skill development, then to purposeful activity, and finally to resumption of life roles.[23] The treatment continuum identifies the concerns of OT practice within the context of performance of occupation and is compatible with the model of human occupation.

Stage 1: Adjunctive Methods

Adjunctive methods are used within OT to prepare the patient to engage in activity.[6] These methods may include exercise, facilitation and inhibition techniques, positioning, sensory stimulation, selected physical agent modalities, and devices such as braces and splints.[31] Adjunctive methods are used not only by OT practitioners but also by physical therapists, physiatrists, chiropractors, and massage therapists. It is the application of these methods as a preparation for purposeful activity that differentiates OT from other professions.

Adjunctive methods are often used in, but are not limited to, the acute stages of illness or injury. During this stage the occupational therapist is likely to be most concerned with evaluating and remediating problems in body structures and functions. The occupational therapist plans the progression of treatment so that adjunctive modalities are used to prepare the patient for purposeful activity and are directed toward the achievement of maximal independence in the performance skills and areas of occupation. Many adjunctive methods require the advanced education and training of the occupational therapist and are not appropriately performed by the entry-level OTA.[1,3,7,8] Hot and cold packs, fluidotherapy, and paraffin may be administered by the service-competent OTA. The OTA may also construct and modify splints, under supervision, and may conduct exercise programs as directed.

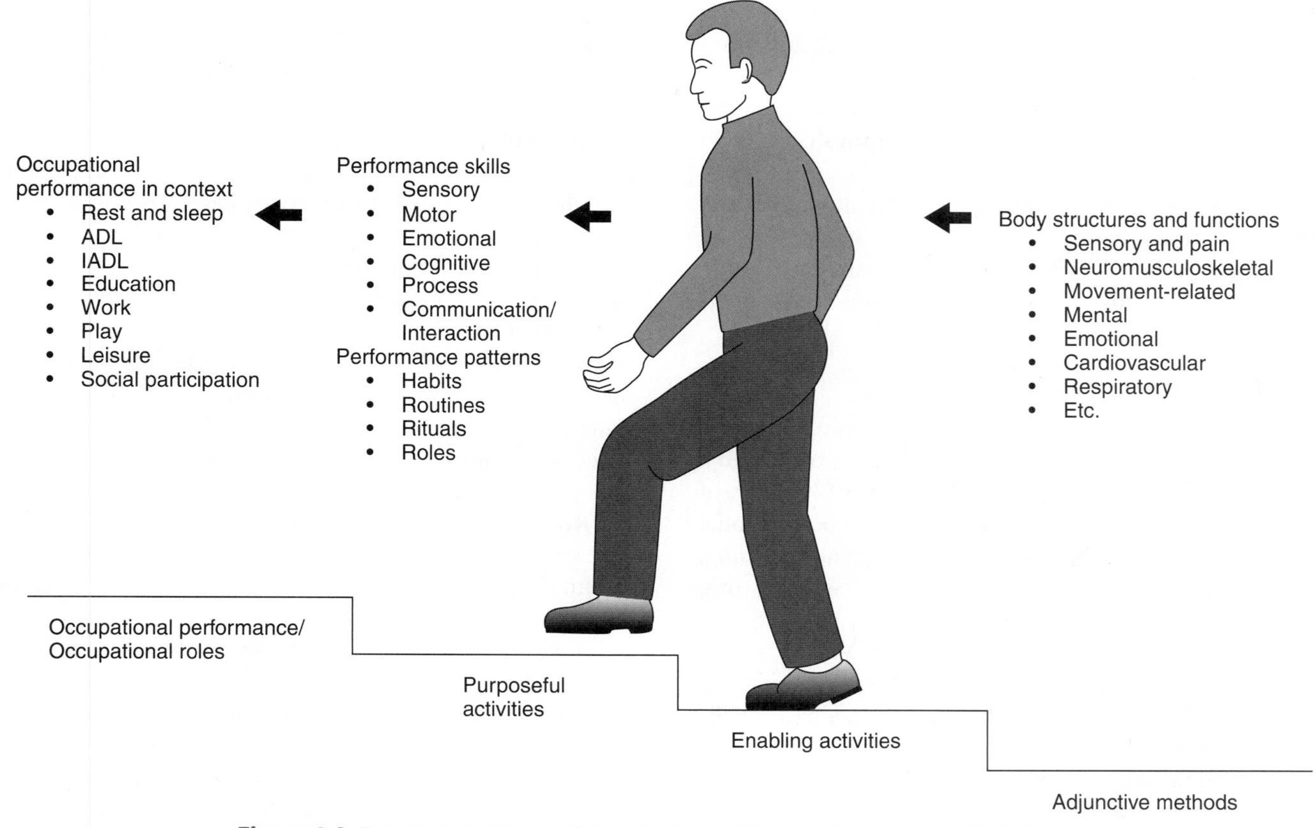

Figure 1-3 Treatment continuum for physical disabilities practice. (Courtesy Karin Boyce.)

To illustrate the treatment continuum, we use the example of a patient who has recently suffered a stroke, or cerebrovascular accident (CVA). The most obvious effect of a stroke is paralysis or weakness on one side of the body. (Other effects of this condition are addressed in Chapter 24.)

The patient is unable to move his arm or leg. Without the stimulation of normal movement and exercise, the muscles will contract, and motion will be limited in the future. To prevent this, the therapist moves the patient's limbs passively (passive range of motion), maintaining as normal a range as possible. Passive ROM is a body function needed for development of skills.

At stage 1 the therapist is mainly concerned with maintaining or remedying the functions of the body.

Stage 2: Enabling Activities

Occupational therapists have created many enabling methods for simulating purposeful activities. Examples are sanding boards, skateboards, stacking cones or blocks, practice boards for mastery of clothing fasteners and hardware, driving simulators, work simulators, and tabletop activities such as pegboards for training perceptual-motor skills. These methods cannot be considered purposeful activity. Such activities are not likely to be as meaningful to the patient or to stimulate as much interest and motivation as purposeful activities. However, they may be necessary as a preparatory or ancillary part of the treatment program to train specific sensory, motor, perceptual, or cognitive functions necessary for performance skills and occupations.

Enabling activities require more patient involvement than do adjunctive methods. Whereas the therapy practitioner usually applies adjunctive methods to the patient who passively receives them, the patient carries out enabling activities. Enabling activities meet two of the three characteristics of purposeful activity: (1) the patient participates actively; and (2) the activity requires and elicits coordination of sensory, motor, psychosocial, and cognitive systems.[11]

However, enabling methods fail to meet the third characteristic of purposeful activity: the presence of an autonomous or inherent goal beyond the motor function required to perform the task.[10] In other words, getting exercise should not be the *only* reason for doing the activity. Although enabling methods might not be considered purposeful, they are often used as a necessary step toward the ability to perform purposeful activities.

Special equipment such as wheelchairs, ambulatory aids, assistive devices, special clothing, communication devices, and environmental control systems may also be necessary to enable independence in the performance areas and assumption of occupational roles.

Returning to our example, the patient at this stage may have some voluntary movement of his arm and leg. However, spasticity makes the movement too weak and uncoordinated for performance that would satisfy the patient's self-esteem needs. In other words, the patient might be able to pick up and place large mosaic tile pieces, but the result would be uneven and unattractive. An activity such as stacking cones or pegboard designs may be given to the patient at stage 2 to allow him to practice motions and skills (lifting, calibrating) that later will be applied to purposeful activities.

In stage 2 the therapist is still concerned with evaluation and remediation of skills and the body functions that support skills. Flexible conditions for using skills may be added at this stage, with the patient experiencing the different weights and textures of materials handled. The OTA may safely carry out most stage 2 enabling activities but must be careful to obtain guidance on the purpose, objectives, procedures, and precautions that apply to each patient situation.

Stage 3: Purposeful Activity

Purposeful activity has been the core of OT since its inception. Purposeful activity has an inherent or autonomous goal and is relevant and meaningful to the patient.[9,10] It is part of the daily life routine and occurs in the context of occupational performance.[4,5,9] Examples are feeding, hygiene, dressing, mobility, communication, arts, crafts, games, sports, work, and educational activities.

The purposefulness of an activity is determined by the individual performing it and the context in which it is performed. OT practitioners use purposeful activities to evaluate, facilitate, restore, or maintain a person's ability to function in life roles.[5] Purposeful activity can be carried out in a health care facility or in the patient's home.

Returning to our example, the patient at this stage has achieved more control of his arm and leg. Weakness and spasticity may remain, but significant improvement has occurred. The occupational therapist or OTA at this point would teach the patient techniques for dressing, self-feeding, toileting, and transfer from the wheelchair. The patient might participate in crafts or games that have been adapted to improve performance skills in, for example, reaching and holding and pinch and release.

In stage 3 the therapist is concerned with evaluating and remediating deficits in the performance of skills related to occupations. The OTA can expect to be involved prominently in the patient's treatment at this point because performance skills and engagement in occupation are the focus of the assistant's treatment skills.

Stage 4: Occupational Performance and Occupational Roles

In the final stage of the treatment continuum, the patient resumes or assumes occupational roles in the living environment and in the community. Appropriate tasks in activities of daily living, work, education activities, play, leisure, and social participation are performed to the patient's maximal level of independence. This level is defined by each client or patient according to personal capacities and limitations and values, interests, and goals. Residual disability may remain, but the person has learned compensatory techniques. Formal OT intervention is decreased and ultimately discontinued.

The stroke patient at this stage has achieved most of the motor return that is believed medically possible. He has learned some sensorimotor techniques to counteract the effects of abnormal spastic tone so that he can dress and feed himself. He has practiced and relearned the many performance skills and habits that make up his daily life. Working with the occupational therapist and OTA, he has identified his needs in work and home life and has selected and been trained with adaptive devices appropriate to his situation. He resumes his life in the community, shaping this new occupational life with the strategies and techniques he has learned in therapy.

In stage 4 the therapist is concerned with assisting the patient in the transition to community life. Both the OTA and the occupational therapist would be involved in this stage.

A particular OT practitioner may be responsible for only one or two phases in the continuum. In fact, the continuum may occur over two or more treatment settings, such as an acute care hospital and an intermediate care facility and finally in the community.

Evidence-Based Practice

Health care providers today are looking carefully at what evidence exists to support their practice; outcomes are usually the focus.[13] Generally, this takes the form of asking a question: "In a case such as this one, which approach is more likely to yield the best outcome?" To give an example, "In a 26-year-old man with C-6 spinal cord injury, what OT procedures will result in the best return to maximum functional independence?" Finding an answer to such a question is not so easy, however, because the quantity of published OT research is limited and has not yet increased to the level needed to support evidence-based practice (EBP).[12]

Within the field of OT, much of the lore and custom of practice has been passed down from therapist to therapist but has not always been well documented or researched in a controlled way before being published in a peer-reviewed journal. Consumers and insurers are asking how we can justify our practices. Consequently, research and outcome studies have become important. The OTA of the twenty-first century should expect to take a role in asking and answering questions for outcomes research. This requires a thoughtful approach to practice, one that relies less on rote procedures from a textbook or classroom and more on reflective analysis of what happens in therapy. This involves considering the consumer's perspective, as well as the practitioner's. It requires that the OTA adopt an inquiring attitude and develop a tolerance for ambiguity and "not knowing." Being able to pose clinical questions and search for information in electronic databases and print sources is also necessary. The OTA may gather data and publish outcomes studies, document and write for publication a single case study report, or work with a group of OT practitioners on a large study. All of these efforts add to the knowledge base of the profession.

Summary

The OTPF-2E (ref 2) provides a guiding structure for the focus of OT—namely to assist or enable individuals to participate in occupations within contexts. The model of human occupation is a frame of reference for occupational performance. This model has three subsystems: volition, habituation, and performance capacity. People with physical dysfunction experience the most direct and visible disruption of their occupational lives at the level of performance capacity and the lived body.

Three treatment approaches commonly applied in physical disabilities practice are the biomechanical, sensorimotor/motor learning, and rehabilitation approaches. These approaches apply to specific types of disabling conditions.

The treatment continuum in physical disabilities practice is a process of four stages through which the patient gradually acquires the abilities to resume occupational life after disability. The OTA is most involved in the final two stages of purposeful activity and resumption of occupational roles.

The goal of OT intervention is to develop maximal functioning in occupational roles, as defined for each individual in consideration of that person's capacities and limitations. Recognizing that the client or patient is the starting point, we shape our interventions toward the individual's goals, values, and interests throughout the OT process. At the same time, we must remember to research and document best practices and to consider the evidence that supports our interventions.

Selected Reading Guide Questions

1. On a separate piece of paper, outline the main elements of the *OTPF-2E.*
2. Discuss the relationship of body structures and functions (client factors) to task demands and performance skills.
3. Differentiate "holistic" from "reductionistic."
4. List and describe the three subsystems of the MOHO.
5. Relate *role change or role transition* to the MOHO.
6. How does the MOHO relate to the *OTPF-2E?*
7. List the typical evaluation and treatment methods used in the biomechanical approach.
8. Identify the conditions for which the biomechanical approach is most appropriate.
9. Identify the conditions for which the sensorimotor approach is most appropriate, and explain why this approach is preferred for these conditions.
10. Discuss the relationship between the sensorimotor approach and purposeful activity.
11. How is the motor learning approach different from the sensorimotor approach?
12. Define *rehabilitation* and state the goal of the rehabilitation approach.
13. List some intervention methods of the rehabilitation approach.
14. List reasons why the three practice approaches used in physical disabilities practice have been criticized for providing an incomplete view of the patient.
15. Discuss why each of the four stages in the OT treatment continuum requires a different level of patient involvement.
16. Explain what is meant by "evidence" to support practice, and discuss the roles of the OTA with regard to gathering and documenting evidence.

References

1. American Occupational Therapy Association: Guidelines for supervision, roles, and responsibilities during the delivery of occupational therapy services, *Am J Occup Ther* 63:797–803, 2009.
2. American Occupational Therapy Association: *Occupational therapy practice framework: domain and process*, ed 2, Bethesda, MD, 2008, the Association.
3. American Occupational Therapy Association: Physical agent modalities, a position paper, *Am J Occup Ther* 62(6):691–693, 2008.
4. American Occupational Therapy Association: Position paper: purposeful activity, *Am J Occup Ther* 47:1081–1082, 1993.
5. American Occupational Therapy Association: Purposeful activities: a position paper, *Am J Occup Ther* 37:805, 1983.
6. American Occupational Therapy Association: Resolution 532-79 (1979): occupation as the common core of occupational therapy, Representative Assembly minutes, Detroit, April 1979, *Am J Occup Ther* 33:785, 1979.
7. American Occupational Therapy Association: Roles and responsibilities of the occupational therapist and the occupational therapy assistant during the delivery of occupational therapy services, *Am J Occup Ther* 58(6):663–667, 2004.
8. American Occupational Therapy Association: Standards of practice for occupational therapy, *Am J Occup Ther* 59(6): 663–665, 2005.
9. American Occupational Therapy Association: Statement: fundamental concepts of occupational therapy: occupation, purposeful activity, and function, *Am J Occup Ther* 51(10):864–869, 1997.
10. Ayres AJ: Basic concepts of clinical practice in physical disabilities, *Am J Occup Ther* 12:300, 1958.
11. Di Joseph LM: Independence through activity: mind, body, and environment interaction in therapy, *Am J Occup Ther* 36:740, 1982.
12. Dirette D, Rozich A, Viau S: Is there enough evidence for evidence-based practice in occupational therapy? *Am J Occup Ther* 63:782–786, 2009.
13. Holm MB: The 2000 Eleanor Clarke Slagle Lecture. Our mandate for the new millennium: evidence-based practice, *Am J Occup Ther* 54:575–585, 2000.
14. Kielhofner G, Burke JP: A model of human occupation: 1. Conceptual framework and content, *Am J Occup Ther* 34:572–581, 1980.
15. Kielhofner G, editor: *A model of human occupation: theory and application*, Baltimore, 1985, Williams & Wilkins.
16. Kielhofner G, editor: *A model of human occupation: theory and application*, ed 3, Baltimore, 2002, Lippincott Williams & Wilkins.
17. Kielhofner G, editor: *A model of human occupation: theory and application*, ed 4, Baltimore, 2008, Lippincott Williams & Wilkins.
18. Lopez-De Fede A, Haeussler-Fiore D: *An introduction to the culture of the Dominican Republic for rehabilitation service providers*, Buffalo NY, 2002, Center for International Rehabilitation Research Information and Exchange (CIRRIE). Available on the web at *http://cirrie.buffalo.edu/monographs/domrep.pdf.* Accessed October 27, 2010.
19. Merleau-Ponty M: *Phenomenology of perception,* (C. Smith, trans.) London, 1945, Routledge & Kegan Paul, originally published, *Phénoménologie de la perception*, Paris: Gallimard.
20. Mosby: *Mosby's medical, nursing, and allied health dictionary*, ed 6, St. Louis, 2005, Mosby.

21. Mosey AC: *Occupational therapy: configuration of a profession*, New York, 1981, Raven.
22. Oxford University Press: *Pocket Oxford American dictionary*, ed 2, New York, 2008, Oxford University Press.
23. Pedretti LW: The compatibility of treatment methods in physical disabilities with the philosophical base of occupational therapy. Paper presented at the American Occupational Therapy Association National Conference, Philadelphia, May 1982.
24. Phipps SC, Roberts PS: Motor learning. In Pendleton HM, Schult-Krohn W, editors: *Pedretti's Occupational therapy—practice skills for physical dysfunction*, ed 6, St. Louis, 2006, Mosby.
25. Reed KL: *Models for practice in occupational therapy*, Baltimore, 1984, Williams & Wilkins.
26. Rogers JC: The spirit of independence: the evolution of a philosophy, *Am J Occup Ther* 36:709, 1982.
27. Schmidt RA, Lee T: *Motor control and learning*, Champaign IL, 1999, Human Kinetics.
28. Schultz-Krohn W, Royeenm CB, McCormack G, Pope-Davis SA, Jourdan JM: Traditional sensorimotor approaches to intervention. In Pendleton HM, Schult-Krohn W, editors: *Pedretti's Occupational therapy—practice skills for physical dysfunction*, ed 6, St. Louis, 2006, Mosby.
29. Shumway-Cook M, Woollacott M: *Motor control: theory and practical applications*, Baltimore, 2001, Lippincott Williams & Wilkins.
30. Smith LK, Weiss EL, Lehmkuhl LD: *Brunnstrom's clinical kinesiology*, ed 5, Philadelphia, 1996, FA Davis.
31. Trombly CA: Include exercise in purposeful activity, *Am J Occup Ther* 36:467, 1982:(letter to the editor).

CHAPTER 2

The Disability Experience and the Therapeutic Process

MARY BETH EARLY

Key Terms

Person with a disability (PWD)
Personal causation
Locus of control
Values
Social supports
Identity versus role confusion
Generativity versus stagnation
Intimacy versus isolation
Person-first perspective
Apparent acceptance
Persons without a disability (PWOD)
Spread factor
Anxiety
Fear of falling (FoF)
Depression
Denial
Displacement
Dependency
Regression
Passing
Body image
Compromise body image
Therapeutic mode
Advocating
Collaborating
Empathizing
Encouraging
Instructing
Problem solving
Self-definition
Emotional intelligence
Self-help groups
Milieu therapy
Substance abuse
Disability rights movement
Independent living model
Architectural barriers
Universal design

Chapter Objectives

After studying this chapter, the student or practitioner will be able to do the following:

1. Relate the personal and social experience of physical disability to the model of human occupation and to human development.
2. Discuss possible personal reactions to the experience of physical dysfunction.
3. Describe the "person-first perspective" and how this frames the therapist's interactions with the patient.
4. Describe common societal reactions to physically disabled persons, and discuss the origins of these reactions.
5. Describe the process of adjustment to the experience of physical disability, and list some possible stages of the adjustment process.
6. Identify and discuss factors that may help or hinder the process of adjustment.
7. Name and describe specific interventions used in occupational therapy to help disabled individuals cope with and adjust to personal and social effects of physical dysfunction.
8. Discuss substance abuse in relation to physical disability.
9. Describe negative societal attitudes toward persons with disabilities and how the occupational therapy assistant (OTA) may help address these.
10. Discuss the role of the OTA as advocate for the person with a disability.

Imagine this scenario: you are a novice occupational therapy assistant (OTA) student and your supervisor has asked you to choose and talk to any one of four patients in the therapy clinic.* You see an older Caucasian man in a wheelchair with a distorted face and a slumped posture; an older Latina woman sitting in a regular chair trying to do arm exercises with some weights and bands, though she seems to have multiple upper extremity injuries; an African-American man who seems to be in his 20s, in a power wheelchair and learning to use some kind of complicated splint; and a South Asian woman wearing a sari, who has burn scars and is wearing bilateral splints (she is accompanied by her young daughter, who is helping her remove the splints). Which client do you choose to approach? Why? What do you think the person expects from OT? And how do you expect the person to respond to you?

When first encountering a client, the OTA student or novice practitioner (who is without personal experience of disability) may struggle to appreciate the experience and perspective of the person with the disability. Most of us, before entering the OT field, are not even aware of how our ideas of disabled individuals have been formed. Popular culture and the media generate and promulgate images and stereotypes that may not represent the client at all and act as barriers to a genuine helping relationship.

The effects of physical disability extend beyond the physical body. To be truly effective, occupational therapists must consider the psychological, social, and spiritual person, as well as the presenting physical problem. OT practitioners must accustom themselves to approaching the situation from the patient's point of view, to helping individuals process and integrate what has happened to them, and to involving them as much as possible in setting goals.

Physical dysfunction is initially an experience of loss: loss of function of a physical part, loss of body image dependent on the "normal" functioning of that part, and loss of social roles, normal occupations, and personal identity. Independence, self-sufficiency, and autonomy may be diminished, partially or totally and permanently or temporarily.[13]

The content and quality of daily life change dramatically; for inpatients and residents in long-term care the new environment and lifestyle of the health care facility enforce passivity and dependence. The schedule, people, and activities are new and are not self-chosen. Privacy must be surrendered, and strangers must be allowed to probe the body. Familial, social, and vocational roles are interrupted and may be seriously altered by the disability experience.

Not only is the **person with a disability** (PWD) affected but also the others with whom the person has contact. The responses of the PWD and significant others affect the outcome of rehabilitation.[13] The person with the disability must first learn to survive, then to regain essential physical skills, and finally to resume meaningful life roles. These are monumental tasks that require significant adjustment.[45]

This chapter considers the relationship between the psychosocial and the physical self in the context of physical disease and disability. The reader will gain an appreciation of the disability experience, examining individual response, societal expectations, and environmental factors. The personal and social reactions to disability and the nature of adjustment to disability are examined. The chapter concludes with guidance for the clinician and some interventions and techniques to facilitate psychosocial adjustment and optimal functioning in the community. Therapeutic use of self with so-called "difficult clients" is discussed.

We begin with a review of concepts from the model of human occupation (MOHO) and from human developmental theory, which will frame the rest of the chapter. The MOHO is described in Chapter 1, which the reader is encouraged to review. The following is only a summary, with particular emphasis on physical disability and its effects.

A Context: The Model of Human Occupation

Physical disability disrupts the occupational life of the individual in many ways and on many levels.[34] Initially (and most obviously) the disability impairs the performance capacity—the skills and foundation of skills used in activities of daily living (ADL). However, this disruption reverberates into habituation; the loss of skills prevents or alters the performance of habits (e.g., bathing, dressing) and occupational roles (e.g., homemaker, worker, student). Because of physical disability, the person may be able to handle only a few roles, and these may be different from those previously held.[16] Interestingly, OT assessment of role changes has been relatively rare in physical dysfunction settings, where therapists have focused predominantly on physical restoration.[83]

Effects on volition (**personal causation**, values, and interests) may be profound. Physical disability occurs most often as a result of some external agent (e.g., accident, infection, disease) rather than any personal action (e.g., suicide attempt, recklessness, substance abuse). The power of an outside agency to alter a person's life so dramatically may challenge the individual's sense of self-direction (locus of control). Being unable to perform in customary roles may engender uncertainty about long-held values (e.g., economic self-sufficiency, social productivity) and may prevent realization of valued goals (e.g., to hike the length of the Appalachian Trail during retirement). Previously held interests may be incompatible with physical restrictions. All these consequences are potentially negative and damaging but can be ameliorated by intrapersonal, social, and environmental factors.

Intrapersonal Factors

Evidence strongly indicates that the individual's premorbid personality, particularly a strong sense of locus of control and social efficacy, may promote positive adjustment to physical disability.[20,25,28,61] In other words, people who have an internal orientation of **locus of control** (a strong sense that they,

*This chapter uses the word "patient" to refer in general to the recipients of OT services. We caution the reader that persons with disabilities are not always "patients"; they are sometimes "clients," "residents," or simply "persons with disabilities."

rather than fate, are in control of their lives) are more likely to tackle their limitations and to achieve the maximal possible quality of life. In some individuals, physical disability becomes a challenge to meet, and the effort involved reinforces and may increase the personal sense of competence and efficacy.

Values will also play a role. A sense of obligation to others, a desire to contribute productively, or a willingness to accept loss and change will differently affect the person's orientation toward disability. Although society generally devalues disability, assigning PWDs to a lower social status and marginalized economic position, some PWDs have come to identify their disability situation positively and are vocal in advocating for social and political change.[34]

Social Factors

The family and other close social supports are critical in adjustment to physical dysfunction. To rebuild a meaningful occupational life, the individual with physical disability must be able to trust in the helpfulness of other people and to count on the support of others to compensate for lost skills and roles.[61] Previously able to provide for personal needs in areas such as bathing and dressing, the person with severe disabilities may need assistance (permanently or temporarily) from others. The availability and willingness of significant others to perform these functions are crucial. The psychological messages (e.g., acceptance, curiosity, interest, irritation, resentment, revulsion) sent consciously or unconsciously by the caregiver will affect the patient's psychosocial adjustment. Stigma and marginalization by society at large will adversely affect the PWD.

Environmental Factors

The human-made environment is designed for able-bodied people. Although legislative and social pressures have introduced accessible features into banks, sidewalks, restaurant toilets, and other public environments, disabled individuals must still determine how to move and communicate in a world that in some instances only minimally meets their needs. Altering physical features (e.g., installing ramps and handrails) and providing appropriate communication devices (e.g., computers) and adaptive equipment often make adjustment easier. Even with modifications and equipment, PWDs will feel constrained in their ability to move about and negotiate their environments freely.[66] Despite functional benefits, new devices can be stressful to learn and may cause the person to feel somewhat "odd," especially in comparison with the premorbid self; the sense of the lived body has been profoundly disturbed.[34]

Organizing Questions

Human occupation is a useful model for considering the effects of disability on an individual. The OT practitioner who frames the approach to the patient around this model asks questions such as the following:

- What skills, habits, and roles has this person lost or reduced as a result of this disability?
- What is the person's sense of personal causation?
- What values and interests does the person have?
- What is the person's social and object environment?
- Most importantly, which interventions will assist in increasing the person's sense of personal causation and in putting the environment more within his or her control?

Another Context: Developmental Stages

Psychological consequences of physical disability depend on many factors. The range of personal reactions varies from one individual to another. Some factors that may influence the person's response to the dysfunction are (1) life stage in which the disability was acquired; (2) the extent and location of the defect; (3) whether it is visible; (4) the social definition of the defect; (5) the attitudes of significant others toward the individual and the defect; (6) the extent to which the disability interferes with functioning; and (7) the disruption of valued goals.

Physical disability may be congenital (from birth) or may occur at any time of life, with its effects varying with the developmental stage. Table 2-1 summarizes the stages of psychosocial development according to Erikson.[19] Without reviewing all of human development, this section briefly uses as examples just two stages, adolescence and middle adulthood, and the possible effects of disability occurring at these stages. The reader is cautioned that these are *possible* effects and that experiences of individuals differ.

Adolescence is the stage of identity versus role confusion. The adolescent is learning, comparing, and "trying on" various adult roles. Vocational choice, gender identification, and identification with peers rather than the family are key issues. Many of the OT studies of psychosocial adjustment to disability have focused on adolescence,[28,35,54] perhaps because of the dramatic effects of disability on personal identity. Reactions of peers and authorities, perceived lack of romantic appeal, worries over scholastic competence, and continued dependence on parents are some of the concerns of PWDs at this developmental stage.[35,54]

Each developmental stage carries its own tasks and will be affected differently by disability. A spinal cord injury occurring in later life is devastating but usually does not affect the *development* of personal identity, because this task has been achieved normally during adolescence. Rather, the current developmental task is challenged while previously achieved tasks are revisited and reevaluated. For example, a married 56-year-old male schoolteacher is typically in Erikson's stage of generativity versus stagnation, with an emphasis on contributing to the future through work, community activity, and raising children (who may be college age or older). A spinal cord injury to this individual requires an adjustment in the way generativity is addressed, perhaps with retirement from employment and a shift in ADL, often to a more sedentary, intellectual, computer-based lifestyle. However, each preceding developmental task is also reevaluated.

For example, the adolescent task of developing an identity may reemerge as individuals consider their new role of "patient" or "PWD" and ponder who they will "be" now that they cannot perform the activities they once identified as part of their "being."[59] They also question their sexual identity and

Table 2-1 Erikson's Eight Stages of Psychosocial Development

Approximate Age	Psychosocial Stage	Explanation
Birth-18 mo	Basic trust versus mistrust	Infant needs nurturance from mother. If infant perceives mother as reliable, infant will develop the capacity to trust others. If not, infant will tend to mistrust others, will feel anxious about their willingness to meet infant's needs, etc.
2-4 yr	Autonomy versus shame and doubt	During this period, child learns to control bowel and bladder and becomes more independent in exploring the environment. Child's sense of motivation and will are shaped by parents' attitudes toward bodily functions and their willingness to allow child to practice self-control.
3-5 yr	Initiative versus guilt	Preschool and kindergarten child begins to combine skills and plan activities to accomplish goals. Child begins to imitate adult roles and to try out new ways of doing things. Child develops a sense of self-direction.
6-12 yr	Industry versus inferiority	During elementary school, child acquires skills and work habits and compares self with peers. Attitudes about parents, teachers, and other children contribute to child's sense of personal competence.
Adolescence	Identity versus role confusion	Adolescent experiments with a variety of adult roles. Key issues include vocational choice and gender identification. Rebellion against parents is common as teenagers try to assert a separate identity.
Young adulthood	Intimacy versus isolation	Central concern of this period is to find a suitable partner with whom to share the person's life.
Middle adulthood	Generativity versus stagnation	Adult looks toward future and tries to make a contribution to it through work, community leadership, childrearing, etc.
Old age	Ego integrity versus despair	Faced with prospect of death, older adult reviews and evaluates life's choices to determine if what the person meant to do has been accomplished.

Modified from Early MB: *Mental health concepts and techniques for the occupational therapy assistant*, ed 2, New York, 1993, Raven.

performance and their ability to be an intimate partner. Thus the task of intimacy versus isolation resurfaces as well.

The OT practitioner approaching the individual with physical disability must keep in mind the following questions:

- What is this person's developmental stage?
- With what developmental task(s) might this person be grappling?
- Based on this information, what concerns or responses might I expect from this individual?
- How can I assist this person to recognize and state personal goals and achieve them?

With the context of human occupation and human development in mind, we now turn to the personal and social consequences of physical dysfunction.

Psychological and Social Consequences of Physical Dysfunction

Individual Reactions

Reactions to physical dysfunction vary tremendously, and some examples are given next. The "person-first perspective" asks us to see the person rather than the diagnosis. With a "person-first perspective" one never assumes that the disability is the defining characteristic of the person or that a list of adjustment stages would apply to every patient. People react in different ways; one should never assume that a given individual will respond in any particular way. Reactions depend on the psychological meaning of the specific dysfunction in relation to the individual's personality and life history.[24] For example, paraplegia is likely to have a different meaning to an athlete (who has experienced self-worth in terms of physical performance and physique) than to an office worker (whose sense of self may be defined more in terms of using mental and hand activities).[37]

Paradoxically, some persons may evaluate the physical disability as positive. A dysfunction viewed as a well-deserved punishment may lead to a greater sense of well-being. A dysfunction viewed as an opportunity to depend on a caring person may gratify dependency wishes or allow the patient to avoid responsibility.[74]

Productivity and physical attractiveness are highly valued in American culture, as are self-sufficiency and independence. Deficiencies in these areas may generate feelings of low self-worth that tend to be "all or none" in quality. The individual may focus on only one characteristic and generalize from this to a belief that the entire self is worthless. The feelings of low self-worth often infect memories of the past and visions of the future so that the person can neither conceive of self as ever having been productive or attractive nor contemplate the possibility of future change.

The conclusion of worthlessness fits society's stereotypes about the self in terms of productivity and attractiveness, and for this reason may be deeply held. This perception is a distortion because it bases self-worth on deficits and neglects remaining assets and intrinsic worth. Although the concept of intrinsic worth (i.e., the person valued for self alone without external comparisons) is desired and ideal, it is probably difficult or impossible to achieve for most people. In general, people in American society value themselves according to external standards of attractiveness, productivity, and achievements.

Some PWDs may conclude that they are worthless and of negative value. They may expect and think that they deserve the rejection of others based on that notion. If they are not of any value to themselves, others will not see them as valuable and therefore will reject them. This type of thinking can persist and may lead to withdrawal or an intense search for approval and love. Some persons will draw from this thinking process what seems to be a logical conclusion: They are worth nothing to self or to others; therefore life is meaningless and empty, and they should not exist. This feeling may be especially strong in those who feel intense guilt.[23,69]

The meaning of the disability to the person is the crucial factor in planning a sound intervention approach and in aiding with the adjustment process. Therefore strategies to facilitate psychosocial adjustment must be targeted toward individual reactions to the circumstances rather than focusing on reactions and characteristics assumed to be similar among persons with the same physical disability or the same degree of severity of disability.[67]

Societal Responses

Although the personal or individual perspective is one way to view the disability experience, one cannot ignore the social perspective. Some psychologists and social scientists in the area of disability studies traditionally view disability as a social construction, a problem in the way society views disability and responds to it.[46] Historically, American culture's predominant reaction to disabled persons has been negative. Political action including the passage of the Americans with Disabilities Act (ADA) of 1990 and an increasingly active consumer movement and social justice orientation have somewhat altered public perceptions of acceptable behavior toward the disabled.[2,46] Since 2002, the ABC television program *Extreme Makeover: Home Edition* has shown the home lives of PWDs including those with spinal cord injuries.[79] Such media attention helps dispel some of the negative stereotypes but perhaps may create others. Prejudices and stereotypes persist, even among health care providers, and may significantly affect the PWD.

Avoidance and Rejection

Attitudes of others toward physical disability affect attitudes of PWDs toward themselves. In newly disabled individuals, devaluing attitudes toward the disabled population, once an out-group, may now be directed to the self, with serious consequences.[67,69] Few people have much experience with or are really comfortable with individuals who have disabilities or visible deformities. The presence of PWDs confronts nondisabled persons with their own vulnerability. To avoid feeling threatened, nondisabled individuals ignore or avoid PWDs.[74]

The appearance of the injury or disability also engenders nonacceptance. If the disability is unsightly, this perception tends to be overestimated by nondisabled persons and is a factor that prompts rejection or avoidance. Padilla, an occupational therapist, writes about reacting to a brain-injured woman with a "preconscious expectation that the appearance of her body was a representation of her mind."[59] Meeting a person with a visible disability, the nondisabled person may display pity or excessive curiosity. The PWD feels set apart from most "normal" people and is constantly striving to fight the negative implications of the physical dysfunction and to gain genuine social acceptance.[41] Paradoxically, disabilities that are not immediately visible may cause additional problems; if the person does not appear to be disabled, others may believe they are making it up or exaggerating the situation (Box 2-1).

Box 2-1

Perspective on Hidden Disability: Rheumatoid Arthritis

"The outside world doesn't seem to be able to grasp that you can look OK on the outside but maybe feel ah . . . washed out on the inside. They can't see that. I think society on the whole needs to see you missing an eyeball or missing a limb to understand a handicap or a disability."[17]

Nonacceptance

Nonacceptance by nondisabled persons stems from negative attitudes. The PWD feels ostracized when others are resistant or reluctant to interact socially.

Apparent acceptance by nondisabled persons is equally disturbing. In this case the person conveys the socially correct forms of acceptance and inclusion, but this attitude does not necessarily represent genuine social acceptance. Apparent acceptance may be motivated by pity or duty and to the person with the disability will feel devoid of meaning or real pleasure in the interchange. In both nonacceptance and apparent acceptance, PWDs sense the underlying inability or unwillingness of **persons without disability (PWODs)** to know them as they really are.

Individuals with disabilities perceive a lack of patience on the part of nondisabled persons toward slowness and difficulties in performance. Whether this attitude is maintained by the nondisabled population or is projected by the disabled population, it engenders the same feeling of nonacceptance in the PWD.[41]

Spread Factor

PWODs also tend to judge PWDs not only in terms of the apparent physical limitation but also in terms of psychological factors assumed to be associated with the disability.[41] PWODs may treat PWDs as if they are limited mentally and emotionally as well.[62] The person with the disability may internalize this devalued condition. The evaluation of the visible disability is "spread" to other characteristics that are not necessarily affected. The common assumption that a person who has cerebral palsy is also mentally retarded and the practice of speaking loudly to blind persons as if they are also deaf are examples of this phenomenon. This **spread factor** is generally a devaluing process, and the PWD is thereby stigmatized and considered of lower social status and unworthy of acceptance[41] (Box 2-2).

Nondisabled persons also tend to view limitations as more severe and restrictive than they actually are. They may judge that a given physical dysfunction prevents the PWD's participation in a given activity or social situation; however, the

Box 2-2

Perspective on Perceptions of Others: Head Injury

"I don't know if it is my family and friends who can't get past my disability or if it is me. I watch them talk to each other with such ease, and then turn to me and talk to me like a child. They can't understand my horrible voice and turn away as though I had said all I needed. Why try anymore? I am used to being marooned. I don't want to look at their faces when they cannot understand my voice."[59]

nondisabled person cannot know the PWD's capabilities. It is better for nondisabled persons to invite individuals who have disabilities to participate and to allow them to determine whether participation is feasible. Even when the situation appears totally impossible, an invitation still signals acceptance and allows for the person to participate in restructuring the situation. The changes required may be simple or complex but should be left to the discretion of the person and not structured by the preconceived notions of nondisabled persons.[41]

Labeling

Words that have a stigmatizing effect on the PWD exist throughout American English. Expressions such as "retard," "crip," and "psycho" are examples. Within the language of the medical and allied health professions, these terms become formalized to "mentally retarded," "physically disabled," and "mentally ill." These terms have value for the classification of persons into diagnostic categories, but they stigmatize as well.[62] It follows that when rehabilitation workers refer to their patients as a diagnosis or disability (e.g., "quad" or "hemi"), they are contributing to the stigmatization of those they set out to help.

Minority Group Status

Stigma may be considered as negative perceptions or behaviors of "normal" people toward PWDs or toward all persons different from themselves. Socially, PWDs in general are regarded in much the same way as other minority groups in the population. They are subject to both overt and covert stereotyping and a reduced social status. Stigmatization is a basic fact of life for almost all PWDs. Interpersonal relationships between nondisabled and disabled people tend to follow a superior-inferior pattern or not to exist at all. Nondisabled persons tend to demonstrate stereotyped, inhibited, and overcontrolled behavior in interactions with persons who have disabilities. They tend to show less variable behavior, terminate interactions sooner, and express opinions less representative of their actual beliefs.[54,62] The stereotyped feedback the PWD receives from the nondisabled person becomes another barrier to be overcome.

Segregation

The physically disabled population is still substantially segregated, despite the 1990 ADA. Although some of this segregation is necessary (e.g., institutionalization, special schools) and designed to assist PWDs, it nevertheless sets them apart psychologically and environmentally and evokes feelings of inferiority in relation to nondisabled peers.

Unfounded Positive Images

In some instances, PWDs are also subjected to unfounded positive images. The belief that blind people have sharpened senses to compensate for the loss of vision is such an example. This is the myth of "automatic compensation." The fact is that blind and deaf individuals learn to use their other senses more efficiently.[25]

Attitudes in the Health Care System

The health care system can be considered a microcosm of society. Health care workers tend to believe that societal prejudices toward persons with disabilities do not exist. The assumption is that rehabilitation personnel are immune from discriminatory attitudes and that patients are accepted as persons when they are accepted as patients.[24]

The attitudes of the professionals involved with the rehabilitation of disabled individuals are of great importance and may be highly influential in the person's response to rehabilitation. Negative reactions will result in a negative response in the patient. Such reactions increase the patient's suffering and decrease motivation, leading to uncooperative behavior and labeling the person as "difficult."[10]

Although the staff may hold the view that prejudice does not exist in the facility, in reality the staff's view is that the patient is a person to be helped, a malleable individual who can be shaped and educated into a specific health status and behavior. Convictions of superiority are reinforced by the emergence of a teacher-student relationship, a superior-inferior pattern.[24] Practitioners seeking to protect themselves from the pain experienced by those in their care may engage in "distancing behaviors."[60] This pattern is further reinforced in inpatient settings by segregated dining areas, staff uniforms, and the institution's organizational hierarchy.

Patients may come to view themselves as disabled and unable to perform, perceiving themselves as applicants asking the knowledgeable, powerful, and authoritative others if they can regain the characteristics and skills of nondisabled persons. The patients confront a closed, self-sufficient subculture with an unfamiliar value system and are actually outsiders in the facility seeking acceptance from omnipotent persons in authority. The patients occupy the lowest level in the status hierarchy of the institution and are manipulated by many forces over which they have no control. Individual life goals may be partly or completely determined by others and by choices and decisions imposed under a facade of personal involvement and self-determination.

To change this, the OT practitioner must shed the role of teacher and authority figure to engage authentically with the patient as an equal and to assume the role of facilitator and guide. Segregation in residential facilities needs to be abandoned to the extent possible, for example, in the dining and recreation areas. Recognition and respect for different needs, goals, and value systems can change the attitudes of health care workers toward patients. Involvement of the patient in the decision-making process for treatment and in patient government can also be helpful in reducing prejudice and equalizing the status of residents of long-term care settings.[55,57]

Origins of Attitudes toward Persons with Physical Disabilities

Aversion to persons with disability is not natural or instinctive as has been thought. Studies by animal psychologists and cultural anthropologists suggest that the existence of instinctive hostile attitudes toward disabled individuals is a myth.[12]

History

All societies probably have discriminated positively or negatively against disabled persons (as they may against individuals who are different in height, skin color, etc.). Examples of extreme forms of prejudice are the attribution of supernatural powers to physically different individuals on the positive end and the elimination of physically deformed infants on the negative end. More modern societies have expressed their prejudice in more subtle ways such as excluding persons with disabilities from employment opportunities and social interactions.

The popularity of "freak" shows in circuses was testimony to paradoxical repulsion-attraction of nondisabled people toward persons with disabilities and deformities. Negative attitudes toward people with disabilities are rooted in ancestral superstitions and mythologies and have evolved into the sophisticated bigotry of the present age.[26]

Because of the primacy of group survival, "primitive" societies did not tolerate those who were physically impaired. The physically weak individuals were expendable, and the law of survival of the fittest prevailed.[26]

Superstitions and folklore guided primitive peoples before the advent of organized religions. Evil spirits were thought to reside in the bodies of those who were sick or deformed. Therefore such individuals were to be avoided. Mental illnesses and physical afflictions were thought to be the work of evil spirits. If the spirits did not exit the afflicted body after considerable effort, it was believed that the individual was being punished; therefore such individuals were avoided or killed.[26]

In discussing the history and psychology of amputation, Friedmann[22] noted that in ancient civilizations, self-mutilation was practiced to appease the gods and thus was a form of "religious rehabilitation." Few civilizations encouraged the survival of deformed infants. In some societies, transgressions of rules or crimes are even today punished by the amputation of a limb or part. Thus the concepts that disability is a deserved punishment for misdeeds, that disabled persons are not acceptable in society, and that disability is reparation for sin have ancient (and enduring) roots.

As societies became more civilized, methods of dealing with people who had disabilities began to change. In a few societies, they were accepted and treated well. During the Middle Ages, blind persons occupied a privileged position in France. In both Asia and the Mediterranean regions, progressive physicians called for humane treatment of the disabled population. In most countries, however, inhumane treatment of the disabled individual persisted. Infants with disabilities were abandoned, drowned, or killed. Infanticide was practiced by nobility to maintain the purity of the bloodline. Children who escaped the fate of death roamed the country as beggars; some were subjected to slavery or forced into prostitution.[26]

During the Renaissance, more tolerant attitudes toward and improved treatment of physically different persons developed. The Elizabethan English Poor Laws (1597-1601) were the legal foundation for the protection of poor and disabled people from degrading treatment and provided financial support for unemployed persons including those with disabilities. Gradually the perception of the disabled individual began to shift from one of total worthlessness to one of marginal productivity in society.[26]

Despite this progress, early American historical records indicate little knowledge of and few resources available to persons with disabilities. Medical care was limited in the colonies but began to improve in the nineteenth century. Medical personnel began to demand better facilities to treat patients who had disabilities. However, this attitude was not widespread, and many physicians continued to demonstrate negative attitudes toward and inhumane treatment of physically disabled persons. The myth that such afflictions were the result of evil spirits continued, as did treatment with "bleeding," potions, and ostracism.[26]

A few hospitals in New York and Philadelphia provided treatment to physically disabled persons before the Civil War; the first sheltered workshop was established in 1837. At the end of the nineteenth century, the Cleveland Rehabilitation Center was established and was the forerunner of present-day rehabilitation centers. Among private organizations to help persons with disabilities that began during this period were The Salvation Army (1880) and Goodwill Industries (1902).[26]

Literature and Media

Ancient myths and stereotypes persist. Many people still associate disabilities with sin and the Devil or with evil.[21] Disability becomes associated with *bad* and able-bodied with *good*. Metaphorical use of these associations appears in the Bible as well as in both ancient and contemporary literature. This concept is communicated to children through books, television, and religious training.[26]

Media images of persons with disabilities are molded from early childhood through fairy tales and classical literature. Physical deformity, illness, and unattractiveness often symbolize inner defects, evil natures, and villainous behavior.[85] Some of the oldest and best known children's stories convey these prejudices. These stories subtly teach children scorn for PWDs. Characters such as Cinderella's stepsisters (who were obese and unattractive), Captain Hook of *Peter Pan* (who wore a prosthesis), the wicked witch of *Hansel and Gretel* (who was aged, arthritic, and had a kyphosis), and the evil character in *Jack and the Beanstalk* (afflicted by gigantism) set up an association between physical difference and evil.[85]

An examination of these and other well-known stories suggests that physical attractiveness, health, and intactness of the body are usually features of the heroes and heroines, the noble, and the good person. Conversely, villains are often portrayed with some infirmity or unattractive feature such as large noses, wrinkles, and warts. Moral character and personality are thus associated with external appearance.

Some stories show physical disability as a consequence of a misdeed. Pinocchio's nose grew as a result of his failure to tell the truth, and pirates lost eyes and limbs as a result of their violent behavior.[85] There have been almost no average, ordinary physically abnormal individuals in children's stories in the past. More recently, several children's books that portray disabled persons in a more favorable and matter-of-fact manner have been published.*

Although classical children's literature has value and will always be enjoyed, parents and others reading this literature to children need to be aware of the biases that may be conveyed and to discuss and reflect on them with children to minimize the unquestioned acceptance of these portrayals. Fortunately, children today are much more matter-of-fact about disability because they are likely to have disabled classmates and because disability is openly discussed in the classroom.

Persons with disabilities are portrayed in television programs, movies, cartoons, comic strips, and adult fiction. Some of these characters excel beyond the expectations of others around them.[36] For example, little Dumbo (the elephant with big ears that are ridiculed by others) turns out to be able to fly; and in *Finding Nemo,* the small clownfish who has mismatched fins (one quite small) becomes a good swimmer.[36] In reality television shows we may see a heroic farmer or construction worker with bilateral above-knee amputations driving a piece of construction equipment in an aggressive manner, as if to showcase his overcoming of disability. In the film *How to Train Your Dragon*, the young boy Hiccup discovers how to befriend and train dragons rather than kill them. He is slender and appears weak in comparison with his peers. In a battle near the end of the film, he loses his leg and then wears a prosthesis that looks much like the modern versions worn by twenty-first century amputees. Dumbo, Nemo, and Hiccup exemplify the stereotype of *supercrip*, a character who overcomes disability and becomes more capable and able than some "normal" people.[68] This stereotype is hard to live up to and puts pressure on PWDs to perform in exemplary ways.

Increasingly, however, disabled persons are often portrayed in movies, television programs, and television advertising in more natural and positive and less dramatic ways, performing ordinary life roles. And in some films, older adults who have accepted and are living with disabilities provide guidance and give examples to the younger characters.[36]

Religion

The image of the individual with physical disabilities varies from society to society, and the dominant religion in a society may translate the disability into spiritual terms. The disability may be assigned a spiritual cause such as possession, the consequences of sin, a special sign of God's grace, or a blessing.[12]

Many people have grown up with the notion that God is all-wise, all-loving, and all-powerful. He is seen as a parent figure who rewards obedience and disciplines disobedience. He protects those in His favor from harm and arranges for each person to receive what that individual deserves in life. If this premise is accepted, the question must be considered: "Why do bad things happen to good people?"[39] This question is raised when personal tragedy is experienced and when print and broadcast media present seemingly senseless tragedies that occur everywhere and to all types of people. It is troubling to know that suffering is distributed unfairly in the world. For many, this awareness raises questions about the goodness and even the existence of God. Kushner[39] outlines various popular explanations of suffering based on this notion of God and discusses the faulty reasoning in each.

Some of the most common notions of the causes of suffering that are based on scripture are that (1) suffering is punishment for sin (Isaiah 3:10-11, Proverbs 3:7-8); (2) suffering is for personal growth or testing of spiritual strengths (Genesis 22); and (3) suffering is a cure for personality flaws (Proverbs 3:11-12).[8,39]

The New Testament introduces the concept of suffering as a share in the glory of Jesus Christ (Romans 8:17). Illness and disability are also sometimes shown as associated with the presence of demons (Matthew 8:16, 8:28; Luke 9:37-43, 11:14, 13:10-14). However, there are also many accounts of healings in which no association with sin or evil spirits exists (Matthew 8:8-13, Mark 8:22-26, Luke 17:11-18).[8]

Someone who believes that suffering is punishment for sin will believe that the sufferers have received what they deserve. The difficulty arises when the individual cannot find a misdeed that deserves the punishment and may become angry at God or repress that anger to protect the perceived reputation of God as the fair and just parent.[39]

If a person accepts the notion that suffering is for the ennoblement of people to repair faulty aspects of the personality, it follows that suffering is for the individual's own good. Associated ideas are that God teaches a lesson with suffering and that everything happens for a purpose, although that purpose may be obscure and known only to God. Another explanation of suffering is that God tests only those whom he knows are strong of spirit.[39] This generates the idea that those with afflictions are privileged or chosen by God for a special role and are therefore elevated in God's sight. This idea does not explain all those who break under the strain of their suffering or those who do not appear strong enough to deal with it.[39]

If the presence of demons as a cause of illness and disability is accepted, it may follow that some spiritual illness or defect exists. Therefore if the demons are driven out with healing prayers, the sufferer will surely get well. Although accounts of sudden and unexplained healings have been documented, a "formula" cannot be said to work in every instance.

All these responses or attempts at explaining tragedy assume that God is the cause of suffering. They attempt to explain why God would mete out suffering. Is it for the individual's own

*References 5, 42, 44, 52, 58, 64, 65, 67, 80, 81.

growth; is it divine punishment; or is it that God does not care what happens to humans? Some approaches lead the believer to self-blame and foster the denial of reality and repression of true feelings. Kushner[39] asks his readers to consider the possibility that God does not cause suffering and that maybe it occurs for reasons other than the result of the will of God. Perhaps God does not cause bad things to happen, and the question is not "Why me?" but rather, "God, see what is happening to me, can you help?" (Psalms 121:1-2).[8,39] God may not control some events. Some misfortunes that befall people may be the result of "bad luck," bad people, human weakness, random events, and the inflexible laws of nature.[39] Any health care worker or patient who is wrestling with this question is advised to read Kushner's book *When Bad Things Happen to Good People.*[39]

Spiritual counseling is a necessary aspect of the treatment program for many patients. OT practitioners should recognize this need and make the appropriate referrals.

Adjustment to Physical Dysfunction

Physical illness or injury resulting in disability is a significant life stressor to which the individual brings a unique repertoire of coping mechanisms and response patterns.[61] Physical dysfunction may cause minimal or no prolonged effect on personality. However, behavior and emotions may be temporarily disordered by the crisis of physical change. Fluctuations in physical recovery and psychosocial adaptation, rather than a direct and sustained movement toward adjustment, should be expected.[9] Over time, the personality appears to be capable of drawing on its resources and integrating the crisis experience.[72]

The individual with physical dysfunction is faced with the problem of coping with fears and anxieties and maintaining a balance between conflicting needs and tendencies at a time when defenses are weakened and it is most difficult to cope. Anxieties are typically managed through a variety of coping mechanisms.

Reactions and Coping Mechanisms

Anxiety

Uneasiness and concerns about the future are common responses to recent physical dysfunction. Anxiety may take the form of vague feelings of tension and fears but also may be manifest in physical signs such as restlessness, increased perspiration, shallow and fast breathing, and pressured speech. Some fears such as fear of falling (FoF), which may arise following an injury from falling or a stroke or head injury, may be specific and seemingly rational.[70] Combined with depression (see next), FoF may severely impair the person's return to valued occupations. The individual may restrict activities and therefore decline in physical and mental health and social participation. Recovery from stroke may be impaired by FoF and its resultant inactivity.[70]

Depression

Mourning the loss of function or loss of a part invariably occurs after the onset of physical dysfunction. Depression is a feeling of sadness often accompanied by changes in behavior such as sleeplessness or excessive sleeping and disinterest in previously enjoyed activities.[3] Depression often occurs with the realization of the limitations imposed by the disability and may last a year or longer.[59,75] The individual realizes that recovery will not be complete and that returning to "normal" is not possible. This confrontation with reality is likely to evoke a depression, which may occur early or late in the course of the illness or injury. It may have occurred before the patient entered the rehabilitation phase of the treatment regimen. Depression may lead to suicidal behavior, and those with physical disability have a higher lifetime risk of suicide.[69] Russell and colleagues, in a study of more than 1700 disabled and nondisabled participants, showed that "disability status is a strong predictor of suicide ideation risk."[69]

While the patient is depressed, energy is low and progress in rehabilitation is limited. During this time, OT personnel must maintain good communication with the person. Areas for discussion are the patient's emotional pain, self-concept and self-esteem, goals and potential capabilities, and plans for the OT program. Such discussions need to be reinforced often and should focus on both the present and the future.[26] At the same time, the OT practitioner must be an empathic listener, not "rushed or impatient."[59] Patients with depression may respond to treatment with antidepressant drugs, psychotherapy, and stress management.[43] Clinicians should be alert to the possibility of suicide and must take appropriate steps when suicidal intent is suspected.

Denial

The person with an acquired disability may unconsciously deny its reality as a means of reducing its impact. Initially, the individual may believe that the situation will turn out to be just a bad dream. As the disability persists and is recognized as reality, the person may deny the permanence of the disability.[12] Denial may be manifested by cheerfulness and an unrealistic lack of concern about the disabling condition.

The failure to accept the reality of the circumstances may lead to unproductive behavior such as shopping for miracle cures or the "right" experts. Patients in this stage may be difficult to work with in OT.[12,26] They do not accept the role of the disabled person and see little relevance in working toward restorative and compensatory activities that would lead them to a productive life.[26]

Denial can also be helpful. It may assist the patient to restore some emotional equilibrium and is usually followed by a more realistic attitude toward the disability.[26]

Repression

Repression is the mechanism that removes painful memories from awareness. This mechanism may be necessary in the readjustment of some PWDs. Selective forgetting of one's former attitudes toward the disabled may be necessary to self-acceptance.[12] On the other hand, discussion of painful thoughts and memories may be necessary for achieving progress in restoring psychic equilibrium and in OT. Such discussion should be carried out only by well-trained persons.[26]

Projection

The unconscious mechanism of projection allows what is unacceptable to the self to be shifted onto others. The person with an acquired disability may project previously held negative attitudes about PWDs onto OT personnel and family. An important goal in rehabilitation is helping patients to acknowledge their feelings and to accept responsibility for them so that they can gain control of their rehabilitation.[12,26,59]

Displacement

In displacement, energy associated with one object or person is directed to a secondary target. For example, anger about the cause of the disability may be directed to the OT practitioners, who had nothing to do with its onset. The PWD does not know whom to blame and asks, "Why did this happen to me?" Negative energy associated with such inner conflict is often released on family, friends, and OT personnel. Sometimes the anger is internalized and leads to depression. Vacillation between anger and depression may occur.

Patients displaying displacement should be confronted about their behavior and made aware of its negative effect on significant others and those engaged in their therapy efforts. A disability does not give anyone the right to be rude or uncivil to others.[26]

Sublimation

Sublimation is the process of channeling energy from prohibited goals to more socially acceptable ones. In OT, anger and aggression should be channeled into constructive activities. However, it is important to leave time and opportunity for interaction with others as well. Resolution of interpersonal conflict is an important part of the OT process.[26]

Aggression

Bravado and aggressiveness may be used to cover helplessness and dependency and to hide deep fears and anxieties. Aggression can be directed inward to self or outward to others. As a coping style, it may take one of two forms: hostile aggression or aggressive behavior. Hostile aggression is not constructive in the therapeutic process and is disruptive. Aggressive behavior, on the other hand, can be productive, as in aggressively pursuing rehabilitation goals. Aggressive behavior can be a way of asserting the self. Because this is a useful coping skill, assertive behavior and self-advocacy should be encouraged.[26]

Dependency

Dependency as discussed here is an unwillingness to take actions for oneself and an unnecessary reliance on others. This is in contrast to natural dependence in that all people are interdependent to some extent; no person is capable of meeting all needs without some outside assistance. A person may show pathologic dependence by keeping family and personnel close by and having more attendant care than is realistically necessary. The individual who uses dependency may rely unnecessarily on others to perform ADL. This behavior symbolizes a helpless attitude. Dependent persons may be thought of as lazy or lacking in initiative, but dependency is really surrendering independent problem solving and looking to others to find solutions to problems.[26]

Some patients react against expectations for independence after some rehabilitation gains have been made. Late adolescents and young adults and those with longstanding, latent conflicts of dependency versus independence in the developmental phase of separation and individuation may be more at risk for this reaction. The OT staff must understand the patient's developmental issues to plan appropriate intervention strategies.

Individuals whose premorbid personalities tended to be passive and dependent may have difficulty in therapy and may resist efforts to end the sick role and associated dependency. For these patients, limits must be placed on regression and the staff must consistently express clear expectations for cooperation and participation in the OT program.[37]

Some persons with disabilities present themselves as unable to do anything about their problems. OT practitioners must guard against allowing patients to become overly dependent on them. A balance between control and assistance must be maintained because the ultimate goal of OT is to assist self-help.[26]

Regression

Reverting to feelings, thoughts, and behaviors that worked well for coping in the past is sometimes used to relieve anxiety. Regression is a way of denying reality. Helpers may be seen as parents, lovers, or friends who met the patient's needs earlier in life. If the patient does not accept helpers for who they really are, the disability is not accepted and the OT process is delayed. OT practitioners must be careful not to think that they can replace others in the patient's life.[26] When some of the more significant problems are solved, the person may regain enough confidence to resume more mature behavior.[12]

Rationalization

Rationalization is the unconscious justification of thoughts or behavior with reasons that are more acceptable to the ego than are the actual reasons. Rationalization may take four forms: (1) blaming incidental causes for problems; (2) devaluing unobtainable goals; (3) finding some advantage in an undesirable situation; and (4) mentally balancing negative and positive traits. An example of the first form occurs when PWDs believe others do not like them because they are disabled. In the second form, an example is persons who convince themselves that it was alright to lose a job because the salary was too low. An example of the third form can be found in the fable of the blind man who stated that being blind made him a better person because he no longer judged others by external factors such as clothing or skin color. Beliefs such as "pretty women are dumb" or "disabled persons have more human understanding" are examples of the fourth form.[12]

Compensation

Compensation is a way of making up for a deficit in one area by capitalizing on strengths in another. For example, a PWD may excel in academics to compensate for the inability to excel in sports. Compensation is often an unconscious decision.

Deliberately bringing it to consciousness can help the individual make a self-assessment of strengths and weaknesses. Compensation may be helpful and wholesome if adjustment is personally and socially satisfying.[12,26]

Fantasy

Fantasy substitutes imaginary activities for actual activities.[26] It is a way to gain satisfactions not available in real life.[12] Continuous fantasy can be a sign of serious problems, and the health care provider must be careful about encouraging patients to abandon the actual world for fantasy.[12,26] Nonetheless, the disabled person can use fantasy to cope until other solutions are found.[26] The use of fantasy can be channeled constructively in role-playing situations. The PWD who is afraid to be seen in public or of participating in social situations can become desensitized by role-playing possible scenarios. Fantasy can be used to help the individual develop a repertoire of functional behaviors.

Passing

The denial of difference and attempts to conceal it are known as **passing**. This conscious behavior is not a true defense mechanism. Passing may indicate shame and can be a source of interaction strain. It requires constant vigilance; denying the disability becomes a central focus of life. Acceptance, rather than denial, of the disability frees the person to use internal and external resources toward maximal functioning.[26] Those whose disabilities are not apparent to others, such as persons with epilepsy or cardiac dysfunction, can use passing to some advantage. It allows the person to manage the initial stages of social interaction so that essential personal traits make the first impression in relationships (Box 2-3).

When a disability is visible, passing is impossible. The person must manage tension in social encounters. The person who uses passing must cope with tension, as well as hide information about the disability. If the hidden disability is ultimately revealed, the person must deal with the discomfort when others learn the truth.[12]

Whether passing is a negative or positive coping strategy depends on why one adopts it. If it serves a practical purpose and does not reinforce a negative self-concept, it can signal adjustment to disability and concern for the discomfort of others. If it is used because the person is ashamed of the disability, it can be a sign and source of low self-esteem.[12]

Box 2-3

Perspective on "Passing": Chronic Pain

"I had long ago mastered the ability to keep my pain hidden in concert with performing everyday roles as a student and friend. Only with immediate family did I show, through crying or clutching my side, how much I suffered. My performance in roles outside my family was so successful that it became an impediment for communicating how I felt to physicians. ... My outer appearance (well groomed and pleasant) created an impression to practitioners that I did not appear in distress."[56]

Body Image

Body image is formed from multiple perceptions of the body based on experience, current sensations, and the attitudes and values of the culture. Parental attitudes contribute significantly, as do the comments and fantasies of peers and others. Particular body parts may be overvalued, and the body may be perceived as good or bad, attractive or repugnant, and lovable or unlovable. A person needs only to glance at the magazine covers on a newsstand to absorb the prevailing ideal body image of American culture (young, physically fit, slim, toned, with symmetric features).

For persons with new disabilities, comparisons of their bodies with those of others may lead to self-denigration. The more severe the disability and the more altered the appearance, the greater the vulnerability. Increased risk-taking behavior and substance abuse may follow.[75] Shame, anxiety, and disgust may provoke defenses such as denial and repression. Depression and mourning for the lost body part or function may ensue. Research suggests that as the person lives longer with the disability, body self-image does not generally improve.[75] Men are more vulnerable than women, though older women also suffer impaired body image. The use of positive coping mechanisms such as compensation and sublimation can improve adjustment, but for many persons with physical disability the body image is severely damaged and does not recover. If the person copes well and develops a **compromise body image** (combining disabled body image with preinjury body image), then psychic energy may be freed for new activity including OT efforts.[74]

Stages in Adjustment to Newly Acquired Physical Dysfunction

Kerr[32] and others[27,35,37] have described adjustment to physical dysfunction as progressing through five stages. The adjustment process is analogous to the grief process described by Kübler-Ross.[38]

OT practitioners must remember that the stages are points on a continuum and that all stages are not inevitable for all persons who have a disability. They must also understand the adjustment process because a relationship seems to exist between the person's attitude toward the physical disability and the success of rehabilitation.

The stages as described by Kerr[32] are as follows:

1. Shock: "This isn't me."
2. Expectancy of recovery: "I'm sick, but I'll get well."
3. Mourning: "All is lost."
4. Defensive A—healthy: "I'll go on in spite of it." Defensive B—pathologic: Marked use of defenses to deny the effects of the disability.
5. Adjustment: "It's different but not bad."

Shock

Shock is an immediate reaction to trauma and occurs during the early diagnostic and treatment period. It includes a sense of numbness and the inability to integrate or comprehend the magnitude of the event.[37]

The person can neither understand that the body is ill nor comprehend the extent of the seriousness of the illness or injury. Because of these factors, the person may show an apparent lack of anxiety that appears to be unrealistic. As the reality of the situation becomes more apparent to the person, the reaction is, "This can't be me. It's a bad dream. I'll wake up, and this will all be gone." The PWD is likely to blame the hospital and medical personnel for the lost ability to function. The feeling is, "If I could only get out of here, I'd be all right." Psychologically, the person is still a normal, able-bodied person, pursuing the same goals and doing the same things as before the onset of the disabling condition.

The person's real physical situation and the mental image are incompatible. This incompatibility may account for the person's apparently inappropriate references to the disability, situation, recovery, and future performance. At this stage, perceptions incompatible with the self-image are rejected.

Expectancy of Recovery or Denial[27,33]

This stage may last from a few days to some months. The patient may maintain that recovery will be quick and complete. This is a defense mechanism against the sudden, drastic change in functioning and the realization that the condition is permanent. Denial of the severity and irreversibility of the situation is maintained, and the person hopes that the situation will be reversed in the future.[37] The person may make regular references to getting well or being whole again and may discuss future plans in which full recovery or a normally functioning body is essential.

The individual's only goal is to get well. This aim may lead to the search for a cure and "shopping" from one physician or health care agency to another. The person is preoccupied with the physical condition. Small improvements may be overestimated or misinterpreted. The person will do anything perceived as helpful to recovery because that is his or her primary goal. The person believes that recovery will take place, so motivation toward learning to function with a disability is minimal.[33]

The person believes that the disability is a barrier to everything in life that is important and worthwhile. A whole body is necessary to attain important personal goals. Therefore full recovery must be achieved before anything else can be undertaken.[33]

Family, friends, and medical personnel may unwittingly encourage denial by urging the individual not to think of the losses and may make false promises of recovery. Persistent denial delays the healing process of grief.[27]

A change in this belief system or progress toward the next stage occurs when the person is moved toward a condition more similar to normal living. Being transferred from an acute care setting to the OT unit, being discharged in a wheelchair, having therapy terminated, having therapy redirected to learning to live with the disability, or being told that full recovery will not occur are some of the events that may precipitate mourning.[33]

Mourning or Depression

Mourning occurs when expectancy of recovery shifts to the realization that the disability is permanent. This realization may be overwhelming, may lead to "chronic sorrow," and may require the intervention of specialists in psychiatry or psychology.[33,45] Depression is a response to a sense of helplessness and a loss of self-esteem (Box 2-4). Anxiety, sadness, and grief are natural and appropriate and are to be expected in the adjustment process. Self-esteem may be low, and the individual may feel helpless and like a burden to others. The initial depression involves difficulty in integrating the residual disability into a new self-concept.[37] All seems lost, and all former goals seem unattainable. Frustrations with daily activities remind one that the disability is incapacitating. Motivation to cope with the disability vanishes. The person wants to give up and may contemplate suicide.[69]

The patient may believe that any overt expression of sadness is childish or will be seen that way. OT practitioners must assure the patient that such sadness is normal and natural and should be expressed if the patient is to move beyond this stage. The person in mourning for lost abilities needs the opportunity to work out such feelings.[27] If the individual is not allowed to express grief for the lost function or part because of the reprimands and attitudes of OT practitioners and others, discussion of these feelings may be avoided. Hostility toward those who limit the expression of feelings may result in a "problem patient" who will not work and who spends much time complaining about the health care agency procedures and personnel.[33]

Some individuals may subsequently externalize hostility and blame for the loss to family, friends, physicians, and other clinicians. The OT practitioner can help the person make functional gains by channeling hostility and anger into productive activity.[37]

Patients may become resigned to depression, believing they are worthless and inadequate, and may remain at this stage. They may adopt the role of the invalid and become permanent residents of a health care institution.[40] The disability is now seen as an impenetrable barrier to important life goals, and unlike the hope for recovery that characterized the previous stage, the goal of recovery is now seen as unrealistic.

To assist progress to the next stage, the therapist must help the patient evaluate the "disability barrier" differently, as a challenge. Further, the therapist must provide opportunities to experience the self as competent. Creating situations in which previously held goals can be attained is helpful in some situations. Goals chosen by the patient are much preferred over goals routinely identified for disabilities. For example, self-care activities were probably taken for granted and adults may not view their accomplishment as a positive goal.[33] However, a person might be more motivated by the

Box 2-4

Perspective on Frustration and Depression: Hand Injury

"There is [sic] a lot of little things and if you are used to being on your own then you really get frustrated. That for me was the depressing part of having to rely on somebody always to be there to help me."[9]

possibility of return to a previously valued productive or leisure activity.

The person in this stage may also begin to mourn the loss of some psychological characteristics. Patients may believe they have lost their "fight," "pride," or "faith," which can be more distressing than the physical loss. In this situation, exposing the person to PWDs who demonstrate these qualities may be important. The person can then begin to realize that the disability is irrelevant for the attainment of more basic goals.[33]

Defensive A—Healthy

The defensive stage may be considered healthy if the person begins to deal with the disability. Motivation to learn to function with the disability increases significantly. The person is pleased with accomplishments and takes an active interest in being as normal as possible.

The disability barrier is being reduced and becomes less impenetrable. The person attains some goals that were held as a nondisabled person. Some treasured experiences, although altered are still possible. Although the barrier remains, ways to circumvent it are discovered. The person learns to achieve previously held goals by other routes. Other goals may remain unattainable, and the person may remain distressed by the areas perceived to be unachievable.[33]

The movement toward adjustment comes through a changed need system. The need for a whole or normal body may be relinquished when important goals can be attained despite the disability. The goals are attainable, so the disability becomes less relevant. When physical impairment does interfere with goal attainment, the person must relinquish the goals and discover equally satisfying ways of meeting important needs[33] (Box 2-5).

Defensive B—Pathologic

The defensive stage may be considered pathologic if the person uses defense mechanisms to deny the continued existence of a partial barrier imposed by the disability. Diverse behavior may be displayed, depending on the defense mechanisms used. Patients may attempt to conceal the disability; may rationalize and say they do not want the things that are now unattainable to them; may project negative feelings to others, claiming that others cannot accept the disability although the patients have; and may try to convince others that they are well adjusted. The existence of barriers imposed by the disability is denied. A new compromise body image that can be accepted both consciously and unconsciously fails to develop. Psychotic reactions may occur. Passive, dependent reactions may be manifested by a complete loss of motivation and a surrendering of all ambition. Psychological regression may become apparent, and pathologic denial may be manifested by an inability to express negative feelings and by a repression of anger.[74]

Under some additional stress, the person may regress to an earlier stage and remain there permanently, or the person may progress to adequate adjustment after a temporary regression.

Adaptation or Adjustment

After grief, mourning, and hope of return are relinquished, new roles based on new functions can be achieved. An understanding of the person's defense mechanisms and coping strategies will help assist the process of adaptation to functioning with a physical difference. The therapist or assistant can assess coping strategies by learning how the person customarily managed stresses in the past. Coping strategies tend to be consistent, and stresses are handled by intensified use of previous strategies. Once identified, those strategies that can be used to enhance OT efforts can be maximized, whereas those that deter such efforts can be rechanneled.[37] If an adequate adjustment is attained, the person considers the disability as merely one of many personal characteristics. The disability is no longer considered a major barrier to be overcome, because satisfying ways to meet personal needs and goals have been found.

Practitioners cannot assume that teaching the disabled individual to perform activities will automatically lead to an adequate adjustment. Two other goals, held by many (but not all) people, may need to be attained before adjustment is possible. The first goal lies in religion or personal philosophy. The person with religious beliefs must feel "right with God." All the beliefs about the role of suffering in relation to God's influence on life must be resolved. The disability will be a barrier between the person and God if the person regards it as a punishment or believes that God will heal those who love Him. The second goal involves achieving a feeling of personal adequacy. Because of the tendency in society to relegate the PWD to an inferior status, this person must be helped to discriminate between adequate and inferior based on intrinsic worth rather than physique and productivity[33,82] (Box 2-6).

Box 2-5

Perspective on New Ways of Being in the World: Post Polio Syndrome and Low Back Pain

"I wasn't tired when I got home, I'd managed to have a look in all the shops. ... Wonderful! That's when I sort of got over it [the idea of using a wheelchair in public]."[6]

Box 2-6

Perspective on Self-Acceptance: Head Injury

"When I got to the office I had to call [my sister]. It dawned on me that all these years she has seen in me the potential to let go. I tried, I really tried hard all those years—I tried to do everything people told me would be good for me, but I didn't realize that it wasn't important what I did or even how I did it. What was important wasn't 'doing' at all. It was that through doing I could realize I could be myself and be someone who, like others, continues to live and change and grow. So I called her and we both cried on the phone."[59]

Sexual Adjustment

After pain, fear of death, and major discomforts of the disability have subsided, persons with newly acquired disabilities begin to reassess life and relationships. Social concerns become more intense. Questions about attractiveness and the possibility of sexual relationships arise.[12,51] The sex-related limitations imposed by the disability and sexual taboos and prohibitions generate anxiety in the disabled person. Anxiety can be intensified by misunderstanding and misinformation. Anxiety increases if the person's questions are not answered or concerns are not discussed. If such silence prevails, patients receive the message that they are asexual beings and that sex should not be a concern. Uncertainties about sexual matters are influenced by the attitudes of health care professionals and the premorbid beliefs of the disabled individual about the sexuality of disabled persons.[12]

Practitioners who are reluctant to address the patient's sexual concerns send the message that these concerns are well founded and that interest or efforts that do not focus directly on the disabling condition are of minor interest.[12,14,51] The predisability attitudes of disabled persons make them aware that others may regard them as asexual or incapable of any satisfying sexual activity.[12] Because sexual matters are regarded as personal and private, people are reluctant to discuss them. The patient may consider sexual concerns as separate from the disability and think that they are to be borne in silence and handled without assistance.[14]

Chapter 16 discusses sexuality and sexuality counseling of PWDs.

Psychological and Social Considerations in Treatment of Physical Dysfunction

Assessment and Evaluation

Psychological and social aspects should be considered as part of the evaluation of the person with physical disabilities.[1] Role assessments and similar tools may be used, although the occupational profile and a discussion with the client should be the first steps and often are sufficient.[15,31] Some instruments may be administered by the service-competent OTA. On a less formal level, the OTA may obtain much useful information about the patient's life context, goals, and interests through casual conversation during treatment activities.

Interpersonal Approaches in Treatment

Attitudes toward the Patient

The patient must be regarded as a whole person. The individual's capabilities, problems, interests, experiences, needs, fears, prejudices, beliefs, cultural influences, and reactions to the physical dysfunction are as important as the physical considerations in planning interaction strategies and the treatment program.[1,31]

To facilitate self-acceptance, the OT practitioner can demonstrate to patients that they are accepted. The clinician reacts to the patient as a person who happens to have a disability. Such an approach reduces the fear and anxiety associated with being different. The OTA should demonstrate genuineness, empathy, and concern for the patient as a unique human being.[1,31]

Becoming disabled alters a person's social interactions with others. The person with a newly acquired disability feels to be the same person inside but may find that responses from others are very different from what they had been in the past. These responses may cause questioning of personal identity, appropriate roles, and expectations in performance ability. The early answers to such questions come from the OT practitioners in everyday treatment situations. By their words and actions, clinicians may communicate answers to critical and perhaps unspoken questions from the person with the disability[32] (Box 2-7).

Behavior of practitioners that reflects respect for the rights, capabilities, and abilities of the person to make judgments and be involved in the OT process communicates faith in the individual as a human and a fully functioning adult. The OTA should accord patients equal status and avoid treating them as dependent children. The communication of a belief in the patient's capacities is essential. An attitude of helping the person to explore and discover possibilities in performance skills and social interchange is essential.

Clinicians should guard against preconceived notions and conclusions about the patient's capacities.

The focus of therapy and rehabilitation should be on helping the person to reformulate an approving self who wants to continue with life despite important discontinuity with past identity.

Recognizing and Changing Negative Attitudes toward the Patient

Despite the advice given earlier, clinicians may experience negative reactions to patients. Adverse or negative reactions of OT workers toward patients may stem from a number of causes. Lack of experience with persons with disabilities and in particular with disfiguring conditions may lead to an uncontrolled unconscious reaction of horror or revulsion to, for example, the appearance of someone with a severe facial burn. In addition, personality incompatibility or prejudicial reactions to a particular age, gender, ethnic group, or physical dysfunction can evoke a negative reaction. Awareness and admission of adverse reactions are the first steps in coping with them constructively.

Box 2-7

Perspective on the Need for Understanding: Brain Injury

"And [the occupational therapist] said, 'I'd like to come to your [dental] office and watch you work.'... So, at the end of the session, after I'd tried to drill on some teeth, and ... ['the occupational therapist] watched me treat a patient ... he said, 'I've obviously been to the dentist,' and he said, 'I didn't have a clue.' And he said, 'Now I know what you've been trying to do, I don't think,' he said, 'I don't see how you're going to continue.' And that was real hard to hear. But it was nice that somebody was finally honest with me, too. I mean, I had tears in my eyes, and I do again ... 'cause somebody finally understood."[11]

Some signs of adverse reactions to patients are (1) failure to keep appointments; (2) offering less treatment time; (3) regularly arranging for the patient to be treated by an aide, student, or other therapist; (4) unnatural and excessive politeness and service to the patient; (5) a feeling of boredom when the patient is present; (6) a tendency to ignore the patient when others are present; (7) unrealistic optimism or pessimism about the patient's prognosis or potential achievements; and (8) giving the patient inadequate answers and instructions.

OT practitioners who become aware of these reactions may undertake a self-analysis or analysis with the aid of peers or a counselor to identify the underlying cause of the negative reaction, if it is not readily apparent. Discussion of such reactions with the patient who evokes them is sometimes appropriate. If the reaction is caused by an asocial or inappropriate behavior that is within the person's capacity to change and if changed would aid in acceptance by others, discussion of the feeling with the patient may be helpful.

Clinicians may be able to change their reactions and construct more positive interactions with the patient through ongoing counseling with peers or a professional counselor. If these measures fail and the negative reactions cannot be resolved, transferring the patient to another's care is essential to the patient's progress.[74]

Strategies for Effective Engagement with Patients

Taylor[78] has analyzed the interaction styles of effective therapists and has identified six **therapeutic modes:** advocating, collaborating, empathizing, encouraging, instructing, and problem solving. When **advocating,** the clinician ensures that the patient has resources and supports; advocating may extend to political action. When **collaborating,** the therapist partners with the patient and encourages participation and self-determination. When **empathizing,** the occupational therapist or OTA works to understand the patient's perspective and to accept and validate feelings. When **encouraging,** the therapist cheers the patient on, instills hope, and provides praise and feedback. When **instructing,** the occupational therapist or OTA shares knowledge or skills and endeavors to help the patient master these. When **problem solving,** the therapist addresses technical and environmental and social dilemmas the patient has encountered or is likely to encounter. The modes are defined in Table 2-2, which also provides some background on when each mode is best employed. The reader is encouraged to consult the original source and other references for further detail.[76,78]

Every therapist (occupational therapist or OTA) has his or her preferred modes of interaction. Some clinicians are more businesslike and direct their attention to the technical aspects of therapy (instructing and problem solving), whereas others

Table 2-2 Taylor's Therapeutic Modes[76,78]

Therapeutic Mode	Description	Best Used When
Advocating	Promoting client participation in occupation by ensuring client access to resources such as transportation, housing, education, etc.	Immediate needs for remediation have been met, when client problems have already been addressed, and when client is interested in moving forward and addressing barriers.
Collaborating	Involving clients in making decisions, in setting goals, in choosing priorities for treatment	Client is disposed toward collaboration, is able to consider a partnership with therapist, does not view the therapist and the medical community as authorities to be obeyed.
Empathizing	Listening to clients, paying attention to the feelings conveyed, observing nuances of nonverbal expression, validating and reflecting back client perceptions	Client has emotional reactions (especially those that are interfering with the progress of therapy), has feelings that are being expressed in challenging or negative behaviors, or client is in conflict with staff or significant others. Empathizing mode may and should be used frequently and as needed, but clinicians should be careful not to fall into a pattern where empathic discussions take so much time that therapeutic goals and activities are not addressed.
Encouraging	Instilling hope and confidence by praising efforts and achievements, selecting activities that clients value, using feedback and positive reinforcement, using playfulness and humor	Clients will benefit from encouragement, when clients seem to need external motivation, when clients seem resistant. Should not be overused because clients may become dependent on therapist praise. Should be used carefully if clients are suspicious of therapist's intentions.
Instructing	Teaching and educating, instructing and sharing information, explaining research findings and possible outcomes	Clients value professional expertise and need information and explanations, especially about intervention procedures and possible outcomes, about long-term prognosis under different approaches. Should not be used when client's needs are more emotional than informational.
Problem solving	Using logic, reasoning, and analysis to address obstacles to client recovery and participation. Engaging clients in the problem-solving process, in generating and evaluating possible solutions	When clients are comfortable with an analytic approach, when clients have technical problems that need solutions, when clients rely on professional expertise more than empathy from therapist. Should be balanced with empathizing and encouraging mode, or some clients may perceive therapist as unfeeling and only interested in outcomes.

are more naturally drawn to the emotional and relationship aspects (encouraging and empathizing). It would be unusual for a novice therapist to be able to use all six modes well, but it is worth learning about and trying to apply the modes that do not come easily because this puts more tools in the therapist's toolbox of interventions. The most effective therapists interact with patients in a flexible manner, adjusting their behavior as best suits the patient's interpersonal needs at the moment.

Strategies for Working with the So-Called "Difficult Client"

Patients who are uncooperative, who exhibit manipulative or challenging behaviors, or who appear overly dependent or unmotivated are frequently labeled "difficult" by staff. Certainly it is difficult to work with them, but the key to success lies in understanding the barriers to participation from the client's point of view. Costa[10] reports that the OT or OTA must give attention to why the person is engaging in the difficult behavior. Some clients have dysfunctional family histories; others are in unrelenting pain that has not been adequately addressed; and some may have had prior negative experience with health care providers. Asking questions and listening to what the patient says are important first steps. The OTA might employ therapeutic modes such as empathizing, encouraging, and collaborating (see Table 2-2).[77,78]

McCormac[48] lists factors that may be contributing to the behavior of the patient who seems unmotivated:

- Anxiety about the therapy process
- Fatigue
- Communication barriers
- Vision or hearing impairment
- Cognitive deficits
- Fear of failure
- Grief
- Worry over finances or the future
- Frustration over slow progress
- Depression (and associated problems such as poor sleep)
- Problems with social support from family and others[48]

These many factors illustrate again why it is important to evaluate and identify what is at the root of the problem behavior because each factor might call for a different response from the clinician.

As for managing difficult behavior and crafting a therapeutic response, several strategies have been proposed. One is the CALMER approach (Box 2-8) developed by Pomm, Shahady, and Pomm.[63] In this approach, the OTA would first recognize or remind herself that the patient is the one who is responsible for change. The second step is to alter thoughts to change feelings, which helps the OTA identify what he or she is thinking and reflect on personal responses. The third step is to listen in order to understand the problem. The fourth is to make an agreement or contract with the patient, which might be a restatement of a prior agreement or plan. The fifth is to educate the client about what to do between this meeting and the next. And the last is to reach out and discuss feelings with supervisors or other support systems. The CALMER approach provides systematic steps that help the clinician distance herself from the patient's behavior, avoid taking the behavior personally, and place the responsibility for change on the patient.

Box 2-8

The CALMER Approach[61]

Catalyst for change—the patient is responsible, and we cannot change others. The question is how we can support change for the person.

Alter thoughts to change feelings—when uncomfortable feelings arise, take time to reflect on them and the thinking behind them; change the thinking and the feelings will shift.

Listen to determine what the problem is.

Make an agreement, which might be a restatement of the established plan. Make time for the client to rephrase the plan and ask questions.

Educate the client about what he or she should be doing now and before the next visit.

Reach out and discuss your feelings with your supervisor and other professional supports.

Pomm H, Shahady E, Pomm R: The CALMER approach: teaching learners six steps to serenity when dealing with difficult patients. *Family Medicine* 36:467-469, 2004.

It is important for the OTA to understand that difficult behavior that crosses the line into assault or other criminal activity requires a different approach. Costa[10] advises that sexual acting out and violent behaviors should not be tolerated. Instead, the clinician must document the situation; set firm, clear, and consistent limits on behavior; and follow established policies of the health care facility.

Fostering Coping Skills and Positive Adjustment

Self-Definition

Geis[23] stresses self-definition and a sense of personal worth as critical factors in successful rehabilitation and suggests some methods for helping patients to value themselves positively. The PWD cannot adjust and adapt while maintaining an unrealistic self-image.

The individual's definition of self is the crucial factor, determining the degree of sense of worth and self-satisfaction that can be achieved. The goal of OT is to help the patient to change a self-defeating definition to one that is self-enhancing. Fixed beliefs about attractiveness, productivity, or achievement will cause the patient to define the self and measure individual value in terms of these standards. Therapy involves helping the patient to challenge fixed beliefs and to feel worthwhile in other ways. The patient needs to be directed to satisfactions that are attainable and helped to value goals and self preferentially rather than by some absolute standard.

The traditional OT focus has been on assisting the patient to develop better modes of "doing." An emphasis on doing only or becoming efficient at reaching performance goals may focus self-valuation on an extrinsic standard of productivity. Techniques for helping the patient simply to "be" and to value aspects of himself or herself need to be added to treatment modalities.[59] Geis[23] describes "being" as a spontaneous expressive activity that may be purposeless and nonstriving. It exists during such pursuits as fiestas, ballet, dancing, and leisure activities, as well as in enjoying theatrical performances, comic events, and sports events, in which gratification is intrinsic and linked with the process rather than with the goal or result of the activity. In contrast, "doing" activity has its satisfaction linked with the effect or ultimate achievement of the goal of the activity process. Before the onset of physical disability, the person's self-definition and sense of personal worth have usually been based largely on "doing" behavior. With the onset of physical dysfunction, a major loss occurs in the self-satisfaction derived from "doing." This may evoke feelings of reduced self-worth, which can be ameliorated by helping the patient derive gratification from "being" experiences. Padilla asks that OT therapists consider engaging as "co-investigators" in the discovery of the meaning of life experience for the client.[59] Treatment methods that emphasize the individual's exploration, manipulation, personal interests and choices, enjoyment, delight, and play can facilitate self-satisfaction from "being."[23]

Emotional Intelligence

Emotional intelligence is the capacity to understand and manage one's feelings.[25,49] Two components of emotional intelligence are (1) the ability to initiate and maintain activity and (2) the ability to act with purpose and reason. A person who has a high level of emotional intelligence is in control of his or her emotions, rather than being at their mercy. Dealing with physical disability or illness generates high levels of emotion, as well as countless problems to be solved. Emotional intelligence would be an asset to any PWD, but can it be taught? McKenna[49] describes an OT program for training emotional intelligence. The two components of this program are the therapeutic relationship and specific therapeutic activities. In the relationship, the therapist employs a person-first and person-centered perspective. The relationship aims to foster honest communication and evaluation, collaboration, empowerment, and trust. The activities, which may be individual and/or group, are oriented toward personally valued goals and independent functioning in the person's preferred context. Sample activities include role play and rehearsal, emotion identification, impulse and anger management skills, journal keeping and review, communication, and emotion sharing.

Preventing Maladjustment

Pathologic reactions in adjustment may be reduced if OT practitioners can recognize the stage of adjustment that the patient is experiencing and structure approaches and activities to accommodate the individual's particular emotional needs at that point in the adjustment process. Patients should be encouraged to express their fears, anxieties, worries, and sense of loss. This must be done with tact and understanding. Therapists and assistants must expect that the patient has strong emotions and must be prepared to invite the expression of these emotions and cope with them. Practitioners should not minimize the problems or enter into the patient's denial. Attitudes of acceptance of individuals with physical dysfunction will facilitate their self-acceptance. A cheerful and optimistic attitude from the staff is useful, but appropriately expressing irritation and anger may help the patient realize that such expressions are allowed and will be accepted.[74] Confrontation can also be used effectively when a patient is denying or avoiding an issue.[50] Similarly, being quiet and tolerating and using silence can create openings for expression of difficult ideas and feelings.[50]

Early recognition of pathologic reactions is important.[47] OT practitioners should observe for deep depression, suicidal tendencies, undue guilt or preoccupation with symptoms, bizarre behavior, confusion, paranoid symptoms, or other evidence of serious mental disorder.

Therapists and OTAs should share their observations for reality testing and for referral of problems to the appropriate specialists with other members of the rehabilitation team. All should make a concerted effort to deal with the normal adjustment process and minor problems. Assistance and special treatment by psychiatry or psychology specialists may be required to manage pathologic reactions. Counseling of personnel by these specialists may be helpful in dealing effectively with a given patient, coping with feelings toward the patient, and helping the patient progress toward a healthy adjustment.

Enhancing Adjustment to Long-Term Disability

Two goals of OT are (1) to promote ego integrity and feelings of self-worth and (2) to help persons with newly acquired (and in some cases with chronic) disabilities believe that their "inner self" still exists. Functional efforts in the early stages of therapy should be designed to help the patient see that performance is possible and that the future holds some promise. Emphasis on functional achievements as ends in themselves for specific skill development, however, can divert energy and attention from feelings about physical dysfunction that must be manifested and resolved.

Therefore the OT practitioner's proper role is as an assistant to the patient. Unfortunately, most treatment settings are founded on the medical model. The professionals assume the expert and authoritarian role, whereas the patients assume a passive, dependent, and compliant role. Passivity and authoritarian direction are inappropriate for individuals with chronic, permanent conditions. Their role should be primary, and clinicians' roles should be secondary.[73]

The patient's self-enhancement is supported when practitioners see themselves as assistants to patients who are working toward restoring their lives (Box 2-9). The clinician's role must shift from that of active authoritarian to a more receptive mode of professional behavior. The patient's role must shift from passive recipient of services to active doer. This approach is better suited (than the medical model approach) to the needs of PWDs, whose issues are social, emotional, functional, and vocational performance problems to be solved.[73]

The OT practitioner plays an important role in assisting psychosocial adjustment to physical dysfunction, for example, in the frustrations of dealing with minor ADL. The OTA teaches the patient to master ADL and to deal with the problems of everyday life. Through the process of the ADL program, the patient learns to solve problems and gains

Box 2-9

Perspective on Autonomy: Wheelchair User

"Before I got the wheelchair, I really didn't do much at all because it was just too difficult and then if there was stuff on the floor, which there is, you know, that's an added barrier for me ... and I would get the kids to clean up as best as they could so that I could come into their rooms, but the reality is that they weren't very good at doing that and you can tell if you just glance into the kids' rooms, I mean things don't get hung up, they get dropped on the floor. Now that I'm in a wheelchair, I can go into the rooms."[66]

confidence that frustrations associated with the disability can be overcome.[82]

The OTA is in a unique position to observe the person's psychological functioning when working closely together and observing the performance of a variety of tasks. Motivation, initiative, creativity, originality, and persistence can be assessed by performance observation.[47]

Watson[84] described a psychiatric consultation-liaison program in an acute physical disabilities setting. The program's goal was to facilitate adjustment to a lifestyle compatible with the patient's value system, disability, and prognosis. Depression was the most common reason for referral to the program. A team approach was used, and the members were the psychiatrist, psychiatric nurse, and occupational therapist.

The occupational therapist used functional activities to help the patient explore the meaning of the disability or illness. Participation in activity and the accompanying discussion ultimately had a positive outcome, although the patient encountering limitations sometimes directed negative behavior or attitudes toward the therapist. The therapist used informal discussion to address fears, anxieties, feelings of helplessness, and vulnerability. The treatment program helped the patient redefine problems and assets.[83]

The goals of OT were to provide opportunities for mastery and control, reduce emotional distress, promote psychological competence, and help to maintain or establish an active support network. The OT evaluation assessed premorbid competencies and level of functioning; previously used coping methods; roles, responsibilities, values, and goals; past history and interests; available support network; and discharge plans. This information was attained through interviews and observation during participation in activities.

The occupational therapist encouraged the discussion and helped the patient to evaluate the situation.

The therapist's primary concern was to build rapport. This goal was accomplished by meeting the patient on the patient's level, showing an understanding of the patient's emotional distress, and structuring the environment to promote psychological competence. Activities related to the patient's roles, interests, values, and responsibilities were important to promote psychological competence. Patients seemed motivated and pleased with activities such as homemaking, cooking, crafts, games, and work simulations.

Box 2-10

Example Actions Promoting the Good Life following Acquired Physical Disability

Connections to people
- Socializing with others (quality and depth of relationships is important, as well as frequency)
- Social comparisons (e.g., to inspiring role models)
- Helping others

Positive personal qualities
- Finding meaning (perhaps through journaling about the disability experience to explore personal meaning)
- Resilience
- Expressing gratitude (using cognitive strategies such as a list for each letter A through Z)
- Humor
- Savoring (noticing, reflecting on, and enhancing experiences)

Life regulation qualities
- Exercise and creature comforts (napping, meditating, eating, vacations, and recreation) Finding flow ("losing oneself" in an activity, which may require finding new activities if old ones are not possible or not pleasurable in disabled state)
- Special pleasures (getting a seat on the subway, zooming around in a power chair) and self rewards (planned activities that are pleasurable or reflecting on positive experiences)
- Giving back by being generative (associated with Erikson's sixth stage, may involve tutoring, or peer counseling, or volunteer work)

Modified from Dunn DS, Brody C: Defining the good life following physical disability, *Rehabil Psychol* 53:417ff, 2008.

The interventions focused on ability rather than disability. The occupational therapist structured treatment to ensure success. Making objects for others helped the patient resume the role of contributor. Doing and giving were emphasized to help reestablish significant relationships and restore engagement in meaningful activities. The therapist gradually transferred responsibility for choice and control to the patient, keeping in mind the patient's emotional status and changing psychosocial needs. Easily accomplished, pleasant, and familiar activities were presented initially to motivate and engage the patient. As emotional stresses decreased, more demanding physical rehabilitation activities were introduced.[83]

Another approach to adaptation centers on the concept of "right action" detached from expectations of outcomes. This principle is associated with several spiritual and philosophical practices (e.g., Buddhism, Stoicism). It involves doing the right thing and not worrying about how it all turns out.

Although losses and a sense of helplessness associated with physical disability are corrosive to quality of life, applying such principles and using coping strategies and taking action may promote greater well-being. Dunn and Brody[18] list some sample actions that the patient might take to gain a greater sense of well-being. Examples are grouped into three categories: connections to others, positive personal qualities, and life regulation qualities (Box 2-10).[18] Note that many of these actions involve doing and thus are based in occupation.

Group Approaches

Besides interpersonal interaction strategies to facilitate adjustment to physical dysfunction, group approaches (see also Chapter 12) can be applied in OT. Therapeutic communities, **self-help groups**, milieu therapy, group counseling, and sensitivity training may be helpful to facilitate the patient's adjustment and the development of a positive self-image.[73] Coping skills, problem-solving exercises, and role-playing can be used effectively in groups.

Milieu Therapy

Kutner[40] suggested that milieu therapy may offer a solution for acquiring new roles, readapting old ones, and gaining the social and physical skills necessary to reach goals. **Milieu therapy** is particularly appropriate as an OT method because it uses environmental or residential settings as a training situation for persons with disabilities to practice social, interpersonal, and functional skills and to test their ability to deal with problems commonly encountered in the community. Historically this approach has been fundamental to OT practice in mental health, habilitation, and substance abuse settings.

The milieu therapy program engages the patient in a variety of social encounters—both group and individual—and exposes him or her to increasingly challenging problems. This same gradation can be applied simultaneously to performance skills. The experiences test social competence, judgment, problem-solving ability, and social responsibility.

The major therapeutic objective of milieu therapy is maintaining achievements gained in therapy. It aims to provide the patient with social, psychological, and performance skills to overcome frustration, to deal effectively with new or risky social situations, to cope with rebuffs or rejection, and to remain independent.

Most therapeutic efforts for PWDs have been concentrated on physical restoration, with the assumption that personal and social readjustment follows as physical integrity is restored. When adjustment difficulties occur, calling on social, psychological, and psychiatric services to manage these special problems has been customary. In contrast, milieu therapy deals with the problems of adjustment to new or changed roles by structuring situations and environments to allow the patient to adopt and test roles as part of the process.[40]

Self-Help Groups

The self-help group model is another approach to managing psychosocial adjustment to physical dysfunction. The self-help group provides aid for each group member around specific problems or goals. Positive benefits to members of self-help groups include (1) gaining information and knowledge about the dysfunction or the problem; (2) learning coping skills from group members who are living successfully with the condition; (3) gaining motivation and support through communication with others who have similar experiences; (4) modeling the successful problem-solving behaviors of group members; (5) evaluating personal progress; (6) belonging to and identifying with a group; and (7) finding self-help in a situation of mutual concern.[29]

The mutual aid or self-help group is an excellent means of maintaining therapeutic gains and preventing deterioration of function. It provides modeling by members who are coping with stigma and problems of functioning and reintegrating life roles.

Certain operational assumptions are characteristic of the self-help approach. Individuals with shared problems come together. All group members maintain peer status. Peers come together expecting to help themselves or one another. Behavior change is expected in each individual at that person's own pace. Group members identify with the program, are committed to it, and practice its principles in daily life. Group meetings are regularly scheduled, but peers are available to one another as needed outside of group meetings. This practice allows for both individual and group modes of contact. The group process includes acknowledging, revealing, and relating problems; receiving and giving feedback; and sharing hopes, experiences, encouragement, and criticism. Members are responsible for themselves and their behavior. Leadership develops and changes within the group based on giving and receiving help. Status comes from giving and receiving help effectively.

Many persons who were not helped in professional relationships and experiences turned to and received aid in self-help groups, which arose to meet needs that professionals could not meet. The professional process and self-help group models can share experiences with one another under certain conditions. The professional must meet the conditions of common problems, peer relationship, and mutual aid, and those professionals who cannot meet these conditions can act only as visitors or observers. A professional can act as a consultant or speaker to self-help groups if invited to do so by the group; however, professional therapeutic skills would be not used as such within the self-help group.[29] The OTA and other concerned professionals could act as consultants, invited speakers, or group members, if the necessary conditions outlined previously are met.

Group Counseling

Mann, Godfrey, and Dowd have described a group counseling approach to psychological rehabilitation for patients with spinal cord injuries.[47] The group was based on the proposition that self-concept is one of the factors determining psychological adjustment to physical disability. The goals of the group were (1) to assist each patient in increasing self-concept to facilitate total rehabilitation; (2) to overcome depression; (3) to provide a setting where problems with interpersonal relationships could be discussed and plans for their resolution could be made; and (4) to modify perceptual distortions that patients may have about staff or other patients.

In the group, established members assumed leadership roles and assisted new members in coming to terms with their disabilities and planning new lives. Members gave each other feedback about their strengths and assets to correct negative self-evaluation. Group interaction focused on how each patient could make maximum use of remaining function rather than on concentrating on lost abilities. Patients were encouraged to share feelings with the group and reaped the benefit of knowing that others had similar feelings and experiences.

Substance Abuse

National research continues to show that more disabilities result from substance abuse than from any other preventable health condition.[71] The OTA should anticipate encountering both active and former (inactive) substance abusers among persons treated in rehabilitation settings. Substance abuse is a recognized psychiatric disorder.[3] Active substance abuse is often associated with other maladaptive behaviors such as denial, projection, and rationalization, which form the *preferred defensive structure* (PDS) of the patient with alcoholism.[53] In addition, persons with physical disabilities may use alcohol or other substances including prescription medications to cope with anxiety and depression.[43] The PWD who abuses alcohol or other substances requires treatment for both the physical disability *and* the substance abuse disorder. This situation is not usually a focus of OT intervention in physical medicine and rehabilitation settings, but the OTA should be alert to the possibility of substance abuse and should report any suspicions to the OT supervisor and attending physician.

Advocacy, Empowerment, and Changing Societal Attitudes

Disability can be framed from the experience of the person, or it can be framed from the context of the society. Societies build their objects and infrastructures and buildings and tools (the built environment) to meet the needs of the able bodied. Built environments that do not accommodate the needs of the person with an impairment (or variation from "normal") prevent participation and engagement. Thus in this view, it is the society and the environment that disables the person who has an impairment.

Recognition of this situation sparked the disability rights movement in the 1970s and 1980s, in which PWDs began to organize politically to advocate for greater community integration, self-determination, and independent living for those with disabilities.[4] Among the results were several new laws including the 1990 ADA and the Individuals with Disabilities Education Act of 1997. Rather than medicalizing disability status, these laws recognized PWDs as a minority group subject to discrimination and entitled to protection of rights under law. It is understood that the discrimination experienced by PWDs is not intentional and persecutory, but rather it is the product of a lack of accommodation in the built environment and in social customs and beliefs. The intent of the laws is to reduce and if possible eliminate barriers to full participation by PWDs.

One outgrowth of the disability rights movement has been the independent living model, in which the nature of independence is defined by the PWD, who is seen as a consumer of services. Independence in this model is not the concrete self-sufficiency of performing one's ADL without assistance, but rather it is independence in self-determination. The PWD knows what he or she needs to be independent in the community and makes the necessary decisions. This may lead to selecting technology, equipment, housing, personal services, and professional services to obtain the best quality of participation as defined by the PWD.[7] The PWD may choose to employ personal attendants to help with ADL so that he or she has more energy for activities that are more important.

The built environment as experienced by a PWD is an obstacle course of architectural barriers that limit access to desired places and activities. With the passage of the ADA came a mandate to modify the built environment to better accommodate PWDs, but the implementation has been spotty and imperfect. Although curb cuts, large toilet stalls with hand rails, and elevators with Braille signage are common in modern or renovated public spaces, there still exist many significant barriers, particularly in older buildings and cities. For example, in New York City most subway stations do not have elevators, causing many PWDs to rely on buses and Access-A-Ride services (publicly funded taxi services for the disabled). Traffic is typically congested during the daytime hours, resulting in lengthy trips and long delays for PWDs. It may take 5 minutes or more for the bus driver to deploy the wheelchair access mechanism of a public bus. And the person in the wheelchair may need the bus for only a short distance before the bus stops again for 5 minutes to allow the person to exit. Once the wheelchair is back on the sidewalk, the person must navigate around pedestrians, cyclists, children with scooters, parents with strollers, containers for trash and recycling, street trees and protective tree fencing, etc., all on narrow pedestrian walkways that may be broken or cracked or that may contain grates or metal plates. For this reason, it is not unusual to see a person in a wheelchair or power-operated vehicle (POV) scooter using the bicycle lane in the street.

Jenkins[30] points out that even with the best of intentions designers and planners do not imagine and build new environments that accommodate disabilities well because they do not understand the range of disabling conditions or the measurements of people with different disabilities. The dimensions of the human body used for architectural planning are based on populations of young and fit men of military age.[30] Although more studies are under way to more accurately measure the dimensions and performance abilities of a variety of people, these will still not yield data sufficient to describe all the ways in which persons with disabilities need to access environments.[4]

Universal design is an approach to creating built environments and objects that will support individual differences by flexible and clean design that accommodates the needs of PWDs as well as persons who do not have disabilities.[7] Thus for example, if all doors are wide enough for wheelchairs, all doors open with automatic motion sensors, and all room entrances are level (without raised thresholds), then access for a person in a wheelchair does not require additional adaptations. But even universal design does not meet the needs of every PWD. Therefore the person must learn skills of self-advocacy, which the OTA can model. Alternately, self-help groups and partnerships with people with disabilities of long standing can provide role models and advice to the person with a new disability.

The OTA can best help the consumer in this aspect of resolving problems in social and environmental barriers by applying Taylor's therapeutic modes of advocating, educating, problem solving, and encouraging.[77,78] Studies have suggested that society's attitudes and expectations toward PWDs may critically influence their mental health. If this is so, health professionals should seek ways to influence attitudes positively. The natural environments of occupational performance (shopping venues, churches and community centers, parks and playgrounds, workplace environments) provide many opportunities for contact between the disabled and nondisabled populations.

Summary

Psychological and social adjustment is intimately related to the disability experience and must be considered in the OT program for persons with physical dysfunction.[1] Interventions may include using therapeutic relationships, providing training in assertiveness and emotional intelligence, structuring a therapeutic environment, and using group and dyadic interpersonal experiences. Activities should assist the patient in adjusting to the physical dysfunction and in restructuring his or her lifestyle to achieve the maximal independence possible.

OT uses methods that demand the action and involvement of the patient in the rehabilitation process. In the initial stages of adjustment to a new disability, when depression and denial are present and ego strength is poor, formal teaching or discussion groups may fail because the patient cannot integrate verbal material that addresses psychological exploration. Therefore social, recreational, special interest, and activity groups can be used to facilitate participation in therapeutic tasks.

The group process may include discussion of needs and feelings, mutual support, and learning skills for working with the health care agency, its personnel, and the community. The occupational therapist and OTA should plan and structure group experiences that enhance social skills, allow opportunities to test interaction strategies, discover assets and new or modified roles, and practice problem-solving behavior.

The OTA can facilitate a collaborative treatment program through individual and group processes, using a person-first and person-centered focus. The patient's involvement in setting goals is critical because the patient who uses individual skills in planning, sharing, playing, socializing, and making judgments is more likely to want to work toward ADL skills and personally meaningful objectives.

When the patient is involved in setting goals, pointing out that all skills have not been lost and that assets and capabilities still can be used is unnecessary.

Professional health care workers must facilitate the achievement of self-acceptance and the development of coping strategies in their clients with disabilities. Negative public attitudes toward PWDs are a deterrent to successful psychosocial rehabilitation. These attitudes are slowly changing but have not resulted in total acceptance of persons with disabilities; the OTA can serve as an advocate and support as the PWD learns to apply physical and psychological resources to cope in a difficult world.[82]

Selected Reading Guide Questions

1. Why should OT practitioners evaluate and consider the patient's environment including physical, social, and cultural elements?
2. Define the following terms as they apply to societal reactions to PWDs: avoidance and rejection, nonacceptance, spread factor, labeling, minority group status, segregation, and unfounded positive images.
3. Give an example of a distancing behavior by a health care provider.
4. Describe the behaviors that might be seen in a depressed person.
5. Give an example of each of the following, as they may be expressed or exhibited by a patient with a physical dysfunction: denial, repression, projection, displacement, sublimation, aggression, dependency, regression, rationalization, and compensation.
6. Describe *passing* as a strategy used by PWDs. Is this an effective strategy or not? Explain.
7. What is the *compromise body image,* and how does it develop?
8. Name and describe Taylor's six therapeutic modes.
9. Discuss the relationship of emotional intelligence to coping with disability.
10. Why is it important for OT practitioners to be aware of their own reactions to patients and disabilities?
11. Explain what the OTA should do when a patient becomes emotional and upset about the disabling condition.
12. Why is this the correct response?
13. Give three reasons why group approaches are useful in treating patients with physical disabilities.
14. Discuss the independent living model and the role of the OTA as advocate.

Exercises

1. Using a case example from your own clinical experience or one provided by the instructor, identify the patient's chronological age and expected psychosocial stage (according to Erikson). Discuss the effects of the disability on the achievement of the developmental task of this stage.
2. Imagine that you had a severe and disfiguring impairment such as an extensive facial burn. Discuss with a peer partner how you would feel about yourself (self-image), your relationships with others, and your expectations for the rest of your life (e.g., relationships, work, social roles).
3. Temporarily disable yourself for a few hours by strapping your dominant arm to your side using a scarf. Continue

your normal activities as best you can. When the time is up, write about the feelings you experienced while "disabled." Share these in class.

References

1. American Occupational Therapy Association: *Occupational therapy services in the promotion of psychological and social aspects of mental health.* Retrieved May 1, 2011, from http://www.aota.org/Practitioners/Official/Statements/40878.aspx?FT=.pdf.
2. American Occupational Therapy Association: White paper: occupational therapy and the Americans with Disabilities Act, *Am J Occup Ther* 45:470–471, 1992.
3. American Psychiatric Association: *Diagnostic and statistical manual of mental disorders, text revision (DSM-IV-TR)*, ed 4(TR), Washington, DC, 2000, American Psychiatric Press.
4. Beaulaurier RL, Taylor SH: Social work practice with people with disabilities in the era of disability rights. In Dell Orto AE, Power PW, editors: *The psychological and social impact of physical disability*, ed 5, New York, 2007, Springer.
5. Blume J: *Deenie*, Scarsdale, NY, 1973, Bradbury.
6. Bontje P, Kinébanian A, Josephsson A, Tamura Y: Occupational adaptation: the experiences of older persons with physical disabilities, *Am J Occup Ther* 58:140–149, 2004.
7. Burnett SE: Personal and social contexts of disability: implications for occupational therapists. In Pendleton HM, Schultz-Krohn W, editors: *Pedretti's occupational therapy practice skills for physical dysfunction*, ed 6, St. Louis, 2006, Mosby Elsevier.
8. Catholic Biblical Association of America: *Bishops' Committee of the Confraternity of Christian Doctrine: The New American Bible*, Nashville, Tenn, 1971, Nelson.
9. Chan J, Spencer J: Adaptation to hand injury: an evolving experience, *Am J Occup Ther* 58:128–139, 2004.
10. Costa DM: Working with the "difficult" client, *OT Practice* 13(13):15–18, July 28, 2008.
11. Darragh AR, Sample PL, Krieger SR: "Tears in my eyes 'cause somebody finally understood": client perceptions of practitioners following brain injury, *Am J Occup Ther* 55:191–199, 2001.
12. De Loach C, Greer BJ: *Adjustment to severe disability*, New York, 1981, McGraw-Hill.
13. Dell Orto AE, Power PW, editors: *The psychological and social impact of physical disability*, ed 5, New York, 2007, Springer.
14. Diamond M: Sexuality and the handicapped. In Marinelli RP, Dell Orto AE, editors: *The psychological and social impact of physical disability*, ed 2, New York, 1984, Springer.
15. Dickerson AE: The role checklist. In Hemphill-Pearson BJ, editor: *Assessments in occupational therapy mental health*, ed 2, Thorofare NJ, 2008, Slack.
16. Dickerson AE, Oakley F: Comparing the roles of community living persons and patient populations, *Am J Occup Ther* 49:221–228, 1995.
17. Dubouloz C-J, Laporte D, Hall M, Ashe B, Smith CD: Transformation of meaning perspectives in clients with rheumatoid arthritis, *Am J Occup Ther* 58:398–407, 2004.
18. Dunn DS, Brody C: Defining the good life following physical disability, *Rehabilitation Psychology* 53(4):413–425, 2008.
19. Erikson E: *Childhood and society*, New York, 1963, Norton.
20. Fine SB: 1990 Eleanor Clarke Slagle Lecture. Resilience and human adaptability: who rises above adversity? *Am J Occup Ther* 45:493–503, 1991.
21. Frank G: Life histories in occupational therapy clinical practice, *Am J Occup Ther* 50:251–264, 1996.
22. Friedmann LW: *The psychological rehabilitation of the amputee*, Springfield, Ill, 1978, Thomas.
23. Geis HJ: The problem of personal worth in the physically disabled patient. In Marinelli RP, Dell Orto AE, editors: *The psychological and social impact of physical disability*, New York, 1977, Springer.
24. Gellman W: Roots of prejudice against the handicapped, excerpted from *J Rehabil* 25:4, 1959. In Stubbins J, editor: *Social and psychological aspects of disability*, Baltimore, 1977, University Park.
25. Goleman D: *Emotional intelligence*, New York, 1995, Bantam.
26. Henderson G, Bryan WV: *Psychological aspects of disability*, Springfield, Ill, 1984, Thomas.
27. Hughes F: Reaction to loss: coping with disability and death. In Marinelli RP, Dell Orto AE, editors: *The psychological and social impact of physical disability*, ed 2, New York, 1984, Springer.
28. Janelle S: Locus of control in nondisabled versus congenitally physically disabled adolescents, *Am J Occup Ther* 46:334–342, 1992.
29. Jaques ME, Patterson K: The self-help group model: a review. In Marinelli RP, Dell Orto AE, editors: *The psychological and social impact of physical disability*, New York, 1977, Springer.
30. Jenkins GR: The challenges of characterizing people with disabilities in the built environment, *OT Pract* 16(9):CE1–CE8, May 23, 2011.
31. Kannenberg K: Evaluating psychological and social concerns in physical disability settings, *OT Pract* 16(7):21, April 25, 2011.
32. Kerr N: Staff expectations for disabled persons: helpful or harmful. In Marinelli RP, Dell Orto AE, editors: *The psychological and social impact of physical disability*, New York, 1977, Springer.
33. Kerr N: Understanding the process of adjustment to disability. In Stubbins J, editor: *Social and psychological aspects of disability*, Baltimore, 1977, University Park.
34. Kielhofner G, editor: *A model of human occupation: theory and application*, ed 4, Baltimore, 2008, Lippincott Williams & Wilkins.
35. King GA, et al: Self-evaluation and self-concept of adolescents with physical disabilities, *Am J Occup Ther* 47:132–140, 1993.
36. Kirkpatrick SR: *The Disney-fication of disability: the perpetuation of Hollywood stereotypes of disability in Disney's animated films, 2009.* At http://etd.ohiolink.edu/send-pdf.cgi/Kirkpatrick%20Stephanie%20Renee.pdf?akron1248051363, retrieved May 3, 2011.
37. Krueger DW: Emotional rehabilitation: an overview. In Krueger DW, editor: *Emotional rehabilitation of physical trauma and disability*, New York, 1984, Medical and Scientific Books.
38. Kübler-Ross E: *On death and dying*, New York, 1969, Macmillan.
39. Kushner HS: *When bad things happen to good people*, New York, 1981, Avon.
40. Kutner B: Milieu therapy. In Marinelli RP, Dell Orto AE, editors: *The psychological and social impact of physical disability*, ed 2, New York, 1984, Springer.
41. Ladieu-Leviton G, Adler DL, Dembo T: Studies in adjustment to visible injuries: social acceptance of the injured. In Marinelli RP, Dell Orto AE, editors: *The psychological and social impact of physical disability*, New York, 1977, Springer.
42. Lasker J: *He's my brother*, Morton Grove, IL, 1974, Whitman.
43. Leary WE: As fellow traveler of other illnesses, depression often goes in disguise, *New York Times*, Jan 17, 1996.
44. Lewis B: *In Jesse's shoes*, Bloomington, 2007, Minn, Bethany House.

45. Livneh H, Antonak RF: Psychological adaptation to chronic illness and disability. In Dell Orto AE, Power PW, editors: *The psychological and social impact of physical disability*, ed 5, New York, 2007, Springer.
46. Lutz BJ, Bowers BJ: Understanding how disability is defined and conceptualized in the literature. In Dell Orto AE, Power PW, editors: *The psychological and social impact of physical disability*, ed 5, New York, 2007, Springer.
47. Mann W, Godfrey ME, Dowd ET: The use of group counseling procedures in the rehabilitation of spinal cord injured patients, *Am J Occup Ther* 27:73, 1973.
48. MacCormac BA: Reaching the unmotivated client, *OT Pract* 15(4):15–19, March 8, 2010.
49. McKenna J: Emotional intelligence training in adjustment to physical disability and illness, *Int J Ther Rehabil* 14(12):551–556, 2007.
50. McKenna J: Psychosocial support. In Curtin M, Molineux M, Supyk-Mellson J, editors: *Occupational therapy and physical dysfunction—enabling occupation*, Edinburgh, 2010, Churchill-Livingstone Elsevier.
51. Miller E, Marini I: Female sexuality and spinal cord injury: counseling implications. In Dell Orto AE, Power PW, editors: *The psychological and social impact of physical disability*, ed 5, New York, 2007, Springer.
52. Moran G: *Imagine me on a sit ski*, Morton Grove, Ill, 1995, Whitman.
53. Moyers PA: An organizational framework for occupational therapy in the treatment of alcoholism, *Occup Ther Ment Health* 8:27–46, 1988.
54. Mulcahey MJ: Returning to school after a spinal cord injury: perspectives from four adolescents, *Am J Occup Ther* 46:305–312, 1992.
55. Nelson CE, Payton OD: The issue is … a system for involving patients in program planning, *Am J Occup Ther* 45:753–755, 1991.
56. Neville-Jan A: Encounters in a world of pain: an autoethnography, *Am J Occup Ther* 57:88–98, 2003.
57. Northen JG, et al: Involvement of adult rehabilitation patients in setting occupational therapy goals, *Am J Occup Ther* 49:214–220, 1995.
58. Osofsky A: *My buddy*, New York, 1992, Holt.
59. Padilla R: Clara: a phenomenology of disability, *Am J Occup Ther* 57:413–423, 2003.
60. Peloquin SM: The depersonalization of patients: a profile gleaned from narratives, *Am J Occup Ther* 47:830–837, 1993.
61. Persson L, Ryden A: Themes of effective coping in physical disability: an interview study of 26 people who have learnt to live with their disability, *Scand J Caring Sci* 20:355–363, 2006.
62. Phemister AA, Crewe NM: Objective self-awareness and stigma. In Dell Orto AE, Power PW, editors: *The psychological and social impact of physical disability*, ed 5, New York, 2007, Springer.
63. Pomm H, Shahady E, Pomm R: The CALMER approach: teaching learners six steps to serenity when dealing with difficult patients, *Family Med* 36:467–469, 2004.
64. Powers ME: *Our teacher's in a wheelchair*, Morton Grove, Ill, 1986, Whitman.
65. Pranghofer M, Hubby C: Ally's busy day, the story of a service dog, *Trafford Publishing*, 2006.
66. Reid D, Angus J, McKeever P, Miller K-L: Home is where their wheels are: experiences of women wheelchair users, *Am J Occup Ther* 57:186–195, 2003.
67. Robinson V: *David in silence*, Philadelphia, 1956, Lippincott.
68. Roper L: *Disability in media.* From http://www.mediaed.org.uk/posted_documents/DisabilityinMedia.htm, retrieved May 3, 2011.
69. Russell D, Turner RJ, Joiner TE: Physical disability and suicidal ideation, *Suicide and Life-Threatening Behavior* 39(4):440–451, August 2009.
70. Schmid AA, Van Puymbroeck MV, Knies K, Spangler-Morris C, Watts K, Damush T, Williams LS: Fear of falling among people who have sustained a stroke: a 6-month longitudinal pilot study, *Am J Occup Ther* 65:125–132, 2011.
71. Schneider Institute for Health Policy, Brandeis University: *Substance abuse: the nation's number one health problem—key indicators for policy*, Princeton, NJ, 2001, Robert Wood Johnson Foundation.
72. Shontz F: Six principles relating disability and psychological adjustment. In Dell Orto AE, Power PW, editors: *The psychological and social impact of physical disability*, ed 5, New York, 2007, Springer.
73. Siller J: Psychological situation of the disabled with spinal cord injuries. In Stubbins J, editor: *Social and psychological aspects of disability*, Baltimore, 1977, University Park.
74. Simon JI: Emotional aspects of physical disability, *Am J Occup Ther* 15:408, 1971.
75. Taleporos G, McCabe MP: The relationship between the severity and duration of physical disability and body esteem, *Psychol Health* 20(5):637–650, Oct 2005.
76. Tamm-Seitz A: Evidence-based strategies for engaging clients with physical disabilities, *OT Pract* 15(22):9–13, December 20, 2010.
77. Taylor RR: *Pain, fear and avoidance: Therapeutic use of self with difficult occupational therapy populations* (Continuing Education on CD), Bethesda, MD, 2008, AOTA.
78. Taylor RR: *The intentional relationship: Occupational therapy and use of self*, Philadelphia, 2008, FA Davis.
79. The Anderson Family: *Season 2, Episode 12, ABC television.* http://abc.go.com/primetime/xtremehome/bios/families/the_anderson_family.html, retrieved February 3, 2005.
80. Thomas P, Harker L: Don't call me special: a first look at disability, *Barron's Education Series*, 2005.
81. Thurer S: Cited in Burtoff B: Fairy tale stereotypes can harm, *San Jose Mercury News*, Jan 26, 1980.
82. Vargo JW: Some psychological effects of physical disability, *Am J Occup Ther* 32:31, 1978.
83. Vause-Earland T: Perceptions of role assessment tools in the physical disability setting, *Am J Occup Ther* 45:26–31, 1991.
84. Watson LJ: Psychiatric consultation-liaison in the acute physical disabilities setting, *Am J Occup Ther* 40:338, 1986.
85. Zipes J: *Breaking the magic spell: radical theories of folk and fairy tales*, Lexington, Ky, 2007, University of Kentucky.

Recommended Reading, Study and Viewing

Costa DM: Working with the "difficult" client, *OT Pract* 13(13): 15–18, July 28, 2008.

Early MB: *Mental health concepts and techniques for the occupational therapy assistant*, ed 4, Baltimore, 2009, Lippincott Williams & Wilkins.

French S, Swain J: *Understanding disability: a guide for health professionals*, Edinburgh, 2008, Churchill Livingstone Elsevier.

Hockenberry J: *Moving violations*, New York, 1995, Hyperion.

Kannenberg K: Evaluating psychological and social concerns in physical disability settings, *OT Pract* 16(7):21, April 25, 2011.

Mairs N: *Plaintext: deciphering a woman's life*, New York, 1986, Perennial.

McKenna J: Emotional intelligence training in adjustment to physical disability and illness, *Int J Ther Rehabil* 14(12):551–556, 2007.

McKenna J: Psychosocial support. In Curtin M, Molineux M, Supyk-Mellson J, editors: *Occupational therapy and physical dysfunction—enabling occupation*, Edinburgh, 2010, Churchill-Livingstone Elsevier.

Mullins A: *The opportunity of adversity,* TED Talk, at http://www.ted.com/talks/aimee_mullins_the_opportunity_of_adversity.html, retrieved May 3, 2011.

Price R: *A whole new life*, New York, 1994, Macmillan.

Taylor RR: *Pain, fear and avoidance: therapeutic use of self with difficult occupational therapy populations (Continuing Education on CD)*, Bethesda, Md, 2008, AOTA.

CHAPTER 3 Infection Control and Safety Issues in the Clinic*

LYNN E. JAFFE

Key Terms

Universal precautions
Standard precautions
Decontamination
Sterilization
Disinfectants
Isolation
Protective isolation
Shock
Seizure
Insulin reaction
Acidosis
Cardiopulmonary resuscitation
Fowler position
Turning frame
Ventilator
Endotracheal tube
Electrocardiogram
Pulmonary artery catheter
Intracranial pressure monitoring
Arterial monitoring line
Nasogastric tube
Gastric tube
Intravenous feeding
Total parenteral nutrition
Hyperalimentation
Infusion pump
Intravenous lines
Urinary catheter

Chapter Objectives

After studying this chapter, the student or practitioner will be able to do the following:

1. Recognize the role of occupational therapy personnel in preventing accidents.
2. Identify recommendations for safety in the clinic.
3. Identify standard precautions and recognize the importance of following them with all patients.
4. Describe proper techniques of hand washing.
5. Recognize the importance of having all health care workers understand and follow isolation procedures used in patient care.
6. Identify procedures for handling patient injuries.
7. Describe guidelines for handling various emergency situations.
8. Describe preventive positioning for patients with lower extremity amputations, rheumatoid arthritis, burns, and hemiplegia.
9. Describe the purpose of special equipment.
10. Identify precautions when treating patients who require special equipment.

Safety begins with common sense and continues through adherence to proper protocols. The occupational therapy assistant (OTA) must ensure that patients remain safe within the health care setting. Medical technology and cost-control methods have forced seriously ill patients into the occupational therapy (OT) clinic early in their illnesses and for shorter lengths of treatment. This practice increases the potential for injury to the patient. Occupational therapy personnel are legally liable for negligence if a patient is injured because the staff failed to follow proper procedures.[3]

This chapter reviews safety precautions associated with selected diagnoses. It also identifies precautions to consider for equipment typically found in treatment settings. Guidelines for handling various emergency situations are reviewed. This chapter is only an overview and cannot substitute for training in procedures specific to a particular facility. In

*Wendy Buckner contributed large portions of this chapter to the first edition of this text.

addition to following these procedures, the OTA should teach patients and their families applicable techniques to follow at home.

CASE STUDY

Karen, Part 1

Karen enjoyed the flexibility of working PRN vacation/sick coverage but found herself in some challenging situations. One morning Karen was running late for her next patient. The whole day began late (she couldn't believe the amount of traffic getting to work) and just continued with complications ("Where is Mike? He was supposed to take Mr. Smith back to his room!"). So as she raced into Mrs. Jones' room and found her already in a wheelchair, she hardly had time to say, "Hello, Mrs. Jones, I'm Karen, your OT person for the day" before turning the wheelchair and starting down the hall to the OT clinic. Today was her first time meeting Mrs. Jones, and Karen had glanced quickly at the notes left by the supervising therapist. Noting that Mrs. Jones had some expressive aphasia after her stroke, she took extra care in responding to her when she said, "Hey, girlie, where are you taking me?" Karen stopped the chair in the hall and swung it around so that she was facing the patient.

"I'm sorry, Mrs. Jones, I'm covering for Becky while she's on maternity leave."

"That's nice, but I'm not Mrs. Jones. I was visiting her, but she was in the bathroom."

Reflection: Karen made a few mistakes in her haste. What would have been the correct steps to follow when picking up a patient?

Box 3-1

Safety Recommendations for the Clinic

1. Wash hands for at least 40 to 60 seconds[2,4] before and after treating each patient to reduce cross-contamination.
2. Make sure you are working with the correct patient, under the correct set of medical orders.
3. Make sure adequate space to maneuver equipment is available. Place patients where they may be protected from bumps by equipment or passing personnel. Keep the area free from clutter.
4. Do not attempt to transfer patients in congested areas or in areas where your view is blocked.
5. Routinely check equipment to be sure it is working properly.
6. Ensure that furniture and equipment in the clinic are stable. When not in use, store items out of the way of the treatment area.
7. Keep the floor free of cords, scatter rugs, litter, and spills. Avoid highly polished floors, which may be slippery.
8. Do not leave patients unattended. Use restraint belts properly to protect the patients when they are not closely observed. Follow correct protocols for restraint use.[5]
9. Have the treatment area and supplies ready before the patient arrives.
10. Allow only properly trained personnel to provide patient care.
11. Follow the manufacturer's and facility's procedures for handling and storage of potentially hazardous material. Be sure such materials are marked and stored in a place in clear view. Do not store items above shoulder height.
12. Ensure that emergency exits and evacuation routes are clearly indicated.
13. Have emergency equipment such as fire extinguishers and first-aid kits readily available.

Safety Recommendations for the Clinic

The prevention of accidents and subsequent injuries begins with consistent use of generic safety recommendations for any health care setting, from ensuring you are working with the correct client and washing your hands before and after working with every client, through such actions as knowing the location and use of fire safety equipment (Box 3-1). These recommendations should strike you as common sense, but please understand that following common sense is not as common a practice as it should be. When was the last time you washed your hands today? When was the last time you touched your face? What types of potential contamination occurred between those two events? Common sense tells us we must maintain personal hygiene, yet it is often forgotten in the multiple tasks and demands of our lives and sometimes we suffer the consequences of exposure to germs. We must protect our clients from such careless contamination, as well as provide the safest care we have been trained to do.

Patient Safety

The Joint Commission's *2010 National Patient Safety Goals*[8] begins with the goal of improving accuracy of patient identification before any procedure or treatment. Although OT practitioners do not often engage in life-threatening interventions, ensuring that the therapist is working with the correct client and addressing the required problem is advisable. The rest of the safety goals vary slightly across settings but address improving the effectiveness of communication among caregivers, using medications and infusion pumps, reducing the risk of health care–associated infections or pressure sores, and reducing the risk of patient harm resulting from falls. The complete list of goals and recommendations for performance of them is available from the referenced website.[8]

Infection Control

Infection control procedures are used to prevent the spread of diseases and infection among patients, health care workers, and others.[6] They are designed to interrupt or establish barriers to the infection cycle even when the source of infection is undetermined. The Centers for Disease Control and Prevention (CDC) first established universal precautions to protect the health care worker from infectious diseases such as human immunodeficiency virus (HIV), acquired immunodeficiency syndrome (AIDS), and hepatitis B virus (HBV). The CDC revised that information and now promotes standard precautions[4,7] and transmission-based

Box 3-2

Summary of Standard Precautions

1. Wash hands immediately with soap and water before and after examining patients and after any contact with blood, body fluids, and contaminated item regardless of whether gloves were worn. Soaps containing an antimicrobial agent are recommended. Avoid wearing artificial fingernails.
2. Wear clean, ordinary thin gloves anytime there is contact with blood, body fluids, mucous membrane, and broken skin. Change gloves between tasks or procedures on the same patient. Before going to another patient, remove gloves promptly and wash hands immediately. Then don new gloves.
3. Wear a mask, protective eyewear, and gown during any patient-care activity when splashes or sprays of body fluids are likely. Remove the soiled gown as soon as possible and wash hands.
4. Handle needles and other sharp instruments safely. Do not recap needles. Ensure that contaminated equipment is not reused with another patient until it has been cleaned, disinfected, and sterilized properly. Dispose of nonreusable needles, syringes, and other sharp patient-care instruments in puncture-resistant containers.
5. Routinely clean and disinfect frequently touched surfaces including beds, bed rails, patient examination tables, and bedside tables.
6. Clean and disinfect soiled linens and launder them safely. Avoid direct contact with items soiled with blood and body fluids.
7. Place a patient whose blood or body fluids are likely to contaminate surfaces or other patients in an isolation room or area.
8. To avoid injury or accidental exposure, minimize the use of invasive procedures.

precautions (Box 3-2 and Figure 3-1) to apply to all body fluids, broken skin, and mucous membranes. These precautions are effective only when used with *all* patients, not only those identified as infected.

The U.S. Occupational Safety and Health Administration (OSHA) issues regulations to protect the employees of health care facilities. All treatment settings must comply with the following federal regulations[9]:

1. Educate employees on the methods of transmission and the prevention of HBV and HIV.
2. Provide safe and adequate protective equipment, and teach the employees where it is located and how to use it.
3. Teach employees about work practices used to prevent occupational transmission of disease including but not limited to standard precautions, proper handling of patient specimens and linens, proper cleaning of body fluid spills (Figure 3-2), and proper waste disposal.
4. Provide proper containers for the disposal of waste and sharp items, and teach the employees the color-coding system used to distinguish infectious waste.
5. Post warning labels and biohazard signs (Figure 3-3).
6. Offer the hepatitis B vaccine to employees at substantial risk of occupational exposure to HBV.
7. Provide education and follow-up care to employees who are exposed to communicable disease.

OSHA has also outlined the responsibilities of health care employees, which include the following:

1. Use protective equipment and clothing provided by the facility whenever the employee comes in contact—or anticipates coming in contact—with body fluids.
2. Dispose of waste in proper containers, using knowledge and understanding of the handling of infectious waste and color-coded bags or containers.
3. Dispose of sharp instruments and needles into proper containers without attempting to recap, bend, break, or otherwise manipulate them before disposal.
4. Keep the work and patient care areas clean.
5. Wash hands immediately after removing gloves and at all other times required by hospital or agency policy.
6. Immediately report any exposures (e.g., needle sticks, blood splashes) or any personal illnesses to the supervisor and receive instruction about any further follow-up action.

Although eliminating all pathogens from an area or object is impossible, the risk of infection transmission can be greatly reduced. The largest source of preventable patient infection is contamination from the hands of health care workers.[4] Hand washing (Box 3-3) and gloves are the most effective barriers to the infection cycle. Additional personal protection measures include wearing caps, masks, and gowns and properly disposing of sharp instruments, contaminated dressings, and bed linens. Facial, or fit, masks come in various sizes; therapists should know their own sizes. Be aware if you must wear long-sleeved garments so that the sleeves do not come in contact with pathogens. Hand sanitizers are being used frequently, sometimes placed in every clinic and patient room, and have their own guidelines for use.[2]

In the clinic, general cleanliness and proper control of heat, light, and air are also important for infection control. Spills should be cleaned up promptly. Work areas and equipment should be kept free from contamination.

Decontamination is a physical or chemical process of removing or inactivating pathogens on a surface or item to the point where they will not transmit infectious particles. This makes the surface or item safe for handling, use, or disposal. **Sterilization** is used to destroy all forms of microbial life including highly resistant bacterial spores. Items to be sterilized or decontaminated should first be thoroughly cleaned to remove any residual matter. There are multiple methods used to sterilize items including steam under pressure, ethylene oxide, dry heat, and immersion in sterilizing chemicals.

A variety of **disinfectants** may be used to clean environmental surfaces and reusable instruments. When using liquid disinfectants and cleaning agents, gloves are worn to protect the skin from repeated or prolonged contact. The CDC, local health department, or hospital infection control department can provide information regarding the best product and method to use.

Instruments and equipment used to treat a patient should be cleaned or disposed of according to institutional or agency policies and procedures. Only one client at a time should use small

GLOVE
Before touching blood, body fluids, mucous membranes, non-intact skin or performing venipuncture. Change gloves after contact with each patient.
WASH
Wash hands immediately after gloves are removed. Wash hands and other skin surfaces immediately if contaminated with blood or other body fluids
GOWN/APRON
For procedures likely to generate splashes of blood or other body fluids.
MASK/EYEWEAR
Masks and protective eyewear or face shields for procedures likely to generate splashes of blood or other body fluids.
SHARPS
Dispose of needles with syringes and other sharp items in puncture-resistant container near point-of-use.
NO HAND RECAP
NO
Do not recap needles or otherwise manipulate by hand before disposal.
RESUSCITATION
Mouthpieces or resuscitator bags should be available to minimize need for emergency mouth-to-mouth resuscitation.
WASTE/LINEN
Waste and soiled linen should be handled in accordance with hospital policy and local law.
Universal Precautions apply to blood, visibly bloody fluid, semen, vaginal secretions, tissues and to cerebrospinal, synovial, pleural, peritoneal, pericardial and amniotic fluids.
FORM UNI
BREVIS Corp. 3310 South 2700 East • SLC, UT 84109
© 1994 BREVIS Corp.

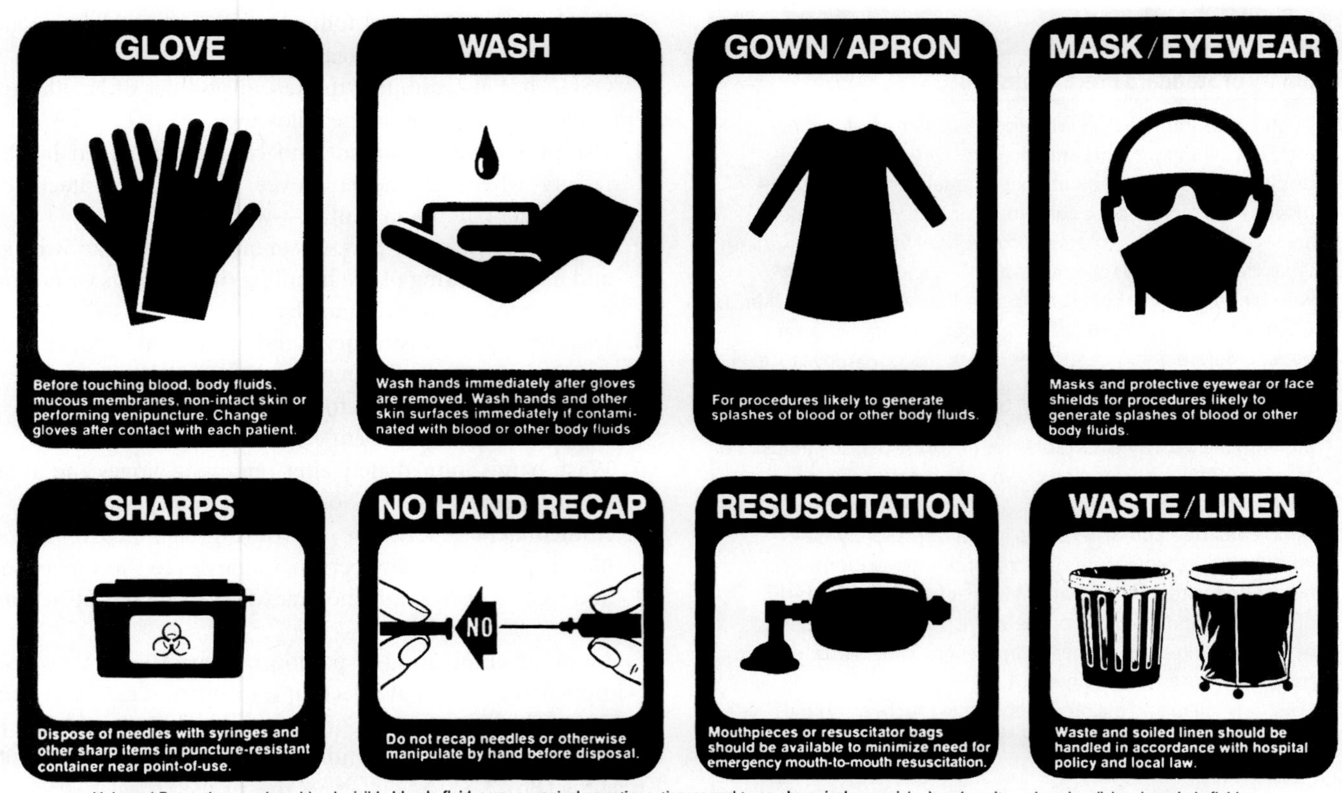

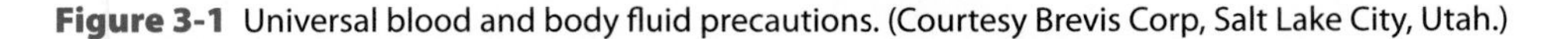

Figure 3-1 Universal blood and body fluid precautions. (Courtesy Brevis Corp, Salt Lake City, Utah.)

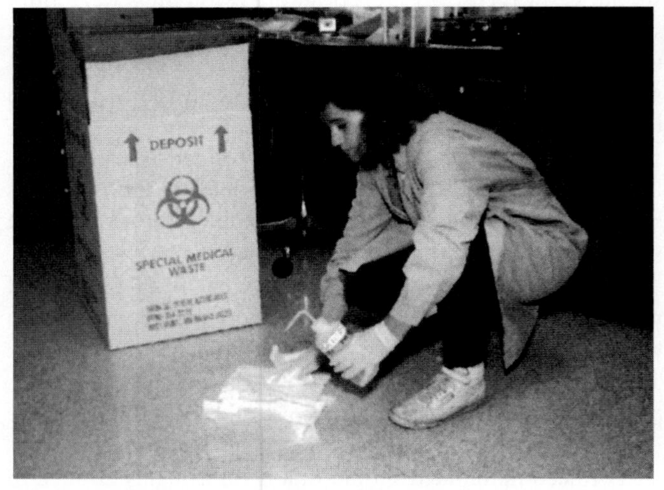

Figure 3-2 Spills of body fluids must be cleaned up by a gloved employee. He or she should use paper towels and dispose of them in an infectious waste container. Then 5.25% sodium hypochlorite (household bleach) diluted 1:10 should be used to disinfect the area. (From Zakus SM: *Clinical procedures for medical assistants,* ed 3, St. Louis, 1995, Mosby.)

BIOHAZARD

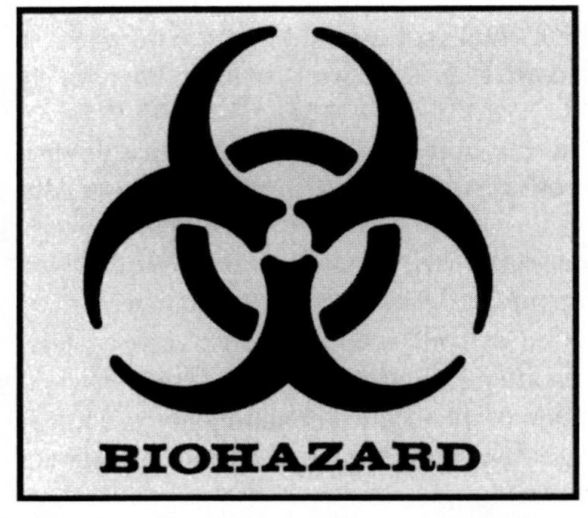

Figure 3-3 Biohazard label. (From Zakus SM: *Clinical procedures for medical assistants,* ed 3, St. Louis, 1995, Mosby.)

equipment/tools such as walkers or gait belts, and the equipment should be cleansed properly. Contaminated reusable equipment should be placed carefully in a specified area or container, labeled, and returned to the appropriate department for sterilization. Contaminated disposable items should be placed carefully in a container, labeled, and disposed of properly.

Contaminated or soiled linen should be disposed of with minimal handling, sorting, and movement. It can be placed in an appropriate bag and labeled before transport to the laundry, or the bag can be color coded to indicate the type or condition of linen it contains. Other contaminated items such as toys, magazines, personal hygiene articles, dishes, and eating utensils should be disposed of or disinfected. Others should not use these items until they have been disinfected. As with all contaminated items, disposable diapers and wipes should be discarded in a secured container and hands should be washed immediately.

Box 3-3

Technique for Effective Handwashing*

1. Remove all jewelry, except plain band rings. Remove watch or move it up the arm. Provide complete access to area to be washed.
2. Approach the sink, and avoid touching the sink or nearby objects.
3. Turn on the water, and adjust it to a lukewarm temperature and a moderate flow to avoid splashing.
4. Wet wrists and hands with fingers directed downward, and apply approximately 1 teaspoon of liquid soap or granules.
5. Begin to wash all areas of hands (palms, sides, backs); fingers; knuckles; and between fingers using vigorous rubbing and circular motions. If wearing a band, slide it up or down the finger and scrub skin underneath it. Interlace fingers and scrub between each finger.
6. Wash for at least 40 seconds, keeping the hands and forearms at elbow level or below and hands pointed down. Wash longer if a patient known to have an infection was treated.
7. Wash as high up wrists and forearms as contamination is likely.
8. Rinse hands, wrists, and forearms well under running water.
9. Use an orangewood stick or nail brush to clean under each fingernail at least once a day (preferably when starting work) and each time hands are highly contaminated. Rinse nails well under running water.
10. Dry hands, wrists, and forearms thoroughly with paper towels. Use a dry towel for each hand. Water should continue to flow from tap as hands are dried.
11. Use another dry paper towel to turn water faucet off. Discard all towels in an appropriate container.
12. Use hand lotion as needed.

*Poster available from http://www.who.int/gpsc/5may/How_To_HandWash_Poster.pdf

Isolation Systems

Isolation systems are designed to protect a person or object from becoming contaminated or infected by transmissible pathogens. Various isolation procedures are used in different institutions. All health care workers must understand and follow the isolation approach used in their facilities to ensure protection.

Generally, patients are isolated from other patients in the hospital environment if they have a transmissible disease. Isolation involves placing the patient in a room alone or with one or more patients with the same disease to reduce the possibility of transmitting the disease to others. All who enter the patient's room must follow specific infection control techniques. These requirements are listed on a color-coded card and placed on or next to the door of the patient's room. Box 3-4 lists transmission risk precautions for the three main forms of transmission. Protective clothing including gown, mask, cap, and gloves may be required. When leaving the patient, the health care professional should remove the garments in the proper sequence.

Occasionally, patients' conditions (e.g., burns, systemic infections) make them more susceptible to infection. They may be placed in protective isolation. With this approach, persons entering the patient's room may need to wear protective clothing to prevent transmission of pathogens to the patient. In this case, the sequence and method of donning the protective garments are more important than the sequence used to remove them.

Box 3-4

Summary of Transmission Risk Precautions

Airborne Transmission

- Place the patient in an airborne infection isolation room (AIIR) where air is not circulated to the rest of the health facility. Make sure the room has a door that can be closed.
- Wear a respirator or other biosafety mask when working with the patient or in the patient's room.
- Limit patient movement from the room to other areas. If possible, place a surgical mask on the patient who must be moved.
- Wash hands thoroughly upon entering and leaving room.

Droplet Transmission

- Place the patient in an isolation room.
- Wear a respirator or other biosafety mask when working with the patient.
- Limit patient movement from the room to other areas. If patient must be moved, place a surgical mask on the patient.

Contact Transmission

- Place the patient in an isolation room and limit access.
- Wear gloves during contact with patient and with infectious body fluids or contaminated items. Reinforce handwashing throughout the health facility.
- Wear two layers of protective clothing.
- Limit patient movement from the isolation room to other areas.
- Avoid sharing equipment between patients. Designate equipment for each patient, if supplies allow. If sharing equipment is unavoidable, clean and disinfect it before use with the next patient.

Modified from Siegel JD, Rhinehart E, Jackson M, Chiarello L, and the Healthcare Infection Control Practices Advisory Committee, 2007 Guideline for Isolation Precautions: Preventing Transmission of Infectious Agents in Healthcare Settings. Retrieved October 28, 2010 from http://www.cdc.gov/ncidod/dhqp/pdf/isolation2007.pdf.

Incidents and Emergencies

OTAs should be able to respond to a variety of medical emergencies and to recognize when it is better to receive assistance from the most qualified individual available such as a physician, emergency medical technician, or nurse. Outside assistance should be easily accessible in a hospital but may require an extended time if the treatment is conducted in a patient's home or outpatient clinic. The assistant should keep emergency telephone numbers close at hand. The OTA needs to determine at the time of the incident whether to call for assistance before or after emergency care. In most cases it is advisable to call for assistance before initiating emergency care, unless the delay would be life threatening.

CASE STUDY

Karen, Part 2

Karen was completely embarrassed and continued to apologize profusely to Mrs. Thomas as she went back to Mrs. Jones' room. She was relieved when Mrs. Thomas assured her she was okay. While Mrs. Thomas wheeled off to her own room, Karen knocked on the bathroom door to find Mrs. Jones but got no response. She cracked the door open slightly and heard a soft moan, so she opened the door farther. Mrs. Jones was on the floor. Karen immediately pushed the call button. She knelt down to Mrs. Jones (noting that her armband said "Mrs. Edna Jones") and asked her if she was all right. Mrs. Jones responded with a smile but looked flustered.

"Does anything hurt?" Karen asked as she scanned Mrs. Jones for obvious bruises.

Mrs. Jones shook her head.

The nurse, Susan Peters, arrived, and Karen explained that she had come to get Mrs. Jones for OT and found her this way in the bathroom.

"Now how did you get out of bed?" asked Susan.

Karen volunteered that Mrs. Thomas had been in the room before Karen got there.

"Not again! I'll tell her one more time not to let down bedrails and to get a nurse instead. It's just not safe!"

Ms. Peters carefully checked Mrs. Jones and then she and Karen helped her back into her bed. She seemed unhurt, but Karen and Susan decided that the OT session could wait until later so that Mrs. Jones could be monitored and have time to settle down.

Reflection: What are your thoughts about the way Karen handled the situation to this point?

Many accidents can be prevented by consistently following safety measures. However, OT practitioners should always be alert to the possibility of an injury and should "expect the unexpected." Most institutions have specific policies and procedures to follow. In general, when a patient is injured, the OTA should do the following:

1. Ask for help. Do not leave the patient alone. Prevent further injury to the patient and provide emergency care.
2. When the emergency has passed, document the incident according to the institution's policy. Do not discuss the incident with the patient or significant others. Do not admit to negligence or provide information that suggests negligence to anyone.[3]
3. Notify the supervisor of the incident, and file the incident report with the appropriate person within the organization.

Falls

Staying alert and reacting quickly when patients lose their balance can prevent injuries from falls. Proper guarding techniques must be practiced. In many instances, trying to keep the patient upright is unwise. Instead, the practitioner should carefully assist the patient to the floor or onto a firm support.

If a patient begins to fall forward, the OTA should do the following:

1. Restrain the patient by firmly holding the gait belt.
2. Push forward against the pelvis, and pull back on the shoulder or anterior chest.
3. Help the patient to stand erect once it is determined that the patient is not injured. The patient may briefly lean against the OTA for support.
4. If the patient is falling too far forward to be kept upright, guide the patient to reach slowly for the floor.
5. Slow the momentum by gently pulling back on the gait belt and the patient's shoulder.
6. Step forward as the patient moves toward the floor.
7. Tell the patient to bend his or her elbows to help cushion the fall when the hands contact the floor.
8. Ensure the patient's head is turned to the side to avoid injury to the face.

If the patient begins to fall backward, the procedure is the following:

1. Rotate your body so that one side is turned toward the patient's back, and widen your stance.
2. Push forward on the patient's pelvis, and allow the patient to lean against your body.
3. Assist the patient to stand erect.
4. If the patient falls too far backward, continue to rotate your body to stay upright until it is turned toward the patient's back and widen your stance.
5. Instruct the patient to lean briefly against your body or to sit on your thigh.
6. Consider lowering the patient into a sitting position on the floor, using the gait belt and good body mechanics.

Burns

Generally, only minor first-degree burns are likely to occur in OT practice. These can be treated with basic first-aid procedures. The OTA should contact skilled personnel for immediate care if skin is charred, missing, or blistered. For first-degree burns, where the skin is only reddened, the following steps are taken:

1. Rinse or soak the burned area in cold (not iced) water.
2. Cover with a clean or sterile dressing or bandage. A moist dressing may be more comfortable for some patients.
3. Do not apply any cream, ointment, or butter to the burn; doing so will mask the appearance and may lead to infection or a delay in healing.

Bleeding

A laceration may result in minor or serious bleeding. The objectives of treatment are to prevent contamination of the wound and to control the bleeding. To stop the bleeding, the OTA should do the following:

1. Wash hands and don protective gloves. Continue to wear protective gloves during treatment of the wound.

2. Place a clean towel or sterile dressing over the wound, and apply direct pressure to the wound. If no dressing is available, use the gloved hand.
3. Elevate the wound above the level of the heart to reduce blood flow to the area.
4. In some cases, consider cleansing the wound with an antiseptic or by rinsing it with water.
5. Encourage the patient to remain quiet and to avoid using the extremity.
6. If arterial bleeding occurs, as evidenced by spurting blood, apply intermittent, direct pressure to the artery above the level of the wound as needed. The pressure point for the brachial artery is on the inside of the upper arm, midway between the elbow and armpit. The pressure point for the femoral artery is in the crease of the hip joint, just to the side of the pubic bone.
7. Do not apply a tourniquet unless you have been trained to do so.

Shock

Excessive bleeding, changing from a supine to an upright position, or excessive heat may induce **shock.** Signs and symptoms of shock include pale, moist, and cool skin; shallow, irregular breathing; dilated pupils; a weak or rapid pulse; and dizziness or nausea. Shock should not be confused with fainting, which would result in a slower pulse, paleness, and perspiration. Patients who faint generally recover promptly if allowed to lie flat. The OT practitioner who notices a patient experiencing symptoms of shock should intervene with the following actions:

1. Determine the cause of shock, and correct it if possible. Monitor the patient's blood pressure and pulse rate.
2. Place the patient in a supine position, with head slightly lower than the legs. If head and chest injuries are present or respiration is impaired, consider keeping the head and chest slightly elevated.
3. Do not add heat, but prevent loss of body heat, if necessary, by applying a cool compress to the patient's forehead and covering the patient with a light blanket.
4. Keep the patient quiet, and ensure the patient avoids exertion.
5. After the symptoms are relieved, gradually return the patient to an upright position and monitor the patient's condition.

Seizures

Seizures may result from a specific disorder, brain injury, or medication. The OTA should be able to recognize a seizure and take appropriate action to keep the patient from being injured. A patient experiencing a **seizure** usually becomes rigid and statue-like for a few seconds, then begins to convulse with a whole-body jerking motion. The person will most likely turn blue and may stop breathing for up to 50 or even 70 seconds. Some patients' sphincter control may be lost during or at the end of the seizure, and they may involuntarily void urine or feces. The OTA who suspects a patient is about to have a seizure should initiate the following interventions:

1. Place the person in a safe location, away from anything that might cause injury. *Do not* attempt to restrain or restrict the convulsions.

Table 3-1 Warning Signs and Symptoms of Insulin-Related Illnesses

Observations	Insulin Reaction	Acidosis
Onset	Sudden	Gradual
Skin	Moist, pale	Dry, flushed
Behavior	Excited, agitated	Drowsy
Breath odor	Normal	Fruity
Breathing	Normal to shallow	Deep, labored
Tongue	Moist	Dry
Vomiting	Absent	Present
Hunger	Present	Absent
Thirst	Absent	Present

Modified from Pierson FM: *Principles and techniques of patient care,* ed 3, Philadelphia, 2002, WB Saunders.

2. Assist in keeping the patient's airway open, but do not attempt to open the mouth by placing any object between the teeth. Never place your finger or a wooden or metal object in the patient's mouth, and *do not* attempt to grasp or position the tongue.
3. If the patient's mouth is open, place a soft object between the teeth to prevent the patient from accidentally biting the tongue. A sturdy cloth object or a tongue depressor wrapped with several layers of gauze and fastened with adhesive tape may be used.
4. When the convulsions subside, turn the patient's head to one side in case he or she vomits.
5. After the convulsions cease, the patient should rest. Covering the patient with a blanket or positioning a screen to provide privacy may be helpful.
6. Obtain medical assistance.

Insulin-Related Illnesses

Many patients seen in OT practice may experience insulin-related episodes. The OTA must be able to differentiate between the conditions of hypoglycemia (insulin reaction) and hyperglycemia (acidosis), as shown in Table 3-1.

An **insulin reaction** can be caused by too much systemic insulin, the intake of too little food or sugar, or too much physical activity. If the patient is conscious, some form of sugar is provided (e.g., candy, orange juice). If the patient is unconscious, glucose may have to be provided intravenously. The patient should rest, and all physical activity should be stopped. This condition is not as serious as acidosis, but the patient should be given the opportunity to return to a normal state as soon as possible.

Acidosis can lead to a diabetic coma and eventual death if not treated. It should be considered a medical emergency requiring prompt action including assistance from qualified personnel. The patient should not be given any form of sugar. An insulin injection is usually necessary, and a nurse or physician should provide care as quickly as possible.

Choking and Cardiac Arrest

All health care practitioners should be trained to treat patients who are choking or experiencing cardiac arrest. Both the American Heart Association and the American Red Cross offer specific training courses. Printable posters are available online (see Resources). The following information is presented as a reminder of the basic techniques and is *not* meant to substitute for training.

The urgency of choking cannot be overemphasized. Immediate recognition and proper action are essential. When assisting a conscious adult or child older than one year, the OTA should do the following:

1. Ask the patient, "Are you choking?" If the patient can speak, or cough effectively, *do not* interfere with the patient's own attempts to expel the object.
2. If the patient is unable to speak, cough, or breathe, check the mouth and remove any visible foreign object.
3. If the patient is unable to speak or cough, position yourself behind the person. Clasp your hands over the patient's abdomen, slightly above the umbilicus but below the diaphragm.
4. Use the closed fist of one hand, covered by your other hand, to give three or four abrupt thrusts against the person's abdomen by compressing the abdomen in and up forcefully (Heimlich maneuver). Continue to apply the thrusts until the obstruction becomes dislodged or is relieved or the person becomes unconscious.
5. Obtain medical assistance.

When assisting an unconscious adult or child older than one year, the OTA should take the following steps:

1. Place the patient in a supine position, and call for medical help.
2. Open the patient's mouth, and use your finger to attempt to locate and remove the foreign object (finger sweep).
3. Open the airway by tilting the head back and lifting the chin forward. Attempt to ventilate using the mouth-to-mouth technique.
4. If step 3 is unsuccessful, deliver up to five abdominal thrusts (Heimlich maneuver), repeat the finger sweep, and attempt to ventilate. It may be necessary to repeat these steps.
5. Be persistent and continue these procedures until the object is removed or medical assistance arrives.
6. Consider initiating cardiopulmonary resuscitation (CPR) techniques to stabilize the patient's cardiopulmonary functions after the object has been removed.

The following procedures, updated in 2010, are recommended for CPR.[1] These guidelines emphasize the life-saving value of compression and distinguish between recommendations for trained versus untrained lay rescuers. All OT practitioners should be trained lay rescuers.

1. Check quickly (within 10 seconds) for absent or abnormal breathing; if necessary, activate emergency response system. Retrieve or send someone for automated external defibrillator (AED).
2. Unresponsive adults should be placed in a supine position on a firm surface.
3. Initiate chest compressions immediately; push hard and fast. Kneel next to the patient, place the heel of one hand on the inferior portion of the sternum just proximal to the xiphoid process, and place your other hand on top of the first hand. Position your shoulders directly over the patient's sternum; keep your elbows extended; and press down firmly, depressing the sternum at least 2 inches (5 cm) with each compression. Relax after each compression, but do not remove your hands from the sternum. The relaxation and compression phases should be equal in duration. This can be accomplished by mentally counting "1001," "1002," "1003," and so on, for each phase. Aim for 30 compressions.
4. Open the patient's airway by lifting up on the chin and pushing down on the forehead to tilt the head back.
5. Pinch the patient's nose closed, and maintain the head tilt to open the airway. Place your mouth over the patient's mouth and form a seal with your lips; perform two full breaths, then proceed to evaluate the circulation. Some persons prefer to place a clean cloth over the patient's lips before initiating mouth-to-mouth respirations. If it is available, a plastic intubation device can be used to decrease the contact between the caregiver's mouth and the patient's mouth.
6. If you are doing all CPR procedures without assistance, perform 30 chest compressions and then two breaths. Compress at the rate of at least 100 times per minute, minimizing interruptions. Continue these procedures until qualified assistance arrives or the patient is able to sustain independent respiration and circulation. If you are alone, get assistance from other persons by calling loudly for help. If a second person is present, the person should contact an advanced medical assistance unit before beginning to assist with CPR. The patient usually requires hospitalization and evaluation by a physician. (NOTE: Extreme care must be used to open an airway in a patient who may have a cervical spine injury. For such patients, use the chin lift, but avoid the head tilt. If the technique does not open the airway, tilt the head slowly and gently until the airway is open.)

These procedures are appropriate for adults and children eight years of age and older. A pamphlet or booklet containing diagrams and instructions for CPR techniques can be obtained from most local offices of the American Heart Association or online (see Resources). Courses of instruction in first aid and CPR are offered through the American Heart Association, the American National Red Cross, and other organizations. OT practitioners in clinical practice should make every effort to update and maintain service competency in basic first aid, CPR, and emergency measures.

Preventive Positioning for Specific Diagnoses

Many patients require special positioning to prevent complications and maintain function. Staying in one position for a long time can lead to the development of contractures and bedsores (decubitus ulcers).

Specific patient conditions such as impaired sensation, paralysis, poor skin integrity, poor nutrition, impaired circulation, and spasticity require special attention. The patient's skin, especially bony prominences over the sacrum, ischium, trochanters, elbows, and heels, should be inspected. Reddened areas may develop from pressure within 30 minutes. Other indicators of excessive pressure are complaints of numbness or tingling and localized swelling.

CASE STUDY

Karen, Part 3

Later in the day, when Karen came to check on Mrs. Jones, she saw a note on the door stating that isolation precautions were in effect.

"What's going on with Mrs. Jones?" Karen asked Susan, who was still on duty.

"Oh, we got the labs back on Mrs. Thomas and she has MRSA. You said she had been in to see Mrs. Jones, and we're afraid there may have been transmission."

"Oh no," thought Karen. In the hubbub surrounding the fall Karen had totally forgotten standard precautions. She was sure she had touched her own face before washing her hands. As her thoughts retraced her steps during those hours she was relieved to recall washing her hands as she entered her next patient's room. But was that enough?

"When we helped Mrs. Jones back into bed we weren't gowned; do you think that will matter?"

"Good point," said Susan, "We'd better make a list of everyone you saw today and put them on the watch list."

"After I do that I'll need to gown up and check on Mrs. Jones. If she is going to stay in her bed, I'd like to check her positioning."

Reflection: How can one remember to use standard precautions for all people at all times?

Pillows, towel rolls, or similar devices may be used to provide comfort and stability but should be used cautiously to prevent secondary complications. The following examples of patient conditions demonstrate the need for specific positioning techniques. It is important to review these with both the patient and caregiver.

Patients with above-knee lower extremity amputations should avoid hip flexion and hip abduction. The time the patient may sit is limited to 30 minutes per hour. When the patient is supine, the stump is elevated on a pillow only for a few minutes. The patient should lie in a prone position to avoid contracture of the hip flexor muscles.

Patients with below-knee lower extremity amputations should avoid prolonged hip and knee flexion to prevent contractures. Again, the patient may sit only 30 minutes per hour, and when supine, the patient should not keep the stump elevated for more than a few minutes. When it is elevated, the knee is maintained in extension. The patient is instructed to keep the knee extended throughout the day. Lying prone is recommended.

To avoid contractures resulting from muscle spasticity, patients with hemiplegia should avoid the following positions for prolonged periods: shoulder adduction and internal rotation, elbow flexion, forearm supination or pronation, wrist flexion, finger and thumb flexion and adduction, hip and knee flexion, hip external rotation, and ankle plantar flexion and inversion. Both the arm and the leg should be moved through the available range of motion (ROM) several times per day.

Patients with rheumatoid arthritis should avoid prolonged immobilization of the affected extremity joints. Gentle active range of motion (AROM) or passive range of motion (PROM) of the joints should be performed several times per day if the joints are not acutely inflamed.

As burns heal, scars and contractures are likely to form. Therefore avoiding prolonged static positioning of the joints affected by the burn or skin graft, especially positions of comfort, is important. The positions comfortable to the patient do not produce the stress or tension needed to maintain mobility of the wound area. When the burn is located on the flexor or adductor surface of a joint, positions of flexion and adduction should be avoided. Passive or active exercise should be done frequently to both the involved and the uninvolved joints. The patient will probably have to endure significant pain to restore normal joint function.

Precautions with Special Equipment

When seeing patients at the bedside, the OTA first should contact the nurses' station to determine whether any specific positioning instructions exist. For example, a patient may need to follow a turning schedule or may be limited in time allowed to remain in one position. If the patient's current position in bed is not suitable for treatment, the treatment might be rescheduled. Other options would be to change the patient's position temporarily or to treat the patient as much as possible in the current position. If the patient's position is changed, the OTA ensures that the patient is returned to the preferred position at the end of treatment. The OTA should use common sense with any equipment. Note the position of the patient and any tubes and wires before, during, and after treatment to ensure that nothing is disconnected or disturbed to the extent that its function is impaired.

Hospital Beds

Two of the more commonly used beds in hospitals are the standard manually operated bed and the electrically operated bed. Both beds are designed to make it easier to support the patient and to change a patient's position. Other more specialized beds are necessary for patients with more traumatic conditions. Whatever type is used, the bed should be positioned so that the patient is easily accessed and the OT practitioner can use good body mechanics (see Chapters 11 and 15).

Most standard adjustable beds are adjusted by using electrical controls attached to the head or the foot of the bed or to a special cord that allows the patient to operate them. The controls are marked according to their function and can be operated by hand or foot. The entire bed can be raised and lowered, or its upper portion can be raised while the lower portion remains unchanged. When the upper portion is raised slightly, the patient's position is called the **Fowler position.** Most beds allow the lower portion to be adjusted to provide knee flexion, which in turn causes hip flexion.

Side rails were once common on most beds as a protective measure but are now considered a form of restraint. The Resource site on *Hospital Beds* contains multiple website links addressing this issue and safety alternatives. Where safety rails are in use, the OTA should be aware that some rails are lifted upward to engage the locking mechanism, whereas others are moved toward the upper portion of the bed until the locking mechanism is engaged. If a side rail is used for patient security, the practitioner ensures that the rail is locked securely and has not compressed or stretched any intravenous (IV) lines or other tubing before he or she leaves the patient.

Some beds are specifically designed to provide support and mobility for a patient, such as the **turning frame** (e.g., Stryker wedge frame), which has a front and back frame covered with canvas. The support base allows the head or foot ends or the entire bed to be elevated. One person can easily turn the patient horizontally from prone to supine or from supine to prone positions. This bed is used most commonly for patients with spinal cord injuries who require immobilization. The turning frame allows access to patients and permits moving them from one place to another without removing them from the frame. The skin of patients using this type of bed must be monitored frequently because the bed allows only two basic positions. Another bed for support and mobility is a post-trauma mobility bed that maintains alignment through adjustable bolsters yet can rock from side to side to reduce pressure on the patient's skin.[5]

Other beds that specifically address the skin-related complications of prolonged immobility have been developed. The air-fluidized support bed (Clinitron) is a heavy, expensive bed that contains silicone-coated glass beads that simulate the properties of a fluid when heated. Pressurized air flows through the mattress to suspend a polyester cover that supports the patient. Patients feel like they are floating on a warm waterbed. The risk of developing skin problems is reduced because of the minimal contact pressure of the patient's body against the polyester sheet. This bed is used with patients who have several infected lesions or who require skin protection and whose position cannot be altered easily or who cannot on their own change positions easily. Caution should be used to prevent puncturing the polyester cover, which would cause the silicone beads to leak.[5] Another similar bed is the low air loss bed, which relies on air bladders rather than glass beads to adjust pressure; this bed was developed to reduce the incidence of pressure ulcers.

Ventilators

A **ventilator** (respirator) moves gas or air into the patient's lungs and maintains adequate air exchange when normal respiration is decreased. Two frequently used types are volume-cycled ventilators and pressure-cycled ventilators. Both ventilators deliver a predetermined volume of gas ("air") during inspiration and allow for passive expiration. The gas from the ventilator is usually delivered to the patient through an **endotracheal tube (ETT)**. When the tube is in place, the patient is considered to be *intubated.* Insertion of the ETT prevents the patient from talking. When the ETT is removed, the patient may complain of a sore throat and may have a distorted voice for a short time. It is important to avoid disturbing, bending, or kinking the tubing or accidentally disconnecting the tube of the ventilator from the ETT. A patient using a ventilator can perform various bedside activities including sitting and ambulation, as long as the tubing is long enough. Because the patient has difficulty talking, the occupational therapist or OTA should ask questions that can be answered with head nods or other nonverbal means. A patient using a ventilator may have reduced tolerance for activities and should be monitored for signs of respiratory distress such as a change in the respiration pattern, fainting, or blue lips.

Monitors

Various monitors are used to observe the physiologic state of patients who require special care. Patients who are being monitored can perform therapeutic activities if care is taken to avoid disrupting the equipment. Many of the units have an auditory and/or visual signal that is activated by a change in the patient's condition or position or by a change in the equipment's function. A nurse will need to evaluate and correct the cause of the alarm unless the OTA has received special instruction.

The **electrocardiogram (ECG, EKG)** monitors the patient's heart rate, blood pressure, and respiration rate. Acceptable or safe ranges for the three physiologic indicators can be set in the unit. An alarm is activated when the upper or lower limits of the ranges are exceeded or the unit malfunctions. A monitoring screen provides a graphic and digital display of the values for observation of the patient's responses to treatment.

Various catheters and monitors do not impede treatment as long as care is taken to leave them undisturbed by avoiding activities in muscles or joints close to the insertion point. The OTA should employ common sense and due diligence with the following devices. The **pulmonary artery catheter (PAC)** is a long, plastic IV tube inserted into the internal jugular or the femoral vein and passed through to the pulmonary artery to provide accurate and continuous measurements of pulmonary artery pressures and detect subtle changes in the patient's cardiovascular system including responses to medications, stress, and activity. The **intracranial pressure (ICP) monitor** measures the pressure exerted against the skull by brain tissue, blood, or cerebrospinal fluid (CSF). It is used to monitor ICP in patients who have experienced a closed head injury, cerebral hemorrhage, brain tumor, or an overproduction of CSF. Some of the complications associated with this device are infection, hemorrhage, and seizures. Physical activities should be limited when these monitors are in place. Avoid activities that would cause a rapid increase in ICP such as isometric exercises. Positions to avoid include neck flexion, hip flexion greater than 90 degrees, and the prone position. The patient's head should not be lowered more than 15 degrees below the horizontal plane. The **arterial monitoring line** (A line) is a catheter inserted into an artery to measure blood pressure continuously or to obtain blood samples without repeated needle punctures. Treatment can be provided with an A line in place, but care should be taken to avoid disturbing the catheter and inserted needle.

Feeding Devices

Special feeding devices may be necessary to provide nutrition for patients who are unable to chew, swallow, or ingest food. Some of the more common devices are the nasogastric tube, gastric tube, and IV feeding tube.

The nasogastric (NG) tube is a plastic tube that is inserted through a nostril and terminates in the patient's stomach. The tube may cause the patient to have a sore throat and an increased gag reflex. The patient cannot eat food or drink fluids through the mouth while the NG tube is in place. Movement of the patient's head and neck, especially forward flexion, should be avoided.

The gastric tube (G tube) is a plastic tube inserted through an incision in the patient's abdomen directly into the stomach. During treatment the OT practitioner must avoid disturbing or removing the tube.

Intravenous feeding, total parenteral nutrition (TPN), and hyperalimentation devices are used to infuse the total calories or nutrients (hyperalimentation) needed to promote tissue growth without going through the digestive system. A catheter is inserted directly or indirectly into the subclavian vein. The catheter may be connected to a semipermanently fixed cannula or sutured at the point of insertion. The OTA should carefully observe the various connections to be certain they are secure before and after treatment. A disrupted or loose connection may cause an air embolus, which could be life threatening to the patient.

The system usually includes an infusion pump, which administers fluids and nutrients at a preselected, constant flow rate. An audible alarm is activated if the system becomes imbalanced or the fluid source is empty. Treatment activities can be performed as long as the tubing is not disrupted, disconnected, or occluded and if undue stress on the infusion site is avoided. Motions of the shoulder on the side of the infusion site, especially abduction and flexion, may be restricted. Medication infusion pumps are specifically mentioned in the JCAHO safety goals.

Most intravenous (IV) lines are inserted into superficial veins. Various sizes and types of needles or catheters are used, depending on the purpose of the IV therapy, the infusion site, the need for prolonged therapy, and site availability. During treatment the OTA must be careful to avoid disrupting, disconnecting, or occluding the tubing. The infusion site should remain dry; the needle should remain secure and immobile in the vein; and no restraint should be placed above the infusion site (e.g., no blood pressure cuff applied above the site). The total system should be observed to ensure it is functioning properly when treatment begins and ends. The patient who ambulates with an IV line in place should be instructed to grasp the IV support pole so that the infusion site will be at heart level. If the infusion site is allowed to hang lower, blood flow may be affected. Similar procedures to maintain the infusion site in proper position should be followed when the patient is treated in bed or at a treatment table. The patient should avoid activities that require the infusion site to be elevated above the level of the heart for a prolonged period. Problems related to the IV system should be reported to nursing personnel. Simple procedures such as straightening the tubing may be performed by the properly trained OTA.

Urinary Catheters

A urinary catheter is used to remove urine from the bladder when the patient is unable to control its retention or release. The urine is then drained through plastic tubing into a collection bag, bottle, or urinal. Any form of trauma, disease, condition, or disorder affecting the neuromuscular control of the bladder sphincter may require the use of a urinary catheter. The catheter may be used temporarily or for the remainder of the patient's life.

A urinary catheter can be applied internally (indwelling catheter) or externally. Female patients require an indwelling catheter inserted through the urethra and into the bladder. Two commonly used internal catheters are the Foley and suprapubic catheters. The Foley catheter is held in place in the bladder by a small balloon that is inflated with air, water, or sterile saline solution. To remove the catheter, the balloon is deflated and the catheter withdrawn. The suprapubic catheter is inserted directly into the bladder through incisions in the lower abdomen and bladder. The catheter may be held in place by adhesive tape, but care should be taken to avoid its removal, especially during self-care activities. Males may use an external catheter. A condom is applied over the shaft of the penis and is held in place by an adhesive applied to the skin or by a padded strap or tape encircling the proximal shaft of the penis. It is connected to a drainage tube and bag.

When treating patients with urinary catheters, the OTA must remember the following precautions:

1. Avoid disrupting or stretching the drainage tube, and do not put tension on the tubing or the catheter.
2. Do not allow the bag to be placed above the level of the bladder for more than a few minutes.
3. Do not place the bag in the patient's lap when the patient is being transported.
4. Observe the production, color, and odor of the urine.
5. Report the following observations to a physician or nurse: foul-smelling, cloudy, dark, or bloody urine or a reduction in the flow or production of urine.
6. Be sure to empty the collection bag when it is full.

Infection is a major complication for persons using catheters, especially indwelling catheters. Everyone involved with the patient should maintain cleanliness during treatment. The OTA should not attempt to replace or reconnect the tubing unless properly trained. Health care settings that routinely treat patients with catheters have specific protocols for catheter care. (See CDC Guideline in Resources, *Infection Control.*)

Summary

All OT personnel have a legal and professional obligation to promote safety for self, the patient, visitors, and others. The OTA should be prepared to react to emergency situations quickly, decisively, and calmly. The consistent use of safe practices helps to reduce accidents to patients and workers and decreases the time and cost of treatment.

Selected Reading Guide Questions

1. Why is it important to teach the patient and significant others guidelines for handling various emergency situations?
2. Describe at least four behaviors the OTA can adopt to improve patient safety.
3. Describe the consequences of improper positioning of patients.
4. Define the following: IV line, NG tube, TPN, hyperalimentation, and ventilator.
5. Describe standard precautions.
6. Why is it important to follow standard precautions with all patients?
7. Describe the proper technique for handwashing.
8. How should the OTA respond to a patient emergency?
9. How would you help a patient who is falling forward? A patient who is falling backward?
10. What emergency situations might require obtaining advanced medical assistance, and what situations could an OTA handle alone?

References

1. American Heart Association: *Highlights of the 2010 American Heart Association Guidelines for CPR and ECC.* Retrieved October 30, 2010 from: http://www.heart.org/idc/groups/heart-public/@wcm/@ecc/documents/downloadable/ucm_317350.pdf.
2. Centers for Disease Control and Prevention: *Hand Hygiene Basics, How to Wash Your Hands Poster.* Retrieved October 28, 2010 from: http://www.who.int/gpsc/5may/How_To_HandWash_Poster.pdf and How to Rub Your Hands Poster http://www.who.int/gpsc/5may/How_To_HandRub_Poster.pdf.
3. Kornblau BL: The ethical and legal implications of the use of aides in occupational therapy practice, *Admin & Manag SIS Quar* 15(3):1–6, 1999.
4. Nazarko L: Standard precautions: how to help prevent infection, *Br J Healthcare Assistants* 2(3):119–123, 2008.
5. Pierson FM, Fairchild SL: *Principles and techniques of patient care*, ed 3, Philadelphia, 2002, WB Saunders.
6. *State of Arizona publication on OSHA Bloodborne Pathogens Standard.* Retrieved October 28, 2010 from: http://gocyf.az.gov/Children/Policy/manual/FORM_OSHA_bloodborne_pathogen.pdf.
7. Tarrac SE: Application of the updated CDC isolation guidelines for health care facilities, *AORN J* 87(3):534–542, 2008.
8. The Joint Commission: *2010 National Patient Safety Goals.* Retrieved October 21, 2010, from: http://www.jointcommission.org/PatientSafety/NationalPatientSafetyGoals/.
9. United States Department of Labor: Occupational Safety & Health Administration, Safety and Health Topics. Retrieved October 28, 2010 from: http://www.osha.gov/SLTC/healthcarefacilities/index.html:(links to all regulations).

Resources

Adult Basic Life Support

American Heart Association Guidelines/video: http://www.youtube.com/americanheartassoc

JAMA reference article link: http://www.emergencydispatch.org/articles/lifesupport1.htm

Resuscitation Council (UK) Poster of guidelines: http://www.resus.org.uk/pages/blsalgo.pdf

University of Washington, Learn CPR: http://depts.washington.edu/learncpr/

First Aid

American Heart Association Guidelines/CPR & First Aid links http://www.heart.org/HEARTORG/CPRAndECC/CPR_UCM_001118_SubHomePage.jsp

American Heart Association local offices, American National Red Cross: Contact for information on first aid, choking, and CPR.

Hand Washing

CDC Hand Hygiene in Healthcare Settings, http://www.cdc.gov/handhygiene/

World Health Organization: *WHO Guidelines on Hand Hygiene in Health Care (an evidence based guide to everything you would want to know about handwashing).* Retrieved October 28, 2010 http://whqlibdoc.who.int/publications/2009/9789241597906_eng.pdf.

Hospital Beds

U.S Department of Health & Human Services: *U.S. Food and Drug Administration: Medical Devices*, http://www.fda.gov/MedicalDevices/ProductsandMedicalProcedures/GeneralHospitalDevicesandSupplies/HospitalBeds/default.htm.

Infection Control and Universal Precautions

Centers for Disease Control and Prevention (CDC): The "An Ounce of Prevention" Campaign. http://www.cdc.gov/ounceofprevention/Contains link to downloadable poster and brochure for Infection Control in the home.

CDC Guideline for infection control in health care settings. http://www.cdc.gov/hai/

CDC Guideline for infection control in health care personnel. http://www.cdc.gov/ncidod/dhqp/pdf/guidelines/InfectControl98.pdf

CDC Guideline for prevention of catheter-associated urinary tract infections, 2009, http://www.cdc.gov/hicpac/cauti/003_cauti2009_execSum.html.

OSHA Hazard Information Bulletins: *potential for occupational exposure to bloodborne pathogens from cleaning needles used in allergy testing procedures*, http://www.osha.gov/pls/oshaweb/owadisp.show_document?p_table=FEDERAL_REGISTER&p_id=16265.

Restraint Use

CDC Injury Center: Falls in nursing homes, http://www.cdc.gov/ncipc/factsheets/nursing.htm.

PART II

Process

CHAPTER 4

Occupational Therapy Process: Evaluation and Intervention in Physical Dysfunction

PATTY COKER-BOLT AND MARY BETH EARLY

Key Terms

Referral
Screening
Evaluation
Clinical reasoning
Treatment planning or intervention planning
Treatment implementation or intervention
Reevaluation
Discharge planning
Transition services
Occupational profile
Analysis of occupational performance
Occupation-centered interview
Active listening
Daily schedule interview
Participation
Clinical reasoning

Chapter Objectives

After studying this chapter, the student or practitioner will be able to do the following:

1. Identify and describe the major stages in the occupational therapy process.
2. Describe the "flow" of the occupational therapy process, and give examples to illustrate this concept.
3. Identify and contrast the roles of the occupational therapist and the occupational therapy assistant in the evaluation and intervention planning stages of the occupational therapy process.
4. Explain how the medical record can assist the practitioner in preparing for evaluation of the client.
5. Discuss the importance of an occupational profile client interview in the evaluation process.
6. Describe the skills and behaviors of an effective interviewer.
7. Differentiate standardized and nonstandardized tests.
8. Discuss how to use practice models to guide planning of an occupation-centered treatment plan.
9. Define treatment or intervention planning and describe the process.
10. Differentiate the roles of the occupational therapist and the occupational therapy assistant in intervention planning.
11. Write clear, measurable, relevant treatment goals and objectives.

Occupational dysfunction due to physical limitations is a common problem for persons with physical disabilities. For these individuals, occupational therapy (OT) is a bridge back to everyday life, maintaining or restoring the ability to function with maximal independence in occupational roles and daily life activities. The OT process is a team effort between the occupational therapist and the occupational therapy assistant (OTA), who work together with the client. The occupational therapist is responsible for client evaluations and determining the initial intervention plan. The occupational therapist, with input from the OTA, is also responsible for the continuation and termination of the OT services throughout the clients' rehabilitation process. This chapter provides an overview of the OT process and the evaluation and treatment planning stages with particular emphasis on the role of the OTA and the relationship between the client, OTA, and occupational therapist. Each step in the process requires a positive working relationship among all members of the OT team.

Steps or Stages in the Occupational Therapy Process

When a client begins to receive OT services in a hospital, nursing home, or outpatient clinic, the treating therapists follow a series of stages or steps. The *Guide to Occupational Therapy Practice* describes the steps in OT services that are client centered, effective, and reimbursed[4]:

1. Referral: The physician or another legally qualified professional requests OT services for the client. The initial referral may be oral, but a written record is also necessary. In most instances, a written referral from a physician is required for reimbursement from a third-party payer.
2. Screening: The occupational therapist obtains data to determine the need for evaluation and intervention. The occupational therapist performs a brief, general assessment to determine whether OT services would benefit the client.

3. **Evaluation:** The OT team attempts to discover the nature of the client's problems or to evaluate a specific area of concern listed by a physician, parent, or other caregiver in the referral. The two major parts of evaluation are the occupational profile and an analysis of occupational performance.[5] Under supervision of the occupational therapist, the OTA may carry out elements of the evaluation. The occupational therapist analyzes the evaluation data to identify the client's specific strengths and deficits.
4. **Treatment planning or intervention planning:** A plan that will guide actions is developed in collaboration with the client (and the client's caregivers, as appropriate).[5] Considering research evidence of effective treatment principles and methods, the occupational therapist develops the initial treatment plan based on selected theories and intervention approaches.
5. **Treatment implementation or intervention:** Intervention is the process of ongoing therapeutic activities that will influence and support client occupational performance. Interventions are directed toward identified outcomes or goals developed in the intervention plan. The client's response to the intervention is monitored and documented on a regular basis, as determined by the clinical facility. The OTA may have significant responsibilities for this part of the process.
6. **Reevaluation:** Reevaluation of a client is the process of evaluating the client's progress toward the goals of the treatment plan and modifying the treatment plan and goals as needed.[4] Measurement of the outcomes of treatment is critical in showing the effectiveness of the therapy intervention. The treatment plan may be modified or continue toward the set plan based on the reevaluation results.
7. **Discharge planning:** The OT team may provide recommendations for further interventions at such time as a client is discharged from a health care facility. Additional OT services may be necessary as a result of the client's change in functional status, living situation, workplace, caregiver, technology, development, personal interest, or age.[4] Working with the client, the client's family, and the treatment team, the occupational therapist and assistant develop a plan for the client to follow after discharge.

Process and Flow

Despite the discrete stages just listed, the OT more closely resembles a flowing or fluid current (like a river) rather than a stepwise progression (like climbing a mountain). Although referral generally comes first, in some cases the OT practitioner (therapist or assistant) may consult with the physician to recommend a client who would benefit from OT services. Some physicians rely on OT staff to identify those clients who are most likely to benefit; these physicians may issue referrals at the therapists' suggestion.

Similarly, evaluation and treatment are interwoven. The client is seen for a short period of time in the first evaluation, and intervention may begin that same day. As the client's skills and needs change, the OT team continuously reevaluates the client's functional performance status and updates the intervention plan. For example, the client's initial evaluation may include the occupation of dressing because at that time the client requires moderate assistance to complete dressing. The goal is to increase the client's independence with specific dressing tasks and decrease the level of assistance the client requires. As the client becomes more independent with dressing, the OT team will evaluate his or her functional status, document any improvement, and update the intervention plan. The OTA must notify the occupational therapist if a client needs to be reevaluated. The OTA who has achieved service competency may assume some responsibility for updating intervention plans in activities of daily living (ADL) and other areas of occupation.

The rapid pace of today's health care environment requires occupational therapists to consider discharge planning during the initial evaluation process. Restrictions on reimbursement demand quick discharge, making early planning essential. Occupational therapists historically have viewed their clients in the context of their occupational lives and have engaged clients in thinking of themselves as occupational beings. Thus the client and therapist(s) create a vision of future performance that guides the OT treatment process from beginning to end.

Role of the Occupational Therapist

In keeping with the most recent *Standards of Practice for Occupational Therapy* issued by the American Occupational Therapy Association (AOTA),[3] the authors remind the reader that the occupational therapist has the leadership role in the OT process. The occupational therapist is responsible for accepting and acting on referrals and for designing and supervising individual or group screenings.

The occupational therapist is the manager, director, and analyst. The therapist documents the OT evaluation, which forms the scientific foundation for the decisions in the treatment plan.[9] The therapist must be knowledgeable about the dysfunction and its causes, course, and prognosis; be familiar with a variety of evaluation procedures, their uses, and proper administration; and be able to identify evaluation procedures suitable to the client and the dysfunction.

The occupational therapist selects the areas to be evaluated, chooses appropriate evaluation instruments and procedures, and administers those evaluations or delegates their administration to another therapist or qualified OTA.

The occupational therapist designs, develops, and documents the treatment plan of care. A treatment plan of care should include the following[3]:

- An occupational profile with the client's goals for OT treatment
- A list of client's strengths and weaknesses
- An estimation of the client's rehabilitation potential
- Measurable short-term and long-term goals
- Documentation of collaboration with the individual, family members, other caregivers, and professionals
- Identification of support systems and community resources
- Selection of media, methods, environment, and personnel needed to accomplish the intervention goals

- Determination of the frequency and duration of OT services
- Identification of a plan for reevaluation
- Recommendation for discharge plan after therapy services are completed

The occupational therapist may delegate some aspects of treatment planning to the OTA. However, the occupational therapist retains legal and supervisory responsibility for the plan and its implementation.

The occupational therapist manages and documents treatment implementation and reevaluation. Major portions of implementation may be delegated to the OTA. Nevertheless, the occupational therapist is responsible for overseeing and supervising treatment and reevaluating and documenting progress.

The occupational therapist determines when service should be discontinued and develops the client's discharge plan. Parts of discharge planning may be delegated to the OTA. The occupational therapist documents all outcomes and recommendations for follow-up in the final OT report.

Role of the Occupational Therapy Assistant

The OTA is a co-participant in the entire OT process, at the discretion of the supervising occupational therapist and depending on the experience and service competencies of the particular OTA. The 2010 *Standards of Practice* employs the term OT practitioner, referring to both the occupational therapist and the OTA.[3] Thus the training and qualifications of the OTA are recognized as consistent with significant responsibilities in the OT process. The occupational therapist and the OTA need to review individual state licensure laws to ensure compliance. Some state licensure laws provide specific guidelines for the roles and responsibilities of the OTA.

With regard to referral, the OTA can educate physicians and other potential referral sources about how to initiate OT referrals. The OTA may administer parts of the screening under OT supervision.[3]

Once the occupational therapist has selected appropriate evaluation instruments, the OTA may administer some of the assessments used in the evaluation process.[3] As a general rule, the more standardized and structured the instrument, the more quickly the OTA can acquire adequate service competency for administration. The OTA must be able to communicate the results, both orally and in writing, of assessments he or she administers. The OTA may be given responsibility for educating the client and family about the purposes of the evaluation.

OTAs may administer evaluation procedures for which they have achieved service competency. Such evaluations are performed with the guidance and supervision of the occupational therapist. OTAs can perform these procedures with only general supervision once they have demonstrated consistent and reliable administration techniques. When performing evaluation procedures, the assistant must approach the client with openness and without preconceived ideas about the client's limitations or personality. The assistant must have good observation skills and be able to build rapport with the client in a short time.[2]

Occasionally, OTAs may encounter pressure to administer evaluation procedures for which they are not qualified. Administrators or other staff may even ask the OTA to conduct an entire evaluation. To do so would be inappropriate and exceed the scope of practice and expertise of the OTA role. The OTA who encounters such pressure may take several courses of action. The first is to explain as clearly as possible the difference between the occupational therapist and OTA roles. The OTA also must contact the OT supervisor for guidance. If pressure continues or the employer threatens the OTA with loss of a job or other penalties, the OTA should contact the local and state practice associations and the AOTA. Under no circumstance should OTAs ever attempt any procedure for which they do not have service competency.

The OTA can contribute to the intervention plan,[3] especially in the occupational performance areas of daily living activities (both basic and instrumental), work, education, play, and leisure. The OTA with sufficient experience and skill may work fairly independently in these areas. Generally, interventions directed toward development of motor or process skills or toward remediation of impaired body functions (e.g., perceptual deficit) must be planned by the occupational therapist.

According to the 2010 *Standards of Practice,* the OTA may implement the intervention plan under OT supervision.[3] Responsibilities might include carrying out treatment activities, educating the client and family about treatment, and documenting the services provided. The OTA may also contribute to reevaluation, as directed.

The OTA may have responsibility for **transition services,** which help the client change from one health care facility or environment to another.[3] For example, the client with a head injury may need to move toward independent community living. This transition might require the services of a community agency. Depending on the practice area and personal expertise, the OTA may coordinate or administer a plan for moving the client through such a transition. The occupational therapist generally designs the transition plan.

Experience, Expertise, and Service Competency

As a matter of personal responsibility and professional prudence, the OTA student or recent graduate is required to follow the 2009 *Guidelines for Supervision, Roles, and Responsibility during the Delivery of Occupational Therapy Services.*[2] Further, all students and OTAs must learn and follow applicable state regulations regarding OTA services. New practitioners need and benefit from close supervision and direction in all stages of the OT process. They should undertake independent service provision in evaluation and treatment planning only when service competency is ensured after careful training. For these reasons, the authors strongly advise new graduates to seek their first jobs in a setting with strong supervision; in particular, new graduates are advised to avoid working on a contract basis in settings with limited supervision.

The more experienced OTA may function fairly autonomously, with only general supervision from the occupational therapist, in designated areas of evaluation and treatment planning.[2] Years of experience are not sufficient by themselves. The OTA who desires more autonomy and responsibility must study, learn, and practice service tasks until he or she gains competency in the specific health care setting in which he or she is employed.

The experienced OTA might assume leadership or specialty positions within the OT department, perhaps within an area of practice or administration.[2] Examples might include technology specialist, pain management specialist, administration, or director of student training. Each of these roles requires certain skills and competencies that the OTA can master through supervised experience and/or through specialized training acquired through continuing education. Alternative roles outside the OT field such as director of durable medical equipment or director of adult day care exist as well.

Evaluation Process

The evaluation process begins with the physician's referral and screening (Figure 4-1). Screening typically starts with reviewing the client's medical record to determine the need for further evaluation, the type of assessment tools that may be needed, and specific OT intervention that may be required.[4] During a client screening, the occupational therapist may also interview the client, make observations, and estimate time of treatment and the need to coordinate treatment with other services.[4]

After the screening the occupational therapist will determine whether a full OT evaluation would be beneficial to the client. The OT team must gather information to develop a plan of intervention. The goal of the OT evaluation is to complete an occupational profile of the client and analyze occupational performance in both basic and instrumental activities of daily living (ADL). The **occupational profile** describes the client's occupational history, patterns of daily living, interest, and therapy needs. The **analysis of occupational performance** looks at the client's observable performance in carrying out desired occupational tasks and ADL. The occupational therapist observes the client's performance skills (motor skills, process skills, and/or communication and interaction skills) and evaluates client factors (such as cognitive-mental factors, physical factors, social-emotional factors) that can interfere with occupational performance. The client-centered evaluation process analyzes client factors that support or hinder occupational performance. Client goals and limitations in occupational performance become the basis for developing treatment goals or objectives and strategies to remediate or compensate for problems in occupational performance.

Evaluation provides specific information that can be communicated to other members of the rehabilitation team. Evaluation data may indicate which treatment techniques are most suitable and show the effectiveness of OT intervention.

The occupational therapist, considering the general picture of the client's situation, selects a practice model suited to determining the cause of limitations in occupational performance. The model helps identify the range of evaluation procedures that might be used to gather the information needed

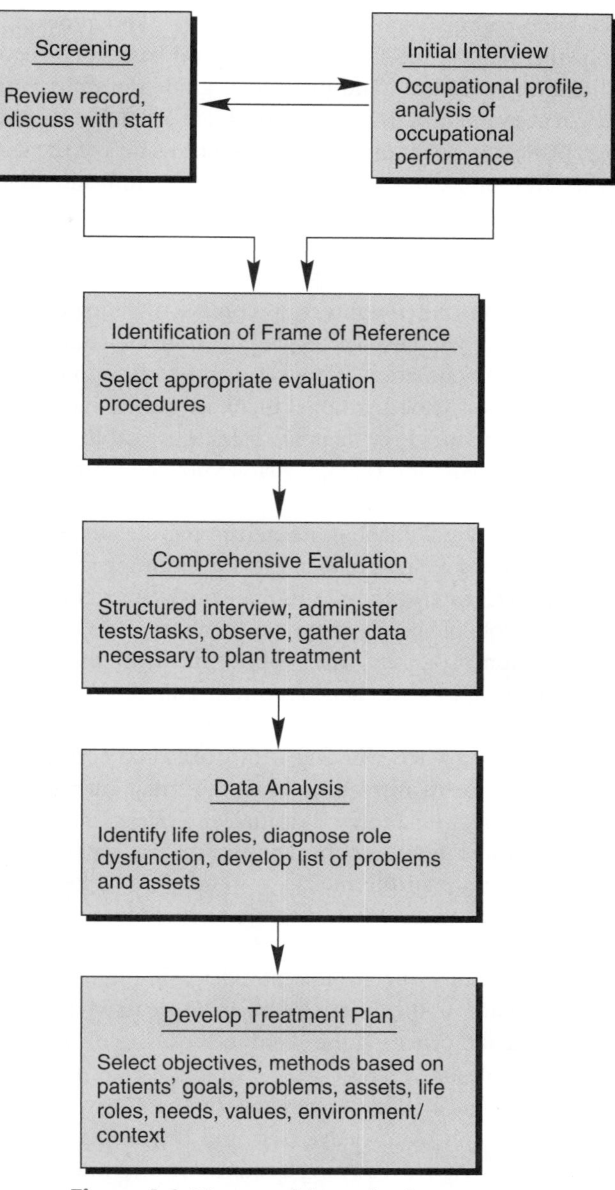

Figure 4-1 Diagram of the evaluation process.

for planning treatment. The therapist selects and administers (or directs the OTA to administer) specific tests, clinical observations, structured interviews, standardized tests, performance checklists, and activities and tasks. The therapist gathers, interprets, and analyzes the information from the evaluation procedures.[5] Some typical evaluation techniques that an occupational therapist will assign or use are discussed in this chapter.

Medical Chart Review

A comprehensive review of the medical chart or the client's medical record is completed by the OT or OTA. Information can include the client's occupational and medical history, age, sex, family situation, education, occupation, work history, leisure habits, self-care habits, social relationships, cultural background, diagnosis, and medical and/or psychiatric history. Daily notes from nurses and physicians list current medications and the client's reactions and responses to the facility, treatment regimen, staff, and other clients.[9] The information from the medical record serves as a good basis for selecting evaluation procedures and provides a guide for approaching the client evaluation. It indicates problem areas and helps the therapist focus attention on the pertinent factors of the case.[8] Generally, an occupational therapy evaluation should not occur until after a review of the client's medical record.

Occupation-Centered Interview

An occupation-centered interview consists of asking the client or family member questions relating to occupational habits and life roles, family situation, home setup, interests, values, and/or therapy goals. The occupational therapist gathers information on how clients perceive their life roles, physical dysfunction, health care needs, and therapy goals. Knowing the client's life roles, interests, and activities is most helpful for diagnosing role dysfunction. It is valuable for determining the client's values and establishing realistic possibilities for resuming former roles following OT intervention. Simultaneously, clients can learn about the role of the occupational therapist and OTA in the rehabilitation program.[9] The rapport and trust that develop between therapist and client are important outcomes of the initial occupation-centered interview. In certain settings and situations (e.g., when working with occasional consultation) the OTA may be required to conduct the initial interview.

The occupation-centered initial interview should take place in a quiet environment that ensures privacy. The practitioner should plan the interview in advance to know what information must be obtained and to have some specific questions prepared. A specified period of time, identified by the therapist and client before the interview, should be set aside. The first part of the interview may be devoted to getting acquainted and orienting the client to the OT clinic or service and to the role and goals of OT.

The two essential characteristics of the successful interviewer are a solid knowledge base and the use of active listening skills. Active listening requires study, practice, and preparation. The therapist's knowledge will influence the selection of questions or topics to be covered in the interview. Although the OTA follows a structured format in any interview, a knowledge base is still helpful for deciding which questions to skip and which to repeat, expand, or rephrase.

The interviewer who actively listens demonstrates respect for and interest in the client.[14] During active listening, the receiver (interviewer) tries to understand what the sender (client) is feeling or the meaning of the message. An interviewer then rephrases the responses into his or her own words and feeds it back for verification by saying, for example, "This is what I believe you mean. Have I understood you correctly?" While listening actively, the interviewer does not send a new message such as an opinion, judgment, advice, or analysis. Rather, an interviewer relates back only what he or she thinks the client meant.

Throughout the interview the practitioner should listen to understand the client's attitude toward the physical dysfunction. A client should be encouraged to express what he or she sees as the primary problems and goals for rehabilitation. Client beliefs and preferences may differ substantially from what the therapist believes, but a client must be given careful consideration in order for the OT team and client to set realistic treatment goals together. As the interview progresses, the client should have an opportunity to ask questions about therapy intervention and goals. The OT practitioner must have good listening and observation skills to gather maximum information during this interview process.

The rapport and trust that develop between the client and the OT practitioner are based on their open and honest communication. The communication in the interview and observation phases of the evaluation are critical to all subsequent interactions and thus to the effectiveness of treatment. Clients need to sense that they have been heard and understood by someone who is caring and empathetic. Clients must be able to trust that a therapist has the skills necessary to facilitate a successful rehabilitation plan. The practitioner needs to project self-confidence in his or her own skills and in the OT profession. This attitude will set the tone for all future client interaction. It will enhance the development of the client's trust in the practitioner and in the potential effectiveness of OT intervention.[17]

The therapist will take notes and record the occupation-centered interview. The client should be advised of this fact in advance and told that the interview will be used to complete a comprehensive OT plan of care. The client will have access to the OT evaluation as part of the medical record.[9,17]

During the initial phase of the interview, the OT practitioner should explain the role of OT, the respective roles of the therapist and the therapy assistant, the purpose of the interview, and how the information is to be used. As the interview progresses, the interviewer may seek the desired information by asking appropriate questions and guiding the responses and ensuing discussion so that relevant topics are addressed. (In general, this sort of unstructured or semistructured interview is conducted by the therapist; the OTA follows a structured interview protocol with specific questions to be asked.) The interview can be concluded with a summary of the major points covered, information gained, estimate of current strengths and functional problems, and plan for further OT evaluation and treatment.

The occupational therapist may want information about the client's family and friends, community and work roles, education and work histories, leisure and social interests and activities, and living situation. Information about how the client spends and manages time is important. The therapist or assistant should interview the client to obtain a detailed account of his or her activities for a typical day (or week) before the onset of physical dysfunction. This information can be determined with a tool such as the daily schedule interview, the Activities Configuration described by Watanabe,[21] or another similar instrument. The OTA can administer these structured assessments. Information that should be elicited in the daily schedule interview includes the following:

- Time when client wakes and gets out of bed
- Morning activities
- Typical hygiene and dressing tasks

- Breakfast routine
- Work/leisure/home management
- Childcare
- Lunch
- Afternoon activities
- Work/leisure/home management
- Rest
- Dinner
- Evening activities
- Leisure and social activities
- Preparation for retiring to bed (i.e., bathing/hygiene)
- Bedtime

The amount of time spent (hours and fractions thereof) on each activity should be recorded carefully. During the interview, the OT practitioner should cue with appropriate questions so that the client will not gloss over or omit any of the daily activities. The interviewer might ask, "What time do you wake up?"; "What is the first thing that you do in the morning?"; "When do you eat lunch?"; and "Who fixed lunch for you?"

The therapist or assistant helps the client review the daily life schedule as it was before the physical disability. The client may share information freely, giving many recollections of social, community, vocational, and leisure activities. At times, allowing discussion to stray from the schedule itself is desirable to elicit a well-rounded picture of the client's roles and relationships. The client's needs, values, and personal goals should be revealed in a good occupation-centered interview. However, it is important to keep the discussion focused and to redirect the client if it becomes tangential. The interviewer should focus the client's attention on the specific daily schedule. If the client cannot remember or communicate his or her schedule, the OT practitioner should seek information from friends or family members to reconstruct the client's daily activities patterns.

The therapist then helps the client to construct a new daily schedule of activities, focusing on the current situation in the treatment facility (or at home if the client is being seen in an outpatient clinic or at home). The interviewer must remember to ask the client who helps with each activity and how much assistance is needed and received. The therapist and client can discuss and compare the two schedules. This process will yield valuable information about the client's occupational needs, values, satisfaction/dissatisfaction with the activities pattern, primary and secondary goals for change, interests, motivation, interpersonal relationships, and fears. This information gives a basis for treatment objectives that meet the client's needs and values. Conducting an occupation-centered interview in this manner will assist the therapist in planning intervention that is meaningful to the client.

The daily schedule reveals how clients view themselves in their occupational and life roles. The practitioner can see the client as a functioning human rather than someone with a diagnosis or disability. The client's individual needs become the basis for intervention (rather than standard evaluation and treatment regimens established for a given disability).

Observation

A skilled clinician relies heavily on structured and unstructured observations of the client during the interview, evaluation, and treatment. By carefully watching, looking, and seeing, the practitioner learns much about the client's functioning during unstructured observation. Consider what can be learned by observing clients during the evaluation. What is the posture, mode of ambulation, and gait pattern? How is the client dressed? Is there obvious motor dysfunction? Are musculoskeletal deformities apparent? What is the facial expression, tone of voice, and manner of speech? How does the client use the affected and nonaffected extremities? Does the client demonstrate any pain mannerisms such as protection of an injured part or grimaces and groans?

In addition to these unstructured observations, which can be made during the first few minutes of the initial contact with the client, OT practitioners use structured observation to evaluate performance of self-care, home management, mobility, and transferring. These structured observations, which may be performed by the OTA, are usually carried out by observing the client performing real tasks in real or simulated environments. Data from these observations yield information about the client's level of independence, speed, skill, and need for special equipment and the feasibility for further training.

Standardized Tests

Standardized tests generally follow a strict protocol or set of administration procedures. It is common for a standardized test to have been normed, or tested against a sample population, to demonstrate the normal ranges (norms) and abnormal ranges. This procedure allows the score of the person being evaluated to be compared with those of a normed group.[6,7]

Standardized tests also have known reliability and validity. Reliability refers to the consistency of results. For example, two different evaluators should be able to obtain similar results on the same client; this demonstrates interrater reliability. Also, an evaluator should be able to administer a test in the same way to each person and in the same way to the same person on two different occasions (i.e., pretest and posttest). Assuming conditions are similar, the test should yield similar results. Validity is concerned with the degree to which the test measures what it is supposed to measure (construct validity). For example, a test of cognitive skills is more valid when it measures just those skills, uncontaminated by psychosocial factors or motor skill or communication/interaction factors.

Occupational therapists have been encouraged to use standardized tests to record information obtained from clients. Because such assessments yield quantitative (numeric) results, they are useful in showing outcomes of treatment. Results of the initial evaluation and follow-up evaluations can be reported in a consistent, objective, and reliable manner.[22]

Standardized tests are considered superior to nonstandardized tests, and most clinicians would prefer to use standardized tests. However, relatively few standardized evaluation procedures are available in OT. Many evaluation procedures in use have unknown reliability and validity. Many are informal instruments developed by occupational therapists to suit the needs of their own practice settings. Still others are adaptations of existing evaluation instruments and are used with clients other than those for whom they were designed.

Some of the standardized tests used by occupational therapists were designed by professionals in other disciplines.[19,23] These include tests for measuring achievement, development, intelligence, manual dexterity, motor skills, personality, sensorimotor function, and vocational skills.[6,12] Several excellent sources of information about standardized tests are available.[6,9] Current health care journals and psychological abstracts discuss standardized evaluations that may be relevant to OT.[7] Although having standardized and objective measures is desired, professional judgment and interpretation are also essential to evaluation.

To participate in the administration of standardized tests, the OTA needs certain skills. The assistant should be capable of the following:

- Understanding the theory that supports using the standardized tests for a specific client
- Administering standardized tests only as directed by the occupational therapist
- Following directions of the standardized tests including guidelines to administration and scoring of the tests
- Accurately communicating and documenting the information for the occupational therapist to interpret

While administering a standardized test, the OTA must scrupulously follow the procedures outlined in the test instruction. Typically this information can be found in the guide to administration booklet for each test. Varying from the standard testing procedure will yield unreliable results, and the results of the testing will be invalid. The OTA communicates the results to the occupational therapist, who interprets the results and may select additional tests.

One of the most widely used standardized evaluation tools in physical disabilities is the Functional Independence Measure (FIM).[12] This evaluation measures 18 functional items on a scoring scale ranging from 1 to 7. The main areas evaluated by the FIM are self-care, toileting, mobility, locomotion, communication, and social cognition; the FIM is first typically used when the client is first referred for OT services in an acute care setting. As with other standardized scales, the client is first scored during the initial evaluation on the FIM scale, is rescored at discharge, and then is rescored at follow-up about 1 month after discharge. Scores on repeat administrations are used to verify a client's functional progress during therapy and to provide the medical team with an indication of how the client will be able to function at home after discharge. The FIM administered at home measures the client's ability to carry over skills learned during the rehabilitation process after discharge from an inpatient hospital or rehabilitation stay.

Specific training is required to administer the FIM accurately. Health care facilities using the FIM scale typically offer this training to clinicians. The FIM scale norms are maintained through a national database so that facilities and clinicians can pool their scores. Information from sites across the country is analyzed and sent back to the facilities that use the scale. The rehabilitation sites can see how the outcomes of clients in their program compare with outcomes of clients in other rehabilitation programs within the FIM system. The OTA can have a major role in gathering FIM outcomes data. Once the OTA receives training and certification for using the FIM scale, the OTA can report data to the national database. It is important that the guidelines for the FIM scale are followed strictly because the scores generate national ranges that affect many things beyond individual client care.

Nonstandardized Tests

In contrast to a standardized test, a nonstandardized test is subjective and often has no specific instructions for administration of items, no criteria for scoring, and no information on interpreting results of the test. Nonstandardized tests are valued and continue to be used because they provide subtle information that is not necessarily quantifiable but is nonetheless helpful for planning treatment. The quality of the information from such a test depends on the clinical skill, experience, judgment, and bias of the evaluator.[7] Some nonstandardized evaluation procedures provide broad criteria for scoring and interpretation but still require considerable subjective professional judgment. The manual muscle test, described in Chapter 8, is one such test.

The information from the various evaluation tools provides a comprehensive picture of the client that is based on his or her goals and occupational profile and the OT practitioner's analysis of occupational performance. Limitation in occupational performance as measured against client goals becomes the basis for developing treatment goals and for selecting strategies to remediate or compensate for obstacles in performance. The therapist considers the individual's occupational roles and any role dysfunction and generates a list of client strengths and limitations relevant for planning OT intervention.

Information-Gathering Strategies

The skilled clinician combines two different approaches to gather evaluation information. Using the top-down approach, the therapist focuses on the client's report of the important occupational performance issues limiting abilities to engage successfully in ADL, IADL, work, education, leisure, and social participation. Using the bottom-up approach, the therapist focuses on evaluating the client's body structure and function deficits, as well as developing a plan to compensate for individual performance skills or client factors that interfere with occupational performance. Clinicians working in a strong medical model environment such as a hand therapy clinic or traditional rehabilitation unit may use a bottom-up approach. Clinicians in a community-based practice or home health setting may emphasize the top-down approach. However, experienced clinicians will use both approaches. Taking a simultaneously top-down and bottom-up approach illuminates the client's goals (top-down) and the body functions and deficient performance skills (bottom-up) that limit participation in occupation.[24] The OTA uses observation and active listening to gather information that will contribute to both the top-down and bottom-up approach to treatment.

Clinical Reasoning

Given the various practice models and many tests and procedures that might be used in evaluation, it may seem incredible that the therapist "knows" which ones to select and can remember and assemble all the information to determine an effective analysis and treatment plan. In fact, the therapist does not "know" in a conscious and preordained way, but rather works through a series of decisions in a process known as clinical reasoning. Clinical reasoning is defined in the allied health literature as the many modes of thinking and decision making associated with clinical practice.[19] Specifically cited in the *Standards of Practice* document, it is the occupational therapist's responsibility to "use sound clinical judgment when selecting, measuring, documenting, and interpreting expected or achieved outcomes that are related to the client's ability to engage in occupations." [3] Fleming[12] defined clinical reasoning as "the many types of inquiry that an occupational therapist uses to understand clients and their difficulties." Further, she stated that clinical reasoning includes—but is not limited to—hypothetical reasoning and problem solving. Clinical reasoning refers to the complex processes used when the occupational therapist thinks about the client, the disability, the circumstances, and the meaning of the disability to the client.

Clinical reasoning has been the focus of much study in the past several decades.[8,14,18,20] Clinical reasoning develops professional expertise, a form of knowing that comes from doing or action. Such knowledge is difficult to articulate and in a sense exceeds the knowledge that can be expressed verbally. Clinical reasoning includes expression of theoretical reasons for clinical decisions, but it is more than that. Based on expertise gained from hands-on experience working with clients, it embodies the tacit knowledge and habitual ways of seeing and doing things and dealing with clients. Tacit knowledge is information the novice clinician learns from observing and participating in therapist-client interactions. It develops from entry-level practice and builds with each client interaction. This knowledge determines appropriate action for the particular client at a particular time in a specific circumstance. It is not merely the response to a technical question or theoretical hypothesis. In essence, clinical reasoning is a process of deciding how to act and what to do in a specific circumstance involving the client's well-being.[16]

OT theory can provide a starting place for clinical reasoning but cannot provide all the answers for the course of action in a particular case. Because each client is unique and complex, treatment must be individualized, which requires judgment, creativity, and improvisation. Mattingly[16] proposed that clinical reasoning in OT be primarily directed to the "human world of motives and values and beliefs—a world of human meaning," rather than to a biological world of disease. "Occupational therapists' fundamental task is treating … the illness experience"—that is, what the disability means to the individual person.[16]

OT practitioners teach everyday activities such as dressing skills and toilet transfers to increase self-care independence. In teaching, they confront the client's experiences of profound life changes resulting from the disability—the loss of capacities taken for granted and the necessity to reorient to the world as a person with physical and functional limitations. The practitioner treats not only the physical dysfunction but also the person experiencing the dysfunction. The therapist and assistant must help the client confront the limitations, "claim the disability," reclaim a changed body and different kind of functioning, and develop a new sense of self with meaning, purpose, and value. Thus the simple application of theoretical constructs to arrive at answers to questions about appropriate intervention strategies is only a part of the clinical reasoning process. When planning OT intervention, the therapist must consider the unique meaning of the disability to the client, beyond the physical impairments that result from the disability.[16]

A pilot study of clinical reasoning found that occupational therapists in physical disabilities practice used the following six stages of clinical reasoning during the initial evaluation[17]:

1. Obtaining available information from the medical record, referral statement, and medical team reports before meeting the client
2. Selecting evaluation procedures based on medical diagnosis, prognosis, and the client's ability to cooperate and participate in the evaluation
3. Implementing the evaluation plan by interacting with the client and carrying out selected evaluation procedures
4. Defining problems and possible causes
5. With the client's involvement, defining treatment objectives based on the problem list
6. Selecting treatment tasks and a plan to carry out additional evaluation
7. Evaluating the effectiveness of the evaluation plan and the reliability of evaluation results

In the pilot study of clinical reasoning, therapists used the medical diagnosis to select evaluation procedures, recall standard problem lists for the diagnoses, and select objectives and methods of treatment.[18] This use of clinical reasoning skills reflects a medical model that focuses on the diagnosis.[11] It is a formula approach that bypasses important considerations about the client as a person—considerations that are essential for client-centered OT treatment.[16,17] The medical model approach has value as an element of clinical reasoning, but it omits the complex needs, unique situation, and meaning of the disability in the client's life—all important considerations for OT treatment planning. The occupational therapist may use a medical model of reasoning when considering the physical disability and the body structure and function limitations to client participation in daily activities. However, this model is inadequate for individualizing treatment, facilitating independence, and creating a new future.[9,16]

Fleming[16] proposed occupational therapists use three types of reasoning. The first is *procedural reasoning*, used to consider physical problems; an example is evaluating and analyzing the extent and possible causes of limited range of motion (ROM). *Interactive reasoning* is used to guide interactions with the client (e.g., when trying to obtain information, elicit cooperation, or develop rapport). Finally, *conditional reasoning* is used to consider clients within their personal and social contexts and futures.[10,11] Conditional reasoning uses a "what if..." approach. The therapist considers what might happen if different treatment methods, approaches, techniques, and goals were applied. Clinical reasoning is a complex, changing process for meeting the individual's unique needs for reclaiming a valued sense of self and a meaningful life.[14]

Intervention Planning

Setting up the initial treatment plan for the client provides a design or proposal for an overall plan of care and therapeutic program. The intervention plan is based on the client's stated goals, the therapist's analysis of performance deficits, the unique circumstances of the individual client, and the treatment setting. Intervention planning presents a challenge because of the complexity and variety of circumstances, goals, and problems seen in clients.

The occupational therapist is responsible for the treatment plan, to which the OTA can contribute. The OTA may play a major role in intervention planning for areas of occupation included in the *Occupational Therapy Practice Framework Domain and Process,* edition 2,[5] such as ADL, IADL, rest and sleep, education, work, play, leisure, and social participation.[5] Although the OTA may become more practiced, skilled, and independent with experience, the final responsibility for planning treatment rests with the occupational therapist.

An effective treatment or intervention plan should provide (1) objective and measurable goals with a specific time frame; (2) OT intervention based on theory and current evidence; and (3) a statement describing the mechanisms for service delivery.[5] The plan should indicate who will provide the intervention services and the types, frequency, and duration of interventions. The importance of having a written treatment plan cannot be overstated. Specific objectives or goals must be outlined in an orderly and sequential manner so that these will be clear to the therapist, therapy assistant, client, family, and health care team. The treatment plan helps OT practitioners initiate intervention. It also provides a standard for measuring the client's progress in therapy so that the plan's effectiveness can be measured. For the OTA, a written treatment plan is essential to provide a clear structure and sequence for treatment interventions. Without a written plan, the OTA is not likely to have a clear understanding of the occupational therapist's intended direction and focus of treatment. This lack can lead to inconsistent client services that could jeopardize reimbursement and client outcomes. It is the OTA's responsibility to understand the treatment plan provided by the occupational therapist. Understanding the treatment plan may require asking for clarification of information about the client's intervention and directions on how to implement the plan.

In writing the treatment plan, the therapist formally documents and analyzes the proposed course of action. Some questions considered in the planning process are listed in Box 4-1.

Box 4-1

Questions to Be Considered in the Planning Process

- What is the most appropriate frame of reference or practice model on which to base the treatment plan?
- What are the client's goals, capabilities, and assets?
- What are the client's limitations and deficits?
- What does OT have to offer this client?
- What are the goals of treatment?
- What are specific long-term and short-term objectives or goals?
- Are the treatment objectives consistent with the client's needs and personal aspirations?
- If objectives are not compatible, how do they need to be modified?
- Which treatment methods are available to meet these objectives?
- When should the client have met the objectives?
- What standards will be used to determine when the client has reached an objective?
- How will the effectiveness of the treatment plan be evaluated?
- What is the estimated length of treatment?

The written treatment plan affirms the need for OT services to the client and the medical team. It documents the purposes and effectiveness of OT services and can provide a structure for gathering research data. Most importantly, it guides the OTA and occupational therapist in implementing treatment.

Identifying Problems and Imagining Solutions

The OT treatment planning process (Figure 4-2) requires identifying problems and finding their solutions. The goal is to promote health, well-being, and optimal participation in occupation in desired contexts by persons who are ill or disabled. Treatment planning is a problem-solving process that follows a logical progression. The first step is evaluation, analysis, and identification of problems. The therapist uses data gathered in evaluation to identify functions and dysfunctions in terms of areas of occupation and performance skills. A list of the client's strengths and limitations is developed. This analysis of strengths and limitations becomes the basis of the treatment plan. The therapist then explores prospective solutions and develops treatment objectives, often in close collaboration with the client. From these goals or objectives, the therapist designs and implements a plan of action—the treatment plan.

Selecting a Frame of Reference or Practice Model

The OT treatment plan derives its logic and rationale from an OT frame of reference or a specific practice model. The model or frame of reference structures which evaluation procedures, objectives, and methods will be most appropriate for the client.[9] The process of identifying problems and imagining solutions is influenced by the frame of reference or practice model being used. Each model has its particular philosophy, body of knowledge, and methods of evaluation and treatment, although some overlap exists. Each provides some guidelines for the clinical reasoning process in treatment planning.[19]

The client's motivation and goals must also be considered in planning treatment. For this reason, a frame of reference

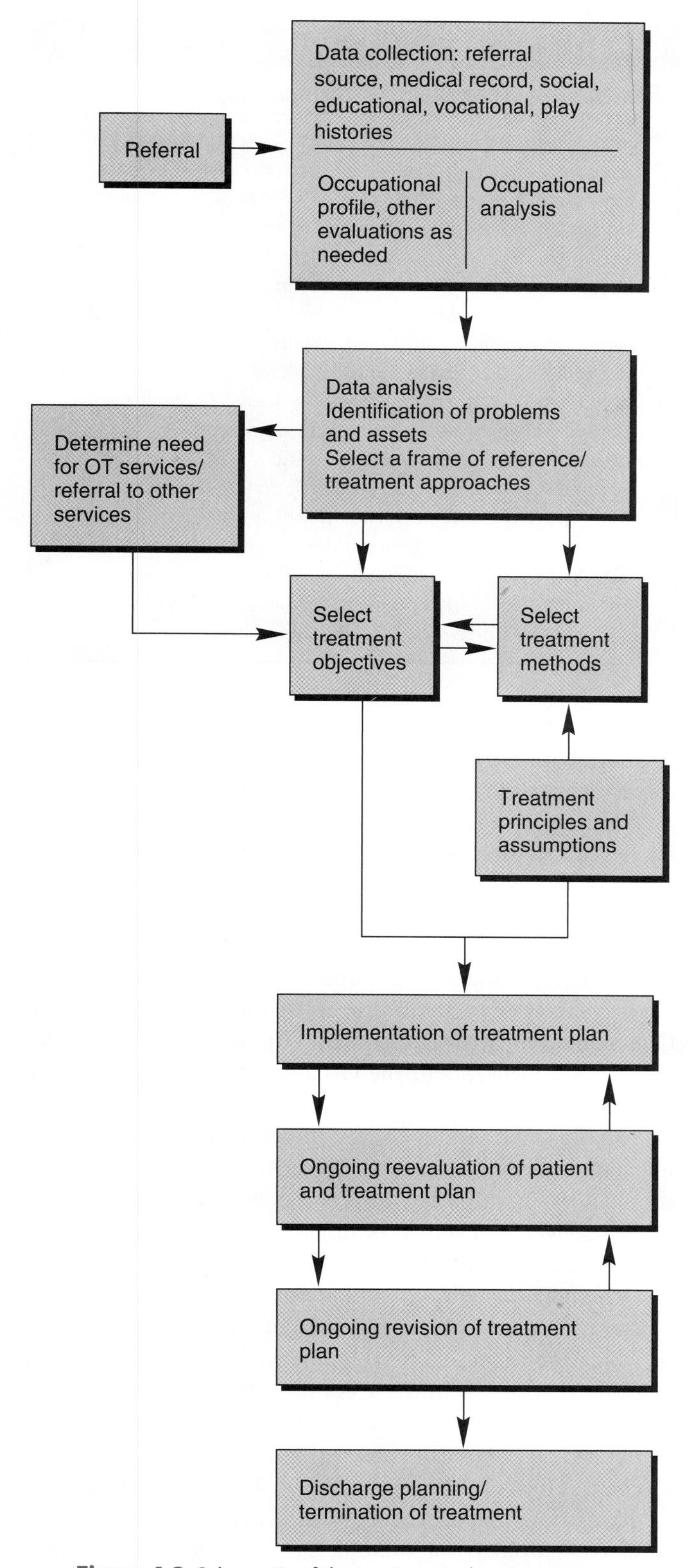

Figure 4-2 Schematic of the treatment planning process.

such as the Model of Human Occupation is helpful. As noted in Chapter 1, some practice models typically used in physical dysfunction practice neglect this important element of the treatment process. (See Chapter 1 for discussions of the Model of Human Occupation and the biomechanical, rehabilitation, sensorimotor, and motor learning practice models.) A current

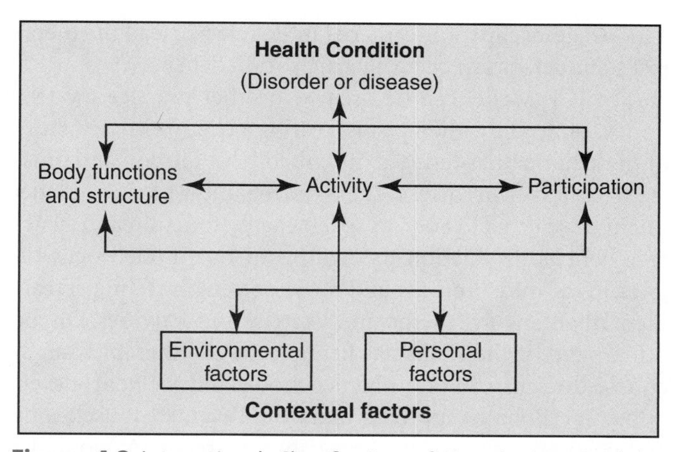

Figure 4-3 International Classification of Functioning, Disability and Health (ICF Model). (From World Health Organization. International Classification of Functioning, Disability and Health (ICF Model). Retrieved on August 20, 2011 at http://www.who.int/classifications/icf/en/.)

model used by therapists to evaluate and treat clients with physical dysfunction that highly values client's interests and overall life goals is the International Classification of Functioning, Disability and Health (ICF Model)[17,25](see Figure 4-3).

The ICF Model emphasizes health and participation in the context of a client's disability. The first version was published by the World Health Organization for trial purposes in 1980, and the ICF has become a multipurpose classification intended for a wide range of uses in client-centered rehabilitation. The ICF is a classification of health and health-related domains—those that provide a guide to help the therapist describe changes in a client's body function and structure, determine what a client with a health condition can do in a standard environment (his or her level of capacity), and what a client can actually do in his or her usual environment (level of performance). These domains are classified from body, individual, and societal perspectives by means of two lists: a list of body functions and structures and a list of domains of activity and participation. In the ICF model, functioning refers to all body functions, activities, and participation, whereas disability is an umbrella term for physical impairments, activity limitations, and participation restrictions. The ICF Model also considers the environmental factors that interact with all of these components. For example, a patient recovering from spinal cord injury may have several body function and structure impairments including motor and sensory impairments below the level of the spinal cord injury. One potential activity limitation could be related to easy use of transportation in the community. This could lead to participation limitations because lack of transportation limits a client's ability to resume normal roles and interests (e.g., going to church, a grocery store, or a job). A therapist using the ICF model would take a top-down approach to treatment planning in order to focus on the client's health and participation in important life activities. This will include treatment of the patient's physical deficits but also problem solving the client's transportation limitations in order to help the client resume normal daily life roles. Again, a thorough occupation-centered interview will lead the therapist to understand a client's participation deficits.

The ICF Model can be used with other practice models. For example, if the therapist is treating a client with a fracture of the arm that has resulted in limited joint motion and muscle weakness from disuse, the biomechanical practice model might be selected to address specific body function and structure deficits. Evaluation procedures in this model focus on joint ROM measurement and muscle strength testing. Treatment might involve therapeutic exercise and activities. On the other hand, if the client has hemiplegia, the therapist might choose the sensorimotor practice model and the neurodevelopmental (Bobath) approach and would evaluate muscle tone and postural mechanisms. Sensorimotor treatment would be directed toward normalizing tone through positioning, handling techniques and special movement patterns, and facilitating a more normal postural mechanism through activities that demand weight shifts and weight bearing. A therapist using an ICF Model would also consider how the body function and structure limitations affect the client's daily tasks and participation in community activities. Is the client able to grasp objects in the kitchen in order to cook meals? Can the client go back to work or resume her role as a mother with the deficits resulting from the arm fracture? A therapist incorporating the ICF Model with other practice models would attach a treatment plan related to body function and structure limitations to important and valued activity and participation goals.

Selecting and Writing Treatment Goals and Objectives

The therapist writes treatment goals and objectives to address the specific client problems identified in the OT evaluation. At the same time, the therapist considers potential treatment interventions that could be used to improve the client's overall function in daily activities. Writing objectives and selecting treatment methods are mutually dependent elements of the treatment planning process.

Novice or entry-level OT practitioners can get confused with the terminology of treatment plan writing. The terms *goal* and *objective* sometimes are used interchangeably; some facilities use one, while some use the other. A treatment objective or goal states what new functional activity a client will be able to perform as a result of OT intervention. A well-written goal or objective will convey clearly the change in function, performance, or behavior that the client will demonstrate when the treatment intervention or program has been completed successfully. The goal or objective will include an occupation-based functional outcome that is clear to the reader. Whenever possible, the therapist (and assistant) should involve the client in selecting objectives and planning. Both therapist and client must consider whether objectives or goals are attainable within the time limits of the treatment program. Objectives or goals should reflect the client's life roles and interests and should be consistent with the general needs of the client as stated on the referral and determined by the occupation-centered interview and evaluation. The OT goals and/or objectives should complement those of other rehabilitation services (i.e., physical therapy, speech language pathology, nursing, and recreational therapy).When clearly defined objectives have not been stated, no sound basis for selecting appropriate treatment methods exists and evaluating the effectiveness of the treatment program is impossible.

Box 4-2

Elements of a Comprehensive Treatment Objective

Occupation-based functional outcome. Describes the "real-life" occupation or occupational task that the client will be able to engage in as a result of achieving the goal. Example: *To participate in religious services.* The statement may include the context if this makes the outcome clearer (e.g., *to cope with cognitive demands of receptionist job in a medical office*).

Statement of terminal behavior. Specifies the physical changes, type of behavior, or performance skill that the patient is expected to display. The terminal behavior consists of an action verb and the object receiving the action. Example: The patient will *don* (action verb) a *shirt* (object).

Conditions. States the circumstances required for the performance of the terminal behavior. Example: *Given verbal prompts* (condition), the patient will don a shirt.

Criterion. States the degree of competence or the performance standard by which the patient's behavior is to be measured. Example: Given verbal prompts, the patient will don a shirt *in 5 minutes with no errors* (criterion).

Writing Treatment Objectives

Writing clear treatment objectives is not difficult. However, it does require time, thoughtfulness, and thoroughness. Having a method or structure to guide the process is helpful. One method for writing treatment objectives, described next, includes the concepts of the Occupational Therapy Practice Framework (OTPF).[5]

The objective should convey the client's future functioning and performance once the objective has been achieved. It should do so in simple language and should be understandable to anyone who reads it. A comprehensive treatment objective has the following four elements (Box 4-2):

1. *Occupation-based functional outcome.* The functional outcome describes the occupation or occupational task in which the client will be able to engage after achieving the goal. Many goals in the areas of occupation already have implied functional outcomes that are occupational in nature (e.g., getting dressed, eating, transferring from bed to chair). However, these goals can be strengthened by adding occupations that the client identifies as being of high importance. Consider, for example, *to dress for work.* Another example is *to participate in religious services.* The statement may include the context if this makes the outcome clearer (e.g., *to dress for work as a high-school teacher*).

Including an occupation-based functional outcome is especially important for goals that focus primarily on body function and structure limitations such as ROM, muscle strength, and coordination. The emphasis should be placed on occupation—the goal within the domain of OT.

A goal that emphasizes shoulder external rotation might have a functional outcome such as *in order to brush and style hair.*

2. *Statement of terminal behavior.* Terminal behavior specifies the observable physical change, the type of behavior, or performance skill that the patient is expected to display following treatment.[6] The terminal behavior comprises an action verb and the object receiving the action. Consider, for example, *to remove the blouse. Remove* is the action verb, and the *blouse* is the object of the action.
3. *Conditions.* Conditions are the circumstances required for the performance of the terminal behavior. The conditions answer questions such as, "Is special equipment needed?"; "Are assistive devices necessary?"; "Is supervision or assistance necessary?"; "Are special cues necessary?"[1,6] An example would be: "When given verbal cues, the patient will remove the blouse." This statement indicates that the client will only be able to remove the blouse when someone is present to provide verbal cues. The phrase *when given verbal cues* represents a special circumstance or condition that enables adequate performance of the terminal behavior. Another example would be: "When using a built-up handle spoon, the patient will feed self. ... " The patient may only be able to feed self if given special equipment. In this case, the adaptive equipment is an important condition needed to meet the client goal.

Clients achieve many treatment objectives without any special devices, equipment, environmental modification, or human assistance. Therefore the statement of conditions is not always necessary. *Conditions should be used only when some special circumstance is required to enable the performance of the terminal behavior.* The treatment methodology and the treatment program's time frame are *not* considered conditions.

4. *Criterion.* The criterion is the performance standard or degree of competence the patient is expected to achieve, stated in measurable or observable terms.[1,6] The criterion answers questions such as, "How much?"; "How often?"; "How well?"; "How accurately?"; "How completely?"; and "How quickly?"[1] It is important to include a criterion or performance standard that estimates the patient's potential level of competence. Only in this way can the therapist determine achievement of the stated terminal behavior with certainty.

Here is an objective that contains a criterion: "If given verbal cues, the patient will don the blouse within 1 minute." The criterion or performance standard indicates that the task will be completed *within 1 minute.* This specification might be a necessary criterion in a long-term care facility in which an aide supervises the patient's dressing; speed of performance is important so that the aide can attend to other tasks and patients.

Stating a performance standard is important to show incremental progress of a functional task over time. For example, a patient may be able to complete a transfer to the toilet with moderate assistance at the initial evaluation. The occupational performance objective may be *the patient will complete the toilet transfer with minimal assistance.* Once this goal has been achieved, each new functional goal would be one step closer to *the patient completing the transfer to the toilet independently.* In fact, the therapist may have set the client's long-term goals for this much desired functional outcome.

Changes in muscle grades, increases in joint ROM, degree of competence in task performance, and speed of performance are possible measures for criteria.

Critiquing Sample Objectives

Studying sample objectives and analyzing their elements can help the beginner refine skills in writing clear objectives. Consider the following examples:

1. *Given assistive devices, the patient will eat independently in 30 minutes.* In this objective the terminal behavior is the statement *the patient will eat,* and *eat* is the action verb. No object needs to be named because the object (food) of the action is implicit. The condition is *given assistive devices.* This statement indicates the special circumstances—in this case devices—that will make eating possible. The performance standards are *independently in 30 minutes.* This statement reflects that the patient will be able to eat without human assistance and will complete eating a meal within 30 minutes, a reasonable amount of time for this activity. The occupation-based functional outcome is not stated separately because eating independently is an occupational task, as well as a statement of behavior.
2. *The joint ROM of the left elbow will increase.* As written, this objective is a good statement of terminal behavior. It indicates the type of change in physical function that is expected as a result of the treatment program. Conditions are not necessary because no special circumstances are required for the patient to demonstrate or perform the increased ROM. However, the objective does need a criterion because the amount of increase in ROM is not indicated, making it difficult to measure progress. The objective can be improved as follows: *The joint ROM of the left elbow will increase from 0-120 to 0-135 degrees.* This adds the criterion of a 15-degree increase in ROM, which is measurable. More critically, the occupation-based functional outcome is missing. The objective could be further improved: *The joint ROM of the left elbow will increase from 0-120 to 0-135 degrees so that the client can prepare for return to work as a licensed practical nurse.*
3. *The patient will operate the control systems of the left above-elbow prosthesis without hesitation so that he can begin practicing skills for job as auto-supply parts clerk.* In this objective, *operate the control systems* is the terminal behavior. *Operate* is the action verb, and *control systems* is the object of the action. This outcome is the skill (behavior) that is expected as a result of the prosthetic training program. Conditions are not necessary because the desired goal is for the patient to perform this skill under any circumstances. *Without hesitation* is the criterion. It is an observable level of skill indicative of automatic performance. The phrase *job as auto-supply parts clerk* conveys the occupational outcome.

4. *Given assistive devices, the patient will dress herself in less than 20 minutes so that she can participate in group outings. Dress* is the action verb that indicates the terminal behavior. The indirect object of the action (herself) is stated; the direct object (in clothes) does not need to be stated because it is implied in the action verb. The availability of assistive devices is a necessary condition for this patient to perform this task; thus the statement of conditions, *given assistive devices,* is necessary. The criterion or performance standard is stated in terms of speed and indicates that dressing within 20 minutes is a reasonable expectation for this patient and for this task. Other standards could be added if formal neatness or appropriateness for a given occasion were important for the patient's life roles. The occupation-based functional outcome is *participating in group outings.*
5. *Given equipment setup and assistive devices, the patient will use mobile arm supports to feed himself independently.* The equipment setup and the availability of assistive devices constitute the conditions for this objective. The criterion for performance under these circumstances is *independently,* which indicates that once the equipment and devices are provided, the task of eating can be performed without further human assistance. Eating is an occupational task.

Many variables and unknowns exist in the performance and functions of persons with physical dysfunction. Therefore the degree to which they can benefit from, participate in, or succeed at rehabilitation programs cannot be predicted with certainty. This fact often makes it difficult for OT practitioners to write comprehensive treatment objectives. However, the therapist and assistant should attempt to write such objectives, using past experience with similar patients and knowledge gained during the evaluation process to describe desired terminal behavior, conditions, and criteria for each treatment objective. If the conditions and criteria cannot be predicted, practitioners should use a specific statement of terminal behavior until applicable conditions and criteria become apparent. The stated terminal behaviors can then be modified, as treatment progresses, to become comprehensive objectives. Unless the behavior itself is an occupational task, an occupation-based functional outcome should always be included in the OT plan of care.

Selecting Treatment Methods or Interventions

Selecting treatment methods or interventions is a challenging aspect of the treatment planning process. Therapists select a treatment method based on a principle or theory related to the problem being treated and its cause. The underlying principle may come from a frame of reference or a practice model.[10] For example, nerves regenerate after peripheral nerve injury and repair. Increasing movement and strength of reinnervated muscles helps to maintain or increase the performance of the muscles in functional tasks. Improvement of function through use is a principle of the biomechanical model. This principle guides the therapist to select graded therapeutic activity or exercise as the method of choice to affect the desired goals.

Box 4-3

Questions to Ask While Selecting a Treatment Method

What is the goal for the client?
What are the precautions or contraindications that affect the OT program?
What is the prognosis for recovery?
What were the results of evaluations in OT and other services?
What other treatment is the client receiving?
What are the goals of other treatment programs, and are the OT goals compatible with these goals?
How much energy does the client expend in other therapies?
What is the state of the client's general health?
What are the client's interests, vocational skills, and psychological needs?
What is the client's physical and sociocultural environment?
What roles will the client assume in the community?
What kinds of activities or exercises will be most useful and meaningful to the client?[5]
How can treatment be graded to meet the client's changing needs as progression or regression occurs?
What special equipment or adaptations of therapeutic equipment are necessary for the client to perform maximally?
What can be provided under the terms of the reimbursement source and the facility policy?
What other means exist for providing needed interventions if the primary sources refuse to reimburse?

Many other factors that influence the selection of treatment methods are listed in Box 4-3.

When treatment methods are selected and written, others reading the treatment plan should understand exactly how the methods will be used to reach specific objectives. Sometimes several methods may be necessary to achieve one objective, or the same methods may be used to reach several objectives.

Another aspect of treatment planning and documentation of treatment intervention concerns the requirements of the different reimbursing companies and agencies. The guidelines for writing treatment goals may need to be adjusted to suit the standards of the reimbursing entity, as illustrated in Box 4-4.

Implementing the Treatment Plan

The treatment plan can be implemented when at least one objective or goal and one or more treatment method have been selected. During implementation, the therapist and assistant guide the client as he or she engages in the procedures that have been designed. The comprehensive treatment plan may evolve over time. For example, over the days in which a lengthy evaluation procedure (e.g., complete evaluation of basic self-care skills) is in progress, the client may begin a program of therapeutic activity to strengthen specific muscle groups. As the evaluation continues, an increasing number of problems may be identified and additional objectives or goals and methods may be added to the treatment plan. Thus the OTA should not be surprised by continual changes in the plan.

Box 4-4

Writing Treatment Goals to Satisfy Reimbursing Agencies

To ensure that OT services are reimbursed, practitioners must suit their documentation to the demands of insurers and Medicare and Medicaid. The following is a treatment plan that would be accepted by Medicare.

Long-Term Goals (LTGs)

1. Client will independently dress self in 3 weeks.
2. Client will demonstrate functional transfers to and from bed and toilet with equipment in 3 weeks.
3. Client will complete simple household mobility tasks with equipment in 3 weeks.

Short-Term Goals (STGs)

1. Client will require only minimal assistance for UE dressing tasks in 1 week.
2. Client will demonstrate bed mobility with minimal assistance in 1 week.
3. Client will demonstrate wheelchair transfer to and from toilet with moderate assistance in 1 week.

Intervention

Client will be seen five times a week for trunk control, postural alignment, sitting balance, transfer, and dressing training.

The long-term goals are written in terms of what the occupational therapist believes the client will be able to perform after 3 weeks of OT intervention. The short-term goals are small components or steps toward meeting the long-term goals. Short-term goals are written as components of the long-term goal to show the client's gains in functional recovery. For example, the long-term goal *client will demonstrate dressing independently in 3 weeks* may be broken down into several steps such as UE dressing with minimal assistance, LE dressing with minimal assistance, and dressing independently. During the first week of treatment the short-term goal identified earlier is *client will require only minimal assistance for UE dressing in 1 week.* If the client can meet this goal within a week, the occupational therapist or OTA revises the plan. The long-term goal stays the same; however, the short-term goal may change to *client will require only minimal assistance for LE dressing in 1 week.* If this goal is met the following week, what might be another short-term goal that continues to lead to the long-term goal?

The next component of the treatment plan is the intervention. The purpose of the intervention is to identify clearly the occupational therapist's professional assessment of how often the client will need treatment and the focus and methods of the proposed treatment. A clear link between the goals and the intervention exists. The services provided should directly reflect what the therapists will do with the client to develop the client's abilities to meet the identified goals.

Beginning therapists frequently get confused as to the difference between an **intervention** and a goal. A **goal** is what the client will be able to do, and an intervention is what the therapist will do with the client to foster functional performance. Discussion or statement of intervention should not be included in a client's goal.

Reevaluating the Client, Revising the Plan

Once the treatment plan is implemented, its effectiveness is evaluated on an ongoing basis through continuous observation and reevaluation. The therapist and assistant must be alert observers and ask the following questions:

- Are the treatment goals and/or objectives suitable to the client's needs and capabilities?
- Are the treatment interventions most appropriate for fulfilling the treatment plan?
- Does the client engage in the treatment interventions and see them as worthwhile and meaningful?
- Are the treatment objectives realistic and are they consistent with the client's personal goals and interests?

The therapist may choose to reevaluate physical functions and performance skills with the same evaluation procedures used in the initial evaluation. Improvements and continued limitations can then be compared with baseline functions recorded at the initial evaluation. Such comparisons validate the treatment plan and provide the objective evidence of change required for reimbursement of OT services. Scrutinizing the treatment plan in this way enables the therapist to modify the plan as the need arises. The client's progress toward the stated objectives is the criterion for determining the treatment plan's effectiveness.

The therapist may recognize a need to revise or modify the initial treatment plan based on information gained from observations and reevaluation of the client, as just outlined. For example, the client's progress may be significant enough that increasing the duration, complexity, or resistance of the activity is beneficial. Conversely, the gradual decline of physical resources may necessitate a decrease in resistance, duration, and complexity of activity. This situation applies in degenerative diseases, in which a primary objective is to maintain optimal function despite declining strength and coordination.

If the client cannot see the therapeutic program as helpful or meaningful, a change in treatment approaches and methods may also be necessary. On the other hand, if the client is highly motivated and progressing well in treatment, the plan can be accelerated. The initial plan is continually revised according to the client's needs and progress. This process of reevaluation, revision, and reimplementation of the treatment plan continues throughout the course of the therapeutic program.[4,9]

Discharge Planning and Discontinuation of Treatment

Ultimately, the OT treatment plan is directed to preparing the client to return to daily life roles and interests, which may include living at home or to another suitable living arrangement. Discharge planning is a continual process that starts at the initial evaluation and continues throughout the treatment program. A therapist will begin to consider possible discharge recommendations during the client's occupation-centered interview. All treatment is directed to preparing the client to return to the community. Therapy often will continue on a less intensive basis at home or in another living environment.

Discharge Planning

Discharge planning should be initiated as the client's treatment program in the primary health care facility is progressing. Discharge planning is a team effort that involves the client, the family, and all the rehabilitation specialists concerned with the client's care. Preparation for discharge includes discussing the client's goals for discharge, medical considerations, needs for assistive devices and mobility equipment, and considering caregiver and community support systems. This information will help the rehabilitation team recommend an appropriate discharge placement and plan a home activity or exercise program. Many times a visit to the client's home will allow a therapist to assess architectural barriers in the environment. Discharge planning should include education and training of the client and caregivers for a smooth transition. Arrangements for homecare referral for continued therapies and appropriate community support agencies are also important.

The client and family must be prepared emotionally and psychologically for discharge. Therapists should not assume that clients are emotionally prepared for (or functionally capable of) managing the transition to the new environment. Generalization (transfer) of learning from a health care facility to the home may be difficult for the client. The family may not know the client's capabilities or how best to give assistance. Emotional support, education, training, counseling, and information about resources are helpful measures in easing the transition. The family needs information about the client's ADL status and performance expectations; solutions to accessibility problems in the home, workplace, and community; information on home modification; how to obtain, use, and care for assistive devices or mobility equipment; and availability of community resources such as emergency care, self-help groups, respite care, and independent living centers.[2] Maintaining contact with the primary care facility as a resource for information or further treatment can be reassuring and helpful.[13]

Termination of Treatment

Termination of treatment requires a final reevaluation of the client. The clinician should clearly indicate objectives achieved, partially achieved, or not achieved in the treatment program. The assistant may be directed to perform parts of this evaluation. The therapist writes a discharge summary based on these data. The summary should indicate expected future performance of the client and potential for further rehabilitation. Termination of OT services can affirm the success of the treatment program. In reality, however, meeting all therapy goals set at the initial evaluation is not always achieved; clients may be discharged before objectives of treatment are met and treatment is concluded.[15] The client may be referred to another facility or to homecare, with another therapist continuing the treatment program. Careful communication between therapists and agencies is necessary to ensure a smooth transition and continuity of care.

Case #
Personal data
- **Name**
- **Age**
- **Diagnosis**
- **Disability**
- **Occupations**
- **Treatment goals stated in referral**

Other services
Frame of reference, practice model
OT Evaluation
- Occupational profile
  - Occupations of concern
  - Occupational tasks of concern to client
  - Performance patterns
  - Contexts

Analysis of occupational performance
- **ADL**
- **IADL**
- **Work**
- **Leisure**
- Education
- Social participation

Performance skill deficit areas
1. Motor
2. Process
3. Communication/interaction

Client factors, body functions and structures
1. Mental
2. Sensory
3. Neuromusculoskeletal and movement-related
4. Cardiovascular, respiratory, immunological
5. Voice and speech
6. Genitourinary
7. Skin

Evaluation summary
Assets
Problem list
Outline treatment plan (OTA focuses on performance of occupational tasks)
1. Problem
2. Occupation-based functional outcome
3. Objective
4. Treatment methods
5. Grading and adaptations

Figure 4-4 Treatment plan model. Sections appropriate for the entry-level occupational therapy assistant are shown in **boldface.**

Treatment Plan Model

The model provided in Figure 4-4 and in a more extended version in Figure 4-5 is useful for learning what goes into treatment planning. Figure 4-4 shows in boldface the areas that the OTA might complete. Both the model and the extended version are limited in their range; actual clinical practice will demand planning that is highly specific to the individual and that is focused on the main areas of need. In other words, in Figure 4-5, every possible area for evaluation is noted; however, with an actual client or patient, only a small portion of

EXTENDED TREATMENT PLAN GUIDE

PERSONAL DATA

Fill in the requested information from the medical record or case study (occupational and medical history, education, occupation, work history, leisure habits, self-care habits, social relationships, cultural background).

- Name
- Age, Gender, Marital Status, Family
- Occupation(s)
- Diagnosis(es)
- Disability(ies)

OTHER SERVICES

List and describe briefly other services the client is using.

- Physician
- Psychology/psychiatry
- Nursing
- Respiratory therapy
- Social service
- Speech pathology
- Community social groups/day care
- Vocational counseling
- Supported employment
- Educational services
- Spiritual counseling
- Physical therapy
- Home health care

FRAME OF REFERENCE/TREATMENT APPROACH

State the frame of reference and treatment approach on which the treatment plan is based. More than one may be necessary.

OT EVALUATION

Occupational profile: State how this is obtained, which interviews or other assessments are or were used.
Analysis of occupational performance: State which occupations, occupational tasks are to be evaluated, including context as relevant.

- Activities of daily living
  - Bathing and showering
  - Bowel and bladder management
  - Dressing
  - Eating
  - Feeding
  - Functional mobility
  - Personal device care
  - Personal hygiene and grooming
  - Sexual activity
  - Sleep/rest
  - Toilet hygiene
- Instrumental activities of daily living
  - Care of others (include supervising caregivers)
  - Care of pets
  - Child rearing
  - Communication device use
  - Community mobility
  - Financial management
  - Health management and maintenance
  - Home establishment and management
  - Meal preparation and cleanup
  - Safety procedures and emergency responses
  - Shopping
- Work
  - Employment interests and pursuits
  - Employment seeking and acquisition
  - Job performance
  - Retirement preparation and adjustment
  - Volunteer exploration
  - Volunteer participation
- Leisure
  - Leisure exploration
  - Leisure participation
- Education
  - Formal educational preparation
  - Exploration of informal personal interests
  - Participation in informal personal education
- Social interaction
  - Community
  - Family
  - Peer/friend

Performance skills: For each category selected, list the specific skills, using the OTPF[4] as a guide

- *Motor skills*
  - Posture
  - Mobility
  - Coordination
  - Strength and effort
  - Energy
- *Process skills*
  - Energy
  - Knowledge
  - Temporal organization
  - Organizing space and objects
  - Adaptation

Figure 4-5 Extended treatment plan guide. (Use of categories from American Occupation Therapy Association: Occupational therapy practice framework: domain and process, *Am J Occup Ther* 56:608-639, 2002.)

EXTENDED TREATMENT PLAN GUIDE

Communication/interaction skills
- Physicality
- Information exchange
- Relations

Performance patterns
- Habits
- Routines
- Roles

Contexts: Discuss relationship of contexts to occupations affected by disability.

Client factors: From the list below, select the areas that are or were evaluated. For each area selected, list the specific factors, using the OTPF[4] as a guide. Indicate whether evaluation was determined by testing or by observation.

BODY FUNCTIONS

Global mental functions
- Level of arousal
- Orientation
- Motivation

Specific mental functions
- Memory
- Attention
- Perception
- Body schema
- Motor planning
- Stereognosis
- Spatial relations
- Position in space
- Figure/background
- Perceptual constancy
- Judgment
- Safety awareness
- Problem-solving ability
- Sequencing
- Abstract thinking
- Functional language skills
- Comprehension of speech/writing
- Ability to express ideas
- Reading
- Writing
- Functional mathematical skills
- Mental calculations
- Written calculations
- Self-esteem
- Self-concept
- Coping skills
- Maturity (developmental level)
- Adjustment to disability
- Reality functioning
- Rigidity
- Self-control
- Emotional expression

Sensory functions and pain
- Seeing and related functions
- Visual perception
- Visual fields
- Visual-motor coordination
- Depth perception

Figure 4-5, cont'd

EXTENDED TREATMENT PLAN GUIDE

- Perception of vertical/horizontal elements
- Eye movements

Hearing and vestibular functions
Sensations of touch, pain, temperature, proprioception, taste, smell
Pain
Neuromusculoskeletal and movement-related functions

- ROM
- Muscle strength
- Physical endurance
- Standing tolerance
- Walking tolerance
- Sitting balance
- Involuntary movement
- Movement speed
- Level of motor development
- Equilibrium/protective responses
- Coordination/muscle control
- Spasms
- Spasticity
- Stage of motor recovery (stroke client only)
- Postural reflex mechanism
- Functional movement patterns
- Hand function
- Swallowing/cranial nerve functions

Cardiovascular functions
Respiratory functions
Voice and speech functions
Skin integrity, wound healing, other skin functions

EVALUATION SUMMARY
Summarize findings from tests and observations.

ASSETS
List the assets of the client and his or her situation that can be used to enhance progress toward maximum independence.

PROBLEM LIST
Identify and list the problems that require occupational therapy intervention.

OBJECTIVES
Write specific treatment objectives in comprehensive form. Each should relate to a specific problem in the problem list and be identified by the corresponding number.

METHODS OF TREATMENT
Describe in detail appropriate treatment methods for the client.

GRADATION OF TREATMENT
Briefly state how treatment methods will be graded to enhance the client's progress.

Figure 4-5, cont'd

this would be relevant based on the client's specific life roles and interests. Today's health care environment demands rapid assessment and treatment, focusing on functional outcomes and improvements made by OT services. The OTA student and new graduate face a great challenge in learning how to apply treatment planning principles with flexibility and focus so that objectives can be met within the time frame allowed by insurance.

A case study with an example of a treatment plan for a hypothetical client follows at the end of the chapter.

Summary

The OT process begins with referral and ends with termination of therapy services. Although the process includes discrete stages that can be named and described, the process is not stepwise but rather fluid, with the stages intermingled at times.

The occupational therapist and OTA have specific responsibilities and areas of emphasis within the OT process. The occupational therapist is the manager and director of the process and delegates specific tasks and steps to the qualified OTA. With time, study, and experience, OTAs can develop sufficient service competency to take on additional responsibilities and specialty roles.

The OT process begins with evaluation, in which information about the patient is gathered and analyzed to identify problems and assets in the patient's life and to plan appropriate treatment strategies. Occupational therapists have developed many informal evaluation procedures that are useful in particular treatment facilities including tests, checklists, and rating scales. Some of these have been developed into standardized tests. The need for reliable standardized tests pertinent to OT continues, however, as occupational therapists have recognized the need to identify and employ discipline-specific evaluation procedures to help establish the scientific basis of the profession.

Treatment planning involves the identification of goals, objectives, and methods directed toward resolving the limitations in areas of occupation noted in the evaluation stage. The occupational therapist is responsible for the treatment plan, to which the OTA can contribute significantly, especially with regard to performance of occupational tasks. Treatment plans should be written so that staff members have a clear procedure to follow and effectiveness can be measured.

The client's motivation cannot be underestimated as a factor in treatment success. Treatment goals should coincide with the client's own goals. Goals are broad descriptive statements of how the client might function at some future time following OT intervention (e.g., "The client will be independent in ADL"). Goals may be broken down into component objectives, each of which is a step toward the ultimate goal (e.g., "The client will transfer from the wheelchair to the toilet without assistance"). A comprehensive treatment goal contains an occupation-based functional outcome, a terminal behavior, a statement of conditions, and a criterion (or set of criteria) for measuring accomplishment. When the terminal behavior describes an occupational task such as dressing or eating, an occupation-based functional outcome need not be stated. Methods are chosen based on the objectives, practice model or frame of reference, client's values and motivations, and performance context.

The OTA is encouraged to study and practice writing clear and comprehensive treatment goals and objectives and to learn as much as possible about different intervention methods. Such study will yield great rewards: clinical clarity, effective communication, and professional self-confidence.

CASE STUDY

Sample Intervention Plan

The following plan presents a sampling of parts of a proposed intervention program; it is not a comprehensive plan. The reader is encouraged to add objectives and methods to address additional problems to make the plan more comprehensive.

Case Study

Mrs. R. is 49 years old. She has been a homemaker and mother to her two sons; one is 26 and married, and the other is 17. Mrs. R. is divorced. Before the onset of her illness, Mrs. R. lived in an apartment with her younger son. At present, she and her younger son live with her married son, his wife, and their 4-year-old boy.

Mrs. R. had Guillain-Barré syndrome. She has been left with residual weakness of all four extremities. Mrs. R. uses a standard wheelchair for mobility.

Mrs. R. appears thin and frail. She speaks in a weak voice and appears to be passive and discouraged. She says she cannot accomplish anything. The home situation is poor. Mrs. R. does not communicate with her daughter-in-law, and the couple and Mrs. R. disagree over management of the teenage son. Mrs. R. feels unable to assert her authority as his mother or to express her needs and feelings. The disability has brought about the loss of her independence and has changed her role in relation to her younger son.

Her daughter-in-law reports that Mrs. R. is dependent for self-care, never attempts to help with homemaking, and isolates herself in her room much of the time. She believes that her mother-in-law is capable of more activity "if only she would try." She says she is willing to allow Mrs. R. to do some of the household work.

Mrs. R. was referred for outpatient OT services for restoration or maintenance of motor functioning and increased independence in ADL.

Personal Data

Name: Mrs. R.
Age: 49
Diagnosis: Guillain-Barré syndrome

Continued

CASE STUDY—cont'd

Disability: Residual weakness, upper and lower extremities
Treatment aims stated in physician referral: restoration or maintenance of motor functioning; increased independence in ADL

Other Services

Physician: prescription of medication, maintenance of general health, supervision of rehabilitation program
Physical therapy: muscle strengthening, ambulation and transfer training
Social service: individual and family counseling
Community social group: socialization

Frame of Reference

Model of Human Occupation

Treatment Approaches

Biomechanical
Rehabilitative
Cognitive-behavioral

OT Evaluation

Occupational profile
Occupational history (short interview)
Canadian Occupational Performance Measure
Occupational performance observation and interview
Self-care
Home management
Performance skills (to be observed in execution of occupational tasks such as dressing or housework)
Motor Skills
Posture
Mobility
Coordination
Strength and effort
Energy (physical)
Process skills
Energy (mental)
Knowledge
Temporal organization
Organization of space and objects
Adaptation, adjustment, accommodation
Communication/interaction skills
Physical communication: observe gestures, eye contact, body language
Exchange of information: observe for assertiveness
Relations: observe naturally occurring interactions with family
Evaluation of client factors
Sensory and movement-related functions
Muscle strength: test
Passive ROM: test
Physical endurance: observe, interview
Walking tolerance: observe, interview
Movement speed: observe
Coordination: test, observe
Functional movement: test, observe
Sensation (touch, pain, thermal, proprioception): test
Mental functions
Energy, drive, motivation: observe, interview
Judgment: observe
Safety awareness: observe
Motor planning, sequencing movement: observe
Regulation of emotions, coping skills: observe
Adjustment to disability: observe, interview

Evaluation Summary

Before onset of illness, Mrs. R. lived independently with her 17-year-old son. Since her illness, she and her son have moved in with her 26-year-old son, his wife, and their 4-year-old son. This arrangement has proved less than ideal. Little communication occurs between Mrs. R. and her daughter-in-law. Conflicts between the couple and Mrs. R. about the management of her teenage son are a problem.

The disability has caused the loss of Mrs. R.'s independence and has changed her roles as homemaker and mother. She says she has no authority as mother of her 17-year-old; she also says she does not know how to express her needs and feelings anymore. On the Canadian Occupational Performance Measure, Mrs. R. identified the following four goals as immediately important to her. She expressed low satisfaction with her ability at present to perform in all of the following four goals:

1. To be able to dress independently
2. To be able to help with housework, laundry, and dishes
3. To talk with and guide her teenage son
4. To get out more to see friends as she did in the past

Mrs. R. was observed while dressing with assistance from her daughter-in-law. She needs some physical help with dressing and has difficulty with buttons and zippers. Mrs. R. reports that she manages some personal care such as washing her face, hair care, and dental care. She requires an adaptive toothbrush and needs assistance in toilet transferring and showering. Mrs. R. does not perform any home management tasks but is potentially capable of light activities such as setting the table, dusting, and folding laundry. Mrs. R.'s daughter-in-law is willing to allow her mother-in-law some household activities if an understanding about their respective roles can be established.

Throughout the interview and observation, Mrs. R. made limited eye contact, sighed deeply, and appeared passive and discouraged about her disability. She said several times that she cannot accomplish anything. She agreed with her daughter-in-law's statement that she tends to stay in her room alone.

Muscle testing revealed that all muscles are the same grades bilaterally: scapula and shoulder muscles are F+ to G (3+ to 4), elbow and forearm muscles are F+ to G (3+ to 4), and wrist and hand musculature is graded F+ (3+). Trunk muscles are G (4);

CASE STUDY—cont'd

all muscles of the hip are G (4) except adductors and external rotators, which are F+ (3+). Knee flexors and extensors are G (4). Ankle plantar flexors and dorsiflexors are F (3), and all foot muscles are F– (3–) to P (2).

All joint motions are within normal to functional range. Physical endurance is limited to 1 hour of light activity of the upper extremities, with some ambulation, before rest. Mrs. R. uses a wheelchair for energy conservation and propels it with both arms and legs. Slight incoordination, evident in fine hand function, is caused by muscle weakness.

Sensory modalities of touch, pain, temperature, and proprioception are intact. No cognitive deficits were observed.

Assets

Can identify own goals
Potential for good living situation
Presence of able-bodied adults who can assist
Potential for some further recovery
Some functional muscle strength
Good joint mobility
Good sensation

Problem List

1. Muscle weakness
2. Low physical endurance
3. Limited walking tolerance
4. Mild incoordination
5. Self-care dependence
6. Homemaking dependence
7. Dependent transferring
8. Isolation, apparent depression
9. Reduced social interaction
10. Lack of assertiveness

Problem 1

Muscle weakness (shoulders)

Objective

Muscle strength of shoulder flexors will increase from F+ (3+) to G (4) to allow patient more independence in self-care and resumption of a portion of homemaking tasks and role.

Method

Light progressive resistive exercise to shoulder flexion: client is seated in a regular chair, wearing a weighted cuff one half the weight of her maximum resistance above each elbow. Lifts arms alternately through 10 repetitions and then rests. The activity is repeated using three-quarters' maximum resistance, then full resistance. Activities: reaching for glasses in overhead cupboard and placing them on the table, replacing glasses in cupboard when dry; rolling out pastry dough on a slightly inclined pastry board; wiping table, counter, and cupboard doors, using a forward push-pull motion; Turkish knotting project with weaving frame set vertically in front of her and tufts of yarn on right and left sides, at hip level.

Gradation

Increase resistance, number of repetitions, and length of time as strength improves.

Problem 1

Muscle weakness (fingers and wrists)

Objective

Strength of wrist flexors and extensors and finger flexors will increase from F+ (3+) to G (4) to allow patient more independence in self-care and resumption of a portion of homemaking tasks and role.

Method

Light progressive resistive exercises for wrist flexors and extensors: client is seated, side to table, with pronated forearm resting on the table and hand extended over edge of table; a hand cuff, with small weights equal to one half of her maximum resistance attached to the palmar surface, is worn on the hand; client extends the wrist through full ROM against gravity for 10 repetitions, then rests. The exercise is repeated with three-quarters' maximum resistance and then full resistance. The same procedure is used to exercise wrist flexors, except that the forearm is supinated on the table, and the weights are suspended from the dorsal side of the hand cuff. Activities to improve finger flexors: tearing lettuce to make a salad; handwashing panties and hosiery. Progress to kneading soft clay or bread dough.

Gradation

Increase resistance, repetitions, and time.

Problem 5

Self-care dependence

Objective

Given assistive devices, Mrs. R. will be able to dress herself independently within 20 minutes.

Method

Putting on bra: Using a back-opening stretch bra, pass bra around waist so that opening is in front and straps are facing up; fasten bra in front at waist level; slide fastened bra around at waist level so that cups are in front; slip arms through straps and work straps up over shoulders; adjust cups and straps. Putting on shirt: Place loose-fitting blouse on lap with back facing up and neck toward knees; place arms under back of blouse and into arm holes; push

Continued

CASE STUDY—cont'd

sleeves up onto arms past elbows; gather back material up from neck to hem with hands and duck head forward and pass garment over head; work blouse down by shrugging shoulders and pulling into place with hands; use button hook to fasten front opening. Putting on underpants and slacks: Sitting on bed or in wheelchair, cross legs, reach down, and place one opening over foot; cross opposite leg, place other opening over foot; uncross legs, work pants up over feet and up under thighs (a dressing stick may be used to pull pants up if leaning forward is difficult); shift hips from side to side and work pants up as far as possible over buttocks; stand, if possible, and pull pants to waist level; then sit and pull zipper up with prefastened zipper pull; use Velcro at waist closure on slacks. Putting on socks: Using stretch socks and seated, cross one leg, place sock over toes and work sock up onto foot and over heel; cross other leg and repeat. Putting on shoes: With slip-on shoe with Velcro fasteners, use procedure for socks.

Gradation

Progress to more difficult tasks such as pantyhose, tie shoes, dresses, pullover garments.

Problem 6

Homemaking dependence

Objective

Given assistive devices, Mrs. R. will perform homemaking activities.

Method

Using a dust mitt, client dusts furniture surfaces easily reached from wheelchair such as lamp tables and coffee table; sits at sink to wash dishes; practices folding small items of clothing such as panties, nylons, and children's underwear while sitting at kitchen table; have Mrs. R.'s daughter-in-law observe activities at treatment facility; work out an acceptable list of activities and a schedule with both women. Discuss how Mrs. R. could make some contributions to home management routines; ask Mrs. R. to keep activity diary, noting any performance difficulties and successes for review at next visit.

Gradation

Increase number of household responsibilities. Increase time spent on household activities.

Problem 8

Isolation, depression

Objective

Mrs. R. will reduce time spent alone from 6 waking hours to 3 waking hours.

Method

Engage Mrs. R. in self-reflection about precursor events that discourage participation. Help Mrs. R. to restructure thinking about her own ability to participate. Establish acceptable graded activity schedule between Mrs. R. and son and daughter-in-law; include homemaking tasks and socialization with family through playing games, watching TV, preparing and eating meals, and conversing; family members encourage Mrs. R. to be with them but will be accepting if she refuses; have Mrs. R. keep activity diary for self-reflection and review; determine how time is spent and discuss how it could be more productive and enjoyable. Initiate a vocational activity such as needlework or tile mosaics to complete at home; set goals for where and how much activity will be performed.

Gradation

Increase time spent out of own room; include friends, neighbors, and family in household social activities; plan a community outing for shopping or lunch.

Selected Reading Guide Questions

1. List and describe the stages or steps in the OT process.
2. Describe and contrast the roles of the occupational therapist and the OTA with regard to each stage of the OT process.
3. Give at least one example that shows the "flow" of the OT process.
4. Summarize what the OTA must do to achieve greater responsibility for the OT process.
5. Define *evaluation.*
6. Discuss the purposes of *OT evaluation.*
7. Describe the role of the occupational therapist and the OTA in evaluation.
8. What skills must the OT practitioner possess to be an effective evaluator?
9. Define and discuss *clinical reasoning.*
10. List and differentiate three types of clinical reasoning.
11. Which specific areas of occupation and performance skills does the occupational therapist generally evaluate while setting up a treatment plan for patients with physical dysfunction?
12. Describe four methods of evaluation that the occupational therapist may use in the evaluation process.
13. Describe the daily schedule interview including the information to be covered and the recommended ways of obtaining this information.
14. Discuss how the International Classification of Functioning, Disability and Health (ICF Model) is used to develop client-centered OT treatment.
15. Define *treatment plan.*

16. Describe the roles of the occupational therapist and the OTA in treatment planning.
17. Why should a treatment plan be written down?
18. Why should a treatment plan be based on a specific frame of reference or treatment approach?
19. List the steps in developing a treatment plan.
20. List, define, and give examples of the three elements of a comprehensive treatment objective or goal.
21. List six factors to consider while selecting treatment methods.
22. Is it necessary to develop a comprehensive treatment plan before treatment can begin? Explain.
23. Is it ever necessary to change the initial treatment plan? Why?
24. What criterion is used to evaluate the effectiveness of a treatment plan?
25. How does the therapist know when to modify or change the plan?
26. What are some of the concerns and preparations involved in termination of treatment?

References

1. AJOT: Special issue on clinical reasoning, *Am J Occup Ther* 45(11), 1991.
2. American Occupational Therapy Association: Commission on Practice: Guidelines for supervision, roles, and responsibilities during the delivery of occupational therapy services, *Am J Occup Ther* 63(6):797–803, 2004.
3. American Occupational Therapy Association: Commission on Practice: Standards of practice for occupational therapy, *Am J Occup Ther* 64(6):415–420, 2010.
4. American Occupational Therapy Association: Commission on Practice: The guide to occupational therapy practice, *Am J Occup Ther* 53(3), 1999.
5. American Occupation Therapy Association: Occupational therapy practice framework: domain and process, ed 2, *Am J Occup Ther* 62(6):6625–6637, 2008.
6. Asher IE: *An annotated index of occupational therapy evaluation tools*, ed 2, Rockville, Md, 1998, American Occupational Therapy Association.
7. Atchison B: Selecting appropriate assessments, *Phys Disabil Special Interest Section Newsl* 10:2, 1987.
8. Coker P: The effects of an experiential learning program on the clinical reasoning and critical thinking skills of occupational therapy students, *J Allied Health* 39(4):280–286, 2010.
9. Cohn ES, Schell BA, Neistadt ME: Overview of evaluation. In Crepeau EB, Cohn ES, Schell BAB, editors: *Willard and Spackman's occupational therapy*, ed 10, Philadelphia, 2003, Lippincott.
10. Day D: A systems diagram for teaching treatment planning, *Am J Occup Ther* 27:239, 1973.
11. Fleming MH: Clinical reasoning in medicine compared with clinical reasoning in occupational therapy, *Am J Occup Ther* 45(11):988, 1991.
12. Fleming MH: The therapist with the three-track mind, *Am J Occup Ther* 45(11):1007, 1991.
13. Hamilton BL, Laughlin JA, Fiedler RC, et al: Interrater reliability of the 7-level functional independence measure (FIM), *Scand J Rehabil Med* 26:115–116, 1994.
14. Henry AD: The interview process in occupational therapy. In Crepeau EB, Cohn ES, Schell BAB, editors: *Willard and Spackman's occupational therapy*, ed 10, Philadelphia, 2003, Lippincott.
15. Lederer J: Disposition toward critical thinking among occupational therapy students, *Am J Occup Ther* 61(5):519–526, 2007.
16. Mattingly C: What is clinical reasoning? *Am J Occup Ther* 45(11):979, 1991.
17. Noonan V, Kopec J, Noreau L, et al: Comparing the content of participation instruments using the International Classification of Function, Disability and Health, *Health Qual Life Outcomes* 7(93), 2009. doi:10.1186/1477-7525-7-93.
18. Rogers JC, Masagatani G: Clinical reasoning of occupational therapists during the initial assessment of physically disabled clients, *Occup Ther J Res* 4:195, 1982.
19. Schell BAB: Clinical reasoning: the basis of practice. In Crepeau EB, Cohn ES, Schell BAB, editors: *Willard and Spackman's occupational therapy*, ed 10, Philadelphia, 1993, Lippincott.
20. Unsworth C: Using a head-mounted video camera to explore current conceptualizations of clinical reasoning in occupational therapy, *Am J Occup Ther* 59(1):31–40, 2005.
21. Watanabe S: *Activities configuration*, 1968 Regional Institute on the Evaluation Process, Final report RSA-123-T-68, New York, 1968, American Occupational Therapy Association.
22. Watson M: Analysis: standardized testing objective, *Phys Disabil Special Interest Sect Newsl* 6:4, 1983.
23. Watts JH, Kielhofner G, Bauer DF, et al: The assessment of occupational functioning: a screening tool for use in long-term care, *Am J Occup Ther* 40:231, 1986.
24. Weinstock-Zlotnick G, Hinojosa J: The issue is: bottom-up or top-down evaluation: is one better than the other? *Am J Occup Ther* 58(5):594–599, 2004.
25. World Health Organization: International Classification of Functioning, Disability and Health (ICF Model) http://www.who.int/classifications/icf/en/ Retrieved on August 20, 2011.

CHAPTER 5

Documentation of Occupational Therapy Services*

MICHELLE MAHONE

Key Terms

HIPAA
SOAP notes
Narrative notes
Flow sheets
Functional outcomes
EHR/EMR
Classification codes
Occupational Therapy Practice Framework 2E
Clinical reasoning
Referral
Initial evaluation report
Intervention plan/treatment plan
Daily notes
Progress notes
Discharge summary

Chapter Objectives

After studying this chapter, the student or practitioner will be able to do the following:

1. Describe the purposes of documentation for occupational therapy services.
2. Describe the legal implications for complete and accurate documentation.
3. List fundamental elements of documentation.
4. Differentiate occupational therapy assistant and occupational therapist documentation responsibilities.
5. List the sequential steps in the clinical reasoning process for documentation.
6. Describe the reporting process including initial evaluation reports, intervention plans, progress reports, and discharge summaries.
7. Discuss the value of the *Occupational Therapy Practice Framework, 2nd Edition* to the documentation process.
8. Describe the opportunities and challenges of using an electronic health record.

Documentation is an essential element in the day-to-day practice of occupational therapy (OT). Although most practitioners choose this profession because they want to work with people and assist in improving their quality of life, the documentation of treatment is necessary to provide a record and to justify the therapy. As an OT practitioner, one can provide the highest quality of care, but if it is undocumented, there is nothing to reflect the progress and efforts made by both the client and the practitioner. The occupational therapy assistant (OTA) plays a valuable role in the documentation of the ongoing treatment of the client.

Documentation is a continuous process that begins immediately on receipt of the initial referral. The written record should include clarification of the referral, initial evaluation results, and ongoing daily and/or weekly progress notes. These notes should document the interactions between the client and the OT practitioner including the type of intervention and the client's response.[2] Any periodic reevaluation reports and discharge summary are also included. The complete medical record contains pertinent information about the client's history, status, progress, and performance as described by all health care practitioners involved in the client's care.

No standard or single method for documenting OT intervention exists within the profession. The types of records and reports to be written are determined by the treatment facilities and the funding agencies. Regardless of the method used, all documentation should be clear, concise, objective, accurate, complete, timely, and legible.

Purposes of Documentation

According to the Guidelines for Documentation of Occupational Therapy, the purposes of documentation are to[2]:

1. Articulate the rationale for provision of OT services
2. Reflect the OT practitioners' clinical reasoning
3. Communicate information about the client from the OT perspective
4. Create a chronologic record of client status, OT services provided to the client, and client outcomes

*Janet Jabri and Janna M. Dreher contributed large portions of this chapter to the first edition of this book.

Occupational Therapist Practitioner Roles in Documentation

According to the *Standards of Practice for Occupational Therapy,* the occupational therapist and the OTA each have their own roles and responsibilities with regard to documentation.[5] The occupational therapist has overall responsibility for all documentation including the evaluation results, the intervention plan, modifications to the intervention plan, outcomes, transitions, and discontinuations.[5] The OTA has complete responsibility for preparing certain reports as delegated by the occupational therapist.[2] Documentation of the client's response to intervention, as well as of communications between the OTA and the client during intervention, is important and can contribute to the decision-making process of the occupational therapist as updates are made to the client's outcomes, transitions, and discharge plans. The OTA may also assist in the preparation of the intervention plan, document progress, report any necessary revisions in the intervention plan based on reevaluation, and complete the discharge summary in collaboration with the occupational therapist.[4]

No matter the type of documentation, all OT practitioners are responsible for documenting within the time frames, formats, and standards established by their practice facility, federal and state laws, payer sources, and various other regulatory programs.

Documentation and Ethics

The *Occupational Therapy Code of Ethics and Ethics Standards* discusses the idea of truth, which is one of the seven core concepts of OT.[6] Truth means that the information OT practitioners provide both verbally and in writing is accurate. The *Code of Ethics* also discusses the concept of veracity, which is based on the virtues of truthfulness, candor, and honesty.[6] According to the concept of veracity, an OT practitioner should record and report in an accurate and timely manner and ensure that documentation for reimbursement purposes is completed in accordance with applicable laws, guidelines, and regulations.

Competent documentation effectively communicates a client's response to therapy and also educates other health care providers and fiscal intermediaries about the value of OT. Ongoing financial constraints have motivated reimbursement intermediaries to scrutinize the need for OT services. To pass scrutiny, OT practitioners must provide a clear rationale for service through competent, ethical, and truthful documentation.

Legal Aspects of Documentation

OT practitioners must know the laws that affect their practice and must meet the requirements of these laws in their documentation. They must also be familiar with the laws on protecting the private identifying information of their clients. The Health Insurance Portability and Accountability Act of 1996 (HIPAA) includes the Privacy Rule, which became effective in 2003.[13] The Privacy Rule is designed to allow health care providers to share information regarding their clients yet still protect this sensitive information from the general public.

Facilities must provide clients a Notice of Privacy Practices and must gain written authorization from the client before giving out health information not related to treatment or payment. Although the practice is optional under the Privacy Rule, most facilities have clients sign a consent form that allows for the release of relevant medical information related to their treatment. In addition, the client has the right to know what is in his or her medical record and can ask for this information. Thus the OTA must know the practices of the facility so that documentation can be disseminated in ways that protect the client's right to privacy.

Because documentation is part of the legal record and may be used in court, the services that the OT practitioner documents must accurately reflect the treatment given. The legal written record is the only acceptable proof of the treatment intervention. In court, the content of the documentation within the chart will be deemed far more reliable than the memory of the OT practitioner. The standard phrase of "If it was not written, it did not happen" holds true, especially with outside reviewers looking at the documentation. The OT practitioner has to rely on what is actually documented. Therefore completeness and accuracy of the record are essential.

Some documentation guidelines that may be used to ensure meeting the therapist's legal and ethical obligations include the following[12]:

- Date all entries for accurate sequencing of the treatment
- Document length of treatment with times and treatment codes/descriptions
- Document missed treatments including a reason why missed
- Document at the time of treatment so that the entry will completely and accurately reflect the treatment session
- Document using specific facts rather than general terms
- Include all supportive documentation such as physicians' treatment orders or consents for release of information
- Do not criticize another health care provider in the written record
- Do not change a legal record after the fact without clarifying the time and nature of the change

To promote uniformity in OT documentation and to improve continuity of legal records, the American Occupational Therapy Association (AOTA) has provided guidelines that include the fundamental elements of documentation.[2] These are helpful regardless of the method used to document the OT intervention. Box 5-1 lists 13 elements of the documented record.

Accrediting bodies include the Joint Commission, the Commission on the Accreditation of Rehabilitation Facilities (CARF), and the Comprehensive Outpatient Rehabilitation Facilities (CORF). Medicare, Medicaid, and other third-party payers also have documentation requirements. In addition, state laws related to licensure, registration, and certification

Box 5-1

Fundamental Elements of Documentation

1. Client's full name and case number on each page of documentation
2. Date and type of OT contact
3. Identification of type of documentation and department name
4. OT practitioner's signature, with a minimum of first name or initial, last name, and professional designation
5. Signature of the recorder directly at the end of the note, without space left between the body of the note and the signature
6. Cosignature by an occupational therapist on documentation written by students and OTAs when required by law or the facility
7. Compliance with confidentiality standards
8. Facility-approved terminology
9. Facility-approved abbreviations
10. Errors corrected by drawing a single line through the mistake and the correction initialed or facility requirements followed; liquid correction fluid and erasures are not acceptable
11. Adherence to professional standards of technology when documenting
12. Disposal of records within law or agency requirements
13. Compliance with agency or legal requirements for storage of records

Modified from American Occupational Therapy Association: Guidelines for documentation of occupational therapy, *Am J Occup Ther* 62:199-204, 2008.

may also have specific requirements for documentation such as cosignature of the OTA's documentation by the occupational therapist. OTAs must be familiar with the documentation requirements of the facility, third-party payers, and the state within which they practice.

Quality of Documentation Content

The quality of the documentation content is significant. Documentation must be well organized, contain only pertinent information, and be objective and accurate. Conciseness and brevity are critical because both the OTA and the reader have other demands on their time. Consideration must be made to who will read the OT documentation. This will have a direct influence on what needs to be reported and how the report will be written. An audience of clinicians, insurance payers, or laypersons may determine the type of medical terminology or accepted medical abbreviations used and the amount of detail needed for accurate understanding of the report.

Many facilities will undergo a quality management process for documentation. In this process, charts are audited by internal staff. The audit team will typically pull a random number of charts from each team member and will check for standard elements to make sure these items are included in the documentation. For the OT practitioner, these chart audits can be a learning opportunity regarding one's own documentation strengths and weaknesses.

Permanent Legal Record

The documents contained in the permanent record are considered the only official records related to that client. Each facility determines the official contents of this record. This may be based on requirements set by internal systems, licensing agencies, accrediting bodies, and third-party payers. The treatment team uses the record internally to understand the total client treatment plan, and reviewers use it to determine justification for continued treatment. Moreover, quality assurance teams use the record to assess overall client outcomes and services. Externally, third-party payers may use records to determine payment for services, the court system uses them for hearings and litigation, and outside agencies use the documents for continued treatment or services after discharge from the facility.

Occupational Therapy Record

The OT documents contained in the permanent legal record comprise the physician's referral, initial evaluations and assessments, daily notes, ongoing weekly and monthly progress notes, reevaluation reports, and discharge summary. These records identify all tests and observations, intervention outcomes, intervention plans, and progress toward the established outcomes. The OT practitioner may also be required to provide entries in other sections of the permanent record such as the interdisciplinary care plan or the client care conference note.

In some facilities OT will maintain separate departmental files or soft charts. These files include supporting records, communication logs, notes, and worksheets, as well as copies of the reports prepared for the permanent legal record. The supporting data may include assessment results (e.g., muscle test form), treatment observations (e.g., activities of daily living checklist), informal therapy team conference notes, or intervention plan approaches. The supporting data form the basis for the reports that become part of the permanent legal record.

Methods of Documentation

SOAP notes are often used for communicating daily or weekly information within facilities. The value of SOAP note charting is that it gives the writer a logical way to organize thoughts and the reader an easy way to review the information. The original SOAP format has been adapted by many professionals in medical and allied health fields.[9] Each section of the SOAP note includes specific information, as described in the following[9]:

Subjective: what has been said subjectively by the client or what has been reported by significant others

Objective: observable and measurable data derived from evaluation and treatment results

Assessment: the opinion, interpretation, or assessment of the results of the client's functional performance and anticipated outcomes including a problem list and long- and short-term goals

Plan: the treatment plan including the frequency and duration of treatment

Narrative notes are less structured than the SOAP format. Narrative notes can be used to document client contact that

Table 5-1 Definitions of Levels of Assistance (Figure 5-5)

Level of Assistance	Abbreviation	Definition
Independent	Ind.	Client requires no assistance or cueing in any situation and is trusted in all situations 100% of the time to do the task safely.
Supervision	Sup.	Caregiver is not required to provide any hands-on guarding but may need to give verbal cues for safety.
Contact guard/standby	Con. Gd./Stby	Caregiver must provide hands-on contact guard to be within arm's length for client's safety.
Minimum assistance	Min.	Caregiver provides 25% physical and/or cueing assistance.
Moderate assistance	Mod.	Caregiver assists client with 50% of the task. Assistance can be physical and/or cueing.
Maximum assistance	Max.	Caregiver assists client with 75% of the task. Assistance can be physical and/or cueing.
Dependent	Dep.	Client is unable to assist in any part of the task. Caregiver performs 100% of the task for client physically and/or cognitively.

is not necessarily during treatment.[13] Narrative notes can be used to document conversations with a client when the client cancels an OT treatment session. They can also be used to document training with caregivers or when instructions specific to an activity or task are given outside of the treatment session.

Flow sheets are another form of documentation that can be used. Progress flow sheets are typically in the form of a grid. They will have a slot for the dates of OT intervention and a slot for specific activities performed. Flow sheets are an efficient way to quickly document numbers of reps of an exercise or level of independence for a functional activity but have only room for objective data to be recorded and leave little room for descriptive phrases of how the client performed.[13]

Functional Outcomes

Current trends, as dictated by payer sources such as Medicare, require that goals or outcomes be functional.[8] Functional outcomes have four main components. First, the outcome must address performance. What is it that the client must perform? This part of the outcome should be written using positive language. It should also be objective and observable.[8] Second, the outcome must have measurable criteria to indicate when the outcome has been met. Third, the outcome will need to specify specific conditions under which the performance should be completed. See Table 5-1 for a list of levels of assistance that can be used to define conditions.

Finally, the outcome will need to give a time frame for completion.

Consider the following outcome: "The client will be able to independently climb three flights of stairs within 90 seconds for 4 of 5 treatment sessions while maintaining a heart rate less than 80% of max while wearing 50 pounds of protective gear so that he can return to work by 1/31/2011." This functional outcome can be broken down as follows:

- Performance—"climb three flights of stairs while wearing 50 pounds of protective gear"
- Criteria—"within 90 seconds for 4 of 5 treatment sessions while maintaining a heart rate less than 80% of max"
- Condition—"independently"
- Time frame—"by 1/31/2011"

Functional outcomes can be achieved through a series of short-term intervention goals or objectives that are designed to move the client through the intervention process, week by week. The OT evaluation will determine baseline for the client and functional outcomes will be developed to identify the end process. The short-term objectives will then identify step-by-step progression from baseline to discharge. For example, in the previously stated functional outcome, a short-term objective may be that "While carrying 25 pounds, the client will be able to climb one flight of stairs within 30 seconds with a heart rate less than 80% of max within 1 week." It is important to remember that even short-term objectives must still be measurable and must continue to describe expected performance as a result of OT treatment.[12]

Electronic Health Record

As part of the American Recovery and Reinvestment Act of 2009, Congress passed the Health Information Technology for Economic and Clinical Health (HITECH) Act of 2009.[10] One of the provisions of this act is to provide incentive payments to eligible health care professionals and hospitals who adopt electronic health record (EHR) technology. There are many obstacles along the path to fully implementing the EHR. However, there are also many opportunities for both the client and the OT practitioner with the use of the EHR or the electronic medical record (EMR). Box 5-2 outlines both the advantages and disadvantages to using the EHR.[7]

Digital documentation can take many forms, from the simple to the complex. Using a word processing program to type notes is the simplest form. Templates that form the basic structure of the documentation can be built; the OTA then types the required data in the appropriate section. More advanced programs will allow the OT practitioner to enter the information into a database and then merge the data into a report form. Software developed for personal data assistants and tablet-sized personal computers make the documentation process more mobile, thus allowing for documentation wherever the client may be.

With the release of the iPad by Apple and the numerous medical applications and interfaces that go along with it, the idea of the EHR is more a reality than ever before.[11] Health care workers can have instant access to client history including medications, xrays, etc. Client information can be carried by

Box 5-2

Electronic Health Record

Advantages

- Improved access to medical records
- Easier to read
- Take less time to locate
- Decrease the duplication of information
- Streamline the billing process
- Reduce the amount of paper used
- Decrease storage space needed
- Track staff productivity
- Identify referral patterns
- Alert to duplicate physician orders
- Identify potential adverse drug reactions and conflicting medications

Disadvantages

- High cost in time and money for hardware and software
- The need to back up the systems in case of power outages and system crashes
- The use of templates that can limit information entered
- Resistance and anxiety of the staff
- Training staff with varying degree of computer skill
- Extensive time needed for design of system and implementation
- The potential for privacy breaches

Modified from Arabit L: Preparing for electronic documentation, *OT Practice* 12:13-15, 2010.

the health care provider from room to room, and information can be updated via touch screen using a writing stylus or by using a keyboard. However, this approach can distract from the human touch if practitioners become more involved in interacting with technology and spend less time focused on their clients. Regardless of the type of digital documentation used, the OT practitioner who possesses basic keyboarding and word-processing skills is well prepared for the increasing use of digital documentation systems.

Classification Codes for Billing of Services

OT practitioners who work in facilities where Medicare, Medicaid, other major insurance plans such as Blue Cross/Blue Shield, and managed care organizations are billed for services must be familiar with classification codes known as the *Health Care Financing Administration* (HCFA) *Common Procedure Coding System* (HCPCS).[14] These codes are used in reimbursement programs to classify the various types of services rendered. As part of this coding system, the Physician's Current Procedural Terminology (CPT) lists descriptive terms and identifying codes for reporting medical services and procedures performed by physicians and nonphysician practitioners. The terminology provides a uniform language that designates medical, surgical, and diagnostic services and accurately and effectively provides a means of reliable, nationwide communication among health care practitioners, clients, and third parties.

Services rendered by OT practitioners must be classified according to the terminology used in the coding systems. These codes provide uniform language related to OT and aid in the reimbursement process. OT practitioners have been instrumental in collaboratively revising the physical medicine section of the CPT to better reflect the procedures performed in practice.

Box 5-3

Eight-Step Process of Clinical Reasoning for Documentation

1. After referral to OT and evaluation, predict functional outcomes on the basis of groups of people with similar problems.
2. Consider the client, present and past functional abilities, and occupational history.
   a. Collaborate with the client on activities that are meaningful and achievable.
   b. Set client outcomes.
3. Observe performance.
4. Establish a sequence for short-term objectives.
5. Consider the timing of outcomes and short-term objectives, and prioritize and sequence treatment methods.
6. Reassess performance and complete daily and/or weekly notes.
7. Reexamine outcomes and short-term objectives, and complete the monthly summary.
8. Complete the discharge summary.

Modified from Allen C: Clinical reasoning for documentation. In Acquaviva JD, editor: *Effective documentation for occupational therapy*, ed 2, Rockville, MD, 1998, American Occupational Therapy Association.

Occupational Therapy Practice Framework

OT practitioners should become familiar with the document *Occupational Therapy Practice Framework: Domain and Process (OTPF) 2nd Edition.*[3] An official document of the AOTA, the *OTPF, 2nd Edition* provides an outline of the domain of OT and describes evaluation and intervention processes involving the use of occupation. The author recommends that the OT practitioner refer to the *OTPF, 2nd Edition*, available from the AOTA, for further understanding.

Overview of the Reporting Process

Documentation and Clinical Reasoning

Creating accurate documentation that reflects effective OT intervention requires a step-by-step process of clinical reasoning.[1] The process provides useful information for treatment planning and note writing. The OTA completes an eight-step process collaboratively with the occupational therapist (Box 5-3).

Referral

OT evaluation and treatment is usually initiated by receipt of a client referral. This referral is generally (but not always) received from the physician and may specify the reason for requesting OT services. It is sometimes called a *prescription* or *physician's orders.* When a physician's referral is required, it should include the OT treatment diagnosis, the onset date of the treatment diagnosis, a request for evaluation and other specific treatment orders, the date, the physician's signature, and frequency and duration of OT services.[13] Figure 5-1 provides an example of a physician's orders form that includes the entire treatment team.

When one or more of the required items for a physician's order is missing from the referral, it is important to clarify the order. Figure 5-2 shows one type of form that can be used to clarify a physician's therapy order. The occupational therapist fills out this form after the initial evaluation is complete. The clarification order has all the required components. This order is sent to the physician along with the initial evaluation for the physician's signature.

The first entry into the client's permanent record may be to document receipt of the referral and the initial plan of action, for example, "10/1/2011 OT referral received and client contacted by phone. OT evaluation scheduled for 10/4/2011 at 1:00 pm" or "10/1/2011 OT initial evaluation completed today with instruction in activity pacing techniques. Refer to evaluation for intervention plan." The response time is established by each facility but is usually within 24 to 48 hours after the referral is received.

Evaluation Process

The evaluation process should be client centered in that it focuses on the needs and wants of the client. The initial evaluation process comprises two basic steps. The first step is to identify the client's occupational profile. This is where the client's needs, problems, and concerns are identified with priorities set.[3] The second step is analysis of the client's occupational performance. In this step, factors that interfere with performance of functional activity are identified, and treatment goals are established.[3]

Occupational Profile

The occupational profile addresses the client's interests, values, and needs. The occupational therapist focuses on gaining an understanding of the client to identify strengths and limitations. This information is collected not only during the initial evaluation but also during subsequent therapy visits. Outcomes are continuously modified based on information learned about the client's occupational profile. Box 5-4 outlines a list of questions that will assist in gathering data related to the occupational profile.

Specific information that may be collected includes the client's name and address; important phone numbers; family members; third-party payers; family history; educational and work history; learning style and preferences; pertinent medical, physical, and mental status information related to specific primary and secondary diagnoses; and other information related to the client's prior level of functioning. Information regarding expected treatment outcomes and discharge plans is also pertinent. The initial evaluation process begins with the occupational therapist reviewing available data obtained from the existing permanent record and interviewing referral sources, the client, and family members.

Occupational Performance

The occupational therapist will take the information gathered during the occupational profile and analyze it for specific performance areas and/or components that will need to be evaluated. Then, using specific assessments, the occupational therapist identifies facilitators and barriers to performance. These assessments can address specific performance skills or client factors such as range of motion (ROM) measurements; manual muscle testing; sensory testing; perceptual/cognitive assessment results; and activities of daily living (ADLs), functional mobility, home management, vocational, and leisure assessment findings.

Many facilities and third-party payers require the occupational therapist to perform the initial evaluation. However, after demonstrating service competency, the OTA, working under the supervision of an occupational therapist, may contribute to the initial evaluation by administering certain structured or standardized tests.[4] The OTA may also complete interviews, general observations, and behavioral checklists; score test protocols; and report these findings orally and in writing.

The occupational performance analysis is a process for establishing the client's baseline status. Accuracy in administering and recording evaluation results is critical. All future evaluation reports will compare progress to this initial baseline status, and the degree of improvement may determine the course and amount of treatment that physicians and third-party payers approve.

Outcomes are created based on the evaluative data gathered. These outcomes are developed in conjunction with the client and should address the client's areas of weakness, as well as his or her identified priorities. While outcomes are client centered, it is also important to be aware of payer sources when establishing outcomes. For example, a client injured on the job may want to be able to play ball with his child. However, because workman's compensation is the payer source for this particular client, outcomes will need to be worded and focused on return to work. After outcomes are established, the treatment plan or intervention process is identified.

Initial Evaluation Report

The occupational therapist has primary responsibility to complete the initial evaluation. The **initial evaluation report**, whether it is a form (Figure 5-3) or a narrative, can be divided into four sections as follows[2]:

1. Description of the client's occupational profile
2. Analysis of the client's occupational performance
3. Prioritizing areas of occupation and occupational performance
4. Intervention plan

Description of the Client's Occupational Profile

Basic client identifying information includes the client's name, medical record or account number, the referring physician's name, the referral, and evaluation dates. This first section details pertinent medical history including the primary treatment diagnosis and any related secondary diagnoses and their onset dates. This section should list any precautions or contraindications that need to be observed during treatment. The client's prior level of functioning, previous living situation, and prior vocational and leisure status are also noted. The client's priorities and desired outcomes are also identified in the section.

Patient Information

Name ______________________ ***Goals (functional expectations)*** ______________________

Phone: H __________ ***W*** __________ ______________________

Date of Onset/Exacerbation ______________________ ***Previous Therapy Results*** ______________________

Diagnosis ______________________ ______________________

______________________ ***Post Op:*** ____ ***Yes*** ____ ***No*** ***Date of Surgery*** ______________________

PHYSICIAN SERVICES

- ☐ Consult Physical Medicine Physician
- ☐ Impairment Rating __________
- ☐ EMG/NCV __________
- ☐ NCV __________
- ☐ EMG __________
- ☐ Injections/type __________
- ☐ Other (Specify) __________

PHYSICAL THERAPY

- ☐ Evaluate & Treat
  - ☐ Exercise
  - ☐ Heat/Ice Modalities
  - ☐ Massage
  - ☐ Aquatics
  - ☐ Electrical Stimulation
  - ☐ TENS
  - ☐ Ultrasound
  - ☐ Phonophoresis
    - __ with 10% Hydrocortisone Cream (Provider initials)
  - ☐ Traction
  - ☐ Iontophoresis
    - __ Acetic Acid (MD initials)
    - __ Dexa 4 mg/ml (MD initials)
  - ☐ Whirlpool
  - ☐ Whirlpool/Wound Care
  - ☐ Gait Wt. Bearing
  - __________
  - ☐ Vestibular Rehabilitation
  - ☐ Manual Therapy
  - ☐ Other

NUMBER OF VISITS __________

BEGINNING FREQUENCY __________

OCCUPATIONAL THERAPY

- ☐ Evaluate & Treat
- ☐ Splint: Type/Revision
  - __________
  - __________
  - __________
- ☐ Hand Therapy Program
  - __________
  - __________
  - __________
- ☐ Modalities __________
- ☐ Desensitization
- ☐ Upper Extremity Activities/Exercise
- ☐ Activities of Daily Living
- ☐ Other __________
- ☐ Community/Work Integration

NUMBER OF VISITS __________

BEGINNING FREQUENCY __________

SPEECH THERAPY

- ☐ Evaluate & Treat
- ☐ Speech/Language Therapy
- ☐ Dysphagia Evaluation/Therapy
- ☐ Modified Barium Swallow
- ☐ Fiberoptic Endoscopic Evaluation of Swallow
- ☐ Augmentative Device Evaluation
- ☐ Voice Therapy
- ☐ Other (Specify) __________

NUMBER OF VISITS __________

BEGINNING FREQUENCY __________

SPECIALTY PROGRAMS

- ☐ Adapted Driving
- ☐ Amputee Clinic
- ☐ Incontinence Program
- ☐ Low Vision Clinic
- ☐ Lymphedema Program
- ☐ Day Treatment – A Neurocognitive Development Program
- ☐ Orthotics Clinic
- ☐ Osteoporosis Clinic
- ☐ Spasticity Clinic
- ☐ Spinal Cord Follow-Up Clinic
- ☐ TBI Follow-Up Clinic
- ☐ Wheelchair Positioning Clinic
- ☐ Urodynamics
  - ☐ Uroflow
  - ☐ CMG
  - ☐ EMG
  - ☐ Erectile Dysfunction Study

NEUROPSYCHOLOGY

- ☐ Evaluate & Treat
- ☐ Neuropsych Battery (8 hour testing)
- ☐ Cognitive Therapy
- ☐ Adjustment Counseling

WORK INJURY PROGRAM

- ☐ Work Hardening
- ☐ Work Conditioning
- ☐ Functional Capacity Evaluation
- ☐ Post Rehab Conditioning

SPECIAL PRECAUTIONS: ______________________

____

Verbal/Written Order for Dr./Provider ______________________ **Taken By** __________

I hereby certify these services as medically necessary for the patient's plan of care.

Physician Signature ______________________ **Date** __________ **Office Ph.** __________

Other Provider Signature ______________________ **Date** __________ **Office Ph.** __________

Pre-Certification ______________________

Figure 5-1 Physician's orders form. (Courtesy Baylor University Medical Center, Dallas.)

Rehabilitation Clarification Orders	
Date	Primary Diagnosis: ______ Treatment Diagnoses: ______ ______ Date of Onset: ______ Treatment Frequency: ______ Treatment Duration: ______ Treatment Plan:
	Physician's Signature:

Figure 5-2 Clarification order request form. (Courtesy Baylor University Medical Center—The Tom Landry Center, Dallas.)

Analysis of the Client's Occupational Performance

This section identifies the types of assessments used and summarizes the results of each client assessment. The occupational therapist selects specific assessments depending on the diagnosis and the individual client. For example, a brain-injured client may require a physical assessment (ROM, motor and sensory function) and perceptual and cognitive testing, while a client with a distal radius fracture may require only a physical assessment. The OTA completes certain aspects of the evaluation as identified by the occupational therapist.[4] It is helpful to use standardized results or standardized rating scales for easy interpretation by others. Standardized scales also permit reliable replication of the evaluation process at reevaluation and discharge times.

Also included in this section is the evaluation of the client's functional performance, or how well the client performs in essential activities. A standardized scale (Table 5-1) is used so as to ensure reliable results. The focus and scope of the OT evaluation depend on the defined roles of the various professional departments in the facility. In the sample form (see Figure 5-3), bed mobility, transfers, wheelchair mobility, and daily living skills are assessed.

Prioritizing Areas of Occupation and Occupational Performance

This section is the most important section of the report. It is a summary of the evaluation process and sets up the transition of the OT evaluation report for the intervention plan. The occupational therapist completes the evaluation summary, and the OTA, under the occupational therapist's direction, contributes to it. In this section the previously recorded information is analyzed, and a problem list is developed. The problems listed are those that will impede the client from obtaining maximal independence. This list may include problems that OT intervention may or may not directly affect; these problems will influence the OT practitioner's treatment approach. This section also includes the occupational therapist's judgment of the appropriateness of the client for OT services and is based on the clinical reasoning of the occupational therapist.

Box 5-4

Data Gathering Questions for the Occupational Profile

Who is the client?

Why is the client seeking service, and what are the client's current concerns relative to engaging in occupations and in daily life activities?

What areas of occupation are successful, and what areas are causing problems or risks?

What contexts support engagement in desired occupations, and what contexts are inhibiting engagement?

What is the client's occupational history?

What are the client's priorities and desired targeted outcomes?

Modified from American Occupational Therapy Association: Occupational therapy practice framework: domain and process, ed 2 *Am J Occup Ther* 62:625-683, 2008.

Intervention Plan

Using this problem list, the occupational therapist, the OTA, and the client will set realistic and functional therapy outcomes that focus the intervention plan. This section will include these functional outcomes and the short-term objectives and, if necessary, referrals or recommendations to other professionals.[2] Intervention approaches will also be identified, as well as service delivery options. Service delivery options will include the frequency and duration of the OT service. Other important entries in the intervention plan may include a potential discharge plan and a section noting that the stated goals have been discussed with and reflect the goals of the client and his or her family. Finally, if the initial physician's order was for an evaluation only or was not specific for the treatment intervention now planned, a physician's review of the plan and verifying signature may be necessary (see Figure 5-2).

Intervention Process

The intervention process is divided into three phases. First there is the intervention plan. The intervention plan is created as part of the initial evaluation report and has been previously discussed. The second phase of the intervention process is intervention implementation. During this phase the OTA will carry out the intervention plan and document through the use of daily notes and progress notes the client's response to treatment. The third and final phase of the intervention process is intervention review. During the review process, the plan and its implementation are reviewed and modified as needed.

Intervention Plan

As briefly described earlier, the intervention plan or treatment plan involves organizing and interpreting the data previously gathered during the evaluation to establish a clear plan of action. This process identifies the problems impeding function and then applies clinical reasoning skills to specify predictable functional outcomes. The result is a clear set of functional outcomes and short-term objectives with an established plan of treatment to accomplish those outcomes. An intervention approach is also chosen at this time and is based on the established outcomes of therapy. The occupational

Name: John Doe
Doctor: Dr. J. Smith
Therapist: J. Gomez, OTR S. Johnson, COTA
Referred for: OT THA protocol including eval + tx for ADLs
DOB: 12/30/27 Date: 7/2/11
Diagnosis: THA
Precautions: THA precautions
Frequency: 3x/week
Duration: 1 week
Rehab potential: Good

PROBLEMS:	SHORT-TERM GOALS:	LONG-TERM GOALS:	APPROACHES:
↓ ADL: Dressing Hygiene Bathing Functional mobility	• Provided assistive devices & instructions & following THA precautions, patient will dress L/E c̄ min. assist in 3 days. • Provided raised toilet seat, patient will transfer from standing ↔ toilet c̄ min. assist following THA precautions within 3 days. • Provided tub chair and grab bars, patient will transfer from standing ↔ tub chair c̄ min. assist following THA precautions within 3 days.	• Patient will perform ADLs independently in order to return to ADL at home by D/C.	• Instruct and demo THA precautions. • Train in use of assistive devices including: reacher, dressing sticks, sock aid, long-handled shoe horn, elastic shoe laces, raised toilet seat, tub chair, grab bars. • Instruct in tub/shower, toilet and car transfers. • Provide options for work simplification, meal preparation, & item transport. • Assist in obtaining equipment as needed.

Figure 5-3 Occupational therapy evaluation form. (Courtesy Occupational Therapy Department, Santa Clara Valley Medical Center, San Jose, Calif.)

therapist will need to determine if the outcome is to create or promote a new habit or skill, to establish or restore routines, to maintain current levels of functioning, to modify behaviors, or to prevent disability or injury.[3] Finally, the occupational therapist will determine which interventions can be provided by the OTA, and which by the occupational therapist.

It is important to involve the client (or, when necessary, a client advocate) in planning treatment. The occupational therapist must consider goals that the client finds personally meaningful, valuable, and culturally relevant. Involvement in outcomes development increases client motivation and improves rehabilitation potential. Figure 5-4 provides an example of an OT intervention plan.

Intervention Implementation

Once the implementation of the OT plan begins, the OTA will be responsible for documenting his or her interactions with the client. This documentation can take various forms and will be determined by the facility in which the OTA works. It is important to document all contact between the client and the OTA, which may include telephone conversations between the OTA and the client; case consultations between the OTA and the occupational therapist or other professionals; and OT interventions.

OT practitioners must complete daily records on client attendance and the treatment provided. Generally, daily notes are brief and reflect the treatment provided, the client's response to treatment, and progress noted. Revision of the treatment plan and outcomes or objectives is not always necessary. These records are provided to insurance payers to verify that charges and treatment interventions are consistent. Many different formats are available to record daily documentation. Some facilities use a SOAP format, whereas others use a narrative. Figures 5-5 and 5-6 provide some example of daily treatment records while Box 5-5 is a sample of a brief narrative daily note.

Critical Pathway

Physician: Dr. J. Smith
Nurse case manager: M. Ryan, RN
PT: R. O'Hearn, RPT; B. Crowell, PTA
OT: J. Gomez, OTR; S. Johnson, COTA
Speech: M. Swor, SLP
Psych: G. Stallig, MALP
Ther. rec.: T. Chang, TRS
Social worker: B. Kucinski, MSW
Dietician: F. Wood, RD
Additional team members:

Diagnosis: Right CVA Left Hemiplegia
Admission date: 7/6/11
Discharge date: 8/2/11
Length of stay: 1 month

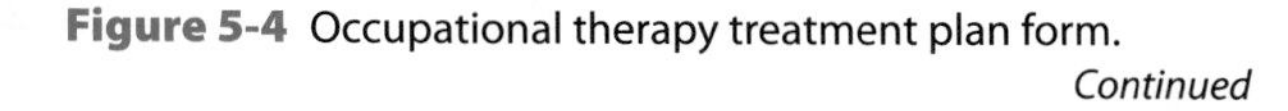

Figure 5-4 Occupational therapy treatment plan form.

Continued

Moderate-Severe
(Right CVA Left Hemi)

Admission date: 7/6/11

1	2	3	4	5	6	7
Establish bowel and bladder program Establish skin program Begin eval Oriented to unit/room Oriented to rehab program Bedside dysphagia screen Swallow risk ID band DNR/DNI status	W/C fitted Assess for positioning equipment Assess need for referral to DRS and/or CIL	Evaluations complete Assess transfers w/team Assess for dining grp Assess need for psych eval Conference	Assess need for CD referral Assess need for TR Foley out	Assess self-transport Stroke films Referral to Stroke Club		Family Day Members attended ____ ____ ____ ____ ____ Review patient goals with patient and family
8	**9**	**10**	**11**	**12**	**13**	**14**
Assess need for adaptive equipment Reassess dysphagia Re-evaluate bowel and bladder program Re-evaluate skin program			Assess phone skills, check writing, money skills Dry run	Assess simple meal prep Assess appropri-ateness for self-meds	Assess need for positioning equipment/splints	Family Day Members attended ____ ____ ____ ____ Assess car transfer Assess light housekeeping skills W/E pass
15	**16**	**17**	**18**	**19**	**20**	**21**
Community re-entry activity Reassess dysphagia Re-evaluate bowel and bladder program Re-evaluate skin integrity		Assess anticipated equipment needs Assess home adaptation needs	Equipment ordered Wet run			Family Day Members attended ____ ____ ____ ____ Begin instruction in home program Assess need for DPA W/E pass
22	**23**	**24**	**25**	**26**	**27**	**28**
	D/C FIM complete Referral call to O.P. therapist					

Figure 5-4, cont'd

SANTA CLARA VALLEY MEDICAL CENTER
OCCUPATIONAL THERAPY DEPARTMENT
page 1 of 2

OCCUPATIONAL THERAPY

Service ______________________ ☐ Inpatient ☐ Outpatient

☐ Initial ☐ Interim ☐ Discharge
(Rating scale on back of form)

INFORMATION

Onset Date: ____________ Referral Date: ____________ Sex: M F Language: ____________
Diagnosis

Medical History:

Precautions/Diet:

Living Situation:

A/Vocational History:

UPPER EXTREMITY

Range of Motion
☐ Refer to range of motion form

Muscle Picture
☐ Refer to muscle test form

Sensation
(Light touch, pain, kinesthesia, other)

Hand Function
Dominance: ☐ Right ☐ Left

Splinting:

	Right			Left		
	Grip	3 point	Lateral	Grip	3 point	Lateral
Initial						
Interim/DC						
Norm						

OTHER MOTOR
(Endurance, head/trunk posture and control, sitting/standing balance, reflexes, LE picture, functional ambulation)

VISUAL PERCEPTUAL SKILLS

VISUAL	Initial	Interim/DC	PERCEPTUAL	Initial	Interim/DC
Visual attention			Motor planning		
Near acuity			Graphic praxis		
Distance acuity			Body scheme		
Pursuits			R/L discrimination		
Saccades			Form		
Ocular alignment			Size		
Stereopsis			Part/whole		
Visual fields			Figure ground		
Visual neglect			Position in space		

SCALE: 0 = intact; 1 = impaired; 2 = severely impaired; 3 = unable to perform
COMMENTS:

Wears corrective lenses ☐ Y ☐ N Testing not indicated ☐

COGNITION AND BEHAVIOR
(Orientation, initiation, direction following, memory, judgment, organization, problem solving, impulsivity, attention span)

DISPOSITION - White - MEDICAL RECORD Yellow - O.T. Chart Therapist's Signature: ____________

9502 SCVMC 6628-17

Figure 5-5 Occupational therapy daily documentation and treatment record.

SANTA CLARA VALLEY MEDICAL CENTER
OCCUPATIONAL THERAPY DEPARTMENT
page 2 of 2

OCCUPATIONAL THERAPY

Service ______________________ ☐ Inpatient ☐ Outpatient

☐ Initial ☐ Interim ☐ Discharge
(Rating scale on back of form)

	ACTIVITY	Initial	Interim D/C	Goal	
BED MOBILITY	Rolling R				Bed: Positioning: Caregiver Training: Comments:
	Rolling L				
	Bridging				
	Scooting				
	Long sit				
	Sidelying to sit				
TRANSFERS	Bed				Type: Equipment: Caregiver Training: Comments:
	Toilet				
	Tub/shower				
	Car/van seat				
	Furniture				
WHEELCHAIR	Management				Type: Weight Shift Type: Positioning/Cushion: Caregiver Training: Comments:
	Weight shift				
	Home				
	Community				
	In/out of car				
DAILY LIVING SKILLS	Eating				Equipment: Home Environment: A/Vocational/Driving Skills: Caregiver Training: Comments:
	Upper body dressing				
	Lower body dressing				
	Hygiene/ grooming				
	Bathing				
	Toileting				
	Kitchen				
	Homemaking				
	Community				
	Communication tasks				

Problems:

Goals/Recommendation: ☐ Patient/Caregiver participated in goal setting

X / /
Frequency/Session Length/Duration of Treatment

Therapist's Signature Date Physician's Signature

DISPOSITION - White - MEDICAL RECORD Yellow - O.T. Chart 9502 PAGE 2 of 2 SCVMC 6628-17

Figure 5-5, cont'd

Occupational Therapy
Outpatient Treatment Record

Demographics

Place Patient Label Here

Eval Date: ______________________

Dx: ______________ **Injury Date:** __________

Order Date: ______________________

Freq/Duration: ______________________

Treatment/Supplies

Date	Start Time/ Stop Time												Additional Comments

Date	Treatment Notes

Figure 5-6 Occupational therapy treatment record form. (Courtesy Occupational Therapy Department, Unity Hospital, Fridley, Minn.)

Box 5-5

Brief Daily Note Sample

12/10/2011, 1:00-1:43 P.M. Client participated in 15 minutes of right upper extremity passive ROM and was instructed in self-mobilization techniques, followed by 28 minutes of ADL retraining to address upper body dressing. Donned pullover shirt with minimal assistance and button-front, long-sleeve shirt with moderate assistance.

Progress notes may be required on a weekly or biweekly basis. Weekly progress notes are more thorough and should summarize the treatment, its frequency, the client's response, and progress toward outcomes (or lack of progress, with justification). The short-term objectives should be updated and the intervention plan revised. The new objectives and intervention plan are usually considered short-term and reflect the expected outcomes for the upcoming week's treatment regimen.

The SOAP note is one format commonly used to ensure consistency of the progress notes' content. Figure 5-7 is one example of a form that can be used for either a progress or a discharge note. Boxes 5-6 and 5-7 provide some examples of progress notes.

Intervention Review

If treatment occurs over an extended period, the occupational therapist may need to complete a full reevaluation. Again, the OTA contributes to this process. The format is often the same as the initial evaluation. The primary difference is that this report reflects the differences between the initial baseline of evaluation results and the client's present clinical status. The reevaluation report reflects progress made toward the predicted goals and is a measure of success of the treatment intervention. Based on the new evaluation results, initial outcomes and treatment timelines can be revised. The reevaluation is an important tool for the ongoing utilization review process. It allows the OT practitioner to justify continued intervention by clearly quantifying the effectiveness and efficacy of the OT intervention.

Outcomes Process

According to the *OTPF, 2nd edition*, outcomes are the end result of the OT process.[3] Outcomes can be subjective adjustments by the clients when ideal return of function is not achieved. More commonly, outcomes are phrased as measurable objective progress related to occupational performance. Outcomes are continuously addressed throughout the OT process and have been discussed in relation to the evaluation and intervention processes. Outcomes are continually modified and adapted throughout the interactions between the client and the OT practitioner.

Discharge Summary Report

The discharge summary report is part of the outcomes process and is a summary of the OT services provided for the client, as well as a summary of the overall outcomes of the OT intervention. At completion of the OT intervention regimen, the client's status must be documented. Insurance or facility requirements may stipulate that the occupational therapist complete the discharge summary. Again, the format can be the same as that used for the initial evaluation and reevaluation. The discharge summary describes the client's final status on discharge from the facility. The progress made from the initial evaluation to discharge must be accurately outlined. Some key elements may be added including a statement of which outcomes were and were not achieved, with a reason given for those not achieved. Discharge recommendations clearly indicate the additional interventions and follow-up that may be required to ensure continued functional improvement or maintenance of the functional gains made during OT. Any home program plans or referral plans are also described.

The discharge summary is the key document that reflects the client's total progress and all the accomplishments achieved. The data can be used for many purposes. Quality assurance committees may use the data to evaluate the effectiveness of treatment. The data may also be used for outcome studies to prove overall effectiveness of treatment within certain diagnostic categories. Insurance payers may use the report to determine payment for the service. Other service agencies such as outpatient clinics will use the data to help establish continued outcomes and intervention plans in the new treatment setting. Figures 5-7 and 5-8 provide sample forms for the discharge summary.

Medicare Reports

Medicare is the largest single payer for OT services.[14] For this reason, OT practitioners are often required to complete reports for Medicare, Part A: Hospital Insurance Program, which pays for hospital inpatient, skilled nursing facility, home, and hospice care, and Part B: Supplemental Medical Insurance Program, which covers hospital outpatient, physician, and other professional services. Certain requirements apply to Medicare; therefore records may include prior authorizations, certifications, and recertifications. The OT practitioner must become familiar with Medicare regulations as they pertain to documentation. Figure 5-9 provides an example of a Medicare B form.

Summary

Documentation of OT services produces written records and reports that contain pertinent information about the client's status, progress, and performance. The OT practitioner is responsible for keeping accurate records to document the client's evaluation results, the identified problems, the treatment outcomes and intervention plan, and the client's progress toward the established plan.

OT documentation includes the referral, evaluation data, initial evaluation, daily notes, progress notes, reevaluation, and discharge summary. Records and reports should reflect clear, concise, accurate, and objective information about the client. Documentation should be well organized and developed according to an agreed-upon system for internal consistency of the record.

OCCUPATIONAL THERAPY

IP/OP Room ________

Month															
Date															
9705 OT eval/re-eval 1-15															
0959 ADL training 1-15															
0977 OT consult/care conf 1-15															
9707 Cognitive treatment 1-15															
973 Develop treatment 1-15															
9877 Environmental stim 1-15															
0970 Motor skills 1-15															
0972 Preventive skills 1-15															
0971 Sensory integration 1-15															
9785 Therapeutic adapt 1-15															
9712 Initial out/pt ADL 30															
0967 Out/Pt no show 1-15															
0968 OT eval/hand 1-15															
0969 Motor skills/hand 1-15															
0963 Preventive skills/hand 1-15															
0960 Therap adapt/hand 1-15															
0962 Splint (prefab-hand)															
0965 Splint (fabricated-H)															
97832 Splint-prefab															
609610 Splint-fabricated															
610063 2/Piece formfit TLSO															
9798 In/Pt OT adapt equip															
0964 O/P hand equip															
1008 O/P occ therapy supply															

B, Bedside; C, clinic; H, hold treatment; S, surgery; DC, discontinued; D, discharged.

Therapist's signature ________________________________

OCCUPATIONAL THERAPY TREATMENT RECORD

Figure 5-7 Occupational therapy progress report or discharge note. (Courtesy Baylor University Medical Center—The Tom Landry Center, Dallas.)

Box 5-6

Weekly Progress Note Sample

12/10/2011. Client seen 3 times this week for instruction in home exercise program, passive ROM, and ADL retraining. Upper body dressing improved from maximum assistance to moderate assistance. Continues to perform lower body dressing independently with assistive device. Short-term goal: Client will dress upper body with minimum assistance in 1 week.

Box 5-7

SOAP Note Sample

12/10/2011

S: Client expressed frustration with her inability to fully dress herself independently.

O: Dressing lower body independent using assistive device, dressing upper body with moderate assistance for button-front shirt. Right shoulder flexion and abduction improved to 45 degrees; elbow active ROM remains at minus 30 degrees extension to 50 degrees of flexion.

A: Decreased active ROM of right elbow and shoulder due to tightness related to humerus fracture continues to limit upper extremity ADL independence. Short-term goal: Client will dress upper body in long-sleeve, button-front shirt with minimum assistance in 1 week.

P: Continue current plan of care, 3 times a week for 2 more weeks to address ADL deficits related to decreased active ROM.

Selected Reading Guide Questions

1. Think back to 1 year ago from today. At 9:30 A.M., who were you with, what were you doing, where were you, why were you there? Now do the same for 6 months ago, 1 month ago, yesterday, 1 hour ago. Discuss this memory exercise in relation to the requirement that OT services be documented in a timely fashion, generally the same day.
2. Write a functional outcome and a possible short-term objective for each of the following:
   a. Your client would like to be able to dress himself in a button-up shirt for church on Sunday.
   b. Your client would like to be able to open the lid on a water bottle.
   c. Your client would like to be able to take a shower without getting short of breath and having to stop.
3. Observe someone in your household complete a daily task such as cook a meal or get dressed.
   a. Write a narrative note about what you observed.
   b. Write a SOAP note based on your observations.

References

1. Allen C: Clinical reasoning for documentation. In Acquaviva JD, editor: *Effective documentation for occupational therapy*, ed 2, Rockville, MD, 1998, American Occupational Therapy Association.
2. American Occupational Therapy Association: Guidelines for documentation of occupational therapy, *Am J Occup Ther* 62:199–204, 2008.
3. American Occupational Therapy Association: Occupational therapy practice framework: domain and process, ed 2, *Am J Occup Ther* 62:625–683, 2008.
4. American Occupational Therapy Association: Guidelines for supervision, roles, and responsibilities during the delivery of occupational therapy services, *Am J Occup Ther* 63:797–803, 2009.
5. American Occupational Therapy Association: Standards of practice for occupational therapy, *Am J Occup Ther* 64, 2010:(pages).
6. American Occupational Therapy Association: Occupational therapy code of ethics and ethics standards, *Am J Occup Ther* 64, 2010:(online supplement) Retrieved from http://www.aota.org/Practitioners/Ethics/Docs/Standards/38527.aspx, Accessed January 15, 2012.
7. Arabit L: Preparing for electronic documentation, *OT Practice* 15(12):13–15, 2010, July 12.
8. Brennan C, Robinson M: Documentation: Getting it right to avoid Medicare denials. [Electronic Version], *OT Practice* 11(14): 10–15, 2006.
9. Borcherding SJ, Morreale MJ: *The OTA's guide to writing soap notes*, ed 2, Thorofare, NJ, 2007, Slack.
10. Hitchon J: Electronic health records update, *OT Practice* 15(5):6, 2010, April 5.
11. News MacDaily: *Doctors can now use ipads with macpractice emr, digital radiography, practice management, and more [Web log message]*, 2010, April 16, Retrieved from http//macdailynews.com/index.php/weblog/comments/24831/.
12. McCann KD, Steich T: Legal issues in documentation: fraud, abuse and confidentiality. In Acquaviva JD, editor: *Effective documentation for occupational therapy*, ed 2, Rockville, MD, 1998, American Occupational Therapy Association.
13. Sames KM: *Documenting occupational therapy practice*, ed 2, Boston, 2010, Pearson.
14. Thomas VJ: Evolving health care systems: payment for occupational therapy services. In Acquaviva JD, editor: *Effective documentation for occupational therapy*, ed 2, Rockville, MD, 1998, American Occupational Therapy Association.

Recommended Reading

American Occupational Therapy Association: Occupational therapy practice framework: domain and process, ed 2, *Am J Occup Ther* 62:625–683, 2008.

Occupational Therapy
Hand Clinic Progress Report/Discharge Note

Patient Name: ____________________ Date: ____________

Diagnosis: ____________________ Physician: ____________

Treatment: ____________________

Number of visits: attended ________ cancelled ________ no shows ________

Treatment results/comments

____

____

____

____

____

____

Range of Motion: Active/Passive

Wrist	Right	Left
Ext./Flex.		
RD/UD		
Sup./Pro.		

Strength:

	Right	Left
Grip		
Lateral Pinch		
Tripod Pinch		
Tip Pinch		

	Thumb	Index	Long	Ring	Small
MP ext./flex.					
PIP ext./flex.					
DIP ext./flex.					
Palmar abd.					

STG'S ______________________________

____

____

____

Established Goals

Increased range of motion	met	not met	continue
Increased strength/endurance	met	not met	continue
Decreased swelling/pain	met	not met	continue
Patient education	met	not met	continue
Improved functional activities:			
ADL self-care	met	not met	continue
ADL home management	met	not met	continue

Recommendations

I would like to request this patient:

______ Be discharged from Occupational Therapy

______ Continue present treatment for ______ days/week for ______ weeks.

______ Other______________________________.

Thank you for your referral.

Therapist ______________________________ phone ____________

Figure 5-8 Discharge summary form. (Courtesy Occupational Therapy Department, Unity Hospital, Fridley, Minn.)

DATE DISCONTINUED:	REASON:	REFERRAL OBJECTIVES:	LENGTH OF TIME PT WAS SEEN:
DIAGNOSIS:			

GOALS	MET	NOT MET	REASON
STG: ___			
___			
___			
Pt/family will make DC plans based on level of independence at time of DC.			
LTG: ___			
___			

PATIENT'S HOME SITUATION PRIOR TO ADMIT:	PATIENT DISCHARGED TO: ☐ Home ☐ Rehab ctr ☐ NH ☐ Other ___	LIST HELP AVAILABLE IF DC HOME:

PATIENT'S ADL STATUS AT THE TIME OF DISCHARGE

	INDEP.	ASSIST	COMMENTS
TRANSFERS			
SELF CARE			
DRESSING			
EATING			
COOKING			

ADAPTIVE EQUIPMENT (RECOMMENDED FOR) WITH PATIENT

☐ Long handled reacher ☐ Bath sponge ☐ Sock aide ☐ Dressing stick ☐ Elastic shoe laces ☐ Walker bag

☐ Elevated toilet seat ☐ Leg lift device ☐ Tub grab bar ☐ Other ___

WRITTEN MATERIAL SENT WITH PATIENT

☐ Ortho restrictions & transfer instructions
☐ Crutch/walker safety instructions
☐ Dressing equipment instructions
☐ Adaptive equipment list & purchase information
☐ Joint protection/arthritis exercises
☐ Brain trauma information
☐ One handed ADL techniques
☐ Back saving ADL techniques
☐ Low vision adaptation/safety techniques
☐ Carpal tunnel prevention
☐ U/E strengthening instructions
☐ U/E coordination instructions
☐ Adaptive dressing techniques
☐ Cognitive worksheets/instructions
☐ Range of motion instructions
☐ Other ___

COMMENTS: ___

RECOMMENDATIONS FOR FURTHER TREATMENT OR SUPERVISION

☐ None needed ☐ Outpatient OT is recommended ☐ OT at new facility ☐ Other: ___

AREAS OF CONCERN: ___

Occupational therapist signature ___ Date ___

61-00206 REV. 7/93

OCCUPATIONAL THERAPY DISCHARGE SUMMARY

OCCUPATIONAL THERAPY DISCHARGE SUMMARY

Figure 5-9 Occupational therapy information and plan of treatment form. (Courtesy Blue Cross/Blue Shield of Minnesota, St. Paul, Minn.)

PART III

Assessment

CHAPTER 6

Assessment of Motor Control and Functional Movement

JEAN W. SOLOMON AND JANE O'BRIEN

Key Terms

Motor control
Dynamical systems theory
Postural mechanisms
Postural tone
Muscle tone
Hypotonicity
Hypertonicity
Spasticity
Manual muscle testing
Rigidity
Primitive reflexes
Protective extension reactions
Righting reactions
Equilibrium reactions
Sensory processing
Selective movement
Brunnstrom's stages of motor recovery
Neurodevelopmental treatment (NDT)
Coordination
Occurrence of incoordination

Chapter Objectives

After studying this chapter, the student or practitioner will be able to do the following:

1. Delineate occupational therapy assistant/occupational therapist roles with regard to assessing motor control and functional motion.
2. Describe the dynamical systems theory of motor control.
3. Discuss how OT practitioners use dynamical systems theory when assessing motor control.
4. Understand how postural control affects motor control and functional motion.
5. Define *normal* and *abnormal* muscle tone.
6. Describe specific primitive reflexes and how to assess for the presence of such reflexes.
7. Describe the influence on function when primitive reflexes persist after neurologic damage in the adult patient.
8. Define protective extension, righting, and equilibrium responses and how to assess for the presence of these responses.
9. Describe the functional significance of these responses while a patient is engaged in activities.
10. Describe expected motor recovery patterns in the adult with central nervous system dysfunction.
11. Define levels of assistance, and give examples of functional use of an involved extremity in the adult with central nervous system dysfunction.
12. List and describe simple structured tests used by the occupational therapy practitioner to evaluate coordination and dexterity.
13. Define the occurrences and types of incoordination that might affect the adult with central nervous system dysfunction.
14. Identify how incoordination affects one's occupational performance.

Occupational therapy (OT) practitioners help clients engage in their desired occupations. Motor control is required to perform tasks and activities necessary for independence and life fulfillment. Therefore practitioners must understand how clients control movement, the factors involved in skilled movement, and how to remediate motor control deficits. Knowledge of abnormal motor patterns and how to help clients who exhibit impaired motor control is essential for helping clients engage in occupations.

This chapter begins with a definition of motor control and an overview of dynamical systems theory. A description of the multiple systems involved in motor control is provided, with a detailed analysis of postural mechanisms and a review of reflexes that underlie movement. The authors describe stages of recovery and present theories for intervention including Brunnstrom's stages of motor recovery and Bobath's neurodevelopmental treatment.

Motor Control

Motor control is necessary for a person to function independently during occupational performance tasks. Motor control refers to the "ability to regulate or direct movement."[44] Information is relayed to the central nervous system to organize the musculoskeletal system and create coordinated movements and skilled actions. Movement involves perception (making sense of the input), motor planning (processing input), motor execution (carrying out movement), feedback (internal and external), and biomechanics (relationship of muscles and joints to each other). Impairment or dysfunction in any of these areas results in motor control deficits interfering with function. Many times clients will exhibit difficulties in all areas, as may be observed in clients who have had a cerebrovascular accident (CVA).

A 62-year-old male had a CVA (stroke) on the left side of his cerebral cortex. Four weeks after the stroke, he is unable to use his preferred right arm for self-feeding or simple oral hygiene activities because of the loss of motor control on the right side of his body. He has difficulty dressing and engaging in his leisure activity of fishing. The OT practitioner works with him to help him regain motor function in his right arm so that he can return to previous activities.

Complex neurologic systems work together to make motor control possible. When an insult to the central nervous system (CNS) occurs (e.g., stroke) or a progressive, neurologic disease develops (e.g., multiple sclerosis), motor control is affected. Functional recovery depends on the extent of the damage to the CNS and the expected neurologic recovery for a particular diagnosis.

Dynamical Systems Theory

Dynamical systems theory proposes that movement is a function of interactions among the neuromuscular system, environment, cognition, and the task itself.[35] These systems interact with each other to influence movement. For example, the male client mentioned earlier who had a stroke may be able to complete a motor task such as preparing his fishing rod, in the supportive environment at the clinic, but not be able to perform while standing on the riverbank in the outdoors. In this example, the change in environment altered the motor demands. The goal of OT intervention is for clients to perform the motor tasks in multiple environments and especially the environments of choice.

Consequently, OT practitioners evaluate multiple systems to determine how they influence the patient's ability to carry out occupational performance such as feeding, dressing, personal hygiene activities, leisure, work, and social participation. Intervention may consist of remediating a deficit area or changing the requirements of the task so that the person can be successful. The practitioner may decide that assistive technology is necessary for the client to succeed. The practitioner may decide to target one system or work within all systems to address motor control issues. In acute care or rehabilitation settings practitioners often begin by examining the neuromusculoskeletal system so that they can address areas of deficiency that may be influencing motor control.

Neuromusculoskeletal System

The neuromusculoskeletal system includes the nervous system, muscular system, and skeletal systems, which interact to influence and produce movement. Disruptions in any of these systems (such as a CVA) may result in motor control dysfunction.

When examining the neuromusculoskeletal system, practitioners evaluate:

- Physical appearance
- Postural mechanism
    - Postural tone
    - Muscle tone
    - Reflexes
- Coordination

Physical Appearance

Practitioners evaluate a client's physical appearance in terms of limb and skeletal symmetry because this may interfere with movement. Clients who have deformities or injuries (e.g., burns, scarring, edema) may not be able to move in certain ways. The following questions may guide the practitioner's observation of the client:

- Does the client lean to one side when sitting? Standing? Walking?
- Are there any physical anomalies observed?
- Does the person have any swollen joints?
- Are both sides of the body symmetrical?
- Are the limbs of equal size?
- Are there any skeletal or muscular deficits that may interfere with movement?

Postural Mechanism

The postural mechanisms include postural tone, muscle tone, integration of the primitive reflexes and mass patterns of movement, righting reactions, equilibrium reactions, protective extension, and selective voluntary or intentional movement.[8,13] By the time a person reaches adulthood, he or she has developed postural support sufficient to provide stability and allow functional movement. Normal postural mechanisms are automatic, involuntary (nonintentional) movements that together provide stability and mobility during activity.[13] These automatic reactions develop early in life. The postural mechanisms allow for the development of head control (stability) and mobility, trunk control and mobility, midline orientation of self and symmetry, weight bearing and weight shifting in all directions, balance during transitional movements, controlled voluntary limb movement, and coordination.[8,13]

In patients who have sustained CNS damage secondary to a CVA or traumatic brain injury, the normal postural mechanism is disrupted. Abnormal muscle tone and mass patterns dominate the patient's movements, which may be slow and uncoordinated. OT practitioners assess the degree of damage to the postural mechanism in patients with CNS trauma or disease. The OT practitioner also assesses the effect of abnormal postural mechanism on the patient's occupational performance activities.

Postural Tone

Postural tone refers to *tonus* (muscle tension) in the neck, trunk, and limbs. Postural tone must be high enough to resist gravity, thus enabling persons to be upright against gravity yet low enough to allow movement.[8] Tone allows persons to adjust automatically and continuously to their movements or to movements imposed on them externally. Postural tone provides the necessary proximal stability (close to the body center) to enable distal (away from the body center), voluntary, selective movements. Abnormal muscle tone may be too low, resulting in poor stability, or too high, resulting in rigidity. High or low muscle tone interferes with normal selective movement. The occupational therapist evaluates postural tone.

If he or she has achieved service competency, the occupational therapy assistant (OTA) may help evaluate the status of the postural mechanism (and selective movement and coordination) with simple structured tests or checklists to guide in the clinical observations. Both the occupational therapist and the OTA observe how impaired motor control affects the patient's functional abilities and independence during activities.

CLINICAL PEARL

Observe the client sitting and performing simple weight shifting from side to side as a way to determine general postural tone. This can be done during the initial interview.

Normal Muscle Tone

Normal muscle tone, a component of the normal postural mechanism, is a continuous state of mild contraction, or state of readiness of a specific muscle.[42] Muscle tone is the resting state of a muscle in response to gravity and emotion. It depends on the integrity of the peripheral nervous system (PNS) and the CNS mechanisms and the properties of muscles. While passively manipulating the head, trunk, or limbs, the therapist can feel the tension between the origin and insertion of the muscle. In other words, when they are passively stretched, muscles offer a small amount of involuntary resistance.

Normal muscle tone varies from one individual to another and depends on factors such as age, gender, occupation, and exercise regimen. A normal range is characterized by the following (Figure 6-1):

1. Effective coactivation (stabilization) at axial (neck and trunk) and proximal shoulder and pelvic girdle joints
2. Ability of a limb to move against gravity and resistance
3. Ability to maintain the limb's position if it is placed passively by the therapist and then released
4. Equal amount of resistance to passive stretch between the *agonist* (muscle that contracts to create movement at a joint) and the *antagonist* (muscle that relaxes, or elongates, to allow movement at a joint), for example, equal amount of resistance in the biceps and triceps muscles or in the wrist flexors and extensors
5. Ease of ability to shift from stability to mobility, and vice versa, as needed, for example; ability to raise arm above head and then to maintain that position while reaching for a glass in a high cabinet
6. Ability to use muscles in groups or selectively, if necessary,[19] for example, opening the hand to release an item versus pointing the index finger while keeping the other digits flexed
7. Slight resistance to passive movement[17]

Assessing Muscle Tone

OT practitioners assess muscle tone in patients presenting with a variety of diagnoses affecting the musculoskeletal and nervous systems. Normal muscle tone is dynamic. Objective evaluation of muscle tone in the patient with CNS dysfunction is difficult because of its continuous fluctuation and its relationship to the postural mechanism.[8,23] For example, when he or she is lying supine, a patient's level of muscle tone is lower than when the patient is sitting or standing upright against gravity. The level and distribution of muscle tone change as the position of the patient's head in space changes.[8] The emergence of primitive reflexes and associated reactions alters muscle tone. Therefore muscle tone must be evaluated with regard to the postural mechanism, synergies present, the specific task, and other factors related to motor control. The occupational therapist is responsible for evaluating muscle

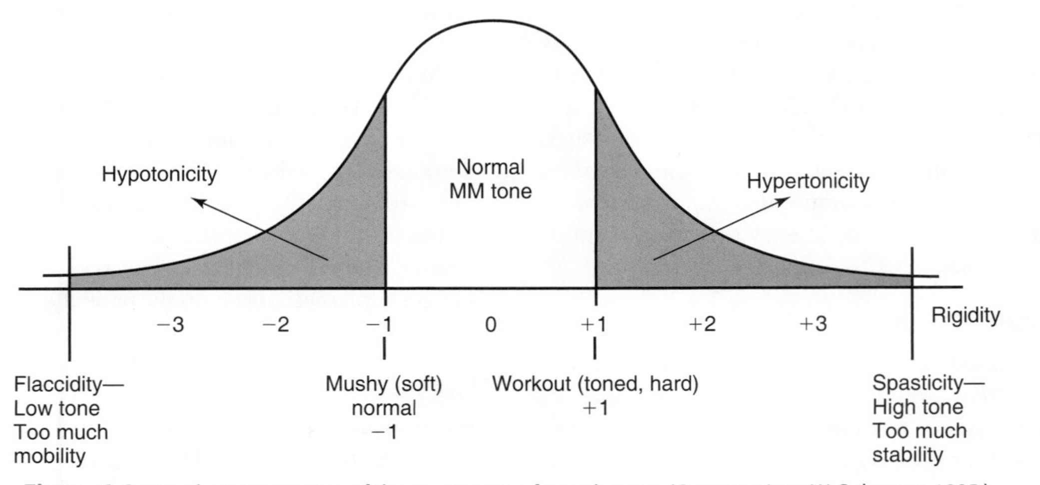

Figure 6-1 Visual representation of the continuum of muscle tone. (Courtesy Jean W. Solomon, 1995.)

tone and its distribution. The OTA and occupational therapist observe how abnormal muscle tone interferes with activities.

The occupational therapist follows guidelines for assessing muscle tone in the patient with CNS damage. The preferred position of the patient for assessment of muscle tone is upright, either sitting or standing, because these positions are most often used for occupational performance tasks. The therapist grasps the patient's arm proximally and distally to the joint on which the muscle acts. The joint is moved slowly through the full range of motion (ROM). The occupational therapist notes how freely and readily the limb passively moves through ROM. The type and distribution of muscle tone are recorded for various muscle groups or movements. These notes provide a framework for formal assessment. Abnormal muscle tone is described as hypotonicity, hypertonicity, or rigidity. The therapist must be able to identify clinically the type and distribution of abnormal muscle tone to select appropriate intervention techniques.

CLINICAL PEARL

Practice assessing muscle tone on a variety of people to begin to "feel" the range of muscle tone.

CLINICAL PEARL

Muscle tone increases with stress or difficulty. Observe muscle tone when a client is performing an activity to better understand what types of activities are suitable for intervention.

Abnormal Muscle Tone

Hypotonicity

Hypotonicity, also called *flaccidity,* is a decrease in muscle tone. Hypotonicity is usually the result of a peripheral nerve injury, cerebellar disease, or frontal lobe damage and is found temporarily in the shock phase after a stroke or spinal cord injury. The muscles feel soft and offer no resistance to passive movement. Usually a wide or excessive passive ROM is present.[51] The flaccid limb feels heavy when moved passively. The patient cannot hold a position once the limb is placed and released by the therapist. The hypotonic limb cannot resist the pull of gravity and therefore drops.[6] Deep tendon reflexes (reflexive contractions of muscles when their tendons are tapped) are diminished or absent.[16,21] In clients who have CVA and spinal cord injuries, flaccidity is usually present initially but is soon replaced by hypertonicity.

Hypertonicity

Hypertonicity, also called spasticity, refers to increased muscle tone. It is commonly defined as an increased resistance to passive stretch caused by an increased or hyperactive stretch reflex.[42,47] Any neurologic condition that alters upper motor neuron pathways may result in hypertonicity.[23]

Hypertonicity is characterized by hyperactive deep tendon reflexes and *clonus* (quick, repetitive, alternate contraction of the agonist and antagonist muscles).[36] Hypertonic muscles offer greater than normal resistance to passive ROM. Hypertonicity usually occurs in patterns of flexion or extension.[8,27,36] The patterns of hypertonicity typically occur in the antigravity muscles of the limbs. Flexor hypertonicity is more commonly apparent in the upper extremity and extensor hypertonicity in the lower extremity.

Hypertonicity varies with the site of the insult to the nervous system. Hypertonicity associated with cerebral damage, as occurs with stroke or head injury, is often seen in combination with other motor deficits such as rigidity or ataxia. Such hypertonicity is influenced by the patient's position and the components of the postural mechanism.[23] Spinal cord hypertonicity is often violent, with severe episodic muscle spasms in muscle groups normally innervated below the level of the lesion.[23,43]

Hypertonicity is often found in patients with upper motor neuron disorders such as multiple sclerosis, CVA, head injury, brain tumors or infections, and spinal cord injury or disease.

Influencing Factors

The postural mechanism influences the degree and patterns of hypertonicity. Therefore the positions of the body and head in space and the head in relation to the body influence the degree and distribution of abnormal muscle tone.[8] Extrinsic factors that influence the degree of hypertonicity include environmental temperature extremes, pain, infection, and emotional stress.[20,23] Therapeutic intervention focuses on empowering the patient to reduce, eliminate, or cope with these extrinsic factors.

CLINICAL PEARL

Loud noises, bright lights, cool temperatures, and bright-colored cluttered walls may stimulate muscle tone. Practitioners may want to reduce these stimuli with clients who have hypertonicity.

Method of Evaluation

Because hypertonicity fluctuates, accurate measurement can be difficult. The occupational therapist can clinically judge the degree and distribution of hypertonicity while assessing a patient with CNS dysfunction. The occupational therapist must remember the dynamic aspect of muscle tone and the factors that might influence a patient's muscle tone. While observing a patient performing occupational tasks such as feeding or dressing, the occupational therapist or OTA notes the influence of abnormal muscle tone. The ultimate purpose of evaluating hypertonicity is to determine how function is impaired by the abnormal muscle tone.

The modified Ashworth Tone Scale[9] provides a uniform way to measure muscle tone in adults. This scale can be completed by experienced practitioners and may provide some reliability in measuring muscle tone (Figure 6-2).

Measurement of Degree

Following the general guidelines for muscle tone assessment, the occupational therapist can determine whether hypotonicity, hypertonicity, or rigidity is present. With hypertonicity

GRADE	DESCRIPTION
0	No increase in muscle tone
1	Slight increase in muscle tone, manifested by a catch and release or by minimal resistance at the end of the ROM when the affected part(s) is moved in flexion or extension
1	Slight increase in muscle tone, manifested by a catch, followed by minimal resistance throughout the remainder (less than half) of the ROM
2	More marked increase in muscle tone through most of the ROM, but affected part(s) easily moved
3	Considerable increase in muscle tone, passive movement difficult
4	Affected part(s) rigid in flexion or extension

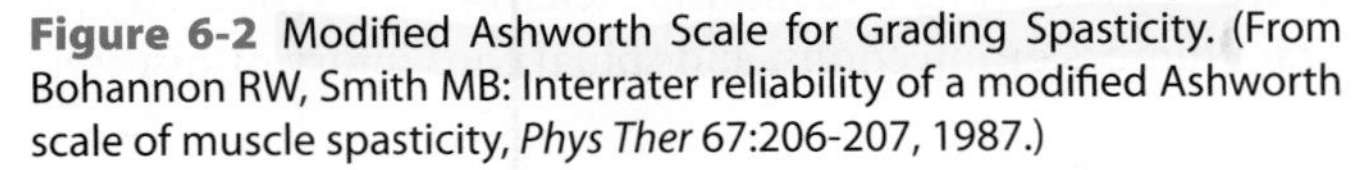

Figure 6-2 Modified Ashworth Scale for Grading Spasticity. (From Bohannon RW, Smith MB: Interrater reliability of a modified Ashworth scale of muscle spasticity, *Phys Ther* 67:206-207, 1987.)

the occupational therapist determines the degree of increased muscle tone, which may be mild, moderate, or severe. In a patient with mild hypertonicity, resistance during passive movement of a joint through full ROM may be felt; however, full ROM is readily attainable. The patient with mild hypertonicity may have difficulty performing functional activities at a normal speed. A patient with moderate hypertonicity demonstrates consistent resistance during passive movement of a joint through full ROM; however, full ROM is attainable. The patient actively demonstrates observable deviations while performing occupational performance tasks. For example, the patient may be unable to incorporate forearm supination (palm up) and wrist extension (wrist in upward position) during self-feeding because of hypertonicity in the forearm pronator and wrist flexor muscles. The patient with severe hypertonicity demonstrates strong resistance during passive movement of a joint through full ROM. A patient with severe hypertonicity is significantly limited in the ability to actively control the involved extremities.

Manual muscle testing is inappropriate for patients who demonstrate abnormal muscle tone. Hypotonic patients are at risk of subluxation or dislocation of joints during manual muscle testing. Hypertonic and rigid muscles may appear "strong" because of resistance during movement. The increased resistance to movement is involuntary. With severe hypertonicity the application of resistance in an effort to stretch the hypertonic muscle may tear or cause other injuries to the muscle.[8]

Rigidity

Rigidity is an increase in muscle tone in the agonist and antagonist muscles simultaneously. Both muscle groups contract continually, resulting in increased resistance to passive movement in any direction and throughout the joint ROM.[18,31] *Lead-pipe rigidity* is identified in patients who demonstrate a constant resistance throughout the joint ROM when a limb is passively moved in any direction. With *cogwheel rigidity* a rhythmic "give" occurs in the resistance throughout the ROM, similar to the feeling of turning a cogwheel. In rigidity the deep tendon reflexes are normal or only moderately increased.[18,31]

Occurrence

Rigidity results from lesions of the extrapyramidal system such as in Parkinson's disease, certain degenerative diseases, encephalitis, tumors,[17] and traumatic brain injury. Cogwheel rigidity occurs in some types of parkinsonism and in some cases of carbon monoxide poisoning. Rigid *decerebrate posturing* (full body extension) and *decorticate posturing* (full body flexion) may occur with diffuse brain injury or anoxia. Rigidity and hypertonicity of muscles often occur simultaneously in a patient with CNS dysfunction.

Muscle tone is only one component of the postural mechanism. The occupational therapist must also assess for the presence of primitive reflexes and automatic reactions.

CLINICAL PEARL

When assessing ROM, move slowly, hold and wait to "feel" a release. Do not pull on extremities.

CLINICAL PEARL

Always inform the client of what is happening and the process. This will ensure the best movement.

Reflexes

Reflexes are innate motor responses elicited by specific sensory stimuli. In normal development, primitive reflexes are observed in the infant and are involuntary. The primitive reflexes help to elongate muscle groups in preparation for voluntary control. In normal development the reflexes occur only under stress (e.g., infant is hungry or tired) and are never seen in the total complement or pattern. The primitive reflexes become integrated as the infant gains voluntary motor control. The occupational therapist and, in certain situations, the OTA on the establishment of service competency may assess for the presence of primitive reflexes. Formal reflex testing is typically performed with the patient in the sitting or supine position. The therapist provides the specific sensory stimulus and observes for the expected motor response, as described in Table 6-1. The emergence or persistence of primitive reflexes in an adult will interfere with the recovery of the automatic protective extension, righting, and equilibrium reactions. The functional significance of the presence of specific reflexes is described next.

CLINICAL PEARL

For clients who have persisting reflexes, the goal of therapy is to increase a person's ability to function in daily activities despite the influence of reflexes. Practitioners may suggest strategies to help clients be successful such as requesting caregivers present food at midline so as not to elicit the asymmetrical tonic neck reflex (ATNR).

Table 6-1 Functional Implications with Persistence of Primitive Reflexes*

Reflex	Stimulus	Response	Examples of Potential Impact†
Suck/swallow reflex	Light touch to lips or gums	Suckling (immature protrusion and retraction of tongue as observed in neonate)	Difficulty performing oral hygiene activities Excessive tongue protrusion during eating and drinking Difficulty creating negative pressure to suck from a straw
Asymmetrical tonic neck reflex (ATNR)	Head turned to one side with chin over shoulder	Extension of arm and leg on face side; flexion on arm and leg on skull side	Difficulty performing self-maintenance activities if head turned to one side
Symmetrical tonic neck reflex (STNR)	Flexion of neck Extension (hyperextension of neck)	Flexion of arms and extension of legs Extension of arms and flexion of legs	Difficulty bridging (lifting buttocks off supporting surface with hips and neck flexed) Difficulty crawling reciprocally Difficulty using arms to reach over head
Tonic labyrinthine reflex (TLR)	Supine position Prone position	Extension of trunk and extremities or increased extensor postural tone Flexion of trunk and extremities or increased flexor postural tone	Difficulty performing all transitional movements that require dissociation between upper and lower body (flexion of upper body with extension of legs—e.g., moving from supine to long sitting in bed)
Positive supporting reflex (PSR)	Pressure to ball of foot	Extension in leg stimulated (hip and knee extension with plantar flexion of ankle—i.e., toe pointing downward)	Difficulty bridging Difficulty donning shoes or keeping them on Difficulty with swing-through phase of walking as it precedes toe-off phase Difficulty climbing stairs
Crossed extension reflex (CER)	Flexion of one leg	Extension of opposite leg	Difficulty bridging with both legs flexed simultaneously Difficulty walking with a reciprocal arm/leg gait pattern
Palmar grasp reflex	Pressure in palm of hand	Flexion of digits into palmar grasp	Difficulty releasing objects from a palmar grasp (e.g., drinking glass, hairbrush, mop)
Plantar grasp reflex	Pressure to ball of foot	Flexion of toes	Curling of toes in shoes Difficulty walking with foot flat Absence of equilibrium responses in foot

*In adults who have sustained an insult to the central nervous system (CNS), the emergence of primitive reflexes may interfere with motor control recovery. Typically, these reflexes are assessed while the patient is sitting or supine with the head initially in midline, with the exception of the tonic labyrinthine reflexes.
†In adults with CNS dysfunction while engaged in occupational performance tasks.

Suck/Swallow Reflex

The patient with a suck/swallow reflex has difficulty eating. The involuntary protrusion and retraction of the tongue make it difficult to keep food and liquids in the oral cavity. The patient will not be able to suck from a straw.

Asymmetrical Tonic Neck Reflex

The patient with a persistent asymmetrical tonic neck reflex (ATNR) may have difficulty maintaining the head in midline while moving the eyes toward or past midline.[7] The patient may be unable to extend or flex an arm without turning the head.[7,16] In addition, the patient may be unable to bring the hands to midline. Thus the presence of the ATNR impedes bringing an object to the mouth, holding an object in both hands, or simultaneously looking at and grasping an object in front of the body.

Symmetrical Tonic Neck Reflex

The patient with a persistent symmetrical tonic neck reflex (STNR) cannot support the body weight on hands and knees, maintain balance in quadruped, and creep normally.[8] The patient struggles to move from the supine to sitting position because bending the head forward (flexed) to initiate the task increases extension in the legs. The patient is unable to bend at the hips to sit upright. The patient has difficulty with moving from sitting to standing. Because the arms and head are extended to initiate the movement, one or both legs may flex. Also, the patient who has had a CVA may demonstrate total flexion of the affected leg, resulting in an inability to bear weight.[16]

Tonic Labyrinthine Reflex

The patient who exhibits a poorly integrated tonic labyrinthine reflex (TLR) has severely limited movement. Examples of functional limitations are inability to lift the head in the supine position, to move from supine to sitting position using flexion of trunk and hips, to roll supine to prone (and vice versa), and to sit in a wheelchair for long periods.[8,16] When the patient attempts to move from supine to sitting position, extensor tone is initially dominant until halfway up, when flexor tone begins to take over. Flexor tone continues until full sitting is reached, when the head falls forward, the spine flexes, and then the patient falls forward.[7] Sitting in a wheelchair for extended periods can result in increased extensor tone as the patient hyperextends the neck to view the environment. With the increased extensor tone the patient slips into a semisupine position with feet off footplates[16] (Figure 6-3).

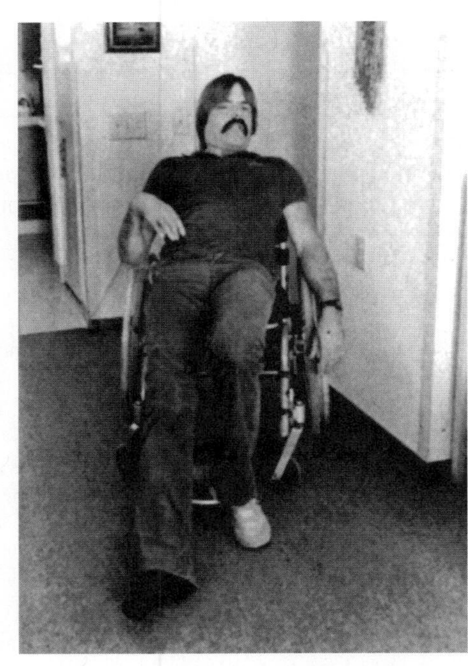

Figure 6-3 Functional influence of tonic labyrinthine reflex (TLR) on sitting up in a wheelchair.

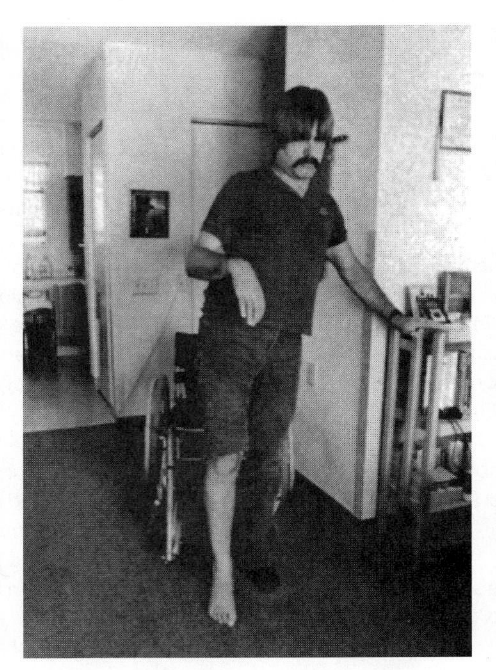

Figure 6-4 Positive supporting reflex (PSR).

CLINICAL PEARL

For clients who still have the TLR, be sure to tilt their chairs forward (slightly so as not to get too much flexion) during feeding to encourage flexion required for swallowing.

CLINICAL PEARL

Caregivers may need to be reminded to cleanse and dry the palms thoroughly and completely to avoid skin breakdown in clients with palmar grasp reflex who may hold hands fisted tightly.

Positive Supporting Reflex

The patient who exhibits a positive supporting reflex (PSR) has difficulty placing the heel on the ground for standing and walking. A persistent PSR interferes with foot-flat lower extremity weight bearing and weight shifting.[8,16] The patient has difficulty arising from a chair and descending steps because the leg remains stiffly in extension. The rigid leg can carry the patient's body weight but cannot adjust in any balance reactions. Therefore all balance reactions are compensated with other body parts[7] (Figure 6-4).

Crossed Extension Reflex

The patient who exhibits the crossed extension reflex (CER) has difficulty with developing a normal gait pattern because strong extension occurs in the affected leg as the unaffected leg is flexed. The patient has difficulty bridging (lifting buttocks while supine with both legs flexed) in bed.[7,16]

Palmar Grasp Reflex

The patient with a poorly integrated grasp reflex cannot release objects placed in the hand, even if active finger extension is present.[16]

CLINICAL PEARL

Clients who have a persisting palmar grasp may benefit from using built-up handles for utensils and implements.

Plantar Grasp Reflex

The patient with a poorly integrated plantar grasp reflex has difficulty keeping toes from curling in the shoes. Normal equilibrium responses in the foot do not develop if the plantar grasp reflex is present.

Functional Significance

The OT practitioner must observe for the influence of primitive reflexes as a part of the motor control evaluation. Observing a patient during his or her occupational performance tasks enhances the practitioner's understanding of the functional significance of the persistence of these reflexes in patients with CNS damage.

As the primitive reflexes become integrated in normal development, higher-level protective extension, righting, and equilibrium reactions emerge. In clients with CNS dysfunction, the OT evaluates automatic reactions, which are a part of the postural mechanism.

Automatic Reactions

Protective Extension Reactions

Protective extension reactions (extending the arms) are used to protect the head and face when a person is off balance or falling.[19,21] Without these reactions, the patient may fear moving or hesitate to bear weight on the affected side during bilateral or two-handed activities such as getting dressed, cutting meat with a knife and fork, or playing a game of pool.

Righting Reactions

The automatic righting reactions maintain or restore the normal position of the head in space (eyes parallel to the horizon) and its normal relationship with the trunk and limbs. Without effective righting responses, the patient has difficulty moving from one position to another such as going from the supine position to sit or stand in order to arise from bed.[8]

Equilibrium Reactions

Equilibrium reactions maintain and restore a person's balance in all activities.[8,26] They ensure sufficient postural alignment when the body's supporting surface is changed, thus altering a person's center of gravity. In mature equilibrium responses the patient's trunk elongates on the weight-bearing side. Without equilibrium responses, the patient has difficulty maintaining and recovering balance in all positions and activities. The patient with inadequate equilibrium reactions may be unable to sit unsupported while performing dressing activities or standing at a sink while performing oral hygiene activities.

Testing

Formal testing of protective extension, righting, and equilibrium reactions may be difficult because of the patient's cognitive and physical limitations. The OTA develops observational skills to note the absence or presence of righting, equilibrium, and protective extension during transfers and self-maintenance activities. Equilibrium and protective extension reactions can be observed when the patient shifts farther out of midline during functional activities. The OTA observes whether the patient can regain balance efficiently and effectively to complete the functional activity. Alternately, if the patient is unable to regain balance, the OTA observes whether protective responses are used to break a fall. The OT practitioner should be positioned to protect the patient if these responses fail. If reflexes or stereotypical patterns are not integrated and if protective extension, righting, and equilibrium reactions are impaired, the patient will have difficulty using the limbs for functional self-maintenance activities.

The Berg Balance Test[2,3] and Tinetti Test of Balance[48] provide convenient protocols to measure balance in adults. These tests are easy to administer and require little equipment. They can provide practitioners with techniques to measure outcomes.

Upper Extremity Motor Recovery

In addition to evaluating a patient's postural mechanism, the OT practitioner assesses upper extremity functional motion. The practitioner identifies where and to what extent stereotypical patterns of movement dominate the patient's motor control and where and under what conditions isolated movement is present. The therapist notes the degree to which the patient's abnormal postural mechanism interferes with selective volitional movement and determines in which direction of movement hypertonicity occurs and its effects on function.

The upper extremity motor recovery evaluation begins with observation of the patient's overall posture.

- Is the patient's posture symmetrical with equal weight on both hips (if sitting) or on both feet (if standing)?
- Is the head in midline or tilted to one side?
- Is one shoulder higher than the other (elevated)?
- Is the trunk twisted or long on one side and short on the other?
- How does the patient move in general?
- What is the quality of the movement?
- How does the client sequence and time movements?

Asymmetries impede the patient's ability to move the limbs normally and efficiently. Clients may lean to one side and exhibit unequal muscle tone or strength. They may tilt the head to the side. Keeping one's head to the side and elevating one shoulder are signs of asymmetry and may indicate a neurologic deficit.

Asymmetrical head position may interfere with movement because the person may not perceive his body in space accurately. It may be that one shoulder is actually depressed because of hypotonicity or flaccidity. Trunk elongation on one side also indicates discrepancies in muscle tone or muscle strength.

Trunk involvement suggests that postural control is impaired. Clients with trunk involvement may experience difficulty remaining upright. Absence of sufficient stability interferes with mobility as the client is unable to position the body effectively for coordinated movement. Over time, disuse of one side of the body may lead to muscle atrophy interfering with functional movement.

Quality of movement requires stability and precision. Clients who move in smooth coordinated patterns with ease show good quality of movement and can move as desired. A variety of factors may interfere with quality of movement: muscle tone abnormalities, neurologic processing deficits, musculoskeletal deficits, poor body awareness, and sensory processing difficulties. Clients who are trying to move an extremity experience changes in muscle tone that interfere with the coordinated muscle contractions of the agonist and antagonist, resulting in an uncoordinated movement. Neurologic processing deficits may cause poor timing and sequencing of muscle contractions, resulting in poor movements. These deficits may be subtle, resulting in slower reaction times (as found in clients with low cognitive abilities) or more severe as found in clients who have experienced a CVA. Many clients show poor quality of movement associated with musculoskeletal deficits such as those noted after orthopedic injuries. These quality-of-movement issues may arise as the client struggles with understanding the new sense of his or her body. Poor body awareness and sensory processing difficulties including poor kinesthesia (awareness of movement), proprioception (awareness of muscles and joints), and tactile awareness (feeling one's body) result in poor quality of movement. All of these systems may interfere with the timing and sequencing of movements and result in poor quality of movement.

Examining how the patient moves can provide insight into areas in need of remediation. Smooth coordinated movements and an easy transition from movement to movement are the hallmarks of functional movement. Slow movements with uneasy transitions indicate processing difficulties and/or underlying motor deficits. For example, some clients who have experienced CNS damage may experience difficulty planning movements. They may appear awkward or clumsy. They may underreach or overreach. Some clients forget how to do the movement altogether.

CLINICAL PEARL

Observe clients in a variety of environments and performing a variety of activities. This helps the practitioner understand the client's volition for activities and his or her reaction to different environments. Clients will perform better when doing activities that are meaningful to them or give them identity.

CLINICAL PEARL

Providing a mirror so that the client can see her performance may help her adjust movements. Providing tactile cues and simple brief verbal feedback may be effective in improving movement.

Intervention

OT focuses on achieving functional motion to the extent possible to achieve maximal independence while being engaged in occupational performance. The first step in intervention involves assessing the current abilities of the client. The patient usually sits during testing. However, observing upper extremity control in a standing patient may provide the OT practitioner with a better indication of the degree of impairment, especially if the patient will eventually be ambulatory. Functionally speaking, many occupational performance tasks (e.g., donning slacks, sweeping the floor) are performed while standing.

After general observations of the patient's functional motion and posture, the practitioner assesses more specifically the amount and type of motor recovery present in the upper extremities. Assessment and intervention may occur simultaneously. For example, if asymmetry is noted, the OT practitioner attempts to correct the asymmetry before continuing with the assessment. This process provides valuable information about the patient's ability to respond to therapeutic touch and how the patient's posture affects muscle tone and movement.

Understanding the client's goals and occupational performance desires is fundamental to intervention planning and execution. Once the practitioner identifies the direction of therapy, the practitioner determines the underlying motor control factors that may need to be addressed for intervention. Therapy includes developing activities that will challenge the motor control of the client and provide the client with practice in a supported environment. The goal of therapy is for the client to perform the desired occupation in the specific contexts in which the client lives and acts. For example, the goal may be for the client to dress himself at home. The practitioner analyzes the motor control movements that are required to make this happen. The goal is smoothly coordinated and effective movement patterns.

Dynamical systems theory proposes that movement is the result of many systems working collaboratively with each other. Earlier theories took a more hierarchical and linear approach toward motor recovery.[10] Brunnstrom's stages of motor recovery were developed specifically for examining clients with CVA. Brunnstrom's stages do not consider multiple systems, but they provide a developmental progression that may be helpful to consider along with more current motor control concepts. OT practitioners may find it helpful to develop intervention using meaningful occupations while addressing the stages of motor recovery in clients after a CVA.

CLINICAL PEARL

The *Model of Human Occupation Screening Tool* (MOHOST)[37] provides an occupation-based screening that allows practitioners to objectively examine a client's volition for occupations. Using this helps practitioners better understand their clients and design meaningful intervention.

Brunnstrom's Stages of Motor Recovery

In the 1950s and 1960s Brunnstrom observed progressive changes in motor function and behavior during the motor recovery process after a CVA (Box 6-1).[10] Figure 6-5 provides a framework for assessing motor recovery as described by Brunnstrom. The various stages of motor function, as adapted from Brunnstrom, are detailed in the following discussion.

No Motion

No motion can be elicited from the involved upper extremity.

Reflex Responses

These movements are limited to generalized or localized motor responses to specific sensory stimuli.[24] For example, a patient with a positive palmar grasp reflex involuntarily holds an object placed in the palm of the hand. Table 6-1 provides additional examples.

Associated Reactions

Abnormal increases in muscle tone in the involved extremities occur when activity requires intensive effort of the unaffected limbs. The involved extremities often move in a synergistic, mass pattern. Associated reactions can be elicited by resisting motion at a joint in an uninvolved limb or by having the patient squeeze

Box 6-1

Brunnstrom's Stages of Motor Recovery

1. No motion
2. Reflex responses
3. Associated reactions
4. Mass responses (synergistic)
5. Deviation from pattern
6. Wrist stability
7. Individual finger movement
8. Selected pattern with overlay
9. Selective movement

III. SENSORY MOTOR ASSESSMENT (continued)

OCCUPATIONAL THERAPY EVALUATION

F. Mass Pattern Responses: key: 0 = zero, W = weak, M = moderate, S = strong.
Observe active R.O.M. and effect of heat and trunk position on motion.

	ADMISSION		DISCHARGE	
1. FLEXION PATTERN	Right	Left	Right	Left
Shoulder abduction/elevation				
Elbow flexions				

Comments: Note any motion occurring at forearm, wrist and hand.

	ADMISSION		DISCHARGE	
2. EXTENSION PATTERN	Right	Left	Right	Left
Shoulder Adduction/Internal Rotation				
Elbow Extension				

Comments: Note any motions occurring at forearm, wrist and hand.

Key: N = normal, WE = with ease, WD = with difficulty, U = unable, NT = not tested

G. Deviation from Patterns

	ADMISSION		DISCHARGE	
	Right	Left	Right	Left
Shoulder add./Int. rot. with Elbow flexion				
Shoulder abduction with Elbow extension				
Forearm pronation with Elbow flexion				
Forearm supination with Elbow extension				

Comments:

H. Wrist and Hand Recovery: record grasp and pinch measurements

	ADMISSION		DISCHARGE	
	Right	Left	Right	Left
Stable Wrist During Grasp				
Mass Grasp: Notch #				
Mass Release (3 inch cube)				
Lateral Pinch				
Palmar Pinch				
Individual Finger Motions				

Comments:

I. Selective with Pattern Overlay

	ADMISSION		DISCHARGE	
	Right	Left	Right	Left
Integrate prox. to distal control (stack cones)				
Reciprocal total U.E. motion (tether ball)				
Rapid elbow flexion–extension				
Rapid wrist flexion–extension				

Comments:

HAND FUNCTION: (Functional Use Test)

Class #

Involved Side:

Describe highest function:

Figure 6-5 Upper extremity motor control assessment, part of the Occupational Therapy Stroke Evaluation. (Courtesy Occupational Therapy Department, Ranchos Los Amigos, Downey, Calif.)

an object with the unaffected hand. These reactions can also be observed during the patient's performance of transfers and other self-maintenance activities that require effort (Figure 6-6).

Mass Responses (Synergistic)

Voluntary motion is limited to total limb movements in flexion or extension. The patient is unable to isolate individual joint motion or deviate from the stereotypical movement pattern.[10,24] This situation can be evaluated by asking the patient to move at only one joint and observing where the motion actually occurs. Patients with synergistic movement responses cannot move one joint in isolation. The stereotypical patterns of movement may be seen partially or in full complement. The *flexion pattern response* consists of scapular adduction and elevation, humeral abduction and external rotation, elbow flexion, forearm supination, wrist flexion, and digit flexion (Figure 6-7, *A*). The *extension pattern response* consists of scapular abduction and depression, humeral adduction and internal rotation, elbow extension, forearm pronation, and wrist and finger flexion or extension (Figure 6-7, *B*).

Deviation from Pattern

Voluntary motor control deviates from the synergy through movement and is patterned predominantly when functional tasks are attempted. For example, a patient may be able to

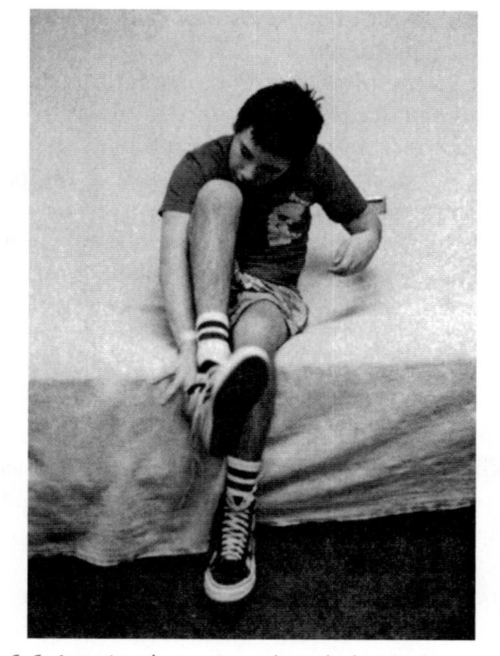

Figure 6-6 Associated reaction elicited during lower extremity dressing.

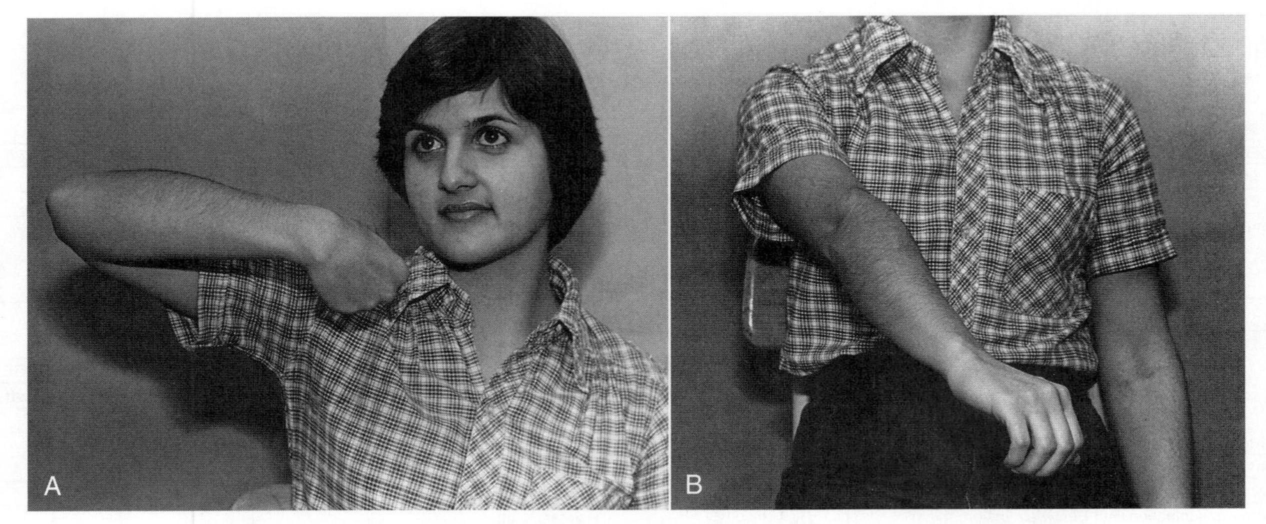

Figure 6-7 **A,** Flexion synergy in upper extremity. **B,** Extension synergy in upper extremity.

actively extend the wrist when asked but unable to use wrist extension while the shoulder is flexed (e.g., reaching for an item above the head). Testing involves asking the patient to perform movements that deviate from the synergies and observing the patient's ability to accomplish such movements successfully. The techniques are described in the following list[24]:

1. Ask the patient to touch the back of the uninvolved shoulder with the involved hand (requires scapular abduction and humeral horizontal adduction or scapular abduction with elbow flexion).
2. Ask the patient to touch, using the involved hand, the therapist's finger, which is held out to the patient's involved side (requires shoulder or humeral abduction with elbow extension).
3. Ask the patient to use the involved hand to pick up an object from the therapist's hand, positioned approximately 4 inches (10 cm) above the patient's involved knee (requires elbow flexion with forearm pronation).
4. Ask the patient to reach out in front of the body using the involved hand to receive an object in the palm (requires elbow extension with forearm supination).

The OT practitioner can detect whether the patient is beginning to deviate from mass patterns by observing the patient performing these movements. Also, observations of the patient engaged in occupational performance tasks indicate when a patient is beginning to deviate from these patterns.

Wrist Stability

The OT practitioner asks the patient to make a fist and observes for stability of the wrist joint in extension. The patient must also be observed while performing tasks such as grasping a toothbrush or holding a spoon during self-feeding.

Individual Finger Movements

The OT practitioner asks the patient to touch the tip of each finger with the tip of the thumb or to perform a tapping motion with the fingers against the table or the patient's leg. The practitioner observes for isolated selective movements. If muscle tone is normal, grasp and pinch strength can be measured by using a dynamometer, bulbometer, or pinch gauge.

Selective Pattern with Overlay

Joint movement in the affected limb may be isolated with voluntary control, and motion may occur in a variety of planes and directions. However, when the limb is functionally stressed (e.g., patient attempting to button small buttons on a shirt sleeve), synergistic patterns may be seen. The OT practitioner observes for compensatory movements during functional activities if the patient is in this stage of motor recovery. The patient may lean to the uninvolved side to raise the involved hand over the head. Shoulder elevation may be used to increase shoulder joint ROM on the involved side. The patient in this stage has difficulty performing rapid reciprocal motions such as alternating wrist flexion and extension. During evaluation of rapid reciprocal movements, the patient's uninvolved limb should be compared with the involved limb.[24]

Selective Movement

Selective movement is the ability to control movements at each individual joint. The OT practitioner observes for selective movement and control while the patient engages in functional activities.

In summary, Brunnstrom provided a framework for anticipated motor recovery in stroke patients. The last stage of motor recovery is selective movement. However, not all patients will reach this level of recovery. An understanding of Brunnstrom's stages of motor recovery of the upper extremity after a CVA may help practitioners develop intervention strategies. Combining this information with dynamical systems theory suggests that practitioners should engage clients in occupation-based activities to promote the use of the upper extremity. Practitioners may develop activities that work for each stage and promote the progression through the stages this way. Clients will participate in activities with more intensity if they are motivated and see the activities as meaningful to them.

CLINICAL PEARL

Constraint-induced therapy helps clients regain motor functioning by promoting the use of the affected extremity in daily activities. Practitioners are urged to examine this intervention technique.

Evaluating Functional Use of the Limbs

The OT practitioner helps clients regain upper extremity functioning to return to purposeful and meaningful activities within their physical and social environments. After interviewing the client to understand the client's occupational needs, evaluating the functional status of the involved limb helps the practitioner design realistic and functional goals.

If he or she has achieved service competency, the OTA may assess a patient's functional abilities with simple, structured tests. For example, the *Functional Test for the Hemiplegic/Paretic Upper Extremity* assesses the patient's ability to use the involved arm for occupational performance tasks. It contains items ranging from basic stabilization to more difficult tasks requiring distal fine manipulation with proximal stability. Examples of specific tasks include holding a pouch, stabilizing a jar, wringing a wet washcloth, interlocking and zipping a zipper, folding a sheet, and installing an overhead light bulb. This test provides objective data of the patient's functional abilities and is administered in 30 minutes or less.[52]

The OT practitioner also observes the patient during self-maintenance to determine functional use and potential for functional use of the involved extremities. Whether the practitioner uses a simple structured test or observations from a checklist for activities of daily living (ADL), the level of functional assist of the involved limb must be established to set realistic goals. The following descriptors are suggested[1]:

- *Minimal stabilizing assist.* The patient can use the involved upper extremity to stabilize objects being manipulated by the uninvolved extremity. The involved extremity is placed, and stabilization accomplished by the limb's weight. For example, the involved upper extremity is placed on a piece of paper to stabilize it while the patient writes.
- *Minimal active assist.* The patient can use the involved upper extremity to assist actively in a single part of an activity (e.g., actively placing the hand on a piece of paper for writing, actively holding the involved arm away from the body for dressing or hygiene activities).
- *Maximal active assist.* The patient can use the involved arm and hand in all activities that require motor control for pushing or pulling, stabilizing, and gross grasp and release. For example, while writing a letter, the patient can push the paper upward with the involved arm and hand.
- *Incorporation of involved upper extremity in all bilateral tasks.* The patient can use the involved upper extremity to assist the uninvolved extremity in most occupational performance tasks, although speed and coordination may be impaired. For example, the patient can move both arms above the head to put on a pullover shirt, but movements are slow and cautious on the involved side.

The Functional Independence Measure (FIM)[50] is used to determine the client's ability to complete activities of daily living. The FIM measures the type and amount of assistance required for the individual to perform activities effectively. The FIM subscales include self-care, sphincter control, transfers, locomotion, communication, and social cognition. Degrees of independence are graded on a scale of 1 (total assistance with a helper) to 7 (complete assistance with no helper).

OT practitioners also use the Physical Performance Test (1999)[41] as a measure of functioning. This test provides an overview of balance, manipulation, and basic motor skills. Although the test is not standardized, it provides a format to review performance and is readily available to clinicians. It consists of the following tasks: writing a sentence, simulated eating, lifting a book to a shelf, putting on a jacket, picking up a penny, turning 360 degrees, and walking.

Occupational Therapy Considerations Based on Results of Functional Motion Assessment

The OT practitioner bases treatment on the patient's overall evaluation results, including cognition, vision, sensation, psychological aspects, and occupational needs,[38] and the motor control evaluation. Chapter 21 describes one approach to motor control treatment in detail; others are discussed in Chapter 10. The following discussion offers some general guidelines for treatment.

Occupation-Based Activity

Current motor control theories suggest practitioners evaluate the client's current functioning and design activities to meet their occupational needs. Practitioners should consider focusing on postural control and upper extremity functioning while designing tasks that are meaningful to the client. The goal is for the client to complete activities that are closest to the actual occupations they will engage in on discharge from therapy. Participating in whole occupations results in the best carryover and will produce muscle coupling and better co-contraction.

Practitioners may also want to help clients perform the actual occupation as successfully as possible, which may include adapting the activity or providing assistive technology. Success using adaptations serves as a motivator to clients and allows them to regain occupations more quickly resulting in better motor outcomes through participation. For example, instead of waiting to gain postural control before beginning a fine motor task, practitioners may decide to provide adaptive seating (external postural control) to allow the client to engage in the desired occupation. The practitioner would continue to work on postural control, but in the meantime the client would be able to engage in the fine motor task.

Abnormal muscle tone is frequently considered an impairment to functional movement. Therefore practitioners may address muscle tone abnormalities by providing facilitation (increasing muscle tone) or inhibition (decreasing muscle tone) techniques. These techniques are supported in the neurodevelopmental treatment (NDT) frame of reference, which argues that clients must achieve typical muscle tone before moving.[8]

NDT proposes that practitioners first normalize muscle tone and then help clients engage in typical movement patterns by providing gentle cueing techniques at key points of control. Key points of control include the hips, pelvis, shoulders, hands, or trunk. Practitioners who understand typical movement patterns help clients move in the typical pattern. This may involve facilitating or inhibiting specific muscle groups as the client moves.

Facilitation

For hypotonia and limited to no motion in the upper extremities, the OT practitioner must facilitate increased muscle tone necessary for stability. Weight bearing, as well as tactile and proprioceptive input, may be used to increase muscle tone. The practitioner provides input in such a way as to avoid overstimulating specific muscles or encouraging abnormal patterns of movement.

Therapeutic activities for improving strength may be used if motion is selective (i.e., not patterned) in the involved upper extremity. A primary goal of intervention should be to establish a balance of strength and tone between the agonist and antagonist muscles.[11] The involved arm can be positioned as normally as possible to provide appropriate sensory feedback while the patient is performing occupational tasks. Patient and family education in proper positioning and joint protection is important to prevent trauma to joint structures.

Inhibition

For hypertonia the OT practitioner uses inhibitive techniques to decrease the abnormal muscle tone and patterns of movement. The motor learning and sensorimotor approaches described in Chapters 10 and 21 may be appropriate, depending on the disability, severity, and distribution of the hypertonia and the associated problems. The goal of treatment is to balance the muscle tone for more normal movement. This requires inhibition of the hypertonic muscles and facilitation of the antagonist muscles, using one of the sensorimotor approaches.

Casting or Orthoses

In some patients, hypertonicity is severe enough to require progressive inhibitory casting or orthoses.[5,32,38,46] Casting provides the circumferential pressure necessary to prevent soft tissue contractures and maintain the muscle's normal length for functional ROM.[28,34]

Serial casting is most successful when a soft tissue contracture has been present for less than 6 months. A series of casts is applied to obtain the maximal end range of a contracted muscle. The final cast may be bivalved (cut into two halves) and used as a night positioner. However, many clinicians prefer bivalving *all* casts in the series to prevent skin breakdown.[5] A bivalved cast also allows the practitioner to remove the cast for therapy on a regular basis. Various types of casts can be used to decrease hypertonicity in the adult with CNS damage.

A combination of peripheral nerve blocks and casting or orthoses is often used.[5,28,31] The physician can administer short-acting lidocaine blocks before applying an inhibitory cast to make limb positioning easier. Phenol nerve blocks, also given by a physician, can last up to 3 months. Nerve blocks allow the therapist to increase antagonist control and strength to achieve a balance of muscle control between the agonist and antagonist muscles.[28,49]

Physical Agent Modalities

Physical agent modalities such as cold, heat, and neuromuscular electrical stimulation can be used in preparation for or along with purposeful activity. These modalities can help to reduce hypertonicity temporarily so as to allow for the development of antagonistic control; modalities must be provided by a practitioner with established service competency.

Patients who experience severe pain with hypertonicity may require evaluation of the cause of pain. Drug therapy (as prescribed by the physician) and other pain management techniques may be included in the program plan. If a patient has a drug therapy regimen, the OT practitioner must recognize the potential side effects. The practitioner must communicate to the medical staff any observed side effects that interfere with the patient's overall function.

Although motor control may be adequate for the performance of occupational tasks, sensory and perceptual deficits may limit the patient's success in performing functional activities. Perceptual deficits may alter the patient's abilities, thus requiring the occupational therapist to lower expected goals.[4] (See Chapters 9 and 23 for further discussions on perception.)

Coordination

Coordination is the harmonious interaction of muscles throughout the limb that allows for the production of accurate controlled movement. Such movement is characterized by smoothness, rhythm, and appropriate speed. Voluntary control of muscle tone, postural tone, and balance among muscle groups is necessary for coordinated movement.

Coordinated movement requires that all the elements of the neuromuscular structures and functions be intact. Coordinated movement depends on the contraction of specific agonist muscles with the simultaneous relaxation of the corresponding antagonist muscles, anchored by co-contraction of the joint-stabilizing muscles. Proprioception, kinesthesia, and body schema also must be intact. The patient must be able to judge space accurately and to direct body parts through space to the desired target with correct timing.[6]

Occurrence of Incoordination

Coordination of muscle action is controlled by the cerebellum and influenced by the extrapyramidal tracts. Coordinated movement also requires knowledge of body schema and body-to-space relationships. Because of these multiple sources of control, many types of lesions can result in disturbances of coordination.[6] Causes include diseases and injuries of muscles and peripheral nerves, lesions of the posterior columns of the spinal cord, and lesions of the cerebral cortex. Limb paralysis due to a PNS lesion prevents coordination testing even though CNS mechanisms are intact.[31]

Common signs of incoordination seen by the OT practitioner include the following:

- *Ataxia* is impaired gross coordination and gait. The patient with ataxia may have visible tremorlike movements. Ataxia is seen in the delayed initiation of motor responses, in errors in range and force of movement, and in errors in rate and regularity of movement. For example, an ataxic patient cannot calibrate the force of grasp and might crush a Styrofoam cup. The patient's gait demonstrates a wide base of support (legs far apart) with a reduced or absent arm swing. Step length may be uneven, and the patient may tend to fall toward one side. Ataxia results in a lack of postural stability; patients tend to fixate or tighten specific muscle groups to compensate for the instability.[14,22,30]
- *Adiadochokinesia* ("not moving together") is an inability to perform rapidly alternating movements such as forearm supination and pronation or elbow flexion and extension.[17] For example, a patient has difficulty dusting or washing windows.
- *Dysmetria* ("faulty distance between two points") is an inability to estimate the ROM necessary to reach the target of movement. It is evident when touching the finger to the nose or placing an object onto a table.[17] A patient has difficulty judging distances and may knock a cup while reaching for it.
- *Dyssynergia* ("faulty working together") is a decomposition of movement in which voluntary movements are broken into their component parts and appear jerky. Problems in articulation (see dysarthria entry below) and phonation may be present.[17]
- *Tremor* is an involuntary shaking or trembling motion. Tremors are classified according to their type. An *intention tremor* occurs during voluntary movement, is often intensified at the termination of movement, and is often seen in patients with multiple sclerosis. The patient with an intention tremor may have difficulty performing tasks that require accuracy and precision of limb placement (e.g., drinking from a cup, inserting a key in a door). A *resting tremor* is present in the absence of voluntary movement (occurs while the patient is not moving). A *pill-rolling tremor,* in which the individual appears to be rolling a pill between the thumb and index and middle fingers, is a type of resting tremor often seen in patients with Parkinson's disease.
- *Rebound phenomenon of Holmes* ("to bounce or spring again") is a lack of the *check reflex,* or the inability to stop a motion quickly to avoid striking something. For example, if the patient's arm is bent against the resistance of the therapist and the resistance is suddenly and unexpectedly removed, the patient's hand will hit the face or body.[14,17]
- Nystagmus is an involuntary movement of the eyeballs in an up-and-down, back-and-forth, or rotating direction. After rotation or spinning of the body and head in space, nystagmus is the normal response that helps a person regain balance and orientation. Nystagmus can interfere with head control and fine adjustments required for balance.[17]
- *Dysarthria,* or faulty speech production, is explosive or slurred speech caused by the incoordination of the speech mechanism. The patient's speech may also vary in pitch, may appear nasal and tremulous, or both.[14,17]
- *Choreiform movements* are uncontrolled, irregular, purposeless, quick, jerky, and dysrhythmical movements of variable distribution that may also occur during sleep.[17]
- *Athetoid movements,* or movements without stability, are slow, wormlike, arrhythmical movements that primarily affect the distal portions of the extremities. *Athetosis* occurs in predictable patterns in the same subject and is not present during sleep.[17]
- *Spasms* are sudden, involuntary contractions of a muscle or large groups of muscles.[14] In a patient with a spinal cord injury, spasms often cause violent and involuntary straightening of the legs.
- *Dystonia* is faulty muscle tension or tone. Dystonic movements tend to involve large portions of the body and produce grotesque posturing with bizarre writhing movements.[6,14]
- *Ballism,* or projectile movement, is a rare symptom produced by continuous, gross, abrupt contractions of the axial and proximal musculature of the extremity. It causes the limb to fly out suddenly and occurs on one side of the body.[14,17]

Clinical Assessment of Coordination

Incoordination consists of errors in rate, rhythm, range, direction, and force of movement.[22] Observation is an important element of the evaluation. The neurologic examination for incoordination may include the nose-finger-nose test, the finger-nose test, the knee pat (pronation-supination) test, and the finger wiggling test.[6,31] Such tests can reveal dysmetria, dyssynergia, adiadochokinesia, tremors, and ataxia. The neurologist usually performs these examinations.

Occupational Therapy Assessment of Coordination

Engagement in occupation is the ultimate goal of OT; therefore the OT practitioner seeks to translate the clinical evaluation to a functional one. Selected activities and specific performance tests can reveal the effect of incoordination on function, which is the OT practitioner's primary concern. The practitioner can observe for coordination difficulties during the patient's self-maintenance evaluation and training. The practitioner should observe for irregularity in the rate or force of the movement and sudden corrective movements in an attempt to compensate for incoordination. Movement during the performance of functional activities may appear irregular and jerky and may overreach the target.[31]

The following general guidelines and questions can be used when the practitioner is evaluating incoordination:

1. The occupational therapist evaluates the patient's muscle tone and joint mobility.
2. The occupational therapist and the OTA provide manual stability to joints proximally to distally during functional tasks and note any differences in performance with and without stabilization.

Table 6-2 Tests for Upper Limb Function

Test	Reference	Testing Method
Functional Tests		
Motor Assessment Scale: Upper Limb Items	Carr et al, 1985; Poole and Whitney, 1988; Malouin et al, 1994	The test consists of eight separate motor items, each measured on a 7-point scale. Three items measure upper limb function: upper arm function, hand movements, advanced hand activities. Administration is strictly standardized. For patients who achieve top scores, additional tests of dexterity such as the NHPT need to be performed.
Nine-Hole Peg Test (NHPT)	Mathiowetz et al, 1985	A measure of dexterity. Time taken to complete the test is measured as the patient grasps nine pegs and places them in holes on a board.
Grip Force	Mathiowetz, 1990; Bohannon et al, 1993; Hermsdorfer and Mai, 1996	Grip-force dynamometer.
Spiral Test	Verkerk et al, 1990	A measure of coordination. Patient draws a line as quickly as possible between two spirals, separated by a distance of 1 cm, without touching either spiral. Particularly useful for a patient with cerebellar ataxia.
Arm Motor Mobility Test (AMAT)	Kopp et al, 1997	Measures ability to perform 13 activities of daily life composed of one to three component parts. The time taken to perform each task is measured with a stopwatch; the actions are videotaped and rated on 6-point scales.
Action Research Arm Test (ARA)	Van der Lee et al, 2001	The ability to grasp, move, and release objects of different size, weight, and shape is tested by measuring three subtests (grasp, grip, pinch) on a 4-point (0-3) scale. Points 2 and 3 are qualitative in the original scale, but subjectivity can be overcome by setting time limits for each item.
Functional Independence Measure	Uniform Data System for Medical Rehabilitation	Measures the types and amount of assistance a person requires to perform basic life activities effectively (self-care, sphincter control, transfers, locomotion, communication, social cognition): 1 (total assistance, helper) to 7 (complete independence, no helper).
Measures of Real-Life Arm Use		
Motor Activity Log: Amount of Use Scale (AOU)	Taub et al, 1993	Provides information about actual use of the limb in life situations. Patient reports at semistructured interview whether and how well, on a 6-point (0-5) scale, 14 daily activities were performed during a specified period.
Actual Amount of Use Test	Taub et al, 1993	Measures actual use of the limb on 21 items using a 3-point rating scale. Patients are videotaped.
Biomechanical Tests	Trombly, 1993	Kinematic analysis of reaching.
Shoulder ROM Tests	Mngoma et al, 1990	Isokinetic dynamometry: LIDO Active System†, a valid and reliable measure of resistance to passive external rotation of the glenohumeral joint. Goniometer plus hand-held dynamometer (to standardize force).
Tests of Isometric Strength		Handheld dynamometry, grip force‡ dynamometry, pinch force‡ dynamometry
Tests of Sensation	Lincoln et al, 1998; Carey 1995	Nottingham Sensory Assessment Tactile Discrimination Test Proprioceptive Discrimination Test

From Carr JH, Shepherd RB: Stroke rehabilitation: guidelines for exercise and training to optimize motor skill, St Louis, 2003, Butterworth Heinemann.
*Conditions of testing must be standardized.
†Loredan Biomedical Inc., 3650 Industrial Boulevard, West Sacramento, CA, 95691, USA.
‡Digital Pinch/Grip Analyser, MIE Medical Research, Leeds, United Kingdom (see Sunderland A et al: Enhanced physical therapy improves recovery of arm function after stroke: a randomised controlled trial. *J Neurol Neurosurg Psychiatry*. 1992;55:530-535. 1989).

3. The occupational therapist and the OTA observe for resting or intention tremor during functional activities.
4. The occupational therapist and OTA observe for any noticeable signs of incoordination during therapy sessions.
5. The occupational therapist and the OTA observe whether the patient becomes more uncoordinated in distracting environments.

Several standardized tests of motor function and manual dexterity are available, as outlined by Smith.[45] These include the Purdue Pegboard,[40] the Minnesota Rate of Manipulation Test,[33] the Lincoln-Oscretsky Motor Development Scale,[29] the Pennsylvania Bi-Manual Work Sample,[39] the Crawford Small Parts Dexterity Test,[15] and the Jebsen-Taylor Hand Function Test.[25] The occupational therapist and the OTA with established service competency may administer one or more of these tests during the evaluation of coordination. For additional tests of upper limb function, see Table 6-2.[12]

CLINICAL PEARL

OT philosophy is based on the premise that meaningful activity helps clients reengage in their occupations. Therefore meaningful activities are both a means and an end product of therapy. Research shows that clients perform movements more efficiently and with better coordination when they are engaged in a meaningful task-oriented activity. Furthermore, clients engage in more repetitions of movement. Therefore the OT practitioner working to help clients improve motor function must first identify the activities and occupations that are meaningful to the individual client. Finding activities that are closely related to the client's occupations will help with motor recovery.

Summary

Motor control is the ability to make continuous postural adjustments and to regulate body and limb movements in response to functional situations. It results from the interaction of complex neurologic systems. Evaluation of motor control includes assessment of the postural mechanism, selective movement, and coordination.

The presence of abnormal elements of motor control affects the quality of movements and the ability to perform functional tasks in all areas of occupation. The occupational therapist evaluates muscle tone and upper extremity motor recovery. The OTA may assess aspects of the postural reflex mechanism and coordination using simple structured tests. The OTA also observes for abnormal motor control while the patient is engaged in functional activities. The results of the motor control evaluation along with an occupation-based interview guide the practitioner in selecting the appropriate treatment approaches including sensorimotor approaches or rehabilitative and compensatory methods.

Selected Reading Guide Questions

1. What are the roles of the occupational therapist and the OTA in the evaluation and treatment of an adult with CNS dysfunction who has a motor control deficit? How do these roles change with the establishment of service competency and with experience in a particular setting?
2. What are the components of the normal postural reflex mechanism?
3. Define *normal* muscle tone.
4. Describe the characteristics of normal muscle tone. Give an example of how normal muscle tone varies depending on the type of occupational performance task.
5. Describe the characteristics of hypotonicity.
6. Describe the characteristics of hypertonicity.
7. Diagrammatically depict the spectrum of normal and abnormal muscle tone.
8. Define *specific primitive reflexes,* and describe how the OT practitioner would assess for their presence.
9. Describe the functional difficulties encountered when the following primitive reflexes persist during the performance of functional activities in the adult who has sustained a CNS insult: (a) asymmetrical tonic neck reflex; (b) symmetrical tonic neck reflex; (c) tonic labyrinthine reflex; (d) crossed extension reflex; and (e) grasp reflex.
10. Define the expected stages of motor recovery in an adult after CNS dysfunction caused by a CVA.
11. Describe the upper extremity flexion and extension pattern responses typically observed in the patient who has sustained a CVA.
12. Define fine coordination.
13. Analyze the stability and mobility necessary to perform specific occupational performance tasks such as feeding and dressing.
14. List five types of incoordination, and describe the functional impact on an adult's performance of ADL. For example, "Ataxia would interfere with self-feeding because ... "

References

1. Andric M: Projecting the upper extremity functional level. *In Professional Staff Association of Rancho Los Amigos Medical Center: Stroke rehabilitation: state of the art, 1984,* Downey, CA, 1984, Los Amigos Research and Education Institute.
2. Berg K, Wood-Dauphinee S, Williams J, Gayton D: Measuring balance in the elderly: preliminary development of an instrument, *Physiother Can* 41:304–311, 1989.
3. Berg KO, Maki BE, Williams JI, et al: Clinical and laboratory measures of postural balance in an elderly population, *Arch Phys Med Rehabil* 73(11):1073–1080, Nov 1992.
4. Bernspang B, Viitanen M, Erickson S: Impairments of perceptual and motor functions: their influence on self-care ability 4-6 years after a stroke, *Occup Ther J Res* 9:27–37, 1989.
5. Berrol S: The treatment of physical disorders following brain injury. In Wood R, Eames P, editors: *Models of brain injury rehabilitation,* Baltimore, 1989, Johns Hopkins University Press.
6. Bickerstaff ER: *Neurological examination in clinical practice,* ed 3, London, 1973, Blackwell.
7. Bobath B: *Abnormal postural reflex activity caused by brain lesions,* ed 2, London, 1975, Heinemann.
8. Bobath B: *Adult hemiplegia: evaluation and treatment,* ed 2, London, 1978, Heinemann.
9. Bohannon RW, Smith MB: Interrater reliability of a modified Ashworth scale of muscle spasticity, *Phys Ther* 67:206–207, 1987.
10. Brunnstrom S: *Movement therapy in hemiplegia,* New York, 1970, Harper & Row.
11. Carr JH, Shepherd RB: *A motor relearning program for stroke,* ed 2, Rockville, MD, 1987, Aspen.
12. Carr JH, Shepherd RB: *Stroke rehabilitation: guidelines for exercise and training to optimize motor skill,* St. Louis, 2003, Butterworth Heinemann.
13. Charness A: *Stroke/head injury: a guide to functional outcomes in physical therapy management,* Rockville, MD, 1986, Aspen.
14. Chusid JG: *Correlative neuroanatomy and functional neurology,* ed 18, Los Altos, CA, 1982, Lange.
15. Crawford Small Parts Dexterity Test, New York, 1981, Psychological Corporation.
16. Davies PM: *Steps to follow: a guide to treatment of adult hemiplegia,* New York, 1985, Springer Verlag.
17. deGroot J: *Correlative neuroanatomy,* ed 21, East Norwalk, Conn, 1991, Appleton & Lange.
18. DeMyer W: *Technique of the neurologic examination: a programmed text,* ed 2, New York, 1974, McGraw-Hill.

19. Farber S: *Neurorehabilitation: a multisensory approach*, Philadelphia, 1982, WB Saunders.
20. Felten DL, Felten SY: A regional and systemic overview of functional neuroanatomy. In Farber S, editor: *Neurorehabilitation: a multisensory approach*, Philadelphia, 1982, WB Saunders.
21. Fiorentino M: *Normal and abnormal development: the influence of primitive reflexes on motor development*, Springfield, IL, 1972, Thomas.
22. Ghez C: The cerebellum. In Kandel ER, Schwartz JH, Jessel TM, editors: *Principles of neural science*, ed 3, New York, 1991, Elsevier.
23. Griffith ER: Spasticity. In Rosenthal M, Griffifth ER, Bond MR, Miller JD, editors: *Rehabilitation of the head-injured adult*, Philadelphia, 1983, FA Davis.
24. Hazboun V: *Occupational therapy evaluation guide for adult hemiplegia*, Downey, CA, 1991, Los Amigos Research and Education Institute.
25. Jebsen RH, et al: An objective and standardized test of hand function, *Arch Phys Med Rehabil* 50:311–319, 1969.
26. Jewell MJ: Overview of the structure and function of the central nervous system. In Umphred DA, editor: *Neurological rehabilitation*, ed 2, St. Louis, 1990, Mosby.
27. Johnstone M: *Restoration of motor function in the stroke patient*, ed 2, New York, 1983, Churchill Livingstone.
28. Keenan MA: The orthopedic management of spasticity, *J Head Trauma Rehabil* 2:62, 1987.
29. Lincoln-Oseretsky Motor Development Scale: Chicago, 1954, Stoelting Co.
30. Marsden CD: The physiological basis of ataxia, *Physiotherapy* 61:326, 1975.
31. Mayo Clinic and Mayo Clinic Foundation: *Clinical examinations in neurology*, ed 5, Philadelphia, 1981, WB Saunders.
32. McPherson JJ, Kreimeyer D, Aalderks M, Gallagher T: A comparison of dorsal and volar resting hand splints in the reduction of hypertonus, *Am J Occup Ther* 36:664, 1982.
33. Minnesota Rate of Manipulation Test: Circle Pines, MN, 1969, American Guidance Service.
34. Newton RA: Motor control. In Umphred DA, editor: *Neurological rehabilitation*, ed 2, St. Louis, 1990, Mosby.
35. O'Brien J, Lewin J: Part I; Translating motor control and motor learning principles into occupational therapy practice with children and youth, *AOTA CEU article. Invited paper*, November 2008.
36. Okamoto GA: *Physical medicine and rehabilitation*, Philadelphia, 1984, WB Saunders.
37. Parkinson S, Forsyth K, Kielhofner G: *Model of Human Occupation Screening Tool (MOHOST), Version 2.0, Model of Human Occupation Clearinghouse*, 2006, University of Illinois at Chicago.
38. Pelland MJ: Occupational therapy and stroke rehabilitation. In Kaplan PE, Cerrillo LJ, editors: *Stroke rehabilitation*, Boston, 1986, Butterworth.
39. Pennsylvania Bi-Manual Work Sample, Circle Pines, MN, Educational Test Bureau, American Guidance Service.
40. Pegboard Purdue: Chicago, 1948/1961/1987, Science Research Associates.
41. Reuben DB, Siu AL: An objective measure of physical function of elderly outpatients: the Physical Performance Test, *J Am Geriatr Soc.* 38:1105–1112, 1990.
42. Ryerson S: Hemiplegia resulting from vascular insult or disease. In Umphred DA, editor: *Neurological rehabilitation*, ed 2, St. Louis, 1990, Mosby.
43. Schneider F: Traumatic spinal cord injury. In Umphred DA, editor: *Neurological rehabilitation*, ed 2, St. Louis, 1990, Mosby.
44. Shumway-Cook A, Woollacott M: *Motor control: theory and practical applications*, ed 2, Philadelphia, 2001, Lippincott Williams & Wilkins.
45. Smith HD: Occupational therapy assessment and treatment. In Hopkins HL, Smith HD, editors: *Willard and Spackman's occupational therapy*, ed 8, Philadelphia, 1993, Lippincott.
46. Snook JH: Spasticity reduction splint, *Am J Occup Ther* 33:648, 1979.
47. Thilmann AF, Fellows SJ, Garms E: The mechanism of spastic muscle hypertonus, *BRN* 114:233–244, 1991.
48. Tinetti ME: Performance oriented assessment of mobility problems in elderly patients, *J Am Geriatric Soc* 34:119–126, 1986.
49. Tomas ES, et al: Nonsurgical management of upper extremity deformities after traumatic brain injury, *Phys Med Rehabil State Art Rev* 7, 1993.
50. Uniform Data System for Medical Rehabilitation (2008). The FIM System.
51. Urbscheit NL: Cerebellar dysfunction. In Umphred DA, editor: *Neurological rehabilitation*, St. Louis, 1990, Mosby.
52. Wilson DJ, Baker LL, Craddock JA: *Functional Test for the Hemiplegic/Paretic Upper Extremity*, Downey, CA, 1984, Los Amigos Research and Education Institute.

Recommended Reading

Boehme R: *Improving upper body control*, Tucson, Ariz, 1988, Therapy Skills Builders.

Cech D, Martin ST: *Functional movement development across the life span*, ed 2, Philadelphia, 2002, WB Saunders.

Pedretti LW, Early MB: *Occupational therapy practice skills for physical dysfunction*, ed 5, St. Louis, 2001, Mosby.

Shumway-Cook M, Woollacott M: *Motor control: theory and practical applications*, Baltimore, 2001, Lippincott Williams & Wilkins.

CHAPTER 7 Assessment of Joint Range of Motion*

CINDY LISKA AND TERRI R. GONZALEZ

Key Terms

Range of motion
Joint movement
Active range of motion
Passive range of motion
Functional range of motion
Planes of movement
Goniometer
Stationary bar
Movable bar

Chapter Objectives

After studying this chapter, the student or practitioner will be able to do the following:

1. Define goniometry in relation to range of motion.
2. Describe functional range of motion in relation to activities of daily living.
3. State 11 basic principles for joint measurement.
4. Determine range-of-motion measurements of the major upper extremity joints.
5. Contrast active and passive range of motion.
6. Describe basic goniometry testing positions of the upper extremity.
7. Recommend a therapeutic exercise program based on goniometric measurements.
8. Describe the three cardinal planes of movement.

Range of motion (ROM) is the extent of movement that occurs at a joint. The human body contains several types of joints, muscle tissue, tendons, and other supporting structures that allow for a high degree of joint mobility. Many factors (e.g., disease processes, trauma, periarticular changes) can adversely affect joint movement. Development and maintenance of the greatest ROM maximize function. The study of joint range is the foundation for understanding how movement—or the lack of movement—affects how people engage in occupation.[3] From an anatomic standpoint, normal joint movement and muscular strength facilitate effortless movement in life activities, from simple to complex. Joint measurement is an important tool in the assessment of physical dysfunction in conditions such as cerebrovascular accident (CVA, stroke); arthritis; fractures; and general debility.

Joint measurement data assist the occupational therapy (OT) practitioner in evaluating progress or lack of progress toward treatment outcomes. Many patients are motivated by seeing concrete improvement based on recorded ROM measures. ROM data are important for establishing a baseline database, but this information must be linked to occupation-based activity.[3] Increases in motion are not significant unless the person has gained in function such as in the ability to dress independently because of increased ROM.[2] Simply put, ROM is joint movement: active, passive, or a combination of both. Motion occurs in an arc; the joint acts as the axis or pivot of the arc (Figure 7-1). Active range of motion (AROM) is the arc of motion through which the joint passes when voluntarily moved by muscles acting on the joint. Passive range of motion (PROM) is the arc of motion through which the joint passes when moved by an outside force. Normally, PROM is slightly greater than AROM.[9] ROM is measured by an instrument or tool known as a *goniometer.*

Role of the Occupational Therapy Assistant in Joint Measurement

The extent of the occupational therapy assistant's (OTA's) involvement in ROM assessment is determined by the supervising occupational therapist in agreement with the applicable laws and professional practice standards of the particular state.[4,6] In many clinical practices the OTA performs basic goniometry of the upper extremity. The role of the OTA in this area should be based on competency level, and the OTA must consider legislation and restrictions governing the practice setting.

General Principles of Joint Measurement

The OT practitioner must have complete understanding of (1) the degree and type of motion that will occur at a specific joint; (2) average or normal ROM[7]; and (3) how to position himself or herself and the patient during measurement.[10] Establishing good habits for approaching the patient

*Lorraine Williams Pedretti and Michael K. Davis contributed large portions of this chapter to the first edition of the book.

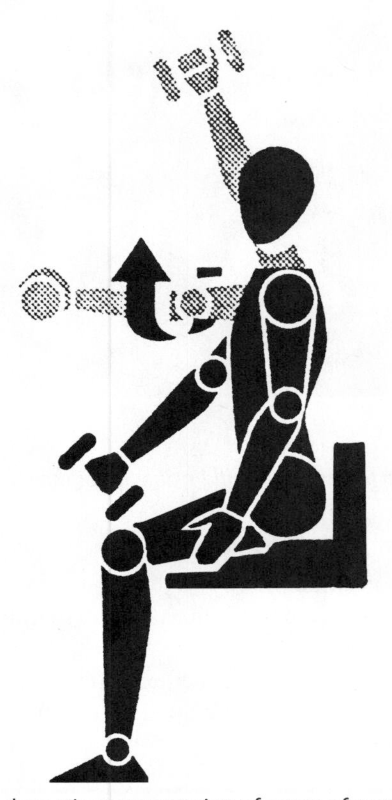

Figure 7-1 Schematic representation of range of motion occurring around the axis of the glenohumeral joint in shoulder flexion. (Courtesy Jerry L. Pettis, VA Medical Center, Los Angeles.)

for assessment early is important. That is, the occupational therapist or OTA should take a few minutes to establish rapport and to instruct the patient about the nature and purpose of the particular assessment.[1] Before measuring, the clinician should ask the patient to move the extremity through a comfortable ROM. After aligning the goniometer, he or she notes any discomfort, unusual restriction or freedom of movement, or audible noise *(crepitation)* from the joint.

Formal joint measurement is not necessary for all patients. The OT practitioner can measure joint movement informally by asking the patient to place the affected extremity in a variety of normal positions. Comparing the movement of the affected extremity to that of the opposite extremity allows the examiner to detect any gross limitations. The practitioner should always check the medical record for any causes that may predispose the patient to joint limitations (e.g., fused joints, previous injuries, arthritis). Pain may limit ROM, and crepitation may be heard on movement in some conditions. Joints should not be forced when resistance is met on PROM.

Clinicians are generally concerned with functional range of motion. This term typically describes the minimum ROM needed to execute performance in essential areas of occupation without the use of special equipment.[8] Performance in occupation is a primary goal of OT. If the patient is completely independent in all areas of occupation and has adequate ROM to perform these functions, treatment to increase ROM is generally not indicated, even though the patient may have less than "normal" ROM. ROM for any individual is affected by age, gender, and other factors including lifestyle and occupation.[9]

Method of Joint Measurement

Joint ROM is measured with a goniometer calibrated from 0 degrees to 180 degrees. In this system, 0 degrees is the starting position. The system increases toward 180 degrees for almost all joint motions. In general, measurements are performed with the patient in the anatomic position. In the anatomic position, the person stands erect with the face directed forward; the arms are at the sides, and the palms of the hands are facing forward.

Measurement of rotation is an exception to this rule. Basically, motions of the body occur in three cardinal planes of movement: sagittal, frontal, and horizontal (Figure 7-2). A semicircle of 180 degrees is superimposed on the body in the plane, with degrees increasing in the direction in which movement will occur. The axis of the joint is the axis of the semicircle, or arc of motion.

Goniometer

The universal goniometer is the tool most widely used to measure joint ROM in the clinical environment. The word *goniometer* is derived from the Greek *gonio,* which means "angle," and *metron,* which means "a measure."[7] Made of either plastic or metal, goniometers come in a variety of sizes and shapes and may be purchased from medical supply houses or through medical catalogs.

The goniometer consists of a stationary (proximal) bar and a movable (distal) bar. The body of the stationary bar includes a small protractor (half circle) of 0 degrees to 180 degrees or a full circle printed with a scale from 0 degrees to 360 degrees. The movable bar is attached at the center or axis of the protractor and acts as a dial. As the dial rotates around the protractor, the number of degrees is indicated on the scale (Figure 7-3).

One important feature of the goniometer is the *axis,* or *fulcrum.* The rivet that acts as the fulcrum must move freely but hold tightly enough to keep the arms at the measured position when the goniometer is removed from the body.

Two scales of figures are printed on the half circle. Each starts at 0 degrees and progresses toward 180 degrees, but in opposite directions. The key to reading the goniometer is common sense. Once the movement of the body part has exceeded 90 degrees, the larger numbers are read. A common error for beginners is to position the patient and goniometer correctly and then *misread* the actual measurement. Many practitioners align the two arms first and then center the axis point over the exact anatomic landmark as an easier method to maneuver the goniometer.

Figure 7-4 shows five styles of goniometers. The first (Figure 7-4, *A*) is a full-circle goniometer. The longer arms are for use on the long bones or large joints of the body. The goniometer in Figure 7-4, *B* is radiopaque and can be used during x-ray examinations. The notched dial allows an accurate

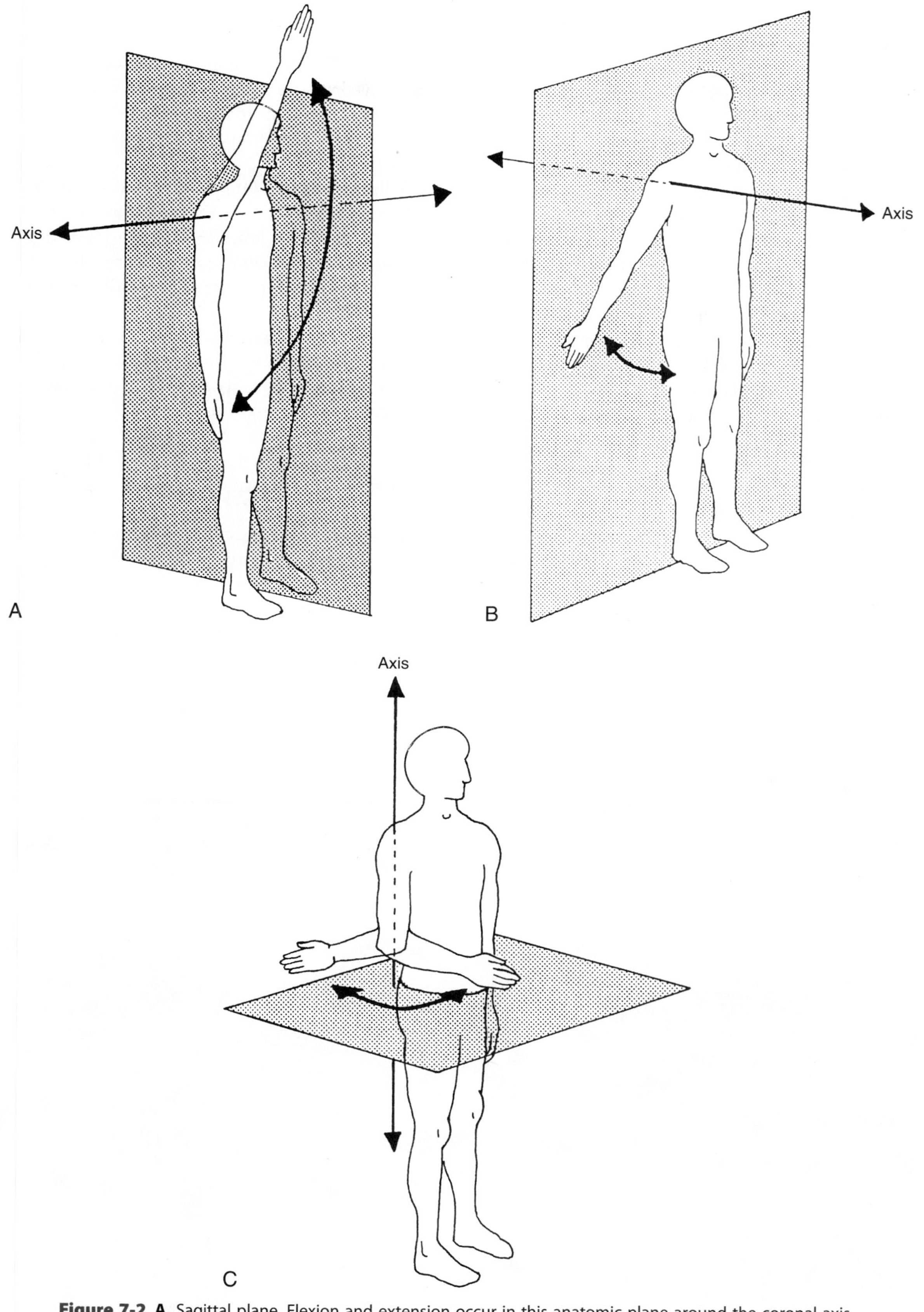

Figure 7-2 **A,** Sagittal plane. Flexion and extension occur in this anatomic plane around the coronal axis. **B,** Frontal plane. Abduction and adduction occur in this anatomic plane around the anteroposterior axis. **C,** Horizontal plane. Shoulder internal rotation and external rotation occur in this anatomic plane. (Courtesy Jerry L. Pettis, VA Medical Center, Los Angeles, CA.)

reading of the motion regardless of whether the convexity of the half circle is directed toward or away from the direction of motion. The finger goniometer in Figure 7-4, *D* has short, flattened arms designed to be used over the finger joint surfaces rather than along their sides. Small plastic goniometers are shown in Figure 7-4, *C* and *E*. These devices are inexpensive and easy to carry. The longer one can be used with both large and small joints. The dials of both goniometers are transparent and are marked and notched in two places similar to the goniometer in *B*. The smaller of these two goniometers is simply a larger one that has been cut to be adapted as a finger goniometer.

Other goniometers use fluid with a free-floating bubble that provides the reading after the motion is completed. Digital types have a liquid crystal display (LCD) readout. Others can be attached to a body segment and have dials that register rotary motions such as pronation and supination.

Recording Measurement Results

The OT practitioner records ROM testing results using a form similar to that shown in Figure 7-5. Table 7-1 lists average normal ranges of motion with the 180-degree method. The practitioner must remember that these ranges are only representative. Often the patient's unaffected extremity provides the closest approximation of what is normal for that individual. The following simple rules of thumb should clarify situations that arise during measurement:

1. Alternate methods of recording ROM are possible, and the OT practitioner should adapt to the method required by the facility.[5]
2. A limitation in ROM is indicated when the start position is not 0 degrees. Examples are (1) extension limitation at elbow joint 15-degree to 140-degree; flexion limitation at the elbow joint 0 degrees to 110 degrees and (2) abnormal hyperextension of elbow joint 20 degrees to 140 degrees.
3. Glenohumeral mobility depends greatly on scapular mobility. If the scapular musculature is spastic, contracted, or orthopedically restricted, glenohumeral ROM will be affected.
4. When joint measurements may be performed in more than one position (e.g., shoulder internal and external rotation), the practitioner should note the position used on the ROM form.
5. The practitioner should observe and proceed with caution when spasticity, pain, or abnormal pathology is present.
6. ROM measurements are usually indicated in 5-degree increments. For example, if elbow flexion measures 0 degrees to 128 degrees, the measurement would be recorded as 0 degrees to 130 degrees. Similarly, if elbow flexion is 0 degrees to 122 degrees, the recorded measurement should be 0 degrees to 120 degrees.

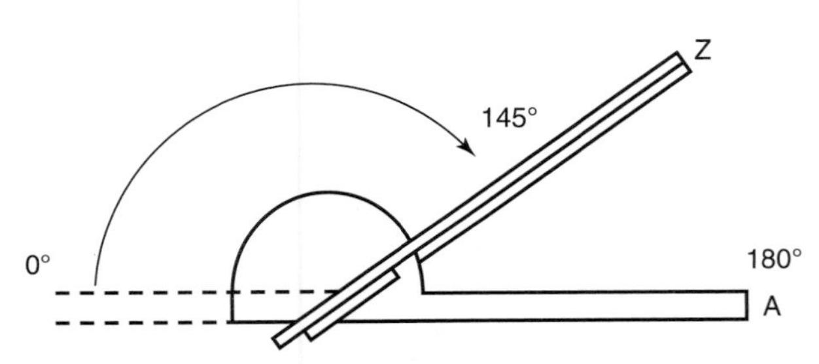

Figure 7-3 Universal goniometer measuring 145 degrees, using the 180-degree joint measurement system. Point *A* represents the stationary bar and *Z* the movable bar.

> The practitioner must use caution in measuring ROM when spasticity, pain, or abnormal pathology is present. Seek advice from a qualified supervisor before proceeding.

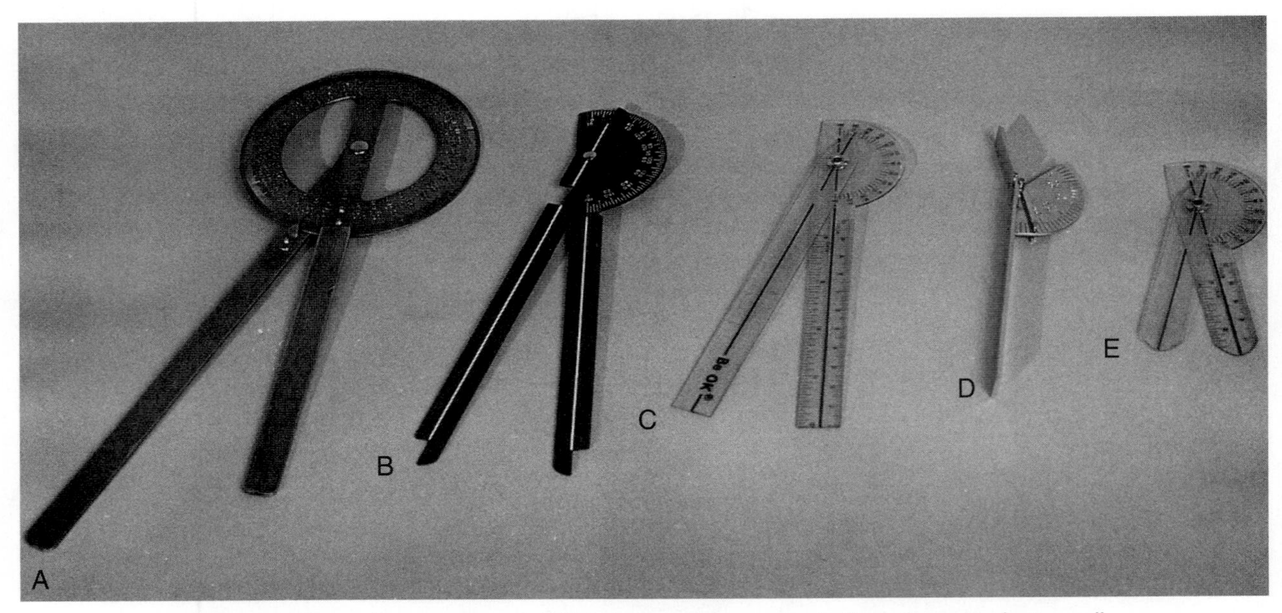

Figure 7-4 Types of goniometers. **A,** Full circle; **B,** radiopaque; **C,** plastic; **D,** finger; **E,** plastic small.

JOINT RANGE MEASUREMENTS

Patient's name ______________________ Chart number ______________

Date of birth ______________ Age ________ Sex ______________

Diagnosis ______________________ Date of onset ______________

Disability ______________________________________

LEFT 3	LEFT 2	LEFT 1			RIGHT 1	RIGHT 2	RIGHT 3
			SPINE				
			Cervical spine				
			Flexion	0 to 45			
			Extension	0 to 45			
			Lateral flexion	0 to 45			
			Rotation	0 to 60			
			Thoracic and lumbar spine				
			Flexion	0 to 80			
			Extension	0 to 30			
			Lateral flexion	0 to 40			
			Rotation	0 to 45			
			SHOULDER				
			Flexion	0 to 170			
			Extension	0 to 60			
			Abduction	0 to 170			
			Horizontal abduction	0 to 40			
			Horizontal adduction	0 to 130			
			Internal rotation	0 to 70			
			External rotation	0 to 90			
			ELBOW AND FOREARM				
			Flexion	0 to 135-150			
			Supination	0 to 80-90			
			Pronation	0 to 80-90			
			WRIST				
			Flexion	0 to 80			
			Extension	0 to 70			
			Ulnar deviation	0 to 30			
			Radial deviation	0 to 20			
			THUMB				
			MP flexion	0 to 50			
			IP flexion	0 to 80-90			
			Abduction	0 to 50			
			FINGERS				
			MP flexion	0 to 90			
			MP hyperextension	0 to 15-45			
			PIP flexion	0 to 110			
			DIP flexion	0 to 80			
			Abduction	0 to 25			
			HIP				
			Flexion	0 to 120			
			Extension	0 to 30			
			Abduction	0 to 40			
			Adduction	0 to 35			
			Internal rotation	0 to 45			
			External rotation	0 to 45			
			KNEE				
			Flexion	0 to 135			
			ANKLE AND FOOT				
			Plantar flexion	0 to 50			
			Dorsiflexion	0 to 15			
			Inversion	0 to 35			
			Eversion	0 to 20			

Figure 7-5 Form for recording joint range-of-motion measurements.

Table 7-1 Average Normal Range of Motion (180-Degree Method)

Joint	Range of Motion	Associated Girdle Motion
Cervical Spine		
Flexion	0-45 degrees	---
Extension	0-45 degrees	---
Lateral flexion	0-45 degrees	---
Rotation	0-60 degrees	---
Thoracic and Lumbar Spine		
Flexion	0-80 degrees	---
Extension	0-30 degrees	---
Lateral flexion	0-40 degrees	---
Rotation	0-45 degrees	---
Shoulder		
Flexion	0-170 degrees	Abduction, lateral tilt, slight elevation, slight upward rotation
Extension	0-60 degrees	Depression, adduction, upward tilt
Abduction	0-170 degrees	Upward rotation, elevation
Adduction	0 degrees	Depression, adduction, downward rotation
Horizontal abduction	0-40 degrees	Adduction, reduction of lateral tilt
Horizontal adduction	0-130 degrees	Abduction, lateral tilt
Internal rotation		Abduction, lateral tilt
Arm in abduction	0-70 degrees	---
Arm in adduction	0-60 degrees	---
External rotation		
Arm in abduction	0-90 degrees	---
Arm in adduction	0-80 degrees	---
Elbow		
Flexion	0 to 135-150 degrees	---
Extension	0 degrees	---
Forearm		
Pronation	0 to 80-90 degrees	---
Supination	0 to 80-90 degrees	---

Joint	Range of Motion	Associated Girdle Motion
Wrist		
Flexion	0 to 80 degrees	
Extension	0 to 70 degrees	
Ulnar deviation (adduction)	0 to 30 degrees	
Radial deviation (abduction)	0 to 20 degrees	
Thumb		
DIP flexion	0 to 80-90 degrees	
MP flexion	0-50 degrees	
Adduction, radial and palmar	0 degrees	
Palmar abduction	0-50 degrees	
Radial abduction	0-50 degrees	
Opposition		
Fingers		
MP flexion	0-90 degrees	
MP hyperextension	0 to 15-45 degrees	
PIP flexion	0-110 degrees	
DIP flexion	0-80 degrees	
Abduction	0-25 degrees	
Hip		
Flexion	0-120 degrees (bent knees)	
Extension	0-30 degrees	
Abduction	0-40 degrees	
Adduction	0-35 degrees	
Internal rotation	0-45 degrees	
External rotation	0-45 degrees	
Knee		
Flexion	0-135 degrees	
Ankle and Foot		
Plantar flexion	0-50 degrees	
Dorsiflexion	0-15 degrees	
Inversion	0-35 degrees	
Eversion	0-20 degrees	

Data from American Academy of Orthopedic Surgeons: *Joint motion: method of measuring and recording,* Chicago, 1965, The Academy; and Esch D, Lepley M: *Evaluation of joint motion: methods of measurement and recording,* Minneapolis, 1974, University of Minnesota Press.
DIP, Distal interphalangeal; *MP,* metacarpophalangeal; *PIP,* proximal interphalangeal.

Joint Limitation and Disease Processes

Joint limitations develop for a variety of reasons. A person with a CVA might have spasticity that restricts ROM. Individuals with significant burn injuries often develop skin adhesions and scar formations that decrease joint movement. Trauma and disease processes such as rheumatoid arthritis mechanically restrict ROM.

Future loss of ROM is expected with many disease processes. Treatment planning must incorporate measures to maintain ROM for as long as possible. For example, arthritis can cause joint stiffness and deformity. A primary therapeutic objective is to preserve function via splints, positioning, exercise, joint protection principles, and assistive devices.

A variety of exercises and activities can be incorporated into a therapy program to increase ROM. Active and passive stretching, resistive exercise, and exercises using equipment such as pulleys can play a significant part. Functional activities such as reaching, catching a ball, table-top activities, and throwing a bean bag can be used. Alternative methods such as yoga, Pilates, and Tai Chi can provide added stretching exercises to promote flexibility and ROM. These activities, using slow movements, can be highly motivating. Whatever the approach, the OT practitioner should develop creative and enjoyable activities that increase ROM.

Procedure for Joint Measurement

The illustrations that accompany the directions for measurement of each motion in the next section show both goniometer placement and general orientation of the examiner in relationship to the patient. In most cases the examiner is squared off directly with the patient so that the examiner can position the goniometer and read the result.

Factors such as degree of muscle weakness, presence or absence of joint pain, and whether PROM or AROM is being measured determine how the examiner holds the goniometer and supports the body part being measured. The examiner and patient should be positioned for greatest degree of comfort, correct placement of the goniometer, and adequate stabilization of the part being measured in correct anatomic plane of movement.

Box 7-1 lists principles for practitioners performing ROM testing that can be applied to the following section on measurement of upper extremity motions. The measurement section indicates the starting position and "normal" final position. Practitioners should record the patient's final position on the form.

Procedures for Goniometric Measurement and Testing of Selected Upper Extremity Motions

Shoulder

Flexion: 0 Degrees to 170 Degrees (Figure 7-6)

Position of subject: Seated or supine with humerus in neutral position.

Box 7-1

Basic Principles for Range of Motion (ROM) Testing

1. Have the patient comfortable and relaxed in testing position.
2. Explain and demonstrate the what, why, and how of goniometry to the patient.
3. Establish body landmarks for the measurement.
4. Stabilize joints proximal to the joint being measured.
5. Move the part passively through ROM to estimate available ROM and get a feel for joint mobility.
6. Return the part to the starting position.
7. At the starting position, place the axis of the goniometer over the axis of the joint. Place the stationary bar on the proximal or stationary bone and the movable bar on the distal or moving bone.
8. Record the number of degrees at the starting position.
9. Depending on what type of measurement is being taken (AROM or PROM), move or have the patient move the part to obtain the measurement desired (e.g., shoulder flexion).
10. Reposition the movable arm of the goniometer, checking that the axis is still accurately placed, and note the number of degrees at final position.
11. Record the reading to the nearest 5 degrees, and make any other appropriate notations on the form (e.g., pain, crepitation).

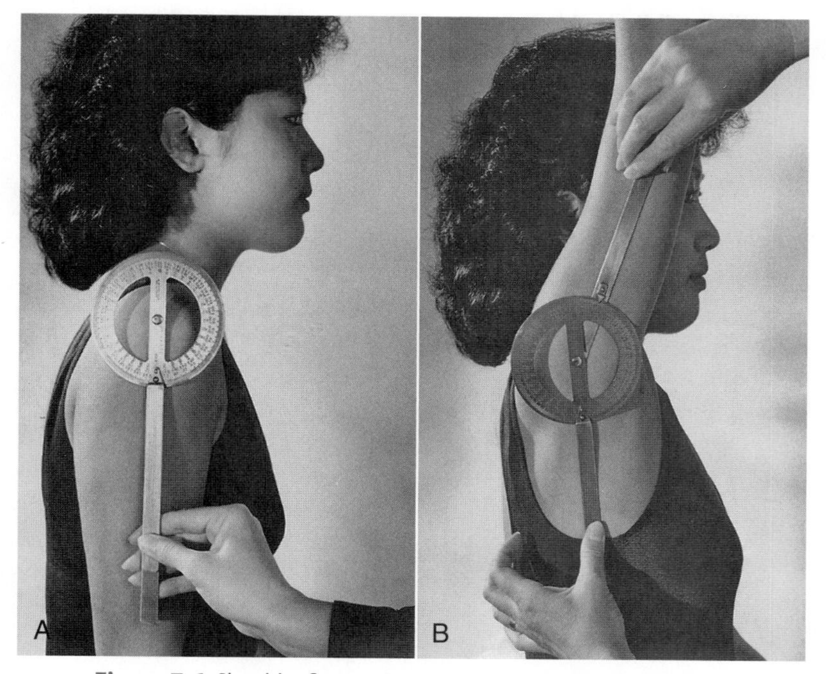

Figure 7-6 Shoulder flexion. **A,** Starting position. **B,** Final position.

Position of goniometer: Axis is center of humerus just distal to acromion process on lateral aspect of humerus. Stationary bar is parallel to trunk, and movable bar is parallel to humerus.

Direction of movement: Patient's arm is raised in front of body in a sagittal plane of movement.

Extension: 0 Degrees to 60 Degrees (Figure 7-7)

Position of subject: Seated or prone, with no obstruction behind humerus. Humerus is in neutral position.

Position of goniometer: Same as for shoulder flexion.

Direction of movement: Patient's arm is to be brought in back of the body in a sagittal plane of movement. Excessive scapular motion should be avoided.

Abduction: 0 Degrees to 170 Degrees (Figure 7-8)

Position of subject: Seated or prone with humerus in adduction and external rotation.

Position of goniometer: Axis is on acromion process on posterior surface of shoulder. Stationary bar is parallel to trunk, and movable bar is parallel to humerus.

Direction of movement: Patient's arm is raised to side of body in a frontal plane of movement.

Horizontal Abduction: 0 Degrees to 40 Degrees (Figure 7-9)

Position of subject: Seated with the shoulder to be tested abducted to 90 degrees, the elbow extended with the palm facing down. The patient's arm may be supported in abduction.

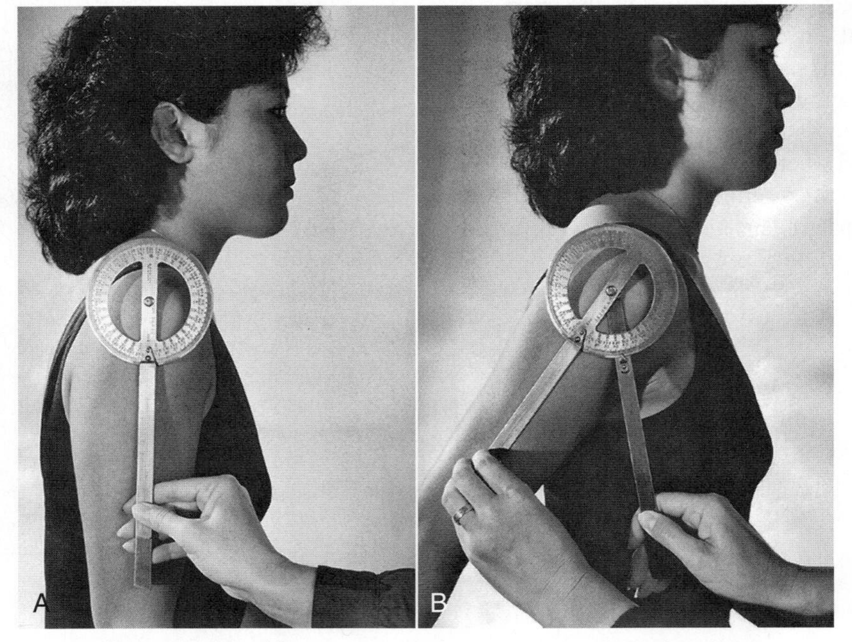

Figure 7-7 Shoulder extension. **A,** Starting position. **B,** Final position.

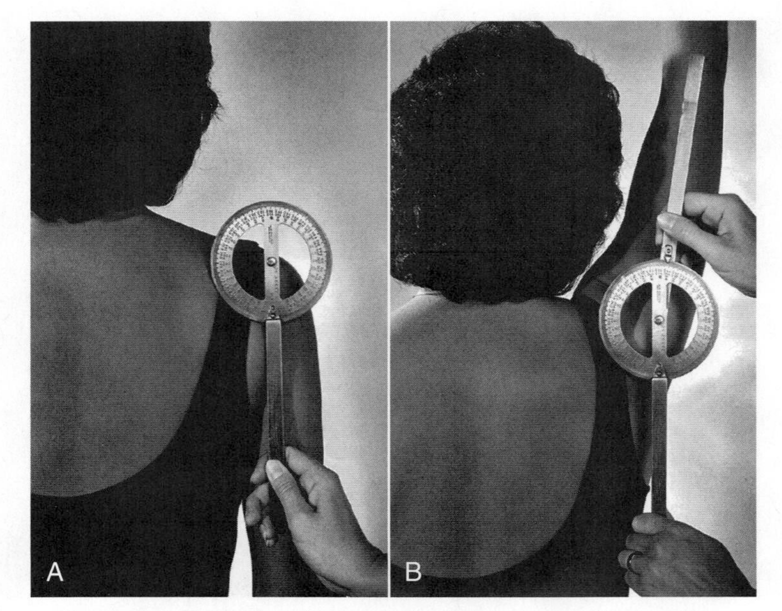

Figure 7-8 Shoulder abduction. **A,** Starting position. **B,** Final position.

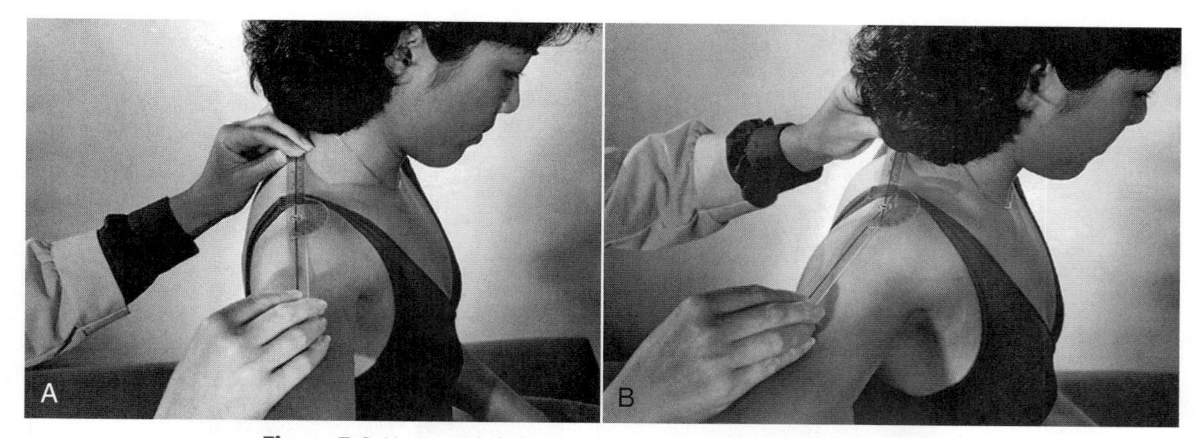

Figure 7-9 Horizontal abduction. **A,** Starting position. **B,** Final position.

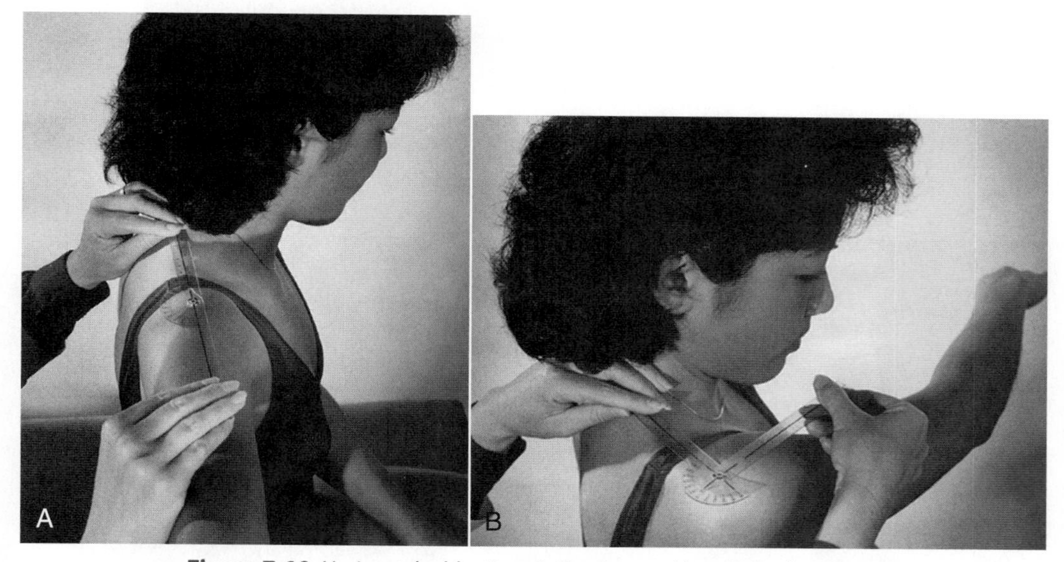

Figure 7-10 Horizontal adduction. **A,** Starting position. **B,** Final position.

Position of the goniometer: The axis is over the acromion process. The stationary bar is parallel over the shoulder toward the neck, and the movable bar is parallel to the humerus on the superior aspect.

Direction of movement: Patient's arm is moved toward the back of the body in the horizontal plane of movement.

Horizontal Adduction: 0 Degrees to 130 Degrees (Figure 7-10)

Position of the subject and goniometer: Same as for horizontal abduction.

Direction of movement: Patient's arm is moved in front of the body in the horizontal plane of movement.

Internal Rotation: 0 Degrees to 60 Degrees (Figure 7-11)

Position of subject: Seated with humerus adducted against trunk, elbow at 90 degrees, and forearm in midposition and perpendicular to body.

Position of goniometer: Axis is on olecranon process of elbow, and stationary bar and movable bar are parallel to forearm.

Direction of movement: Patient's forearm is swung toward body through a horizontal plane of movement. Humerus must remain adducted.

Internal Rotation: 0 Degrees to 70 Degrees (Figure 7-12)

(Alternate position: Used in some practice settings or as preference of supervising occupational therapist.)

Position of subject: Seated or supine with humerus abducted to 90 degrees and elbow flexed to 90 degrees.

Position of goniometer: Axis is on olecranon process of elbow, and stationary bar and movable bar are parallel to forearm.

Direction of movement: Patient's forearm is swung down gently, keeping humerus parallel to floor.

External Rotation: 0 Degrees to 80 Degrees (Figure 7-13)

Position of subject: Humerus adducted, elbow at 90 degrees, and forearm in midposition, perpendicular to body.

Position of goniometer: Axis is on olecranon of elbow, and stationary bar and movable bar are parallel to forearm.

Direction of movement: Patient's forearm is swung out from body through a horizontal plane of movement. Humerus must remain adducted.

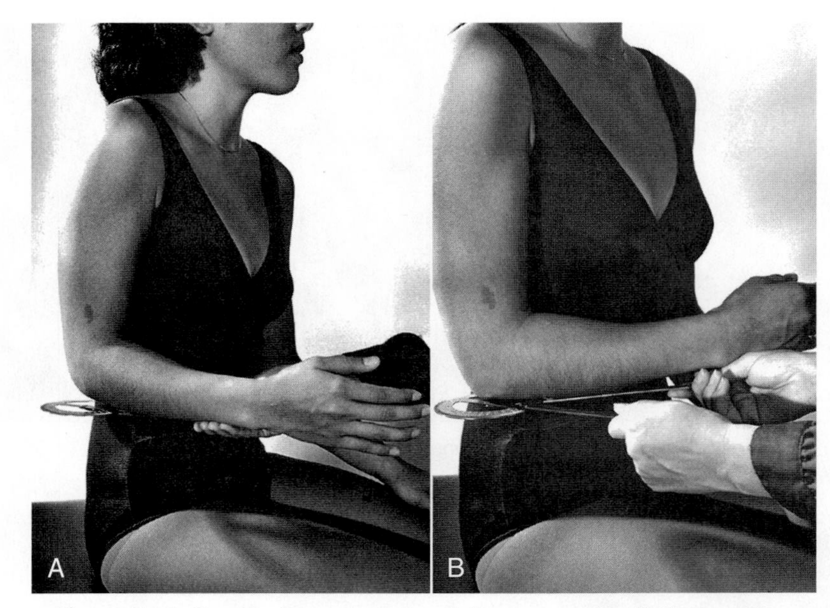

Figure 7-11 Shoulder internal rotation. **A,** Starting position. **B,** Final position.

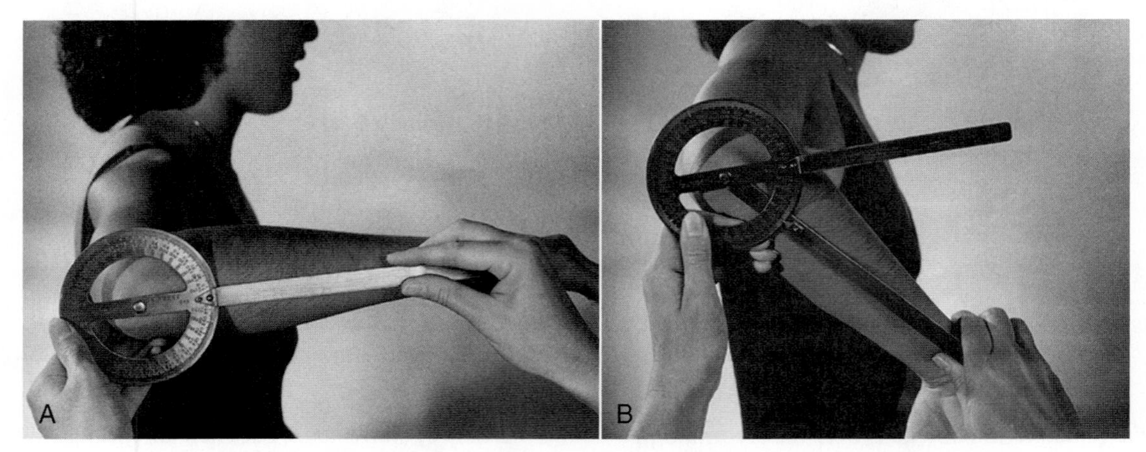

Figure 7-12 Shoulder internal rotation, alternate position. **A,** Starting position. **B,** Final position.

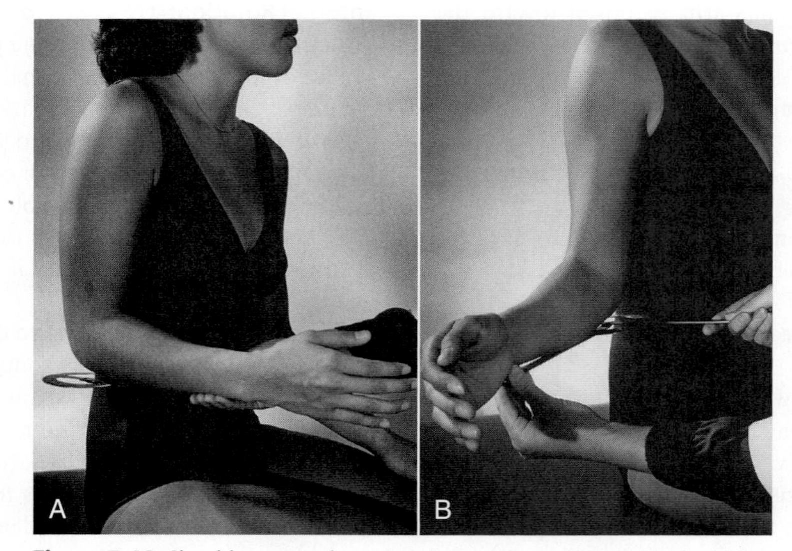

Figure 7-13 Shoulder external rotation. **A,** Starting position. **B,** Final position.

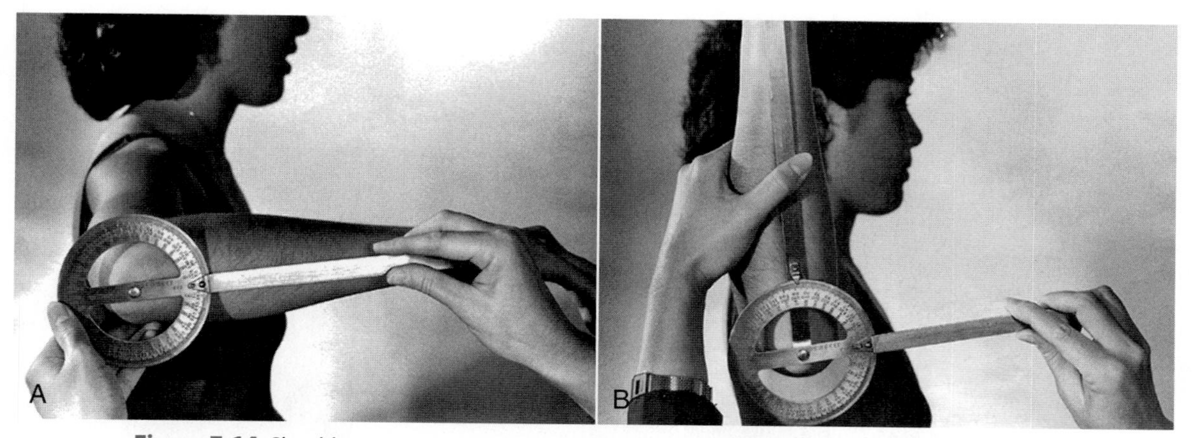

Figure 7-14 Shoulder external rotation, alternate position. **A,** Starting position. **B,** Final position.

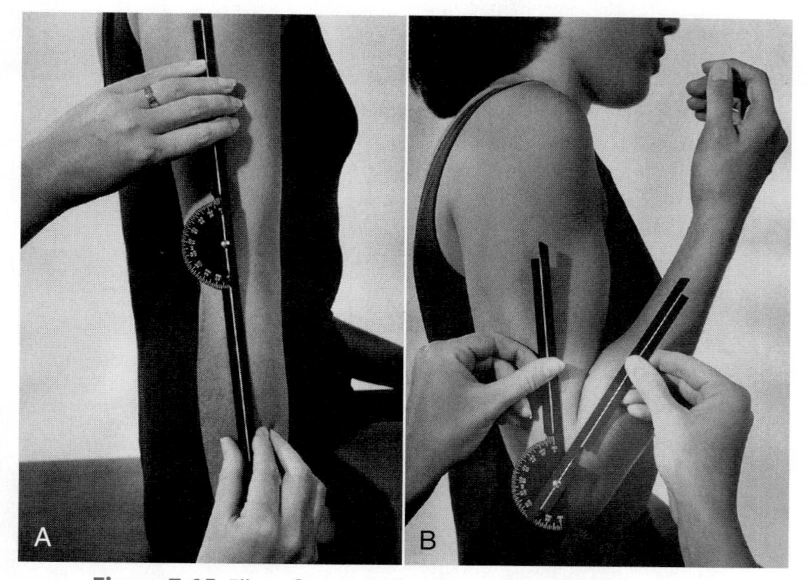

Figure 7-15 Elbow flexion. **A,** Starting position. **B,** Final position.

External Rotation: 0 Degrees to 90 Degrees (Figure 7-14)

(Alternate position: Used in some practice settings or as preference of supervising occupational therapist.)

Position of subject: Seated or supine with humerus abducted to 90 degrees, elbow flexed to 90 degrees, and forearm pronated.

Position of goniometer: Axis is on olecranon process of elbow, and stationary bar and movable bar are parallel to forearm.

Direction of movement: Patient's forearm is swung up gently, keeping humerus parallel to floor.

Elbow

Extension to Flexion: 0 Degrees to 135 to 150 Degrees (Figure 7-15)

Position of subject: Standing, sitting, or supine with humerus adducted and externally rotated and forearm supinated.

Position of goniometer: Axis is placed over lateral epicondyle of humerus at end of elbow crease. Stationary bar is parallel to midline of humerus, and movable bar is parallel to radius.

Direction of movement: Patient's forearm begins in extended position and is raised in a sagittal plane of movement.

Forearm

Supination: 0 Degrees to 80 to 90 Degrees (Figure 7-16)

Position of subject: Seated or standing with humerus adducted, elbow at 90 degrees, and forearm in midposition.

Position of goniometer: Axis is at ulnar border of volar aspect of wrist, just proximal to ulna styloid. Stationary bar is perpendicular to the floor, and movable bar is resting against volar aspect of wrist.

Direction of movement: Patient's forearm is rotated laterally around ulna.

Supination: 0 Degrees to 80 to 90 Degrees (Figure 7-17)

(Alternate position: Used in some practice settings or as preference of supervising occupational therapist.)

Position of subject: Seated or standing with humerus adducted, elbow at 90 degrees, and forearm in midposition. A pencil is placed in subject's hand and held perpendicular to the floor.

Position of goniometer: Axis is over midshaft of third proximal phalanx. Stationary bar is perpendicular to floor, and movable bar overlays shaft of pencil.

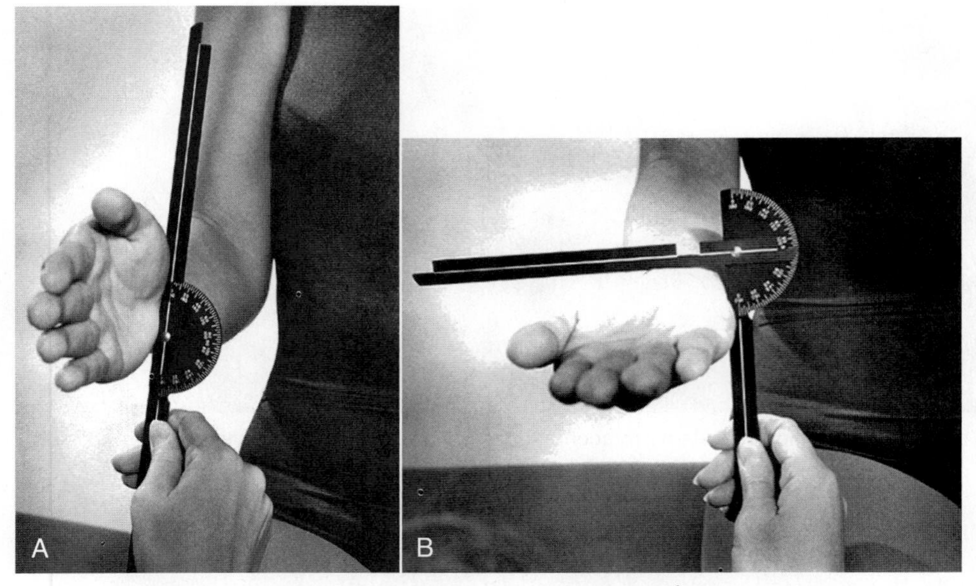

Figure 7-16 Forearm supination. **A,** Starting position. **B,** Final position.

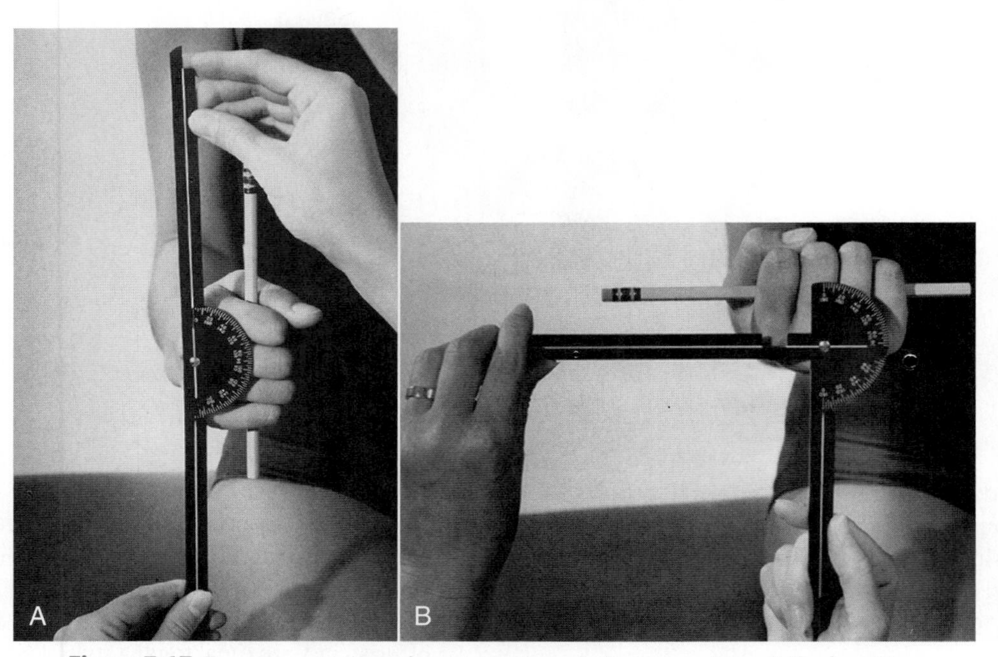

Figure 7-17 Forearm supination, alternate position. **A,** Starting position. **B,** Final position.

Direction of movement: Patient's forearm is rotated laterally around the ulna.

Pronation: 0 Degrees to 80 to 90 Degrees (Figure 7-18)

Position of subject: Seated or standing with humerus adducted, elbow at 90 degrees, and forearm in midposition.

Position of goniometer: Axis is at ulnar border of dorsal aspect of wrist, just proximal to ulna styloid. Stationary bar is perpendicular to floor, and movable bar is resting against dorsal aspect of wrist.

Direction of movement: Patient's forearm is rotated medially around ulna.

Pronation: 0 Degrees to 80 to 90 Degrees (Figure 7-19)

(Alternate position: Used in some practice settings or as preference of supervising occupational therapist.)

Position of subject: Seated or standing with humerus adducted, elbow at 90 degrees, and forearm in midposition. A pencil is placed in subject's hand and held perpendicular to the floor.

Position of goniometer: Axis is over third proximal phalanx. Stationary bar is perpendicular to floor, and movable bar overlays shaft of pencil.

Direction of movement: Patient's forearm is rotated medially around ulna.

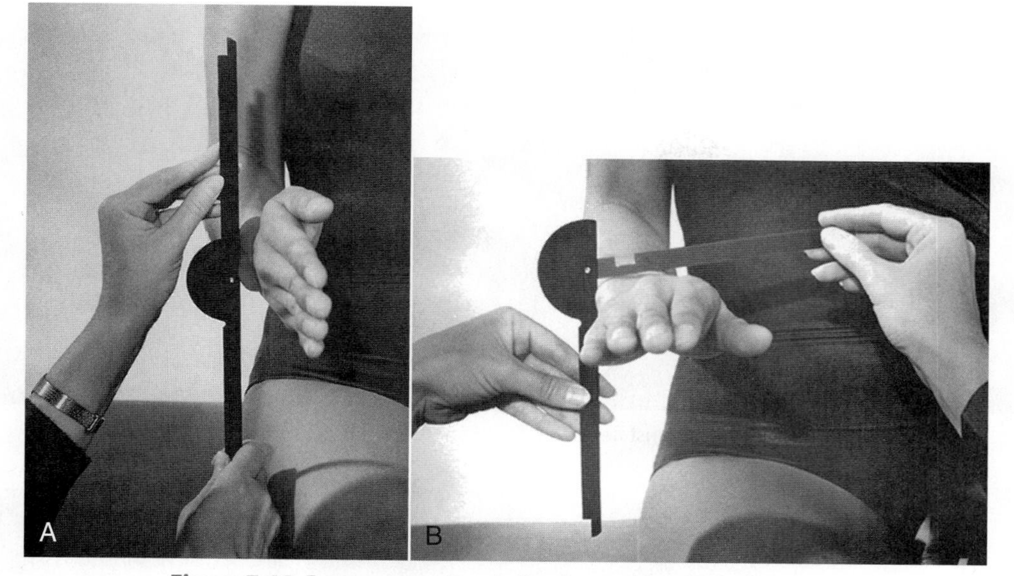

Figure 7-18 Forearm pronation. **A,** Starting position. **B,** Final position.

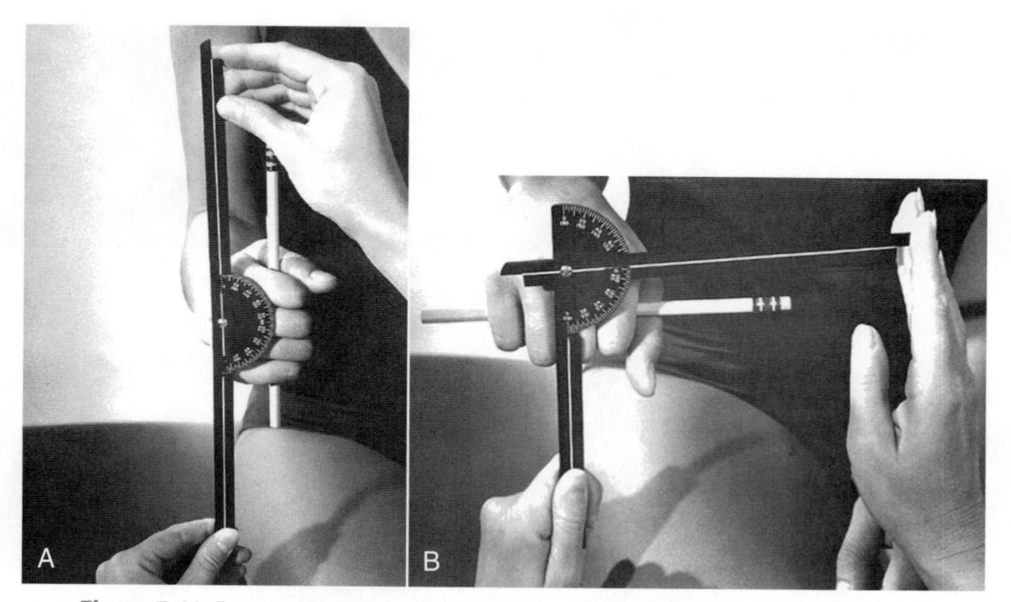

Figure 7-19 Forearm pronation, alternate position. **A,** Starting position. **B,** Final position.

Wrist

Flexion: 0 Degrees to 80 Degrees (Figure 7-20)

Position of subject: Seated with forearm in midposition and hand and forearm resting on table on ulnar border.

Position of goniometer: Axis is on lateral aspect of wrist just distal to radial styloid in anatomic snuffbox. Stationary bar is parallel to radius, and movable bar is parallel to metacarpal of index finger.

Direction of movement: Patient's hand is flexed down so that palm moves closer to volar aspect of forearm.

Extension: 0 Degrees to 70 Degrees (Figure 7-21)

Position of subject: Same as for wrist flexion except fingers should be flexed.

Position of goniometer: Same as for wrist flexion.

Direction of movement: Patient's hand is raised up so that back of hand moves closer to dorsal aspect of forearm.

Ulnar Deviation: 0 Degrees to 30 Degrees (Figure 7-22)

Position of subject: Seated with forearm pronated and palm of hand resting flat on table surface. Goniometer is positioned so that the third finger lines up with center of forearm.

Position of goniometer: Axis is on dorsum of wrist at base of third metacarpal. Stationary bar is positioned in center of forearm, and movable bar is parallel to third metacarpal.

Direction of movement: Patient's hand is laterally extended in a horizontal plane of movement.

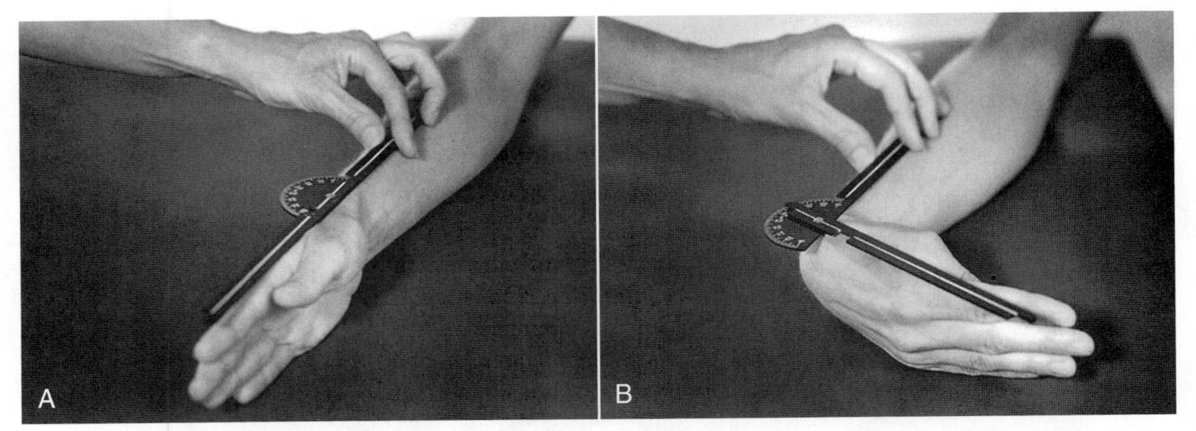

Figure 7-20 Wrist flexion. **A,** Starting position. **B,** Final position.

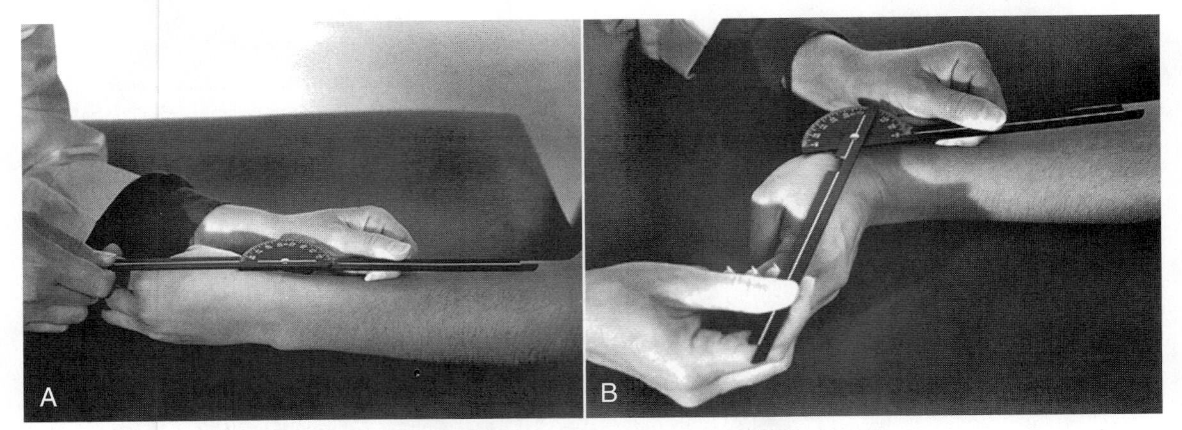

Figure 7-21 Wrist extension. **A,** Starting position. **B,** Final position.

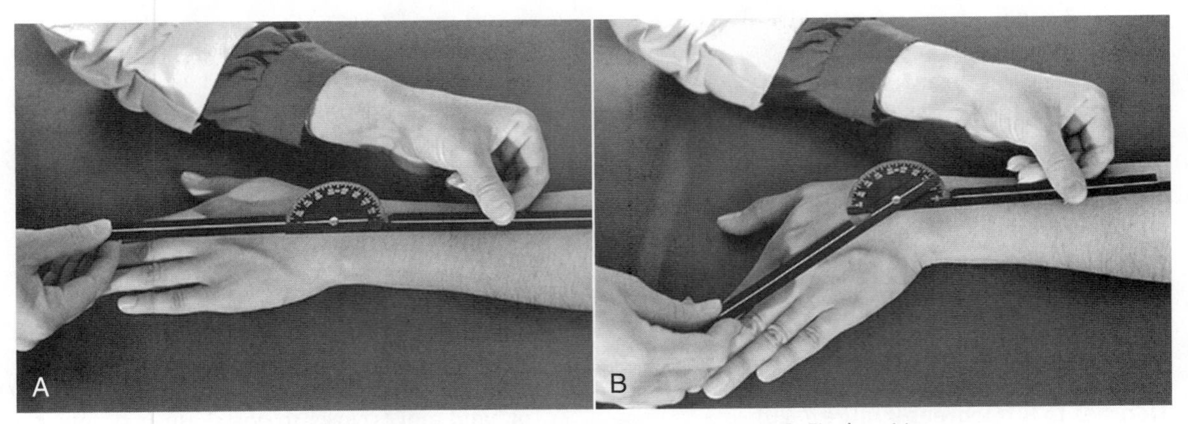

Figure 7-22 Wrist ulnar deviation. **A,** Starting position. **B,** Final position.

Radial Deviation: 0 Degrees to 20 Degrees (Figure 7-23)

Position of subject and goniometer: Same as for ulnar deviation.

Direction of movement: Patient's hand is medially extended in a horizontal plane of movement.

Fingers

Metacarpophalangeal (MP) Flexion: 0 Degrees to 90 Degrees (Figure 7-24)

Position of subject: Seated with forearm in midposition, wrist at 0 degrees neutral, and forearm and hand supported on a firm surface on ulnar border.

Position of goniometer: Axis is centered on top of middle of MP joint. Stationary bar is on top of metacarpal, and movable bar is on top of proximal phalanx.

Direction of movement: Patient's finger distal of MP joint is flexed down in a sagittal plane.

MP Hyperextension: 0 Degrees to 15 to 45 Degrees (Figure 7-25)

Position of subject: Seated with forearm in midposition, wrist at 0 degrees neutral, and forearm and hand supported on a firm surface on ulnar border.

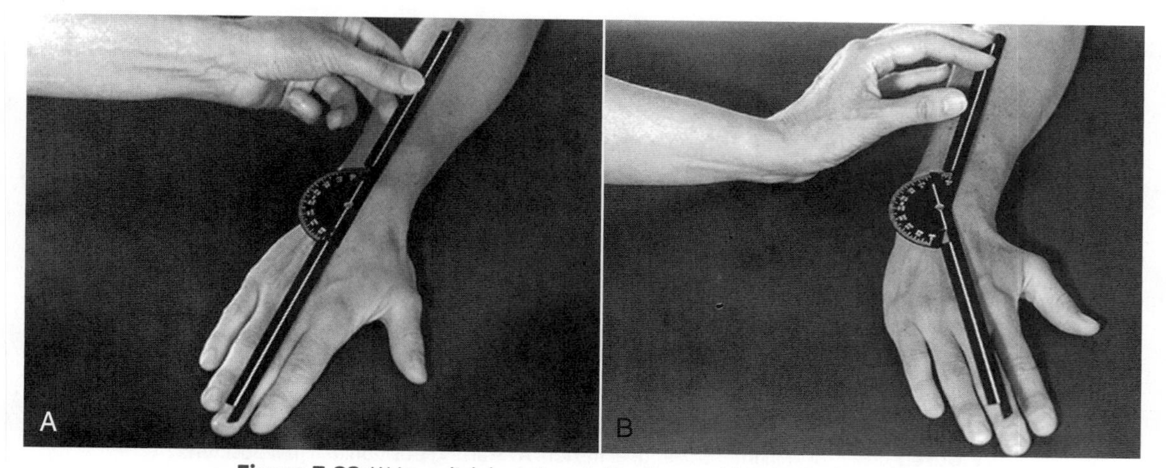

Figure 7-23 Wrist radial deviation. **A,** Starting position. **B,** Final position.

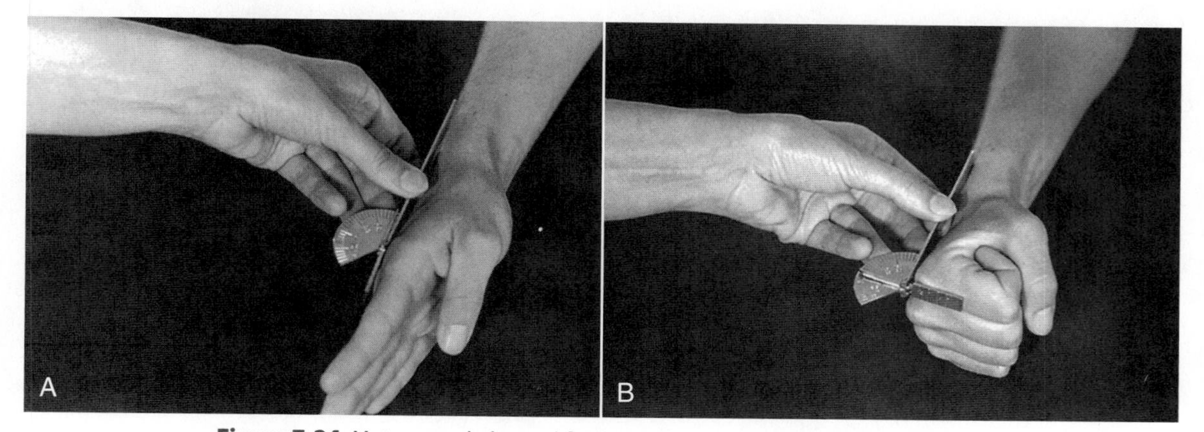

Figure 7-24 Metacarpophalangeal flexion. **A,** Starting position. **B,** Final position.

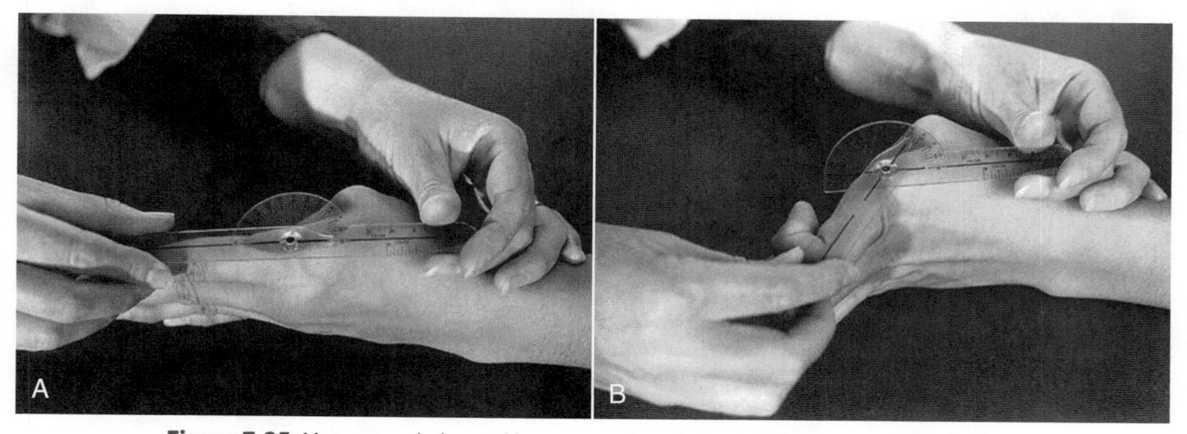

Figure 7-25 Metacarpophalangeal hyperextension. **A,** Starting position. **B,** Final position.

Position of goniometer: Axis is over lateral aspect of MP joint of index finger. Stationary bar is parallel to metacarpal, and movable bar is parallel to proximal phalanx. MP joint of fifth finger may be measured similarly. ROM of third and fourth fingers can be estimated by comparison.

Direction of movement: Patient's finger distal of MP joint is extended up in a sagittal plane of movement.

Proximal Interphalangeal (PIP) Flexion: 0 Degrees to 110 Degrees (Figure 7-26)

Position of subject: Seated with forearm in midposition, wrist at 0 degrees neutral, and forearm and hand supported on a firm surface on ulnar border.

Position of goniometer: Axis is centered on dorsal surface of PIP joint being measured. Stationary bar is placed over proximal phalanx, and movable bar is over middle phalanx.

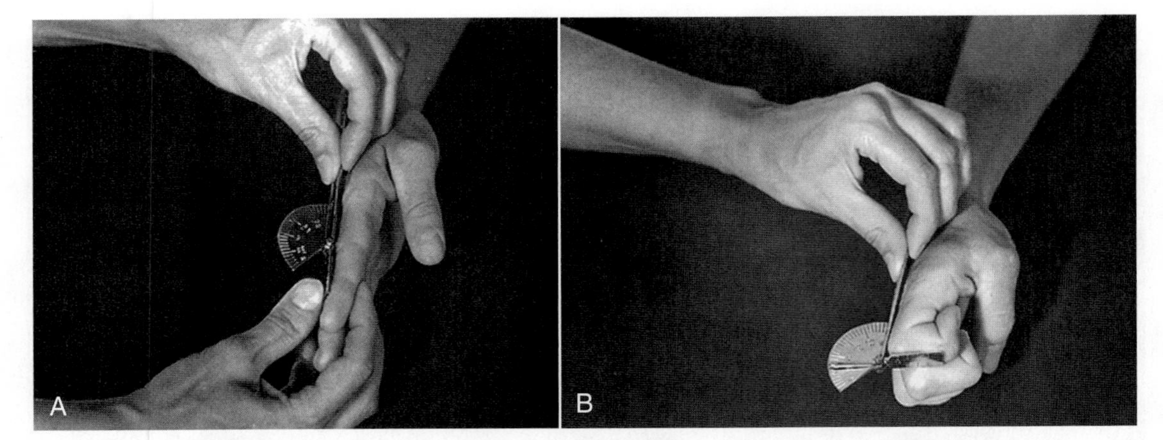

Figure 7-26 Proximal interphalangeal flexion. **A,** Starting position. **B,** Final position.

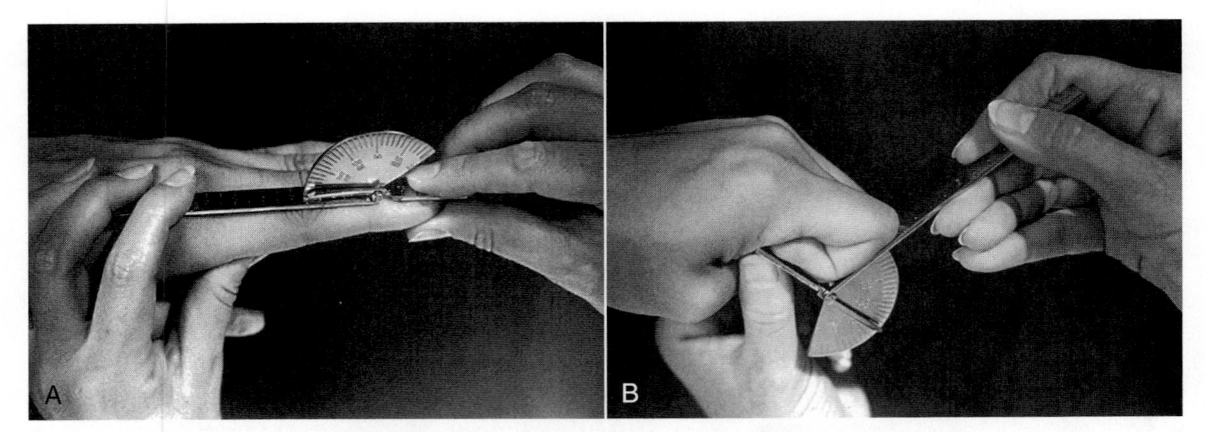

Figure 7-27 Distal interphalangeal flexion. **A,** Starting position. **B,** Final position.

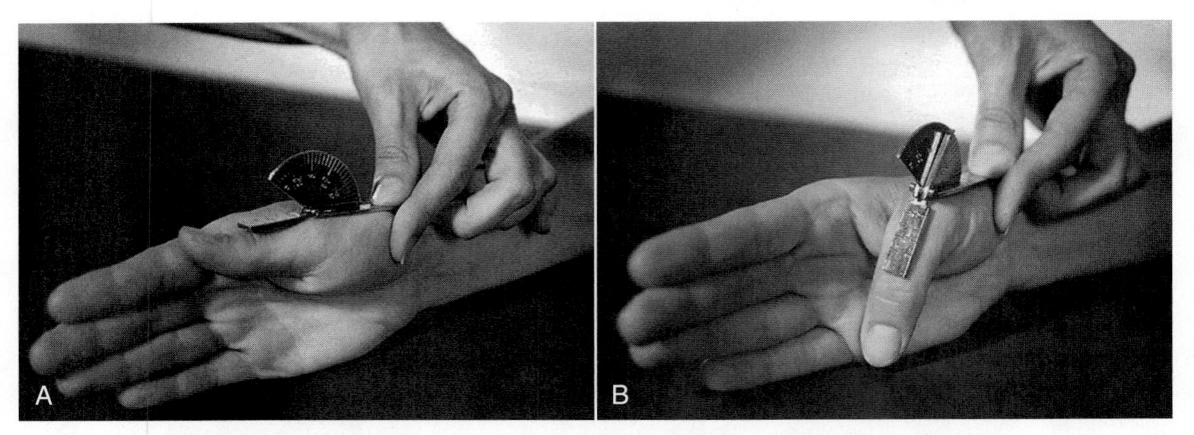

Figure 7-28 Thumb metacarpophalangeal flexion. **A,** Starting position. **B,** Final position.

Direction of movement: Patient's finger distal of PIP joint is flexed down in a sagittal plane of movement.

Distal Interphalangeal (DIP) Flexion: 0 Degrees to 80 Degrees (Figure 7-27)

Position of subject: Seated with forearm in midposition, wrist at 0 degrees neutral, and forearm and hand supported on a firm surface on ulnar border.

Position of goniometer: Axis is on dorsal surface of DIP joint. Stationary bar is over middle phalanx, and movable bar is over distal phalanx.

Direction of movement: Patient's finger distal of DIP joint is flexed down in a sagittal plane of movement.

Thumb

MP Flexion: 0 Degrees to 50 Degrees (Figure 7-28)

Position of subject: Seated with forearm in 45 degrees of supination, wrist at 0 degrees neutral, and forearm and hand supported on a firm surface.

Position of goniometer: Axis is on dorsal surface of MP joint. Stationary bar is over thumb metacarpal, and movable bar is over proximal phalanx.

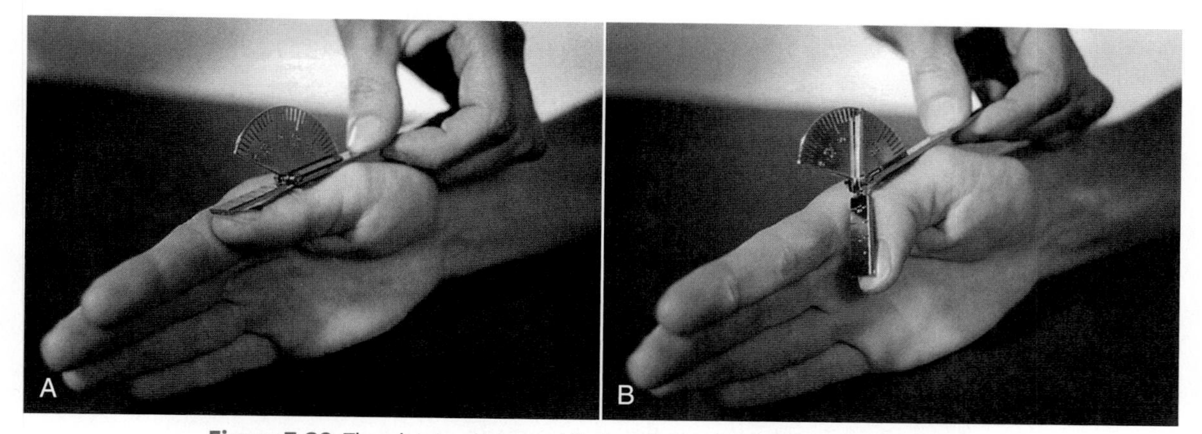

Figure 7-29 Thumb interphalangeal flexion. **A,** Starting position. **B,** Final position.

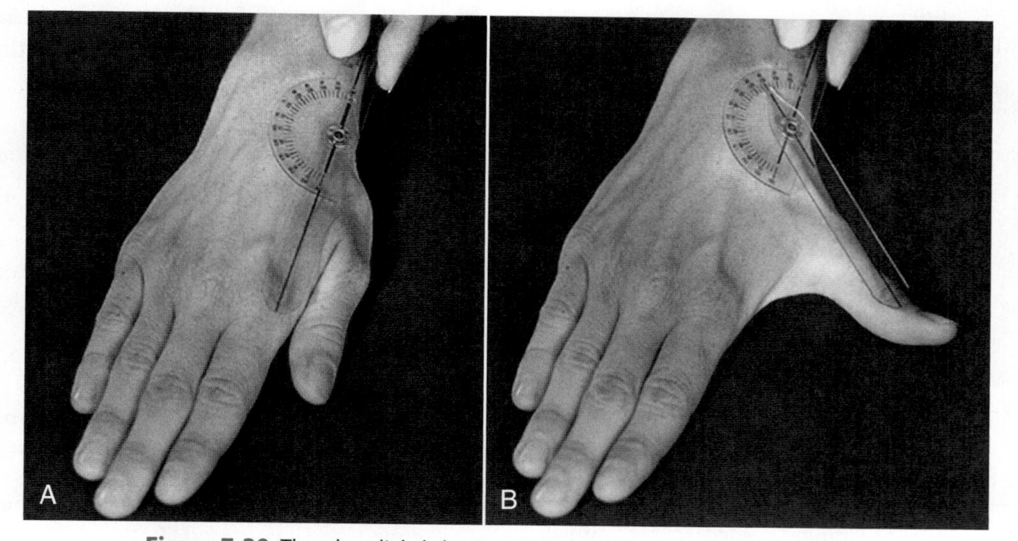

Figure 7-30 Thumb radial abduction. **A,** Starting position. **B,** Final position.

Direction of movement: Patient's thumb distal of MP joint is flexed down.

Interphalangeal (IP) Flexion: 0 Degrees to 80 to 90 Degrees (Figure 7-29)

Position of subject: Same as for PIP/DIP finger flexion.

Position of goniometer: Axis is on dorsal surface of IP joint. Stationary bar is over proximal phalanx, and movable bar is over distal phalanx.

Direction of movement: Patient's thumb distal of IP joint is flexed down.

Radial Abduction (Carpometacarpal [CMC] Extension): 0 Degrees to 50 Degrees (Figure 7-30)

Position of subject: Seated with forearm pronated and hand palm down, resting flat on a firm surface.

Position of goniometer: Axis is over CMC joint at base of thumb metacarpal. Stationary bar is parallel to radius, and movable bar is parallel to thumb metacarpal.

Direction of movement: Patient's thumb is abducted in a horizontal plane of movement.

Palmar Abduction (CMC Flexion): 0 Degrees to 50 Degrees (Figure 7-31)

Position of subject: Seated with forearm at 0 degrees midposition, wrist at 0 degrees, and forearm and hand resting on ulnar border. Thumb is rotated and placed at right angles to palm of hand.

Position of goniometer: Axis is over CMC joint at base of thumb metacarpal. Stationary bar is over radius, and movable bar is over thumb metacarpal.

Direction of movement: Patient's thumb is abducted in a horizontal plane of movement while forearm is in midposition.

Thumb Opposition: (Figure 7-32)

Position of subject: Seated with palmar aspect of hand exposed.

Position of goniometer: Distance between thumb and fifth finger pads is measured with a centimeter ruler.

Direction of movement: Patient's thumb and fifth digit are opposed to one another.

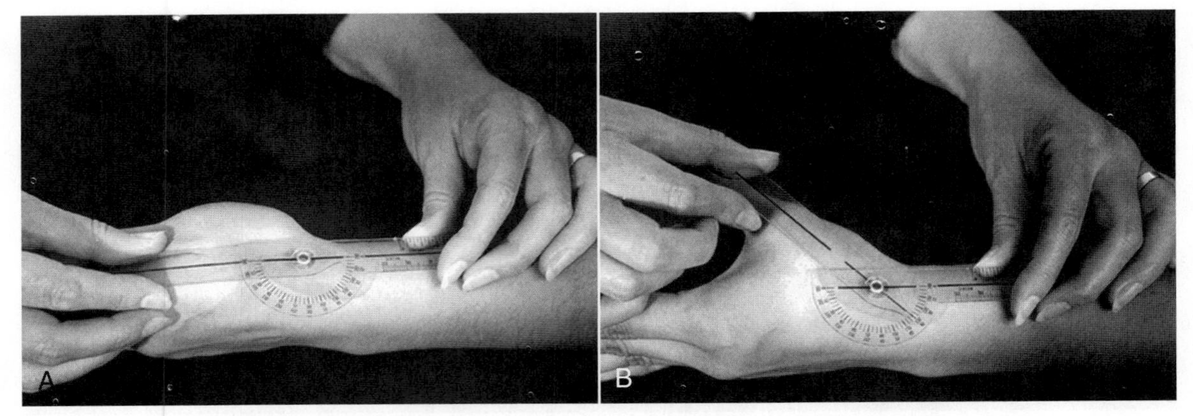

Figure 7-31 Thumb palmar abduction. **A,** Starting position. **B,** Final position.

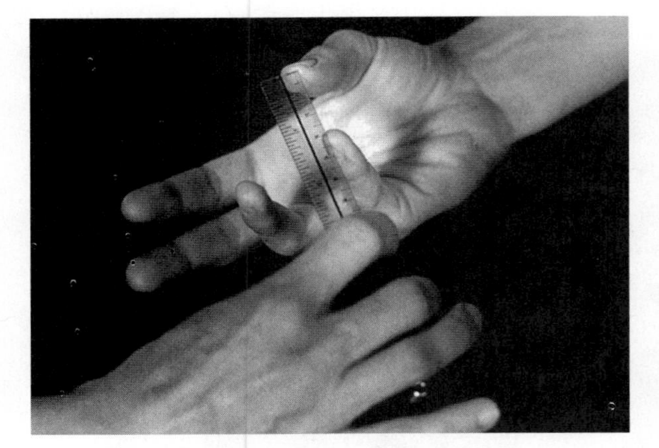

Figure 7-32 Thumb opposition to fifth finger.

Screening for Functional Range of Motion

Functional ROM refers to the range needed to accomplish typical and ordinary daily life activities such as self-feeding, hygiene, dressing, and grooming. This functional range is always less than the "normal" range given for standard measurements with a goniometer. There are many situations in which it is desirable to briefly screen a patient for functional ROM. If deficits are noted in the functional range, the standard evaluation of ROM can be used to obtain more information.

The procedure for testing functional ROM is generally demonstrated by the experienced clinician to the novice or the student on fieldwork (Box 7-2). The sequence and positioning may vary. For example, testing of forearm, wrist, and finger motions of subjects who do not have the strength to maintain shoulder abduction may be done with the forearms resting on a tabletop or the arms of a chair.

Box 7-2

Brief Screening for Functional Range of Motion

S is generally seated, preferably in a chair without arms. For each of the bold-faced motions, E gives directions (in quotes) and should also demonstrate. Alternately, E may demonstrate, saying at the same time, "Do this."

Trunk forward flexion and trunk extension: "Reach down to your toes. Come back up."

Trunk lateral flexion: "Reach down to the floor on the left with your left hand. Come back up. Reach down to the floor on the right with your right hand. Come back up."

Shoulder flexion: "Raise your arms straight up in front of you as far as you can."

Shoulder external rotation: "Place your hands behind your neck."

Shoulder internal rotation: "Reach behind your back."

Shoulder abduction: "Raise your arms out to the side."

Pronation and supination: S keeps arms in shoulder abduction position and is instructed, "Turn your palms up. Now turn your palms down."

Elbow flexion and extension: S keeps arms in shoulder abduction position and is instructed, "Bend and straighten your elbows."

Finger flexion and extension: S keeps arms in shoulder abduction position and is instructed, "Make a fist and then straighten your fingers."

Thumb opposition: S keeps arms in shoulder abduction position and is instructed, "Touch the tip of your thumb to the tips of each of the other fingers."

Wrist flexion and extension: S keeps arms in shoulder abduction position and is instructed, "Bend your wrist up. Bend your wrist down."

Wrist radial and ulnar deviation: S places hands and forearms on lap or table top and is instructed, "Turn your hands out. Turn your hands in."

Summary

The medical professions have evolved to a point where positive *functional outcomes* are the benchmark of sound clinical practice. The assessment process is the foundation that enables the OT practitioner to target the type and scope of therapy services specific to each patient's needs.[3,4] The assessment of ROM cannot be based on hunches relative to the patient's deficits.

The measurement of ROM is an essential aspect of the assessment process. ROM measurement documents objectively the biomechanical changes in joint mobility that result from trauma, disease, or aging. ROM measurement lays the foundation for documenting increases in function proportional to increases in joint ROM.

CASE STUDY

Mr. R

Mr. R., a retired automobile industry executive, recently fractured his right shoulder during a fall. Mr. R. was evaluated at an urgent care center. X-ray films revealed a nondisplaced fracture of the right proximal humerus. The physician ordered fabrication of a full cast, medications for pain, and a follow-up visit to the center. After 6 weeks, Mr. R. lacked independence in dressing his upper body and complained of pain around the elbow joint. The physician removed the cast and, using the SOAP format, noted the following information in the medical record (see Chapter 5):

S/O

62 y/o, male, SP (R) Humeral fracture. Pt. c/o pain at elbow joint with generalized stiffness. Elbow ROM measurements show AROM 45° to 135°, PROM 30° to 150°. Strength is graded 4/5.

A

Limited ROM and strength noted in right upper extremity ([R]UE) along with impaired activities of daily living (dressing).

P

Occupational therapy 2 × week, × 2 weeks for assessment and treatment of (R)UE dysfunction.

Mr. R. was scheduled at a local OT clinic. After careful assessment, the occupational therapist and OTA collaborated in developing the following course of treatment:

- PROM and AROM and progressive strength exercises for elbow extension
- Adaptive equipment (reacher and dressing stick)
- Functional activities such as bilateral reaching, balloon volleyball, and tabletop activities
- Dynamic elbow extension splint for night use and overhead pulleys for clinic and home use.

After a 2-week course of therapy, Mr. R. had regained normal motion of his (R)UE, became independent in dressing, and was continuing a home program of general conditioning.

Selected Reading Guide Questions

1. Describe upper extremity joint motions of the shoulder flexion, extension, external rotation, and internal rotation.
2. Identify major anatomic landmarks associated with joint measurements of elbow flexion and wrist flexion and extension.
3. Describe three types of functional activities that can increase ROM in shoulder flexion.
4. List two medical conditions that can negatively influence ROM in the upper extremity.
5. Describe why the evaluation of joint ROM is an important assessment tool.
6. Describe how crepitation and discomfort can influence ROM.
7. Describe the concept of *functional range of motion* in relation to activities of daily living.
8. Contrast AROM and PROM.
9. List the four components of a goniometer.
10. Explain the reason for the OT practitioner recording goniometric data in 5-degree increments. (HINT: Interrater reliability.)

References

1. American Occupational Therapy Association: The Association: clarification of the use of the terms assessment and evaluation, *Am J Occup Ther* 49:1072–1073, 1995.
2. American Occupational Therapy Association: *Effective documentation for occupational therapy*, ed 2, Bethesda, MD, 1998, the Association.
3. American Occupational Therapy Association: *Occupational therapy practice framework: domain and process*, ed 2, Bethesda, MD, 2008, the Association.
4. American Occupational Therapy Association: Standards of practice for occupational therapy, *Am J Occup Ther* 59(6):663–665, 2005.
5. Asher IE: *An annotated index of occupational therapy evaluation tools*, Rockville, MD, 1989, the Association.
6. Asher IE, editor: *Occupational therapy assessment tools: an annotated index*, ed 2, Bethesda, MD, 2007, the Association.
7. Greene WB, editor: *Clinical measurement of joint motion*, Chicago IL, 1994, American Academy of Orthopedic Surgeons.
8. Killingworth A: *Basic physical disability procedures*, San Jose, CA, 1987, Maple.
9. Norkin CC, White DJ: *Measurement of joint motion: a guide to goniometry*, ed 4, Philadelphia, 2009, Davis.
10. Pendleton H, Schultz-Krohn W, editors: *Pedretti's occupational therapy: practice skills for physical dysfunction*, ed 6, St. Louis, 2006, Mosby.

Recommended Reading

Cole T, Tobis J: Measurement of musculoskeletal function: goniometry. In Kottke FJ, Lehmann JF: *Krusen's handbook of physical medicine and rehabilitation*, ed 4, Philadelphia, 1990, Saunders.

Everett T: *Human movement: an introductory text*, ed 6, St. Louis, 2010, Elsevier.

Moore ML: Clinical assessment of joint motion. In Basmajian JV, editor: *Therapeutic exercise*, ed 3, Baltimore, 1978, Williams & Wilkins.

Stedman's medical dictionary for the health professions and nursing, ed 6, Baltimore, 2007, Lippincott Williams & Wilkins.

CHAPTER 8

Assessment of Muscle Strength*

CINDY LISKA AND TERRI R. GONZELEZ

Key Terms

Range of motion
Passive range of motion
Manual muscle test
Muscle endurance
Muscle coordination
Palpation
Hypertrophy
Atrophy
Resistance
Gravity eliminated
Substitution
Muscle grades
Break test

Chapter Objectives

After studying this chapter, the student or practitioner will be able to do the following:

1. Identify the six general purposes of muscle strength measurement.
2. Identify the three methods of evaluating muscle strength.
3. Discuss the relationship between joint range of motion and muscle strength measurement.
4. Define manual muscle testing.
5. Identify the four primary limitations of the manual muscle test.
6. Identify and describe the two primary factors influencing muscle function.
7. Identify and define the muscle grades.
8. Describe the six steps of the standard procedure for manual muscle testing.
9. Describe the break test.
10. Demonstrate muscle testing procedures for each of the upper extremity muscle groups including positioning, stabilization, palpation, observation, and application of resistance.

The human body is capable of infinitely complex and varied movements. Muscle strength is critical for these movements. The power for the human body comes from muscles as tiny as those that surround the eyes and from others as massive as those in the legs.

Muscle function is the product of strength, endurance, and coordination. The manual muscle test allows the occupational therapy (OT) practitioner to assess, plan treatment, and perhaps predict functional changes in the musculoskeletal system.

Manual muscle testing can be approached in several ways. Simple observation of the patient interacting in the immediate environment allows the practitioner to note any obvious difficulties. However, a more precise assessment of muscle strength is often undertaken to assess primary conditions such as general debility; spinal cord injuries; Guillain-Barré syndrome; primary muscle and neurologic disease processes; and traumatic conditions resulting from contractures, burns, amputation, arthritis, and fractures, as well as a variety of other orthopedic conditions.

Chapter 7 examined the movements of the body. This chapter discusses the muscles, especially in relation to movement, and explores how muscle function affects the ability to perform our daily occupations.

Role of the Occupational Therapy Assistant in Evaluating Muscle Strength

The supervising occupational therapist, in accordance with the applicable laws and professional practice standards of the particular state, determines the extent of the occupational therapy assistant's (OTA's) involvement in data collection and measurement for muscle testing. In many clinical practices the OTA performs basic gross muscle testing of the upper extremity. The role of the OTA in this area is based on demonstrated service competency and must be within the legislation and restrictions governing the practice setting. The American Occupational Therapy Association (AOTA) has defined *service competency* as whether the occupational therapist and OTA can perform the same assessments or tests in the same manner and achieve the same results.

Limitations Resulting from Muscle Weakness

Muscle weakness can restrict performance in self-care, vocational, leisure, and social activities. Documentation of strength limitations must be linked to function. The OT

*Lorraine Williams Pedretti and Michael K. Davis contributed large portions of this chapter to the first edition of this book.

practitioner must assess and monitor the degree of improvement in strength as it relates to occupation—for example, in performance skills required for different aspects of activities of daily living (ADL) such as the ability to carry an object and sustain an activity over time.

Given good to normal endurance, the patient with good (G) to normal (N) muscle strength can perform all ordinary ADL without undue fatigue.[6] The patient with fair plus (F+) muscle strength usually has low endurance and fatigues more easily than one with G or N strength. The patient can perform many ordinary ADL independently but may require frequent rest periods. The patient with the muscle grade of fair (F) can move parts against gravity and perform light tasks that present little or no resistance.[4,6]

Low endurance is a significant problem that limits activity. As a general rule, for every day of hospitalization, 3 days are necessary to recondition back to prehospitalization status. The patient with low endurance probably can self-feed finger foods and perform light self-hygiene but may do so slowly, requiring rest periods to reach their goals.[6] If muscle strength in the lower extremities is only F, ambulation is not possible.[4] Poor (P) strength is considered below functional range, but the patient can perform some ADL with mechanical assistance, and **range of motion (ROM)** can be maintained independently.[4] Patients with muscle grades of trace (T) and zero (0) are completely dependent and can perform ADL only with the aid of externally powered devices. Some activities are possible with special controls on equipment such as electric wheelchairs, communication devices, and hand splints.[6]

General Purposes of Muscle Strength Measurement

The evaluation of muscle strength helps the examiner to assess the strength of a given movement. The purposes for evaluating muscle strength are as follows[6]:

1. Determine the amount of muscle power available and thus establish a baseline for treatment.
2. Assess how muscle weakness is limiting performance of occupation.
3. Prevent deformities that can result from imbalances of strength of agonist and antagonist muscles.
4. Determine the need for assistive devices to compensate for reduced strength.
5. Aid in the selection of activities within the patient's capabilities.
6. Evaluate the effectiveness of treatment.

Methods of Evaluation

As mentioned earlier, muscle strength can be evaluated in several ways. The most precise method, if possible, is a test of individual muscles. In this procedure the muscle is carefully isolated through proper positioning, stabilization, and careful control of the movement pattern. This type of muscle testing, as described by Kendall and McCreary,[5] is not expected of the OTA.

A second and more practical means of measuring function is to assess the strength of groups of muscles that perform specific functions at individual joints, as initially described by Daniels and Worthingham.[4] A third way to evaluate muscle strength is by observing the performance of ordinary activities.[4] During the patient's self-care assessment, for example, the OT practitioner can note difficulties and movement patterns that may signal weakness, muscle imbalance, poor endurance for activity, or substitute motions. The ADL evaluation can be used together with muscle strength evaluation. The functional muscle test is often used to screen for general muscle strength.[8] The OT practitioner performs this screening and can assess effectiveness of treatment interventions based on the patient's gross improvements. *Functional muscle testing* is presented at the end of this chapter.

Relationship between Joint Range of Motion and Muscle Testing

One measure of muscle strength is the movement of the joint on which the muscle acts—that is, did the muscle move the joint through complete, partial, or no ROM? Another criterion is the amount of resistance that can be applied to the part once the muscle has moved the joint through available ROM. Available ROM is not necessarily the full average normal ROM for the given joint. Rather, available ROM is the ROM available to the individual patient. When the practitioner is measuring joint motion (see Chapter 7), the **passive range of motion (PROM)** is the measure of the range available to the patient. PROM does not, however, indicate muscle strength.

The OT practitioner must know the patient's available PROM to assign muscle grades correctly. PROM may be limited or less than the average for a particular joint motion, but the muscle strength may be normal. For example, the patient's PROM for elbow flexion may be limited to 0 degrees to 110 degrees because of a previous fracture. If the patient can flex the elbow joint to 110 degrees and hold against moderate resistance during the muscle test, the grade would be good (G). In such cases the examiner should record the limitation with the muscle grade, for example, 0 degrees to 110 degrees/G. If the patient's available ROM for elbow flexion is 0 degrees to 140 degrees and the patient can flex the elbow against gravity through 110 degrees, the muscle would be graded fair minus (F−) because the part moved through only partial ROM against gravity.

Manual Muscle Testing

The **manual muscle test** is a means of measuring the maximal contraction of a muscle or muscle group. Muscle testing is used to determine the amount of muscle power and to record gains and losses in strength. The muscle test is a primary evaluation tool for patients with lower motor neuron disorders, primary muscle diseases, and orthopedic dysfunction. The criteria used to measure strength are (1) evidence of muscle contraction; (2) amount of ROM through which the joint passes; and (3) amount of resistance against which the muscle can contract including gravity as a form of resistance.[4]

Limitations

The limitations of the manual muscle test are the inability to measure the patient's **muscle endurance** (number of times the muscle can contract at maximum level), **muscle coordination** (smooth, rhythmic interactions of muscle function), or motor performance capabilities (use of the muscles for functional activities).

The manual muscle test cannot be used accurately with patients who have spasticity caused by upper motor neuron disorders such as cerebrovascular accident (CVA, stroke) and cerebral palsy, for the following reasons[2,3,7]:

1. In these disorders, muscles are often hypertonic.
2. Muscle tone and ability to perform movements are influenced by primitive reflexes and the position of the head and body in space.
3. Movements tend to occur in gross synergistic patterns (several muscles and joints working together), which makes isolating muscle action and joint movement impossible for most patients, as demanded in manual muscle-testing procedures.

Examiner's Knowledge and Skill

Validity of the manual muscle test depends on the examiner's knowledge and skill in using the correct testing procedure. Careful observation of movement, careful and accurate **palpation** (detecting muscle activity by placing the fingers over the muscle), correct positioning, consistency of procedure, and the examiner's experience are factors critical to accurate testing.[4,5]

To be proficient in manual muscle testing, the examiner must have detailed knowledge about all aspects of muscle function. Joints and joint motions, muscle innervation, origin and insertion of muscles, action of muscles, direction of muscle fibers, angle of pull on the joints, and the role of muscles in fixation and substitution are important considerations. The examiner must be able to locate and palpate the muscles; recognize whether the contour of the muscle is normal, atrophied, or hypertrophied; and detect abnormal movements and positions. Knowledge and experience are necessary to detect substitutions and to interpret strength grades accurately.[5]

The examiner must acquire skill and experience in testing and grading muscles of normal persons of both genders and all ages. Some muscles in normal individuals may seem to be weak, but this status may be normal for the particular person. Experience in considering the subject's age, gender, body build, and lifestyle can help the examiner differentiate normal strength from slight muscle weakness.[8]

General Principles

Preparation

The examiner should always perform a visual check to assess the general contour, comparative symmetry, and any apparent **hypertrophy** (overdevelopment) or **atrophy** (wasting away) of the muscle(s). When assessing the passive ROM, the examiner can estimate the muscle tone and determine resistance to that motion. During the active ROM the examiner can observe the quality of movement (speed, smoothness, rhythm, abnormal movements such as tremors).

Positioning

Correct positioning of the subject and body part is essential to effective and correct muscle evaluation. The subject should be positioned comfortably on a firm surface. Testing muscles while the subject is seated or in a wheelchair is common. Clothing should be arranged or removed so that the examiner can see the muscle or muscle groups being tested. If this accommodation is not possible, the examiner must exercise clinical judgment in approximating muscle grades.[8] Moreover, correct positioning, careful stabilization, and palpation of the muscle(s) and observation of movement are essential to test validity.[4]

Factors Influencing Muscle Function

Gravity

Gravity provides **resistance** to muscle power[5] that is used as a grading criterion in tests of the neck, trunk, and extremities. Therefore muscle grade must consider whether a muscle can move the part against gravity.[5]

Movements against gravity and applied resistance are performed in a vertical plane (i.e., moving up). Graded manual resistance is used with fair plus (F+) to normal (N) grades. Tests for weaker muscles (0, T, P, and P– grades; see Table 8-1) are often performed in a horizontal plane (i.e., moving sideways).

Table 8-1 Muscle Grades in Manual Muscle Testing

Number Grade	Word (Letter) Grade	Definition
0	Zero (0)	No muscle contraction can be seen or felt.
1	Trace (T)	Contraction can be felt, but there is no motion.
2	Poor minus (P–)	Part moves through incomplete ROM with gravity decreased.
2	Poor (P)	Part moves through complete ROM with gravity decreased.
2+	Poor plus (P+)	Part moves through incomplete ROM (<50%) against gravity or through complete ROM with gravity decreased against slight resistance.[4]
3	Fair minus (F–)	Part moves through incomplete ROM (>50%) against gravity.[4]
3	Fair (F)	Part moves through complete ROM against gravity.
3+	Fair plus (F+)	Part moves through complete ROM against gravity and slight resistance.
4	Good (G)	Part moves through complete ROM against gravity and moderate resistance.
5	Normal (N)	Part moves through complete ROM against gravity and full resistance.

The term gravity eliminated is often used to describe this position of testing, which reduces the resistance to muscle power by eliminating the effect of gravity.

Substitution

The brain "thinks" in terms of movement and not contraction of individual muscles.[4] Thus a muscle or muscle group may attempt to compensate for the function of a weaker muscle to accomplish the desired movement. This act of compensation is termed substitution.[5] To test the muscle or muscle group accurately, the examiner must eliminate substitutions in the testing procedure by correct positioning, stabilization, and palpation of the muscle being tested. He or she must also perform the test motion carefully, without extraneous movements. The correct body position should be maintained and movement of the part performed without shifting the body or turning the part to allow substitutions.[5] The examiner must palpate contractile tissue (muscle fibers or tendons) to detect subtle tension in the muscle group under examination. Only through correct palpation can the examiner ensure that the motion is being performed by the target muscle and not by substitution.[4] Detecting substitutions is a skill gained with experience.

Positioning for movement in the correct plane may not be possible with some patients because of confinement to bed, generalized weakness, trunk instability, immobilization devices, and medical precautions.

Muscle Grades

Although the definitions of the muscle grades are standard, the assignment of muscle grades during the manual muscle test depends on the examiner's clinical judgment, knowledge, and experience.[4] The examiner determines slight, moderate, or full resistance based on clinical expertise. The patient's age, gender, body type, occupation, and avocations all influence the amount of resistance that the examiner perceives to be appropriate.

The amount of resistance that can be given also varies from one muscle group to another.[4] For example, the flexors of the wrist take much more resistance than the abductors of the fingers. The examiner must consider the size and relative power of the muscle(s) or muscle group and accordingly adjust the leverage used when giving resistance.[6] When assessing dysfunction in a given part of the body, the examiner often uses the patient as his or her own control standard by comparing the affected side with the unaffected side when possible.

Because weak muscles fatigue easily, results of muscle testing may not be accurate if the subject is tired. Pain, swelling, or muscle spasm in the area being tested may also interfere with the testing procedure. The examiner should note such problems on the assessment form. Psychologic factors must also be considered. The examiner must assess the subject's motivation, cooperation, mood, cognitive ability, and effort when interpreting strength.[4]

In manual muscle testing, muscles are graded according to the criteria in Table 8-1.[4,10]

The purpose of using plus and minus designations with muscle grades is to "fine-grade" the muscle strength grades. The experienced examiner will probably use these designations. The results attained by two examiners testing the same subject may vary up to a half grade, but they should not disagree by a whole grade.[8]

Procedure for Manual Muscle Testing

Testing should be performed according to a standard procedure to ensure accuracy and consistency. Each test is conducted following the same basic steps: (1) position; (2) stabilize; (3) palpate; (4) observe; (5) resist; and (6) grade.

First, the subject (S) should be positioned for the specific muscle test. The examiner (E) should *position* in relation to S. Then E *stabilizes* the part proximal to the part being tested to eliminate extraneous movements, isolate the muscle group, ensure the correct test motion, and eliminate the chance of substitution. E demonstrates or describes the test motion to S and asks S to perform the desired test motion. E makes a general observation of the form and quality of movement, checking for substitutions or difficulties that may require adjustments in positioning and stabilization. E then places fingers to *palpate* one or more of the prime movers, or the tendinous insertion(s), in the muscle group being tested and asks S to repeat the test motion. E again *observes* the movement for possible substitution and the amount of range completed. When S has moved the part through the available ROM, S is asked to hold the position at the end of the available ROM. E removes the palpating fingers and uses this hand to *resist* in the opposite direction of the test movement. E usually must maintain stabilization when resistance is given. These muscle tests use the break test—that is, the resistance is applied *after* S has reached the end of the available ROM and attempts to break the contraction.

S should be allowed to establish a maximal contraction (set the muscles) before the resistance is applied.[4,6] E applies the resistance after preparing S by giving the command "hold." Resistance should be applied gradually in the direction opposite to the line of pull of the muscle or muscle group being tested.

The break test should not evoke pain, and resistance should be released immediately if pain or discomfort occurs.[4] Finally, E *grades* the muscle strength according to standard definitions of muscle grades (see Table 8-1). This procedure is used for the tests of strength of grades F and above. Resistance is *not* applied for tests of muscles from P to 0. Slight resistance is sometimes applied to a muscle that has completed the full available ROM in a gravity-decreased plane to determine if the grade is P+. Figure 8-1 is a sample form for recording muscle grades. The following protocol does *not* include tests for the face, neck, trunk, and lower extremities and does not consider muscle grades below fair (F). Refer to Kendall and McCreary[5] or Daniels and Worthingham[4] for these tests.

Manual Muscle Testing of the Upper Extremity

Again, note that all the following procedures apply to testing *only* muscle grades fair (F) to normal (N).

BRIEF FUNCTIONAL MUSCLE EXAMINATION OF THE UPPER EXTREMITY

Patient's name ______________________ Chart no.

Date of birth ______________ Name of institution ______________

Date of onset ______________ Attending physician ______________ MD

Diagnosis:

KEY

5	N	Normal	Complete range of motion against gravity with full resistance.
4	G	Good*	Complete range of motion against gravity with some resistance.
3	F	Fair*	Complete range of motion against gravity.
2	P	Poor*	Complete range of motion with gravity eliminated.
1	T	Trace	Evidence of slight contractility. No joint motion.
0	0	Zero	No evidence of contractility.
S or SS			Spasm or severe spasm.
C or CC			Contracture or severe contracture.

*Muscle spasm or contracture may limit range of motion. A question mark should be placed after the grading of a movement that is incomplete from this cause.

LEFT							RIGHT			
					Examiner's initials					
					Date					
				SHOULDER	Flexor	Anterior deltoid				
					Extensors	Latissimus dorsi Teres major				
					Abductor	Middle deltoid				
					Horiz. abd.	Posterior deltoid				
					Horiz. add.	Pectoralis major				
					External rotator group					
					Internal rotator group					
				ELBOW	Flexors	Biceps brachii Brachioradialis				
					Extensor	Triceps				
				FOREARM	Supinator group					
					Pronator group					
				WRIST	Flexors	Flex. carpi rad. Flex. carpi uln.				
					Extensors	Ext. carpi rad. l. & br. Ext. carpi uln.				
				FINGERS	MP flexors	Lumbricales				
					IP flexors (first)	Flex. digit. sub.				
					IP flexors (second)	Flex. digit. prof.				
					MP extensor	Ext. digit. com.				
					Adductors	Palmar interossei				
					Abductors	Dorsal interossei				
					Abductor digiti quinti					
					Opponens digiti quinti					
				THUMB	MP flexor	Flex. poll. br.				
					IP flexor	Flex. poll. l.				
					MP extensor	Ext. poll. br.				
					IP extensor	Ext. poll. l.				
					Abductors	Abd. poll. br. Abd. poll. l.				
					Adductor pollicis					
					Opponens pollicis					

Additional data:

Figure 8-1 Sample form for brief functional muscle examination of the upper extremity. (Modified from March of Dimes—Birth Defects Foundation.)

LEFT							RIGHT			
				Examiner's initials						
				Date						
				SCAPULA	Abductor	Serratus anterior				
					Elevator Depressor	Upper trapezius Lower trapezius				
					Adductors	Middle trapezius Rhomboids				
				SHOULDER	Flexor	Anterior deltoid				
					Extensors	Latissimus dorsi Teres major				
					Abductor	Middle deltoid				
					Horiz. abd.	Posterior deltoid				
					Horiz. add.	Pectoralis major				
					External rotator group					
					Internal rotator group					
				ELBOW	Flexors	Biceps brachii Brachioradialis				
					Extensor	Triceps				
				FOREARM	Supinator group					
					Pronator group					
				WRIST	Flexors	Flex. carpi rad. Flex. carpi uln.				
					Extensors	Ext. carpi rad. l. & br. Ext. carpi uln.				
				FINGERS	MP flexors	Lumbricales				
					IP flexors (first)	Flex. digit. sub.				
					IP flexors (second)	Flex. digit. prof.				
					MP extensor	Ext. digit. com.				
					Adductors	Palmar interossei				
					Abductors	Dorsal interossei				
					Abductor digiti quinti					
					Opponens digiti quinti					
				THUMB	MP flexor	Flex. poll. br.				
					IP flexor	Flex. poll. l.				
					MP extensor	Ext. poll. br.				
					IP extensor	Ext. poll. l.				
					Abductors	Abd. poll. br. Abd. poll. l.				
					Adductor pollicis					
					Opponens pollicis					
				FACE						

Additional data:

Figure 8-1, cont'd

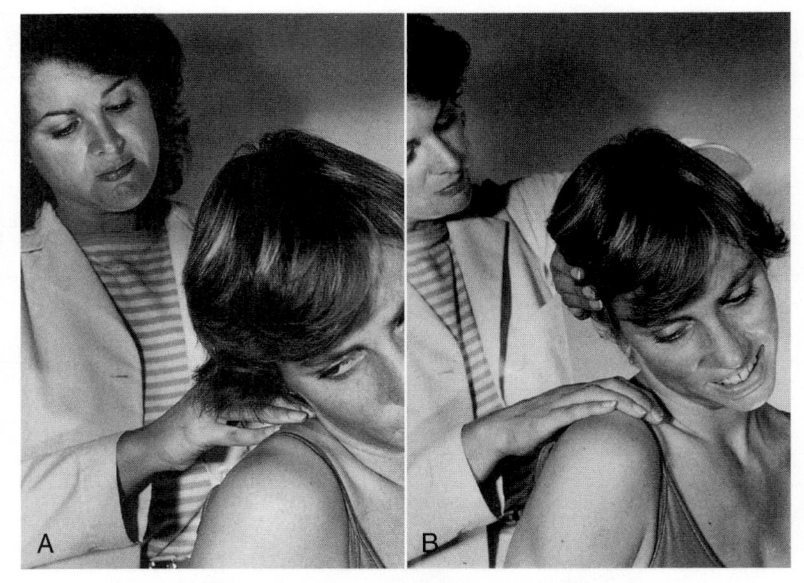

Figure 8-2 Scapula elevation. **A,** Palpate and observe. **B,** Resist.

Motion: Scapula Elevation, Neck Rotation, and Lateral Flexion

Muscles[4]	Innervation[4]
Upper trapezius	Accessory nerve (n.), C2 to C4
Levator scapula	Dorsal scapular n., C3 to C5

Position: S seated erect with arms resting at the sides of the body. E stands behind S toward the side to be tested.
Stabilize: A chair back can offer trunk stabilization, if necessary.
Palpate: The upper trapezius parallel to the cervical vertebrae, near the shoulder neck curve.
Observe: Elevation of the scapula as S shrugs the shoulder toward the ear and rotates and laterally flexes the neck toward the side being tested at the same time (Figure 8-2, *A*).
Resist: With one hand on top of the shoulder toward scapula depression and with the other hand on the side of the head toward derotation and lateral flexion to the opposite side (Figure 8-2, *B*).

Motion: Scapula Abduction and Upward Rotation

Muscles[4]	Innervation[4]
Serratus anterior	Long thoracic n., C5 to C7

Position: S lying supine with the shoulder flexed to 90 degrees and slightly abducted, elbow extended or fully flexed. E stands next to S on the side being tested.
Stabilize: The weight of the trunk or over the shoulder.
Palpate: The digitations of the origin of the serratus anterior are on the ribs, along the midaxillary line and just distal and anterior to the axillary border of the scapula. Note that muscle contraction may be difficult to detect in women and overweight subjects.
Observe: S reaches upward as if pushing the arm toward the ceiling, abducting the scapula (Figure 8-3, *A*).
Resist: At the distal end of the humerus and push the arm directly downward toward scapula adduction (Figure 8-3, *B*). If there is shoulder instability, E should support the arm and not apply resistance. In this instance only a grade of F (3) can be tested.

Motion: Scapula Adduction

Muscles[4]	Innervation[4]
Middle trapezius	Spinal accessory n., C3 and 4
Rhomboids	Dorsal scapular n., C4 and 5

Position: Lying prone with one shoulder abducted to 90 degrees and externally rotated and the elbow flexed to 90 degrees, the shoulder is resting on the supported surface. E stands on the side being tested.
Stabilize: The weight of the trunk on the supporting surface is usually adequate stabilization, or over the midthorax to prevent trunk rotation.
Palpate: The middle trapezius between the spine of the scapula and the adjacent vertebrae in alignment with the abducted humerus.
Observe: S lifts the arm off the table. Observe for movement of the vertebral border of the scapula toward the thoracic vertebrae (Figure 8-4, *A*).
Resist: At the vertebral border of the scapula toward adduction (Figure 8-4, *B*).

Motion: Shoulder Flexion

Muscles[4]	Innervation[4]
Anterior deltoid	Axillary nerve, fifth and sixth cervical nerves (C5, C6)
Coracobrachialis	Musculocutaneous n., C6, C7

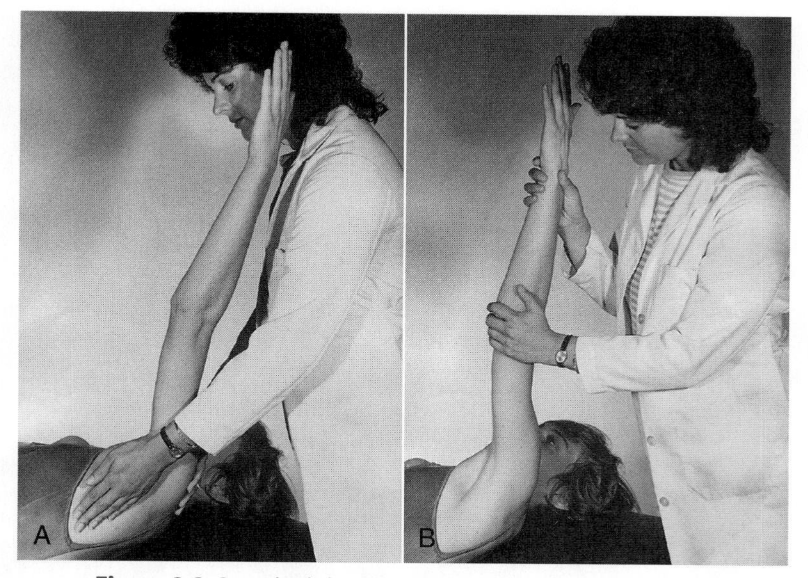

Figure 8-3 Scapula abduction. **A**, Palpate and observe. **B**, Resist.

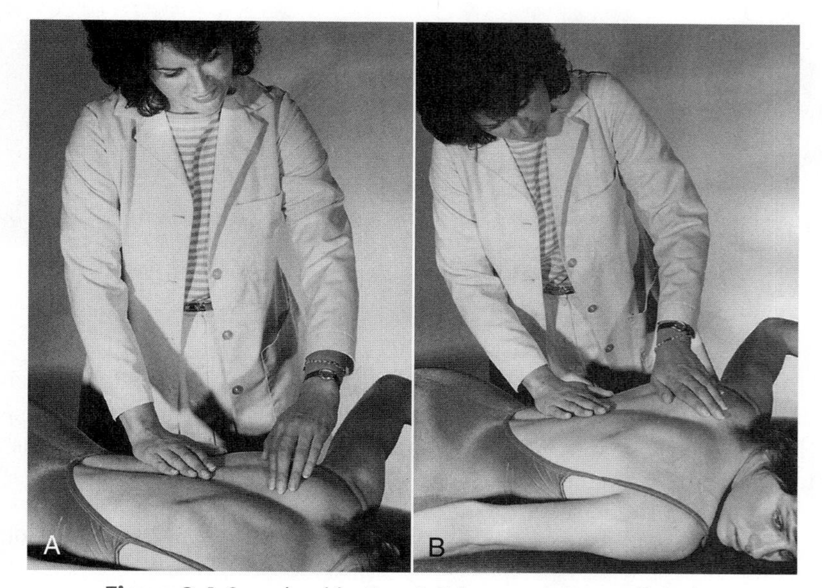

Figure 8-4 Scapula adduction. **A**, Palpate and observe. **B**, Resist.

Position: S seated with arm relaxed at side of body with hand facing backward. A straight-back chair may be used to offer maximum trunk support. E stands on the side being tested and slightly behind S.[4,10]

Stabilize: Over shoulder being tested but allowing normal abduction and upward rotation of scapula that naturally occurs with this movement.[4]

Palpate: Anterior deltoid just below clavicle on anterior aspect of humeral head.

Observe: S flexes shoulder joint by raising arm horizontally to 90 degrees of flexion (parallel to floor) (Figure 8-5, *A*).[4]

Resist: At distal end of humerus downward toward shoulder extension (Figure 8-5, *B*).

Motion: Shoulder Extension

Muscles[4]	Innervation[4]
Latissimus dorsi	Thoracodorsal n., C6, C7, or C6 to C8
Teres major	Inferior subscapular n., C5, C6
Posterior deltoid	Axillary n., C5, C6

Position: S lying prone with shoulder joint adducted and internally rotated so that palm of hand is facing up. E stands on opposite side.

Stabilize: Over scapula on the side being tested.

Palpate: Teres major along axillary border of scapula. Latissimus dorsi may be palpated slightly below this point

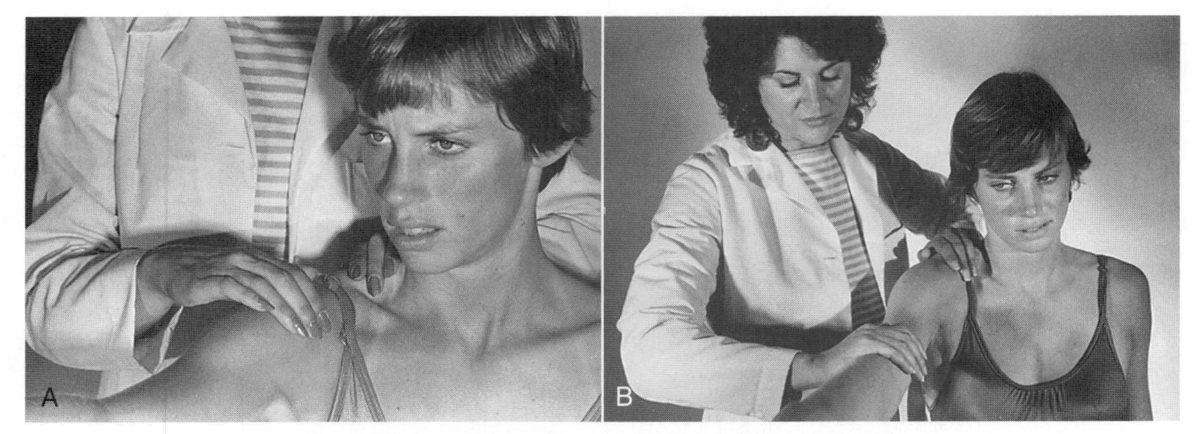

Figure 8-5 Shoulder flexion. **A,** Palpate and observe. **B,** Resist.

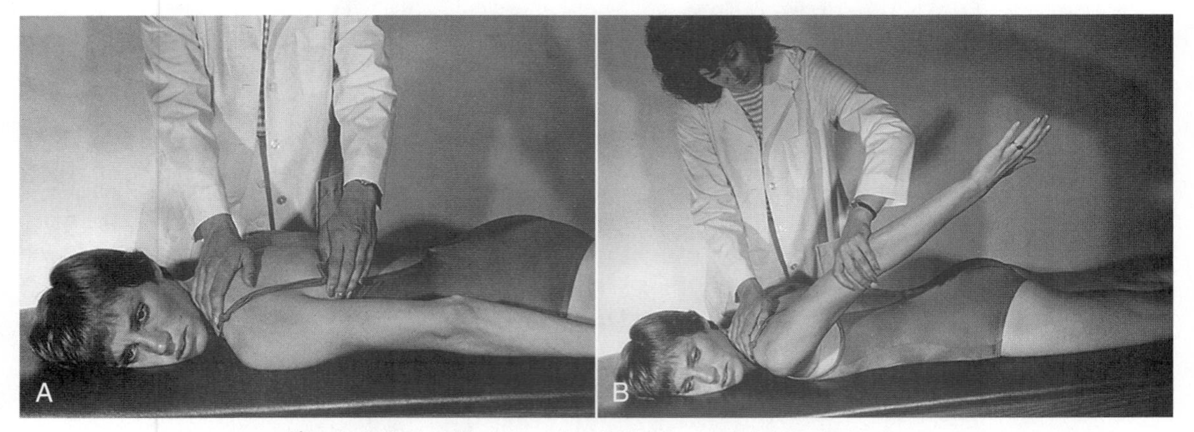

Figure 8-6 Shoulder extension. **A,** Palpate and observe. **B,** Resist.

or closer to its origin parallel to thoracic and lumbar vertebrae.[4] Posterior deltoid may be found over posterior aspect of humeral head (Figure 8-6, *A*).

Observe: S lifts up arm off table, extending shoulder joint.

Resist: At distal end of humerus in a downward and outward direction, toward flexion and slight abduction (Figure 8-6, *B*).[4,5]

Motion: Shoulder Abduction

Muscles[4]	Innervation[4]
Middle deltoid	Axillary n., C5 to C8
Supraspinatus	Suprascapular n., C5

Position: S seated with arms relaxed at sides of body. Elbow on side to be tested should be slightly flexed with palms facing body. E stands behind S.

Stabilize: Over scapula on the side being tested.[4,5]

Palpate: Middle deltoid over middle of shoulder joint from acromion to deltoid tuberosity.[4-6]

Observe: S abducts shoulder to 90 degrees. During movement, S's palm should remain down, and E should observe that no external rotation of shoulder or elevation of scapula occurs.[4-6] Supraspinatus may be difficult to palpate because the muscle lies under the trapezius muscle, but may be palpated in supraspinatus fossa (Figure 8-7, *A*).[4]

Resist: At distal end of humerus as if pushing arm down toward adduction (Figure 8-7, *B*).

Motion: Shoulder External Rotation

Muscles[4]	Innervation[4]
Infraspinatus	Axillary n., C5, C6
Teres minor	Axillary n., C5, C6

Position: S lying prone with shoulder abducted to 90 degrees, humerus in neutral (0 degrees) rotation, and elbow flexed to 90 degrees. Forearm is in neutral rotation, hanging over edge of table, perpendicular to the floor. E stands in front of supporting surface toward side being tested.

Stabilize: At distal end of humerus by placing hand under arm on supporting surface.[5]

Palpate: Infraspinatus muscle just below spine of scapula, on body of scapula, or teres minor along axillary border of scapula.[4]

Observe: Rotation of humerus so that back of hand is moving toward ceiling (Figure 8-8, *A*).[4,5]

Resist: On distal end of forearm toward floor in direction of internal rotation (Figure 8-8, *B*).[4,5]

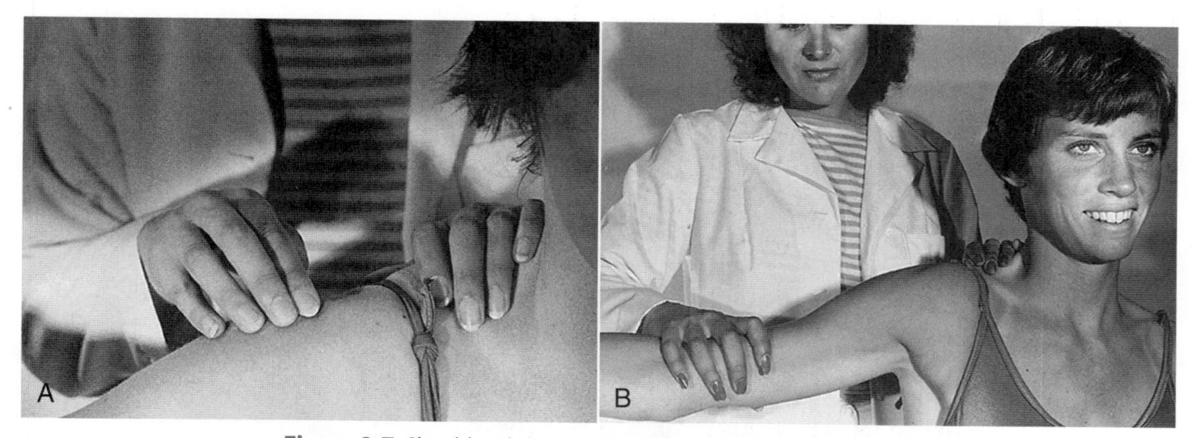

Figure 8-7 Shoulder abduction. **A,** Palpate and observe. **B,** Resist.

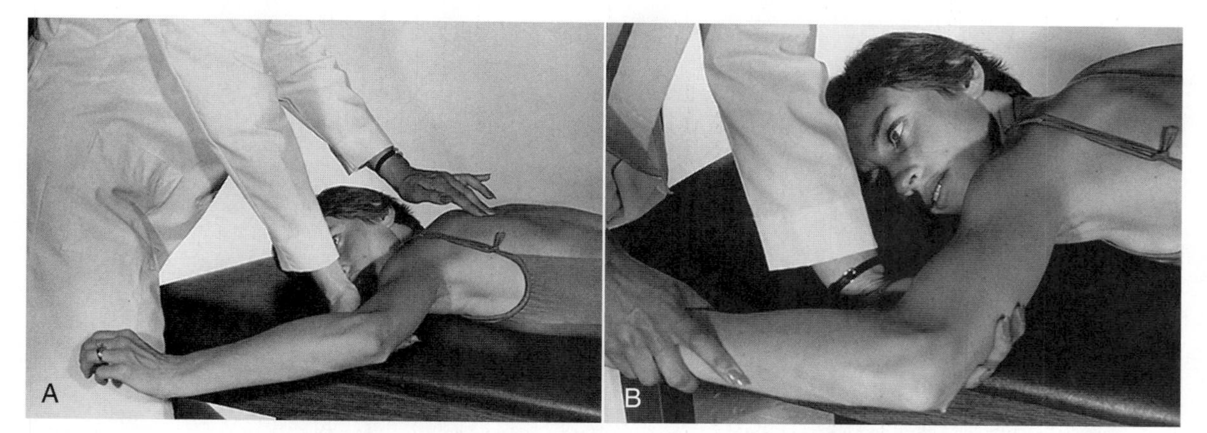

Figure 8-8 Shoulder external rotation. **A,** Palpate and observe. **B,** Resist.

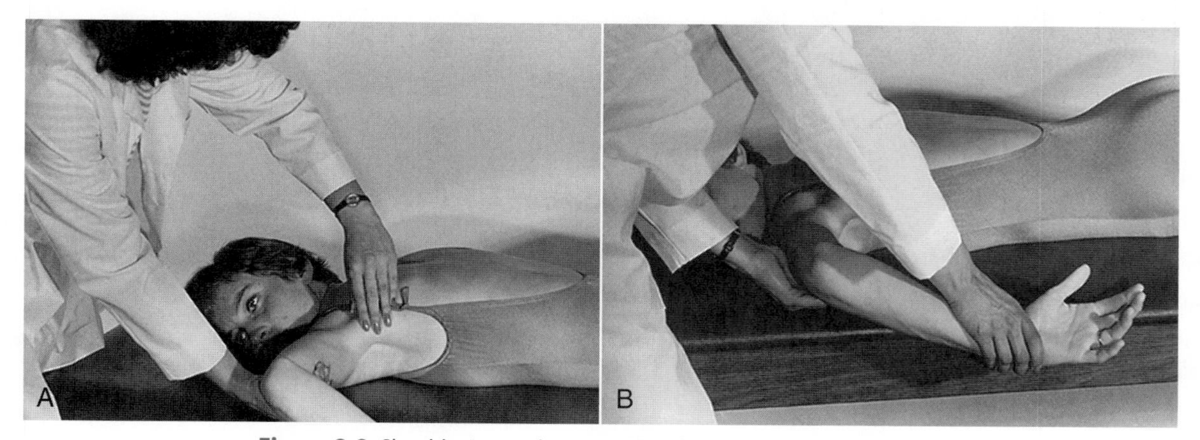

Figure 8-9 Shoulder internal rotation. **A,** Palpate and observe. **B,** Resist.

Motion: Shoulder Internal Rotation

Muscles[4]	Innervation[4]
Subscapularis	Subscapular n., C5, C6
Pectoralis major	Anterior thoracic n., C5 through first thoracic nerve (T1)
Latissimus dorsi	Thoracodorsal n., C6 to C8
Teres major	Subscapular n., C5, C6

Position: S lying prone with shoulder abducted to 90 degrees, humerus in neutral (0 degrees) rotation, and elbow flexed to 90 degrees. Forearm is perpendicular to floor. E stands on the side being tested, just in front of S's arm.

Stabilize: At distal end of humerus by placing hand under arm and on supporting surface, as for external rotation.[4,5]

Palpate: Teres major and latissimus dorsi along axillary border of scapula toward inferior angle.

Observe: Movement of palm of hand upward toward ceiling, internally rotating humerus (Figure 8-9, *A*).[4]

Resist: At distal end of volar surface of forearm anteriorly toward external rotation (Figure 8-9, *B*).[4,5]

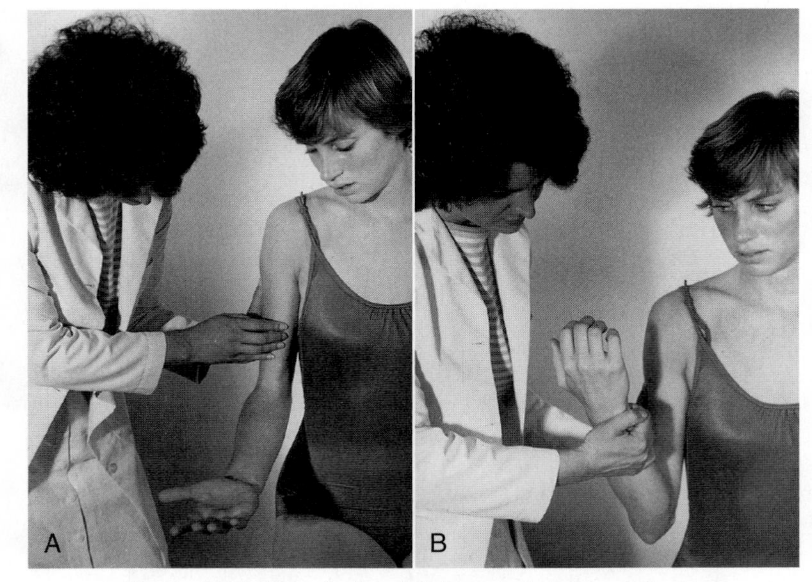

Figure 8-10 Elbow flexion. **A,** Palpate and observe. **B,** Resist.

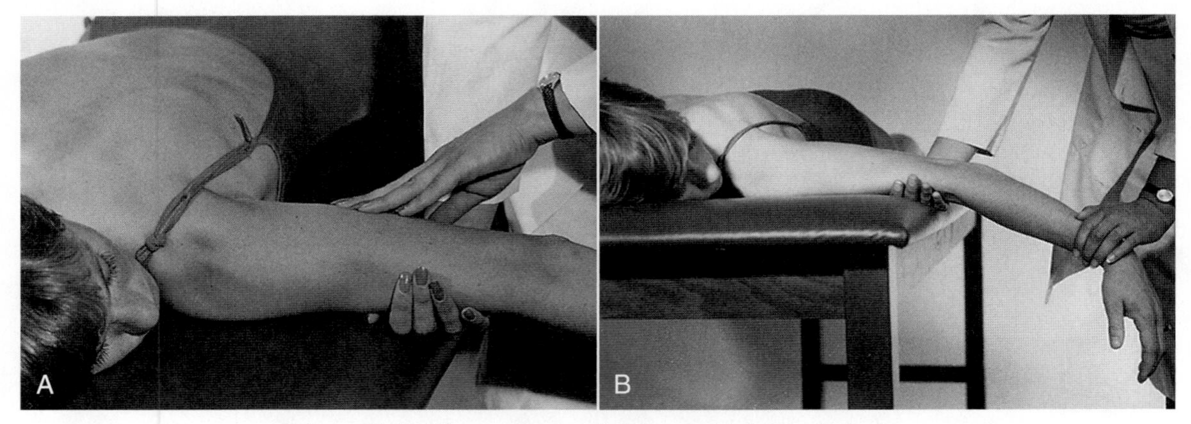

Figure 8-11 Elbow extension. **A,** Palpate and observe. **B,** Resist.

Motion: Elbow Flexion

Muscles[4]	Innervation[4]
Biceps brachii	Musculocutaneous n., C5, C6
Brachialis	Musculocutaneous n., C5, C6
Brachioradialis	Radial n., C5, C6

Position: S sitting with arm adducted at shoulder and extended at elbow, held against side of trunk. Forearm is supinated to test primarily for biceps. E stands next to S on the side being tested or directly in front of S.

Stabilize: Humerus in adduction.

Palpate: Biceps brachii over muscle belly on middle of anterior aspect of humerus. The tendon may be palpated in middle of antecubital space.[4] Brachioradialis is palpated over upper third of radius on lateral aspect of forearm just below elbow. Brachialis may be palpated lateral to lower portion of biceps brachii, if elbow is flexed and in pronated position.[6]

Observe: Elbow flexion and movement of hand toward face. E should observe for maintenance of forearm in supination (Figure 8-10, *A*).[6]

Resist: At distal end of volar aspect of forearm, pulling downward toward elbow extension (Figure 8-10, *B*).[4,5]

Motion: Elbow Extension

Muscles[4]	Innervation[4]
Triceps	Radial n., C7, C8
Anconeus	Radial n., C7

Position: S prone with humerus abducted to 90 degrees and in neutral rotation, elbow flexed to 90 degrees, and forearm in neutral position perpendicular to floor. E stands next to S just behind arm being tested.[5,10]

Stabilize: Humerus by placing one hand for support under it, between S's arm and table.[5]

Palpate: Triceps over middle of posterior aspect of humerus or triceps tendon, just proximal to elbow joint on dorsal surface of arm.[4,6]

Observe: Extension of elbow to just less than maximum range. Wrist and fingers remain relaxed (Figure 8-11, *A*).

Resist: In same plane as forearm motion at distal end of forearm, pushing toward floor or elbow flexion. Before

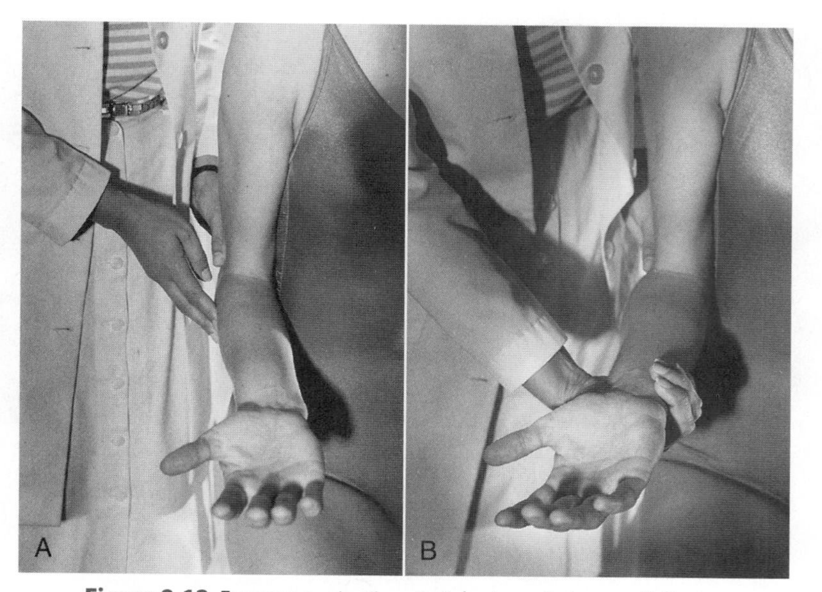

Figure 8-12 Forearm supination. **A,** Palpate and observe. **B,** Resist.

resistance is given, E ensures elbow is not locked. Resistance to a locked elbow can cause joint injury (Figure 8-11, *B*).[4]

Motion: Forearm Supination

Muscles[4]	Innervation[4]
Biceps brachii	Musculocutaneous n., C5, C6
Supinator	Radial n., C6

Position: S seated with humerus adducted, elbow flexed to 90 degrees, and forearm in full pronation. E stands next to S on the side being tested.[4]

Stabilize: Humerus just proximal to elbow.

Palpate: Over supinator on dorsolateral aspect of forearm, below head of radius. Muscle can be best felt when radial muscle group (extensor carpi radialis and brachioradialis) is pushed up and out of the way.[11] E may also palpate biceps on middle of anterior surface of humerus.

Observe: Supination, turning hand up. Gravity may assist the movement after the 0-degree neutral position is passed (Figure 8-12, *A*).

Resist: By grasping around dorsal aspect of distal forearm with fingers and heel of hand, turning arm toward pronation (Figure 8-12, *B*).

Motion: Forearm Pronation

Muscles[4]	Innervation[4]
Pronator teres	Median n., C6
Pronator quadratus	Median n., C8, T1

Position: S seated with humerus adducted, elbow flexed to 90 degrees, and forearm in full supination. E stands beside S on the side being tested.[4]

Stabilize: Humerus just proximal to elbow to prevent shoulder abduction.[4,5]

Palpate: Pronator teres on upper part of volar surface of forearm, medial to biceps tendon and diagonally from medial condyle of humerus to lateral border of radius.[4-6]

Observe: Pronation, turning hand palm down (Figure 8-13, *A*).

Resist: By grasping around dorsal aspect of distal forearm with fingers and heel of hand, turning arm toward supination (Figure 8-13, *B*).[4]

Motion: Wrist Extension with Radial Deviation

Muscles[4]	Innervation[4]
Extensor carpi radialis longus	Radial n., C5 to C8
Extensor carpi radialis brevis	Radial n., C5 to C8
Extensor carpi ulnaris	Radial n., C6 to C8

Position: S seated or supine with forearm resting on supporting surface in pronation, wrist in neutral position, and fingers and thumb relaxed. E sits opposite S or next to S on the side being tested.[6,7]

Stabilize: Over volar aspect of middle to distal forearm (Figure 8-14, *B*).[6,7]

Palpate: Extensor carpi radialis longus and brevis tendons on dorsal aspect of wrist at bases of second and third metacarpals, respectively.[4,6] Tendon of extensor carpi ulnaris may be palpated at base of fifth metacarpal, just distal to head of ulna (Figure 8-14, *A*).[4,6,11]

Observe: Wrist extension and radial deviation, lifting hand up from supporting surface and moving medially (to radial side) simultaneously. Movement should be performed without finger extension, which could substitute for wrist motion (Figure 8-14, *B*).[4,6]

Resist: Over dorsum of second and third metacarpals toward flexion and ulnar deviation (Figure 8-14, *C*).

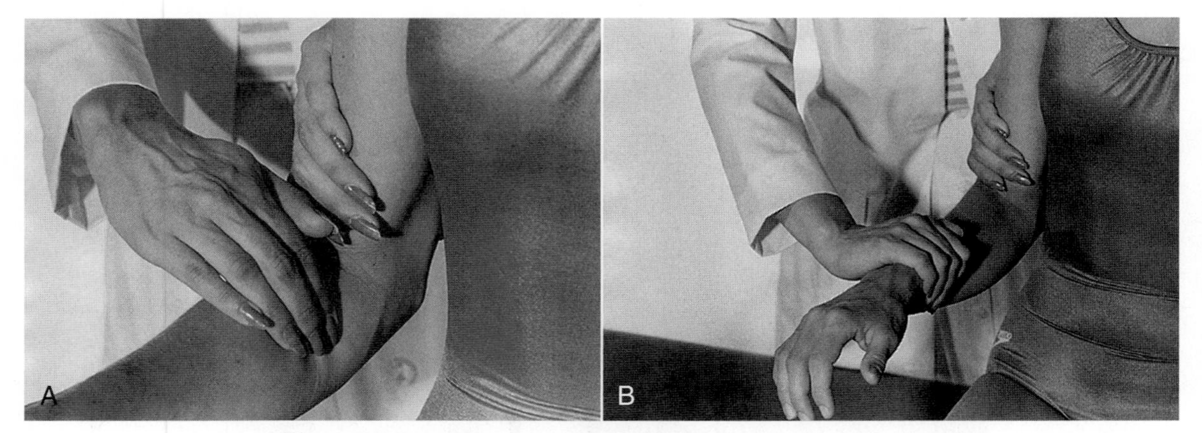

Figure 8-13 Forearm pronation. **A,** Palpate and observe. **B,** Resist.

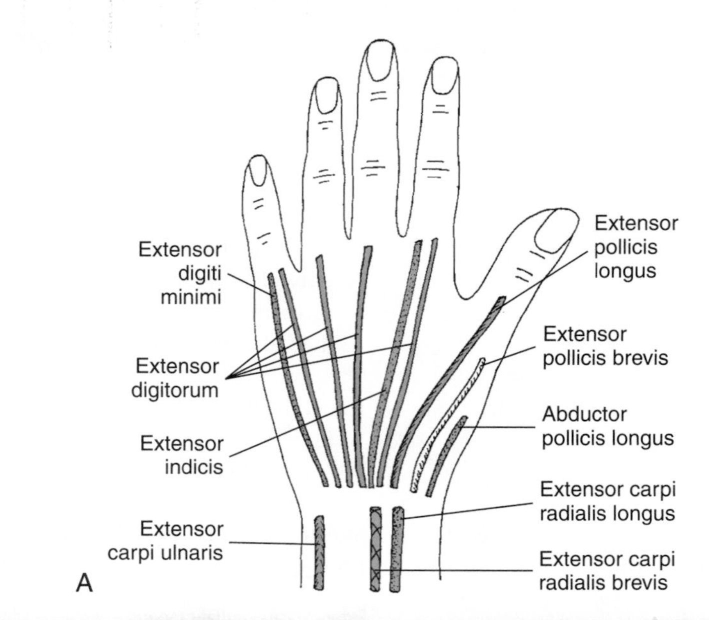

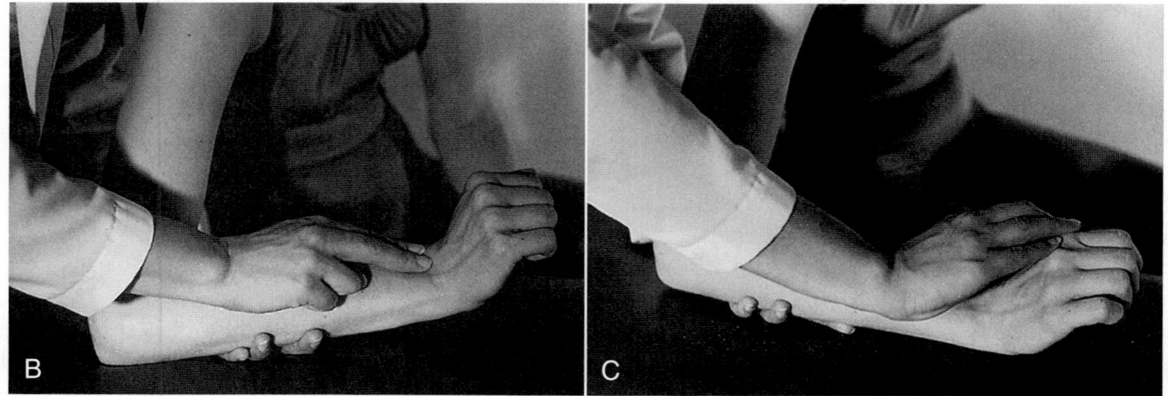

Figure 8-14 **A,** Arrangement of extensor tendons at wrist. **B,** Wrist extension with radial deviation. Palpate and observe. **C,** Resist.

Motion: Wrist Extension with Ulnar Deviation

Muscles[4-6]	Innervation[5]
Extensor carpi ulnaris	Radial n., C6 to C8
Extensor carpi radialis longus	Radial n., C5 to C8
Extensor carpi radialis brevis	Radial n., C5 to C8

Position: S seated with forearm in pronation, wrist in neutral position, and fingers and thumb relaxed. E sits opposite or next to S on the side being tested.

Stabilize: Over volar aspect of middle to distal forearm.[4,5]

Palpate: Extensor carpi ulnaris tendon at base of fifth metacarpal, just distal to head of ulna, and extensor carpi radialis

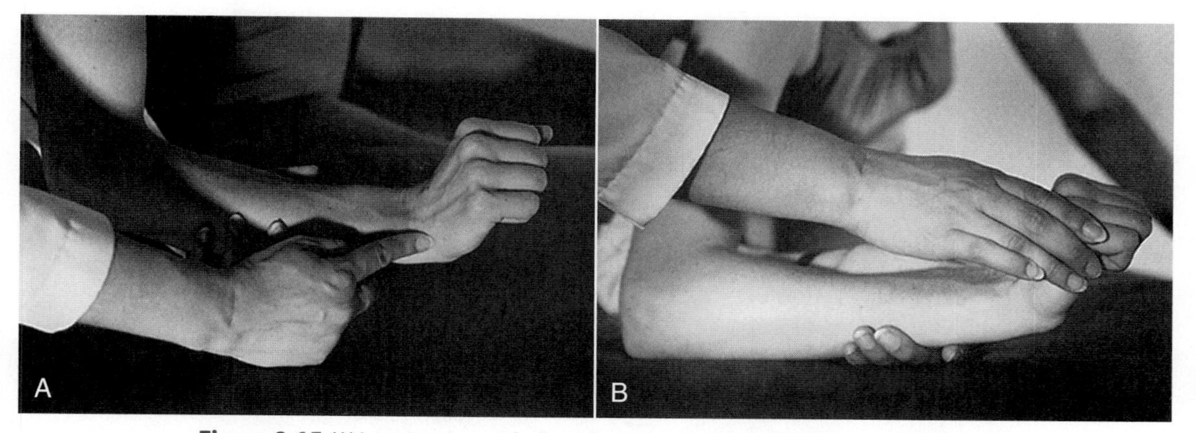

Figure 8-15 Wrist extension with ulnar deviation. **A,** Palpate and observe. **B,** Resist.

longus and brevis tendons at bases of second and third metacarpals.

Observe: S brings hand up from supporting surface and moves laterally (to ulnar side) simultaneously. E should observe that movement is not preceded by thumb or finger extension (Figure 8-15, *A*).[4,6]

Resist: Over dorsolateral aspect of fifth metacarpal toward flexion and radial deviation (Figure 8-15, *B*).[4,5]

Motion: Wrist Flexion with Radial Deviation

Muscles[5]	Innervation[4,5,9]
Flexor carpi radialis	Median n., C6 to C8
Flexor carpi ulnaris	Ulnar n., C8, T1
Palmaris longus	Median n., C7, C8, T1

Position: S seated or supine with forearm resting in almost full supination on supporting surface and fingers and thumb relaxed. E sits next to S on the side being tested.

Stabilize: Over volar aspect of midforearm.[4,5]

Palpate: Muscle tendons. Flexor carpi radialis tendon can be palpated over wrist at base of second metacarpal bone. Palmaris longus tendon is at center of wrist at base of third metacarpal, and flexor carpi ulnaris tendon can be palpated at ulnar side of volar aspect of wrist at base of fifth metacarpal (Figure 8-16, *A*).[11]

Observe: S brings hand up from supporting surface toward face, deviating hand toward radial side simultaneously. E should observe that fingers remain relaxed during movement (Figure 8-16, *B*).

Resist: In palm at radial side of hand over second and third metacarpals toward extension and ulnar deviation (Figure 8-16, *C*).

Motion: Wrist Flexion with Ulnar Deviation

Muscle[4]	Innervation[4,5,9]
Flexor carpi ulnaris	Median n., C8, T1
Flexor carpi radialis	Median n., C6 to C8
Palmaris longus	Median n., C7, C8, T1

Position: S seated or supine with forearm resting in almost full supination on supporting surface and fingers and thumb relaxed. E sits opposite or next to S on the side being tested.[4,5]

Stabilize: Over volar aspect of middle of forearm.[4,5]

Palpate: Flexor tendons on volar aspect of wrist, flexor carpi ulnaris at base of fifth metacarpal, flexor carpi radialis at base of second metacarpal, and palmaris longus at base of third metacarpal.[11] Flexor carpi radialis tendon can be palpated over wrist at base of second metacarpal bone. Palmaris longus tendon is at center of wrist at base of third metacarpal.

Observe: S brings hand up from supporting surface, simultaneously flexing wrist and deviating to the ulnar side (Figure 8-17, *A*).

Resist: In palm of hand over hypothenar eminence toward extension and radial deviation (Figure 8-17, *B*).[5]

Motion: Metacarpophalangeal (MP) Flexion with Interphalangeal (IP) Extension

Muscles[1,11]	Innervation[4]
Lumbricales manus 1 and 2	Median n., C6, C7
Lumbricales manus 3 and 4	Ulnar n., C8, T1
Interossei dorsales manus	Ulnar n., C8, T1
Interossei palmares	Ulnar n., C8, T1

Position: S is seated with forearm in supination resting on supporting surface and wrist in neutral position.[4] MP joints are extended, and IP joints flexed.[11] E sits next to S on the side being tested.

Stabilize: Over palm to prevent wrist motion.

Palpate: First interosseus dorsales just medial to distal aspect of second metacarpal on dorsum of hand. The rest of these muscles are not easily palpable because of their size and deep location in hand.

Observe: S flexes MP joints and extends IP joints simultaneously (Figure 8-18, *A*).[5]

Resist: Each finger separately by grasping distal phalanx and pushing downward on finger into supporting surface toward MP extension and IP flexion, or apply pressure first against dorsal surface of middle and distal phalanges toward flexion, followed by pressure to volar surface of proximal phalanges toward extension (Figure 8-18, *B*).[5]

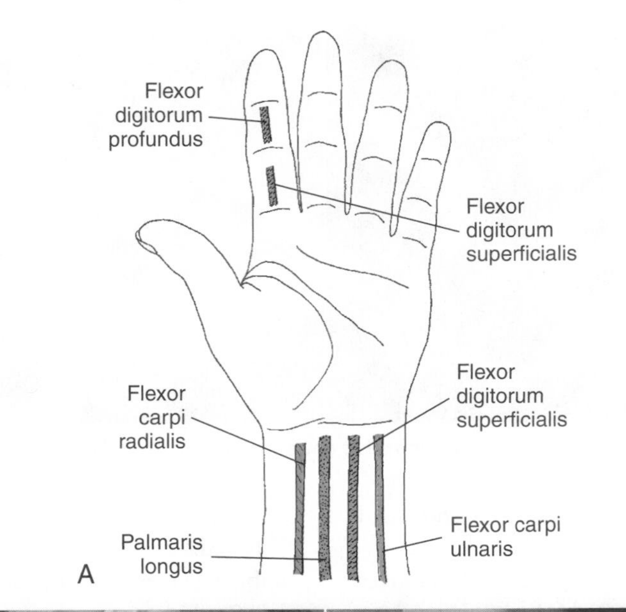

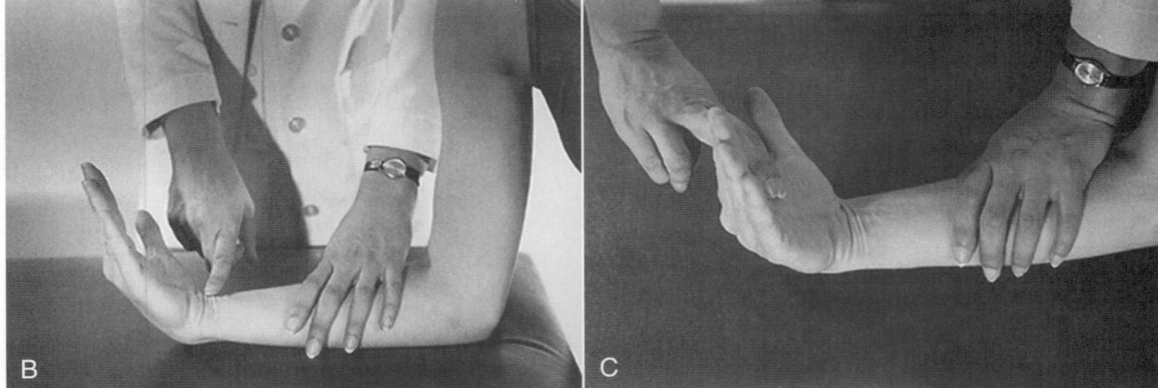

Figure 8-16 **A,** Arrangement of flexor tendons at wrist. **B,** Wrist flexion with radial deviation. Palpate and observe. **C,** Resist.

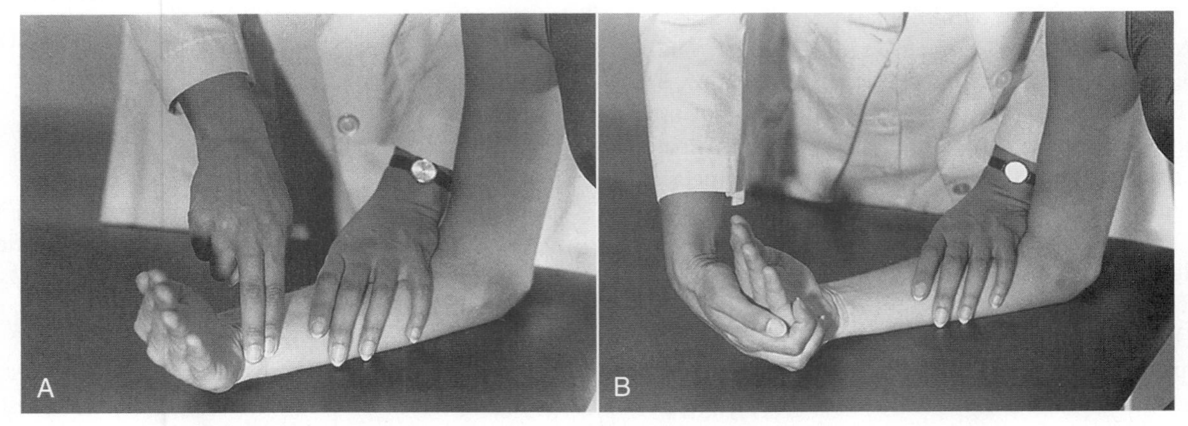

Figure 8-17 Wrist flexion with ulnar deviation. **A,** Palpate and observe. **B,** Resist.

Motion: MP Extension

Muscles[4-6]	Innervation[4]
Extensor digitorum	Radial n., C6 to C8
Extensor indicis	Radial n., C6 to C8
Extensor digiti minimi	Radial n., C6 to C8

Position: S seated with forearm pronated and wrist in neutral position, with MP and IP joints partially flexed.[4] E sits opposite or next to S on the side being tested.

Stabilize: Wrist and metacarpals slightly above supporting surface.[4,5]

Palpate: Extensor digitorum tendons where they course over dorsum of hand.[4] In some people, extensor digiti minimi

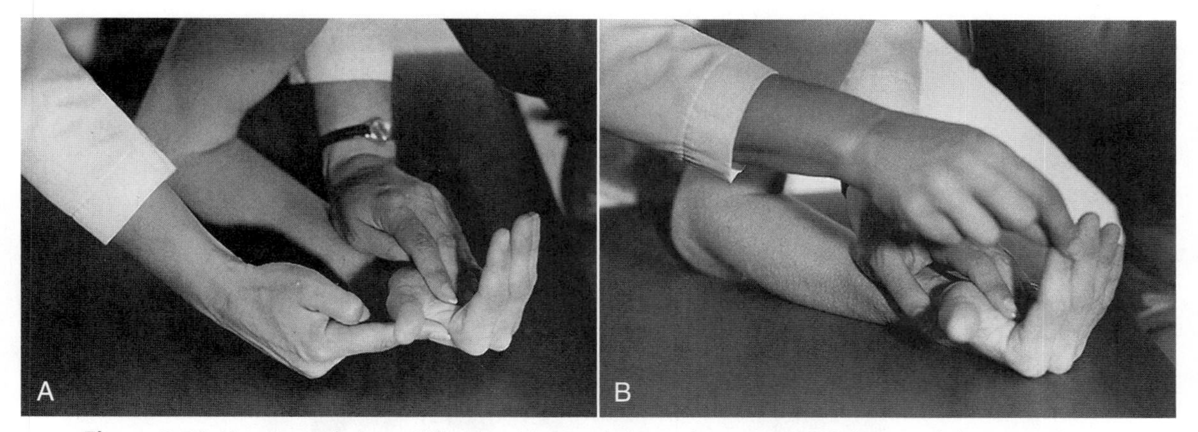

Figure 8-18 Metacarpophalangeal flexion with interphalangeal extension. **A,** Palpate and observe. **B,** Resist.

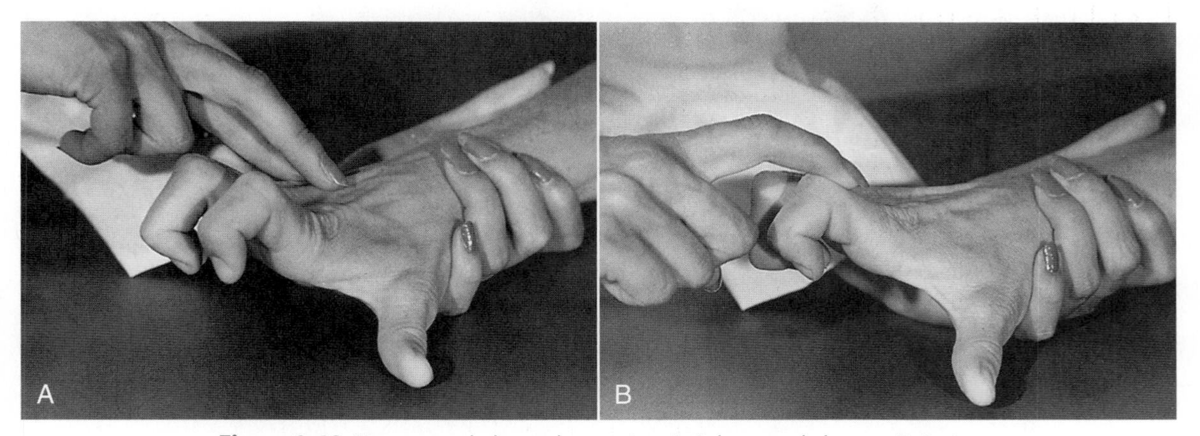

Figure 8-19 Metacarpophalangeal extension. **A,** Palpate and observe. **B,** Resist.

tendon can be palpated or visualized just lateral to extensor digitorum tendon to fifth finger. Extensor indicis tendon can be palpated or visualized just medial to extensor digitorum tendon to first finger.

Observe: S raises fingers away from supporting surface, extending MP joints but maintaining IP joints in some flexion (Figure 8-19, *A*).

Resist: Each finger individually over dorsal aspect of proximal phalanx toward MP flexion (Figure 8-19, *B*).[4,5]

Motion: Proximal Interphalangeal (PIP) Flexion, Second Through Fifth Fingers

Muscle[4,6]	Innervation[4,6]
Flexor digitorum superficialis	Median n., C7, C8, T1

Position: S seated with forearm in supination, wrist in neutral position, fingers extended, and hand and forearm resting on dorsal surface.[4] E sits opposite or next to S on the side being tested.

Stabilize: MP joint and proximal phalanx of finger being tested.[4,5]

Palpate: Flexor digitorum superficialis tendon on volar surface of proximal phalanx. A stabilizing finger may be used to palpate in this procedure.[6] Tendon supplying fourth finger may be palpated over volar aspect of wrist between flexor carpi ulnaris and palmaris longus tendons, if desired.[11]

Observe: S flexes PIP joint while maintaining distal interphalangeal (DIP) joint in extension (Figure 8-20, *A*). If isolating PIP flexion is difficult, all fingers not being tested are held in MP hyperextension and PIP extension by pulling back over IP joints. This maneuver inactivates flexor digitorum profundus (FDP) so that S cannot flex distal joint (Figure 8-20, *B*).[10,11] Most individuals cannot perform isolated action of PIP joint of fifth finger even with assistance.

Resist: With one finger at volar aspect of middle phalanx toward extension.[4,5] If index finger is used to apply resistance, middle finger may be used to move DIP joint back and forth to verify that FDP is not substituting (Figure 8-20, *C*).

Motion: Distal Interphalangeal (DIP) Flexion, Second through Fifth Fingers

Muscle[4]	Innervation[4]
Flexor digitorum profundus	Median n., ulnar n., C8, T1

Position: S seated with forearm in supination, wrist in neutral position, and fingers extended. E sits opposite or next to S on the side being tested.[4]

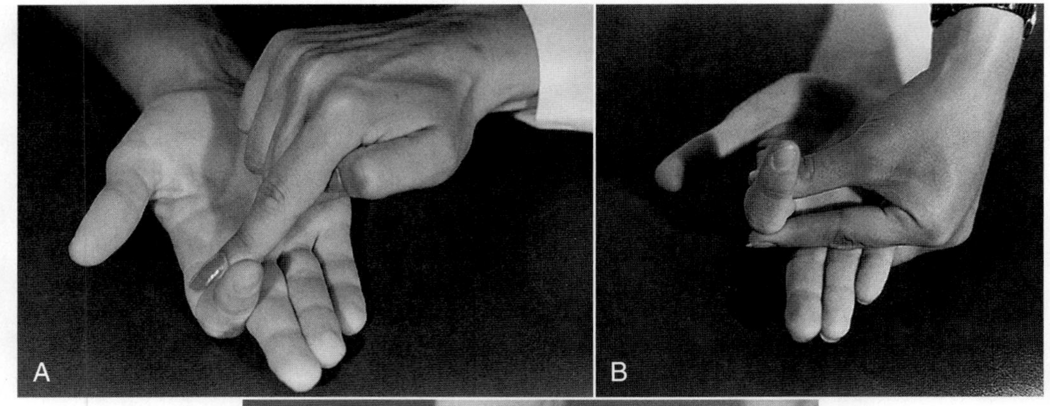

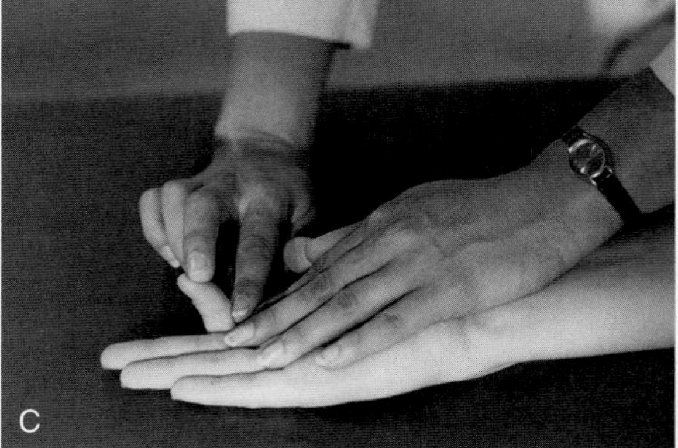

Figure 8-20 Proximal interphalangeal (PIP) flexion. **A,** Palpate and observe. **B,** Position to assist with isolation of PIP joint flexion. **C,** Resist. Examiner checks for substitution by flexor digitorum profundus.

Stabilize: Wrist at neutral position and PIP joint and middle phalanx of finger being tested.[10]

Palpate: Finger stabilizing middle phalanx used to simultaneously palpate FDP tendon over volar surface of middle phalanx.[4,6]

Observe: S brings fingertip up and away from supporting surface, flexing DIP joint (Figure 8-21, *A*).

Resist: With one finger at volar aspect of distal phalanx toward extension (Figure 8-21, *B*).[4,5]

Motion: Finger Abduction

Muscles[4]	Innervation[4]
Interossei dorsales	Ulnar n., C8, T1
Abductor digiti minimi	Ulnar n., C8, T1

Position: S seated or supine with forearm pronated, wrist in neutral position, and fingers extended and adducted. E sits opposite or next to S on the side being tested.[4]

Stabilize: Wrist and metacarpals slightly above supporting surface.

Palpate: First interosseus dorsales on lateral aspect of second metacarpal or of abductor digiti minimi manus on ulnar border of fifth metacarpal.[4] Remaining interossei are not palpable.

Observe: S spreads fingers apart, abducting them at MP joints (Figure 8-22, *A*).

Resist: First, interosseus dorsales by applying pressure on radial side of distal end of proximal phalanx of second finger in an ulnar direction (Figure 8-22, *B*); second, interosseus dorsales on radial side of proximal phalanx of middle finger in an ulnar direction; third, interosseus dorsales on ulnar side of proximal phalanx of middle finger in a radial direction; fourth, interosseus dorsales on ulnar side of proximal phalanx of ring finger in a radial direction; finally, abductor digiti minimi manus on ulnar side of proximal phalanx of little finger in a radial direction.[5]

Motion: Finger Adduction

Muscle[4,5]	Innervation[4]
Interossei palmares	Ulnar n., C8, T1

Position: S seated with forearm pronated, wrist in neutral position, and fingers extended and abducted.[4]

Stabilize: Wrist and metacarpals slightly above supporting surface.

Palpate: Not palpable.

Observe: S adducts first, fourth, and fifth fingers toward middle finger (Figure 8-23, *A*).

Resist: Index finger at proximal phalanx by pulling in a radial direction, ring finger at proximal phalanx in an ulnar direction, and little finger likewise (Figure 8-23, *B*).[5] These muscles are small, and resistance must be modified to accommodate to their comparatively limited power.

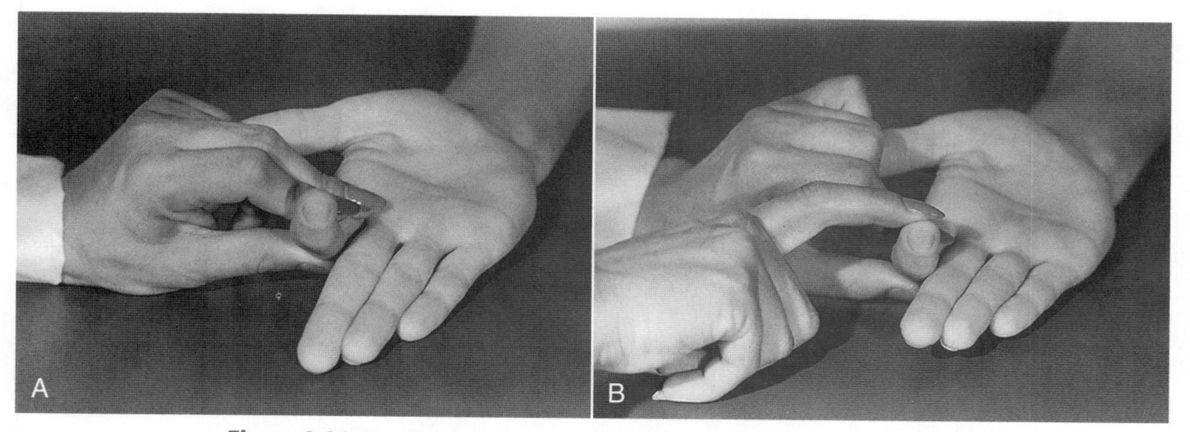

Figure 8-21 Distal interphalangeal flexion. **A,** Palpate and observe. **B,** Resist.

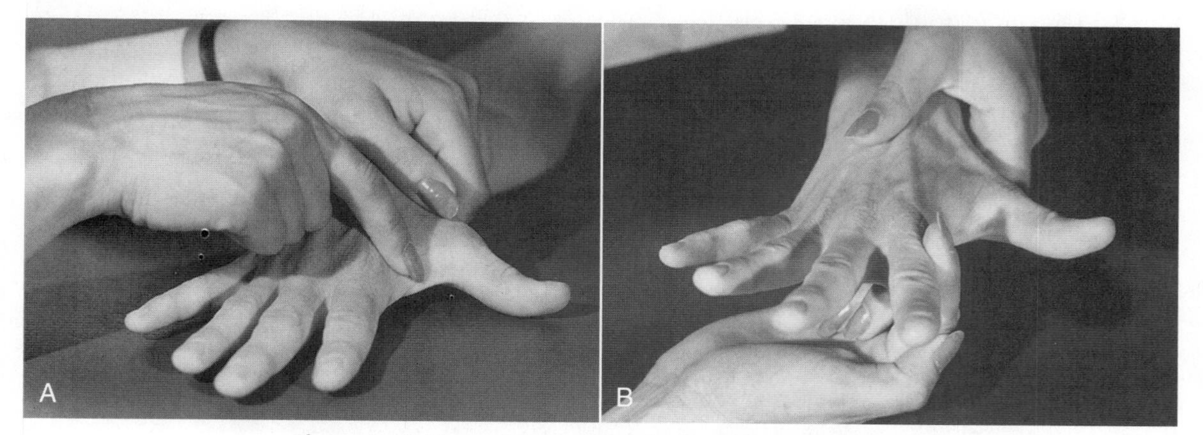

Figure 8-22 Finger abduction. **A,** Palpate and observe. **B,** Resist.

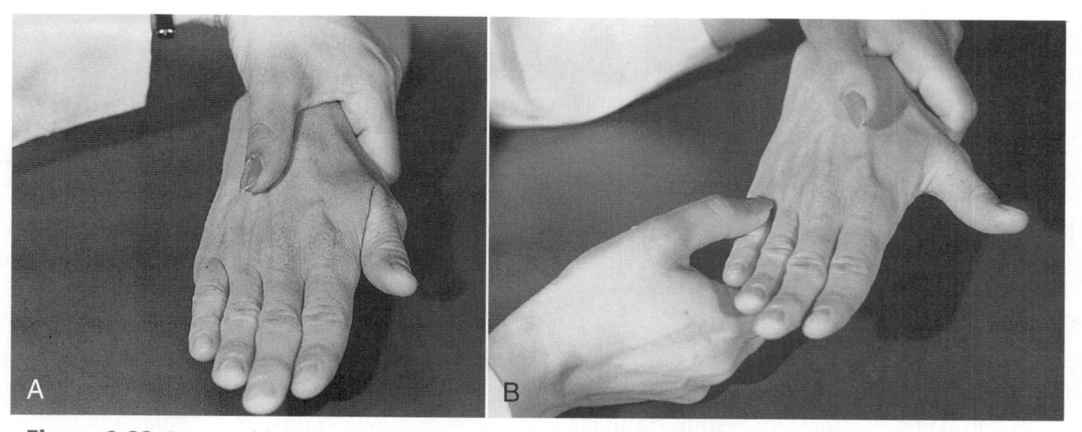

Figure 8-23 Finger adduction. **A,** Examiner observes movement of fingers into adduction. Palpation of these muscles is not possible. **B,** Resist.

Motion: Thumb MP Extension

Muscle[4,5]	Innervation[4,5]
Extensor pollicis brevis	Radial n., C6 to C8

Position: S seated or supine, forearm in midposition, wrist in neutral position, and hand and forearm resting on ulnar border.[4] Thumb is flexed into palm at MP joint, and IP joint is extended but relaxed. E sits opposite or next to S on the side being tested.

Stabilize: Wrist and thumb metacarpal.

Palpate: Extensor pollicis brevis (EPB) tendon at base of first metacarpal on dorsoradial aspect. The tendon lies just medial to abductor pollicis dorsoradial longus tendon on radial side of the anatomic snuffbox, which is hollow space between extensor pollicis longus (EPL) and EPB tendons when thumb is fully extended and radially abducted.[11]

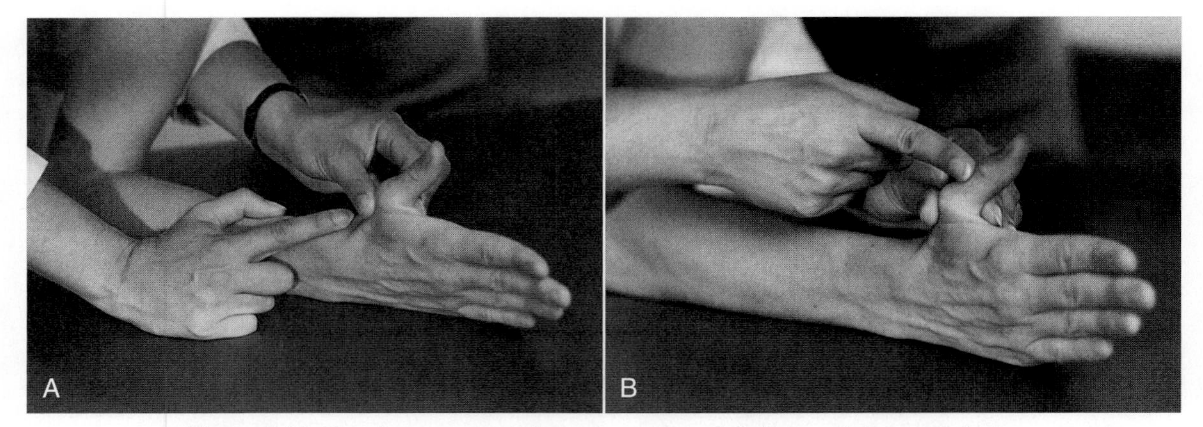

Figure 8-24 Thumb metacarpophalangeal extension. **A,** Palpate and observe. **B,** Resist.

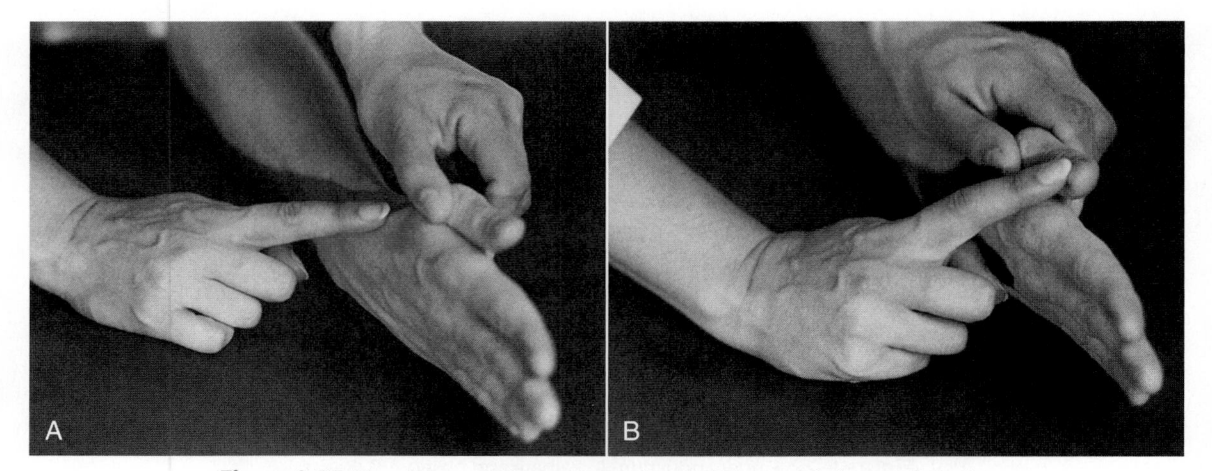

Figure 8-25 Thumb interphalangeal extension. **A,** Palpate and observe. **B,** Resist.

Observe: S extends MP joint. IP joint remains relaxed (Figure 8-24, *A*). Many people have difficulty isolating this motion.
Resist: On dorsal surface of proximal phalanx toward MP flexion (Figure 8-24, *B*).[4,5]

Motion: Thumb IP Extension

Muscle[4-6]	Innervation[4,5]
Extensor pollicis longus	Radial n., C6 to C8

Position: S seated or supine, forearm in midposition, wrist in neutral position, and hand and forearm resting on ulnar border.[4] MP joint of thumb is extended or slightly flexed, and IP joint is flexed fully into palm. E sits opposite or next to S on the side being tested.
Stabilize: Wrist in neutral position, first metacarpal, and proximal phalanx of thumb.
Palpate: EPL tendon on dorsal surface of hand medial to EPB tendon, between head of first metacarpal and base of second metacarpal on ulnar side of anatomic snuffbox.[4,11]
Observe: S brings tip of thumb up and out of palm, extending IP joint (Figure 8-25, *A*).
Resist: On dorsal surface of distal phalanx, down toward IP flexion (Figure 8-25, *B*).[4,5]

Motion: Thumb MP Flexion

Muscle[4,5]	Innervation[4,5]
Flexor pollicis brevis	Median n., ulnar n., C6 to C8, T1

Position: S seated or supine, forearm fully supinated, wrist in neutral position, and thumb in extension and adduction. E sits next or opposite to S.[4,5]
Stabilize: First metacarpal and wrist.
Palpate: Over middle of palmar surface of thenar eminence just medial to abductor pollicis brevis.[4] Hand used to stabilize may also be used for palpation.
Observe: S flexes MP joint while maintaining extension of IP joint (Figure 8-26, *A*). Some individuals may be unable to isolate flexion to MP joint. In this case, both MP and IP flexion may be tested together as a gross test for thumb flexion strength and graded according to E's judgment.
Resist: On palmar surface of first phalanx toward MP extension (Figure 8-26, *B*).[4,5]

Motion: Thumb IP Flexion

Muscle[4-6]	Innervation[5]
Flexor pollicis longus	Median n., C7, C8, T1

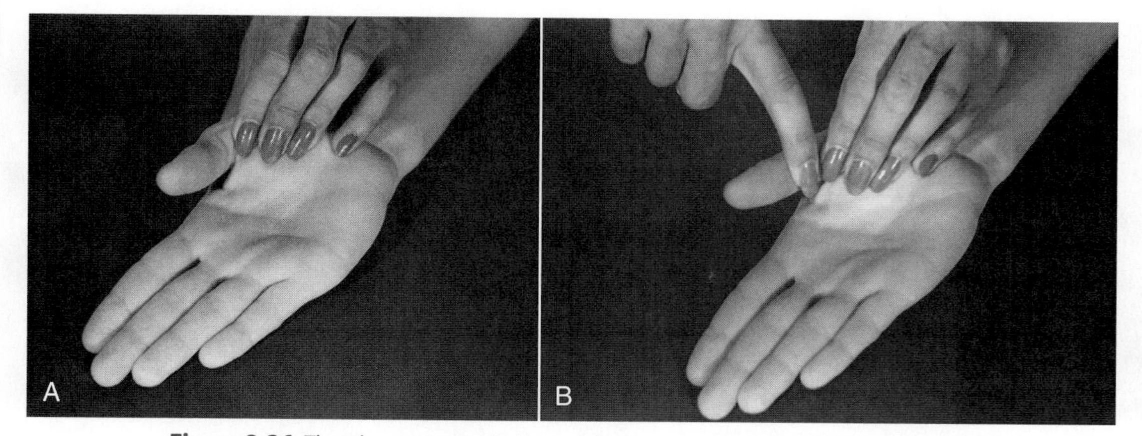

Figure 8-26 Thumb metacarpophalangeal flexion. **A,** Palpate and observe. **B,** Resist.

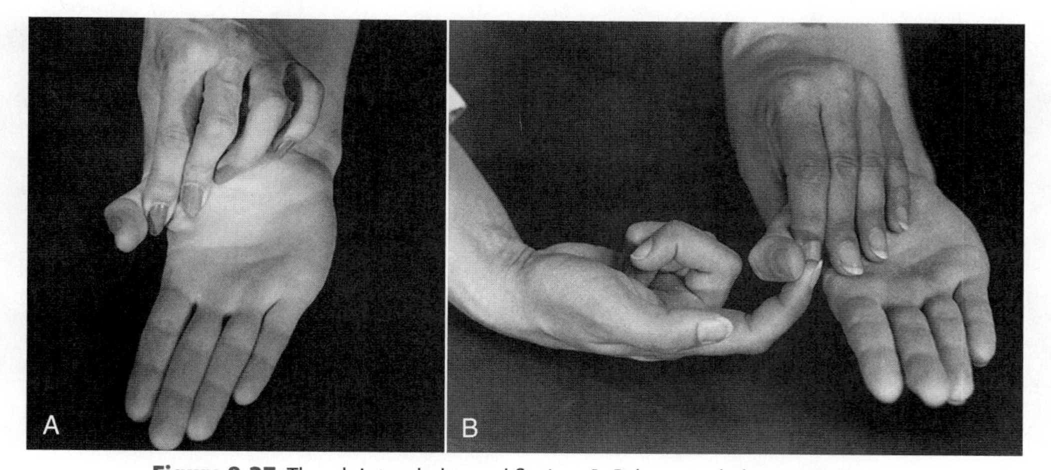

Figure 8-27 Thumb interphalangeal flexion. **A,** Palpate and observe. **B,** Resist.

Position: S seated with forearm fully supinated, wrist in neutral position, and thumb in extension and adduction.[4] E sits next to or opposite from S.

Stabilize: First metacarpal and proximal phalanx of thumb in extension.[4,5]

Palpate: Flexor pollicis longus tendon on palmar surface of proximal phalanx. In this case, palpating finger may be the same one used for stabilizing proximal phalanx.

Observe: S flexes IP joint in plane of palm (Figure 8-27, *A*).[4]

Resist: On palmar surface of distal phalanx toward IP extension (Figure 8-27, *B*).[4,5]

Motion: Thumb Palmar Abduction

Muscle[5,6]	Innervation[5]
Abductor pollicis brevis	Median n., C6 to C8, T1

Position: S seated or supine, forearm in supination, wrist in neutral position, thumb extended and adducted, and carpometacarpal (CMC) joint rotated so that thumb is resting in a plane perpendicular to palm. E sits opposite or next to S on the side being tested.[4,5]

Stabilize: Metacarpals and wrist.

Palpate: Abductor pollicis brevis on lateral aspect of thenar eminence, lateral to flexor pollicis brevis.[4]

Observe: S raises thumb away from palm in a plane perpendicular to palm (Figure 8-28, *A*).[5]

Resist: At lateral aspect of proximal phalanx, downward toward adduction (Figure 8-28, *B*).[5]

Motion: Thumb Radial Abduction

Muscle[5]	Innervation[5]
Abductor pollicis longus	Radial n., C6 to C8

Position: S seated or supine, forearm in neutral rotation, wrist in neutral position, and thumb adducted and slightly flexed across palm. Hand and forearm are resting on ulnar border.[5] E sits opposite or next to S on the side being tested.

Stabilize: Wrist and metacarpals of fingers.[4,5]

Palpate: Abductor pollicis longus tendon on lateral aspect of base of first metacarpal. The tendon is immediately lateral (radial) to extensor pollicis brevis tendon.[4,11]

Observe: S moves thumb out of palm of hand, abducting in the plane of palm (Figure 8-29, *A*).

Resist: At lateral aspect of distal end of first metacarpal toward adduction (Figure 8-29, *B*).[4,5]

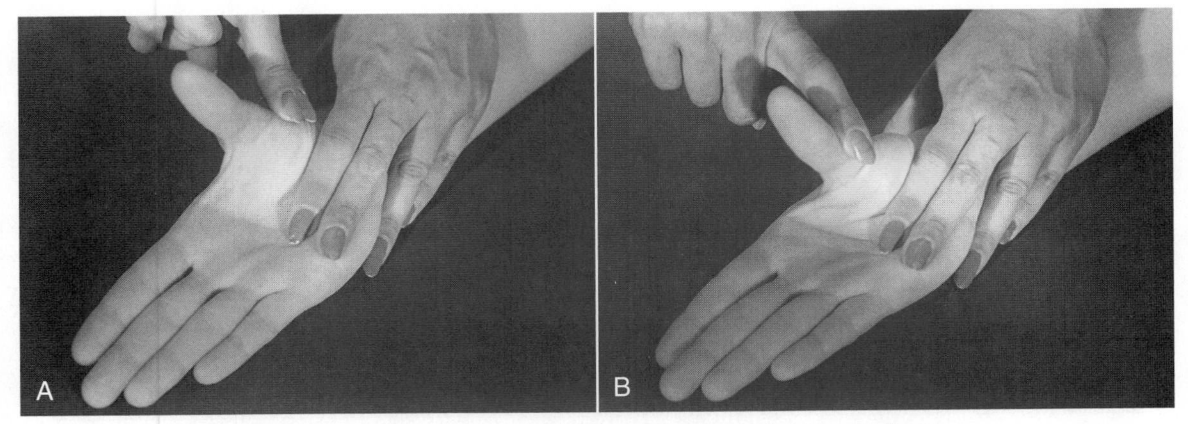

Figure 8-28 Thumb palmar abduction. **A,** Palpate and observe. **B,** Resist.

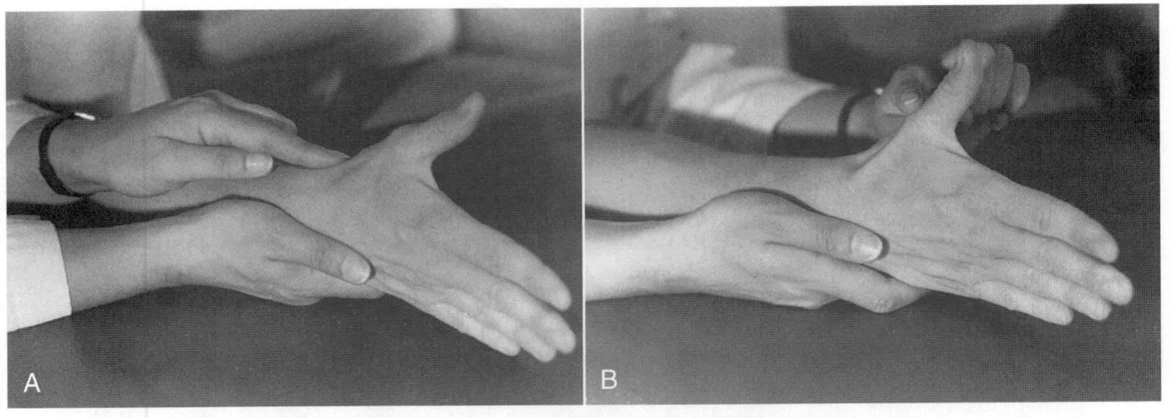

Figure 8-29 Thumb radial abduction. **A,** Palpate and observe. **B,** Resist.

Motion: Thumb Adduction

Muscle[4,5]	Innervation[4,5]
Adductor pollicis	Ulnar n., C8, T1

Position: S seated or supine, forearm pronated, wrist in neutral position, and thumb opposed and abducted.[4,10] E sits opposite or next to S on the side being tested.

Stabilize: Wrist and metacarpals, supporting hand slightly above resting surface.[4]

Palpate: Adductor pollicis on palmar side of thumb web space.[6]

Observe: S brings thumb up to touch palm (Figure 8-30, *A*).[4] (Thumb is turned up in Figure 8-30 to show palpation point.)

Resist: By grasping proximal phalanx of thumb near metacarpal head and pulling downward, toward abduction (Figure 8-30, *B*).[4]

Motion: Opposition of Thumb to Fifth Finger

Muscle[4,5]	Innervation[4,5]
Opponens pollicis	Median n., C6 to C8, T1
Opponens digiti minimi	Ulnar n., C8, T1

Position: S seated or supine, forearm in full supination, wrist in neutral position, and thumb and fifth finger extended and adducted.[4,5] E sits on the side being tested.

Stabilize: Forearm and wrist.

Palpate: Opponens pollicis along radial side of shaft of first metacarpal, lateral to abductor pollicis brevis. Opponens digiti minimi cannot be easily palpated.[4,6]

Observe: S brings thumb out across palm to touch thumb pad to pad of fifth finger (Figure 8-31, *A*).

Resist: At distal ends of first and fifth metacarpals, exerting pressure toward, separating, and rolling away these bones and flattening palm of hand (Figure 8-31, *B*).[4]

Functional Muscle Testing

The functional muscle test is a useful tool when screening muscles for normal strength.[4,8] OT practitioners in some health care facilities use functional muscle testing when specific muscle testing is the responsibility of the physical therapy service. The functional muscle test assesses the general strength and motion capabilities of the patient.

The following functional muscle test should be performed while the subject is comfortably seated in a sturdy chair or wheelchair.

The subject is asked to perform the test motion against gravity. The subject may perform the motion in the gravity-decreased position, if the former is not feasible.

In all of the tests, the subject is allowed to complete the test motion before the examiner applies resistance. The resistance is applied at the end of the ROM while the

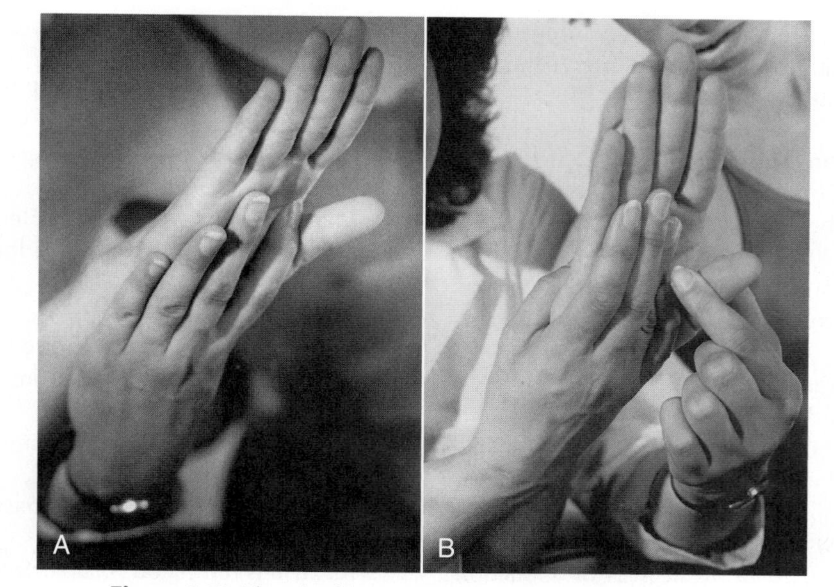

Figure 8-30 Thumb adduction. **A,** Palpate and observe. **B,** Resist.

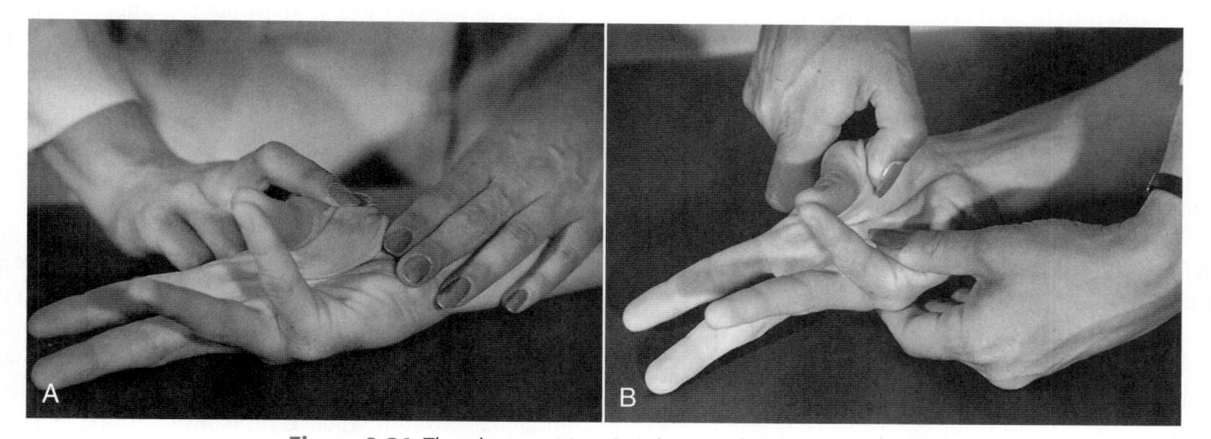

Figure 8-31 Thumb opposition. **A,** Palpate and observe. **B,** Resist.

subject maintains the position and resists the force applied by the examiner. The examiner may make modifications in positioning to suit individual needs. As in the manual muscle tests, the examiner should stabilize proximal parts and attempt to rule out substitutions. The reader should be familiar with joint motions, their prime movers, manual muscle testing, and muscle grades before performing this test. The OTA must establish service competency to ensure accurate and safe testing.

Functional Muscle Test

Shoulder Flexion (Anterior Deltoid and Coracobrachialis)

With S's shoulder flexed to 90 degrees and elbow flexed or extended, E pushes down on arm proximal to elbow into extension.

Shoulder Extension (Latissimus Dorsi and Teres Major)

S moves shoulder into full extension. E pushes from behind at a point proximal to elbow into flexion.

Shoulder Abduction (Middle Deltoid and Supraspinatus)

S abducts shoulder to 90 degrees with elbow flexed or extended. E pushes down on arm just proximal to elbow into adduction.

Shoulder Horizontal Adduction (Pectoralis Major, Anterior Deltoid)

S crosses arms in front of chest. E reaches from behind and attempts to pull arms back into horizontal abduction at a point just proximal to elbow.

Shoulder Horizontal Abduction (Posterior Deltoid, Teres Minor, Infraspinatus)

S moves arms from full horizontal adduction as just described to full horizontal abduction. E pushes forward on arms just proximal to elbow into horizontal adduction.

Shoulder External Rotation (Infraspinatus and Teres Minor)

S holds arm in 90 degrees of shoulder abduction and 90 degrees of elbow flexion, then externally rotates shoulder through available ROM. E supports or stabilizes upper arm proximal to elbow; at the same time, E pushes from behind at dorsal aspect of wrist into internal rotation.

Shoulder Internal Rotation (Subscapularis, Teres Major, Latissimus Dorsi, Pectoralis Major)

S begins with arm as described for external rotation (90 degrees of shoulder abduction and 90 degrees of elbow flexion) but performs internal rotation. E supports or stabilizes upper arm as before and pulls up into external rotation at volar aspect of wrist.

Elbow Flexion (Biceps, Brachialis)

With forearm supinated, S flexes elbow from full extension. E sits opposite subject and stabilizes upper arm against trunk while attempting to pull forearm into extension at volar aspect of wrist.

Elbow Extension (Triceps)

With S's upper arm supported in 90 degrees of abduction (gravity-decreased position) or 160-degree shoulder flexion (against-gravity position), elbow is extended from full flexion. E pushes forearm into flexion at dorsal aspect of wrist.

Forearm Supination (Biceps, Supinator)

S or E stabilizes upper arm against trunk. Elbow is flexed to 90 degrees, and forearm is in full pronation. S supinates forearm. E grasps distal forearm and attempts to rotate into pronation.

Forearm Pronation (Pronator Teres, Pronator Quadratus)

S is positioned as described for forearm supination except that forearm is in full supination. S pronates forearm. E grasps distal forearm and attempts to rotate into supination.

Wrist Flexion (Flexor Carpi Radialis, Flexor Carpi Ulnaris, Palmaris Longus)

S's forearm is supported on the dorsal surface on a tabletop or armrest. Hand is moved up from tabletop, using wrist flexion. E is seated next to or opposite S and pushes on palm of hand, giving equal pressure on radial and ulnar sides into wrist extension or down toward tabletop.

Wrist Extension (Extensor Carpi Radialis Longus and Brevis, Extensor Carpi Ulnaris)

S's forearm is supported on a tabletop or armrest and rests on the volar surface. Hand is lifted from tabletop by wrist extension. E sits next to or opposite S and pushes on dorsal aspect of palm, giving equal pressure at radial and ulnar sides into wrist flexion or down toward tabletop.

Finger MP Flexion and IP Extension (Lumbricales and Interossei)

With forearm and hand supported on tabletop on dorsal surface, E stabilizes palm and S flexes MP joints while maintaining extension of IP joints. E pushes into extension with index finger across proximal phalanges or pushes on tip of each finger into IP flexion and MP extension.

Finger IP Flexion (Flexors Digitorum Profundus and Sublimis)

S is positioned as described for MP flexion. IP joints are flexed while maintaining extension of MP joints. E attempts to pull fingers back into extension by hooking fingertips with those of S.

Finger MP Extension (IP Joints Flexed) (Extensor Digitorum Communis, Extensor Indicis Proprius, Extensor Digiti Minimi)

S's forearm and hand are supported on a table surface, resting on ulnar border. Wrist is stabilized by E in 0-degree neutral position. S moves MP joints from flexion to full extension (hyper-extension) while keeping IP joints flexed. E pushes fingers at PIP joints simultaneously into flexion.

Finger Abduction (Dorsal Interossei, Abductor Digiti Minimi)

S's forearm is resting on volar surface on a table. E may stabilize wrist in slight extension so that the hand is raised slightly off supporting surface. S abducts fingers. E pushes two fingers at a time together at the proximal phalanges into adduction. First, index finger and middle fingers are pushed together. Then ring finger and middle fingers and finally little finger and ring fingers do the same. Resistance is modified to accommodate small muscles.

Finger Adduction (Palmar Interossei)

S is positioned as described for finger abduction. Fingers are adducted tightly. E attempts to pull fingers apart one at a time at the proximal phalanges. First, index finger is pulled away from middle finger. Then ring finger is pulled away from middle finger, and finally little finger is pulled away from ring finger. In normal hand, adducted finger snaps back into adducted position when E pulls into abduction and quickly lets go. An alternate method is for examiner to place index finger between two of S's fingers, and ask S to adduct against examiner's finger.

Thumb MP and IP Flexion (Flexor Pollicis Brevis and Flexor Pollicis Longus)

S's forearm should be supported on a firm surface, with elbow flexed at 90 degrees and forearm in 45-degree supination. Thumb is flexed across palm. E pulls on tip of thumb into extension.

Thumb MP and IP Extension (Extensor Pollicis Brevis and Extensor Pollicis Longus)

S is positioned as for thumb MP and IP flexion. Thumb is extended away from palm. E pushes on tip of thumb into flexion.

Thumb Palmar Abduction (Abductor Pollicis Longus and Abductor Pollicis Brevis)

S is positioned as described for thumb flexion and extension. Thumb is abducted away from palm in a plane perpendicular to palm. S resists movement at metacarpal head into adduction.

Thumb Adduction (Adductor Pollicis)

S is positioned as for all other thumb movements. Thumb is adducted to palm. E attempts to pull thumb into abduction at metacarpal head or proximal phalanx.

Opposition of Thumb to Fifth Finger (Opponens Pollicis, Opponens Digiti Minimi)

S is positioned with elbow flexed to 90 degrees and dorsal surface of forearm and hand resting on a flat surface such as a tabletop or armrest. Thumb is opposed to fifth finger, making pad-to-pad contact. E attempts to pull fingers apart, applying force at metacarpal heads of both fingers.

Summary

Evaluation of muscle strength contributes to the functional assessment of patients with many different physical disorders. Muscle strength is necessary to maintain body posture and to perform activities when gravity or other resistance is a factor. Evaluation of muscle strength objectively documents the physiologic and functional changes in the musculoskeletal system. Functional muscle testing is an important evaluation tool for patients with lower motor neuron dysfunction, orthopedic conditions, and muscle diseases. The role of the OTA in evaluating muscle strength must start with proven service competency and is determined by the supervising occupational therapist, in accordance with practice regulations of the state and the treatment setting.

Selected Reading Guide Questions

1. List two medical conditions in which testing of muscle strength would be appropriate.
2. Define *endurance*, and discuss the relationship of endurance to muscle testing.
3. What is the difference between spasticity and normal muscle strength?
4. What are the purposes of functional muscle testing?
5. Explain why specific positioning is used for testing of specific muscle groups.
6. How does gravity affect the tested strength of a muscle?
7. If joint range is limited, how can strength be tested, and how would this limitation be recorded?
8. Define each of these muscle grades: N (5), G (4), F (3), P (2), T (1), and zero (0).
9. Describe how muscle fatigue, pain, and muscle spasm may affect testing of muscle strength.
10. Explain the importance of knowing the patient's PROM before muscle testing.

Exercise

Demonstrate the muscle testing procedures for the following muscle groups: shoulder flexion, extension, abduction, external rotation, and internal rotation; elbow flexion and extension; forearm supination and pronation; and wrist flexion and extension.

References

1. Basmajian JF: *Muscles alive*, ed 5, Baltimore, 1985, Lippincott Williams & Wilkins.
2. Brunnstrom S: *Movement therapy in hemiplegia*, New York, 1970, Harper & Row.
3. Davis PM: *Steps to follow: a guide to the treatment of adult hemiplegia*, Berlin, 1985, Springer-Verlag.
4. Hislop H, Montgomery J: *Daniels and Worthingham's Muscle testing: techniques of manual examination*, ed 7, Philadelphia, 2002, Saunders.
5. Kendall FP, McCreary EK, Provance PG, Rodgers M, Romani W: *Muscles: testing and function*, ed 5, Baltimore, 2005, Lippincott Williams & Wilkins.
6. Killingsworth A: *Basic physical disability procedures*, San Jose, CA, 1987, Maple.
7. Landen B, Amizich A: Functional muscle examination and gait analysis, *J Am Phys Ther Assoc* 43:39, 1963.
8. Pact V, Sirotkin-Roses M, Beatus J: *The muscle testing handbook*, Boston, 1984, Little, Brown.
9. Pendleton H, Schultz-Krohn W, editors: *Pedretti's occupational therapy: practice skills for physical dysfunction*, ed 6, St. Louis, 2006, Mosby.
10. Rancho Los Amigos Hospital, *Department of Occupational Therapy: Guide for muscle testing of the upper extremity*, Downey, CA, 1978, Professional Staff Association of Rancho Los Amigos Hospital.
11. Smith LK, Weiss EL, Lehmkuhl LD: *Brunnstrom's clinical kinesiology*, ed 5, Philadelphia, 1996, FA Davis.

Recommended Reading

American Occupational Therapy Association: *Occupational therapy practice framework: domain and process*, ed 2, Bethesda, MD, 2008, the Association.

Calais-Germaiin B: *Anatomy of movement*, Seattle WA, 1993, Eastland Press.

Long R, Macivor C: *The key muscles of yoga: scientific keys, Volume I*, Lancaster UK, 2009, Bandha Yoga Publishers.

CHAPTER 9

Evaluation and Observation of Deficits in Sensation, Perception, and Cognition

MARIANA D'AMICO, VICKI SMITH, AND MARY BETH EARLY

Key Terms

Sensation
Feedback
Thermal
Pain
Olfactory
Gustatory
Proprioception
Perception
Stereognosis
Astereognosis
Graphesthesia
Agraphesthesia
Body scheme
Asomatognosia
Praxis
Apraxia
Ideomotor apraxia
Constructional apraxia
Dressing apraxia
Cognition
Orientation
Attention
Memory
Executive functioning
Abstract thinking
Concrete thinking
Problem solving
Reasoning
Insight
Dyscalculia

Chapter Objectives

After studying this chapter, the student or practitioner will be able to do the following:

1. Recognize the supporting role of the occupational therapy assistant in the occupational therapist's evaluation of sensation, perception, and cognition.
2. Define and describe various functions and deficits in the sensory, perceptual, and cognitive systems.
3. Recognize the tests and evaluation principles related to sensory, perceptual, and cognitive dysfunction.
4. Describe the interrelationships among sensory, perceptual, and cognitive functions in the performance of everyday activities.

Occupational therapy (OT) practitioners help clients succeed in their daily life activities. Clients with physical dysfunction experience performance limitations in the areas of activities of daily living (ADL), instrumental activities of daily living (IADL), work, play, leisure, and social participation. These limitations represent the clients' inability to balance the performance skills, performance patterns, context, activity demands, and client factors to successfully participate in the desired areas of occupation.[3]

A client with physical dysfunction who is performing a task such as donning a shirt may have difficulty for reasons as varied as lack of sensation in the arm, neglect of body parts because of perceptual impairment, or an inability to understand the nature of the task. Each reason suggests dysfunction in a different client factor (sensory, perceptual, and cognitive). Identification and correction of problems in client factors are often necessary for the client to achieve success in performance of occupations such as ADL. This chapter aims to describe the client factors that can interfere with performance skills and with a client's ability to engage successfully in areas of occupation. A second purpose is to present a brief discussion of some of the assessments that the occupational therapist might perform. This chapter considers client factors in the areas of sensation, perception, and cognition.

As stated elsewhere in this text, evaluation is the responsibility of the occupational therapist. The occupational therapy assistant (OTA) may assist if the evaluation procedure is structured and the instructions and limitations are well understood. The client factors are generally viewed as complex and require additional advanced study for comprehension. Therefore only the occupational therapist evaluates these factors. Most clinicians agree that even entry-level occupational therapists require supervision and ample experience to gain service competency with some of the tests used to measure client factors dysfunction. A small number of procedures for sensory, perceptual, and cognitive evaluations are simple and straightforward and appropriate for the entry-level practitioner. Consistent with recommendations and policies of the American Occupational Therapy Association,[2,4] directions for evaluations beyond entry-level practice for the OTA are not included here because these tasks should be performed by the occupational therapist. The OTA with several years of experience, as well as advanced skills and the opportunity to attempt more in this area, should do so only under occupational therapist supervision and with the appropriate text references.

This chapter includes directions for some procedures that can be administered by an entry-level OTA who has received the necessary training and supervision. The results of each assessment would be reported to the occupational therapist for interpretation. More involved procedures—which an occupational therapist should administer—are described so that the OTA can appreciate the value of these evaluations in the management of individual patients.

The OTA, who works closely with clients as they attempt tasks of occupational performance, will be able to observe directly many of the deficits discussed in the chapter because these deficits become most apparent when the client performs a task. Observations should be reported to the occupational therapist and to the health care team; they are invaluable as evidence of the client's condition.

Sensation

This section is concerned with somatosensory systems of touch, deep pressure, pain, proprioception, and thermal sensation (Box 9-1) and the special senses of taste and smell. When a person performs an occupation such as brushing teeth, the somatosensory system provides essential information to allow safe and efficient task completion. For example, all the following come into play:

- The sense of touch allows the person to feel the toothbrush.
- Deep pressure helps the person grip the toothbrush.
- Pain alerts the person to avoid brushing a sensitive area in the mouth.
- Proprioception guides the joints of the arm and hand to complete the motion of brushing.
- Thermal sensation lets the person determine if the water is at a desired temperature for rinsing the mouth.

Box 9-1

Sensory Terms

Tactile Referring to sensation received through the skin or hair receptors.
Deep pressure Tactile sensation of force applied to the skin, as in the feeling of the ischial tuberosities pressing into a chair seat.
Pain Unpleasant or noxious tactile sensation.
Thermal sensation Tactile sensation of heat or cold.
Proprioception Information about joint position and motion conveyed at an unconscious level from receptors in the muscles, joints, ligaments, and bone.

The somatosensory system is controlled by peripheral receptors in the skin (and other sense organs). Proprioceptive receptors are located in muscles, tendons, and joint capsules. All sensory information is processed through the spinal cord and brain. Completing the task of brushing teeth uses this entire system. Some sensations may produce a motor response before the brain even registers them. For example, the withdrawal of the hand from a hot object is driven by an automatic motor response or reflex before the object is perceived (by the brain) as being hot.[40]

Sensation and Motor Performance

Sensation is the primary means of learning about the external world. Sensory information can play many roles in the control of movement. As indicated already, sensory stimulation activates reflexive movement. Sensory information is also vital in modulating or regulating movements and controlling movements.[64,65] Sensation provides **feedback** to the brain. During a motor act, a person receives sensory feedback about the effectiveness of the motion through the various sensory systems. Sensations derived from the ongoing movement are sent back to the central nervous system (CNS), where a comparison between intended action and what is actually happening is made. Consider, for example, the act of writing. If the wrong word is used or if misspelling occurs, visual and proprioceptive feedback signals that a motor error has occurred. The CNS processes this sensory feedback and revises the motor response, which is then carried out as the problem is corrected.

Feed-forward control operates more quickly than feedback and is used to plan rapid movements before performing them. It uses sensory information (1) to predict what might happen to disturb movement and (2) to develop the motor plan.[32,33] For example, skiing begins with feed-forward control. The skier must anticipate the sensory experience to plan the motor act of descending the ski run. The slope of the hill, the condition of the snow, the rate of speed, potential obstacles, and the path to be taken must be considered before the descent begins. The skier anticipates the conditions and assumes a specific posture, sets muscles, initiates the motion, makes the appropriate balance responses, and directs movement along a given path toward the destination. As the motor act is being executed, the feedback system operates continuously to correct errors in the intended movement. The feed-forward system operates intermittently to anticipate or reevaluate the required action and to plan movement responses.[32,33,56]

Effects of Sensory Loss on Movement

Proprioception and tactile sensation are essential for feedback and feed-forward control systems. Clients with impaired sensation have deficits in both feedback and feed-forward control. Those with proprioceptive dysfunction cannot sense position and motion of joints; those with tactile dysfunction cannot sense contact with objects. Consequently, motor performance is deficient. Vision can compensate somewhat for the loss of tactile and proprioceptive sensation. However, defects in feedback and feed-forward control still limit the person's ability to use vision effectively. Because the client cannot sense the tension in muscles and tendons or the resistance of the surface on which the hand is moving and because visual feedback is processed slowly, any movement appears jerky and awkward. Errors in direction of movement cannot be corrected in time.[32,33]

When sensation is absent, especially proprioception, the affected part(s) may fail to function, as if paralyzed, even with adequate recovery of muscle function.[36] For example, clients with hemiplegia resulting from a cerebrovascular accident (CVA, stroke) tend not to use the affected hand unless proprioception is intact and two-point discrimination at the fingertip is less than ½ inch (1 cm) apart, thus indicating good discriminative sensation. Even slight sensory deficits result in persistent problems that limit the functional use of the affected hand in performing fine motor activities. The highly motivated client may use visual compensation to engage the affected upper extremity in bilateral activities.[74] It is necessary to understand the client's sensory status to appreciate fully the causes of apparent motor dysfunction and to plan appropriate treatment goals and methods.

Sensory Evaluation

For the purposes of this chapter, the term *sensation* refers to the ability to identify the sensory modality (touch, deep pressure, pain, proprioception, and thermal sensation), its intensity, and its location.

Occupational therapists often evaluate sensation in clients with CNS and peripheral nervous system (PNS) dysfunction. Of utmost concern is whether sensation is adequate for the performance of ADL.[16,45] Clients with CNS dysfunction tend to lose many sensory modalities over generalized areas, whereas those with PNS disorders tend to lose specific sensory modalities in circumscribed areas. Sensory testing may also be indicated in clients with burns (in which sensory receptors in the skin are destroyed), arthritis (in which joint swelling may cause compression of a peripheral nerve), and traumatic hand injuries (in which skin, muscles, tendons, ligaments, and nerves may be involved).

Box 9-2

Purposes of Testing

A complete sensory evaluation[18]:

- Determines the type and extent of sensory loss
- Provides documentation of sensory loss patterns and recovery
- Assists in diagnosis
- Determines impairment and functional limitations
- Provides direction for OT intervention

Other diagnoses that require sensory testing include peripheral nerve injuries and diseases, spinal cord injuries and diseases, brain injuries and diseases, and fractures. In clients with fractures, sensory testing may help to determine whether peripheral nerve involvement is present. Box 9-2 lists the purposes of sensory testing.

Sensory Supply to Specific Areas

Figure 9-1 illustrates the sensory distribution of the major peripheral nerves of the body and limbs. The peripheral nerves (e.g., ulnar nerve) lie outside the CNS. When performing sensory tests for peripheral nerve dysfunction, the therapist focuses on the area(s) supplied by the nerve(s) affected.

Figure 9-1 also shows the segmental or radicular distribution of nerve roots from the spinal cord. Each nerve root that exits from the spinal cord shows a specific area of sensory distribution known as a *dermatome*. When testing clients with spinal cord injury or disease, the therapist follows this dermatomal distribution. This procedure can help to determine the level(s) of spinal cord lesion and to detect any spared spinal cord function.

Results of the sensory evaluation indicate whether the client should be taught to protect against injury and to use compensatory techniques such as visual guidance for movement during activities. Results may also indicate whether a sensory retraining program is feasible.

Sensory loss may affect the use of splints or positioning equipment such as seat cushions and braces because the client may be unaware of pressure points during use. Sensory loss may also affect controlled use of a dynamic splint, which requires good sensory feedback for effective operation.

All those working with the client should keep in mind that sensory testing is purely subjective. Testing results depend heavily on the client's accurate and cooperative responses to the procedures.[40] This fact underscores the importance of evaluating both *functional performance* and sensory functioning. Therapists might use one of the several task-based or occupation-based assessments to observe functional performance or to obtain more reliable evaluation data. OT practitioners should observe the client for spontaneous use of the affected part(s) during ADL. The OTA is in a position to observe patient performance of a variety of tasks and can identify behavioral indicators of sensory deficits (such as failure to protect self from injury).

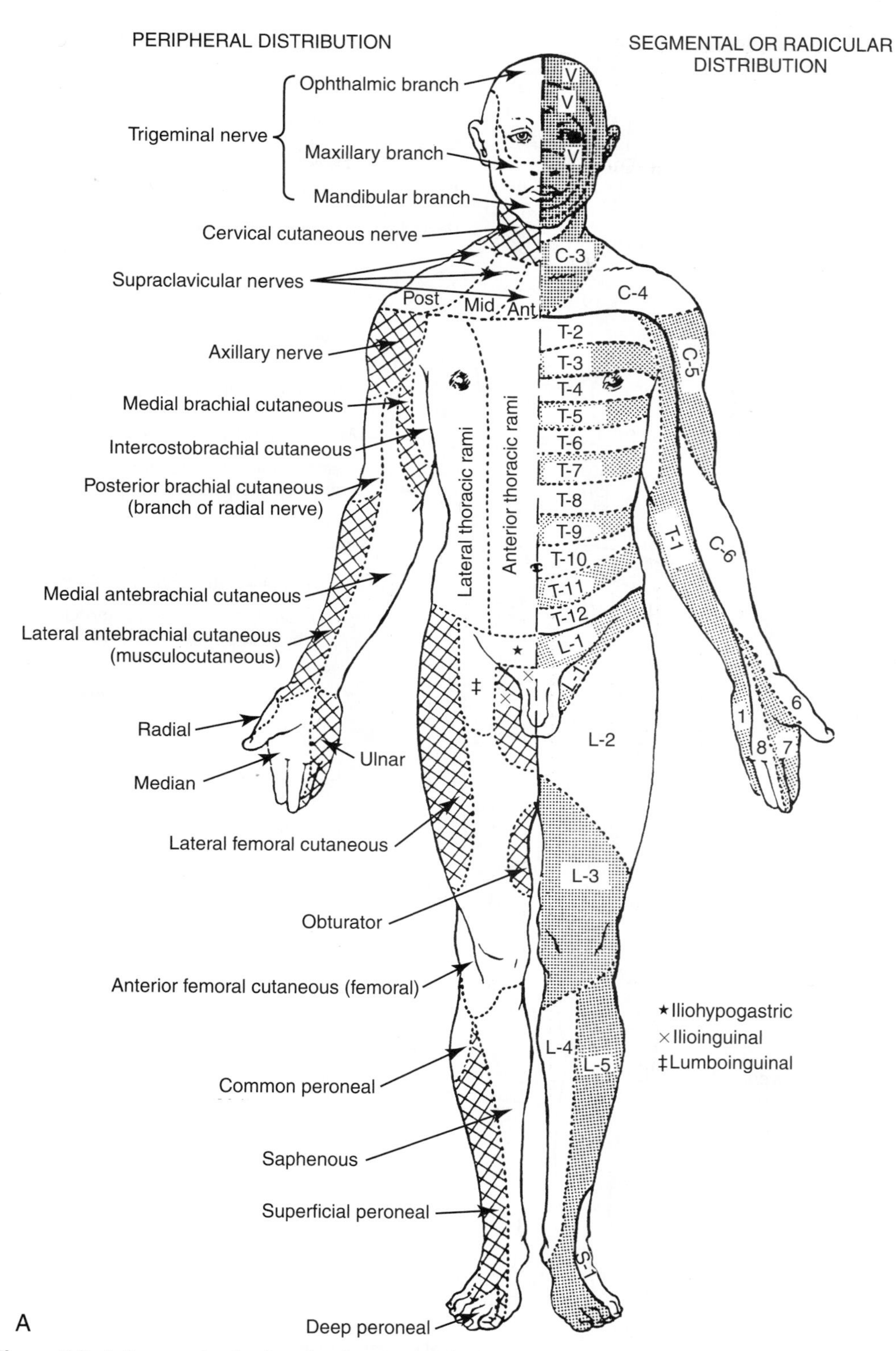

Figure 9-1 **A,** Sensory distribution of major peripheral nerves and dermatomes corresponding to spinal cord segments, anterior view.

Sensory Functions

Light Touch and Pressure Sensation

Tactile sensitivity is critical to the performance of all ADL. Recognizing that there is an object in one's hand depends on intact touch sensitivity, as does the ability to feel clothes on one's body and to recognize whether they are correctly adjusted. Pressure sensation is also important in ADL because it occurs continuously in activities such as sitting, pushing drawers and doors, crossing the knees, wearing belts and collars, and many other activities that stimulate pressure

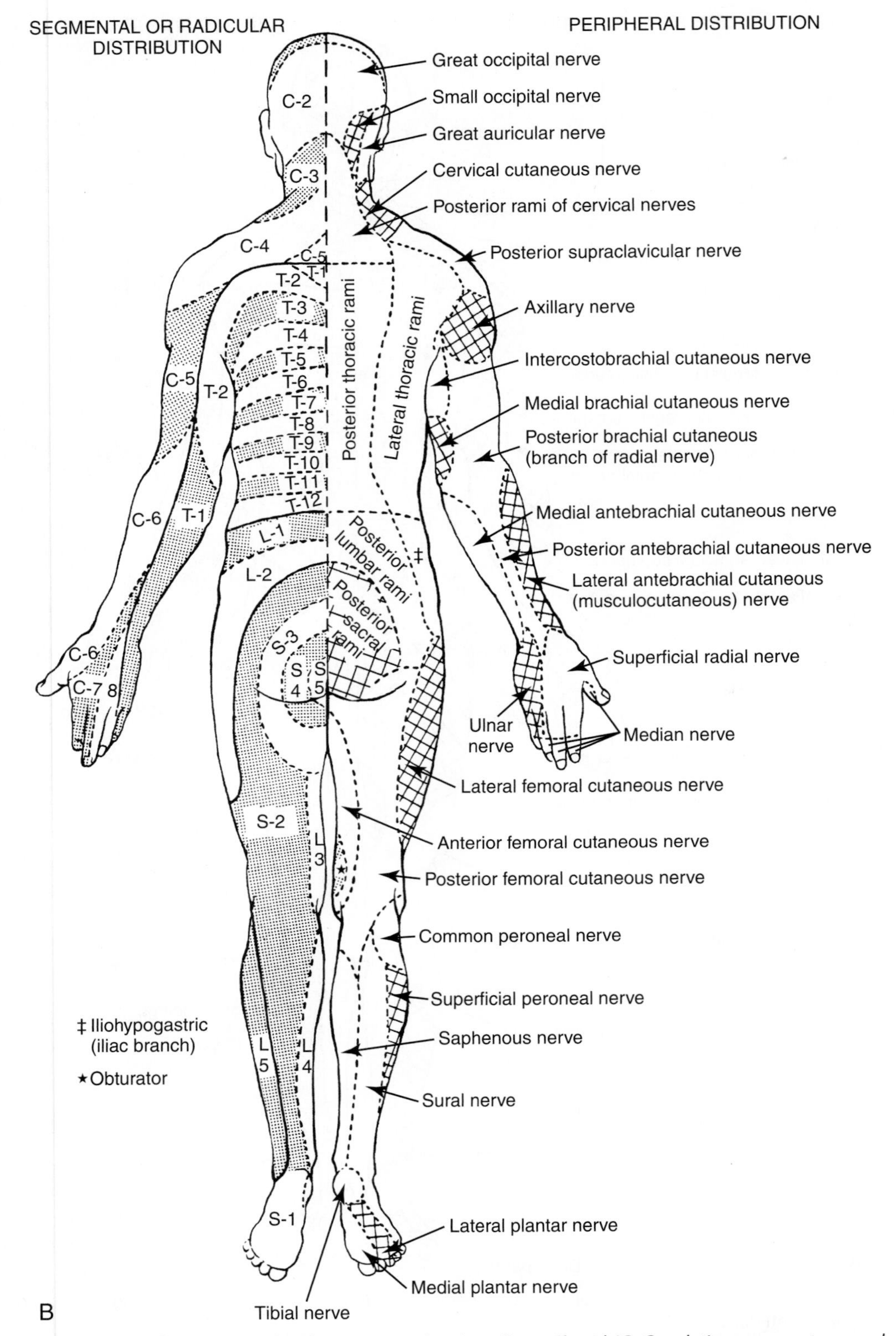

Figure 9-1, cont'd B, Sensory distribution, posterior view. (From Chusid JG: *Correlative neuroanatomy and functional neurology*, ed 19, 1985, Lange Medical Publications.)

receptors. A patient may have intact pressure sensation even when touch is impaired or absent because pressure receptors are in subcutaneous and deeper tissue while touch receptors are in the superficial layers of the skin. Touch sensation is necessary for fine discriminative activities. Pressure is a protective sensation because it warns of deep or repetitive pressure that can lead to injury.[16,45] If touch sensation is impaired, pressure sensation can assist in the performance of ADL and can help to substitute for touch feedback in some activities. Table 9-1 lists some tests for various sensory functions.

Table 9-1 Tests for Various Functions of Sensation, Perception, and Cognition

Function	Test
Light touch	With patient's vision occluded, examiner touches patient's hand lightly with cotton ball, cotton swab, etc. Semmes-Weinstein monofilaments—with patient's vision occluded, examiner touches patient's hand lightly with monofilament according to directions.[24,76]
Deep pressure	With patient's vision occluded, examiner presses hard with cotton swab. Semmes-Weinstein monofilaments—with patient's vision occluded, examiner touches patient's hand with monofilaments according to directions[24, 76]
Thermal sensation	Hot/cold discrimination kit—a thermometer is used to control temperatures of metal probes that contact patient's skin. Patient's vision is occluded. With patient's vision occluded, examiner touches the sides of test tubes filled with hot (110° F) and cool (45° F) water to patient's skin
Pain	With patient's vision occluded, a sterilized safety pin (new for each patient) is used to touch the skin with a light prick. Examination may be contraindicated when *skin atrophy* (wasting of the skin) is present.[16,45] In this case, the end of a straightened paper clip may be used.[13,53,61,68]
Smell (olfactory sense)	With patient's vision occluded, examiner presents various scents (coffee, almond, chocolate, lemon oil, peppermint) on a cotton swab or with the cork of a bottle.[21,53,68]
Taste (gustatory sense)	With patient's vision occluded, examiner presents soft foods with various tastes. Stimulation of the tongue may cause choking and is potentially harmful to dysphagic patients; therefore only the trained occupational therapist administers this test.[59,60]
Stereognosis	With patient's vision occluded, examiner presents one by one various familiar objects for the patient to identify. For patients with aphasia, an array of identical objects is provided so that the patient can point to the same object.
Graphesthesia	With patient's vision occluded, examiner traces letters, forms, etc. on the patient's palm.
Body scheme	Examiner asks patient to carry out motor actions such as pointing to body parts.[51,63,81-85] Draw-a-person test, body and face puzzles.[36,81-85] Examiner asks patient to perform motor actions involving right and left sides of body. Examiner asks patient to name fingers or imitate finger movements.[51,63]
Ideomotor apraxia	The client is asked to carry out motor actions based on spoken instructions.[81] The client is asked to imitate motor actions.
Constructional apraxia	Test of Visual Motor Skills (TVMS)[31,52] Benton Visual Retention Test[67] Rey Complex Figure Test[48] Three-Dimensional Block Construction[8] Observation of tasks such as dressing or setting the table
Dressing apraxia	Observation of client performance of dressing
Cognitive functions	Middlesex Elderly Assessment of Mental State[38] Cognitive Assessment of Minnesota[62] Mini Mental State Examination[29,30] Modified Mini Mental Examination[69] Test of Orientation for Rehabilitation Patients[22] Scales of Cognitive Ability for Traumatic Brain Injury[1] Neurobehavioral Cognitive Status Screening Examination[48] The Arnadottir OT-ADL Neurobehavioral Evaluation (A-ONE)[6] Cognitive Skills Workbook[26]
Memory	Benton Visual Retention Test[67] Rey Complex Figure[49,50] Learning Efficiency Test[75] Rivermead Behavioral Memory Test[77-79] Contextual Memory Test[71] Subjective Memory Questionnaire[10]

Thermal Sensation

Thermal sensation is another example of the protective sensory modalities.[16,45] The ability to detect temperatures is essential for preventing injury in many ADL such as bathing, cooking, and ironing. The ability to detect temperature also contributes to the enjoyment of food and the detection of uncomfortable environmental temperatures. The client who lacks accurate thermal discrimination must be taught burn prevention methods and precautions against injury in ADL. As in the other sensory tests, the results can serve as a baseline for the client's progress. Changes in sensory status may be used to measure recovery or degeneration, depending on the diagnosis.

Superficial Pain Sensation

Pain allows the detection of stimuli potentially harmful to the skin and subcutaneous tissue.[16,45] The ability to detect painful stimuli is critical to avoidance of injury during performance of occupations and to the prevention of skin breakdown while wearing splints and braces and using wheelchairs, crutches, and other adaptive devices. In normal circumstances, pain sensation warns the individual, for example, to move quickly (as when withdrawing a finger from a hot surface), to adjust the position of clothing (as when an elastic leg band is binding), or to remove an offending article of apparel (e.g., a shoe that is rubbing a blister on the foot). The client who lacks the ability to detect such painful stimuli is more likely to be injured. If pain sensation is absent or impaired, the client must learn sensory compensation and safety awareness as part of the treatment program.

Olfactory Sensation (Smell)

The sense of smell is conveyed by receptors that lie deep in the nasal cavity. Individuals with normal olfactory sensation can detect thousands of odors and at low concentrations, making smell discrimination quite extraordinary. Olfactory acuity varies greatly among normal persons and usually declines with age.[15] Olfactory sensation is associated with the pleasure of taste and is important for detection of noxious and pleasant odors. Smell is also connected to neuronal circuits that influence emotional states and evoke memories.

Hyposmia is a diminished sense of smell. It may occur in clients with cystic fibrosis of the pancreas, Parkinson disease, and untreated adrenal insufficiency. Loss of the sense of smell is known as anosmia. Anosmia may be specific—referring to lowered sensitivity to a specific odorant while perception of most others remains intact—or general.[15] *Anosmia* may result from local chronic or acute inflammatory nasal disease or from intracranial lesions that may be the result of a CVA, head injury, tumors, and infections. In some disturbances the sense of smell is distorted. The person may perceive odors that do not exist. Pleasant odors may be distorted or perceived as noxious, a condition known as *parosmia*.[68]

Anosmia interferes with detection of household gas, chemicals, smoke, car exhaust, and noxious environmental odors. Anosmia is a liability for the client who has an occupation in which the sense of smell is critical to safety. The disturbance may interfere with the perception and enjoyment of food odors and taste because decreased sense of smell affects the ability to taste. This may lead to secondary health complications related to nutrition and diet.

Gustatory Sensation (Taste)

Taste receptor cells are located in the taste buds of the tongue; in the palate; and in the pharynx, epiglottis, and esophagus. Taste sensation is conveyed to the brain by way of the facial, glossopharyngeal, and vagus nerves (cranial nerves VII, IX, and X). Generally, four basic tastes—sweet, sour, salty, and bitter—can be detected. Detection of more complex taste sensations is thought to result from activation of combinations of the four basic taste receptors.[15]

Taste is basic to the enjoyment of food and helps to trigger salivation and swallowing.[66] As with smell, taste is connected to neural circuits that control emotional states and trigger specific memories.[15] When the client requires a comprehensive evaluation of oral-motor mechanisms, taste sensation may be a consideration. In planning feeding training programs, evaluation of the sensation of taste is also useful.[66] Disturbances of taste may be caused by PNS or CNS lesions.[16,45] Smokers may demonstrate a decreased sense of taste with aging.[27] The test for gustatory sensation is usually performed by the occupational therapist. Stimulation of the tongue may cause choking or other reactions that are potentially harmful to clients with dysphagia. Pedretti[59,60] provides the directions for this test.

Proprioception (Position and Motion Sense)

Proprioception refers to *unconscious* information about joint position and motion that arises from receptors in the muscles, joints, ligaments, and bone. The *conscious* sense of motion may be referred to as *kinesthesia*. A partial or complete loss of position and motion senses seriously impairs movement, even if muscle function is within normal limits. Therefore to better understand the motor dysfunction, the occupational therapist must know whether the client has a sensory loss. Results of the evaluation suggest whether treatment should employ compensatory methods or sensory retraining. Evaluation of position and motion sense requires specific training and the development of sensitivity in handling and positioning the client. Pedretti[59,60] provides additional information on this component of evaluation.

Perception

Perception is the mechanism by which the brain recognizes and interprets sensory information received from the environment. Perceived information is then further processed by the various cognitive functions. The end result may be a verbal expression or motor act. For example, a man searching for a pen to write something may feel in his pockets. His hand encounters a hard, smooth, cylindrical, oblong object (sensation). These sense data are translated into an image of a pen (perception). The man may then choose (cognition) to remove it (motor action) from his pocket or instead to use a pen provided by someone else.

This section describes the evaluation of perception including higher-level tactile discriminative sensations, body scheme, and praxis. Evaluation of these functions is most accurate when the examiner has a thorough understanding of higher cognitive functions, their anatomic representations, and their interrelationships. For this reason, evaluation of perception is the responsibility of the occupational therapist. Selected tests may be delegated to the experienced OTA with established service competency in administering the test to the particular population being served. Some tests that the OTA may be trained in include the Motor-Free Visual Perception Test (MVPT-3)[19] and the Lowenstein Occupational Therapy Cognitive Assessment (LOTCA-2).[44,46] Administration of these instruments should not be attempted without training and verification of service competency.

Evaluation of Perception

The occupational therapist may evaluate perception separately or in combination with evaluation of ADL performance.[6,81,83,84] The therapist uses a battery of perceptual tests that have varied response modes: verbal response, motor response, or flexible response (either mode). These variations in response mode allow the therapist to determine whether the client has a deficit in the reception of information or in the verbal or motor output. This information will influence the treatment goals and approach. OT practitioners obtain further data on the client's perceptual abilities by observing performance during occupations. Analyzing the perceptual motor demands of the client's functional activities may provide yet more information. The OTA may observe functional performance during the client's execution of ADL and other occupations and may contribute significantly to the evaluation of perception with this information.

The client's age and premorbid status are considered in the interpretation of performance during perceptual testing and ADL. For example, the majority of clients who have sustained a CVA are also elderly. Numerous changes in visual, auditory, perceptual, and cognitive functions are associated with the natural aging process.[28] Similarly, a young, traumatically injured client may have a history of learning disabilities before the head injury. To interpret test results accurately and to establish realistic treatment goals, the therapist requires a clear picture of the client's occupational profile. If the client is unable to supply the necessary information, the practitioner consults the family, friends, and educators.

Perceptual Functions: Evaluation and Observation

Stereognosis and graphesthesia are tactile discriminative skills—that is, they involve discrimination of different touch sensations at a higher level of CNS synthesis than the basic tactile sensory functions of light touch and pressure already described.

Stereognosis

Stereognosis is the ability to identify an object through proprioception, cognition, and the sense of touch. This ability identifies common objects and geometric shapes through touch (without the aid of vision). Stereognosis is essential to daily living because the ability to "see with the hands" is critical to many activities. This skill makes it possible to reach into a pocket or purse and find keys and to reach into a dark room and find the light switch. Stereognosis and proprioception enable the use of hand tools and the performance of hand activities without visual concentration on the implements being used. Examples are knitting while watching television, sawing wood while focusing on the wood rather than the saw, and using a fork during a conversation. A deficit in this stereognostic function is called astereognosis. Clients who have astereognosis but who retain much of their motor function must visually monitor their hands during all activities. Clients become slow and deliberate with their movements and generally tend to be less active.

The OTA can learn the test for stereognosis. Once service competency is ensured, the OTA can administer these tests as the occupational therapist deems appropriate (Box 9-3).

Graphesthesia

An additional test of discriminative sensation that measures parietal lobe function is the test for graphesthesia. This ability allows humans to recognize numbers, letters, or forms written on the skin.[17,36,58,61] The loss of this ability is called agraphesthesia. To test graphesthesia, the occupational therapist occludes vision and traces letters, numbers, or geometric forms on the client's palm with a dull, pointed pencil or similar instrument. The client tells the examiner which symbol was written.[58] If the client is aphasic, pictures of the symbols may be used to indicate a response after each test stimulus.

Body Scheme

An individual's body scheme is an awareness of body parts and the position of the body and its parts in relation to themselves and the environment.[31] It includes knowledge of body construction, the anatomic elements, and their spatial relationships; ability to visualize the body in movement and its parts in different positional relationships; ability to differentiate between right and left; and ability to recognize body health and disease.[31,81-83] During the evaluation, the therapist will be able to identify various body scheme disorders including asomatognosia, right/left discrimination deficits, unilateral inattention or neglect, and finger agnosia.

Asomatognosia refers to a severe loss of body scheme.[34,35,40] The client has a diminished awareness and recognition of a body structure or part and cannot determine the body part's relationship to the rest of his or her body. This condition is usually evaluated by having the client point to body parts on command or by imitation.[51,63,81-85] Figure 9-2 illustrates an impairment in body scheme.

Right/left discrimination deficits can occur in extrapersonal space, intrapersonal space, or both. The most basic testing of right/left discrimination abilities is intrapersonal; the client is asked to point to a body part, specifying the right or left side, on himself or herself. A more advanced (extrapersonal) test is to ask the client to identify right and left body parts on the examiner.[12]

Unilateral inattention or unilateral neglect is a failure to integrate perceptions from one side of the body or one side of body space. Figure 9-3 illustrates evidence of left-sided neglect. The most effective evaluation of unilateral neglect as it relates to a body scheme disorder is direct observation during ADL and IADL. The astute OTA will easily identify such clients simply by watching their ADL performance.

The client with *finger agnosia* has difficulty naming fingers on command or identifying which finger has been touched.[46] The occupational therapist evaluates finger agnosia through finger localization, naming on command, or having the client imitate the therapist's finger movements.[51,63]

Box 9-3

Test for Stereognosis

Purpose
To evaluate a client's ability to identify common objects and perceive their tactile properties.

Materials
Means to occlude client's vision such as a curtain or folder. Any common objects may be used. Typical objects that could be used for identification include a pencil, fountain pen, sunglasses, key, nail, large safety pin, metal teaspoon, quarter, button, and small leather coin purse. The examiner must consider client's social and ethnic background to ensure familiarity with the objects.

Conditions
Test should be conducted in an environment with minimal distractions. The client should be seated at a table in a position that accommodates the affected hand and forearm comfortably. The test can also be completed bedside or in a wheelchair without a table. The examiner should sit opposite the client. If client cannot manipulate test objects because of motor weakness, the examiner should assist the client with the manipulation of the objects.

Method
The client is provided oral instructions and a demonstration within his or her vision on an unaffected area. The client is asked to identify each item visually and verbally. The client's vision is occluded. The dorsal surface of the client's hand is in a resting position. Objects are presented in random order. The client is to use one hand only to identify the object. Manipulation of objects is allowed and encouraged. The examiner assists with manipulation of items if client's hand function is impaired.

Responses
The client is asked to name object, or if unable, to describe its properties. Aphasic patients may view a duplicate set of test objects after each trial and point to a choice.

Scoring
A form may be used to score the client's responses. The examiner marks plus (+) if object is identified quickly and correctly and minus (–) if there is a long delay before identification of object or if the client can only describe its properties (e.g., size, texture, material, shape). The examiner marks zero (0) if the client cannot identify object or describe its properties.

From references 9, 23, 42, 47, 61.

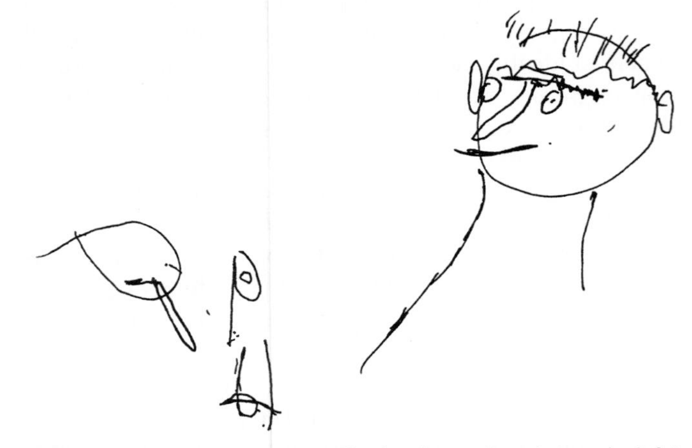

Figure 9-2 Example of impaired body scheme. Drawing on the left is patient's first attempt to draw a face. The therapist asked patient to try again. Patient's second effort is drawing on the right.

Praxis
Praxis is the ability to plan and perform purposeful movement. Apraxia is an impairment in praxis, a deficit in the ability to perform purposeful movement despite normal motor power, sensation, coordination, and general comprehension. Types include ideomotor, constructional, oral, and dressing apraxias.

A client can demonstrate a single form of apraxia or a combination of types. The individual with apraxia faces problems with effective planning and performance of skilled purposeful movement. Evaluation of praxis disorders is reserved for the occupational therapist.

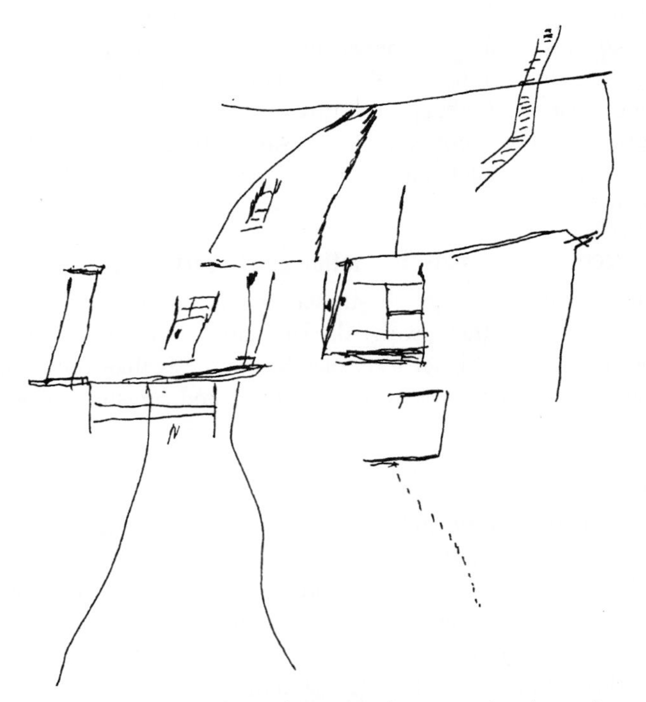

Figure 9-3 Example of two-dimensional constructional apraxia and inattention to the left side in a patient's drawing of a house. The patient was a retired architect.

Ideomotor Apraxia
Ideomotor apraxia is an inability to perform a motor act on command, despite the ability to perform the act automatically. The client may be able to describe the intended motion in words but cannot execute the motor act at will. For

example, the client is asked to stand up and walk across the room but instead looks at the therapist in a puzzled way and does not move. The presence of ideomotor apraxia impairs his understanding of the requested act. Later, the client gets up on his own and walks across the room to get a towel, indicating that the ability to perform the motor act itself is present.

Full test batteries for ideomotor apraxia have been developed.[14,39] Evaluation of apraxia is reserved for the skilled occupational therapist.

Constructional Apraxia

Constructional apraxia is a deficit in the ability to copy, draw, or construct a design, whether on command or spontaneously.[43,81] It is the inability to organize or assemble parts into a whole, as in putting together block designs (three-dimensional) or drawings (two-dimensional). This perceptual motor impairment is often seen in persons with severe head injury or CVA and relates to a dysfunction of the parietal lobes. Constructional apraxia causes significant dysfunction in activities such as dressing, following instructions for assembling a toy, and stacking a dishwasher. Figure 9-3 shows evidence of left-sided neglect and demonstrates constructional apraxia. Constructional apraxia impairs dressing and other sequential ADL and can be observed by the OTA in these functional activities.

Dressing Apraxia

Dressing apraxia, or the inability to plan and perform the motor acts necessary to dress oneself, has been linked with problems of body scheme, spatial orientation, and constructional apraxia.[55,73,81,84] Clinically the client may have difficulty initiating dressing or may make errors in orientation by putting the clothes on the wrong side of the body, upside down, or inside out.[5,81,84]

Box 9-4

Principles of Cognitive Evaluation

1. *Cognition should always be seen in relation to other potential deficit areas.* The client's sensory, language, visual, and perceptual systems affect the observable qualities of cognition. For example, the client may be unable to attend to and concentrate on a particular task because of an underlying deficit in visual scanning.
2. *Discussions of the OT evaluation results with health professionals from other disciplines will enhance the OT practitioner's understanding of the client's capacity.* The speech pathologist, physical therapist, psychologist or neuropsychologist, and the client's family can provide different perspectives.
3. *The testing environment also influences the results of the cognitive evaluation.* A client's behavior in the foreign environment of the hospital or rehabilitation facility may differ from performance in a familiar home setting.
4. *The optimal test battery involves a selection of tests—standardized and normed for the population—and a variety of functional activities (e.g., homemaking).* Therapists need standardized tests to provide objective, quantifiable data to measure the extent of the deficit in comparison with an established norm, to document progress, and to determine discharge planning. Functional activities provide opportunities to observe the practical implications of the deficits revealed by the standardized tests and allow the therapist to better predict the person's functioning in a home environment. Observation of functional performance during occupation is the best way an OTA can contribute to the evaluation of cognitive skills.
5. *When introducing a cognitive test to a client, the examiner should avoid a condescending attitude or a too cheerful, falsely positive approach.* Regardless of the level of functioning, the client should be approached on an age-appropriate level. The therapist should only offer choices that he or she is willing to complete.

Cognition

Cognitive deficits may be the most devastating residual problems of brain damage from a CVA, traumatic brain injury (TBI), or acquired disease (dementia). Within the *Occupational Therapy Practice Framework,* **cognition** is classified under client factors.[3] Cognition includes the following:

- *Global mental functions:* consciousness, orientation, sleep, temperament, personality, energy, and drive.
- *Specific mental functions:* attention, memory, thought, judgment, time management, problem solving, decision making, language, regulation of emotion, and experience of the self.

Cognition relies on information from external sources and internally generated ideas. Cognition allows individuals to use and process sensed and perceived information and thus is intimately connected to sensation and perception.

Clinical evaluation of individual cognitive deficits is challenging and complex. Deficit areas are rarely seen in isolation, and interpreting a client's behavior is difficult. The occupational therapist typically evaluates cognition along with other allied health professionals. The OTA assists by observing client performance in functional activities and reporting observations that demonstrate the presence or absence of cognitive skills and functions.

Cognitive Evaluation

The occupational therapist evaluating cognition must consider several important principles. Because the service-competent OTA may contribute by administering structured evaluation instruments, these principles are included as Box 9-4. When administering standardized tests, the OT practitioner's adherence to the instructions is crucial to attaining valid results.

The process of evaluating a client through observation or during completion of a task can be difficult for a beginner to learn. The therapy practitioner must learn to balance his or her responses to provide assistance only when it is necessary. The novice often assists the client too much or not enough during the task. If the examiner assists too much, he or she will not be gathering accurate information on the client's cognitive functioning. If the examiner does not provide enough assistance, the client will become frustrated with the task and will not experience a positive sense of accomplishment. The

OTA will learn and develop these skills through fieldwork and clinical practice.

Some of the test batteries of cognitive functions that the occupational therapist uses to screen a range of cognitive skills are shown in Table 9-1. Cognitive functions are evaluated in a particular order because certain cognitive skills depend on others. For example, individuals will be unable to display effective problem-solving skills when they cannot attend to or remember a particular task. The following functions are discussed in the order of the recommended progression of testing.

Orientation and Attention

Orientation refers to an individual's ongoing awareness of the current situation, the environment, and the passage of time. Immediately after any traumatic injury, a person must develop an awareness of the events that preceded the accident and those occurring since then. After a CVA, for example, the individual is typically disoriented initially but becomes more aware as healing occurs.[81,84]

Orientation is related to an individual's memory capacity because a person must be able to remember past occurrences to place current events in their proper perspective. After a severe TBI or CVA, a person initially may be confused about personal identity, which indicates a *disorientation to person*.[81] This issue is a more global deficit than an inability to speak one's name, which may occur in the case of aphasia, when a person has difficulty with the verbal expression of any message. The client may also confuse the identities of other individuals, for example, thinking that the therapist or assistant is a family member. *Orientation to place* refers to an individual's awareness of being in a hospital (if appropriate) or knowing the name of the immediate town, city, and state. Difficulty in monitoring the passage of time can result in *time disorientation*. Clients may confuse the sequence of events in time. For example, a client may report that a family member visited the previous day when that person actually came to see him a week earlier.

An unimpaired individual typically can respond to the following questions: (1) What is your name? (or be able to respond to his or her name); (2) Where are you?; and (3) What time is it? (i.e., what year, month, day, and time of day). The client who can respond accurately to all three orientation questions is said to be oriented × three (oriented times three) (the standard abbreviation is written as O × 3), or oriented to person, place, and time. If only able to answer the first two questions, the client is oriented times two, or oriented to person and place (the standard abbreviation is written as O × 2). If he or she can answer only the first question, the client is oriented × one, or oriented to person (the standard abbreviation is O × 1). Because levels of orientation can vary with time of day and other conditions, these questions must be asked several times to determine the consistency of the client's awareness.

Topographical orientation describes an individual's awareness of the position of self in relationship to the environment (e.g., the room, building, city). Functional examples of this disorder are noted when a client becomes confused or lost while attempting to leave a room and locate another therapy department or travel to the cafeteria. These clients may perform better in the familiar environment of home and community, but deficits may still be apparent. Topographical orientation is assessed by observing a client traveling from one place to another or by asking the client to draw a floor plan of the room, the therapy area, or his home. The therapist then verifies the latter with the family. Clients with visual field deficits may appear to have deficits in topographical orientation when, in fact, their difficulty in navigation is caused entirely by a deficit in vision.

Attention is an active process that allows the individual to focus on the environmental information and sensations relevant at a particular time. Attention involves the simultaneous engagement of alertness, selectivity, sustained effort, flexibility, and mental tracking.[70] A client must be alert and awake and able to select a relevant focus of interest. The client must be able to maintain this focus for as long as needed but be able to shift the focus if another event of interest or importance occurs. Consider, for example, attending to the task of dressing until the task is completed and shifting attention to breakfast when it arrives. The client must be able to ignore information if it is not relevant and to track several types of information simultaneously. This need requires, for example, dressing without being distracted by the people in the hall while recognizing when someone brings in the breakfast tray. Because these skills underlie all aspects of cognitive functioning, the deficits can interfere with all areas of occupation, especially in clients who have experienced neurological damage.

The two types of information processing relevant to attention are automatic and controlled processing.[80,81] *Automatic processing* occurs at a subcortical (not deliberately conscious) level. *Controlled processing* is used when new information is being considered. Two disorders, focused attentional deficit and divided attentional deficit, are related to these two types of information processing. A *focused attentional deficit* occurs when an automatic response is replaced by a controlled response. For example, walking (an automatic response) may require focused attention and deliberate control in a client with a CVA who is concentrating on trying to walk.

A divided attentional deficit occurs when the individual cannot process all the information required for task completion. The person becomes "overloaded" and typically responds by reverting to focused attention. For example, if a client with a CVA is asked a question while ambulating, the client may stop movement to engage in conversation.

Concentration requires that an individual sustain focused attention for a period of time. Clients with difficulties in this area may be distracted easily or be sensitive to events in the immediate environment that pull their focus away from the task at hand. Noting which types of stimuli (e.g., visual, auditory, tactile, gustatory) appear to distract the client easily is important. A low-stimulus environment or "quiet room" may be available in the hospital or rehabilitation center.

Other clients have the opposite problem; they can become deeply focused on a given stimulus or activity and have difficulty maintaining general awareness of events occurring around them. Neither extreme is desirable. Effective

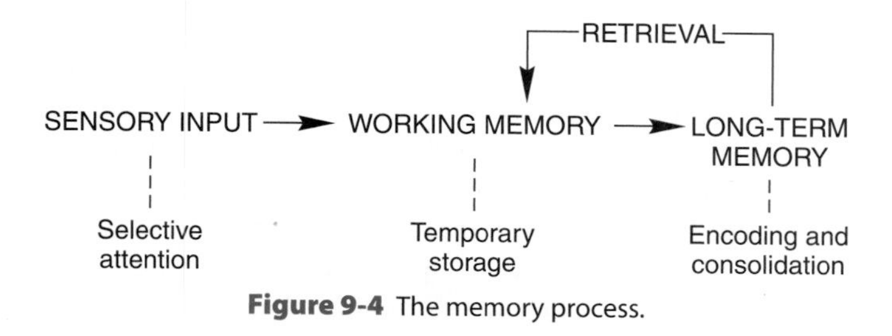

Figure 9-4 The memory process.

functioning in daily life demands the ability to focus, to remain aware of (but not distracted by) peripheral events, and to disengage and reengage concentration as needed.

Memory

Memory is the cognitive function that allows a person to retain and recall information. Figure 9-4 summarizes the memory process. Consider the client who is learning one-handed dressing after experiencing a CVA. The therapist demonstrates and explains the steps in one-handed dressing. The client uses sensory input or the selective attention portion of memory. The information is moved to working memory or temporary storage as the client completes the task one or two times. Finally, after the client has repeated the task several times, the information is stored in long-term memory or encoding and consolidation. After this phase, when the client wants to put on his or her shirt using the one-handed dressing technique, the information is retrieved (from long-term memory) and sent to the working memory. Thus the task can be completed.

A breakdown in the memory process can occur at any level. If a client cannot attend to information, it may never enter the system. Some clients can process information in short-term or working memory but never encode the information into the long-term storage. Still others can store the information but have trouble retrieving it. Clients with memory deficits, who need to expend additional effort to learn new material, may also have difficulty forgetting information when it is no longer needed. For example, the client learning to use a one-handed dressing technique may repeatedly try to use the dressing technique learned before the CVA. A client whose memory is this impaired cannot "learn" the new technique.

A person's ability to recite or reproduce information is generally taken as an indication of recall and is referred to as *declarative memory* or *explicit memory*.[37,59] Tests of declarative memory may require a client to repeat a word list or draw a set of geometric designs. Less formally, the practitioner may ask a client about events occurring earlier in the day. Declarative memory is subdivided into two categories. *Episodic memory* refers to an individual's personal history and lifetime of experiences. *Semantic memory* describes the general fund of knowledge shared by groups of people such as language and rules of social behavior.[41] Episodic memory and semantic memory are types of explicit memory.[37,81]

Some clients may have a significant deficit in declarative memory, but procedural memory (a type of nondeclarative or implicit memory) or memory for a skill or series of actions[37,41,59,81] may be less impaired. For example, a client who cannot tell a therapist the steps to make a sandwich and cup of coffee nonetheless may be able to perform the activity adequately.

Procedural memory may enable a client to learn new self-care techniques despite severe declarative memory deficits on standardized tests. *Everyday memory* refers to a person's ability to remember information pertinent to daily life.[77,78] In the hospital or rehabilitation facility, this term refers to learning the names and faces of the physicians, nurses, and therapy staff who work regularly with the client. Learning a schedule of appointments or the locations of various departments may be difficult and further complicated by frequent changes; therefore the hospital escort staff often assumes this responsibility for the client. Everyday memory also includes the ability to keep track of daily events in their proper sequence. *Prospective memory* refers to the ability to remember events that are set to occur at some future time such as an appointment scheduled for later in the day.[77,78]

Clients with memory deficits may confabulate, or fill in memory gaps with imaginary material.[20,72] They are unaware that they are "making up stories" or adding erroneous information and thus can become confused regarding past events. A client's memories are generally better for specific activities and for topics of interest or of a personal relevance. For this reason the family may minimize a memory deficit, stating for example that "he can remember if he wants to." Staff members need to explain this inconsistent performance and educate family members to the reality of the underlying deficit. For example, a client who has difficulty with the sensory input or working memory will not remember new or recent events or activities. The same client may remember information that has been stored in long-tem memory. Family members may be puzzled by the fact that a client cannot remember them visiting yesterday but can remember every detail of a birthday party last year. This memory is recalled because the birthday party is stored in the unimpaired long-term memory.

Tests (see Table 9-1) can be used to determine where the breakdown in the process occurs. For example, a client may be unable to remember information when he is asked to recall it (with no or minimal cues) but may score high on recognizing the same information. This would suggest that the information was adequately stored, but that the client has a deficit in retrieval. Treatment would then focus on the development of retrieval strategies.

Executive Functioning

Executive functioning includes higher-order reasoning and planning functions such as goal formation, planning, implementing the plan, and effective performance.[49,50] The client who cannot think of anything to fix for breakfast but who responds well to an established routine of making toast and coffee in the morning demonstrates a deficit in goal formation. Occasionally the structured schedule of a hospital or rehabilitation facility may mask goal formation deficits, which then become apparent once the client is discharged home, where externally structured goals and routines are absent. Some clients may be able to verbalize an intended goal and

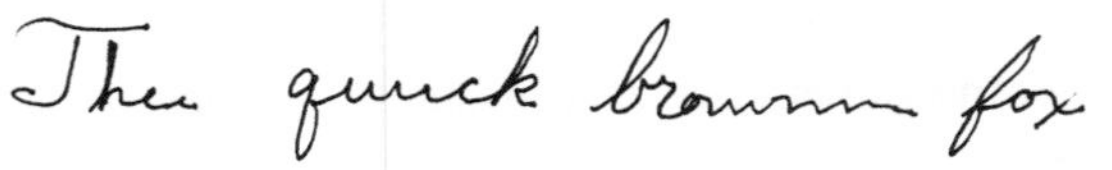

Figure 9-5 Example of writing perseveration.

plan a course of action but are unable to implement it. These clients often seem much more capable than their behavior actually demonstrates.

A client may demonstrate poor mental flexibility, resulting in perseveration or impulsivity. *Perseveration* refers to repeated acts or movements during functional performances as a result of difficulty in shifting from one response pattern to another.[34,35] Perseveration can be seen in motor acts, verbalizations, or thought processes. Figure 9-5 illustrates writing perseveration. Another example is seen with a client buttering toast and then moving on to eating cereal while using the motion of spreading butter with the spoon in the cereal bowl. *Impulsivity* or impulsive behavior is seen when a client begins a task before formulating a plan. The impulsive client will begin a task before receiving instruction or in an unsafe manner because he or she has not generated a plan. A client in a wheelchair who tries to stand up without taking his or her feet off the foot rests is one example.

Effective performance of occupations requires that the clients continually monitor and adjust performance activities throughout the execution of tasks. Some clients cannot perceive their errors, and others may recognize the error but make no effort to correct the mistake.

Family members, nurses, and nursing aides are often the best source of information about the client's executive functioning. A homemaking evaluation that involves planning and simultaneously preparing a variety of dishes for a meal is useful for observing the client's executive functioning. Perseveration or impulsivity would be noted in relation to the specific environment and particular tasks. Perseveration and impulsivity may be related to other clinical deficits such as poor comprehension or apraxia or may be a sign of depression.

Reasoning and Problem-Solving Skills

Abstract thinking enables a person to see relationships among objects, events, or ideas; to discriminate relevant from irrelevant detail; or to recognize absurdities.[49,50,81] Clients with frontal lobe damage often lose this ability and think only in a concrete, literal manner. This concrete thinking is often paired with mental inflexibility. This problem creates difficulty in problem solving and transfer of knowledge to new situations.[81,83,84,85]

The following example illustrates concrete thinking. A client is asked the interview question, "What brought you to this hospital?" The client responds, "My parents' car." The client is interpreting the question literally rather than in reference to the accident that resulted in the brain injury.

Problem solving is a complex process involving many cognitive skills. It requires attention, memory, planning and organization, and the ability to reason and make judgments. Various types of reasoning can be used in the problem-solving process. The client must be able to process complex information in order to plan strategies and to evaluate established strategies.[11] Formal evaluation of problem solving and reasoning is performed by the occupational therapist or the psychologist or neuropsychologist. Evaluation of a client's ability to solve problems requires observation and attention to the process the person uses to complete tasks.

The OTA may be able to apply the following questions to observations of the client's performance of functional tasks. He or she should decide whether the client can do the following:

1. Define the problem or recognize when a problem exists
2. Develop possible solutions to a problem
3. Choose the best solution
4. Execute the solution
5. Evaluate the outcome once the solution has been executed

Insight and Awareness

Consider the paralyzed client with brain damage who falls out of bed trying to walk to the bathroom. This behavior results from a denial or lack of awareness of the paralysis. Limited insight results in impulsive and unsafe behavior. The client with this deficit cannot monitor, correct, and regulate the quality of his behavior.[81,83,84,85] A client's insight may increase as body scheme is modified in response to the changes imposed by the disability. This process is long and complex. Memory deficits may also complicate the client's awareness of the problem or the frequency with which it occurs. The client may remember making only a few errors, when in fact the number of errors was far greater. For example, the client may remember having difficulty recalling a nurse's name two or three times in a given day and thus judge that the memory problem is minimal. However, the incidence actually may be closer to 12 to 15 times a day. The use of a frequency checksheet, recorded by the client under the supervision of the therapist or assistant, may help the client better recognize the severity of the problem.

A client may have a total inability to recognize deficits, termed *anosognosia*.[34,35] A team approach is necessary to distinguish between neurological and psychological (e.g., denial) types of awareness deficits.[7]

Some clients are able to recognize and discuss their mood swings and inappropriate behavior but may be unable to control them. This trait is called *emotional lability*[34,35]; the person is unable to exert the usual level of impulse inhibition. The person may laugh or cry or express other emotions that have no relationship to the actual emotional context of the situation. A related condition exists when the client responds with the correct category of emotion such as laughing at a humorous situation but to an exaggerated, inappropriate extent and forcefulness.

Judgment

Judgment is the ability to make realistic decisions based on environmental information.[34,35] The client with poor judgment cannot use feedback to correct errors. Some typical behaviors that show impaired judgment are transferring without putting on the brakes and dressing inappropriately for the weather. The OTA may struggle to classify a behavior as an example of poor judgment, poor insight, or impulsivity. The OTA is responsible for notifying the occupational therapist regarding a problem behavior so that the occupational therapist can perform select appropriate evaluation techniques to determine the client's deficits.

Sequencing

Sequencing is the ability to organize an activity in logical and timely steps.[34,35] A client with poor sequencing has difficulty organizing a task in a logical sequence. For example, a client making a peanut butter sandwich may take out the peanut butter and a knife and begin to spread the peanut butter before he gets the bread. Clients generally can recognize the problem as it occurs and make corrections using their problem-solving skills. The deficit is in the logical organization of the steps while completing the task. The most effective method of evaluation is to have the client complete familiar tasks that are within physical abilities and observe the performance of sequencing the steps of the task.

Dyscalculia

A deficit in the ability to perform simple calculations, or dyscalculia, can have serious implications for an individual's independent functioning in the community. Various types of calculation disorders have been identified.[54] A client may have difficulty reading *(alexia)* or writing *(agraphia)* the numbers. The speech/language pathologist may evaluate these functions further. *Spatial dyscalculia* refers to a deficit in the spatial arrangement of the numbers.

Summary

Sensation provides the background information to perform essential daily activities. Without intact sensation, motor performance becomes inefficient, fatiguing, and discouraging. Evaluation of sensation is important for clients with CNS disorders and peripheral nerve injuries. The OTA may be asked to assist the therapist in administering some portions of the sensory assessment—but only when the OTA has achieved and verified service competency with independent evaluators (other occupational therapists). The OTA's observations of a client's performance in ADL and other occupations illuminate the functional implications of sensory deficits for the individual.

Deficits in perception and in motor acts dependent on perception (perceptual motor) impair overall function. Problems vary in intensity and diversity, depending on the client's diagnosis and area of brain damage. A systematic, comprehensive evaluation of perceptual motor functions by the occupational therapist is crucial to facilitating achievement of the client's highest functional potential. The OTA contributes to the evaluation of perception by administering structured tests as directed, carefully observing the client's performance of occupational tasks and reporting observations to the occupational therapist.

Cognition is a complex, hierarchical, interwoven process. Many different cognitive functions are involved in performing daily life activities. Assessment of specific cognitive deficits is the responsibility of the occupational therapist and other members of the rehabilitation team such as the psychologist and the speech/language pathologist. By observing the clients performing occupations, the OTA can identify indications of cognitive deficits. These behaviors should be reported to the occupational therapist to enhance evaluation and reevaluation processes and to allow the occupational therapist to provide the OTA with specific treatment techniques that will benefit the client.

Selected Reading Guide Questions

1. Why is sensory and perceptual evaluation necessary and important for OT?
2. Discuss the relationship between sensation and motor performance.
3. In what types of disabilities are sensory evaluations routinely given?
4. What is the functional significance of olfactory sensation?
5. Define *perception* and describe its role in everyday activities.
6. Define *body scheme.*
7. Describe how unilateral neglect can be observed.
8. List four types of apraxia, and discuss how each can affect the ability to perform daily living skills.
9. What are the implications of a deficit in attention and concentration on an individual's functioning in everyday activities?
10. Differentiate between procedural and declarative memory.
11. Define *confabulation* and explain why patients with memory problems may confabulate.
12. What behaviors will the client with poor mental flexibility and abstraction display?

References

1. Adamovich BB, Henderson J: *Scales of cognitive ability for traumatic brain injury (SCATBI)*, Austin, TX, 1992, Pro-Ed.
2. American Occupational Therapy Association: Guidelines for supervision, roles, and responsibilities during the delivery of occupational therapy services, *Am J Occup Ther* 63:797–803, 2009.
3. American Occupation Therapy Association: Occupational therapy practice framework: domain and process, *Am J Occup Ther* 62:625–683, 2008.
4. American Occupational Therapy Association: Standards of practice for occupational therapy, *Am J Occup Ther* 64:S106–S111, 2010.
5. Archibald YM, Wepman JM: Language disturbance and nonverbal cognitive performance in eight patients following injury to the right hemisphere, *Brain* 91:117–130, 1968.
6. Arnadottir G: *The brain and behavior: assessing cortical dysfunction through activities of daily living*, St. Louis, 1990, Mosby.
7. Barco PP, et al: Training awareness and compensation in postacute head injury rehabilitation. In Kreutzer JS, Wehman PH, editors: *Cognitive rehabilitation for persons with traumatic brain injury*, Baltimore, 1991, Brookes.
8. Benton AL, Fogel ML: Three-dimensional constructional praxis: a clinical test, *Arch Neurol* 7:347–354, 1962.

9. Benton AL, Schultz LM: Observations of tactile form perception (stereognosis) in pre-school children, *J Clin Psychol* 5:359–364, 1949.
10. Bennett-Levy J, Powell G: The Subjective Memory Questionnaire (SMQ): an investigation into the self-reporting of "real life" memory skills, *Br J Soc Clin Psychol* 19:177–188, 1984.
11. Bolger JF: Cognitive retraining: a developmental approach, *Clin Neuropsychol* 4:66–70, 1980.
12. Boone P, Landes B: Right-left discrimination in hemiplegic patients, *Arch Phys Med Rehabil* 49:533, 1968.
13. Brand PW, Hollister A: *Clinical mechanics of the hand*, ed 3, St. Louis, 2000, Mosby.
14. Brown J: *Aphasia, apraxia, agnosia*, Springfield, IL, 1972, Thomas.
15. Buck L: Smell and taste: the chemical senses. In Kandel ER, Schwartz JH, Jessel TM, editors: *Principles of neural science*, ed 4, New York, 2000, McGraw-Hill.
16. Callahan AD: Sensibility testing: clinical methods. In Hunter JM, et al: *Rehabilitation of the hand and upper extremity*, ed 5, St. Louis, 2002, Mosby.
17. Chusid JG: *Correlative neuroanatomy and functional neurology*, ed 19, Los Altos, CA, 1985, Lange.
18. Cooke D: Sensibility evaluation battery for the peripheral nerve injured hand, *Austral Occup Ther J* 38:241–245, 1991.
19. Colarusso R, Hammill P: *Motor Free Visual Perception Test*, ed 3, Ann Arbor, MI, 2003, Academic Therapy Publications, (MVPT-3).
20. Darby D, Walsh K: *Walsh's neuropsychology*, ed 5, 2005, Churchill Livingstone.
21. deGroot J: *Correlative neuroanatomy*, East Norwalk, CT, 1991, Appleton & Lange.
22. Deitz T, Beeman C, Thron D: *Test of orientation for rehabilitation patients*, Tucson, AZ, 1993, Therapy Skill Builders.
23. DeJong R: *The neurologic examination*, New York, 1958, Hoeber.
24. Dellon AL: *Evaluation of sensibility and re-education of sensation in the hand*, Baltimore, 1981, Williams & Wilkins.
25. Dodd J, Castellucci VF: Smell and taste: the chemical senses. In Kandel ER, Schwartz JH, Jessel TM, editors: *Principles of neural science*, New York, 1991, Elsevier.
26. Doughtery PM, Radomski MV: *The cognitive rehabilitation workbook*, ed 2, Rockville, MD, 1993, Aspen.
27. Farber SD: *Neurorehabilitation: a multisensory approach*, Philadelphia, 1982, WB Saunders.
28. Feldman R: *Development across the life span*, ed 6, Upper Saddle River, NJ, 2011, Prentice-Hall/Pearson Education.
29. Folstein MF, Folstein SE, McHugh PR: Mini-mental state: a practical method for grading the cognitive state of patients for the clinician, *J Psychiatr Res* 12(3):189–198, 1975.
30. Folstein MF, Folstein SE, White T, Messer MA: *Mini Mental State Examination*, ed 2, Lutz, FL, 2010, PAR, (MMSE-2).
31. Gardner MF: *The Test of Visual Motor Skills (TVMS)*, Burlingame, CA, 1992, Psychological and Educational Publications.
32. Ghez C: The control of movement. In Kandel ER, Schwartz JH, Jessel TM, editors: *Principles of neural science*, New York, 1991, Elsevier.
33. Ghez C, Krakaur J: The organization of movement. In Kandel ER, Schwartz JH, Jessel TM, editors: *Principles of neural science*, ed 4, New York, 2000, McGraw-Hill.
34. Gillen G: *Stroke rehabilitation: a functional-based approach*, ed 3, St. Louis, 2011, Mosby.
35. Gillen G: *Cognitive and perceptual rehabilitation: optimizing function*, St. Louis, MO, 2009, Elsevier/Mosby.
36. Gilroy J, Meyer JS: *Medical neurology*, London, 1969, Macmillan.
37. Glogoski C, Milligan NV, Wheatley CJ: Evaluation and treatment of cognitive dysfunction. In Pendleton H, Schultz-Krohn W, editors: *Pedretti's occupational therapy: practice skills for physical dysfunction*, ed 6, St. Louis, 2006, Mosby.
38. Golding E: *The Middlesex elderly assessment of mental state*, Thames, England, 1989, Thames Valley Testing.
39. Goodglass H, Kaplan E: *Assessment of aphasia and related disorders*, ed 2, Philadelphia, 1972, Thomas.
40. Haines DE: *Fundamental neuroscience*, ed 3, Philadelphia, 2006, Churchill Livingstone.
41. Harrell M, et al: *Cognitive rehabilitation of memory: a practical guide*, Gaithersburg, MD, 1992, Aspen.
42. Head H, et al: *Studies in neurology*, London, 1920, Oxford University Press.
43. Hécaen H, Albert ML: *Human neuropsychology*, New York, 1978, Wiley.
44. Katz N, Itzkovich M, Averbuch S, Elazar B: Lowenstein occupational therapy cognitive assessment (LOTCA) battery for brain-injured patients: reliability and validity, *Am J Occup Ther* 43(3):184–192, 1989.
45. Krotoski JB: Sensibility testing: history, instrumentation and clinical procedures. In Skirven TM, Osterman AL, Fedorczyk J, Amadio PC, editors: *Rehabilitation of the hand and upper extremity*, ed 6, Philadelphia, 2011, Elsevier.
46. Itzkovich M, Averbuch S, Elazar B, Katz N: *Lowenstein occupational therapy cognitive assessment*, ed 2, Wayne, NJ, 2000, Maddak Inc, (LOTCA-2).
47. Kent BE: Sensory-motor testing: the upper limb of adult patients with hemiplegia, *J Am Phys Ther Assoc* 45:550, 1965.
48. Kiernan RJ, et al: The Neurobehavioral Cognitive Status Examination: a brief but differentiated approach to cognitive assessment, *Ann Intern Med* 107(4):481–485, 1987.
49. Lezak MD: *Neuropsychological assessment*, ed 3, New York, 1995, Oxford University Press.
50. Lezak MD, et al: *Neuropsychological assessment*, ed 4, 2004, Oxford University Press.
51. MacDonald J: An investigation of body scheme in adults with cerebral vascular accident, *Am J Occup Ther* 14:72–79, 1960.
52. Martin N: *The Test of Visual Motor Skills (TVMS-3)*, ed 3, Ann Arbor, MI, 2006, Academic Therapy Publications.
53. Mayo Clinic and Mayo Foundation: *Clinical examinations in neurology*, Philadelphia, 1981, WB Saunders.
54. McCarthy RA, Warrington EK: *Cognitive neuropsychology: a clinical introduction*, San Diego, 1990, Academic.
55. Miller N: *Dyspraxia and its management*, Rockville, MD, 1986, Aspen.
56. Montgomery PC: Perceptual issues in motor control. In Contemporary management of motor control problems. Proceedings of the II Step Conference, Alexandria, VA, 1991, Foundation for Physical Therapy.
57. Neistadt ME: Occupational therapy for adults with perceptual deficits, *Am J Occup Ther* 42(7):434–440, 1988.
58. Occupational Therapy Department, *Rancho Los Amigos Hospital: Upper extremity sensory evaluation: a manual for occupational therapists*, Downey, CA, 1985, the Department.
59. Pedretti LW, Early MB: *Occupational therapy: practice skills for physical dysfunction*, ed 5, St. Louis, 2001, Mosby.
60. Pendleton H, Schultz-Krohn W: *Pedretti's occupational therapy: practice skills for physical dysfunction*, ed 6, St. Louis, 2006, Mosby.
61. Reese NB: *Muscle and sensory testing*, ed 2, Philadelphia, 2005, WB Saunders.

62. Rustad RA, et al: *The cognitive assessment of Minnesota*, San Antonio, TX, 1993, Pearson.
63. Sauget J, Benton AL, Hécaen H: Disturbances of the body scheme in relation to language impairment and hemispheric locus of lesion, *J Neurol Neurosurg Psychiatry* 34:496, 1971:52.
64. Shumway-Cook W, Woollacott MH: *Motor control theory and practical applications*, ed 2, Baltimore, 2001, Lippincott Williams & Wilkins.
65. Shumway-Cook W, Woollacott MH: *Motor control theory: translating research into clinical practice*, ed 4, Baltimore, 2011, Lippincott Williams & Wilkins.
66. Silverman EH, Elfant IL: Dysphagia: an evaluation and treatment program for the adult, *Am J Occup Ther* 33(6):382–392, 1979.
67. Sivan AB: *The Benton visual retention test manual*, ed 5, San Antonio, TX, 1991, Pearson.
68. Spillane JA: *Bickerstaff's neurological examination in clinical practice*, ed 6, London, 1996, Blackwell.
69. Teng E, Chui H: The modified mini-mental state (3MS) examination, *J Clin Psych* 48(8):314–318, 1987.
70. Toglia JP: Attention and memory. In Royeen CB, editor: *AOTA self study series: cognitive rehabilitation*, Rockville, MD, 1993, American Occupational Therapy Association, *AU: Please mention in text.*
71. Toglia JP: *The contextual memory test manual*, San Antonio, TX, 1993, Pearson.
72. Walsh K: *Neuropsychology: a clinical approach*, Edinburgh, 1987, Churchill Livingstone.
73. Warren M: Relationship of constructional apraxia and body scheme disorders to dressing performance in adult CVA, *Am J Occup Ther* 35(7):431–437, 1981.
74. Waters RL, Wilson DJ, Gowland C: Rehabilitation of the upper extremity after stroke. In Hunter JM, et al: *Rehabilitation of the hand*, ed 3, St. Louis, 1990, Mosby.
75. Webster RE: *The learning efficiency test*, ed 2, Novato, CA, 1992, Academic Therapy.
76. Werner JL, Omer GE: Evaluating cutaneous pressure sensation of the hand, *Am J Occup Ther* 24(5):347–356, 1970.
77. Wilson B, Cockburn J, Baddeley A: *The Rivermead Behavioural Memory Test*, Suffolk, England, 1985, Thames Valley Testing.
78. Wilson B, Greenfield E, Clare L, Baddeley A, Cockburn J, Watson P, Tate R, Sopena S, Nannery Revermead: *Behavioral Memory Test-Third Edition*, San Antonio, TX, 2008, Pearson, (RBMT-3).
79. Wilson BA, Moffat N, editors: *Clinical management of memory problems*, ed 2, London, 1992, Chapman and Hall.
80. Wood RL: Management of attention disorders following brain injury. In Wilson BA, Moffat N, editors: *Clinical management of memory problems*, Rockville, MD, 1984, Aspen.
81. Zoltan B: *Vision, perception and cognition: a manual for the evaluation and treatment of the adult with acquired brain injury*, ed 4, Thorofare, NJ, 2007, Slack Incorporated.
82. Zoltan B, et al: *Perceptual motor evaluation for head injured and other neurologically impaired adults*, rev ed, San Jose, 1987, Santa Clara Valley Medical Center.
83. Zoltan B: *Vision Perception and cognition: a manual for the evaluation and treatment of the neurological impaired adult*, Thorofare, NJ, 1996, Slack Inc.
84. Zoltan B, Siev E, Freishtat B: *Perceptual and cognitive dysfunction in the adult stroke patient*, ed 2, Thorofare, NJ, 1986, Slack.
85. Zoltan B, Siev E, Frieshtat B: *The adult stroke patient: a manual for evaluation and treatment of perceptual and cognitive dysfunction*, rev ed 2, Thorofare, NJ, 1986, Slack.

Recommended Reading

Army individual test battery: manual of directions and scoring, Washington, DC, 1944, Adjutant General's Office, US War Department.

Beyer BK: *Practical strategies for the teaching of thinking*, Boston, 1987, Allyn & Bacon.

Brand P, Yancy P: *The gift nobody wants*, New York, 1993, Harper Collins.

Brown L, Sherbenou RJ, Johnsen SK: *The test of nonverbal intelligence (TONI)*, Austin, TX, 1982, Pro-Ed.

Callahan AD: Sensibility assessment: prerequisites and techniques for nerve lesions. In Hunter JM, Mackin EJ, Callahan AD, editors: *Rehabilitation of the hand: surgery and therapy*, ed 4, St. Louis, 1995, Mosby.

Giles GM: *Concepts in neuro-rehabilitation self paced course*, Bethesda, MD, 2006, AOTA Press.

Krotoski JB: Sensibility testing: history, instrumentation and clinical procedures. In Skirven TM, Osterman AL, Fedorczyk J, Amadio PC, editors: *Rehabilitation of the hand and upper extremity*, ed 6, Philadelphia, 2011, Elsevier.

De Myer W: *Technique of the neurologic examination: a programmed text*, ed 2, New York, 1974, McGraw-Hill.

Gardner MF: *The Test of Visual Perceptual Skills (TVPS)*, Burlingame, CA, 1992, Psychological and Educational Publications.

Katz N, editor: *Cognitive rehabilitation and occupation in rehabilitation*, Bethesda, MD, 1998, American Occupational Therapy Association.

Likert R, Quasha WH: *The revised Minnesota paper formboard test*, New York, 1970, Psychological Corporation.

Lynch WJ: Ecological validity of cognitive rehabilitation software, *J Head Trauma Rehabil* 7:36, 1992.

Royeen CB, editor: *AOTA self study series: cognitive rehabilitation*, Rockville, MD, 1993, American Occupational Therapy Association.

Ruch FL, Ruch M: *Employee Aptitude Survey*, San Diego, 1963, Educational and Industrial Testing Service.

Shumway-Cook W, Woollacott MH: *Motor control theory and practical applications*, ed 2, Baltimore, 2001, Lippincott Williams & Wilkins.

Shumway-Cook W, Woollacott MH: *Motor control theory: translating research into clinical practice*, ed 4, Baltimore, 2011, Lippincott Williams & Wilkins.

Sohlberg MM: *The Profile of Executive Control System (PRO-EX)*, Puyallup, WA, 1992, Association for Neurological Research and Development.

Stone MH, Wright BD: *Knox's Cube Test*, Wood Dale, IL, 1980, Stoelting.

Strauss AA, Werner H: Disorders of conceptual thinking in the brain-injured child, *J Nerv Ment Dis* 96:153, 1942.

Zoltan B: *Vision, perception, and cognition*, ed 4, Thorofare, NJ, 2007, Slack Incorporated.

PART IV

Intervention Principles

CHAPTER 10

Teaching and Learning Motor Performance in Occupational Therapy*

JANE CLIFFORD O'BRIEN AND JEAN W. SOLOMON

Key Terms

Learning
Motor learning
Procedural learning
Declarative learning
Context
Extrinsic feedback
Intrinsic feedback
Generalization
Blocked (mass) practice
Skill acquisition stage
Skill refinement stage
Distributed practice schedule
Skill retention stage
Random practice schedule
Whole learning
Progressive-part learning
Pure-part learning
Whole-to-part-to-whole learning
Occupation
Contrived activities
Preparatory activities
Transfer
Summary feedback
Reinforcement

Chapter Objectives

After studying this chapter, the student or practitioner will be able to do the following:

1. Define and describe motor learning concepts.
2. Consider the effects of various practice schedules and practice methods on motor learning.
3. Contrast various types of feedback and their effects on learning.
4. Identify the characteristics of an effective teacher.
5. Identify the stages of the teaching/learning process.
6. Name and discuss the four basic steps in good instruction.
7. Contrast various methods of teaching, and match these to characteristics of individual learners.

Teaching and learning are core concepts of the occupational therapy (OT) process. Learning takes place within the learner and can be defined as the acquisition of skills or information that changes a person's behavior, attitudes, insights, or perceptions.[6] Teaching refers to the process of instructing and helping other people acquire information.

The OT practitioner (occupational therapist or occupational therapy assistant) teaches clients motor performance by providing the environment and designing and guiding the experiences that facilitate learning.[15] The practitioner instructs the client or learner in the skills that facilitate independence and occupational performance. OT practitioners working in physical dysfunction settings teach motor skills to help clients engage in desired occupations. This chapter explores the concepts of motor learning as they apply to physical skills taught to clients. The authors describe the stages and

*Lorraine Williams Pedretti and Darcy Ann Umphred contributed large portions of this chapter to the first edition of this book.

types of motor learning and discuss dynamical systems' view of applying motor learning principles in practice. The authors define important motor learning concepts including transfer of learning, feedback, distribution and variability of skill practice, and the use of mental practice. A review of the teaching-learning process as it relates to motor performance is addressed. The steps of instruction to help clients return to desired occupations and methods used to instruct clients with multisensory needs are discussed. Case examples are used to illustrate concepts.

Motor Learning

Motor learning is the acquisition of motor skills. It is "a set of processes associated with practice or experience leading to relatively permanent changes in the capability for responding."[21] The desired outcome of motor learning is a permanent change in motor behavior or skill as a result of practice and experience. This change in behavior leads to the formatting of motor programs (brain blueprint of motor sequences) that are at first highly specific to the activity learned but in time generalize to similar tasks in different environments. The goal of motor learning is for clients to perform the skill in a variety of environments, under a variety of conditions. "Motor learning is the way that techniques of motor control are put into practice and how one teaches movement for retention during occupational performance. Specifically, motor learning is concerned with how one acquires motor skills and includes type and amount of practice, type and amount of feedback, type of activities, and presentation of tasks for learning."[18]

Stages of Motor Learning

CASE STUDY

Han

Han is a 56-year-old man who suffered a traumatic head injury from a shallow dive into a pool. He experiences difficulty getting dressed and feeding himself. The OT practitioner has decided to use a motor learning approach to reteach Han how to perform his daily occupations. Han begins the task of dressing by labeling the clothing, and the OT practitioner provides simple verbal directions. Han verbalizes each step.

OT practitioners work with clients who are at different stages of motor learning (Table 10-1). Each stage requires different intervention strategies. The stages of motor learning discussed here are cognitive, associative, and autonomous.[20] During the beginning stages, individuals rely on cognition to guide movement. Frequently clients in this stage "talk and think through" the steps. In the case example, Han talks himself through each dressing step. This once familiar skill is no longer automatic for him and he must again think it through. This requires more time and effort to complete the task.

Table 10-1 Examples of Stages of Motor Learning

Stage	Example
Cognitive	Adult learning to dance; Older person who had a stroke learning to brush his teeth again; Person with LE amputation learning to move around house
Associative	Adult remembering similar movements in previous dance routine; Older person picking up familiar toothbrush; Person with LE amputation noticing how nice it feels to be back home
Autonomous	Adult dancing routine flawlessly even when the music suddenly skips; Older person quickly adjusting the water temperature; Person with LE amputation moving easily around the house even when the cat passes unexpectedly in front of him

In the associative stage, the learner makes connections to previous experiences. For example, Han may remember that a few days ago the shirt was positioned upside down on the bed which made the process of putting it on easier. At the associative stage, Han makes this connection without talking it through and turns the shirt around without verbalizing the step.

In the final autonomous stage, the learner no longer thinks consciously about the movements but can perform them quickly and efficiently and adjust to changes. For example, Han picks up the clothing without hesitation and adjusts it for directions and variation.

Types of Motor Learning

Practitioners engage clients in motor learning tasks of two types: procedural or declarative. Each type demands different intervention strategies. Procedural learning involves mastering movements or techniques. Procedures are the process and steps of how movements are performed. Examples include transferring from a wheelchair to a bed or putting on a shirt. Practitioners include demonstrative instruction followed by practice and feedback sessions. They first divide the motor performance into simple actions so that they can carefully instruct clients.

Declarative learning, on the other hand, depends more on memory and other analytic skills and refers to the descriptive sequencing of events.[12] Declarative learning can be related as a story ("First, I do this … next, I do that …"). Learning to use a computer is an example of this type of learning. Getting dressed from start to finish is another example.

The areas of the brain involved in the storage and retrieval of procedural learning and declarative learning are different. The environments and teaching procedures that enhance optimal learning vary according to the type of learning desired.[3,21]

Often tasks are first learned in a declarative way and later become procedural. Declarative learning fits well within the cognitive stage of learning because learners can talk themselves through the sequence. For example, tying shoelaces or typing at a keyboard first requires intense concentration on the sequence of the steps and on how and where and when to move each body part. Once learned, however, speed and efficiency of movement are possible only when the person operates on a procedural level, without conscious control or attention.

Dynamical Systems' View

On first meeting the patient, OT practitioners typically analyze movement using a dynamical systems view by examining the individual, task, and environment. The practitioner explores how the characteristics and limitations of each learner influence the content and speed of learning in relationship to the specific task and the context in which the task occurs (Figure 10-1).

Individual

OT practitioners work with clients to help them acquire skills so that they may engage in occupations. Careful assessment or evaluation of the individual's ability to engage in occupations required for activities of daily living (ADL), IADL, work, leisure, and/or social participation is essential. OT intervention focuses on identifying the reasons for deficient skills and helps the client learn or relearn specific functional tasks. The focus of motor learning is on how motor skills are learned, controlled, and retained with the primary focus on the learner. Thus the practitioner examines client factors in terms of physical, cognitive, and social-emotional abilities and how these may influence motor performance.

The physical system involves the interaction of many client factors such as range of motion (ROM), muscle strength, synergy patterns, balance, postural integrity, rate, direction, speed, and endurance. Each factor affects the entire system's performance. For example, if lack of joint stabilization at the shoulder unsteadies the hand, the CNS may increase the firing rate of motor neurons going to muscles that normally would provide this stabilization—that is, the CNS would make the neurons that control the muscles stabilizing the shoulder (e.g., pectoralis minor, trapezius) more sensitive to stimulation so that they would contract with only a small stimulus. In that scenario, a hypertonic muscle or synergy may develop to correct the instability but have the undesirable effect of limiting motor function.

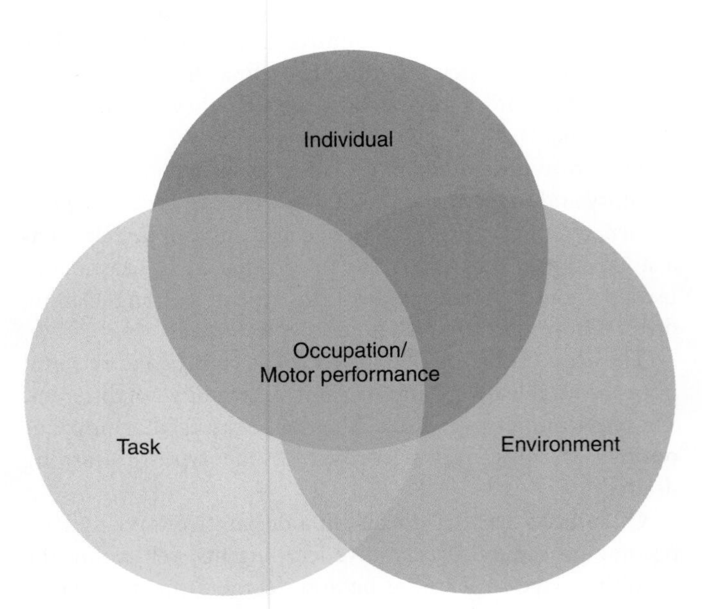

Figure 10-1 Systems model of teaching-learning process.

In such cases, in which the client is using dysfunctional motor components to compensate for instability, the OT practitioner must decide whether to try to change this or allow it to continue. With the dysfunctional pattern, the person may be able to succeed at the task in a limited environmental context. Another approach is for the clinician to give extrinsic feedback and provide a contrived environment so that the client can experience success at the task. However, this approach may lead to dependency on the practitioner for task success unless the clinician at some time relinquishes control of the motor patterns and the client begins to use intrinsic feedback to self-correct. Neither method will automatically lead to better performance or retention of motor learning. With many trials and much practice, the learner refines the muscular organization of the task until the movement can be performed most efficiently and in a variety of ways.[5]

Task

Gilner proposed that purposeful activity is the common ground between the fields of motor learning and OT.[5] The hallmark of functional movement is that the client can perform many variations of the motor skill. The learner discovers appropriate muscular organizations to perform movement. The OT practitioner structures the task using purposeful activity to maximize achievement of occupational performance goals. In considering the purposeful activity for a client, the practitioner analyzes the activity demands in relation to the individual's characteristics. The practitioner works with the client to develop activities that are interesting, motivating, and meaningful to the client. Additionally, the practitioner evaluates the activity to be certain it will help the client achieve stated goals. The tasks within the purposeful activity are challenging enough to maintain the client's interest, while allowing the client to succeed.

The practitioner works toward providing occupation-based intervention (where the client engages in the actual occupation). Intervention also includes purposeful activity that is meaningful to the client, addresses client goals, and frequently includes an end product. Intervention also consists of tasks that refer to the basic units of actions (or steps) to complete an activity.

Environment

The context or environment within which the client learns and practices the task affects the outcome. For example, an older person who has just experienced a cerebral vascular accident may be able to maneuver the clinic space in his wheelchair easily but have difficulty in the grocery store in his home town. This same person may be able to dress himself while in the hospital but find that the lighting in his bedroom makes it difficult to continue when he is at home. Environment includes cultural, physical, virtual, personal, temporal, and social aspects.[1] Completing motor tasks in complex environments increases activity demands and thus may influence the quality of performance.

CASE STUDY

Mrs. C.

Mrs. C. is a 75-year-old woman with diabetes, congestive heart failure, and difficulty walking due to arthritis in both knees. She lives at home with her husband of 50 years, who is accustomed to Mrs. C.'s care; their children live in another state. Mrs. C. will need to learn to prepare meals for her husband and herself. She must time motor actions, as well as the cooking of items.

The OT practitioner considers the home environment, location of the kitchen, meal requirements for a diabetic client, and the meaning that Mrs. C. ascribes to preparing meals for her husband. The context of meal preparation has significant social value for Mrs. C. and her husband. The OT practitioner cannot assume that all clients hold meal preparation to the same standard. For example, Mrs. C.'s daughter requires her husband make his own meal, which typically consists of a microwave dinner.

An activity analysis helps the OT practitioner develop an intervention plan by considering the individual, task, and environment. Mrs. C. must use cognitive processes to select the menu, prepare the recipe, time the cooking, and sequence the steps. Mrs. C. must use motor functions to grip a knife, cut food, stir, spread, lift, and turn. Mrs. C. must show adequate standing balance and move around her kitchen. She must have adequate strength and endurance to complete meal preparation. The OT practitioner carefully considers the individual (what abilities Mrs. C. possesses), the task (steps and client factors required for success), and the environment (social, cultural, personal). The OT practitioner determines whether Mrs. C. requires accommodations, adaptations, or remediation of motor skills for success in her occupation.

Motor Learning Principles

Williams[25] provides an overview of motor learning principles that provides practitioners with strategies to enhance intervention (Box 10-1). Being mindful of these principles can help practitioners practice motor learning techniques supported by research.

Transfer of Learning

In the past, motor performance was observed or measured during the intervention session in the clinic. If performance was successful during therapy, practitioners assumed that the task was learned. However, a return performance during therapy does not ensure retention of skills or generalization of skills to other situational contexts.[8,10] For example, if the client learns to don trousers, can he or she also put on undershorts? If he or she can put on trousers in the hospital room, can he or she also don them at home? If the instruction takes place on Monday, will he or she be able to perform the same skill on Saturday if no opportunity exists to practice during the intervening days?[9,21] To obtain a true measure of learning and skill retention, the therapist must assess performance later, outside of the intervention sessions and in as realistic a setting as possible.[11,19]

Generalization or transfer of learning occurs more reliably with practice in different contexts.[10] Transfer enables an individual to perform similar tasks in a new context by drawing on past experience. This ability indicates not only that the skill was performed in a single situation but also has been acquired and retained; this point would be considered the motor retention stage of motor learning.[19] For example, the client who learns to sponge-bathe the upper body in the hospital lavatory and can perform the task in the bathroom in his or her own home has transferred the learning to a new context. Although the motor skills and the practice environment are not identical in the new context, the memory of performing the required motor skills in a similar environment enables the client to perform the task.

Practice under variable conditions can increase generalization of learning to new situations. Dressing training, for example, can occur in the client's room some of the time and in the OT clinic's ADL area at other times. Various types of clothing requiring similar motor patterns should be used. Undershorts and running shorts could be alternated with trousers, and shirts with cardigan sweaters in dressing practice. Training should occur in the environment most appropriate and most realistic for the task being performed. For example, eating should occur at a table with the appropriate utensils and real food at a regular meal time.[19]

Feedback

Modeling or Demonstration

Practitioners use modeling or demonstration to help clients see the desired action. Research shows that demonstration is most effective when it is given before the client practices the skill and in the early stages of skill acquisition.[25] The demonstration should be given throughout the practice as needed but should not be accompanied by verbal commentary. The practitioner should direct the client's attention to critical cues before the skill is demonstrated.

Verbal Instructions

Verbal instructions should be brief, highlight the main cues, and be carefully timed. Verbal cues should be used for major aspects of the movement and repeated so that the client can use these cues.[25] Practitioners may benefit from practicing limiting verbal cues, especially when the client is performing the movement.

Intrinsic and Extrinsic Feedback

Information about whether a movement has been successful in acting on the environment is a critical ingredient in motor learning.[19,21] If learners do not receive the intrinsic feedback

Box 10-1

Williams' Motor Learning Principles

Transfer of Learning

- Skill experiences need to be presented in logical progression.
- Simple, foundational skills should be practiced before more complex skills.
- Skill practice should include "real" life and simulated settings.
- Skills with similar components are more likely to show transfer effect.

Feedback

Modeling or Demonstration

- Demonstration is best if it is given to the individual prior to practicing the skill and in the early stages of skill acquisition.
- Demonstration should be given throughout practice and as frequently as deemed helpful.
- Demonstration should not be accompanied by verbal commentary as this can reduce attention paid to important aspects of the skill being demonstrated.
- It is important to direct the individual's attention to the critical cues immediately before the skill is demonstrated.

Verbal Instructions

- Verbal cues should be brief, to the point, and involve 1-3 words.
- Verbal cues should be limited in terms of numbers of cues given during or after performance.
- Only the major aspect of the skill that is being concentrated on should be cued.
- Verbal cues should be carefully timed, so they do not interfere with performance.
- Verbal cues can and should be initially repeated by the performer.

Knowledge of Results (KR) and Knowledge of Performance (KP)

- A variety of different combinations of both KR and KP typically helps to facilitate learning.
- KP error information may help performer change important performance characteristics and thus may help facilitate skill acquisition.
- Information about "appropriate" or "correct" aspects of performance helps to motivate the person to continue practicing characteristics of the performance.
- KP feedback can also be descriptive or prescriptive; prescriptive KP is more helpful than just descriptive KP in early or beginning stages of learning.
- KP and KR should be given close in time to but after completion of the task.
- KP and KR typically should not necessarily be given 100% of the time.
- Learning is enhanced if KP/KR are given at least 50% of the time.
- A frequently used procedure for KR/KP is to practice a skill several times and then provide the appropriate feedback.

Distribution and Variability of Skill Practice

- Shorter, more frequent practice sessions are preferable to longer, less frequent practice.
- If a skill or task is complex and/or requires a relatively long time to perform or if it requires repetitive movements, relatively short practice trials/sessions with frequent rest periods are preferable.
- If the skill is relatively simple and takes only a brief time to complete, longer practice trials/sessions with less frequent rest periods are preferable.
- It can enhance skill acquisition to practice several tasks in the same session.

From Williams, H. (2010). Motor control: fine motor skills, In Solomon & O'Brien (Eds). *Pediatric skills for occupational therapy assistants* (3rd ed.), St. Louis: Mosby, p. 475-6.

necessary to estimate the success of their own motor performance, learning may be poor or not occur at all.

Intrinsic Feedback

The learner receives intrinsic feedback as a natural consequence of performing the task.[21] Intrinsic feedback arises from sensory stimulation to tactile receptors, proprioceptors, and visual and vestibular systems while performing the task. Intrinsic feedback occurs during performance of the task (i.e., information about the movements) and after the task is completed (i.e., results of the action).[19] This feedback may not be brought to conscious awareness; it may be processed at a preconscious level within the CNS. Preconscious processing can sort out whether the motor patterns selected for task accomplishment were accurate or needed refinement.

For example, a client putting on a shirt receives knowledge of performance when he or she can feel the movements of joints and muscles and the sensation of the shirt on the skin as the task progresses. The client can sense whether arms and hands are in the correct position to grasp the edge of the shirt or to push an arm through a sleeve. He or she can feel the fabric on the arms and trunk and thus knows whether a sleeve is pulled up over the shoulder. When the task is completed, the client can see the results by looking in the mirror and seeing that the shirt is properly adjusted, the buttons are buttoned, and the collar is lying flat.

Extrinsic Feedback

Feedback about performance from an outside source such as an OT practitioner or a mechanical device is called *extrinsic feedback.* It is used to augment intrinsic feedback.[19,21] Two types of extrinsic feedback are (1) knowledge of performance and (2) knowledge of results.

Knowledge of Performance

Verbal feedback about the process or performance provides the client with information about the movements progressing toward the goal of a motor skill.[11,19,21] The OT practitioner might say, "Raise your arm a little higher" or "Hold onto the edge of the shirt tightly." Such feedback informs the performer about the quality of movement and its effectiveness in achieving the goal.

Knowledge of Results

The OT practitioner provides feedback about the outcome, product, or results of the motor actions.[11,19,21] The practitioner might say, "The shirt is put on correctly; it looks neat, and each button is lined up with its buttonhole." Such feedback can also point out faulty performance and facilitate the revision of movement patterns. The practitioner could point out that the buttons are not aligned with the correct buttonhole or that the body of the shirt is twisted to one side. The client then can revise the movement plan to correct the faulty performance.[19]

Feedback is essential to learning and enhances the learning process. Knowledge of performance is given more frequently than knowledge of results during intervention sessions because knowledge of performance is directed toward correcting faulty movement patterns. Extrinsic feedback is given frequently during the early stages of learning so that the client can correct performance errors.[19] Summary feedback may be given at the end of a series of trials rather than after each attempt. Studies have demonstrated that when enough feedback has been provided for the client to correct significant errors in movement, the feedback should be gradually decreased.

Distribution and Variability of Skill Practice

Blocked Practice

Blocked (massed) practice involves repeated performance of the same motor skill. For example, the client is asked to pick up a cup from the left side and place it on a saucer on the right side of a table. The client needs to solve the motor problem only once or twice and then repeat the same motor skill over and over again. If measured during the therapy session, performance improves faster with blocked practice but does not generalize to other settings. Blocked practice provides limited learning; once he or she learns the skill, the client does not need to attend to the task because it no longer requires novel solutions. No opportunity exists for alternative activities and the reformulation of the solution to the motor problem, a process that enhances long-term learning and retention.[19,21]

In early learning or with confused individuals, blocked practice may be necessary to promote learning. The person needs to practice the same movements over and over to establish the motor pattern. For example, practicing with the same open-front shirt repeatedly before introducing a jacket or housecoat that requires similar movement patterns may be helpful at the outset.[19]

Random Practice

If several tasks are planned for the intervention session, presenting them in random order is most effective. For example, the client may be asked to pick up cubes, buttons, and spheres in random order. The prehension (grasping) pattern for each is different. This variability requires that the client reformulate the solution to the motor problem each time a different object is approached. **Random practice** involves not only repetition of the same motor patterns but also the formulation of plans to solve motor problems.[19] If motor skill acquisition is measured by performance during a random practice session, learning may not be as rapid as with the repetitive or blocked practice. However, the repeated regeneration of the solution to motor problems has been shown to be more beneficial to retention.[21]

Stages of Motor Learning and Practice Schedules

The stages of motor learning are the following: (1) skill acquisition; (2) skill refinement; and (3) skill retention. During the **skill acquisition stage** the client understands the idea of the movement but has not learned it. Errors are common, and performance is inefficient and inconsistent. Frequent repetition and feedback are necessary; therefore a blocked (mass) practice schedule is generally used at this stage. Mass practice is performed frequently, on a daily schedule. Mass practice is necessary for novel tasks. This practice schedule is found in rehabilitation programs.

As the client moves to a **skill refinement stage**, he or she demonstrates improved performance, fewer and less significant errors, and increased consistency and efficiency of the movement. A **distributed practice schedule** includes delays (or breaks) between sessions. For example, clients may receive training one or two times a week as would be the norm in a fixed home program or fixed outpatient program.

During the **skill retention stage**, clients can perform movement and achieve functional goals. A **random practice schedule** is most effective at this stage, which empowers clients to practice at their own pace. The objective at this stage is to retain the skill and transfer that skill to different settings. In these varied contexts, clients must modify the timing, force, sequencing, balance, postural integrity, and ongoing excitation of all the neurons in the brainstem and the spinal motor neurons (the motor pool) to succeed at the task. This achievement may be considered motor problem solving and is a hallmark of true motor learning. Retention is essential in motor learning.[9] Once a motor pattern is learned, encoding for long-term retention and retrieval depends on the context of the activity, the amount and type of practice performed, the motivation and attention of the learner, and the feedback both from the therapist and the learner's intrinsic feedback mechanisms.[17]

Whole versus Part Learning

Simple and discrete tasks usually are learned best through **whole learning**, in which the client practices the entire task at one time. A transfer from wheelchair to bed would be considered a simple task and often can be learned as one procedure. Contrast this with learning the task in the following separate steps: (1) lock the chair; (2) move weight forward to edge of chair; (3) shift weight over feet; (4) stand up; (5) pivot; and (6) sit down. By teaching six different steps or procedural programs as part of the transfer, the clinician may increase the difficulty level unnecessarily. Teaching tasks in steps is called **progressive-part learning**.

Clients may learn intermediate skills and serial tasks more easily through progressive-part learning. For example, a dance step sequence might be considered an intermediate skill. It may require walking or stepping to a beat and various movements between and within limbs while moving on a diagonal and with a partner. If the dance has a specific sequence, learning the first few movements and then adding more steps, always starting from the beginning, would be considered a progressive-part practice schedule.

Some skills can be learned through pure-part learning (the part is learned alone). If the skill is cutting food on a plate, whether the individual cuts the meat or the vegetables first does not matter. All types of cutting are required; thus pure-part learning can be used. Whole-to-part-to-whole learning (learning a part in the context of the whole) generally leads to the best retention when the client must learn a complex skill. Putting on a necktie with one hand is an example of this type of skill. Knowing the whole while working on component parts helps with long-term retention. OT practitioners consider the client and activity demands when determining the learning approach to the task.

CLINICAL PEARL

Clients learn motor skills best when they are performing the actual occupation.

Occupation as Whole Learning

Motor learning research shows that the most useful motor learning occurs when the task resembles the actual task in that it is performed in a similar environment, with similar tools, yet requires adaptations to a variety of situations.[23] Thus OT practitioners are most successful when the tasks performed in therapy are occupation based.[4] Occupation-based activities are those deemed meaningful to the client in terms of desired occupations in desired contexts. Occupation-based activities occur in the actual context and require the client to adapt to real situations.

For example, for a mother of young children, caring for her children is an occupation. Some tasks associated with this may include feeding the children, getting them ready for school, and reading to them. The OT practitioner may visit the mother at home after school and ask that she feed the children a snack. This is considered an occupation-based activity.

Contrived activities may be used in clinical settings when replicating the exact occupation is impossible.[4] For example, the OT practitioner may ask the mother to pretend she is making lunch for the children in the OT clinic. The closer the activity is to the actual experience, the more useful the learning. The OT practitioner might make this activity more real if he or she were to ask the children to come in for lunch at the clinic.

Finally, preparatory activities include those activities that help the client perform the specific components of the motor tasks. These activities are the furthest from the occupation and thus should be used sparingly. Furthermore, clients may struggle to connect these preparatory activities and their goals. For example, the OT practitioner may decide that for the mother to begin to make her children lunch, she must show improved upper extremity control. The OT practitioner may start therapy by performing upper extremity strengthening activities.

Box 10-2

Suggested Strategies for Mental Rehearsal

- Demonstrate the movement in front of client. Ask client to picture completing the movement.
- Record the movement on video. Review the tape with the client, pointing out key aspects.
- Ask the client to reflect on the movement by visualizing self actually performing the activity.
- Work with the client to stop the visualization at key points and 'correct' client's pattern.
- Ask the client to "picture" completing the movement in a variety of conditions.
- Once the client has 'imagined' the movement, follow up with actually completing the movement.
- Intersperse periods of imagery with actual performance.
- Conclude sessions with actually performing the occupation.
- Ask clients which strategies are most appealing to them.

The goal of OT is for the client to perform the occupation in a variety of settings and under a variety of conditions. Thus clients benefit from practicing motor skills in a variety of practice contexts.

Mental Practice

Mental practice involves imagery or rehearsing motor performance mentally. It is sometimes referred to as visualization, imagery, or mental rehearsal. Mental practice can help facilitate the acquisition of new skills and the relearning of old ones. It is most beneficial when combined with physical practice.[14] Mental practice can be accomplished by requiring a client to review a videotape or watch a performance and then reflect on it before attempting it. Mental practice can involve visualizing oneself practicing the movement repeatedly. Athletes use this technique to refine motor skills. Liu, Chan, and Hui-chan[13] found that clients who experienced a stroke who used mental imagery were better able to generalize their skills to untrained tasks than the control group. Practitioners are encouraged to examine this form of practice with clients as it can easily be accomplished and used as an adjunct to therapy (Box 10-2).

Principles and Methods of Teaching

Characteristics of an Effective Teacher

Effective teachers are enthusiastic about the learning content, positive, realistic, accepting, empathetic, and nonjudgmental toward the learners. They are consistent in their approach and expectations. Teachers are flexible, adaptable, attentive, and able to motivate learners. The effective teacher gives positive and honest reinforcement to learners and observes and analyzes their behaviors to evaluate the outcome of learning. Such characteristics enhance the possibility of moving the learner toward independence and thus to successful intervention outcomes.[6]

Thorough knowledge of the skill to be taught and the ability to present it in an understandable way are essential; poor preparation or uncertainty about the skill causes the client to lose confidence in the practitioner.[6]

Clinicians must teach clients how to perform motor skills and how to adapt to challenges associated with their diagnosis or condition. Teaching frequently involves helping clients relearn motor tasks. The practitioner helps the client by:

- Guiding the client through the stages of motor learning
- Directing learning through an interaction that is compassionate, and accepting the individual as a unique and worthwhile person.
- Facilitating movement patterns through repetition
- Grading and adapting activities to ensure successful performance

OT practitioners empower clients to take control over their cognitive, psychosocial, and motor systems. Personal control leads to occupational independence and a better quality of life.[24]

Individual and Group Intervention

The occupational therapist is responsible for planning individual and group instruction; the OTA may handle aspects of this planning. Intervention plans and group protocols, analogous to lesson plans, are designed to include problems, goals, teaching methods, and ways to evaluate intervention outcomes. The occupational therapist assumes responsibility for seeing that treatment goals are achieved.

Most intervention in physical disability settings is carried out on an individual basis. However, group intervention may be used in physical disabilities practice when goals require group interaction or when the OT practitioner is treating two or more clients with similar problems. It can also be cost effective. In group intervention the OT practitioner must understand group structure, process, and function; act as a group leader; and facilitate group roles.

Several types of groups including decision making, discovery, and instructional groups may be used in intervention programs. Decision making and discovery groups are typical in psychosocial and developmental settings. Instructional groups are often used in physical dysfunction settings. In an instructional group the leader teaches or demonstrates a skill, and the members share a common need to learn it.[6] If the skill, task, or activity is practiced within a limited context, skill acquisition and refinement may be appropriate at this time. Instructional groups can be divided into project and parallel types.[5,17]

In a parallel group, members work in the presence of one another with minimal sharing of tasks. Examples are the reality-orientation group and hemiplegia exercise group. In a project group, members are involved in a common short-term or long-term task that requires sharing or interaction with one another. The task may be competitive or cooperative. Little interaction is involved, other than that necessary for completion of the task.[16] Examples are a cooking group or a ball toss game.[22] Client members might be at various stages of motor learning. To perform an altered task in a group context, the client must develop and rely on intrinsic feedback to modify the existing motor plans. These modifications elicit adaptation and should encourage better retention and retrieval of motor plans in the future.

The group size generally should be no less than 4 or more than 20, with some compatibility among members' problems and characteristics. Smaller groups are more practical for motor learning. The environment where the group intervention occurs should be appropriate for the activities to be performed. Space should be adequate, and the comfort of each group member ensured. The style of leadership, group format, group roles, and communication reflect the stated group intervention goals and clients' learning needs.[6]

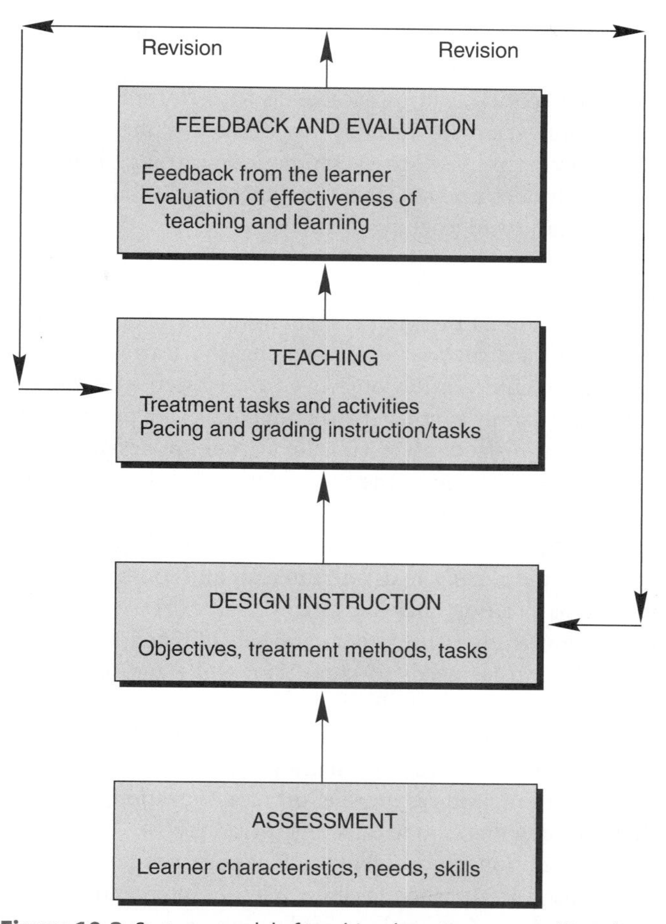

Figure 10-2 Systems model of teaching-learning process. (Data from Kemp JE: The instructional design process, New York, 1985, Harper & Row.)

Teaching/Learning Process

The teaching/learning process is a systematic problem-solving process designed to facilitate learning. The teaching/learning sequence involves four basic elements: assessment, design of the plan, instruction, and feedback/evaluation (Figure 10-2).[11]

Assessment

The OT practitioner (teacher) assesses characteristics of self, learner characteristics, learning needs, learning skills and style, and the situation during the client's evaluation.[6,11] The OT practitioner assesses client factors including cognitive, perceptual, physical, and psychosocial factors. The client's attitudes, feelings, and emotional state in relation to the task, the practitioner who will do the teaching, and the teaching process are also considered.[6] Such information is essential for estimating the client's readiness for learning, planning appropriate intervention activities, and selecting methods of teaching.

Readiness for learning implies that the learner is prepared for the learning process and thus possesses the necessary cognitive, perceptual, and physical skills to perform and master the learning task. Of primary importance is the condition of the brain and CNS to accommodate learning. Therefore the practitioner assesses CNS functions to select appropriate learning tasks and teaching methods.[6]

Design of Teaching Plan

The occupational therapist is responsible for planning intervention or instruction after assessing the learner. Specific learning or intervention objectives are written with the client and/or family's input. Instructional tasks are planned and methods of instruction to suit the learner are designed. The practitioner determines the most appropriate learning environment to foster the client's learning.[6,21]

In selecting intervention activities, the OT practitioner considers the client's goals and interests and sources of motivation. Motivation may be intrinsic or extrinsic. Intrinsic motivation is internally driven and self-initiated and occurs when the learner needs to know something and is ready to learn. Extrinsic motivation, on the other hand, comes from an external stimulus to act such as the therapist deciding what the learner needs to learn and presenting this information. Extrinsic motivation requires more effort, concentration, and time than learning that is motivated intrinsically.

OT practitioners consider the client's age, gender, interests, and cultural group when selecting relevant intervention activities. Clients are involved in the decision-making process, so the task selected will closely match the client's goals. Cultural considerations play a major role in functional carry-over into real-life situations.[15] Selecting activities that are relevant to life roles and meaningful in the client's family or social group ensures a higher level of motivation and participation than activities that seem irrelevant. This relevance needs to be determined by clients and their support systems and not by the practitioner's experience and beliefs. The learner needs to understand why the activity is to be done and how it relates to recovery and resumption of important life activities.[6]

CLINICAL PEARL

Clients perform better and make more significant gains when intervention activities are meaningful to them and occupation-based.

Instruction

The OT practitioner teaches the task or activity to the individual or group in an understandable and meaningful way. Repetition of instruction may be important to the learning process, especially with clients who have cognitive or perceptual limitations. Clients are given opportunities for questions and clarification.[6]

Clients are challenged in task performance but still experience some success. This challenge is often termed the "just right challenge." Tasks that are too easy fail to help the client move to higher levels of accomplishment and those that are too difficult may frustrate the client. Activities can be graded according to the complexity of their physical and cognitive demands and the levels of supervision and assistance provided by the therapist.[6] Tasks are taught in a relevant environment and context. For example, practice in brushing hair is done as part of the normal morning hygiene activities in the client's bathroom rather than in the middle of the afternoon in the OT clinic.[16]

Pacing and Grading Instruction

Pacing refers to structuring the instruction and the practice so that learners can progress at their own speed. Tasks are taught in a manner and at a pace that learners can handle. Once the client is beyond the skill acquisition phase, distributing practice over time and spacing it with intervening rests or alternative activities is more effective for retention than long periods of concentrated practice on the same task.[6,21]

Learning is graded in complexity from simple to complex. Simple tasks are taught as a whole-movement activity. In designing the learning experience, the practitioner analyzes the activity and breaks it down into its component steps. When the type of practice selected is pure-part learning, steps are taught singly, and as each step is mastered, another step in the sequence is added to the learning process until the client masters the whole task.[15,16,21]

One way to grade the client's independent performance of an activity is to use backward or forward chaining as a method of instruction. In backward chaining, the OT practitioner provides assistance through all the steps of the activity and then allows the client to perform the last step independently. The activity is then graded to the last two steps, three steps, and so forth, until the client can perform the whole activity independently. The process would be consistent with a whole-to-part-to-whole type of practice environment. In forward chaining, a similar process is used, except the practitioner allows the client to perform the first step independently and then assists the client in performing the rest of the steps. Then the client performs the first two steps, then three steps, and so on, until the activity can be performed independently. Chaining may be helpful for clients with cognitive or mental deficits.[8] The OT practitioner analyzes the task, considering not only motor plans needed to perform it but also the client factors (e.g., sensory, cognitive, physical, emotional, social abilities).

Active Participation and Repetition

One of the primary principles of OT is for the client to participate actively in the intervention process. The client must be actively engaged in learning, which means that the client helps set intervention goals, plans activities, and participates in the performance processes of learning. Being told or shown an activity is not enough. The client performs it and learns the activity at a tactile and kinesthetic level to ensure retention.[12,15] Active participation enhances learning and enables the client to control the process, as the director of action.

Feedback and Evaluation

Feedback and reinforcement are closely connected. Confirmation of successful responses encourages the person to continue learning.[11] The person also needs feedback during the learning process to recognize mistakes and modify performance.

Correcting the learner as soon as an error is noted is best so that erroneous patterns do not develop.[6]

Reinforcement may be derived intrinsically from the personal satisfaction of observing the results of successful performance or may be provided extrinsically by the OT practitioner. Verbal reinforcement in a cognitive task may be direct and meaningful. In the cognitive arena, behavior that is reinforced tends to be repeated. In a motor task, however, external reinforcement may override the intrinsic mechanism and not allow for innate self-correction. When extrinsic feedback is used to assist in motor learning, feedback should be realistic, honest, and appropriate to the task (i.e., the practitioner does not need to exclaim loudly in superlatives when a shoe has been tied effectively). A more appropriate reinforcer would be a low-key, positive statement that the lace is correctly tied and will effectively keep the shoe on the foot. Similarly, if the motor performance will not reach the identified goal, the practitioner might suggest an alternative plan of action and repeat the instruction, possibly in a different sensory mode.[16]

Constructive criticism is given thoughtfully and tactfully and delivered in a nonthreatening but honest manner. False praise can be just as confusing and insulting as criticism. Constructive suggestions for alternative action that may be more successful are included with any correction.[6] Considerable reinforcement may be necessary in the early stages of learning regardless of whether the task is based on cognitive or motor components. As tasks are mastered, reinforcement can be reduced.[15,21]

In evaluating the effectiveness of the teaching/learning process, the OT practitioner asks the following:

- How did the intervention go?
- Did the client succeed?
- What went well?
- What could have gone better?
- Were treatment objectives achieved?
- What was the extent or quality of achievement of specific objectives?

This evaluation is an opportunity for the occupational therapist or OTA to receive feedback from the learner(s). Feedback can be verbal, reflecting the learners' affective reactions to a group activity, or behavioral, reflecting the ability to perform tasks or behaviors that were not achievable before the instruction.[5] Progress can be evaluated by repeating tests that were administered on the initial evaluation. The results can provide objective evidence of the effectiveness of treatment. A muscle test may show a change in grade of strength, and a self-care reevaluation can demonstrate a change in the level of independent dressing.

The OT practitioner ensures that all measurements submitted for billing and as a part of the medical record are objective and quantifiable. A separate record of descriptive or subjective impressions often helps the practitioner remember behaviors that cannot be measured objectively but that do reflect change in the cognitive, psychosocial, or motor systems.

Instruction: Teaching Process

The instruction phase of the teaching/learning process can be subdivided into four specific steps (Figure 10-3). This process needs to be modified or dramatically altered for a client at a low cognitive level who cannot interact with the external world. The teaching process described in the following discussion applies only to clients who can comprehend and interact with the environment. Assuming this condition is met, the OT practitioner can prepare for intervention systematically, using this process as a guide.

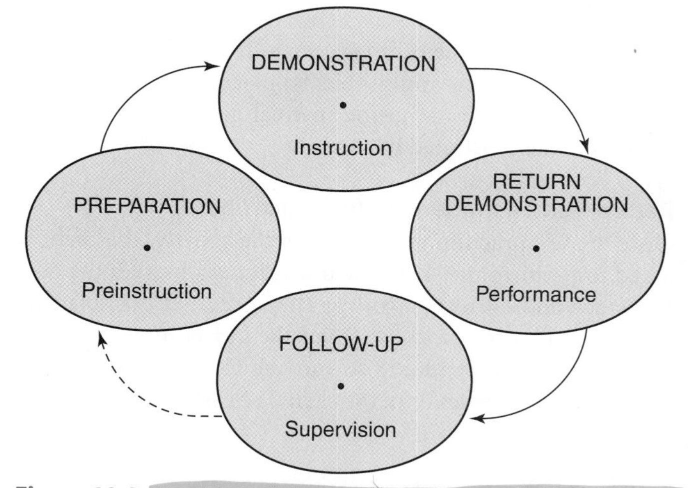

Figure 10-3 Four basic steps in good instruction. Dotted line shows that cycle must begin again for each new activity introduced.

Preparation: Preinstruction Phase

Preparation occurs before instruction. Assuming that the client has been evaluated and problems identified, the practitioner planning instruction selects the purposes and objectives of the intervention with input from the client. The practitioner seeks to answer the following questions: What is the client to learn or achieve? How much skill and competence is the learner expected to acquire? How long will it take to reach each learning objective? The clinician may also analyze potential treatment activities at this stage, considering each activity's physical and cognitive demands and breaking the activity down into its component steps. This analysis helps the OT practitioner estimate the client's potential for learning the activity. Teaching methods are then selected.

The final stage of the preinstruction process is preparation of the environment for the therapy session before the client arrives. Intervention time should not be wasted while the OT practitioner prepares for treatment. Furniture should be arranged, areas cleared, and equipment and materials gathered. On arrival, the client should be positioned comfortably and correctly for the activity.[7]

Demonstration: Motivation and Instruction Phase

Once the preparations are complete, instruction begins. The practitioner puts the client at ease and arouses the client's interest in the activity. Interest is easily aroused when the task matches an occupation of interest to the client. The OT practitioner then demonstrates the activity to the client. The demonstration can take many forms, but in general the practitioner should tell and show the client how to do the activity, illustrating one step at a time. Key points are stressed; instructions are given clearly, completely, and patiently. Repetition and review are often necessary. The clinician does not present any more than the client can successfully master at one time. Words should be few and simple. Some clients require tactile and kinesthetic cues or gentle manual guidance along with verbal and demonstrated instruction.[7]

Return Demonstration: Performance Phase

Once the OT practitioner has shown the activity, the client is asked to perform the skill. The practitioner observes the performance and corrects errors as they occur. If possible, the client should attempt to list aloud the key points while performing the activity; doing so can reinforce understanding. The clinician observes until the client is clearly performing the activity correctly.[7]

Follow-Up: Guided Independence Phase

When the OT practitioner is certain the client is performing the activity in the prescribed manner, the practitioner tapers off contact and periodically observes the client's performance from a distance or attends to the client from time to time to offer assistance and recheck performance. The practitioner corrects faulty performance, gives the client opportunities to ask questions, and provides realistic, positive, and appropriate feedback. The degree of independent performance may be graded by tapering off coaching and close supervision as the client masters the skills.[7]

Methods of Teaching

The methods of instruction that the OT practitioner chooses depend on the client's cognitive level, perceptual functions, physical status, motivation, and the goals of the intervention. Intervention is designed to return the client to engagement in his or her occupations. The teaching methods discussed here require different levels of perceptual and cognitive function and access one or more sensory systems in transmitting data to the cerebral cortex for information processing and execution of the motor plan. In therapy, the methods may be combined. The practitioner finds the method that best suits the client's learning style and level of comprehension.

Teaching through the Auditory System: Verbal Instruction

When using verbal instruction, the clinician gives instructions for the client to carry out. For example, the OTA says, "Brush your hair." The client must understand the words spoken, retain memory of the command, retrieve it from memory, and plan and execute the motor task associated with brushing hair. Furthermore, the client wants to brush the hair. Some clients may have difficulty following verbal instructions only (e.g., individuals with deficits in receptive language, auditory perception, auditory or visual memory, motor planning). Verbal instruction alone is generally the least effective method of teaching.

Teaching through the Visual and Auditory Systems: Verbal Instruction and Demonstration

Demonstrating an activity while giving verbal instruction can enhance learning significantly. The auditory and visual systems are employed as the clinician not only describes or instructs in the steps of the activity but also demonstrates them. For example, OT practitioners may brush their own hair and ask clients to imitate what was shown or may ask them to perform in parallel, one step at a time. This method of instruction relies less on receptive language and auditory memory skills. Instead, the client merely imitates motor acts of another person. Clients with motor-planning deficits (dyspraxia) will have difficulty imitating the clinician's demonstration. Poor visual or auditory memory may also hamper learning through this method of instruction.

Teaching through the Somatosensory and Vestibular Systems: Touch, Proprioception, and Motion

For clients who have difficulty following verbal and demonstrative instructions, the practitioner may have success using tactile, proprioceptive, or movement stimuli to cue the client. The clinician may choose to provide no verbal guidance or to use short, simple commands. Some demonstration may also be appropriate. The practitioner may say, "Brush your hair" and then touch the client's hand and move the hand to the hairbrush. This gesture alone may be enough to cue the client to perform the task. If it is not, the practitioner may lift the client's hand that is holding the hairbrush and simulate the movement pattern of hair brushing on the client's head. The feeling of the correct movements and the tactile cue to pick up the brush augment the auditory and visual input of the demonstration, which in many cases enhances learning.

Guiding is a special form of tactile, proprioceptive, and vestibular input.[2] The client is guided through the activity with the close physical contact of the practitioner throughout the movement process. Little or no verbal instruction is given. The client maintains contact with a reference point of solid support (e.g., table, counter surface) while performing the activity rather than moving through space unsupported. The purpose of guiding is to give the client familiar sensory input.

During the guiding process the client may take over some of the movement as the brain recognizes it from past experience.[2] As learning occurs, the clinician may decrease the amount of guiding and use less intense sensory input. When guiding, the clinician stands behind the client and places the arms along the surfaces of the client's arms. The clinician places the hand over the client's hand and guides it along the surface of the table or vanity to reach the brush. The client's hand, held on the volar surface by the clinician, grasps the brush. The hand is guided back along the vanity surface and to the client's body. The body may be used as a solid surface of support as the arm is guided toward the head. The clinician then guides the client's arm through the brushing movements with the head now as the solid support.

The sensorimotor approaches described in Chapter 21 all use somatosensory input in teaching motor skills. Providing tactile and proprioceptive cues is helpful for clients with apraxia who cannot imitate movements or have forgotten motor patterns associated with common implements (e.g., hairbrush). Clients who have severe tactile and proprioceptive sensory losses or who dislike or resist being touched will not benefit from this approach.

Case Application

Mary, the OT practitioner, is working with Ken, a 35-year-old man who experienced a traumatic head injury resulting in poorly coordinated movements and balance deficits. Ken has three children and enjoys outside activity such as kayaking and hiking. He considers himself an "athlete." When planning his intervention, Mary carefully considers Ken's past occupations and what he finds meaningful. She works with him in OT on gathering the equipment for a hike with his children. Later she accompanies him outside for a short hike, and eventually she invites the children to come along. As Ken improves, Mary reduces her guidance and encourages and allows him to problem solve solutions.

This case illustrates principles of motor learning. Mary has considered Ken's occupations and what he finds meaningful (children and hiking and kayaking). She guides Ken to relearn motor skills by engaging him in the tasks or actions associated with the occupations. For example, she works with him on gathering the equipment for a hike. This requires Ken to use motor skills and problem solve, both important for motor learning and retention.

As they begin the hike, Mary provides physical guidance and verbal cues of the key points to remember. She is careful not to talk the entire way and allows Ken to receive internal feedback of his performance.

Once Ken has succeeded in hiking without distractions, she invites the children to participate. This is close to the actual occupation, but she is still present to help him with his performance.

Mary has skillfully used motor learning principles and integrated Ken's occupations in her sessions.

Summary

The fields of motor learning and OT are concerned with the acquisition and retention of motor skills. It is important to focus on both how the skills are acquired and the end results of performance. OT goals often involve learning motor skills for daily occupations.

Understanding the concepts of motor learning helps practitioners design effective intervention to help clients regain motor performance. For example, motor learning concepts may help a practitioner determine whether and when to provide verbal feedback versus allowing the client to process the feedback internally. Motor learning principles assist OT practitioners in remaining mindful of the type of task they present and in developing intervention plans that lead to occupation-based activity as the key to motor learning. Finally, teaching is an essential component of the intervention process and practitioners benefit from applying the concepts of motor learning into their sessions.

Selected Reading Guide Questions

1. What is the result of learning?
2. Define motor learning.
3. What is the difference between procedural and declarative learning?
4. What is the difference between whole learning and progressive-part learning? Give examples, illustrating when it is appropriate to use each.
5. List and define the stages of motor learning.
6. Identify the different practice schedules, and explain the conditions under which each is most effective.
7. How is learning measured?
8. What is meant by transfer of learning? How is it measured?
9. Describe two methods of practice. What are the advantages and disadvantages of each?
10. What is meant by practice context?
11. Why is feedback/reinforcement important to learning?
12. Identify and contrast two types of feedback.
13. List the components of motor control.
14. List at least eight characteristics of an effective teacher.
15. What are some reasons to use group treatment?
16. List and define the steps in the teaching/learning process.
17. What are some of the important factors a practitioner must consider about the client when designing the instructional (treatment) plan?
18. What is meant by pacing and grading instruction?
19. List three major methods of teaching, accessing the sensory systems used as the mode of instruction. For each method, describe how you would teach a client to use a spoon to eat mashed potatoes.

References

1. American Occupational Therapy Association: *Occupational therapy practice framework: 1. Domain and process - 2nd edition*, Bethesda, MD, 2008, Author.
2. Bonfils K: The Affolter approach. In Pedretti LW, editor: *Occupational therapy: practice skills for physical dysfunction*, ed 4, St. Louis, 1995, Mosby, update.
3. Cai Z: The neural mechanism of declarative memory consolidation and retrieval: a hypothesis, *Neurosci Biobehav Rev* 14: 295–304, 1990.
4. Fisher AG: Uniting practice and theory in an occupational framework: the 1998 Eleanor Clarke Slagle Lecture, *Am J Occup Ther* 52(7):509–521, 1998.
5. Gliner JA: Purposeful activity in motor learning theory: an event approach to motor skill acquisition, *Am J Occup Ther* 39:28, 1985.
6. Hames CC, Joseph DH: *Basic concepts of helping*, ed 2, East Norwalk, CT, 1986, Appleton-Century-Crofts.
7. Hopkins HL, Tiffany EG: Occupational therapy: base in activity. In Hopkins HL, Smith HD, editors: *Willard and Spackman's occupational therapy*, ed 7, Philadelphia, 1988, Lippincott, update.
8. Humphrey R, Jewell K: Developmental disabilities, section 1: mental retardation. In Hopkins HL, Smith HD, editors: *Willard and Spackman's occupational therapy*, ed 8, Philadelphia, 1993, Lippincott.
9. Jarus T: Motor learning and occupational therapy: the organization of practice, *Am J Occup Ther* 48:810, 1994.
10. Kaplan M: Motor learning: implications for occupational therapy and neurodevelopmental treatment, *Dev Disabil Special Interest Sect Newslett* 17:1, 1994.
11. Kemp JE: *The instructional design process*, New York, 1985, Harper & Row.

12. Kupfermann I: Learning and memory. In Kandel ER, Schwartz JH, Jessell TM, editors: *Principles of neural science*, ed 3, New York, 1991, Elsevier.
13. Liu K, Chan C, Lee T, Hui-Chan C: Mental imagery for promoting relearning for people after stroke: a randomized control trial, *Arch Phys Med Rehab* 85:1403–1408, 2004.
14. Malouin F, Richards C: Mental practice for relearning locomotor skills, *Phys Ther* 90(2), 2010:240–251.
15. Mathiowetz V, Haugen JB: Motor behavior research: implications for therapeutic approaches to central nervous system dysfunction, *Am J Occup Ther* 48:734–745, 1994.
16. Mosey AC: *Activities therapy*, New York, 1973, Raven.
17. Newton R: Contemporary issues and theories of motor control: assessment of movement and balance. In Umphred DA, editor: *Neurological rehabilitation*, ed 3, St. Louis, 1995, Mosby.
18. O'Brien J, Lewin JE: Part 2: Translating motor control and motor learning theory into occupational therapy practice for children and youth, *OT Practice* 14:1–8, 2009:CEU article.
19. Poole J: Application of motor learning principles in occupational therapy, *Am J Occup Ther* 45:530, 1991.
20. Posner ML: Orienting of attention, *Q Exp Psychol: Hum Percept Performance* 15:164–169, 1980.
21. Schmidt RA: Motor learning principles for physical therapy. In Contemporary management of motor control problems. Proceedings of the II Step Conference, Alexandria, VA, 1991, Foundation for Physical Therapy.
22. Schwartzberg S: Tools of practice, section 2: group process. In Hopkins HL, Smith HD, editors: *Willard and Spackman's occupational therapy*, ed 8, Philadelphia, 1993, Lippincott.
23. Shumway-Cook A, Woollacott M: Motor control: issues and theories. In Shumway-Cook A, Woollacott M, editors: *Motor control: theory and practical applications*, ed 2, Baltimore, 2002, Lippincott Williams, & Wilkins.
24. Umphred DA: Introduction and overview: multiple interactive conceptual models: frameworks for clinical problem solving. In Umphred DA, editor: *Neurological rehabilitation*, ed 3, St. Louis, 1995, Mosby.
25. Williams H: Motor control: fine motor skills. In Solomon, O'Brien, editors: *Pediatric skills for occupational therapy assistants*, ed 3, St. Louis, 2010, Mosby, pp 475–476.

CHAPTER 11 Habits of Health and Wellness

MARTHA J. SANDERS AND **JESSICA L. KOCH**

Key Terms

Eustress
Stress
Musculoskeletal disorders (MSDs)
Wellness
Body mechanics
Risk factors
Neutral position
Joint protection
Static positions
Ergonomics
Stressors
Stress management
Mind-body interventions
Time management
Assertiveness
Delegation

Chapter Objectives

After studying this chapter, the student or practitioner will be able to do the following:

1. Understand the six dimensions of wellness.
2. Discuss the relationship of risk factors to the development of musculoskeletal disorders.
3. Describe and demonstrate proper body mechanics for performing naturally occurring occupational activities.
4. Describe and use joint protection principles in clinical practice and daily life.
5. Position one's computer workstation for optimum ergonomic use.
6. Describe the components used to adjust an ergonomic chair to fit an individual.
7. Identify the causes and effects of stress.
8. Identify the signs of stress in individuals.
9. Discuss coping strategies to decrease stress for the individual.

CASE STUDY

Jenn

Jenn, a 28-year-old new graduate, began working as an occupational therapy assistant in an outpatient orthopedic clinic shortly after she passed her national examination. She had been a cosmetologist and beautician in her previous career and was eager to get started in a new profession. She was thrilled to get a job in orthopedics; she had been interested in learning splinting techniques and devising creative interventions for clients. Within a few months, she had been trained in basic splinting techniques and had been deemed the "splinting queen," quickly demonstrating the high-level manual and perceptual skills required for splinting. The supervisor recognized Jenn's natural ability and her benefit to the department and began to reorganize the schedules so that Jenn was making most of the splints in the clinic. Jenn saw clients only for splinting interventions.

Jenn's splinting proficiency increased rapidly. However, within 1 year, she began to feel pain in her hands and low back from bending over clients all day. Although she was still flattered that the occupational therapists were so impressed with her splint-making ability, she started to resent the burden of making so many splints. Further, she felt wistful and somewhat bitter that she had no clients of her own, was not learning new interventions, and had to stay late at work to complete postoperative splints. She felt too tired to exercise after work and had abandoned her hobbies of gardening and "surfing the net" because of her hand pain.

Jenn started calling in sick on days when she was scheduled to make many splints; the thought of the work made her hands ache. She started reducing the amount of splinting material she ordered at one time, allowing her the option to cancel clients when she ran out of material for the week. Her annual review was coming up, and she knew that she needed to say something to her supervisor. However, she was not comfortable speaking up and began to complain to other therapists.

Taking Care of Ourselves: Stress and Burnout in Occupational Therapy Practitioners

Occupational therapy practitioners enter the field to help clients function optimally and to promote health. We assume that all clients will want to improve, that colleagues will be kind and courteous, and that work and home life will be separate. However, even our "dream jobs" may have stressors that affect our satisfaction and performance in the job. Stressors range from demanding workloads, to difficult interactions with coworkers, to diminishing interest in daily job tasks (as in Jenn's case). Typically, we find ways to handle these stressors; however, there are times when challenges become frustrations. It is important to examine these frustrations and determine the sources. We then need to develop healthy coping strategies that will enable us to deal with work-related stressors while maintaining a positive attitude in other aspects of our lives. Just as we value the health of our clients, we must value our own health. We must remind ourselves that, in order to be competent therapists, we must take care of ourselves first.

After decades of stress research, we know that stress contributes to dissatisfaction with the job, disease, absenteeism, and lowered productivity in the workplace.[32] Stress is estimated to cost employers and workers 300 billion dollars annually in health care costs and lost time. Stein defines occupational stress as "the cumulative pressures in the workplace that cause psychophysiological symptoms and vulnerabilities to work injuries and disease."[38] Although some stress, known as eustress, motivates us to perform our best, unpleasant stress is more commonly associated with situations in which individuals feel out of control, pressured, or frustrated. Our ability to control our response to stressors and find an optimal state of balance in our lives is essential to promoting our health and our abilities to help others.[28]

This chapter briefly examines how stress affects the body and reviews the literature on stressors and burnout in occupational therapy clinicians. The chapter then addresses specific means by which OTAs can bolster their physical and mental health both during fieldwork experiences and as beginning practitioners. Remember, we can best help others when we are healthy ourselves!

What Is Stress?

Stress is an individual's reaction to perceived threats, demands, or excessive pressures. Each person perceives and reacts to threats differently; thus stress is an individual phenomenon. Hans Selye[37] first described stress as a "fight-or-flight" response in which our bodies become peaked to respond to an emergency situation: sympathetic hormones (such as adrenalin and norepinephrine) are released, which cause one's heart rate and blood pressure to increase, stomach to tense, and muscles to pose ready for action. When the emergency situation is over, body systems should return to a normal, resting state. We all know that numerous demands compete for our attention and emotions today; thus some individuals do NOT return to a resting state and find themselves in a constant state of stress or high alertness.

O'Hara[28] suggests that individuals who remain in constant overdrive lose the ability to "downshift" or return to the original resting state. Chronic stress takes a gradual toll on physical, emotional, mental, and behavioral systems. Physical manifestations of stress include insomnia, frequent colds or sickness, difficulty with digestion, headache or back ache, and anxiety, among others. Emotional and behavioral manifestations include irritability, impatience, difficulty with decisions, forgetfulness, difficulty with concentrating, and negative thoughts. These stress-related symptoms may contribute to more serious conditions such as cardiovascular disease, hypertension, irritable bowel syndrome, tension headaches, and musculoskeletal disorders (MSDs).[17,28]

When Does Stress Become Burnout?

Burnout is an extreme form of stress at work, or even at home. Burnout is a gradual process in which a person becomes emotionally distant and even detached from work or a current situation. Maslach[23] further describes burnout as a syndrome in which individuals feel exhausted emotionally and devalue their own personal accomplishments. Individuals develop a deep cynicism instead of empathy for their clients and begin a downward spiral of physical and emotional exhaustion. Health care workers may be especially prone to burnout due to their desires to improve client functioning, yet they are limited by the realities of health care constraints. Stages of burnout have been described as follows:

Stage 1: Physical and Emotional Exhaustion

Health care professionals can become heavily emotionally involved with clients and overwhelmed by work demands. In extreme cases, they may experience a sense of exhaustion at work and even begin looking for ways to take shortcuts or sidestep typical tasks. Lowered productivity at work may be a beginning sign of burnout.[23]

Stage 2: Depersonalization and Detachment

Beyond feeling exhausted, individuals may begin to pull away from deep client involvement and close contact. They feel less competent at performing their jobs and even feel guilty about their coldness toward others. In order to guard against someone "discovering" their vulnerability, they develop a cynicism or an air of callousness. Others begin to avoid this person who has become short-tempered or even obnoxious. Clearly, this becomes a self-defeating strategy.

Stage 3: Reduced Sense of Accomplishment and Helplessness

In this last phase of burnout, individuals experience little self-efficacy and accomplishment. They feel as failures in their professional jobs and trapped in a "damned if I do, and damned if I don't" situation. Such feelings may exacerbate into depression or ultimately leaving the field.[23]

What Are Typical Stressors?

The term *stressor* refers to the situations or events that arouse stress in individuals. The obvious stressors are major, life-changing events such as changing jobs, major illness, or moving. However, daily pressures at home and at work (such as commuting to work, rushing to get ready for school, getting along with roommates, studying for examinations) seem to be the common stressors that create chronic stress for individuals. In the workplace, stressors may include lack of support from supervisors or coworkers, scheduling conflicts, pressures for productivity, absence of opportunity to use a variety of skills, and lack of opportunity to make decisions or exercise control over aspects of one's job.[17,32]

Stressors may also be embedded in lifestyle (e.g., little sleep, poor organization, unhealthy diet, lack of fitness) or may derive from aspects of one's personality (e.g., perfectionism).[28] Occupational therapy students have additional stressors that may challenge a healthy lifestyle. Such stressors include taking examinations, attending classes, studying, working, and meeting financial responsibilities. Students who are completing fieldwork may experience stress due to anxiety in treating clients, working with complex individuals, and working in a fast-paced work environment. Finally, students must answer to supervisors and other therapists who may all have different communication/teaching styles.[10] Many of these stressors affect the lives of new practitioners as well.

Psychologists suggest that much of the stress we experience is self-generated because it is based on lifestyle choices and our perceptions of events. Neutral events may be conceived as threats (negative) or challenges (positive). In other words, we do not always realistically appraise our life and prioritize the health-maintaining aspects of our lifestyles.[28,32]

Workplace Stressors within the Field of Occupational Therapy

Researchers within the field of occupational therapy (OT) have examined the specific work-related stressors that contribute to strain and emotional exhaustion in occupational therapists. Overall, occupational therapists experience a range of work-related stressors but do not necessarily report higher levels of burnout than other professions. Painter[29] found that at least 40% of a random sample of 492 AOTA members experienced the first level of burnout, emotional exhaustion. Despite this, they reported lower scores on depersonalization and reduced sense of accomplishment (second and third stages) than other health care providers. Other researchers indicate that therapists in long-term rehabilitation, physical rehabilitation, and psychiatry experience higher rates of burnout in all three stages, as do therapists who work with clients who have intellectual disabilities or autism.[9,12,27,29]

The specific stressors in the workplace found to be the most problematic include close and difficult relationships with clients, lack of resources and time pressures due to budget cutbacks, high client caseloads, and limited choice of interventions for clinicians treating clients. Professional factors that contribute to burnout include a lack of professional rewards, a limited structure for career growth, lack of professional identity, lack of supervision and training for newer practitioners, and feelings of ambiguity about the role of OT.[9,21] Edwards and Dirette[9] found that lack of professional identity was associated with the initial phases of burnout in occupational therapy practitioners. Burnout was associated with problems defining the role of OT, feeling undervalued by other professionals, and belief that the scope of practice is too broad.

Gibson, Grey, and Hastings[12] discussed the central role of supervisor support in ameliorating burnout and increasing feelings of efficacy in therapists. Strong supervisor support helped to reduce emotional exhaustion and allow therapists to feel effective even when faced with high work demands. Basset and Lloyd[1] suggest that newer therapists may be at higher risk of burnout because they have fewer established coping skills.

These findings have implications for preparing occupational therapy practitioners to educate the public about the scope of practice of OT and other professionals about the role of OT. As occupational therapists develop the self-assurance to competently explain the role of OT, they will be more likely to receive increased respect from other professions. The next section introduces the broad concept of wellness, a foundation for all principles related to self-care and optimal health maintenance.

Introduction to Wellness

Wellness embraces health as the sum of our mental, emotional, spiritual, and physical well-being; a holistic view of our full human potential. Wellness is a lifestyle approach to managing health that incorporates all these aspects of well-being. Whereas the traditional medical model of health care views health as the absence of disease, wellness reaches far beyond the focus on discrete body systems to identify other factors that contribute to our existence as satisfied, balanced human beings.[3,15]

The traditional medical model (still the dominant form of health care delivery in the United States) and the wellness model differ fundamentally in assigning responsibility for health and in imagining the nature of healing. As summarized in Table 11-1, the medical model holds that physicians (or other health care professionals) are responsible for "curing" the client with medications or techniques that eradicate the disease. In this model, the responsibility for cure rests largely within the medical system; thus health care practitioners mandate the treatment, and clients are expected to comply.

The wellness model is more aligned with Eastern philosophies that assign individual responsibility for health. The practitioner helps the client to heal his or her body and to become aware of the importance of balancing all aspects of life. The wellness model focuses on developing one's strengths to bolster the immune system in order to improve the overall functioning of body and mind rather than changing behaviors after the disease has manifested itself. Wellness emphasizes education for positive health behaviors, strives for a balance of activities, and encourages individuals to actively pursue activities that promote life satisfaction.[15,34]

Six Dimensions of Wellness

Wellness involves at least six dimensions of health, all of which build a foundation of our natural reserves. Although wellness has been primarily associated with physical health, it is just one

Table 11-1 Comparison of Medical and Wellness Models of Health

Features of Model	Medical Model	Wellness Model
Belief system	Health is the optimal state; disease is to be avoided	Health and illness are a continuum; disease is an imbalance of activity
Practitioner-client relationship	Authoritarian relationship	Collaborative relationship
Responsibility for health	Practitioner is responsible for the cure	Client takes responsibility for health
Responsibility for motivation	Practitioner must motivate the client	Client motivates self toward goals
Healing approach	Short-term symptom reduction	Long-term lifestyle plan

Modified from Sanders M, Stricoff R: Management of work-related musculoskeletal disorders: clinical perspective. In Karwowski W, editor: *International encyclopedia of ergonomics and human factors,* Philadelphia, 2001, Taylor-Francis.

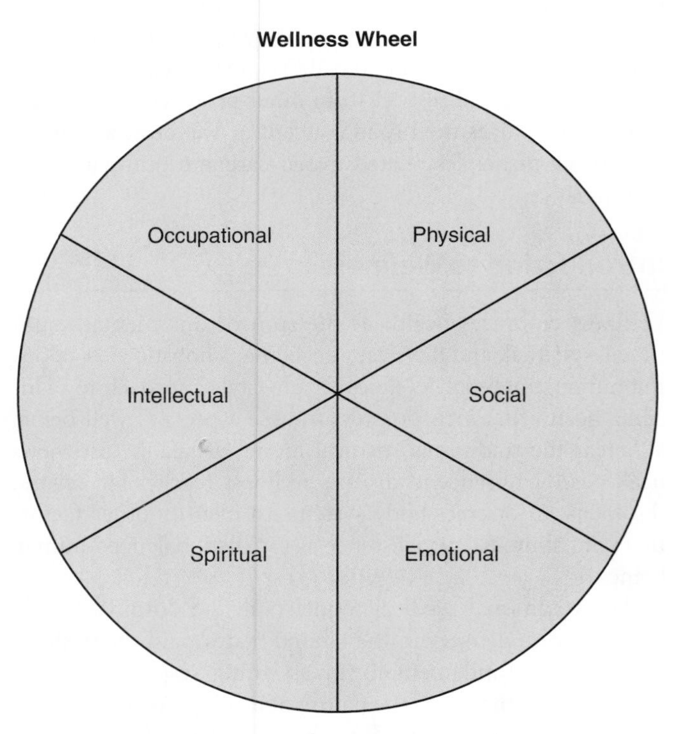

Figure 11-1 Six-Dimension Wellness Wheel. (Modified from Hettler B: *Six dimensions of wellness model*, Stevens Point, Wisc, 1979, National Wellness Institute.)

component of the entire picture. The Six-Dimension Wellness Wheel, a tool used to examine one's balance of health reserves, identifies the six dimensions of well-being (Figure 11-1).

The *physical* dimension refers to maintaining a healthy diet, participating in physical fitness, getting adequate sleep, and learning to relax. Key physical components include the importance of knowing one's own body, one's vital signs, and the physical signs of stress. The physical dimension also acknowledges the importance of safety precautions in preventing injury at work and at home and making efforts to avoid environmental toxins such as pesticides and poor air quality. Interacting with others, belonging to a group, and contributing to the community are elements of the *social* dimension. The *social* dimension emphasizes preserving the natural environment and developing positive social relationships. The *intellectual* dimension refers to the importance of lifelong learning and continual involvement in mental challenges. At work, intellectual stimulation may refer to learning about new diagnoses, intervention techniques, or designing a creative intervention for a client. This dimension cherishes intellectual growth and stimulation throughout one's life.[15]

Assuming a positive outlook on life, managing life's daily stressors, and developing the emotional control to manage conflict within one's personal life contribute to the *emotional* dimension. The *spiritual* dimension is a sense of commitment to an important aspect of one's life. In a greater sense, the spiritual dimension recognizes the search for life purpose.

Involvement in meaningful activities or work is the primary component in the *occupational* dimension. This dimension includes participation in hobbies, volunteering, or work that is interesting and personally satisfying.[15]

The goal of wellness is to achieve balance in all dimensions. When balance exists, the individual is well positioned to heal by drawing on the combined dimensions when illness or injury occurs. Wellness addresses one's present state of health and promotes the maintenance of future health by developing reserves in all dimensions of health.

The National Wellness Institute offers an online self-test called the Holistic Lifestyle Questionnaire that allows an individual to assess his or her level of wellness according to the various dimensions.[12] This test identifies an overall wellness score and provides feedback on the specific component areas: physical, nutrition, safety, environment, sexuality, emotional, intellectual, occupational, spirituality, and self-care.[15]

The wellness approach is a good model for primary prevention (preventing disease), secondary prevention (slowing the progression of disease), and tertiary prevention (maximizing function after onset of disease). The wellness approach suggests that OT practitioners encourage clients to regularly engage in a variety of health-seeking behaviors. It also suggests that OT practitioners model wellness in order to maintain their personal reserves while they participate in positive therapeutic relationships with clients. Because we ascribe to a wellness approach, this chapter addresses the ways that OTs can "practice what we preach" and be role models for good health and wellness lifestyles. This chapter focuses more specifically on the physical, emotional, occupational, and intellectual dimensions of wellness in the workplace.

Maintaining Physical Health: Minimizing the Risk of Musculoskeletal Disorders

Occupational therapy practitioners work in a variety of practice settings that demand physical exertion. Such physical demands may include transferring or transporting clients, playing with children, assisting with ADL, performing range of motion, and restocking inventory. Although the high incidence of low back pain in health care professionals (particularly nurses) is well documented, only recently has the incidence of MSDs in physical and occupational therapists been studied. Among physical therapists, the 1-year incidence rates range from 16.9[7] to 20.7[16] injuries per 100 full-time workers in large random samples of physical therapists. Darragh, Huddleston, and King[7] found that among occupational therapists the 1-year incidence rate is similar, at 16.5 per 100 workers (for 2006), to that of workers in heavy manufacturing.

Some researchers suggest that therapists actually underreport injuries and musculoskeletal discomfort because they assume they "should" not get hurt because they know the principles for body mechanics. They tend to self-treat when they become injured and are likely to continue working even if reporting an MSD. Darragh and colleagues[7] found that 95% of therapists work while injured, even if they have to alter their work habits (74%).

The practice settings with the largest proportion of reported injuries were pediatric clinics, followed by outpatient rehabilitation, hospital acute care and rehabilitation, and skilled nursing facilities.[7,21] The most commonly reported sites of pain were the low back, neck, upper back, thumbs, shoulders, and wrists/hands.[7] For physical therapists, workload issues found to increase the risk of developing an MSD include a high number of clients, transferring more than 6 to 10 clients per day, and lack of rest breaks.[7,21] In occupational therapists, age and weight of therapist were not associated with an increased risk for injury; however, increased hours of work (those with injuries worked 4 hours more per week than those without injuries), and direct client contact increased the chance of injury.[7,29] One may question whether the professional or the organizational culture may have negatively influenced the reporting of work-related conditions because less than half the number of OTs and PTs reported filing a worker's compensation claim. Overall, Darragh and colleagues found that 28% of a random sampling of occupational therapists had considered changing jobs or had changed jobs due to their injuries.[7]

Two of the most important means to prevent MSDs and injuries are to use our bodies properly and to recognize when we are fatigued or strain. Beginning "signs" of an MSD are subtle pain in a particular part of the body that does not go away after rest. Practitioners tend to compensate for bodily discomfort (just like our clients), but self-awareness is key to prevention.

Body Mechanics

One way to prevent injuries is by using proper body mechanics. Body mechanics is a term equated with proper use of the body during daily activities in order to preserve a balance of musculature and minimize strain on body structures.[36] In occupational therapy, body mechanics is commonly taught to workers returning to an industrial job and to OT practitioners in relation to safely positioning clients for transfers.[29] The focus of body mechanics traditionally has been preserving the back during lifting activities and prolonged posturing. However, the focus is now shifting toward proper positions for the entire upper extremity, including the shoulders and arms. OT practitioners routinely assume awkward and repetitive postures in many clinic activities, such as performing manual therapies, retraining clients in activities of daily living, and maintaining clinic equipment. However, little effort has been focused on OT clinicians' care of their own bodies as a means to model self-care for clients and prevent occupational injuries for them.

The importance of training health care professionals in principles of body mechanics to prevent MSDs has been recognized only recently. Licensed massage therapists have found that public demand for more holistic therapies demands a greater number of massages that use deeper, more strenuous bodywork techniques. Not surprisingly, massage therapists are developing upper extremity disorders at an alarming rate.[13]

Concepts in Body Mechanics

Risk Factors for Musculoskeletal Problems

MSDs develop from the cumulative effects of risk factors over a period of months or years. A *risk factor* is an attribute of a situation that increases the chance of a worker developing a particular condition. Risk factors for MSDs include working in awkward positions; using faulty body mechanics; using forceful exertions (to lift, push, pull, or grip); performing repetitive work; and experiencing stressful work conditions.[35] Risks for low back pain relate to lack of flexibility (particularly in the back and legs), a previous history of pain, standing for long periods of time, and an overall lack of physical conditioning.[36] The greater the number of risk factors present, the higher the risk for musculoskeletal problems.

Neutral Position

The concept of neutral position is central to body mechanics. A neutral position is one in which the muscle forces throughout the body are approximately balanced so that the body functions in the most efficient manner.[20] When health care workers use their bodies in positions that deviate from the neutral position, their muscles and tendons must generate much higher forces to accomplish a task than when they work in a neutral posture. For example, when a person carries an object with his or her arms outstretched, significantly more shoulder and low-back effort is necessary to carry the load than if the load is carried close to one's side.

In standing, a neutral posture is one in which the head is upright, shoulders relaxed at one's sides, elbows flexed to 90 degrees, forearm in neutral position (neither supinated nor pronated), wrists straight, back straight (maintaining the natural curves), hips extended, and knees slightly flexed. The ears, neck, shoulders, hips, knees, and ankles should be approximately aligned from a lateral view and the three back curves maintained. A neutral posture in a sitting position is similar for the upper extremity. However, the hips should be flexed to 100 degrees, knees at 90 degrees, and the feet flat on the floor or a supporting surface such as a footrest.[19] Poor posture is the underlying culprit in many MSDs. A chronic, forward head and slouched posture may contribute to decreased circulation, imbalance of musculature (with the chest musculature becoming shortened and the upper back musculature becoming lengthened), and fatigue over time.[25]

All humans move in and out of awkward postures for a short period of time to complete chores, work, and leisure activities. In fact, movement helps to alleviate static loads and promotes blood flow to the extremities. However, when awkward postures are maintained over a prolonged period of time, particularly when combined with excessive force and repetition, the risk of developing a MSD significantly increases. MSDs include low-back pain, shoulder tendonitis, neck strain, lateral epicondylitis, and carpal tunnel syndrome. The awkward postures associated with these MSDs include working in shoulder flexion or abduction greater than 45 degrees, elbow flexion greater than 90 degrees, trunk flexion, and wrist flexion or extension greater than 30 degrees.[19]

Box 11-1

Principles of Body Mechanics for Health Care Professionals

When Moving Equipment

- Keep the load close to the body.
- Move with the feet first.
- Avoid forward bending and twisting at the waist.
- Maintain your three back curves.
- Use a wide base of support and staggered stance.

When Working with Clients

- Position yourself close to the client.
- Move yourself around the client to access body structures.
- Face the client during interventions when possible.
- Adjust your work surface to the appropriate height for the activity.
- Remain upright while performing standing manual therapies.
- Alternate use of the thumb with other parts of the body when creating pressure during manual therapies.
- Keep your joints aligned in your shoulders, elbows, forearms, wrists, and hands.
- Alternate scheduling of hand-intensive interventions.

Principles of Body Mechanics

Principles of body mechanics are used in daily activities to help therapists maintain physical health (Box 11-1). Principles include maintaining an upright posture, using the body in a symmetric manner, and keeping the load close to the body.[36] An upright posture helps maintain the three spinal curves (cervical lordosis, thoracic kyphosis, and lumbar lordosis), thus minimizing compression forces on the spine and reducing effort in low-back muscles. The principle of using the body symmetrically promotes equal distribution of the load across the skeleton and musculature, which decreases compression of the vertebral discs. For example, OTAs should initiate moves with their feet to avoid twisting the back while moving a load.

One of the most important principles of body mechanics is keeping the load close to the body. The farther a load is placed from the body, the more muscle effort the task requires. A diagonal lift combined with a staggered stance allows the load to be positioned and lifted close to the body (see Chapter 15 for a discussion of transfers). Many body mechanics programs emphasize lifting with the knees instead of the back. However, caution must be taken that full knee flexion does not place the load farther from the body. Although most workers initially carry loads close to the body, they may lunge forward or extend their arms to place a load on a surface.

Applications of Body Mechanics

Performing Manual Techniques

The performance of manual techniques including joint mobilization, passive range of motion, massage, and myofascial release may place the OTA in awkward sitting and standing positions if proper body mechanics are neglected. Frye[11] carefully reviewed sitting, standing, and lifting positions that protect the practitioner while he or she is performing manual techniques. From a *sitting position,* the pelvis should be in neutral, the head erect, and the legs slightly separated with the knees at or below the height of the hips. If the practitioner is reaching forward, the pelvis should roll slightly anteriorly (anterior tilt); this position increases the arch in the low-back (lordosis) and further stabilizes the trunk. A rounded low-back posture not only strains the ligaments of the low back but also creates difficulty in raising the arms and maintaining an erect posture of the head. When performing interventions at a table, the OTA should ideally face the client across a narrow table that is of approximately elbow height. When working next to a client, the OTA may consider switching sides in order to avoid constant twisting to the same side.

When performing therapies from the *standing position,* the OTA should take care to avoid a half-leaning posture, with the trunk flexed over the client. This position is common when providing assistance during ADL practice such as dressing training. Practitioners should keep their center of gravity over their feet so that the head remains in alignment with the rest of the body. When moving an extremity (to passively range a joint or perform joint mobilization), practitioners should move their entire bodies with the client's extremity by transferring body weight from the rear to the front foot or by taking small steps. In this manner, the practitioner keeps the extremity (or load) close, prevents awkward forward bending postures of the back, and reduces the muscular strain on the low back and upper extremity (by distributing the load).[11]

When appropriate, OTAs may choose to change the position of the client, change their position relative to the client, and/or change the height of the table. OTAs should move around the client to access specific parts of the body rather than overreaching or bending. OTAs should raise the height of the table or bed so that the client is positioned between waist and elbow height (generally 2 to 4 inches below the elbow). In this position, the OTA can best use the strongest muscles.

In the case presented earlier, Jenn may have been working at a low table that caused her to constantly bend at the waist in order to draw patterns, fit the splint on the clients, and make alterations. Both the splinting surfaces and her surface for client interaction should be adjusted to the proper height. Although most table surfaces are about 29 inches, the surface must be adjusted for each practitioner's overall height and body proportions.

Activities of Daily Living Retraining

During activities of daily living (ADL) retraining OTAs also need to apply principles of body mechanics. For example, to avoid overreaching, OTAs need to position themselves close to the client when they assist with dressing. When working on donning shoes or socks during ADL retraining, the OTA should kneel on one knee and face the client rather than bend down from a standing position. During bathing retraining, the practitioner may consider sitting on a short sturdy stool beside the client (who may be on a bathtub bench) rather than forward bending at the waist to reach the client.[31,33] The more creative the OTA becomes in using and adapting such strategies to prevent injury, the safer he or she will be over a longer period of time.

Client Transfers

The process of transferring clients has inherent biomechanical risks for a practitioner. Holding onto a client at a distance from the body (typically arms' length) creates increased strain on the practitioner's back; difficulty holding a person and maneuvering around furniture makes it challenging to keep the client close. This is the major reason that so many health care professionals develop low back pain from transferring clients. Female nursing aides and orderlies have the highest prevalence of work-related low back injuries due to direct contact lifting and transferring clients.[2,24]

The National Institute of Occupational Safety and Health recommends using mechanical lift devices for transferring clients who are obese, have limited mobility, or those who are largely dependent in transfers.[24] In such circumstances the use of mechanical devices is always preferable despite the extra time needed to locate and transport lifting devices (such as a Hoyer lift). If mechanical devices are not available, the OTA should ask for assistance from other practitioners before transferring a difficult client.

Occupational therapy practitioners also use client transfers as a means to restore function and engage clients in active participation in becoming independent in transfers. Thus client involvement in the transfer process becomes integral to therapy. Even with these goals, equipment to assist OTAs in safely transferring clients and performing bed mobility should be used where available. Height-adjustable beds should be elevated so that clients are approximately at waist height for the OTA performing bed mobility. Other devices should routinely be employed for client and practitioner safety. These include lifting belts, slide boards, sliding surfaces, and mechanical lifting devices. Therapists should incorporate the principles of body mechanics discussed in this chapter. However, OTAs should also be aware of the client's capacities (physical and cognitive), stability of the equipment and environment, and safety devices. The OTA must carefully weigh and analyze the risks of each situation. The practitioner should encourage the client to participate and should provide ongoing cues.[31]

Body Mechanics at Home

Activities performed at home can also place individuals in awkward positions. Practitioners should consider using optimal body mechanics while performing their personal ADL, caring for children, taking out garbage, shoveling snow, raking leaves, doing laundry, and even engaging in leisure activities such as gardening and sports. For example, the simple routine task of brushing one's teeth places stress on the low back as one leans over the sink. The farther one bends, the greater the load of the head and upper body on the back. By supporting upper body weight on the counter with the nondominant hand and staggering one's stance, one can significantly decrease these forces. Similarly, when doing laundry, one should kneel and face the dryer to load or unload clothes rather than forward bending at the waist. Because back injuries most commonly result from an accumulation of small traumas (microtraumas) from both work and home activities, integrating principles of body mechanics while performing common household routines is important.[35,41]

Joint Protection

Joint protection techniques were originally formulated to minimize joint loads for individuals with arthritis in order to prevent further injury, pain, and inflammation.[5] However, joint protection techniques are applicable to all individuals, particularly those who perform hand-intensive work. Joint protection principles emphasize using the strongest parts of the body to accomplish the task and placing the body its most stable, supported position. Adaptive equipment may also ease the task (Box 11-2).

The following are some key joint protection principles:

- *Respect pain.* OTAs need to respect pain and pay attention to the circumstances that evoke painful symptoms. In most cases, painful symptoms will be short-lived if they are addressed in the early stages of a condition. However, if pain lasts more than 1 to 2 hours or is present upon waking, care should be taken to examine the activities performed and to devise an approach less stressful to the body.[5,8]
- *Use the strongest muscles to accomplish the task.* Stronger muscles can absorb higher loads than smaller muscles.[20] Therefore proper use of stronger, more proximal muscles can reduce the daily stress on smaller musculature. The practitioner should (1) use shoulder straps or wheeled carts rather than grasping handles to carry computer cases and therapy bags; (2) move equipment with flexed elbows rather than a heavy hand grasp; and (3) use parts of the upper body other than thumbs or fingers to apply pressure during manual therapy.[13]

- *Distribute the load across several joints.* For similar reasons, OTAs should examine ways to use their hands so as to minimize stress on individual joints. For example, OTAs should (1) carry equipment using both hands instead of one; (2) carry backpacks across both shoulders; (3) perform manual techniques using an open palm when able; and (4) use ergonomic equipment that incorporates larger handle lengths and diameters.
- *Use well-designed tools.* Many tools have been designed to distribute pressure across a larger area of the hand and improve the position of the hand and wrist. Ergonomic pliers, for example, extend the handle through the palm and provide coated rubber padding to the handles. Figure 11-2, *A* shows a person using an ergonomic knife with a pistol grip. This grip design distributes the load over several joints, thus minimizing forces at each joint. This design contrasts with that in Figure 11-2, *B* in which the traditional grip loads the ulnar side of the wrist. As related to the introductory case, Jenn may consider purchasing ergonomic scissors and X-Acto knives (Columbus, Ohio) for the clinic to minimize daily stresses on her hands.
- *Use wrist and fingers in a neutral position.* The strongest, most stable position for most joints is a neutral position, usually midpoint between flexion and extension. In a neutral position the musculature is balanced and can contract effectively.[19] Saws, knives, and other tools are now being designed with a "pistol grip," which includes a vertical handle design that places the wrist in neutral relative to the working area of the tool.[20] Figure 11-2 shows the differences in wrist position using an ergonomic knife versus a traditional knife. The OTA should note his or her wrist position during therapeutic interventions with clients, while handling the computer keyboard and mouse, and when using clinical equipment such as scissors and X-Acto knives.
- *Avoid static positions.* Static positions create high muscle loads and high joint compression forces. OTAs should vary their hand positions and stretch their hands and arms periodically. Manual techniques may compress the finger joints and create overall hand fatigue. Manheim[22] suggests that therapists decompress the joints by loosely gripping each finger between the thumb and first finger and gently stroking the length of each finger, applying light traction. The practitioner should decompress his or her joints periodically during each treatment session and at the end.

Box 11-2

Principles of Joint Protection for Health Care Professionals

- Respect pain.
- Use larger and stronger joints to accomplish the task.
- Distribute the load over as many joints as possible.
- Use wrist and fingers in a neutral position.
- Avoid staying in one position for long periods of time.
- Use the correct technique for manual therapy.
- Rest joints after use.
- Balance between movement and resting a joint.
- Warm hands before manual work with a client.
- Use ergonomic utensils to minimize hand forces.
- Keep scissors and splinting shears sharp and properly lubricated.
- Avoid performing other hand-intensive tasks when treating clients with heavy hands-on care.
- Use the least amount of pressure to get the job done.

From Stamm TA, Machold KP, Smolen JS, et al: Joint protection and home hand exercises improve hand function in patients with hand osteoarthritis: a randomized controlled trial, *Arthritis Care Res* 47:44-9, 2002; Cordery J, Rocchi M: Joint protection and fatigue management. In Melvin JL, Jensen GM, editors: *Rheumatologic rehabilitation series, vol 1*, Bethesda, Md, 1998, American Occupational Therapy Association; and Frye B: *Body mechanics for manual therapists*, ed 2, Stanwood, Wash, 2004, Fryetag Publishing.

Ergonomics in the Occupational Therapy Clinic

Ergonomics incorporates principles of body mechanics and design in work and home environments. Ergonomics is an applied science that addresses the relationship between the work and worker; it promotes productivity while preventing injuries.[19] Ergonomics has traditionally been applied to industrial and corporate environments, but more recently it has been applied to health care and home environments.[33,35]

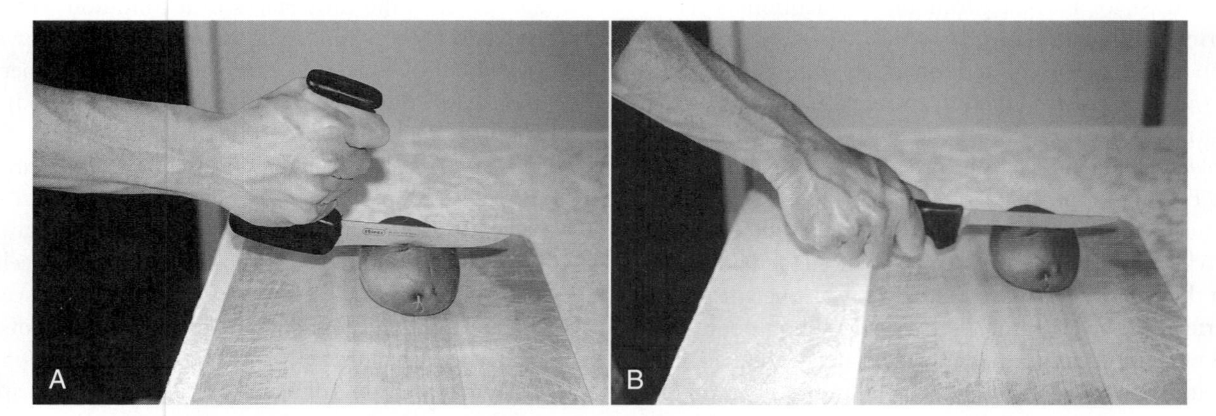

Figure 11-2 **A,** Use of an ergonomic knife with a pistol grip maintains the wrist in a neutral position. **B,** Use of a traditional knife places the wrist in ulnar deviation.

Because OTAs increasingly use computers for work-related functions such as documentation, writing reports, conducting evaluations, performing cognitive retraining, and communication, they need to understand how to arrange their computer workstations to prevent or reduce the risks of musculoskeletal discomfort.

Computer Workstation Ergonomics

A computer workstation consists minimally of a chair, monitor, keyboard, mouse, work surface, central processing unit, light, phone, and peripheral elements such as document holders and wrist rests. Effective use and comfort at a computer workstation depends on the proper configuration of all these components in relation to the person using the computer.

Proper setup of the computer workstation begins with observing the posture of the therapist at the computer workstation and then determining the components of the workstation that are used most frequently. Figure 11-3 is a checklist that identifies optimal posture and provides guidelines for adjusting one's workstation. The most important considerations in computer setup are the following:

- Facing one's computer monitor
- Keying with the shoulders relaxed and wrists straight
- Positioning the mouse close to the keyboard

The individual should view the screen with a downward gaze of about 17 degrees to 18 degrees. The menu bar at the top of the screen should be at or just below eye level. Hip flexion angles should be 100 degrees to 110 degrees to minimize disc pressures; however, some people find this position unreasonable for viewing the screen and prefer a dynamic support that allows them to lean forward and relax backward; people with bifocals and progressive lenses may find that sitting in a more reclined posture with the monitor tilted slightly backwards will enable them to view the monitor without straining their necks.[14] An alternate solution is to use a pair of prescription or reading glasses set for the distance of the monitor from the eyes.

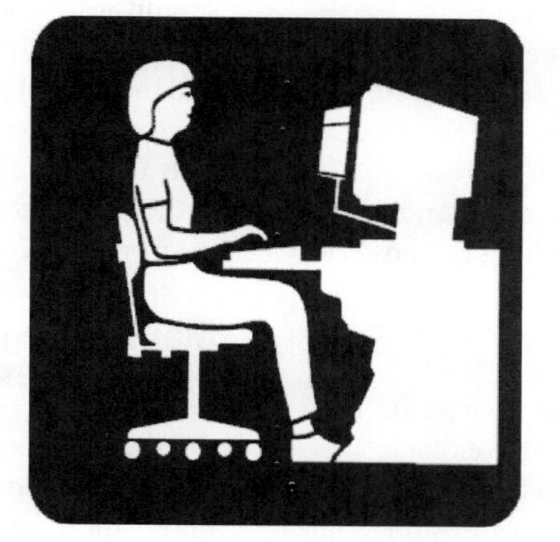

Proper Posture

- ☐ Eyes gaze slightly downward
- ☐ Head and neck upright
- ☐ Shoulders relaxed at one's side
- ☐ Elbows bent to about 90°–100°
- ☐ Hips flexed to 100°–110°
- ☐ Feet flat on floor or footrest
- ☐ Wrists straight

Adjust Your Workstation Keyboard

- ☐ Home row at elbow height
- ☐ Keyboard with a negative tilt
- ☐ Mouse close to keyboard

Monitor

- ☐ Face monitor directly
- ☐ Top of screen at eye level
- ☐ Place an arm's length away
- ☐ Sharpen contrast

Chair

- ☐ Adjust height up or down
- ☐ Adjust back support
- ☐ Adjust seat angle

Lighting

- ☐ Avoid reflections
- ☐ Tilt screen to avoid glare
- ☐ Place monitor perpendicular to window
- ☐ Use task lighting

Figure 11-3 Checklist for comfortable computing. (Modified from Ergonomics and Computer Use Today, Retrieved June 29, 2005, from http://www.quinnipiac.edu/x3925.xml.)

Peripheral equipment may continue to improve the individual's working position. *Keyboards* are commonly positioned in a negative tilt to maintain the wrist in a neutral position (edge of keyboard farthest from body tilts downward). *Document holders* should be used when inputting data or text from a paper. Use of a document holder minimizes eye and neck movements when shifting one's glance between the document and the computer screen. The document holder should be placed as close to the monitor as comfortably possible and at a similar height.

Wrist rests were designed to prevent individuals from placing their wrists on the hard edge of a desk while resting in order to minimize carpal canal pressure. However, people tend to use wrist rests during keying, which actually increases pressure in the carpal canal and increases loads on the finger extensors. People should be careful not to plant their wrists on the wrist rest while computing and instead should float their fingers over the keys.

An ergonomic chair that is properly adjusted to the individual is critical to a comfortable workstation. All ergonomic chairs should have the following *adjustable* features:

- *Chair height:* The chair height should be adjusted so that the elbows are level with the work surface or slightly higher.
- *Seat angle:* A person should be fully seated on the chair with the hips flexed to 100 degrees to 110 degrees.
- *Seat pan:* The seat pan should be wide enough and adjustable to support the thighs without touching the posterior aspect of the knees.
- *Back rest:* The backrest should support both the lumbar curve and thoracic region.
- *Footrests:* Feet need to be resting on the floor or on footrests to relieve pressure on the thigh and lower back.

Laptop computers are increasingly taking the place of conventional desktop computers for both work and home use. Although laptops are convenient, they were originally designed for short periods of computing and are not ideal in terms of ergonomics design. During typical use, the screen is too low and the keyboard too high (when placed on conventional desks or tables) relative to the operator. Thus peripheral accessories should be employed to improve the operator's positions. For long-term use, operators should consider using a laptop stand to raise the height of the screen and an external keyboard to place the wrists in a neutral position.

Use of the telephone may create additional musculoskeletal stress if held between the ear and (elevated) shoulder; this position misaligns the spine and puts pressure on the neck and strain on the cervical nerve roots. Practitioners who use the phone in this manner should consider obtaining a wireless or corded headset to alleviate this problem.

Figure 11-3 could be used as a peer checkout in a clinical setting. Figure 11-4 is a more detailed checklist provided by the Occupational Safety and Health Administration.[26]

Therapist Safety in the Clinic

Although most therapists focus on the safety of their clients, therapists need to acknowledge their own safety when they are at a job site or in the clinic. In the clinic, therapists must acknowledge electrical safety when they are splinting with frying pans filled with water or using multiple appliances plugged into one fuse or circuit (Table 11-2). Ground fault circuit interrupters (GFCIs) should always be installed to prevent faulty equipment from short-circuiting.

Other equipment may cause burns in the absence of precautions. Such equipment includes heat guns, hot packs, and hot water from splinting pans or hydrocollators. Like industrial workers, OTAs should follow safe practices when they are using potentially hazardous equipment. For example, they should use tongs (not fingers) to remove hot packs, turn off a heat gun when not in use, and employ correct positioning when using an X-Acto knife to prevent the knife from injuring the body on a follow-through swipe. Properly maintaining equipment minimizes the risk of mechanical malfunction and thus is safer.

OTAs should remember that proper gloving and handwashing techniques are critical to reducing the spread of germs and infection to practitioners and clients. Practitioners should wash their hands after each client. They should rub soap, preferably antibacterial, thoroughly between the fingers and the back of palms for about 30 seconds (or the duration of the song "Happy Birthday") and finish by drying their hands (see Chapter 3). OTAs should follow proper blood-borne pathogen procedures if dealing with open wounds or sterile environments.

Maintaining Emotional Health: Balance of Work, Rest, and Play

OT practitioners are well versed in the health benefits of maintaining a balance in work, rest, and play. However, casual observation suggests that few practitioners truly exercise this balance on a daily basis. The Wellness Wheel addresses the importance of including many dimensions of being in one's life. Balance begins by examining one's schedule and determining inequities that exist in any of these key areas. Typically, individuals spend more time in chores and work-related activities during the week and save the play for the weekend. However, a more healthful approach may be to interject some "me" time or leisure time into one's daily schedule. One may devise a means to transition from work into home or play activities by exercising, doing short errands, or using a daily commute to transition out of the work mode.[28] One's emotional health is intertwined with physical health. Consequently, stress management techniques include both physical and emotional means to calm one's body in order to face stressors.

Stress Management Approaches

Stress management programs seek to control the effects of stressors by developing individual coping mechanisms to help a person become more resilient to stressors. Stress management programs begin by identifying the individual's pattern of stressors and by teaching individuals to become aware of the physical, behavioral, or emotional signs that indicate stress. Individuals may identify stressors by examining patterns in

WORKING POSTURES–The workstation is designed or arranged for doing computer tasks so it allows your	Y	N
1. Head and neck to be upright, or in-line with the torso (not bent down/back). If "no" refer to Monitors, Chairs, and Work Surfaces.		
2. Head, neck, and trunk to face forward (not twisted). If "no" refer to Monitors or Chairs.		
3. Trunk to be perpendicular to floor (may lean back into backrest but not forward). If "no" refer to Chairs or Monitors.		
4. Shoulders and upper arms to be in-line with the torso, generally about perpendicular to the floor and relaxed (not elevated or stretched forward). If "no" refer to Chairs.		
5. Upper arms and elbows to be close to the body (not extended outward). If "no" refer to Chairs, Work Surfaces, Keyboards, and Pointers.		
6. Forearms, wrists, and hands to be straight and in-line (forearm at about 90 degrees to the upper arm). If "no" refer to Chairs, Keyboards, Pointers.		
7. Wrists and hands to be straight (not bent up/down or sideways toward the little finger). If "no" refer to Keyboards or Pointers		
8. Thighs to be parallel to the floor and the lower legs to be perpendicular to floor (thighs may be slightly elevated above knees). If "no" refer to Chairs or Work Surfaces.		
9. Feet to rest flat on the floor or supported by a stable footrest. If "no" refer to Chairs or Work Surfaces.		
SEATING–Consider these points when evaluating the chair:	Y	N
10. Backrest provides support for your lower back (lumbar area).		
11. Seat width and depth accommodate the specific user (seat pan not too big/small).		
12. Seat front does not press against the back of your knees and lower legs (seat pan not too long).		
13. Seat has cushioning and is rounded with a "waterfall" front (no sharp edge).		
14. Armrests, if used, support both forearms while you perform computer tasks and they do not interfere with movement.		
"No" answers to any of these questions should prompt a review of Chairs.		
KEYBOARD/INPUT DEVICE–Consider these points when evaluating the keyboard or pointing device. The keyboard/input device is designed or arranged for doing computer tasks so the	Y	N
15. Keyboard/input device platform(s) is stable and large enough to hold a keyboard and an input device.		
16. Input device (mouse or trackball) is located right next to your keyboard so it can be operated without reaching.		
17. Input device is easy to activate and the shape/size fits your hand (not too big/small).		
18. Wrists and hands do not rest on sharp or hard edges.		
"No" answers to any of these questions should prompt a review of Keyboards, Pointers, or Wrist Rests.		
MONITOR–Consider these points when evaluating the monitor. The monitor is designed or arranged for computer tasks so the	Y	N
19. Top of the screen is at or below eye level so you can read it without bending your head or neck down/back.		

Figure 11-4 Evaluation for computer ergonomics. (From Occupational Safety and Health Administration: Computer workstations. Accessed June 29, 2005, from http://www.osha.gov/SLTC/etools/computerworkstations/checklist.html.)

20. User with bifocals/trifocals can read the screen without bending the head or neck backward.		
21. Monitor distance allows you to read the screen without leaning your head, neck, or trunk forward/backward.		
22. Monitor position is directly in front of you so you don't have to twist your head or neck.		
23. Glare (for example, from windows, lights) is not reflected on your screen, which can cause you to assume an awkward posture to clearly see information on your screen.		
"No" answers to any of these questions should prompt a review of Monitors or Lighting/Glare.		
WORK AREA–Consider these points when evaluating the desk and workstation. The work area is designed or arranged for doing computer tasks so the	Y	N
24. Thighs have sufficient clearance space between the top of the thighs and your computer table/keyboard platform (thighs are not trapped).		
25. Legs and feet have sufficient clearance space under the work surface so you are able to get close enough to the keyboard/input device.		
ACCESSORIES–Check to see if the	Y	N
26. Document holder, if provided, is stable and large enough to hold documents.		
27. Document holder, if provided, is placed at about the same height and distance as the monitor screen so there is little head movement, or need to re-focus, when you look from the document to the screen.		
28. Wrist/palm rest, if provided, is padded and free of sharp or square edges that push on your wrists.		
29. Wrist/palm rest, if provided, allows you to keep your forearms, wrists, and hands straight and in-line when using the keyboard/input device.		
30. Telephone can be used with your head upright (not bent) and your shoulders relaxed (not elevated) if you do computer tasks at the same time.		
"No" answers to any of these questions should prompt a review of Work Surfaces, Document Holders, Wrist Rests, or Telephones.		
GENERAL	Y	N
31. Workstation and equipment have sufficient adjustability so you are in a safe working posture and can make occasional changes in posture while performing computer tasks.		
32. Computer workstation, components, and accessories are maintained in serviceable condition and function properly.		
33. Computer tasks are organized in a way that allows you to vary tasks with other work activities, or to take micro-breaks or recovery pauses while at the computer workstation.		
"No" answers to any of these questions should prompt a review of Chairs, Work Surfaces, or Work Processes.		

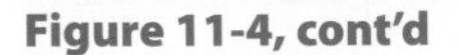

Figure 11-4, cont'd

their lives that seem to create stress (e.g., procrastination, taking on too many responsibilities) or by keeping a stress diary that records the causes and effects of stress. Individuals can then develop strategies to manage stressors that fit their interests and lifestyle. Stress management strategies can be generally grouped into three categories: changing one's thinking (perception of the stressor), changing one's behavior (reaction to the stressor), or changing one's lifestyle (e.g., routines, diet, sleep patterns).[28,32]

Changing Thinking

Cognitive behavioral approaches teach individuals to manage stress by changing their perception of the stressor. *Reframing* is a technique that encourages individuals to alter the way they consciously interpret a particular situation. For example, a person may envision extra work as an opportunity to demonstrate competence to one's supervisor or learn about a new diagnosis rather than as an extra burden in a workday. Driving in daily traffic may be viewed as time alone rather than a

Table 11-2 Safety Precautions Using Splinting Equipment

Splinting Tool	Splinting Technique
Splinting pan	Check to replenish water regularly. Make sure electric cord does not cross the sink. Place a nonstick netting at the bottom of pans. Use a spatula or tongs to remove splinting material. Cool pan before putting away.
Heat gun	Do NOT touch the tip with bare hands. Do NOT reach over the flow of hot air. Do NOT touch splinting material with bare hands. Make sure electric cord does not cross the sink. Do not swing heat gun in someone's direction. Make sure heat gun is sturdy on the stand. Place heat gun on *cool* airflow after use. Cool heat gun before putting away
X-Acto knife	Position your body to the side of where you are cutting. Make sure no body part (i.e., leg) is at the end of your swipe. Make sure no one is behind you while you are cutting. Retract blade when finished.
Scissors	Hand scissors to each other with the handle first. Do not use splinting scissors to cut adhesives. Use right- or left-handed scissors as needed.

Table 11-3 Therapies for Managing Stress

Stress Management Therapy	Examples
Mind-body methods	Progressive relaxation Exercise, dance, leisure sports Biofeedback Deep breathing Massage Yoga *T'ai Chi Chuan* Animal-assisted therapy
Mental approaches to relaxation	Visualization Guided imagery Meditation Hypnotherapy
Complementary techniques	Aromatherapy Reflexology Botanical therapies Naturopathy (among others)

source of frustration on the way home. Reframing does not change the reality of the situation but helps the individual to view the event in a different, less stressful way.[28]

Positive thinking also keeps a person focused on the positive aspects of a situation rather than focusing on elements that fuel stress or negative views of the self. O'Hara[28] recommends identifying common thought distortions (such as exaggerating one's faults, blaming oneself for a situation that is beyond one's control, or creating unrealistic expectations) and replacing those negative thoughts with more positive views. Individuals may find that some stressors cannot be changed. In such cases individuals may decide to let go of that which cannot be controlled.[18]

Changing Behaviors

The ability to change one's response to daily stressors impacts one's ability to manage stress effectively. *Relaxation techniques* are a cornerstone of stress management programs. Relaxation techniques enable the individual to control his or her body by eliciting a "rest and repair" mode rather than a "fight-or-flight" response to a stressor. A relaxed state enables one to think clearly, focus on the issue at hand, and begin to solve problems more clearly and effectively.[28,30]

A myriad of relaxation techniques are available for the OT practitioner (Table 11-3). Some techniques (e.g., deep breathing, humor, or taking a timeout) may be useful for on-the-spot needs; other techniques require spending time in a quiet environment. These techniques include deep relaxation, guided imagery, or the relaxation response. The well known Jacobson's Progressive Muscle Relaxation (PMR) teaches participants to become aware of muscle tension and guides them through a protocol of systematically contracting and relaxing muscles in the body to achieve relaxation. Guided imagery uses creative imagination of the senses through depicting a favorite scene or image. The Relaxation Response, developed by Herbert Benson, relies on repeating a sound or short phrase such as "alert mind, calm body" and assuming a passive state to achieve total body relaxation.[38,39] O'Hara[28] and Payne[30] provide relaxation scripts that can be recorded to calming music. Effective use of each technique requires that individuals practice it regularly.

Changing Lifestyle

A healthy lifestyle includes incorporating stress management techniques into one's day along with eating a balanced diet, getting regular exercise and adequate sleep, planning ahead, and pacing oneself throughout the day. A balanced diet that includes small amounts of protein spread over all meals, plenty of fruits and vegetables, whole grains, and dairy products enables a person to maintain energy for extended periods. Experts advocate exercising at least 30 minutes daily, combining stretching, strengthening, and cardiovascular exercises. Physical activity not only decreases blood pressure, heart rate, and helps maintain weight but is also a potent stress-reliever. Exercise allows one to burn off excess energy generated during a flight-or-fight response and return to a more relaxed state on completion.[28]

Mind-Body Interventions

Mind-body approaches effectively combine changing thoughts, behaviors, and lifestyle to improve stress management and overall well-being. A mind-body intervention is any practice that acknowledges the interconnections between the mind and the body: They are so interconnected that the body and mind reciprocally influence each during all activities. Often, the nervous system is the mechanism through which mind-body connections occur. For example, deep breathing activates the parasympathetic nervous system, which in turn slows and calms the body and the mind. The reverse is true as well—ruminating on anxious thoughts can activate the sympathetic nervous system, which increases heart rate and respiratory rate. Mind-body interventions combine physical and mental practices to bring the nervous system back into balance and in doing this they reduce stress. They also help to reduce stress by allowing us to realize that we may have no control over some stressors themselves, but we do have some control over how we respond to these stressors.[3]

Mind-body interventions are consistent with the wellness model because they recognize the holistic nature of human beings and do not try to divide the mind from the body. They require individuals to be responsible for their own well-being and balance. They are not quick fixes; they are practices that should be done consistently on a daily basis in order to manage stress effectively.

Yoga is one mind-body practice that has been growing in popularity. When the term yoga is mentioned, many people imagine a series of poses or extreme postures. However, yoga is a broad discipline that can be practiced on all levels with benefits for everyone. The "westernized" practice of yoga that we see today originated out of an ancient spiritual practice whose path was focused on achieving enlightenment and union with all creation. Yogic practices can include poses (termed *asanas*), breathing techniques, meditation, deep relaxation, a turning inward of the senses, selfless service, and chanting. At the foundation of yoga is a set of ethical principles. The various yogic practices or tools can be used by anyone to improve stress management and wellness. Although many different styles of yoga are practiced today, all incorporate the mind-body connection and help to bring balance into one's body and mind.[3] Typically, in a yoga class, participants are led through a series of poses and breathing exercises—all of which can be modified to fit an individual's abilities.

Although all yoga classes and styles are different, there are some basic concepts that are true to many yoga styles, which make yoga an extraordinarily beneficial practice for improving overall well-being. Yoga is about the process, not the results, and therefore while practicing yoga it is important to be mindful of the present moment. Yoga is a noncompetitive practice, so an awareness of one's own abilities and limitations is important. Yogic theory also posits that we are all connected, which helps to develop a sense of compassion, empathy, and loving-kindness.

Yoga increases wellness in various ways including increasing flexibility, increasing strength, improving immune function, improving balance, increasing oxygenation of the tissues, relieving pain, improving the functioning of the nervous system, increasing circulation of blood and lymph, improving posture, lowering cortisol levels, and lowering blood pressure.[3] Because yoga helps in all these ways and more, it can help not only to improve well-being in relatively healthy individuals but also to prevent, stop, slow down, and reverse disease processes. However, it is important to remember that in order to see the benefits of yoga, one must practice regularly and have the guidance of a skilled teacher.

Mindfulness

One aspect of yoga that sets it apart from traditional exercise is mindfulness. Mindfulness is awareness and acceptance of the present moment without judgment. All practices in yoga should be done with mindfulness.[3] Mindfulness, however, is not exclusive to yoga. One can also practice mindfulness meditation by focusing awareness on present thoughts, sensations, or emotions. Being mindful of the sensation of the breath, the beauty of nature, or even simple play interactions with children are some examples. Mindfulness can be practiced throughout the day. Mindfulness is a remedy for endless distractions. We may find ourselves going through our days on "auto-pilot" with little awareness of what we are doing; we try to be efficient by multitasking, but because we cannot be mindful of many things at once, we end up making more mistakes and being less efficient, without appreciating the positive aspects of our daily lives.

The process of slowing down and being mindful of the task that we are doing can have many benefits. For example, as OTAs, being mindful of your body position/mechanics while you are working with clients will make you less prone to injury. If you are mindful of bodily sensations while you are documenting on the computer, you are more likely to change a harmful position before developing an MSD. Mindful listening to clients can help to establish a therapeutic connection and may promote observations that you may have missed if you were documenting while listening to the client. Mindfulness will keep you safer and make you a better therapist; in fact, research has shown that health care professionals who practice mindfulness have lower levels of burnout than those who do not practice mindfulness. Box 11-3 provides a mind-body exercise that may help you relax "on the spot."

Maintaining Occupational Health

Managing Workload and Personal Time

Time management techniques can be incorporated into one's lifestyle to manage potential stressors such as meeting deadlines, being on time, meeting productivity standards, and taking on complex projects. Poor organization is one of the most common causes of stress. Therefore time management techniques highlight means to organize one's responsibilities without overload.

Business models of time management previously focused on the efficient use of time. More recently, however, the time management literature has changed its focus to improving effectiveness in daily tasks rather than just increasing efficiency. Planning becomes of utmost importance because one minute of planning is estimated to save 4 minutes of work later. The mantra "work smarter, not harder" embodies the essence of time management skills.[32]

Basic approaches to time management advocate use of *planning tools* to identify and organize demands on individuals' time. Planning tools include "to-do" lists, daily planners, personal calendars, and goal-setting initiatives. The to-do list, the crux of planning, must be prioritized to direct energy toward completing the most important items first. Ideally,

Box 11-3

Mind-Body Exercise, on the Spot

Mindfulness of Breath: Take a moment to stop reading and practice this simple mindfulness exercise. Sit in your chair with a tall but relaxed spine. Allow your shoulders to relax and your hands to rest gently on your lap. Close your eyes. Remember that in the practice of mindfulness we are not trying to change anything, we are just becoming aware of the present moment without judgment. Begin to tune into your breath. Notice its rate, depth, and rhythm. Notice whether you are breathing through your nose or your mouth. Become aware of the sensation of the air passing in and out through your nose or mouth. Notice the temperature of the air. Pay attention to the air as it travels down into your lungs. Notice whether you breathe into your upper chest or into your lower chest and abdomen or both. Although sometimes your breath will automatically change because of your awareness of it, do not try to change anything—just allow your natural breath to flow. Continue to follow each inhalation and exhalation for at least another minute. When you are ready, slowly open your eyes and take a moment to notice how you feel.

important items are completed before they become urgent sources of stress.[32]

Some experts suggest organizing lists according to one's various roles as a parent, clinician, consultant, volunteer, etc. This approach helps to clarify various aspects of one's life. One should check off items on the list to feel a sense of accomplishment but resist the temptation to write routine tasks on the list such as eating lunch. Some individuals find that a master list is helpful to denote everything one needs to do including ongoing projects. Experts recommend using planning tools that allow one to view the entire week rather than just one day.[32]

Additional time management techniques include creating a specific place for all items so that time is not wasted looking for things. Files (hard copy files and file folders on the computer), plastic containers, and labeling systems facilitate locating and organizing daily items. Once activities are completed, the file can be purged. Other techniques include grouping activities together such as answering phones, e-mail, and correspondence during a particular time slot free of interruptions. Finally, experts suggest that individuals break down large projects into smaller tasks so that the projects can be started sooner and completed a little at a time.[32]

Higher-level time management techniques may require social networking and use of more expanded routines. When Cole[4] examined the time management strategies of six highly effective women who were married, worked at least 20 hours per week, and had at least two children, she found that highly established routines were crucial to these women's success. Such routines or habits were so unconscious that this group of women rarely used to-do lists; instead, most of their day flowed from one routine to the next. Successful time management for this group was related to maintaining high motivation to complete tasks, developing a social network to help complete tasks (such as carpooling with neighbors), practicing routines using cues, and grouping common tasks together.[4]

Individuals should realize that time management is not necessarily multitasking. Multitasking may work effectively when at least one task requires little concentration (such as doing dishes while talking on the phone). However, more often, multitasking results in poor execution of several tasks, showing that all would have been better served by completing one job thoroughly in a less stressful, more relaxed manner. OTA students may find that transitioning from the role of a student to the role of a worker presents a good opportunity to fine-tune one's daily organizational skills in order to minimize the daily stressors that affect overall health.

Time Management and Sensible Use of Information Technology

Information and communication technology is everywhere; individuals have access to communication and information updates around the clock. Although one would expect this access to increase our efficacy and efficiency, it sometimes creates information overload that slows our ability to stay focused on the task at hand and decreases our engagement in face-to-face social relationships. Work hours are increasingly blurred into nonwork time, which upsets the balance in one's day. To combat the feeling of being "available" 24/7, individuals may consider organizing their time to answer cell phone calls at appropriate intervals and staying alert to nonproductive behavior patterns such as constantly checking e-mails or surfing the Internet during family or social times. A smart phone, for example, can be used as a scheduling aid rather than constant distraction.

Asserting Oneself

Assertiveness skills help one to state one's needs so that stressors such as work overload, feelings of incompetence, or job task dissatisfaction may be avoided or at least minimized. Assertive individuals stand up for themselves, without hurting, attacking, or compromising the rights of others. Assertiveness skills promote open communication in work relationships and actually increase self-confidence.[6] Assertiveness serves to increase the freedom of the individual. Tillman[40] suggests that many women are socialized to please others and to comply with others' requests. They tend to take on an increasing number of tasks rather than prioritizing and delegating tasks. Assertiveness enables individuals to make choices for themselves rather than allowing others to make decisions for them.

Assertiveness skills include speaking directly, clearly, and positively. Tillman[40] suggests that learning to say "no" can have a positive impact. One may say no explicitly without any further discussion; one may say no with limits (agree to complete part of a job); a person may say no to actually performing the task but agree to delegate and take responsibility; finally, a person may say no with empathy and provide a short explanation. Assertiveness can be used for negotiating, building relationships, and working in a mutually respectful environment. The ultimate goal is to create open dialogue and promote a positive work environment for the future.

Returning to our case study from the beginning of the chapter, Jenn's lack of assertiveness has made her unhappy with her job and she is coping poorly. She has recognized that splinting full-time was not what she expected and does not yield the personal rewards for which she had hoped. She will need to express these concerns to her supervisor and possibly present solutions that may benefit her and her department.

Delegating Tasks

Delegation could be considered an adjunct to time management. Delegation is the capacity to trust another person with responsibilities (at work or at home). The process of delegating may not come easily to individuals who feel guilty not completing all the tasks themselves or uncomfortable asking others to take on more work. However, delegating can benefit all parties involved in the process. The *delegatee* learns new skills, gains experience, demonstrates accountability, and learns to work with the team. The *delegator* can use the time to complete other tasks and to develop leadership and teamwork skills in the process.[17]

Delegating may begin with asking others to perform short-term tasks that are perceived as relatively simple. As the delegator establishes more trust in the delegatee or the process of delegation, tasks may be expanded. At first, the move to delegating may seem awkward because of the following:

- Resistance to asking others to perform tasks (for fear of a negative response)
- Actual rejection from another person
- Ego needs of the delegator to complete all tasks independently
- Impatience at giving directions to others
- Super-martyr syndrome ("I have to do it all")[18]

Nonetheless, delegating can optimize time management when used effectively.

Systems-Level Strategies

Strategies for coping with work-related stressors should incorporate both organizational and individual measures to reduce stress. Managers and employees should regularly review departmental plans and individuals' performance goals to understand how individuals' personal goals may also serve the needs of the department as a whole. For example, if therapists suffer from "boredom" or need "eustress" in their jobs in order to maintain intellectual stimulation, managers may send them to continuing education courses with the long-term goal of developing departmental expertise in a niche area. This process meets the needs of both the individual and the department.

Further, managers may identify the daily operations of the department and the extent to which coworkers support each other. In Jenn's case, the manager may reexamine the allocation of staff resources within the department in order to provide equitable workloads and challenging work responsibilities for all staff. However, this process might not ever begin unless Jenn communicates her frustration to the manager. On an individual level, OT practitioners need to employ strategies to identify and address daily stressors inherent in their jobs in order to ensure long-lasting and satisfying careers.

Summary

Many options exist for OT practitioners to listen to their own advice and take care of themselves. The most simple lifestyle approaches probably yield the most benefit—that is, maintaining a healthy, balanced lifestyle and expressing oneself in a positive manner. If we can model these skills for our clients, everyone will benefit.

In Jenn's case, she has the ability to greatly improve her situation. She can assert herself respectfully and speak to her supervisor about her caseload concerns. Ideally, Jenn could present a solution to the problem such as training others to perform splinting and then gradually rotating herself to another service or splitting her time between splinting and another case focus. Jenn may request attending a continuing education course on a topic other than splinting. For her personal health, she might improve her body mechanics when she is making splints and reflect on her overall approach to managing stress. She may practice a stress management strategy (e.g., yoga, deep breathing) when she gets home (and maybe during lunch), make time for exercise (before or after work), and make sure to eat nutritious meals, get adequate sleep, and spend quality time with friends. Social support is one of the most important keys to reducing stress. So, do you have a plan to maintain balance in your life?

Selected Reading Guide Questions

1. Draw a wellness wheel for yourself. Identify your source of support in each portion of the wheel.
2. Reflect on how you experience stress (fatigue, tight muscles, etc.).
3. Identify the stressors you face at work and at home. Examine how you cope with these stressors.
4. Tell us about one thing you can do for yourself. This will get you one step closer to a balanced life.

References

1. Bassett H, Lloyd C: Occupational therapy in mental health: managing stress and burnout, *Br J Occup Ther* 64(8):408–411, 2001.
2. Bielecki J: *Back injuries in healthcare workers.* Retrieved on October 29, 2010 at: http://systoc.com/tracker/2002/Sum2002/BackInjuries.asp.
3. Carlson J: *Complementary therapies and wellness*, Upper Saddle River, NJ, 2003, Prentice-Hall.
4. Cole MB: Time mastery in business and occupational therapy, *Work* 10:119–127, 1998.
5. Cordery J, Rocchi M: Joint protection and fatigue management. In Melvin JL, Jensen GM, editors: *Rheumatologic rehabilitation series*, vol 1, Bethesda, MD, 1998, American Occupational Therapy Association.
6. Counselling Services University of Victoria: *Assertiveness-analysis and development.* Retrieved on October 29, 2010 at: http://careerplanning.about.com/.

7. Darragh AR, Huddleston W, King P: Work-related musculoskeletal injuries and disorders among occupational and physical therapists, *Am J Occup Ther* 63:351–362, 2009.
8. Duff SL: Treatment of MSD and related conditions. In Sanders MJ, editor: *Ergonomics and the management of musculoskeletal disorders*, St. Louis, 2004, Butterworth-Heinemann.
9. Edwards H, Dirette D: The relationship between professional identity and burnout among occupational therapists, *Occup Ther in Health Care* 24(2):119–129, 2010.
10. Everly J, Poff D, Lamport N, Hamant C, Alvey G: Perceived stressors and coping strategies of occupational therapy students, *Am J Occup Ther* 48:1022–1028, 1994.
11. Frye B: *Body mechanics for manual therapists*, ed 2, Stanwood, WA, 2004, Fryetag Publishing.
12. Gibson JA, Grey IM, Hastings RP: Supervisor support as a predictor of burnout and therapeutic self-efficacy in therapists working in ABA schools, *J Autism Dev Disord* 39:1024–1030, 2009.
13. Greene L: Injury prevention for massage therapists: 10-year retrospective. *Massage & Bodywork*. Retrieved on October 29, 2010 from: http://www.massageandbodywork.com/Articles/FebMar2005/injury.html.
14. Hedge A: *Ergonomic guidelines for arranging a computer workstation: 10 steps for users*. Retrieved on October 29, 2010 from: http://ergo.human.cornell.edu/ergoguide.html.
15. Hettler B: *National Wellness In stitute six dimension wellness model*. Retrieved on October 29, 2010 from: http://www.nationalwellness.org.
16. Holder NL, Clark HA, DiBlasio JM, et al: Cause, prevalence, and response to occupational musculoskeletal injuries reported by physical therapists and physical therapist assistants, *Phys Ther* 79(7):642–652, 1999.
17. Karasek R, Theorell T: *Healthy work: stress, productivity and the reconstruction of working life*, New York, 1990, Basic Books.
18. Khorb-Khalsa KL, Lutenberg EA: *Life management skills IV*, Beachwood, OH, 1996, Wellness Reproductions.
19. Kroemer E, Grandjean E: *Fitting the task to the human: a textbook of occupational ergonomics*, ed 5, Philadelphia, 1997, CRC Press.
20. LeVangie PK, Norkin CC: *Joint structure and function: a comprehensive analysis*, ed 4, Philadelphia, 2005, FA Davis.
21. Lloyd C, King R: Work-related stress and occupational therapy, *Occup Ther Int* 8(4):227–243, 2001.
22. Manheim C: *The myofascial release manual*, ed 2, Thorofare, NJ, 1994, Slack.
23. Maslach C: *Burnout: the cost of caring*, Englewood Cliffs, NJ, 1982, Prentice-Hall.
24. National Institute for Occupational Safety and Health Centers for Disease Control and Prevention: *Safe lifting and moving of nursing home residents*. DHHS (NIOSH) Publication Number 2006-117, Morgantown, PA, 2006, NIOSH.
25. Novak CB, Mackinnon SE: Repetitive use and static postures: a source of nerve compression and pain, *J Hand Surg* 10(2):151–159, 1997.
26. Occupational Safety and Health Administration: *Computer workstations*. Retrieved on October 29, 2010 at: http://www.osha.gov/SLTC/etools/computerworkstations/checklist.html.
27. Oddie S, Osley L: Assessing burnout-out and occupational stressors in a medium secure service, *Br J Forensic Pract* 9(2):32–45, 2004.
28. O'Hara V: *Wellness at work: building resilience to job stress*, Oakland, CA, 1995, New Harbinger Publications.
29. Painter J, Akroyd d, Elliot S, Adams RD: Burnout among occupational therapists, *Occupational Therapy in Health Care* 17(1): 63–78, 2003.
30. Payne RA: *Relaxation techniques: a practical handbook for the healthcare professional*, ed 3, New York, 2005, Churchill Livingstone.
31. Pedretti LW, Early MB: *Occupational therapy practice skills for physical dysfunction*, ed 5, St. Louis, 2005, Mosby.
32. Quick JC, Quick JD, Nelson DL, Hurrell JJ: *Preventive stress management in organizations*, Washington, DC, 1997, American Psychological Association.
33. Rice V: *Ergonomics in health care and rehabilitation*, Woburn, MA, 1998, Butterworth-Heinemann.
34. Rosenfield MS: *Wellness and lifestyle renewal: a manual for personal change*, Bethesda, MD, 1993, American Occupational Therapy Association, Inc.
35. Sanders MJ: *Ergonomics and the management of musculoskeletal disorders*, ed 2, St. Louis, 2004, Butterworth-Heinemann.
36. Saunders D: *For your back: the back care program*, ed 4, Chaska, MN, 1992, The Saunders Group, Inc.
37. Selye H: *The stress of life*, ed 2, New York, 1978, McGraw-Hill.
38. Stein F: Occupational stress, relaxation therapies, exercise and biofeedback, *Work* 17(3):235–245, 2001.
39. Stein F, Cutler SK: *Psychosocial occupational therapy: a holistic approach*, ed 2, San Diego, 2001, Singular Publishing Group, Inc.
40. Tillman L: *Assertiveness in the workplace, the power of saying 'No'*. Retrieved on October, 29, 2010 from: http://www.selfgrowth.com/articles/tillman6.html.
41. Visual Health Information: *Body mechanics resource library*, Tacoma, WA, 1995, Visual Health Information.

CHAPTER 12

Occupations, Purposeful Activities, and Preparatory Activities

ESTELLE B. BREINES

Key Terms

Active occupation
Egocentric realm
Exocentric realm
Consensual realm
Therapeutic exercise
Physical agent modalities
Purposeful activity
Activity analysis
Grading activity
Resistive exercises
Adjunctive modalities
Modality
Active exercise
Passive exercise
Neuromuscular control
Isometric (static) contraction
Isotonic (concentric) contraction
Eccentric contraction
Isotonic resistive exercise
Isotonic active exercise
Active-assisted exercise
Isometric exercise
Isotonic exercise
Conduction
Convection
Conversion
Ultrasound
Cryotherapy
Transcutaneous electrical nerve stimulation (TENS)
Neuromuscular electrical stimulation (NMES)
Simulated or enabling activities

Chapter Objectives

After studying this chapter, the student or practitioner will be able to do the following:

1. Identify mind/body, contextual/environmental, and social influences on active occupation.
2. Discuss the role of activity analysis in the selection of therapeutic activity.
3. Differentiate purposeful activity from other modalities used in occupational therapy.
4. Identify the relationship between physical agent modalities and active occupation in occupational therapy practice.
5. Describe how grading activity can be used to heighten functional performance.
6. Describe how and why simulated and enabling activities and adjunctive modalities are used in occupational therapy practice.
7. Identify the requirements for the use of adjunctive modalities in occupational therapy practice.
8. Perform an activity analysis appropriate for the treatment of physical dysfunction.
9. Contrast biomechanical and sensorimotor approaches to activity analysis.
10. Understand the indications, contraindications, procedures, and precautions for a variety of therapeutic protocols.

CASE STUDY

Mrs. Green

Mrs. Green is a 77-year-old retired bookkeeper, widow, and grandmother whose primary diagnosis is s/p right cerebrovascular accident with residual shoulder/hand pain of her left upper extremity (LUE). The stroke resulted in her hospitalization and subsequent admission to a subacute facility. She has a past medical history of hypertension and has exhibited reactive depression since her recent hospitalization.

Before her recent hospitalization, Mrs. Green lived in her family home in a suburban neighborhood. She was widowed 7 years ago and has been living alone in her home until her daughter moved back into the home 3 years ago for economic reasons. The two women live compatibly with one another. Her other daughter lives nearby and visits weekly. Her son and his two children live within a day's drive. His family visits several times a year.

An occupational profile of "the client's occupational history and experiences, patterns of daily living, interest, values and needs"[4] revealed the following. Since her retirement 10 years ago, Mrs. Green developed several friendships through the senior citizen group she attends in the community. Before the onset of her stroke, she pursued several interests including gardening, cooking, tennis, and traveling. She has been on the boards of several organizations, volunteering as secretary or treasurer of these groups. She also frequently communicated with her grandchildren through social networking computer sites and text messaging. She took yearly vacations, traveling to various locations in the United States for 2 to 3 weeks a year since her retirement. Mrs. Green had also been responsible for managing her personal finances and assisting her children in tax preparation. In all, Mrs. Green had an active schedule before her recent hospitalization. She is anticipating the arrival of her first great grandchild.

Initial evaluation revealed that Mrs. Green is dependent in dressing, is independent in feeding, and exhibits a mild left visual field cut. She has limited active and passive range of motion (ROM) of the left shoulder, with pain on passive flexion of the left shoulder at the end of the range, necessitating the use of a sling. Active ROM is limited in the LUE, but Mrs. Green is able to grasp, pronate her forearm, flex the elbow, and internally rotate the shoulder. Her balance and mobility are impaired. Although her prospects for recovery are positive, Mrs. Green expresses feelings of dejection about regaining her ability to resume her independence, roles, and activities.

Goals for OT intervention included the following:

- Engage in meaningful occupations to reduce depression.
- Adapt and grade activities (activities of daily living [ADL]; assisted, active, and resistive restorative activities) using unilateral, bilateral, and balance activities, to enable participation in life roles.
- Reduce pain associated with movement to enable use of LUE in occupations; use sling intermitttently to support LUE, apply heat to left shoulder, and provide analgesic 20 minutes before active occupation treatment.
- Increase ROM and strength of LUE.
- Improve balance and mobility through participation in activity.
- Prepare Mrs. Green and her resident daughter with skills needed for her to return home.
- Prepare Mrs. Green to resume active and social interactions with family through the use of electronic communication devices and games.

Intervention was initiated at bedside with sitting balance activities in preparation for dressing training. The client was instructed in scanning techniques to compensate for her visual field cut. Mrs. Green learned one-handed techniques for upper extremity dressing, gradually shifting to bilateral dressing as her strength and ROM improved.

The client was further evaluated to identify an intervention activity that she would find meaningful. She decided to pursue a woodworking task, making a step stool for her expected first great grandchild. Because she was not able to use her left arm actively at the initiation of OT services, the therapist set the project on an inclined sanding board. This permitted Mrs. Green to employ first passive, then active-assistive, and then active motion to heighten performance. Before beginning the activity, to reduce pain in her LUE and heighten her tolerance for movement, heat was applied to her shoulder using hot packs. To improve her balance and standing tolerance, the sanding board was placed on a standing table. As her performance improved, Mrs. Green was discharged to home and returned to the clinic as an outpatient three times per week. With encouragement from her family and her therapist, Mrs. Green completed the step stool and expressed great satisfaction in her achievement.

Acting on suggestions from the therapist and input from the patient and family, an intervention plan was developed. The family installed raised garden beds at home, enabling Mrs. Green to participate in an occupation at home that she particularly loved. These efforts resulted in her gradual recognition that she was able to engage in some of her favorite activities, albeit in adapted form. She was introduced to Wii by her teenaged grandson as they engaged in simulated sports activities together. As she recovered motor performance in her left arm and her balance became safer, her depression lifted. She had also been prescribed antidepressant medication. She began to use the Internet to find new recipes that she and her daughter could cook together. She resumed her check writing and returned to volunteer activities on one of the boards she belonged to. She searched the web for potential travel opportunities.

Critical Thinking Questions

1. Identify occupations Mrs. Green engaged in before her stroke, those in which she engaged during intervention, and those she assumed or resumed. Describe how her progress relied on evaluation of her occupational performance.
2. Explore the contextual and environmental factors that influenced Mrs. Green in resuming preferred activities. Describe roles she resumed as a consequence of these influences.

CASE STUDY—cont'd

3. Describe how the activities in which Mrs. Green engaged were adapted to provide an interface between activity demands and client factors.

Wilcock and Townsend stated, "All people need to be able or enabled to engage in occupations of their need and choice, to grow through what they do, to experience independence or interdependence, equality, participation security, health, and well-being."[53] We can best appreciate this foundational belief about the role of active occupation in occupational therapy by analyzing its use in practice.

Active Occupation

Active occupations, those activities in which people engage as part of their life's roles, have been acknowledged since the origins of the profession as the basic tool of occupational therapy (OT) practice. Occupations include personal care; manual tasks that involve the use of hand and mechanical tools; technological activities involving tools such as calculators, computers, electronics, and games of various sorts; and vocational skills. Occupations function together in a complex process, stimulating growth and health throughout the lifespan. When physical disability occurs and the ability to perform occupational roles and activities becomes impaired, OT helps patients regain their skills by engaging in meaningful active occupations. Active occupation is the primary therapeutic modality of OT,

Engagement in activity enhances performance beyond the given task. Learning to perform one activity skillfully leads to skillful performance in other activities. Therefore active occupations are both the objectives and the tools of practice. Activities are both the means and the end to improved performance. Whether related to personal care, work, or leisure, active occupations are an effective and necessary element of any OT program.

Individuals' needs and interests guide the selection of occupations used for therapy. The roles patients and clients play in their worlds govern these choices. To become effective members of society, everyone must acquire the skills needed to perform their particular occupational roles. Persons with disabilities may need to relearn skills or learn to perform in new ways. Therefore the occupational therapy assistant (OTA) must be prepared with a broad knowledge of activities and techniques to use as therapy in a patient-centered approach. OTAs must understand the roles and activities in which people engage to perform their life's tasks as they were experienced before the onset of disability and must comprehend the changes that must be addressed after disability.

As society changes and adapts with the invention of new objects and methods, so do people's activities. As the nature of activities changes over time, the range of OT's treatment methods and modalities has changed and broadened. When the field of OT became formalized in the early 1900s, the nature of human occupation was limited to the scope of activities that had developed up to that time. Therefore handicrafts and early industrial tasks were the models for activity at the outset of the profession. Although handicrafts are commonly described as crafts, these activities can be viewed from an anthropological perspective. These crafts represent the times in which they were developed and in which they met people's personal and social needs. However, times changed and society developed new and different occupations that required OT to incorporate activities and techniques used in the modern era. Many humans no longer manipulate clay as part of their life's work as they did ages ago; today they operate computers.[11]

Today's OT practitioners competently use a wide variety of therapeutic occupations and modalities, both traditional and modern.[2,4] Entry-level through advanced and continuing education, specialty certification, and work experience provide practitioners with the expertise to employ these tools creatively and effectively. The scope of practice is broad and addresses the continuum of treatment from acute care through advanced rehabilitation. The OT practitioner must keep pace with new developments in society and in practice.

Philosophy and Theory

OT practitioners organize treatment by integrating an understanding of the patient's mind and body (the egocentric realm) with knowledge of the tangible or concrete world (the exocentric realm) and social influences (the consensual realm). These relationships interact and change throughout life (Figure 12-1). The holistic relationship between the person and the world reflects the work of John Dewey[18] and the other American philosophers of pragmatism.[12] Dewey's use of

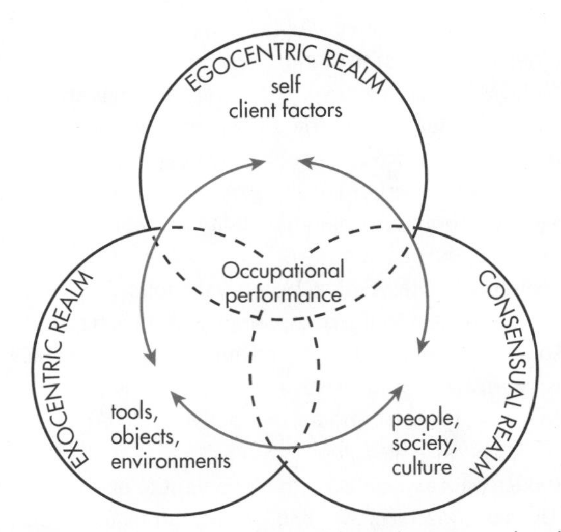

Figure 12-1 The egocentric, exocentric, and consensual realms of occupational therapy's knowledge base are related. (Modified from Breines EB: *Occupational therapy activities from clay to computers: theory & practice,* Philadelphia, 1995, FA Davis.)

the terms *purposive activity* and *active occupation*, along with his concept of learning through doing, are found in his text *Democracy and Education*,[18] which was published in 1916 in Chicago, a year before the National Society for the Promotion of Occupational Therapy was established.

Egocentric Realm

Education and training in the motor, neurologic, and perceptual-cognitive factors that affect people's performance of occupation prepare the OT practitioner to consider the egocentric realm. Human performance of occupation involves the mind and body working together.

Exocentric Realm

OT practitioners also understand the material world in which people live, act, and react. Textures, weights, direction, location, time, and other objective factors regulate performance in the world. The real world is filled with objects and environments that must be manipulated or reacted to in one manner or another. Knowing how to adapt the tangible elements of the world to enhance function is an important aspect of practice. The terms *context* and *environment* represent this realm and are used interchangeably.[4]

Consensual Realm

The occupational therapist must understand social effects on individuals and the groups in which they operate in order to enhance a patient's function in the context of his or her life. The OTA must recognize and value the sociocultural aspects of occupation and their implications for patients.

Relationships among Realms

These three major aspects of OT's knowledge base—the egocentric realm (mind and body), exocentric realm (time and space), and consensual realm (society)—are thoroughly integrated in active performance, regardless of interest, purpose, environment, or era.[11,12] OT uses one or more of these realms to influence or heighten performance in impaired persons. In Mrs. Green's case for example, a sling (exocentric) can be used to stabilize a shoulder to reduce pain (egocentric), thus enabling the patient to prepare a meal for the family (consensual). A walker can be adapted so that a patient can carry her knitting (exocentric), allowing her to prepare gifts for her grandchild (consensual), and heighten her feelings of competence (egocentric).

Development and Evolution

The interaction among these three realms is developmental. They influence one another throughout the lifespan.[10] Interactions among physical and mental performance, the tangible world, and the roles people play in their worlds are reflected in the activities in which people engage throughout their lives—and throughout the history of human occupation.

Intensive preparation in these three realms and their interaction is a foundation in the education and preparation of the OT practitioner. With this preparation, the OT practitioner can skillfully and flexibly use a range of activities and modalities to enhance patient performance and enable patients to meet life needs.

Evolving Practice

Just as society and its occupations have evolved and continue to evolve, OT practice has evolved. New media and modalities enable patients to become skilled in functional performance. In addition to therapeutic exercise and activity and the facilitation and inhibition techniques associated with the sensory-motor approaches to treatment, therapists have added adjunctive therapies to their repertoires, all designed to enhance patients' performance in purposeful occupation.

Although administration of adjunctive therapies such as physical agent modalities (PAM) is not considered an entry-level skill,[2] some occupational therapists and OTAs have become increasingly skilled in the application of these therapies. These modalities traditionally belonged to the field of physical therapy but have established their role in the realm of OT practice. Trained personnel use them to enhance the individual's ability to perform purposeful occupation, the primary objective of OT.

> ***Black Box Warning***
> Physical agent modalities should be employed only in preparation for purposeful active occupation (and not as a substitute).

Purposeful Activity and Active Occupation

Dr. William Rush Dunton, Jr., a founder of the OT profession, stated one of the first principles of OT: Occupation must aim toward some useful end for it to effectively treat mental and physical disability.[48] This principle implies that occupation has a purpose and that purposeful activity has an inherent goal beyond the motor function required to perform the task.[8] An individual engaged in purposeful activity focuses attention on the goal rather than the processes required to reach the goal.[3]

Conversely, nonpurposeful activity has no inherent goal other than the motor function used to perform the activity.[48] A person performing a nonpurposeful activity is likely to focus on the process or movements rather than on a functional or meaningful goal. Therapeutic exercise and enabling activities such as moving cones and stacking blocks cannot be considered purposeful activity when they have no purpose for the patient. Nonetheless, such media occasionally have a place in the treatment continuum. However, treatment planning primarily must consider activities and skills related to the inherent occupational objectives of the patient because these activities are more readily tied to purpose, meaning, and therapeutic value. They constitute the occupational nature of therapy.

Purposeful activity—OT's primary treatment modality—is the cornerstone of the profession.[3,48,50] In a position paper on purposeful activity, the American Occupational Therapy Association (AOTA) defined the term as "goal-directed behaviors or tasks that comprise occupations. An activity is purposeful if the individual is an active, voluntary participant and if the activity is directed toward a goal that the individual considers meaningful."[3] The uniqueness of OT lies in its emphasis on the extensive use of purposeful or meaningful activity. This emphasis gives OT the theoretical foundation for its broad application to psychosocial, physical, and developmental dysfunction, as well as to health maintenance.[3]

Purposeful activity has both inherent and therapeutic goals. For example, sawing wood (Figure 12-2) may have the inherent goal of securing parts for construction of a step stool, in Mrs. Green's case, whereas the therapeutic objectives may be to strengthen the muscles of the shoulder and elbow. The patient's conscious effort is focused on the project's outcome (inherent goal) and not on the movement itself.[8] The patient directs and controls the movement, yet that control is ordinarily outside of the patient's conscious awareness. Performance outside of conscious control distinguishes OT's therapeutic effectiveness. Consciously controlled performance is not effective in producing enhanced levels of skill. To enhance skill building, performance must become automatic.[12] Automatic performance serves as a foundation for more advanced performance; without automatic performance of foundation skills, more advanced performance is almost impossible. For example, Huss[23] suggested that the child who must pay attention to sitting is unable to focus on the task performance that automatic sitting would ordinarily enable. Consequently, the child cannot engage in active occupations essential to growth and the development of social roles.

The importance of purposeful activity is readily observed in goal-directed performance by a person with a physical disability. As the person becomes absorbed in any given activity, affected parts are used more naturally and with less fatigue.[47] Concentrating on motion has a negative effect on that motion; muscles controlled by conscious attention and focused effort fatigue rapidly. Focusing attention on an activity of interest to the patient is of greater therapeutic value than concentrating on the muscles or motions being used to accomplish the activity.[8]

A number of studies have shown the value of purposeful activity.[38] Steinbeck[48] demonstrated that patients performing purposeful activity perform for a longer period than when they are performing nonpurposeful activity. Thibodeaux and Ludwig's[50] study of motivation for product-oriented versus non-product-oriented activity points to the importance of the patient's level of interest in the process and the product. Rocker and Nelson[44] found that not being allowed to keep a project the person has made can elicit hostile feelings in normal subjects. This study demonstrates the importance of tangible productivity for sustaining people's interest. Yoder, Nelson, and Smith[55] studied the effects of added-purpose versus rote exercise in women who lived in a nursing home. The added-purpose exercise resulted in significantly more movement repetitions than did rote exercise.[55] Each of these studies suggest that goal-directed, purposeful activity increases one's motivation for participating in sustained activity.

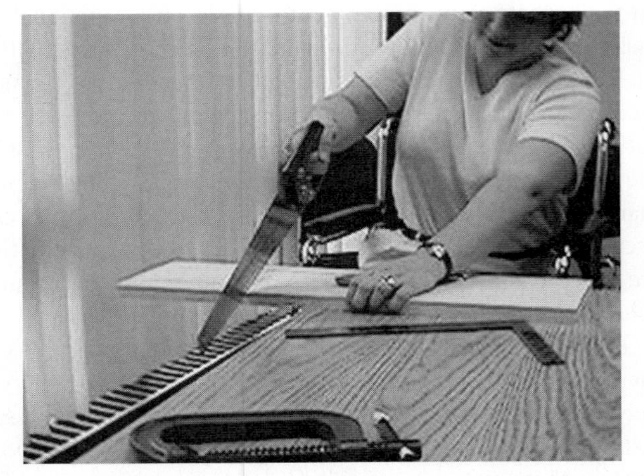

Figure 12-2 Sawing wood to strengthen shoulder and elbow musculature.

When a treatment plan is being developed, the goals of the activity, the patient's level of interest in the activity, and the meaning of the activity and its product are important considerations. Purposeful activities are used or adapted for use to meet one or more of the following therapeutic objectives:

1. To develop or maintain strength, endurance, work tolerance, range of motion (ROM), and coordination
2. To practice and use voluntary and automatic movements in goal-directed tasks
3. To provide for purposeful use of and general exercise to affected parts
4. To explore vocational potential or training in work skills
5. To improve sensation, perception, and cognition
6. To improve socialization skills and enhance emotional growth and development
7. To increase independence in occupational role performance

Unless they relate to function, these objectives alone might not be considered purposeful. Arts, crafts, games, sports, leisure, self-care, home management, purposive mobility, and work-related activities are considered purposeful activities.

Occupation and Health

OT was founded on the concept that human beings have an occupational nature—that is, humans naturally engage in activity. Moreover, occupation contributes to the organism's health and well-being.[4,8,11,16,24] Activity is valuable to maintaining health in the healthy person and to restoring health after illness and disability. When the patient engages in relevant, meaningful, and purposeful activity, change is possible and dysfunction is reversible.[16] The OT practitioner acts as facilitator of the change process.[15] Therefore the effects of physical dysfunction on performance can be ameliorated when the patient participates in goal-directed (purposeful) therapeutic activity.[8]

The value of purposeful activity lies in the patient's simultaneous mental and physical involvement. Activity provides the exercise needed to help develop the use of affected parts and also provides an opportunity to meet emotional, social, and personal gratification needs.[8,47] Cynkin and Robinson[16] pointed out that for the attainment of optimal function and health, the human being must be consciously involved in problem-solving and creative activity—processes that are linked with the use of the hands.[16] Virtually all occupational performance involves the hands or requires the substitution of methods that simulate the use of hands. One adaptation to an activity ordinarily performed with hands is a computer-driven environmental control unit operated by a puff-and-sip mechanism.

Most activities that form the pattern of a person's life are performed routinely and automatically. They are taken for granted until some dysfunction disrupts their performance. The OTA is responsible for adapting activity so that patients can resume performance of life's tasks. Cynkin and Robinson[16] make the following assumptions about activities:

1. A wide variety of activities are important to the individual. Activities fulfill many of a person's needs and wants, and they are essential to physical and psychosocial growth and development and the attainment of mastery and competence.
2. Activities are regulated by the values and beliefs of the culture.
3. Activity-related behavior can change from dysfunctional toward more functional. Persons can change and desire change.
4. Changes in activity-related behavior take place through motor, cognitive, and social learning.[16]

Assessment of Occupational Role Performance

OT assessment establishes the patient's occupational goals and needs. Therapy must be individualized for each patient with evaluative tools such as the interest checklist, activity configuration, occupational history, interview, and activity analysis.[41] A top-down, client-centered approach is recommended. Identifying appropriate and meaningful therapeutic activities should begin with outlining and analyzing the patient's occupational history and interests.[50] The Canadian Occupational Performance Measure[29] and the Activity Configuration[15] are two relevant assessments. See Chapter 4 for more information about assessing occupational performance.

Cost concern may prevent the occupational therapist or OTA from spending time with a patient for the sole purposes of a lengthy interview. However, much can be learned gradually during regular treatment sessions; gathering the information all at once or through a formal interview is not necessary.

Activity Analysis

Activity analysis is the foundational skill for practice. Careful activity analysis is essential to the selection of appropriate treatment activities. Activities should be analyzed from three perspectives: the mental and physical contributions or limitations of the person engaged in the activity, the effects of the physical environment, and the implications of the social environment. These three elements influence one another and form the context for treatment. The importance of context in treatment is widely recognized throughout the profession.[4] Regardless of diagnosis or therapeutic approach, activity analysis should include the contextual aspects of performance. The tangible environment and the social environment guide and dictate occupational performance to the same extent that physical and mental capacities do; therefore they must be considered in developing a treatment plan.

A number of theorists[11,30,51] have developed comprehensive guides to activity analysis that are useful resources. A guide to activity analysis specifically relevant to practice in physical dysfunction follows at the end of the chapter.

Principles of Activity Analysis

A comprehensive activity analysis includes all aspects of performance potentially elicited by specific activities and reveals their potential for therapeutic application. Activities selected for therapy should be (1) goal directed; (2) meaningful to the patient; (3) matched to individual needs in relation to social roles; (4) capable of eliciting the mental or physical participation of the patient; (5) designed to prevent or reverse dysfunction and develop skills to enhance performance in life roles; (6) related to the patient's interests; (7) adaptable, gradable, and age appropriate; (8) selected through knowledge and professional judgment; and (9) selected in cooperation with the patient.[2,4] The educational preparation of the OTA qualifies him or her to consider all of these aspects in preparing a treatment plan.

Adapting and Grading Activity

Adapting Activity

An activity's usefulness in therapy often relies on its adaptation to the special needs of the patient or the environment. An activity may need to be performed in a special way to accommodate the patient's residual abilities (e.g., eating with a special splint with a utensil holder fitted to the hand) (Figure 12-3). An activity may also need to be adapted to the positioning of the person or to the environment—for instance, by setting up a special reading stand and providing prism glasses for a person to read while supine in bed. The problem-solving ability, creativity, and ingenuity of occupational therapists and OTAs in making adaptations are some of their unique skills.

For adaptations to be effective, the patient must be able to use them in a comfortable position. The patient must understand the need and purpose of the activity, as well as the

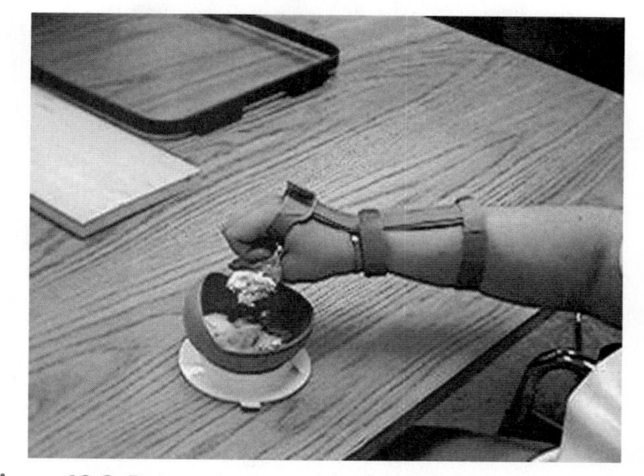

Figure 12-3 Eating using a special splint with a utensil holder fitted to the hand.

adaptations, and be willing to perform the activity with the simple modifications. Peculiar and complicated adaptations that require frequent adjustment and modification should be avoided[41,47] because patients will reject them. If the OT practitioner selects an activity that interests the patient, the patient will be likely to experience enough satisfaction to continue performing the activity.

Grading of Activity

Grading an activity means pacing it appropriately and modifying it to obtain the patient's maximal performance. If movement patterns or degree of resistance cannot be attained when the activity is performed in the usual manner, simple modifications may be made. The patient usually accepts changes if they are not complex and do not require strained and unnatural motions. The novice is cautioned that the value of the activity may be diminished if it is designed to be performed with artificial movements or excessive resistance. Such methods discourage participation and interfere with coordination.[26,47] They also require the patient to focus on movements rather than on the goal of the activity, which reduces satisfaction and defeats the primary purpose of purposeful activity, as described earlier. The skilled practitioner adapts and grades activities so that they are easily accepted by the patient and provide the "just right" demand for performance.

Activities may be graded in many ways to suit the patient's needs and the treatment objectives. Activities can be graded for increasing strength, ROM, endurance and tolerance, coordination, and perceptual, cognitive, and social skills.

Strength

Strength may be graded by increasing resistance. Methods include changing the plane of movement from gravity eliminated to against gravity, adding weights to the equipment or to the patient, using tools of increasing weights, grading the texture of the materials from soft to hard or fine to rough, or changing to another more or less resistive activity.

For example, a weight attached to the wrist by a strap increases resistance to arm movements during needlework or leatherwork (Figure 12-4). A pulley-and-weight system can be attached to an inclined plane sanding board to increase resistance to the biceps when the sanding block is pulled downward, as the patient sands a cutting board for use in one-handed cutting. Springs may be used to increase resistance on a block printing press. When grasp strength is inadequate, grasp mitts can be used to fasten the hand to a tool or equipment handle to assist grip and allow arm motion.

Range of Motion

Activities for increasing or maintaining joint ROM can be graded by positioning materials and equipment to demand greater reach or excursion of joints or by adapting equipment with lengthened handles to facilitate active stretching.

An example of a simple adaptation is placing a weaving project in a vertical position to achieve the desired range of shoulder flexion while working. As the work progresses, the activity itself establishes increased demands on active range. Positioning objects such as tiles used in a mosaic tile project at increasing or decreasing distances from the patient changes the range needed to reach the materials (Figure 12-5). Tool handles such as those used in woodworking can be enlarged with a larger dowel or by padding the handle with foam rubber to accommodate limited ROM or to facilitate grasp (Figure 12-6). Reducing the amount of padding as the range increases grades the tool to the person's increasing ability.

Endurance and Tolerance

Endurance can be graded by moving from light to heavy work and increasing the duration of the work. For example, an initial household task of folding paper napkins can be graded to sorting heavier and heavier objects such as the task of sitting to sort kitchen utensils and then grading to a standing position to organize tools on a pegboard. Standing and walking tolerance can be graded by increasing the time spent standing

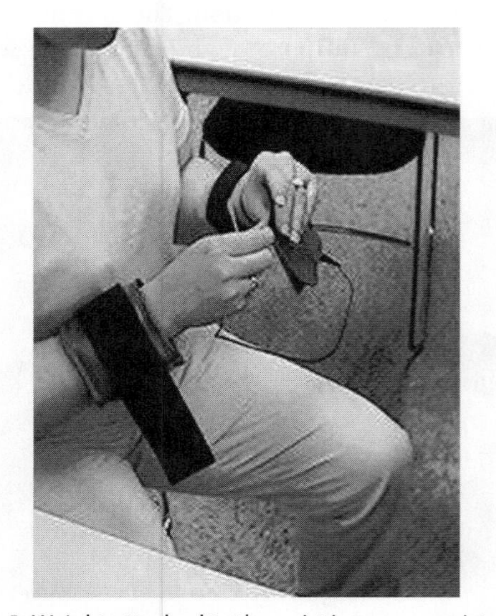

Figure 12-4 Weight attached to the wrist increases resistance during needlework or leatherwork.

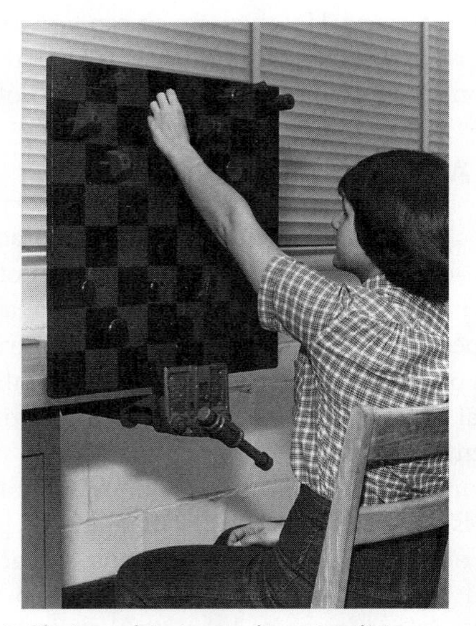

Figure 12-5 Placing objects at alternate distances changes the range needed to reach materials.

to work—perhaps initially at a stand-up table (Figure 12-7)—and increasing the time and distance spent in activities requiring walking—perhaps including home management and workshop activities.

Progressively degenerative conditions such as muscular dystrophy, multiple sclerosis, or Parkinson's disease may require grading endurance in a negative direction to accommodate a diminishing physical condition. In such cases it may be advisable to change the activity to one that requires less effort rather than reducing the demand of an existing project. The latter can have a negative psychologic effect if the patient readily recognizes his or her reduced capability.

Coordination

Coordination and muscle control can be graded by decreasing the gross resistive movements and increasing the fine-controlled movements required. An example is progressing from sawing wood with a crosscut saw to using a coping saw to using a jeweler's saw. Dexterity and speed of movement can be graded by practice at increasing speeds once movement patterns have been mastered through coordination training and neuromuscular education.

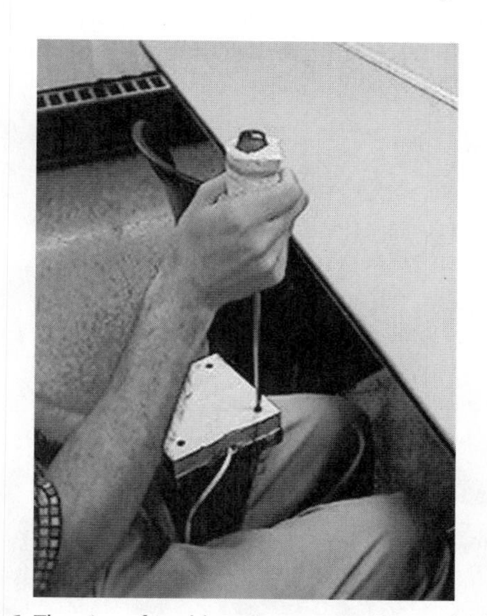

Figure 12-6 The size of tool handles may be increased by padding the handle with foam rubber.

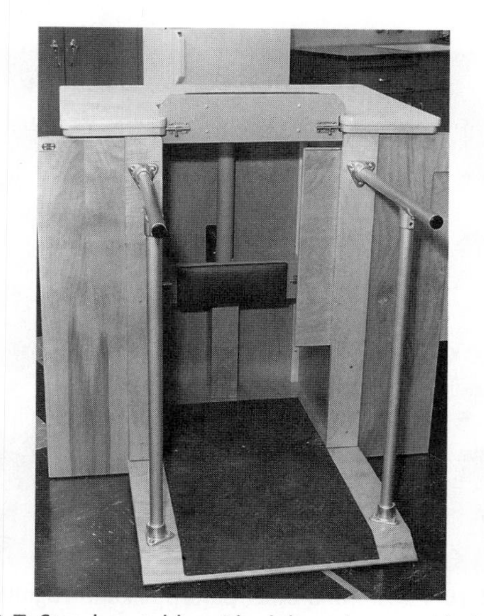

Figure 12-7 Stand-up table with sliding door, padded knee supports, and backrest.

Perceptual, Cognitive, and Social Skills

In grading cognitive skills, the occupational therapist begins with simple one- or two-step activities that require little judgment, decision making, or problem solving and progresses to several-step activities that require some judgment or problem solving. A patient in a lunch preparation group may butter bread that has already been lined up on the work surface. This task could be graded to lining up the bread, then buttering it and placing a slice of lunch meat on it, and ultimately to making sandwiches.

For grading social interaction, the same treatment can begin with an activity that demands interaction only with the occupational therapist or OTA. The patient can progress to activities requiring interaction with another patient and ultimately progress to small group activities. Grading can facilitate the patient's progression from the role of observer to that of participant and then to leader. At the same time, the occupational therapist or OTA decreases his or her supervision, guidance, and assistance to facilitate more independent functioning.

Selection of Activity

Activities for treatment of physical dysfunction are usually selected for their potential to improve functioning in sensory, movement-related, and mental factors to help sustain motivation to engage in activity. Activities selected to improve physical performance should provide desired exercise or purposeful use of affected parts. They should enable the patient to transfer the motion, strength, and coordination gained in adjunctive and enabling modalities to useful, normal daily activities. If activities are to be used for physical restoration, they should have the following characteristics:

1. Activities should provide action rather than merely the position of involved joints and muscles—that is, they should allow alternate contraction and relaxation of the muscles being exercised and allow joints to move through their available ROM.
2. Activities should provide repetition of motion—that is, activities should allow for an indefinite but controllable number of repetitions of movement patterns sufficient to benefit the patient.
3. Activities should allow for one or more kinds of grading such as for resistance, range, coordination, endurance, or complexity.[21,47]

Active and resistive exercises are most often used for purposeful activity.[47] Requirements for passive and active assisted exercise are harder (although not impossible) to apply to purposeful activities. Two examples are bilateral sanding and bilateral sponge wiping. Other important considerations in the selection of activity include the following: the objects and environment required to perform the activity; safety factors;

preparation and completion time; complexity; type of instruction and supervision required; structure and controls in the activity; learning requirements; independence, decision making, and problem solving required; social interaction potential and communication skills required; and potential gratification to the person.

If an activity of interest to the patient is selected, he or she is more likely to experience sufficient satisfaction to sustain performance at the task. It is important to guide the individual to suitable therapeutic activities at just the right level of challenge so that he or she will achieve satisfaction by engaging in the activity.

Simulated or Enabling Activity

When the clinical environment is not fully equipped to meet the exact occupational needs of a patient, simulating appropriate active occupation by adapting the environment or activity to meet the patient's needs may be necessary. OT has developed a variety of methods to simulate active occupation. A number of these activities were devised initially from equipment and found materials used in other activities. For example, common items found in every OT clinic in its earliest days were empty cones that had held the thread used to warp looms. Because of the ready supply, these cones were adapted for many uses in the clinic. Occupational therapists asked patients to move a series of cones from one side of a tabletop to the other or to stack them to increase ROM in the shoulder along with grasp (Figure 12-8). Cones can also be used to train gross coordination and a combined (out of synergy) movement pattern in the Brunnstrom approach, as discussed in Chapter 21.

Another activity is the simulated inclined sanding board (Figure 12-9). The sanding board was designed to incline wood while the wood was being sanded. Therapists began using the board, without the wood, to exercise muscles of the elbow and shoulder. Without the wood there is no end product and thus no inherent purposefulness. However, incorporating wood for a project can turn this activity from a simulated to a meaningful one, such as the project Mrs. Green chose.

Puzzles and other perceptual and cognitive training media are used to develop visual perceptual functions, motor planning skills, memory, sequencing, and problem solving, among other skills (Figure 12-10). Clothing fastener boards and household hardware boards may provide practice in the manipulation of everyday objects before the patient is confronted with the real task (Figure 12-11). At a higher level of technological sophistication, commercial work simulators (see Chapter 17) and computer programs are used to train patients in physical and cognitive skills.

Although many of these items are readily available in clinics, the nature and purpose of OT are best met when the patient can engage in a purposeful activity that is meaningful to him or her. One must consider the needs and interests of the patient in selecting activities rather than rely on available objects that meet only physical needs.

Enabling activities are considered nonpurposeful and generally do not have an inherent goal, but they may engage the

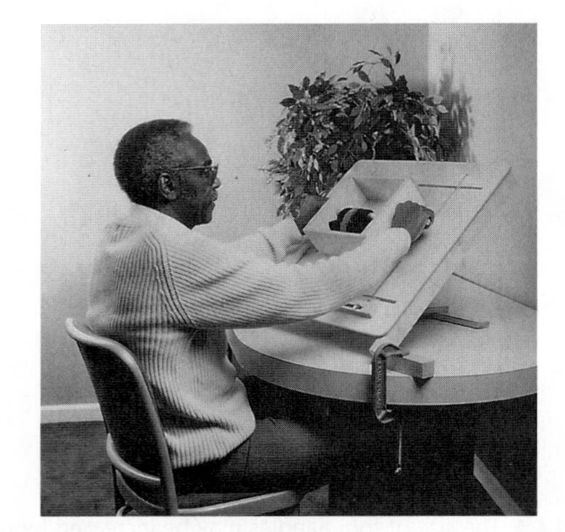

Figure 12-9 Inclined sanding board used to sand wood. (From S & S Worldwide, adaptAbility, 1995.)

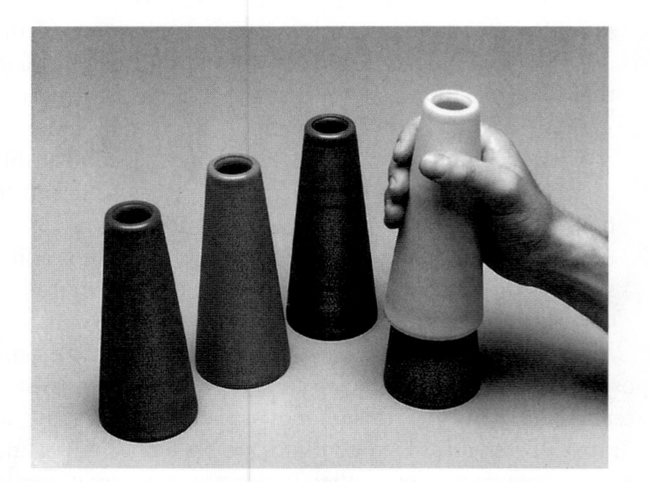

Figure 12-8 Stacking cones are used to train coordination or specific movement patterns such as reaching and grasping. (Courtesy North Coast Medical, Morgan Hill, Calif.)

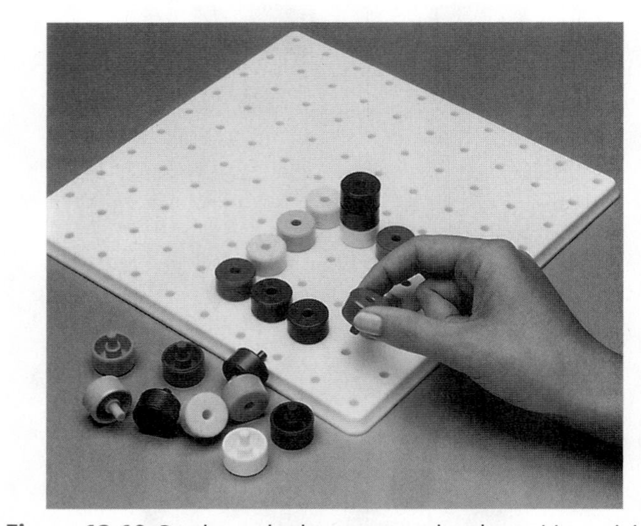

Figure 12-10 Puzzles and other perceptual and cognitive training media are used on the tabletop. (Courtesy North Coast Medical, Morgan Hill, Calif.)

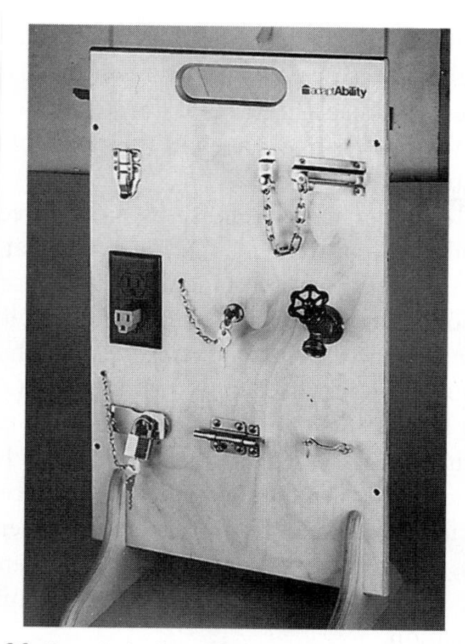

Figure 12-11 Boards built with household fasteners are simulations used for practicing manipulation and management of common household hardware. (Reprinted with permission, S & S Worldwide, adaptAbility, 1995.)

patient mentally and physically. The purposes of enabling activities are to practice specific motor patterns, to train in perceptual and cognitive skills, and to practice motor and process skills necessary for function in the home and community. Indeed, many enabling modalities used in OT practice facilitate perceptual, cognitive, and motor learning. Such activities may be appropriate for skill acquisition, when the patient is getting the idea of the movement and practicing problem solving. Practice should be daily or frequent, and feedback should be given often so that errors are reduced and skills refined to prepare for performance of real-life purposeful activity. These activities should be used judiciously, and their place in the sequence of treatment and motor learning should be well planned. They can be used along with adjunctive modalities and purposeful activities as part of a comprehensive treatment program.

Adjunctive Modalities

Adjunctive modalities can be used as a preliminary step toward purposeful activity preparing the patient for occupational performance. Examples are therapeutic exercise, orthotics, sensory stimulation, and physical agent modalities.[39] Therapeutic exercise and physical agent modalities are described in the following discussion. Many of the principles of therapeutic exercise are readily and customarily incorporated into therapeutic activity and consequently are inherent aspects of OT practice.

The term modality was defined in the AOTA policy statement according to Webster's New World Dictionary [as] "the employment of, or method of employment of, a therapeutic agent."[1] In the context of this chapter, modality includes both media and methods, as defined by Reed.[42] A medium is "the means by which a therapeutic effect is transmitted." [42] For example, a vestibular ball is a medium. Methods are "the steps, sequence or approach used to activate the therapeutic effect of a medium," such as the handling and movements used with the vestibular ball to effect the desired motor responses (Box 12-1).[42]

Modalities chosen for professional practice are influenced by eight factors, according to Reed.[42] These are cultural practices, social acceptance or nonacceptance, economics of health care, available technology, influences of a given theoretical model, historical influences, and research. Chapter 1 reviews the evolution of treatment modalities in physical disabilities practice.

In addition to arts, crafts, and other purposeful activities, therapists and assistants have become increasingly skillful in applications of therapeutic exercise, physical agent modalities, and the facilitation and inhibition techniques associated with the sensorimotor approaches to treatment. Many OT practitioners use these modalities because they promote the development of the individual's abilities to engage in occupational performance—a primary aim of OT. Principles of therapeutic exercise and sensorimotor approaches are also applied to purposeful activities, with adaptations and gradations matched to desired treatment goals.

Today, occupational therapists are qualified in a variety of therapeutic modalities. Their competence is gained through entry-level and graduate education, specialty certification, continuing education, and work experience. OTAs may be exposed to a variety of modalities through their education and clinical fieldwork. Depending on the area in which they practice and the availability of health care services and specialized health care practitioners, OTAs may need to achieve service competency in a number of different modalities.

Box 12-1

Occupational Therapy Modalities

Modality: The employment of—-or method of employment of—a therapeutic agent.[1]

The traditional modalities of OT were its crafts. The term has grown to be understood more broadly and defines active occupation as the primary therapeutic modality of occupational therapy. The term *modality* also includes both media and methods.[42] Media are the means by which therapeutic effects are transmitted. For example, media can include a variety of objects such as an article of clothing, a vestibular ball, or an adapted tool. Methods are the steps, sequence, or approaches used to activate the therapeutic effect of a medium such as the movements required in the creation of a macramé plant hanger to heighten shoulder flexion or reduce edema or those used with the vestibular ball to effect the desired motor responses. The modalities, media, and methods of OT are variable and require considerable expertise to select, modify, adapt, and apply to elicit therapeutic effects.

Black Box Warning

Modalities must be used by practitioners skilled in their use. The OTA should not employ any modality until service competency is established.

Therapeutic Approaches

A variety of therapeutic approaches are available to OTAs. Although these approaches differ in their emphasis, all are consistent with an occupational approach to treatment. Aspects of activity analysis relevant to various therapeutic approaches are listed in the following discussion.

Biomechanical Approach

The biomechanical approach to treatment is likely to be used in the treatment of lower motor neuron and orthopedic dysfunctions. Improvements in strength, ROM, and muscle endurance are the goals of OT for such dysfunctions. Thus the emphasis of activity analysis is on muscles, joints, and motor patterns required for the activity. Steps of the activity must be identified and broken down into the motions required to perform each step. ROM, degree of muscle strength, and type of muscle contraction to perform each step should be identified. The activity analysis format at the end of this chapter is based on the biomechanical approach.

Sensorimotor Approach

Sensorimotor approaches to treatment are likely to be used for upper motor neuron disorders such as cerebral palsy, stroke, and head injury. Activity analysis for these dysfunctions should focus on the sensory perception of the patient and the movement patterns required in the particular treatment approach. The therapist must also consider the effect of the activity on balance, posture, muscle tone, and the facilitation or inhibition of abnormal reflexes and movements. For example, with the proprioceptive neuromuscular facilitation (PNF) approach, one should incorporate PNF patterns in the activity or select activities that use these patterns naturally. For the neurodevelopmental (Bobath) approach, postures and movements that inhibit abnormal reflexes, reactions, and tone are important. Sensorimotor approaches and their applications to activity are discussed in Chapter 21.

Analysis of the perceptual and cognitive requirements of the activity is particularly important for patients with upper motor neuron disorders because these functions are often disturbed. It is important for the therapy practitioner to select activities that not only meet the requirements for motor performance but also can be performed with some success.

Therapeutic Exercise and Activity

Since its beginnings, OT has recognized that the mind and body are completely united in performance. Both the psychological and physical effects of purposeful activity were recognized in the treatment of individuals with mental conditions, as well as in the treatment of persons with physical dysfunction.[9,12,19,24] However, as treatment methods evolved, OT practitioners began to use therapeutic exercise alone to prepare patients for purposeful activity and to expedite treatment in a health care system constrained by budget and time. The treatment of patients in acute stages of illness and disability imposed new demands and role responsibilities on practice. Short treatment sessions in acute care settings, more extensive physical incapacities elicited by medical advances, and shortened length of stay in hospital and rehabilitation facilities caused the profession to expand the range of modalities used in treatment.

The use of therapeutic exercise as an isolated modality raised considerable controversy.[20] Some feared that if OT used exercise or other preparatory modalities, purpose would be forgotten. Some mistakenly saw exercise and activity as mutually exclusive; however, principles of exercise had been applied to purposeful activity from early in the history of OT. Exercise and activity are complementary in the treatment continuum, and both can be used in a single treatment plan. However, if only pure exercise is used, the patient has not received OT.[20] When used in OT, therapeutic exercise should be employed to remediate sensory and motor dysfunction, augment purposeful activity, and prepare the patient for performing a functional occupation.

A comprehensive understanding of the principles of exercise is basic to therapeutic activity. Therapeutic exercise is defined as any body movement or muscle contraction to prevent or correct a physical impairment, improve musculoskeletal function, and maintain a state of well-being.[14,27] A wide variety of exercise options is available; each should be tailored to meet the goals of treatment and the specific capacities and precautions relative to the patient's physical condition.

Exercise can be used to increase ROM and flexibility, strength, coordination, endurance, and cardiovascular fitness.[27] Specific exercise protocols may be used to achieve specific goals. However, exercise without activity is apt to elicit deliberate rather than automatic performance, therefore violating essential principles of OT discussed earlier. Although judicious application of therapeutic exercise may have a limited place in the therapeutic program, the practitioner should structure treatment so that the patient is primarily engaged in activity or occupation so that automatic performance is generated.

Purposes

The general purposes of therapeutic exercise, as with therapeutic activity, are the following:

1. To develop awareness of normal movement patterns and improve voluntary, automatic movement responses
2. To develop strength and endurance in patterns of movement that are acceptable and necessary and do not produce deformity
3. To improve coordination, regardless of strength
4. To increase the power of specific isolated muscles or muscle groups
5. To aid in overcoming ROM deficits
6. To increase the strength of muscles that will power hand splints, mobile arm supports, and other devices
7. To increase work tolerance and physical endurance through increased strength
8. To prevent or eliminate contractures from developing because of imbalanced muscle power by strengthening the antagonistic muscles[41]

Indications for Use

Therapeutic exercise is most effective for orthopedic disorders (such as contractures and arthritis) and lower motor neuron disorders that produce weakness and flaccidity. Examples of the latter are peripheral nerve injuries and diseases such as poliomyelitis, Guillain-Barré syndrome and infectious neuronitis, and spinal cord injuries and diseases.

The candidate for therapeutic exercise must be medically able to participate in the exercise regimen, able to understand the directions and purposes, and interested and motivated to perform. The patient must have available motor pathways and the potential for recovery or improvement of strength, ROM, coordination, or movement patterns. Sensation must be at least partially intact so that the patient can perceive motion and the position of the exercised part and sense superficial and deep pain. Muscles and tendons must be intact, stable, and free to move. Joints must be able to move through an effective ROM for exercises that use joint motion. The patient should be relatively free of pain during motion and should be capable of isolated, coordinated movement. If the patient has any dyskinetic movement, he or she must be able to control it so that the procedure can be performed as prescribed.[40] Exercise selection must consider muscle grade, muscle endurance, joint mobility, diagnosis and physical condition, treatment goals, position of the patient, and desirable plane of movement. Each of these requirements also applies to exercise-focused therapeutic activity and should underlie its selection as a therapeutic tool.

Contraindications

Therapeutic exercise and exercise-focused therapeutic activity are contraindicated for patients who have poor general health or inflamed joints or who have had recent surgery.[40] These therapies may not be useful for patients whose joint ROM is severely limited because of well-established permanent contractures. As defined and described here, they cannot be used effectively for those who have spasticity and lack voluntary control of isolated motion or those who cannot control dyskinetic movement. The latter conditions are likely to occur in upper motor neuron disorders, which are better addressed by the sensorimotor approaches to treatment (see Chapter 21).

> ***Black Box Warning***
>
> Consider the overall health of the patient. Do not use therapeutic exercise or exercise-focused activity where contraindicated by the patient's conditions (see earlier discussion.)

Exercise Programs

Muscle Strengthening

Active-assisted, active, and resistive isotonic and isometric exercises are used to increase strength. After partial or complete denervation of muscle and during inactivity or disuse, muscle strength decreases. When strength is inadequate, substitution patterns, or "trick" movements, are likely to develop.[54] A substitution is the attempt to function with muscle groups and patterns of motion not ordinarily used. Substitution is used in the event of loss or weakness of muscles normally used to perform the movements, or restrictions in ROM because of structural dysfunction. An example is using shoulder abduction to achieve a hand-to-mouth movement if elbow flexors cannot perform against gravity (Figure 12-12). When muscle loss is permanent, some substitution patterns may be desirable to compensate in functional activities such as the use of tenodesis to permit grasp that will enable self-feeding. However, many substitutions are undesirable, and therapeutic exercise often aims to prevent or correct substitution patterns.[54]

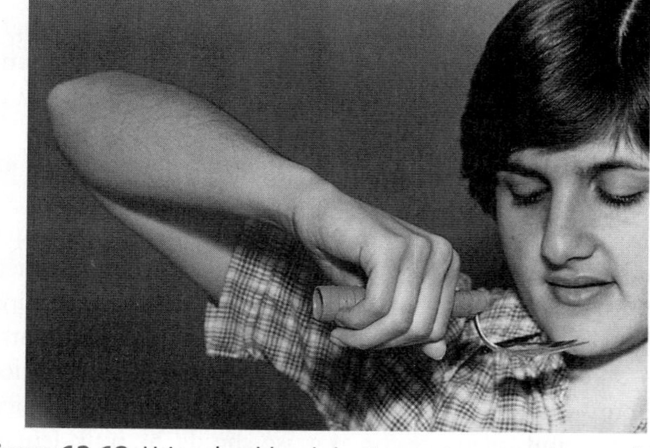

Figure 12-12 Using shoulder abduction as compensation to achieve hand-to-mouth movement.

A muscle must contract at or near its maximal capacity and for enough repetitions and time to increase strength. Strengthening programs are generally based on contracting the muscle against a large resistance for a few repetitions. Strengthening exercises are not effective if the contraction is insufficient.[14,28] Excess strengthening, however, may result in muscle fatigue, pain, and temporary reduction of strength. If a muscle is overworked, it becomes fatigued and is unable to contract. The type of exercise must suit the muscle grade and the patient's fatigue tolerance level. Fatigue level varies from individual to individual, and the threshold for muscle fatigue decreases in pathological states.[28] Many patients may not be sensitive to fatigue or may push themselves beyond tolerance in the belief that this approach hastens recovery. Therefore the patient's muscle power and capacity for performance must be carefully assessed, and the patient must be closely observed for signs of fatigue such as slowed performance, distraction, perspiration, increase in rate of respiration, performance of exercise pattern through a decreased ROM, and inability to complete the prescribed number of repetitions.

Increasing Muscle Endurance

Endurance is the muscle's ability to work for prolonged periods and resist fatigue. Although a high-load, low-repetition regimen is effective for muscle strengthening, a low-load and high-repetition exercise program is more effective for building endurance.[14,17] Having determined the patient's maximum capacity for a strengthening program, the therapist can reduce the resistance load and increase the number of repetitions to build endurance in specific muscles or muscle groups. Strength and endurance training are on a continuum. Resistance and the number of repetitions can be varied from day to day to promote gains in both strength and endurance.[14]

Physical Conditioning and Cardiovascular Fitness

Improving general physical endurance and cardiovascular fitness requires the use of large muscle groups in sustained, rhythmic aerobic exercise or activity. Examples are swimming, walking, bicycling, jogging, and some games and sports. This type of activity is often used in cardiac rehabilitation programs, in which the parameters of the patient's physical capacities and tolerance for exercise should be well defined and medically supervised. For improved cardiovascular fitness, exercise should be done 3 to 5 days per week at 60% to 90% of maximum heart rate or 50% to 85% of maximum oxygen uptake. Fifteen to 60 minutes of exercise or rhythmic activities using large muscle groups are desirable.[14] Meaningful and satisfying active occupations such as gardening can be incorporated into the fitness program.

Range of Motion and Joint Flexibility

Active and passive ROM exercises are used to maintain joint motion and flexibility. Active exercise is performed by the patient without assistance. Passive exercise is provided by an outside force such as the therapist or a device such as the continuous passive motion machine, which can be preset to provide continuous passive motion throughout the joint range.

> ***Black Box Warning***
> Use of any mechanical device requires caution and careful monitoring to prevent mishaps.[14]

Stretching or forced exercise may be necessary to increase ROM. Some type of force is applied to the part when soft tissue (muscles, tendons, and ligaments) is at or near its available length. A low-resistance stretch of sustained duration is preferred. Avoid quick or bouncing movements, which often produce tissue tearing, trauma, and activation of stretch reflexes in hypertonic muscles. Thermal agents or neuromuscular facilitation techniques may enhance static stretching.[14]

> ***Black Box Warning***
> Passive stretch must be administered cautiously and under supervision until service competency is developed. The patient can be harmed if excess force is used or if force is applied incorrectly.

Coordination and Neuromuscular Control

Coordination is the combined activity of many muscles into smooth patterns and sequences of motion. Coordination is an automatic response monitored primarily through proprioceptive sensory feedback. Kottke[26] differentiated neuromuscular control and coordination. Control involves conscious attention to and guidance of an activity. Conscious attention to activity may limit further skill.

A preprogrammed pattern of muscular activity represented in the central nervous system (CNS) has been described as an engram. An engram is formed only if there are many repetitions of a specific motion or activity. With repetition, conscious effort decreases; the motion becomes more and more automatic. Ultimately it requires little conscious attention, as in the case of brushing teeth. It has been hypothesized that when an engram is excited, the same pattern of movement is produced automatically. Coordination training is used to develop preprogrammed multimuscular patterns or engrams.[26]

Types of Muscle Contraction

Isometric or Static Contraction

During an isometric (static) contraction, no joint motion occurs and the muscle length remains the same. The limb is set or held taut as agonist and antagonist muscles are contracted at a point in the ROM to stabilize a joint. This action may be without resistance or against some outside resistance such as the therapist's hand or a fixed object. An example of isometric exercise of the triceps against resistance is pressing down against a tabletop with the ulnar border of the forearm while the elbow remains at 90 degrees flexion. An example of an activity that requires isometric contraction is stabilizing the arm in a locked position to carry a shopping bag slung over the forearm.[22,28]

Isotonic or Concentric Contraction

During an isotonic (concentric) contraction there is joint motion and the muscle shortens. This contraction may be done with or without resistance. Isotonic contractions may be performed in positions with gravity decreased or against gravity, according to the patient's muscle grade and the goal of the exercise or activity. An isotonic contraction of the biceps is used to lift a fork to the mouth for eating.[22,28]

Eccentric Contraction

When muscles contract eccentrically, the tension in the muscle increases or remains constant as the muscle lengthens. This contraction can be performed with or without resistance. An example of an eccentric contraction performed without resistance is lowering the arm to the table when placing a napkin next to a plate. The biceps contracts eccentrically in this instance. An example of eccentric contraction against resistance is the controlled return of a pail of sand lifted from the ground. In this example the biceps is contracting eccentrically to control the rate and coordination of the elbow extension in setting the pail on the ground.[22,28]

Exercise and Activity Classifications

Isotonic Resistive Exercise

Isotonic resistive exercise uses isotonic muscle contraction against a specific amount of weight to move the load through a certain ROM.[14,22,28] One can also use eccentric contraction against resistance. Resistive exercise is used primarily for increasing the strength of fair plus to normal muscles but may also help relax antagonists to the contracting muscles. This purpose can be useful if increased range is desired for stretching or relaxing hypertonic antagonists.

The patient performs muscle contraction against resistance and moves the part through the available ROM. The resistance applied should be the maximum against which the muscle is capable of contracting. Resistance may be applied manually or by weights, springs, elastic bands, sandbags, or special devices. The source of resistance depends on the activity, and resistance is graded progressively with an increasing amount of resistance.[14,22,28] The number of possible repetitions depends on the patient's general physical endurance and the endurance of the specific muscle.

Many types of strength training programs exist; most are based on the principle that to increase strength, the muscle must contract against its maximal resistance. The number of repetitions and rest intervals, frequency of training, and speed of movement vary with the particular approach and with the patient's ability to accommodate to the exercise or activity regimen.[8] One specialized type of resistive exercise is the DeLorme method of progressive resistive exercise (PRE).[17,46] PRE is based on the overload principle: muscles perform more efficiently if given a warm-up period and must be taxed beyond usual daily activity to improve in performance and strength.[17] During the exercise procedure small loads are used initially and increased gradually after each set of 10 repetitions. The muscle is thus warmed up to prepare to exert its maximal power for the final 10 repetitions. The exercise procedure consists of three sets of 10 repetitions each, with resistance applied as follows: first set, 10 repetitions at 50% of maximal resistance; second set, 10 repetitions at 75% of maximal resistance; third set, 10 repetitions at maximal resistance.[14,17,46] The load must be matched to existing strength so that the patient can perform all 10 repetitions. As strength improves, resistance is increased so that 10 repetitions can always be performed.[9] The patient is instructed to inhale during the shortening contraction and exhale during the relaxation or eccentric contraction.[17,46]

An example of a PRE is a triceps, which is capable of 12 pounds maximal resistance, extending the elbow, first against 6 pounds, then against 9 pounds, and the final 10 repetitions against 12 pounds. Maximal resistance, the amount of resistance the muscle can move through the ROM 10 times, is determined by contracting the muscle and moving the part through the full ROM against progressively increasing loads for sets of 10 repetitions, until the maximal load that can be lifted 10 times is reached.

At the beginning of the treatment program it is often difficult for the therapist to determine the patient's maximal resistance. Reasons may be that the patient may not know how to exert maximal effort, may be reluctant to exercise strenuously for fear of pain or reinjury, may be unwilling or unable to endure discomfort, or may have difficulty with the timing of exercises.

The therapist's experience and trial and error determine maximal resistance. The therapist should estimate the amount of resistance the patient can take based on the muscle test results and should add or subtract resistance (weight or tension) until the patient can perform the sets of repetitions adequately.

The exercises should be performed once daily, four or five times a week, and rest periods of 2 to 4 minutes should be allowed between each set of 10 repetitions. The exercise procedure may be modified to suit individual needs. Some possibilities are 10 repetitions at 25% of maximal resistance, 10 repetitions at 50%, 10 repetitions at 75%, and 10 repetitions at maximal resistance. Another possibility is five repetitions at 50% and 10 repetitions at maximal resistance. Still another possibility is to omit the second set of exercises. Adjustments in the first two sets of exercises may be made to suit the patient's capacity.[17]

Another approach is the Oxford technique, essentially a reverse of the DeLorme method. The exercise sequence begins with 100% resistance and decreases to 75%, and then to 50% on subsequent sets of 10 repetitions each.[17,46] The greatest gains may be made in the early weeks of the treatment program, with smaller increases occurring at a slower pace in the subsequent weeks or months. During performance of the exercise, the occupational therapist or OTA should take care with joint alignment of the exercise device; proper fit and adjustment of the device; ruling out of substitute movements; and clear instruction of speed, ROM, and proper breathing.[17,41]

Resistive Exercise—Application to Activity

Many purposeful activities lend themselves well to resistive exercise. For instance, leather lacing can offer slight resistance to the anterior deltoid if the lace is pushed in an upward direction. Sanding wood with a weighted sanding block can offer substantial resistance to the anterior deltoid and triceps if done on an inclined plane. Activities such as sawing and hammering offer resistance to upper extremity musculature. Kneading dough and forming clay objects offer resistance to muscles of the hands and arms. Careful observation of performance is essential for identifying and eliminating substitute motion and for adjusting positioning and directions so that the patient performs the desired motor pattern.

Isotonic Active Exercise

Isotonic muscle contraction is used in isotonic active exercise. Eccentric contraction may also be used. Active exercise is performed when the patient moves the joint through its available ROM against no outside resistance. Active motion through the complete ROM with gravity decreased or against gravity may be used for poor to fair muscles to improve strength, with the added benefit of maintaining ROM. It may be used with higher muscle grades for the maintenance of strength and ROM when resistance is contraindicated. Active exercise is not used to increase ROM because this purpose requires added force not present in active exercise.

In active exercise the person moves the part through the complete ROM independently. If the exercise is performed in a gravity-decreased plane, a powdered surface, skateboard, deltoid aid, or free-moving suspension sling may be used to reduce the resistance produced by friction. The exercise is graded by a change to resistive exercise as strength improves.[22,28]

Isotonic Exercise—Application to Activity

Activities that offer little or no resistance can be used as active exercise. A needlework activity performed in the gravity-decreased plane provides active exercise to the wrist extensors. When a grade of fair or 3 is reached, the activity can be repositioned to move against gravity, as in latch hooking (Figure 12-13).

Active-Assisted Exercise

Isotonic muscle contraction is used in active-assisted exercise. The patient moves the joint through partial ROM, and the therapist or a mechanical device completes the range. Slings, pulleys, weights, springs, or elastic bands may be used to provide mechanical assistance.[46] The goal of active-assisted exercise is to increase strength of trace, poor minus, and fair minus muscles while maintaining ROM. In the case of trace muscles the patient may contract the muscle, and the therapist completes the entire ROM. This exercise is graded by decreasing the amount of assistance until the patient can perform active exercises.[22,28]

Assisted Exercise—Application to Activity

If assistance is required to complete the movement, an activity must be structured so that assistance can be offered by the occupational therapist or OTA, the patient's other arm or leg, or a mechanical device. Various bilateral activities lend themselves well to active-assisted exercise. Bilateral sanding, bilateral sponge wiping, using a sweeper, and sawing are some examples. In bilateral activities the unaffected arm or leg can perform a major share of the work, and the affected arm or leg can assist to the extent possible.

Passive Exercise

In passive exercise there is no muscle contraction. Passive exercise is not used to increase strength. The purpose of passive exercise is to maintain ROM, thereby preventing contractures, adhesions, and deformity. To achieve this goal, the person should perform exercise for at least three repetitions, twice daily.[27] It is used when absent or minimal muscle strength (grades 0 to 1) precludes active motion or when active exercise is contraindicated because of the patient's physical condition. During the exercise procedure the joint or joints to be exercised are moved through their normal ranges manually by the therapist or patient, or mechanically by an external device such as a pulley or counterbalance sling. The joint proximal to the joint being exercised should be stabilized during the exercise procedure.[22]

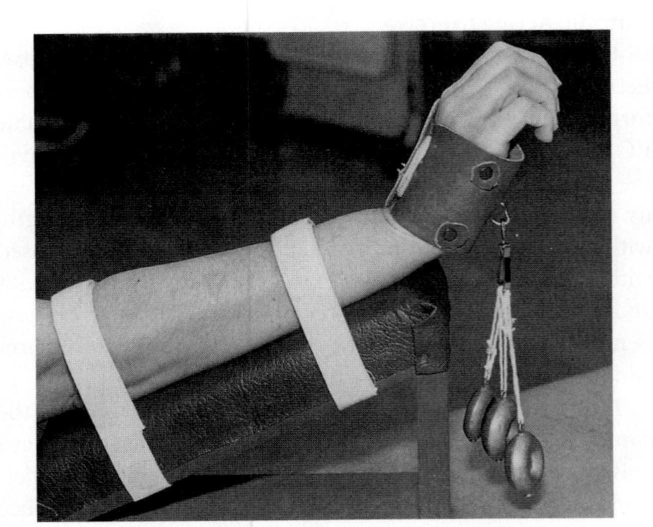

Figure 12-13 Weights may be added during latch hooking to provide active resistive exercise to the wrist extensors.

Passive Exercise—Application to Activity

It is often possible to include a passive limb in a bilateral activity if the opposite limb is unaffected. Several of the activities described previously for active assisted exercise can also be used for passive exercise.

Passive Stretch

For passive stretching, the therapist moves the joint through the available ROM and holds momentarily, applying a gentle but firm force or stretch at the end of the ROM (Figure 12-14). No residual pain should occur when the stretching is discontinued. Passive stretch or forced exercise is meant to increase ROM. It is used with loss of joint ROM and when stretching is not contraindicated. If muscle grades are adequate, the patient can move the part actively through the available ROM and the therapist can take it a little farther, thus forcing or stretching the soft tissue structures around the joint. EXTREME CAUTION AND COMPETENCE MUST BE DEMONSTRATED HERE.

Passive stretching requires a good understanding of joint anatomy and muscle function (Box 12-2). It should be carried out cautiously under good medical and OT supervision and with medical approval. Muscles to be stretched should be in a relaxed state.[28] Muscles should never be forced when pain is present, unless ordered by the physician to work through pain. Gentle, firm stretching held for a few seconds is more effective and less hazardous than quick, short stretching. The parts around the area being stretched should be stabilized, and compensatory movements should be prevented. Incorrect stretching procedures can produce muscle tearing, joint fracture, and inflammatory edema.[27]

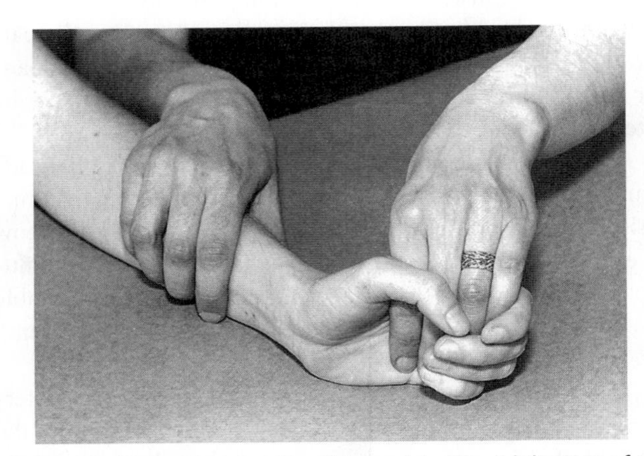

Figure 12-14 Passive exercise of the wrist with stabilization of the joint proximal to the one being exercised.

Active Stretch—Application to Activity

Many activities can be used to incorporate active stretching. For example, slowly sawing wood requires a forceful contraction of the triceps with a concomitant stretch of the biceps.

Box 12-2

Passive Stretching

Guidelines

1. Work under medical supervision and with medical approval.
2. Understand joint anatomy and muscle function.

Procedure

1. Stabilize parts around area to be stretched.
2. Prevent compensatory movements.
3. Make sure muscle is relaxed before stretching.
4. Apply gentle, firm, prolonged stretch, holding for several seconds (up to 45 seconds).

Box 12-3

Active Stretching

Guidelines and Procedure

1. Ensure that antagonist muscles have good to normal muscle strength.
2. Educate patient as to proper position so as to prevent compensatory movements.
3. Observe patient carefully, and correct as needed.
4. Evaluate effectiveness frequently.

Active Stretch

The purpose of active stretch is the same as for passive stretch: to increase joint ROM. In active stretching, the patient uses the force of the agonist muscle to increase the length of the antagonist (Box 12-3). This requires good to normal strength of the antagonist, good coordination, and patient motivation. For example, forceful contraction of the triceps to stretch the biceps muscle can be performed. Because the exercise may produce discomfort, the patient naturally tends to avoid the stretching component of the movement. Therefore supervision and frequent evaluation of its effectiveness are necessary.

Isometric Exercise—Application to Activity

Any activity that requires holding or static posture incorporates isometric exercise. Holding tool handles and holding the arm elevated while painting are examples. This type of exercise can be fatiguing when contraction is sustained.

Isometric Exercise without Resistance

Isometric exercise uses isometric contractions of a specific muscle or muscle group. In isometric exercises a muscle or group of muscles is actively contracted and relaxed without producing motion of the joint that it ordinarily mobilizes. The purpose of isometric exercise without resistance is to maintain muscle strength when active motion is not possible or is contraindicated. It can be used with any muscle grade above trace. It is especially useful for patients in casts, after surgery, and with arthritis or burns.[14]

The patient is taught to set or contract the muscles voluntarily and to hold the contraction for 5 or 6 seconds (Box 12-4). Without offering resistance, the therapist's fingers provide a kinesthetic image of resistance and help the patient learn to set the muscle. If needed, the therapist's fingers may be placed distal to the joint on which the muscles act. If passive motion is allowed, the therapist may move the joint to the desired point in the ROM and ask the patient to hold the position.

Isometric exercise affects the cardiovascular system, which may be a contraindication for some patients. It may cause a rapid and sudden increase in blood pressure, depending on the age of the patient, the intensity of contraction, and muscle mass being contracted. Therefore it should be used with caution.[14]

Box 12-4

Isometric Exercise without Resistance

Guidelines and Procedure

1. Observe precautions because this exercise may increase blood pressure suddenly. Do not use in patients with hypertension or cardiovascular problems.
2. Teach patient to set or hold muscles voluntarily.
3. To increase patient awareness of muscle contraction, apply light fingertip input distal to joint on which muscles act.
4. Instruct patient to hold contraction for specified time and to perform specified number of repetitions.

Isometric Exercise with Resistance

Isometric exercise with applied resistance uses isometric muscle contraction performed against some outside resistance. Its purpose is to increase muscle strength in muscles graded fair+ or 3+ to normal or 5. The patient sets the muscle or muscle group while resistance is applied, and he or she holds the contraction for 5 or 6 seconds. Isometric exercises should be performed for one exercise session per day, 5 days a week. In addition to manual resistance, the patient may hold a weight or resist against a solid surface, depending on the muscle group being exercised. A small weight held in the hand while the wrist is stabilized at neutral requires isometric contractions of the wrist flexors and extensors (Box 12-5).

Exercise is graded by increasing the amount of resistance or the degree of force the patient must hold against. A tension gauge should be used to accurately monitor the amount of resistance applied. Isometric exercises are effective for increasing strength, but isotonic exercise is the method of choice. Isometric exercise has several specific applications, as in arthritis, when joint motion may be contraindicated but muscle strength must be increased or maintained.[22,41]

Black Box Warning

Cardiovascular precautions are particularly important with isometric resistive exercise.

Box 12-5

Isometric Exercise against Resistance

Guidelines and Procedure

1. Observe precautions because this exercise may increase blood pressure suddenly. Do not use in patients with hypertension or cardiovascular problems.
2. Use with muscles graded fair plus (F+) and above.
3. Apply resistance manually, or use weights or other graded resistive devices.
4. Teach patient to set or hold muscles voluntarily at a fixed position (generally neutral).
5. Instruct patient to hold contraction for 5 or 6 seconds and to perform specified number of repetitions.
6. Instruct or supervise patient to perform exercises once a day, 5 days a week.

Box 12-6

Exercise for Neuromuscular Control of Individual Muscles

Guidelines

1. Ascertain that patient is capable of learning and following directions, is cooperative, and can concentrate on muscle retraining.
2. Eliminate distractions in environment.
3. Make sure that patient is calm, alert, and rested.
4. Make sure that sufficient pain-free ROM exists in joint on which targeted muscle acts.
5. Ascertain whether patient has adequate proprioception. If not, compensate through visual and tactile feedback.

Procedure

1. Explain to patient the muscle's location and function, origin and insertion, line of pull, and action on joint.
2. Instruct patient to think about motion while therapist or assistant performs it passively and strokes skin over muscle's insertion, stroking in direction of motion.
3. Instruct patient to assist by contracting muscle while OT practitioner performs passive motion and stimulates skin as before.
4. Instruct patient to move part through ROM with assistance and cutaneous stimulation while therapist or assistant emphasizes contraction of prime mover only.
5. Instruct patient to perform movement independently with prime mover.

Control and Coordination—Application to Activity

OT can be used to develop coordination, strength, and endurance. Active occupations have the advantage of engaging the patient's attention and interest. Activities should be structured to enable the patient to use the precise movement pattern and to work at speeds consistent with the maintenance of precision.

Occupational therapists, often consulting with physical therapists, may initiate coordination training with neuromuscular education and progress to repetitive activities requiring desired coordinated movement patterns. The OTA can acquire service competency in this area, given sufficient information on muscle actions and synergies and sufficient time to integrate and apply this information. Examples of enabling activities that demand repetitive patterns of nonresistive movement are placing small blocks, marbles, cones, paper cups, or pegs. These can later be translated to more purposeful activities such as leather lacing, mosaic tile work, needlecrafts, and repetitive tasks (e.g., sanding, polishing, wiping, sweeping, dusting).

Neuromuscular Control and Coordination

Procedures for the development of neuromuscular control and neuromuscular coordination are briefly outlined in the following paragraphs. The reader is referred to original sources for a full discussion of the neurophysiological mechanisms underlying these exercises. Neuromuscular education or control training involves teaching the patient to control individual muscles or motions through conscious attention. Coordination training is used to develop preprogrammed multimuscular patterns or engrams.[26]

Neuromuscular Control

Teaching control of individual muscles may be desirable when they are so weak that they cannot be used normally. The purpose is to improve muscle strength and muscle coordination for new patterns. To achieve these ends, the person must learn precise control of the muscle.

To participate successfully, the patient must be able to learn and follow instructions, cooperate, and concentrate on the muscular retraining. Before beginning, the patient should be comfortable and securely supported. The exercises should be carried out in a nondistracting environment. The patient must be alert, calm, and rested. He or she should have an adequate pain-free arc of motion of the joint on which the muscle acts and good proprioception. Visual and tactile sensory feedback may be used to compensate or substitute for limited proprioception, but the coordination achieved will never be as great as when proprioception is intact[26] (Box 12-6).

The patient's awareness of the desired motion and the muscles that effect it is first increased by passive motion to stimulate the proprioceptive stretch reflex. This passive movement may be repeated several times. The patient's awareness may be enhanced if the therapist also demonstrates the desired movement and if the movement is performed by the analogous unaffected part. The skin over the muscle belly and tendon insertion may be stimulated to enhance the effect of the stretch reflex. Stroking and tapping over the muscle belly may be used to facilitate muscle action.[26]

The occupational therapist or OTA should explain the location and function of the muscle, its origin and insertion, line of pull, and action on the joint. Then he or she should demonstrate the motion and instruct the patient to think of the pull of the muscle from insertion to origin. The skin over the muscle insertion can be stroked in the direction of pull while the patient concentrates on the sensation of the motion during the passive movement.

The exercise sequence begins with instructions to the patient to think about the motion while the therapist carries it out passively and strokes the skin over the insertion in the direction of the motion. The patient is then instructed to assist by contracting the muscle while the therapist performs passive motion and stimulates the skin as before. Next, the patient moves the part through ROM with assistance and cutaneous stimulation while the therapist emphasizes contraction of the prime mover only. Finally the patient carries out the movement independently with the prime mover.

The exercises must be initiated against minimal resistance if activity is to be isolated to prime movers. If the muscle is very weak (trace to poor), the procedure may be carried out entirely in an active-assisted manner so that the muscle contracts against no resistance and can function without activating synergists. Progression from one step to the next depends on successful performance of the steps without substitutions. Each step is carried out three to five times per session for each muscle, depending on the patient's tolerance.

Coordination Training

The goal of coordination training is achieving multimuscular motor patterns that are faster, more precise, and stronger than those performed when control of individual muscles is used. Coordination depends on repetition. Initially in training, the movement must be simple and slow so that the patient can be consciously aware of the activity and its components. Good coordination does not develop until repeated practice results in a well-developed activity pattern that no longer requires conscious effort and attention (Box 12-7).

Box 12-7

Exercise for Training Coordination of Multiple Muscles

Guidelines

1. Ascertain that patient is capable of learning and following directions, is cooperative, and can concentrate.
2. Eliminate distractions in environment.
3. Make sure that patient is calm, alert, and rested.
4. Divide exercise into component segments that patient can perform correctly. Practice one component at a time.
5. Reduce speed and resistance to keep effort low so that other muscles (outside targeted pattern) are not excited. Keep speed slow.
6. Mental fatigue occurs rapidly because patient is required to concentrate intensely. Provide frequent short rests.
7. Do not permit patient to repeat incorrect or uncoordinated patterns. Instead, have patient rest, determine source of error, and reinstruct.

Procedure

1. Instruct the patient in the movements of the first component segment.
2. Use sensory stimulation and passive movement (see steps 2 through 5 of procedure list of Box 12-6).
3. Assist patient as needed to make sure movement is precise.
4. Add new components as patient masters previous ones. Link components into subtasks or sequences of components by chaining.

Training should take place in an environment in which the patient can concentrate. The exercise is divided into components that the patient can perform correctly. Kottke calls this approach *desynthesis.*[26] The level of effort required should be kept low, by reducing speed and resistance, to prevent the spread of excitation to muscles that are not part of the desired movement pattern. Other theorists offer contrary advice, emphasizing the integration of movements that customarily occurs during activity. The therapist's experience and judgment are important in determining which method to use.

When the motor pattern is divided into units that the patient can perform successfully, each unit is trained by practice under voluntary control, as described previously for training of control. The patient is instructed in the desired movement, and sensory stimulation and passive movement are provided. The patient must observe and voluntarily modify the motion. Slow practice is imperative for monitoring to be effective. Enough assistance is offered to ensure precise movement while allowing the patient to concentrate on the sensations produced by the movements. When the patient concentrates on movement, fatigue occurs rapidly and the patient should be given frequent, short rests. As the patient masters the components of the pattern and performs them precisely and independently, the sequence is graded to subtasks or several components that are practiced repetitively. As the subtasks are perfected, they are linked progressively until the movement pattern can be performed.

The protocol can be graded for speed, force, or complexity, but the increased effort put forth by the patient may result in incoordinated movement. Therefore the grading must remain within the patient's capacity to perform the precise movement pattern. The motor pattern must be performed correctly to prevent the development of faulty patterns. Constant repetition of an incoordinated pattern reinforces faulty patterns, resulting in persistent incoordination. Factors that increase incoordination are fear, poor balance, too much resistance, pain, fatigue, strong emotions, prolonged inactivity,[26] and excessively prolonged activity.

Passive Stretch—Application to Activity

Passive stretching may be incorporated into an activity if an unaffected part guides the movement of the affected part and forces it slightly beyond the available ROM. One example is the passive stretch of wrist flexors during a block printing activity if the block is pressed down with an open hand while the patient is standing.

Physical Agent Modalities

The introduction of PAM into OT practice generated considerable controversy.[49,52] Such modalities were initiated by occupational therapists specializing in hand rehabilitation in which physical agents were expedient in a comprehensive treatment program.[43,45] After much study and discussion, the AOTA published an official statement and a position paper on physical agent modalities.[5,6] In these documents, physical agents were defined, and their use as adjuncts to or preparation for purposeful activity was specified. The position paper stated, "The exclusive use of physical agent modalities as a treatment method during a treatment session without application to a functional outcome is not considered occupational therapy."[6] This statement continues to be included in more recent AOTA position papers.[2] Current AOTA policy states that PAM may be used only by practitioners (OT or OTA) who have acquired the background and training necessary for their safe and effective use.[2] The practitioner must have documented evidence of the theoretical background and technical skills to apply the modality and integrate it into an OT intervention plan.[2,5,6] Practitioners may use a variety of routes to learn about PAM use including continuing education courses, education at conferences, and vendor-specific training.[2] Several states, in their licensure laws, require advanced training for therapists providing PAM.

Strict guidelines exist concerning the use of PAM by OTAs. The OTA does not choose the modalities; rather, the OT must select and delegate the modalities to be used, as is true of other services delivered by the OTA.[7] In addition, the AOTA states that an OTA using PAM must be trained and service competent in the use of PAM. Further, the OTA must be supervised by an OT who has service competency in that area.[2]

Black Box Warning

The OTA using PAM must be supervised by an OT who is service competent in that PAM. In addition, the OTA must have attained verifiable service competency in the PAM before using the PAM on a patient.[2]

PAM are used before or during functional activities to enhance the effects of treatment. This section introduces the reader to basic techniques and when and why they might be applied. Examples of the treatment of upper extremity injuries are presented because modalities are most commonly used for treatment of hand injuries and diseases. The techniques described are not limited to the treatment of hands, however.

Thermal Modalities

Heat is used to increase motion, decrease joint stiffness, relieve muscle spasms, increase blood flow, decrease pain, and aid in the reabsorption of exudates and edema in chronic conditions.[30] Collagen fibers have an elastic component and when stretched will return to their original length. Applying heat before a prolonged stretch, as in dynamic splinting, enables the elongation of these fibers. The blood flow maintains a person's core temperature at 98.6° F. To obtain maximum benefits from heat, tissue temperature must be raised to 105° to 113° F. Precautions must be taken in using temperatures above this range to prevent tissue destruction.

Contraindications to heat include acute conditions, sensory losses, impaired vascular structures, malignancies, and application to the very young or very old. Heat may substantially enhance the effects of splinting and therapeutic activities that attempt to increase ROM and functional abilities.

Black Box Warning

Heat should not be used in acute conditions, or where any of the following factors exist: impaired sensation, impaired circulation, malignancies. Heat should not be used with the very young or the very old, or with persons who are unable to communicate if they are in discomfort from the heat. Tissue damage may result from too much heat.

Conduction

Conduction is the transfer of heat from one object to another through direct contact. Paraffin and hot packs provide heat by conduction. Paraffin is stored in a tub that maintains a temperature between 125° and 130° F. The client repeatedly dips his or her hand into the tub until a thick, insulating layer of paraffin is applied to the extremity. The hand is then wrapped in a plastic bag and towel for 10 to 20 minutes (Box 12-8).[31] This technique provides an excellent conforming characteristic and therefore is ideal for use in hands and digits. Partial hand coverage is possible. The paraffin transfers its heat to the hand, and the bag and towel insulate against dissipation of heat to the air.

Care must be taken to protect insensate parts from burns. To prevent excessive vasodilation, paraffin should not be applied when moderate to severe edema is present. It cannot be used in the presence of open wounds. Paraffin can be used in the clinic or incorporated into a home program. The tubs are small, and the technique is safe and easy to use in the home. It is an excellent adjunct to home programs that include dynamic splinting, exercises, or general activities of daily living (ADL). It may be used in the clinic before therapeutic exercises and functional activities.

Hot packs contain either a silicate gel or bentonite clay wrapped in a cotton bag and submerged in a hydrocollator, a water tank that maintains the temperature of the packs at 160° to 175° F.[31] Because tissue damage may occur at these temperatures, the packs are separated from the skin by layers of towels. As with paraffin, the OT practitioner should take

Box 12-8

Physical Agent Modality: Paraffin

Guidelines

1. Before using this modality, obtain training to ensure service competency.
2. Protect areas of sensory impairment to avoid burns.
3. Do not use on areas with open wounds or moderate to severe edema.

Procedure

1. Verify temperature of paraffin.
2. Instruct patient to dip affected part slowly and repeatedly until desired thickness is obtained.
3. Wrap affected part in plastic bag and towel for 15 to 20 minutes.
4. Peel off paraffin casting, and prepare paraffin for reuse as directed.

precautions when applying hot packs to tissue where sensation is impaired. Hot packs are commonly used for myofascial pain, before soft tissue mobilization, and before any activities aimed at elongating contracted tissue.[13] For a client with a hand injury, the packs may be applied to the extrinsic musculature to decrease muscle tone caused by guarding, without also heating the hand. Unless contraindicated, hot packs can be used (with precautions) when open wounds are present.

Black Box Warning

Paraffin, hot packs, and similar conductive thermal agents may produce burns and tissue damage. Paraffin cannot be used on open wounds and in other situations discussed elsewhere on this page. Hot packs must be separated from the skin by layers of towels. The OT practitioner must monitor the patient and ask the patient to state whether the heat is too much. Patients must be alert and not cognitively impaired.

Convection

Convection supplies heat to the tissues by fluid motion around the tissues. Examples of convection are whirlpool and fluidotherapy. Whirlpool is used more commonly for wound management than for heat application. Fluidotherapy involves a machine that agitates finely ground cornhusk particles by blowing warm air through them. This device is similar to the whirlpool, but corn particles are used instead of water. The temperature is thermostatically maintained, with the therapeutic range extending to 125° F. Studies have shown this technique to be excellent for raising tissue temperature in the hands and feet.[13] An additional benefit is its effect on desensitization. The agitator can be adjusted to decrease or increase the flow of the corn particles, thus controlling the amount of stimulation to the skin. Because an extremity can be heated generally, this technique is effective as a warm-up before exercises, dexterity tasks, functional activities, and work-simulation tasks.

Conversion

Conversion occurs when heat is generated internally by friction (e.g., by means of ultrasound). The sound waves penetrate the tissues, vibrating the molecules. The resulting friction generates heat. The energy of sound waves is thus converted to heat energy. The sound waves are applied with a transducer, which glides across the skin in slow, continuous motions. Gel is used to improve the transmission of the sound to the tissues. Ultrasound is considered a deep-heating agent. At 1 MHz (1 million cycles per second), it can heat tissues to a depth of 5 cm. The previous methods produce heating to 1 cm.[35] Many therapeutic ultrasound machines provide a 3-MHz option for treatment of more superficial structures, with the corresponding heating depth reduced to 3 cm. Ultrasound at frequencies higher than recommended standards can destroy tissue. CAUTION: In addition, precautions must be taken to avoid growth plates in the bones of children, an unprotected spinal cord, and freshly repaired structures such as tendons and nerves. Because of its ability to heat deeper tissues, ultrasound is excellent for treating problems associated with joint contractures, scarring with its associated adhesions, and muscle spasms. When applying the ultrasound, the therapist should apply a stretch to the tissues while they are being heated and should follow with activities, exercises, and splints to maintain the stretch.

Ultrasound can also be used in a nonthermal application in which the ultrasound waves are used to drive antiinflammatory medications into tissues. This process is called *phonophoresis.* Ultrasound is thought to increase membrane permeability for greater symptom relief and can also be used after corticosteroid injections. Ultrasound is an advanced modality that requires additional training.

Black Box Warning

Ultrasound can damage underlying structures. Its use should be avoided over growth plates in children, over the spinal cord, over recently repaired tendons and nerves, and over metal implants.

Cryotherapy, the use of cold in therapy, is often used in the treatment of edema, pain, and inflammation. The cold produces a vasoconstriction, which decreases blood flow into the injured tissue. Cold decreases muscle spasms by decreasing the amount of firing from the afferent muscle spindles. Cryotherapy is contraindicated for clients with cold intolerance or vascular repairs. Cryotherapy can be incorporated into clinical treatment; however, it is particularly useful in a home program.

Cold packs can be applied in a number of ways. There are many commercial packs, ranging in size and cost. An alternative to purchasing a cold pack is to use a bag of frozen vegetables or to combine crushed ice and alcohol in a plastic bag to make a reusable slush bag. Ice packs should be covered with a moist towel to prevent tissue injury. The benefit of commercial packs is that they are easy to use, especially if the client must use them frequently during the day. When clients are working, they should keep cold packs at home and at work to facilitate use. The optimum temperature for storing a cold pack is 45° F.

Other forms of cryotherapy include ice massage and cooling machines. Ice massage is used when the area to be cooled is small and highly specific (e.g., inflammation of a tendon specifically at its insertion or origin). A large piece of ice (water frozen in a paper cup) is used to massage the area in circular motions until the skin is numb, usually for 4 to 5 minutes. Cooling devices, which circulate cold water through tubes in a pack, are available through vendors. These devices maintain their cold temperatures for a long time, but they are expensive to rent or purchase. They are effective in reducing edema immediately after surgery or injury, during the inflammatory phase of wound healing.

Contrast baths combine the use of heat and cold. The physical response is alternating vasoconstriction and vasodilation of the blood vessels. The client is asked to submerge the arm (e.g., alternating between two tubs of water). One contains cold water (59° to 68° F), and the other contains warm water (96° to 105° F). The purpose is to increase collateral circulation, which effectively reduces pain and edema. As with cold packs, contrast baths are a beneficial addition to a home therapy program.

Black Box Warning

Do not use cryotherapy with clients who have vascular disorders.

Electrical Modalities

Electrical modalities are used to decrease pain, decrease edema, increase motion, and reeducate muscles. As with all PAMs, these modalities are used to increase a client's functional abilities. Many techniques are available; those most commonly used are presented here. Electrical modalities should not be used with clients with pacemakers or cardiac conditions. All electrical modalities require additional training.

Transcutaneous Electrical Nerve Stimulation

Transcutaneous electrical nerve stimulation (TENS) employs electrical current to decrease pain. Pain is classified in three categories: physical, physiological, and psychological. When trauma occurs, an individual responds to the initial pain by guarding the painful body part. This guarding may result in muscle spasms and fatigue of the muscle fibers, especially after prolonged guarding. The supply of blood and oxygen to the affected area decreases; soft tissue and joint dysfunction results.[34] These reactions magnify and compound the problems associated with the initial pain response. The goal after an acute injury is to prevent this cycle. In the case of chronic pain the goal is to stop the cycle that has been established. TENS is an effective technique for controlling pain without the side effects of medications. Pain medications are often used in conjunction with TENS, which often reduces the duration of their use. TENS is safe to use, and clients can be educated in independent home use.

TENS provides constant electrical stimulation with a modulated current and is directed to the peripheral nerves through electrode placement. Several attributes of the modulation waveform such as the frequency, amplitude, and the pulse width can be controlled. When TENS is applied at a low-fire setting, endogenous opiates are released. Endorphins, naturally occurring substances, reduce the sensation of pain. The effects of high-frequency TENS are based on the gate control theory, originally proposed by Melzack and Wall in 1965. This theory describes how the electrical current from TENS, applied to the peripheral nerves, blocks the perception of pain in the brain. Nociceptors (pain receptors) transmit information to the CNS through the A, delta, and C fibers. A fibers transmit information about pressure and touch. It is thought that TENS stimulates the A fibers, effectively saturating the gate to pain perception, and the transmission of pain signals via the A, delta, and C fibers is blocked at the level of the spinal cord.[33] TENS can be applied for acute or chronic pain. TENS is often used postsurgically, when it is mandatory that motion be initiated within 72 hours such as in tenolysis and capsulotomy surgeries or when maintaining tendon gliding through the injured area after fractures is important. TENS can be especially helpful with clients who have a low threshold for pain because it makes exercise easier.

TENS can be used to decrease pain from an inflammatory condition such as tendonitis or a nerve impingement; however, the client must be educated in tendon and nerve protection and rest, with a proper home program of symptom management, positioning, and ADL and work modification. Without the sensation of pain, it is possible for the client to overdo and stress the tissues. Other techniques should be tried first to decrease pain for these clients. TENS is also used for treating trigger points, with direct electrode application to the trigger point to decrease its irritability.[36]

Black Box Warning

Electrical modalities (including but not limited to TENS and NMES) must be used only by practitioners who have been educated in the underlying theory and trained in the use of these modalities, and who have demonstrated service competency. These are not entry-level skills.

Neuromuscular Electrical Stimulation

Neuromuscular electrical stimulation (NMES) provides a continuous interrupted current. It is applied through an electrode to the motor point of innervated muscles to provide a muscle contraction. The current is interrupted to enable the muscle to relax between contractions, and the occupational therapist can adjust the durations of the on and off times. Adjustments can also be made to control the rate of the increase in current (ramp) and intensity of the contraction. NMES is used to increase ROM, facilitate muscle contractions, and strengthen muscles.[37] It may be used after surgery to provide a stronger contraction for increased tendon gliding, to strengthen a muscle that has become weakened because of disuse, or during the reinnervation phase after a nerve injury.

Other techniques that use an electrical current include high-voltage galvanic stimulation (HVGS) and interferential electrical stimulation. These techniques are applied to treat pain and edema.[37]

Selection of Appropriate Modalities in the Continuum of Care

Many years ago treatment roles and responsibilities were more specifically delineated. Occupational therapists treated patients only after the patients were capable, at least to some degree, of performing purposeful activity.[20] Evolution of treatment methods, trends in health care, and medical technology have significantly altered the role of the respective therapists and expanded the repertoire of treatment modalities that therapists are competent to practice.

Patients are now referred to OT long before they are capable of performing purposeful activity. Therapists are treating patients in the acute stages of illness and disability. Treatment is directed toward preparing the patient for the time when purposeful activity is possible.

For example, the occupational therapist applies a positioning splint to a patient immediately after hand surgery in anticipation of how the hand will be used later in treatment and in life tasks; the OTA uses sensory stimulation on the comatose patient to elicit arousal and a return to interaction with persons and objects in the environment; and the OT practitioner applies paraffin to decrease joint stiffness and increase mobility of finger joints before performance of a macramé project.

ACTIVITY ANALYSIS MODEL

The activity analysis offers one systematic approach for examining the therapeutic potential of activities. This model includes factors that must be considered regarding the performer, the field of action, and the activity in the selection of purposeful, therapeutic activity. In this example, only two steps (pinch, release) of a multistep activity are analyzed. The reader is encouraged to complete the motor analysis by considering movements of the shoulder, forearm, and wrist that accompany the pinch and release pattern analyzed herein.

I. Preliminary information
  A. Name of activity: pinch pottery
  B. Components of task
    1. Roll some clay into a ball 3 to 4 inches (7.5 to 10 cm) in diameter.
    2. Place ball centered on work table in front of performer.
    3. Make a hole in center of ball with right or left thumb (Figure 12-15, *A*).
    4. With thumb and first two fingers of both hands, pinch around and around hole from base to top of ball.
      a. Pinch by pressing thumb against index and middle fingers.
      b. Release pinch by extending thumb and index and middle fingers slightly.
    5. Continue pinching in this way, gradually spreading walls of clay until a small bowl of the desired size is formed.
  C. Steps of activity being analyzed
    1. Pinch
    2. Release
  D. Equipment and supplies needed
    1. Ball of soft ceramic clay
    2. Wood table 30 to 32 inches (75 to 80 cm) high or wood work surface fastened to table with C clamps
    3. Chair at work table
    4. Sponge and bowl of water
    5. Ceramic smoothing tool
  E. Environment field of action[15]: Occupational therapy workshop or craft activity room. Sink and damp storage area should be available in work area. Ample room should be available around work table so that performer is not crowded and can move freely between table and sink and damp storage closet. Lighting should be adequate for clear visualization of clay object and work area.
  F. Position of performer in relation to work surface/equipment: Performer is seated in chair at table, at a comfortable distance for reaching and manipulating clay and tools. Clay is centered in front of performer, and tool, sponge, and water bowl are to right and near top of work area.
  G. Starting position of performer: Sitting erect with feet flat on floor; shoulders are slightly abducted and in slight internal rotation, bringing both hands to center work surface; elbows are flexed to about 90 degrees; forearms are pronated about 45 degrees; wrists are slightly extended and in ulnar deviation; and thumbs are opposed to index and middle fingers, ready to pinch posterior surface of opened clay ball (Figure 12-15, *B*).
  H. Movement pattern used to perform steps under analysis: Flexion of metacarpophalangeal (MP) and interphalangeal (IP) joints of index and middle fingers; opposition and flexion of thumb (pinch), followed by extension of MP and IP joints of index and middle fingers; and extension and palmar abduction of thumb (release). Repeat pattern around ball of clay until a small bowl of desired size and thickness is formed (Figure 12-15, *C*).

II. Motor analysis[25]
  A. Joint and muscle activity: List joint motions for all movements used during performance of activity. For each, indicate amount of range of motion (ROM) used (minimal, moderate, full), muscle group used to perform motion, strength required (minimal [poor plus to fair], moderate [fair plus to good], full [good plus to normal]), and type of muscle contraction (isotonic, isometric, eccentric). Joints and muscles: (MP, metacarpophalangeal; PIP, proximal interphalangeal; DIP, distal interphalangeal; FDP, flexor digitorum profundus; FDS, flexor digitorum superficialis; FPL, flexor pollicis longus; FPB, flexor pollicis brevis; ED, extensor digitorum; EI, extensor indicis; APL, abductor pollicis longus; APB, abductor pollicis brevis; EPL, extensor pollicis longus; EPB, extensor pollicis brevis)
  B. Grading: Grade this activity for one or more of the following factors:
    1. ROM: Cannot be graded for ROM.
    2. Strength: Grade for strength by stiffening consistency of clay.
    3. Endurance: Grade for sitting tolerance by increasing length of activity sessions; grade for sitting balance by decreasing sitting support.
    4. Coordination: Requires fine coordination as performed. Grade coordination by adding scored or painted designs to surface; grade to sculpture of small clay figures.

ACTIVITY ANALYSIS MODEL—cont'd

Joint Motion	ROM	Muscle Group	Muscle Strength	Type of Muscle Contraction
Motions for Pinch				
Index and Middle Fingers				
MP flexion	Minimal	FDP, FDS, lumbricales	Moderate	Isotonic
PIP flexion	Minimal	FDP, FDS	Moderate	Isotonic
DIP flexion	Minimal	FDP	Moderate	Isotonic
Finger adduction	Maximal	Interossei palmares	Moderate	Isometric
Thumb				
Opposition	Full	Opponens pollicis, FPL, FPB	Moderate	Isotonic
Motions for Release				
Index and Middle Fingers				
MP extension	Minimal	ED, EI	Minimal	Isotonic
PIP and DIP extension	Minimal	ED, EI	Minimal	Isotonic
Finger adduction	Maximal	Interossei palmares	Moderate	Isometric
Thumb				
Radial abduction	Moderate	APL, APB	Minimal	Isotonic
MP and IP extension	Full	EPL, EPB	Minimal	Isotonic

Modified from Killingsworth A: *0T120 activity module*, San Jose State University, San Jose, Calif.

C. Criteria for activity as exercise
   1. Action of joints: Movement localized to flexion and extension of MP and IP joints of index and middle fingers and carpometacarpal (CMC), MP, and IP joints of thumb.
   2. Repetition of motion: Pinch and release sequence is repeated until bowl has reached desired height and thickness.
   3. Gradable: Activity is gradable for strength and endurance.

III. Sensory analysis[32,33]: Check sensory stimuli received by performer. These are any sensory experiences obtained from position, motion, materials, or equipment. Describe how sensation is received, using the following guidelines.

Sensory Modality	How Received during Activity
1. Tactile	Touching clay and tools
2. Proprioception	Awareness of joint position (joint motion, and motion during position sense) pinch/release
3. Vestibular (balance, head motion)	Maintenance of posture in chair while performing sense of body, chair while performing activity
4. Visual	See clay object and environment
5. Olfactory (smell)	May be slight odor of damp clay
6. Pain	0
7. Thermal (temperature)	Coldness of clay felt by hands
8. Pressure	Fingertips pressing against walls of clay bowl
9. Auditory (hearing)	0
10. Other	

IV. Cognitive analysis:[33] Check all that apply and justify your answer, using the following table:

Cognitive Skill	Justification
Memory	Memory for instructions
Sequencing (steps in order)	Perform steps in order
Problem solving	What to do if clay is too wet or too dry and walls of bowl are too thin or too thick
Following instructions:	
Verbal	Ability to comprehend and follow verbal instructions
Demonstrated	Ability to follow demonstrated instructions
Written	0
Concentration/ attention	Moderate: Focusing on bowl and required knowing when its walls are thin enough and high enough

V. Safety factors: What are the potential hazards of this activity? Describe the safety precautions that would be necessary when using this activity, using the following guidelines:

This activity involves few hazards. Ingesting clay and using a smoothing tool inappropriately are possible. Sitting balance must be adequate to maintain upright posture to perform the activity. Precautions to be taken are adequate supervision to ensure appropriate use of clay and tool and having performer accomplish task from a wheelchair with supports if sitting balance is impaired.

ACTIVITY ANALYSIS MODEL—cont'd

VI. Interpersonal aspects of activity[3]
   A. Solitary activity: May be done alone.
   B. Potential for dyadic interaction: May be done in parallel with one other person but does not require interaction.
   C. Potential for group interaction: May be done in a parallel group but does not require interaction.

VII. Psychological/psychosocial factors
   A. Symbolism in performer's culture[15]: Activity may be seen as more feminine than masculine in mainstream American culture. It may be associated with artistic, liberal, naturalist groups of people in American society.
   B. Symbolic meaning of activity to performer: Activity may be seen as a leisure skill rather than work. Some persons may regard it as "child's play."
   C. List feelings/reactions evoked in performer during performance of activity[33]: Soft, moist, pliable, and plastic properties of the clay may evoke soothing feelings in many persons. Others may regard it as messy or dirty. Potential for personal gratification is good because an attractive end product is easy to achieve, creative, individualistic, and useful.

VIII. Therapeutic use of activity
   A. List intrinsic goal of activity: To make a small clay bowl.
   B. List possible therapeutic objectives for the activity.
      1. To increase pinch strength.
      2. To improve coordination of opposition.
      3. To increase sitting tolerance.

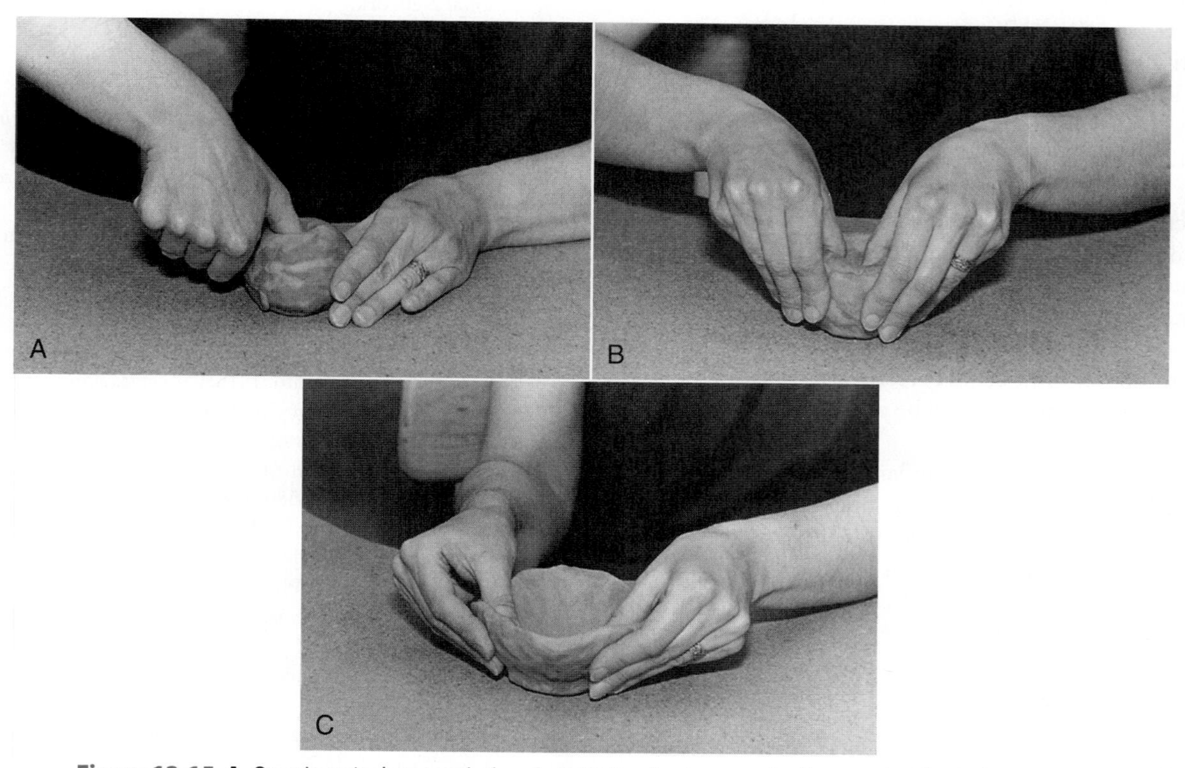

Figure 12-15 **A,** Opening pinch pot with thumb. **B,** Walls of pot are gradually spread with pinching motion of fingers. **C,** Pinching continues in circular direction until desired size of pot is reached.

Summary

Active occupation is the primary tool and objective of OT practice. OT practitioners use purposeful activity, activity analysis, adaptation, grading of activities, therapeutic exercise, simulated or enabling activities, and adjunctive modalities in the continuum of treatment, and they may use these methods simultaneously toward these ends. The breadth of the occupational therapist's or OTA's practice skills, applied to the patient's personal and social needs, helps the patient use newly gained strength, ROM, and coordination for purposeful activity, thus preparing the patient to assume or reassume life roles. Appropriate therapeutic activity is individualized and designed to be meaningful and interesting to the patient while meeting therapeutic objectives.

Therapeutic activity may be adapted to meet special needs of the patient or the environment. It may be graded for physical, perceptual, cognitive, and social purposes to keep the patient functioning at maximal potential at any point in the treatment program. The uniqueness of OT lies in its extensive use of goal-directed purposeful activities as treatment modalities, making use of the mind-body continuum within the tangible and social context. Purposeful activity is the core of OT practice.

In all instances, OTAs must be well trained and well qualified to deliver all aspects of practice. They should not hesitate to refer patients to supervisors and experts for treatment whenever appropriate.

Selected Reading Guide Questions

1. Name two reasons why activity is valuable.
2. List at least five requirements that activities must meet to be used for therapeutic purposes.
3. What is required for an activity to be considered purposeful?
4. What is the "just right" challenge in performance?
5. Grade an activity to accommodate changes in a variety of factors such as strength, ROM, endurance, coordination, and perceptual and cognitive skills.
6. How can activities be adapted to meet specific therapeutic objectives?
7. What are three criteria an activity must meet to be useful for exercise purposes?
8. Identify an activity that can be used to provide resistive exercise, and describe how it could be done.
9. What is meant by substitution patterns? Why do they occur?
10. What demand must be made on a muscle for its strength to increase?
11. List four signs of fatigue from excess exercise.
12. Discuss the appropriate use of enabling activities and adjunctive modalities.
13. State the indications, contraindications, procedures, and precautions for a variety of exercise protocols.
14. What type of exercise should be used if muscle grades are fair plus to good? Why?
15. If a patient has joint pain and inflammation with good muscle strength, what type of exercise should be used? Why?
16. How is passive stretching different from passive exercise?
17. When beginning progressive resistive exercise, how is the patient's maximal resistance determined?
18. How can the application of physical agent modalities enhance the patient's performance of activities?
19. List and describe three physical agent modalities, and discuss their use as preparatory modalities for functional activity.

References

1. American Occupational Therapy Association: Association policy: occupational therapists and modalities (Representative Assembly, April, 1983), *Am J Occup Ther* 37(12):816, 1983.
2. American Occupational Therapy Association: Physical agent modalities, a position paper, *Am J Occup Ther* 62(6):691–693, 2008.
3. American Occupational Therapy Association: Position paper on purposeful activities, *Am J Occup Ther* 37(12):805–806, 1983.
4. American Occupational Therapy Association: *Occupational therapy practice framework: Domain and process - 2nd edition*, Bethesda, MD, 2008, Author.
5. American Occupational Therapy Association: Official AOTA statement on physical agent modalites, *Am J Occup Ther* 45(12): 1075, 1991.
6. American Occupational Therapy Association: Position paper: physical agent modalities, *Am J Occup Ther* 46(12):1090, 1992.
7. American Occupational Therapy Association: Roles and responsibilities of the occupational therapist and the occupational therapy assistant during the delivery of occupational therapy services, *Am J Occup Ther* 58(6):663–667, 2004.
8. Ayres AJ: Occupational therapy for motor disorders resulting from impairment of the central nervous system, *Rehabil Lit* 21: 302, 1960.
9. Barton G: *Teaching the sick: a manual of occupational therapy and reeducation*, Philadelphia, 1919, WB Saunders.
10. Breines EB: Genesis of occupation: a philosophical model for therapy and theory, *Aust Occup Ther J* 37:45–49, 1990.
11. Breines EB: *Occupational therapy from clay to computers: theory and practice*, Philadelphia, 1995, FA Davis.
12. Breines EB: *Origins and adaptations: a philosophy of practice*, Lebanon, NJ, 1986, Geri-Rehab.
13. Cannon NM, Mullins PT: *Manual on management of specific hand problems*, Pittsburgh, 1984, American Rehabilitation Educational Network.
14. Ciccone CD, Alexander J: Physiology and therapeutics of exercise. In Goodgold J, editor: *Rehabilitation medicine*, St. Louis, 1988, Mosby.
15. Cynkin S: *Occupational therapy: toward health through activities*, Boston, 1979, Little, Brown.
16. Cynkin C, Robinson AM: *Occupational therapy: toward health through activities*, Boston, 1990, Little, Brown.
17. DeLateur BJ, Lehmann J: Therapeutic exercise to develop strength and endurance. In Kottke FJ, Stillwell GK, Lehmann JF, editors: *Krusen's handbook of physical medicine and rehabilitation*, ed 4, Philadelphia, 1990, WB Saunders.
18. Dewey J: *Democracy and education: an introduction to the philosophy of education*, Toronto, 1916, Collier-Macmillan.
19. Dunton WR: *Prescribing occupational therapy*, Springfield, Ill, 1928, Charles C Thomas.
20. Dutton R: Guidelines for using both activity and exercise, *Am J Occup Ther* 43(9):573–580, 1989.
21. Hopkins HL, Smith HD, Tiffany EG: The activity process. In Hopkins HL, Smith HD, editors: *Willard and Spackman's occupational therapy*, ed 7, Philadelphia, 1988, JB Lippincott.
22. Huddleston OL: *Therapeutic exercises*, Philadelphia, 1961, FA Davis.
23. Huss AJ: From kinesiology to adaptation, *Am J Occup Ther* 35(9):574–580, 1981.
24. Kielhofner G: A heritage of activity: development of theory, *Am J Occup Ther* 36(11):723–730, 1982.
25. Killingsworth A: *Activity module for OCTH 120, functional kinesiology*, San Jose, California, 1989, San Jose State University, (unpublished).
26. Kottke FJ: Therapeutic exercises to develop neuromuscular coordination. In Kottke FJ, Stillwell GK, Lehmann JF, editors: *Krusen's handbook of physical medicine and rehabilitation*, ed 4, Philadelphia, 1990, WB Saunders.
27. Kottke FJ: Therapeutic exercise to maintain mobility. In Kottke FJ, Stillwell GK, Lehmann JF, editors: *Krusen's handbook of physical medicine and rehabilitation*, ed 4, Philadelphia, 1990, WB Saunders.
28. Kraus H: *Therapeutic exercise*, Springfield, Ill, 1963, Charles C Thomas.
29. Law M, Baptiste S, Carswell A, et al: *Canadian occupational performance measure*, ed 3, Ottowa, Canada, 1998, Canadian Association of Occupational Therapists.

30. Lamport NK, Coffey MS, Hersch GI: *Activity analysis and application: building blocks of treatment*, Thorofare, NJ, 1996, Slack.
31. Lehmann JF: *Therapeutic heat and cold*, ed 3, Baltimore, 1982, Williams & Wilkins.
32. Llorens LA: Activity analysis: agreement among factors in a sensory processing model, *Am J Occup Ther* 40(2):103–110, 1986.
33. Llorens L: Activity analysis for sensory integration (CPM) dysfunction, 1978 (unpublished).
34. Mannheimer JS, Lampe GN: *Clinical transcutaneous electrical nerve stimulation*, Philadelphia, 1990, FA Davis.
35. Michlovitz SL: *Thermal agents in rehabilitation*, ed 2, Philadelphia, 1990, FA Davis.
36. Moran CA, Saunders SR, Tribuzi SM, et al: Myofascial pain in the upper extremity. In Hunter JM, editor: *Rehabilitation of the hand*, ed 3, St. Louis, 1990, Mosby.
37. Mullins PT, et al: Use of therapeutic modalities in upper extremity rehabilitation. In Hunter JM, et al, editors: *Rehabilitation of the hand*, ed 3, St. Louis, 1990, Mosby.
38. Nelson D et al: The effects of occupationally embedded exercise on bilaterally assisted supination in persons with hemiplegia, *Am J Occup Ther* 50(8):639-646.
39. Pedretti LW, Smith RO, Hammel J, et al: Use of adjunctive modalities in occupational therapy, *Am J Occup Ther* 46(12): 1075–1081, 1992.
40. Rancho Los Amigos Hospital: *Muscle reeducation (unpublished)*, Downey, CA, 1963, the Hospital.
41. Rancho Los Amigos Hospital: Progressive resistive and static exercise: principles and techniques (unpublished), Downey, CA, the Hospital.
42. Reed KL: Tools of practice: heritage or baggage? *Am J Occup Ther* 40(9):597–605, 1986.
43. Reynolds C: *OTs and PAMs: a physical therapist's perspective*, OT Week 8(37):17 Bethesda, Md, 1994, American Occupational Therapy Association.
44. Rocker JD, Nelson DL: Affective responses to keeping and not keeping an activity product, *Am J Occup Ther* 41(3): 152–157.
45. Rose H: *Physical agent modalities: OT's contribution*, OT Week 8(37):16–17, Bethesda, MD, 1994, American Occupational Therapy Association.
46. Schram DA: Resistance exercise. In Basmajian JV, editor: *Therapeutic exercise*, ed 4, Baltimore, 1984, Williams & Wilkins.
47. Spackman CS: Occupational therapy for the restoration of physical function. In Willard HS, Spackman CS, editors: *Occupational therapy*, ed 4, Philadelphia, 1974, JB Lippincott.
48. Steinbeck TM: Purposeful activity and performance, *Am J Occup Ther* 40(8):529–534, 1986.
49. Taylor E, Humphrey R: Survey of physical agent modality use, *Am J Occup Ther* 45(10):924–931, 1991.
50. Thibodeaux CS, Ludwig FM: Intrinsic motivation in product-oriented and non-product-oriented activities, *Am J Occup Ther* 42(3):169–175, 1988.
51. Watson DE, Llorens LA: *Task analysis: an occupational performanceapproach*,Bethesda,MD,1997,AmericanOccupationalTherapy Association.
52. West WL, Weimer RB: This issue is: should the representative assembly have voted as it did, on occupational therapist's use of physical agent modalities? *Am J Occup Ther* 45(12):1143–1147, 1991.
53. Wilcock AA, Townsend EA: Occupational justice. In Crepeau EB, Cohn ES, Schell BB, editors: *Willard and Spackman's occupational therapy*, ed 11, Baltimore, 2008, Lippincott Williams and Williams, p 198.
54. Wynn-Parry CB: Vicarious motions. In Basmajian JV, editor: *Therapeutic exercise*, ed 3, Baltimore, 1982, Williams & Wilkins.
55. Yoder RM, Nelson DL, Smith DA: Added-purpose versus rote exercise in female nursing home residents, *Am J Occup Ther* 43(9):581–586, 1989.

Recommended Reading

Ayres AJ: Basic concepts of clinical practice in physical disabilities, *Am J Occup Ther* 12(8):300–302, 1958.

Neistadt ME, et al: An analysis of a board game as a treatment activity, *Am J Occup Ther* 47:154–160, 1993.

Sten DB: Issues affecting PAMs in hand therapy, *OT Week* 6:16–17, 1992.

Zimmerer-Branum S, Nelson DL: Occupationally embedded exercise versus rote exercise: a choice between occupational forms by elderly nursing home residents, *Am J Occup Ther* 49:397–402, 1995.

PART V

Performance in Areas of Occupation

CHAPTER 13 Activities of Daily Living

EMILY HOLZBERG

Key Terms

Activities of daily living
Instrumental activities of daily living
Home management
Community living skills
Functional mobility
Communication management
Community mobility
Performance evaluation
Self-care
Activity analysis
Safety management
Reasonable modifications
Bedside commode
Transfer tub bench
Topographic orientation
Health management
Dressing sticks
Stocking aids
Buttonhooks
Reachers
Swivel spoon
Universal cuffs
Plate guards
Scoop dish
Suction nailbrush
Nonskid mats
Adaptive clothing
Bridging
Rocker knife
Dominance shift
Assistive technology
Nurturing assistance

Chapter Objectives

After studying this chapter, the student or practitioner will be able to do the following:

1. Describe the role of the occupational therapy practitioner in providing activities of daily living services.
2. Discuss the factors that affect the role of the occupational therapy assistant in the practice area of activities of daily living.
3. Name, objectively describe, and contrast differing levels of independence in activities of daily living.
4. Describe the procedures for performing an evaluation of activities of daily living including instruments to be used, techniques, timing, strategies, and reporting procedures.
5. Identify recommended adaptive devices to facilitate participation in and performance of activities of daily living for individuals with specific functional losses.
6. Recommend home modifications to individuals with specific functional losses to enable maximum independence at home.
7. Sequence and carry out training programs to enable individuals with specific functional losses to perform their own activities of daily living to the maximum possible level of independence.
8. Describe techniques and adaptive equipment for individuals with specific functional impairments to increase independence in the occupational role of parent.
9. Describe how a service animal can increase independence in various occupational roles for individuals with physical impairments.

This chapter focuses primarily on activities of daily living skills (ADL—sometimes called *basic ADL,* and instrumental activities of daily living skills (IADL), the skills that support personal independence.[20,27] In addition, the chapter considers the activities associated with education, work, leisure, and social participation. The skills needed to perform ADL and IADL are required for basic survival and integration into the world around us. Self-maintenance, mobility, communication, home management, and community living skills are taken for granted by the average person. For persons with physical dysfunction, losing the ability to care for personal needs and manage the environment can damage self-esteem and provoke feelings of dependence and even infantilism. Family roles may be disrupted, thus requiring partners, other family members, or a personal care attendant to assume caregiving when a person cannot perform basic activities independently.[31]

Occupational therapy (OT) programs provide evaluation and training in ADL and IADL task performance in almost every type of health care setting. OT practitioners assess ADL and IADL performance skills, determine problems that interfere with independence, select treatment objectives, and provide training or equipment to enable a higher level of independence. The OT practitioner may also help reduce or remove physical, cognitive, social, and emotional barriers that interfere with performance. He or she may also recommend devices that enhance performance and independence. A patient's need to learn new methods or to use assistive devices to perform daily tasks may be temporary or permanent, depending on the particular dysfunction, the prognosis for recovery, and the environment. Occupational therapists and occupational therapy assistants (OTAs) may be involved in providing ADL services. In this area, an OTA with proven service competency may function autonomously.

Definitions

Daily activities can be separated into ADL (or basic ADL) and IADL. ADL require basic skills and are oriented toward the care of one's own body or person. IADL require more advanced problem-solving skills, social skills, and complex environmental interactions and are oriented toward life in the community and with others. A breakdown of ADL and IADL categories is shown in Box 13-1.

Some categories of ADL and IADL merit additional detail. **Functional mobility**, part of ADL, includes movement in bed, transfers or moving the body from one surface to another, wheelchair mobility, and ambulation with or without walking aids. **Communication management**, part of IADL, includes all aspects of sending and receiving information, specifically the ability to use tools to write, and to operate a personal computer, read, type, text, or use a telephone, tape recorder, or special communications device. **Community mobility**, part of IADL, refers to the skills used to move around one's neighborhood or community.

If a patient is to be discharged to home under the care of a spouse or partner, the OT practitioner should focus on basic ADL and caregiver training and should defer addressing more complex IADL until later in the rehabilitative process. More definitions and detail can be found in the *Occupational Therapy Practice Framework, 2nd ed.*[2]

Evaluation of Occupational Performance in Activities of Daily Living

ADL represent one of the major areas of activity. A primary purpose of OT is to facilitate performance of these essential tasks of living. Occupational performance evaluation may be conducted either *top-down* or *bottom-up*. In the top-down approach, the therapist focuses on the client's occupational history and interests. The bottom-up approach focuses on identifying problems in specific performance skills. For example, the top-down approach recognizes the client's desire to dress independently. The bottom-up approach identifies a fine motor coordination impairment preventing the patient from independently tying his or her shoelaces. In practice, a blend of both approaches by the therapist is required.

The OT practitioner can begin evaluating the client's performance profile by charting a daily or weekly schedule (see Chapter 4), an activities configuration, an interest checklist, or an occupational role history.[2,12,16,32,36,55] Data about the

Box 13-1

Activities of Daily Living (ADL) and Instrumental Activities of Daily Living (IADL)

ADL
Bathing, showering
Bowel and bladder management
Dressing
Eating
Feeding
Functional mobility
Transfers to/from surfaces
Bed mobility
Transporting objects
Wheelchair mobility
Caring for personal devices
Sexual activity
Toilet hygiene

IADL
Care of others
Supervising caregivers
Care of pets
Child rearing
Communication management
Writing
Typing/computer use
Telephoning
Using special communication devices
Community mobility
Driving
Public transportation
Seated mobility systems
Financial management
Handling money
Banking and budgeting
Shopping for clothing and household goods
Home maintenance
Home organization
Meal preparation and cleanup
Grocery shopping and storage
Knowing health risks
Making medical appointments
Safety procedures
Emergency planning
Fire safety awareness
Ability to call 911
Response to smoke detector
Identification of dangerous situations
Recycling sorting, storage, and management
Access to recreation activities
Windows, doors
Keys, locks, alarm systems
Vacuum cleaner
Faucets
Can opener
Light switches
Stove/oven
Windows/doors
Refrigerator
Microwave oven

client's values, educational history, and work history including current or recent work experience, past work experience, and vocational interests and plans should be sought. The interest checklist indicates degrees of interest in five categories of activities: (1) manual skills; (2) physical sports; (3) social recreation; (4) ADL; and (5) cultural and educational activities.[32] The history of occupational roles gathers data about past and current occupational roles and the balance between work and leisure roles.[16] Although the interest checklist and the occupational role history were developed for a psychiatric population, they can be adapted for application for use with clients with a physical dysfunction.

An interview and performance evaluation can yield a well-rounded picture of the client's performance in activities. Deficits and imbalances will be apparent. The **performance evaluation** is fundamental to a comprehensive treatment plan, which addresses skills and the body structures and functions that support those skills. The performance evaluations addressed in this chapter are for ADL and IADL.

The patient's performance in ADL is critical. Practitioners who focus on remedying specific body functions may lose sight of this important fact. For example, increasing fine motor control cannot be an end in itself. It must be applied to the individual's occupational role performance including independence with handling clothing fasteners, using a computer keyboard, and performing mechanical repairs. The outcome of improving a body function or a performance skill should be linked to a functional task that the patient values.

Factors to Consider in Activities of Daily Living/Instrumental Activities of Daily Living Evaluation and Training

Before ADL/IADL performance evaluation and training can begin, the occupational therapist must assess body structures and functions and consider several factors about the client and the environment. Physical resources such as strength, range of motion (ROM), coordination, sensation, and balance should be evaluated to determine potential skills and deficits in ADL performance and the possible need for special equipment. Perceptual and cognitive functions should be evaluated to determine potential for learning ADL skills. General mobility in a bed or wheelchair or ambulation should be assessed.

In addition to these relatively concrete and objective evaluations, the OT practitioner should be familiar with the client's spirituality, culture, values and beliefs in relation to **self-care**, the sick role, family assistance, and independence. These factors must be considered when the occupational therapist selects objectives and initial activities in the ADL program. The occupational therapist must consider also the prognosis of the disorder—whether it is permanent, temporary, progressive, or unclear. He or she must also estimate or observe the patient's acceptance of the prognosis at the time of treatment. The balance of other activities that demand time and energy in the client's day may influence how many ADL may be performed independently.

The environment to which the client will return is an important consideration. Will the client live alone or with family or a roommate? Will the client go to a skilled nursing facility (SNF) or to a board and care home? If so, will the stay be permanent or temporary? Will the client return to work and community activities? The type and amount of assistance available in the home environment must be considered so that the caregiver can receive proper orientation and training in the appropriate supervision and assistance required.

The finances available for assisted care, special equipment, and home modifications are important considerations. Additional resources include the client's insurance and community-based or philanthropic organizations. The client's case manager or social worker can help determine eligibility for resources. For example, an affluent wheelchair-dependent client may be willing and able to make major modifications in the home such as installing an elevator or lift, lowering kitchen counters, widening doorways, and replacing deep pile carpeting to accommodate a wheelchair lifestyle. A client with fewer financial resources may need the OT practitioner's assistance in making less costly modifications such as removing scatter rugs and door sills, installing a plywood ramp at the entrance, or attaching a handheld shower head to the bathtub faucet.

The ultimate goal of any ADL and IADL training program is for the client to achieve the maximum level of independence. The *maximum level of independence* is defined individually for each client, using clinical guidelines and clinical reasoning. For a client with mild muscle weakness in one arm caused by a peripheral neuropathy, complete independence in ADL may be quite feasible. For the client with high-level quadriplegia, however, self-feeding, oral hygiene, communication via assistive devices, and directing care from a personal care attendant or family member may represent optimal independence. Therefore the potential for independence should be based on each client's unique personal needs, values, capabilities, limitations, and environmental resources.

The therapist will select either a rehabilitative or compensatory approach to guide the training sessions, but a rehabilitative approach is preferred where possible. For example, if the patient is recovering from a recent CVA and is expected to gain trunk control, it is important to challenge the balance during ADL sessions, using a rehabilitative approach. Instead of issuing the patient a long-handled shoe horn to don shoes without forward bending (using the compensatory approach), the OTA should encourage the patient to practice forward bending and weight shifting during the treatment session (a rehabilitative approach). Therapy provides patients the rare opportunity for the affected body parts to experience normal movement and proprioceptive feedback from such movement.

American culture strongly values independence. Rehabilitation personnel and the patient's family or friends may unwittingly push for independence inappropriately. To make independence a goal works only when independence is important to the client and is possible. The physical prognosis and long-term prospects must be considered. The OT practitioner must respect the patient's privacy and cultural beliefs during the training sessions. ADL tasks are normally done privately;

therefore an early discussion about the patient's level of comfort during training sessions is important. One patient may want to be covered while having family members or other practitioners nearby during sessions that include dressing, bathing, or toileting, whereas another patient with cognitive deficits may get confused or distracted by the covering.

Evaluation of Activities of Daily Living/Instrumental Activities of Daily Living

General Procedures

When data have been gathered about the client's physical, psychosocial, and environmental resources, the OT practitioner—together with the client, supervising physician, and other rehabilitation team members—should determine the feasibility of ADL evaluation or training. In some cases, ADL training should be delayed because of client limitations or in favor of more immediate treatment objectives that require the client's energy and participation. For example, a patient with a spinal cord injury may wear an orthosis or halo for 8 to 12 weeks to stabilize the healing spine. This temporary brace may interfere significantly with the patient's ability to bathe independently; therefore training sessions should focus on more feasible skills such as transfers, grooming, dressing, and self-feeding.

The occupational therapist or service-competent OTA may evaluate ADL and IADL performance. Evaluation often begins with an interview, guided by a checklist for questioning the client about individual capabilities and limitations. Several types of living skills checklists and evaluations are available and cover similar categories and performance tasks.[11]

The interview may be used for screening to determine whether further evaluation is necessary. The occupational therapist usually makes this determination. The interview alone can lead to inaccurate assumptions about performance because the client may recall performance before the onset of the dysfunction, may have some confusion or memory loss, or may overestimate or underestimate individual abilities because he or she has had little opportunity to perform routine ADL after the onset of the physical dysfunction. To assess ADL performance accurately, observation of performance is necessary. The phrase "one look is worth a thousand words" applies well here.

Ideally the OT practitioner should evaluate ADL performance when and where the client usually performs the activities. For example, a dressing evaluation could be arranged early in the morning in the treatment facility, where the client may be dressed by nursing personnel, or in the client's home. Self-feeding evaluation should occur at regular meal hours. If normal scheduling is not possible because of personnel and environmental constraints, the evaluation may be conducted during regular treatment sessions in the OT clinic under simulated conditions. However, simulation requires the client to perform routine self-maintenance tasks at artificial times in an artificial environment. Clients who have difficulty generalizing may have problems transferring learning from simulations to actual daily activities.

The practitioner realistically has only one session to evaluate the patient's ADL performance. A quick session simulating various basic ADL tasks should give enough information to infer performance in other ADL. More specific performance information can be obtained during future treatment sessions.

During further evaluative sessions, the OT practitioner should begin by selecting relatively simple and safe tasks from the ADL/IADL checklist and should progress to more difficult and complex items. Those tasks that would be unsafe or obviously unfeasible should be omitted, and the appropriate notation made on the evaluation form.

During the performance evaluation the OT practitioner should observe the methods the client is using or attempting to use to accomplish the task. The occupational therapist should attempt to determine causes of performance problems. Common causes include weakness, spasticity, involuntary motion, perceptual deficits, and low endurance. If problems and their causes can be identified, the clinician has a good foundation for establishing training objectives, priorities, and methods and for determining the need for assistive devices.

Other important aspects of this evaluation that should not be overlooked are the client's need for respect and privacy and the ongoing interaction between the client and practitioner. The client's feelings about having his or her body viewed and touched should be respected. Privacy should be maintained for toileting, grooming, and dressing tasks. The clinician with whom the client is most familiar and comfortable may be the appropriate person to conduct the ADL evaluation and training. As the clinician interacts with the client during performance of ADL, it may be possible to elicit the client's attitudes and feelings about the particular tasks; individual priorities in training; dependence and independence; and cultural, family, and personal values and customs about ADL performance. Respect the patient's desire for family involvement. Training a family member on how to assist the patient may be necessary.

Recording Results

During the interview and performance evaluation the clinician makes the appropriate notations on the checklists. Separate checklists may be used for self-care, home management, mobility, and home environment evaluations. When describing levels of independence, rehabilitation professionals often use terms from the Functional Independent Measurement (FIM) assessment. This assessment includes the following classifications: independent, modified independent (independent with the use of adaptive aids such as a walker), minimal assistance (≤25% help required), moderate assistance (26% to 50% help required), maximum assistance (51% to 75% help required), and dependent (≥76% help required). Such terms must be defined or illustrated by supporting statements to be meaningful and useful descriptors of performance. The practitioner must specify whether the level of independence refers to a single activity; a category of activities such as dressing; or all ADL. In designating levels of independence, an agreed-upon performance scale such as that shown in Figure 13-1 should be used to mark the ADL checklist. Definitions are usually broad

Sample case study

J.V. is a 48-year-old married woman who suffered a cerebral thrombosis resulting in a CVA 6 months ago. She lives in a modest home with her husband and teenage daughter and was a full-time homemaker before the onset of her stroke. She was a cheerful and active woman who enjoyed cooking, baking, gardening, and visiting her neighbors and friends. The stroke resulted in the disturbance of cerebellar and brain stem functions. J.V. has a severe motor apraxia for speech, cannot close her mouth, drools, and walks with a broad-based ataxic gait. Since the onset of her disability J.V. has been very depressed, weeps frequently, is dependent for much of her self-care, and sits idly for long periods of time. She was referred to occupational therapy for evaluation and training in ADL, adjustment to disability, and development of drooling and swallowing control to facilitate feeding.

SAMPLE ADL PROGRESS REPORT

J.V. has attended occupational therapy 3 times weekly for 3 weeks since the initial evaluation. Further evaluation of self-care skills revealed that J.V. is capable of some hygiene skills, except a tub bath, nail care, hair care, and makeup application. However, at home she remains almost entirely dependent on Mr. V. for self-care, while crying and complaining of feeling weak.

Home management evaluation revealed considerable difficulty with most tasks except table setting, dusting, dishwashing, and sweeping, which she can perform if given cues and supervision. Performance of more complex tasks is limited by psychomotor retardation, incoordination, distractibility, inability to sequence a process, and apraxia for fine hand activities. It was necessary to supervise J.V. closely and give step-by-step instructions while she performed household tasks. A few simple homemaking tasks were performed for several training sessions, but performance did not improve.

J.V. appears to be very depressed and lacks intrinsic motivation. It was suggested to her family that they offer less assistance for self-care, and involve her with them in household tasks that she can perform, under their supervision, if possible.

The occupational therapy program will continue with greater emphasis on achieving control of mouth musculature, a primary goal of J.V. ADL training will be delayed until J.V is moving toward the achievement of this primary goal.

A

OCCUPATIONAL THERAPY DEPARTMENT

ACTIVITIES OF DAILY LIVING EVALUATION

Name J.V. Age 48 Diagnosis CVA Dom. Right

Disability Bilateral incoordination, ataxia, apraxia of mouth musculature

Mode of ambulation Independent

Grading key:
I = Independent
MiA = Minimal assistance
MoA = Moderate assistance
MaA = Maximal assistance
D = Dependent
NA = Not applicable
0 = Not evaluated

TRANSFERS AND AMBULATION

	Date	Independent	Assisted	Dependent
Tub or shower	8/1			D
Toilet	8/1		MiA	
Wheelchair	NA			
Bed and chair		I		
Ambulation			MiA	
Wheelchair management	NA			
Car			MiA	

BALANCE FOR FUNCTION

	Adequate	Inadequate
Sitting	I	
Standing	I	
Walking		MiA

B

Figure 13-1 Activities of daily living (ADL) evaluation.

ADL SKILLS

EATING	Date	8/1	8/25			REMARKS
		Grade				
Butter bread		I				
Cut meat		I				
Eat with spoon		I				
Eat with fork		I				
Drink with straw		D				Mouth apraxia
Drink with glass		D				prevents performance
Drink with cup		D				of these activities
Pour from pitcher		D				

UNDRESS	Date	8/1	8/25			REMARKS
Pants or shorts		I				Is physically
Girdle or garter belt		MoA				capable of
Brassiere		MiA				performing the
Slip or undershirt		I				activities as
Dress		I				indicated but
Skirt		I				Mr. V. reports
Blouse or shirt		I				that J.V. is
Slacks or trousers		I				dependent on him
Bandana or necktie		NA				for much assistance,
Stockings		MoA				pleading fatigue,
Nightclothes		I				whining, and
Hair net		NA				crying for help
Housecoat/bathrobe		I				
Jacket		I				
Belt and/or suspenders		I				
Hat		I				
Coat		I				
Sweater		I				
Mittens or gloves		I				
Glasses		NA				
Brace		NA				
Shoes		MoA				
Socks		MoA				
Overshoes		MoA				

DRESS	Date	8/1	8/25			REMARKS
Pants or shorts		MiA				
Girdle or garter belt		MoA				
Brassiere		MoA				
Slip or undershirt		I				
Dress		I				
Skirt		I				
Blouse or shirt		I				
Slacks or trousers		I				
Bandana or necktie		NA				
Stockings		MoA				
Nightclothes		I				
Hair net		NA				
Housecoat/bathrobe		I				
Jacket		I				
Belt and/or suspenders		I				
Hat		I				
Coat		I				
Sweater		I				
Mittens or gloves		I				
Glasses		NA				
Brace		NA				
Shoes		MoA				
Socks		MoA				
Overshoes		MoA				

C

Figure 13-1, cont'd

FASTENINGS	Date	8/1	8/25			REMARKS
		Grade				
Button		I				
Snap		MoA				
Zipper		MiA				
Hook and eye		MaA				
Garters		D				
Lace		D				
Untie shoes		D				
Velcro		MiA				

HYGIENE	Date	8/1	8/25			REMARKS
Blow nose		0	I			
Wash face, hands		0	I			
Wash extremities, back		0	MaA			
Brush teeth or dentures		0	I			
Brush or comb hair		0	I			
Set hair		0	D			
Shave or put on makeup		0	MiA			
Clean fingernails		0	I, D			
Trim fingernails, toenails		0	D			
Apply deodorant		0	I			
Shampoo hair		0	D			
Use toilet paper		0	I			
Use tampon or sanitary napkin		0	NA			

COMMUNICATION	Date	8/1	8/25			REMARKS
Verbal		D				
Read		I				
Hold book		I				
Turn page		I				
Write		I				Writes name and
Use telephone		D				few words
Type		D				

HAND ACTIVITIES	Date	8/1	8/25			REMARKS
Handle money		0				
Handle mail		0				
Use scissors		0				
Open cans, bottles, jars		0				
Tie package		0				
Sew (baste)		0				
Sew button, hook and eye		0				
Polish shoes		0				
Sharpen pencil		0				
Seal and open letter		0				
Open box		0				

COMBINED PERFORMANCE ACTIVITIES	Date	8/1	8/25			REMARKS
Open-close refrigerator		0	I			
Open-close door		0	I			
Remove and replace objects		0	I			
Carry objects during locomotion		0	D			
Pick up object from floor		0	D			
Remove, replace light bulb		0	D			
Plug in cord		0	D			

OPERATE	Date	8/1	8/25			REMARKS
Light switches		0	I			
Doorbell		0	I			
Door locks and handles		0	D			
Faucets		0	I			
Raise-lower window shades		0	D			
Raise-lower venetian blinds		0	D			
Raise-lower window		0	D			
Open-close drawer		0	I			
Hang up garment		0	I			

D

Figure 13-1, cont'd

SUMMARY OF EVALUATION RESULTS

Date 8/1

Intact	Impaired	REMARKS
		SENSORY STATUS
X		Touch
X		Pain
X		Temperature
	X	Position sense More marked on left
	X	Olfaction More marked on left
	X	Stereognosis
	X	Visual fields (hemianopsia)
		PERCEPTUAL/ CONCEPTUAL TESTS
X		Follow directions Verbal
X		Visual spatial (form)
	X	Visual spatial (block design) Minimal impairment
X		Make change
	X	Geometric figures (copy) Some difficulty with triangle and diamond square, circle, triangle, diamond
	X	Praxis Mild apraxia evident on fine hand activities
		FUNCTIONAL RANGE OF MOTION
X		Comb hair-two hands
X		Feed self
X		Button collar button
X		Tie apron behind back
X		Button back buttons
X		Button cuffs
X		Zip side zipper
	X	Tie shoes Poor balance limits
	X	Stoop Reach and bending for these activities
	X	Reach shelf

E

Figure 13-1, cont'd

and general. They can be modified to suit the program plan and approach of the particular treatment facility.

The information is then summarized succinctly for the client's permanent records so that the entire rehabilitation team can refer to it. Figures 13-1 and 13-2 provide a sample case study, ADL and home management checklists, and summaries of an initial evaluation and progress report. The reader should keep in mind that the evaluation and progress summaries relate to the ADL portion of the treatment program only.

Home Management

Home management tasks are IADL and are evaluated similarly to self-care ADL tasks. The client should first be interviewed to elicit a description of the home and former and present home management responsibilities. The tasks that the client will need to perform at home, as well as those the client would like to perform, should be ascertained during the interview. If the client has a communication disorder or a cognitive deficit, assistance from friends or family members may be enlisted to obtain the information needed. The client may also be questioned about the ability to perform each task on the activities list. However, the evaluation is much more meaningful and accurate if the interview is followed by a performance evaluation in the treatment facility's kitchen and simulated living environment or, if possible, in the client's home.

At this point the motor, sensory, perceptual, and cognitive skills have already been evaluated. Therefore the OT practitioner should select tasks and exercise safety precautions consistent with the client's capabilities and limitations. In the beginning, the patient may not be expected to perform the task independently; therefore performing an activity analysis and breaking the task into components that the patient can perform is important. In order to perform an effective activity analysis, the OT practitioner must understand the demands of

OCCUPATIONAL THERAPY DEPARTMENT

ACTIVITIES OF HOME MANAGEMENT

Name J.V. Date 8/25

Address Anytown, U.S.A.

Age 48 Weight 135 Height 5'5" Role in family Wife, mother

Diagnosis CVA Disability Bilateral ataxia, apraxia of mouth musculature

Mode of ambulation Independent, no aids, mild ataxic gait

Limitations or contraindications for activity ______

DESCRIPTION OF HOME

1. Private house ✓
   - No. of rooms 6 - kitchen, dining room, living room, 3 bedrooms
   - No. of floors 2
   - Stairs 14 - bedrooms on second floor
   - Elevators 0

2. Apartment house ______
   - No. of rooms ______
   - No. of floors ______
   - Stairs ______
   - Elevators ______

3. Diagram of home layout (attach to completed form)

Will patient be required to perform the following activities? If not, who will perform?

Meal preparation	No	Daughter
Baking	No	Daughter (J.V. used to bake a lot)
Serving	Yes	
Wash dishes	Yes	
Marketing	No	Husband
Child care (under 4 years)	No	
Washing	Yes	
Hanging clothes	NA	Has dryer
Ironing	No	Daughter
Cleaning	Yes	Light cleaning
Sewing	No	Does not sew
Hobbies or special interest	Yes	Baking and gardening would be desirable activities

Does patient really like housework? No

Sitting position: Chair X Stool X Wheelchair NA

Standing position: Braces NA Crutches NA Canes NA

Handedness: Dominant hand Right Two hands X One hand only ______ Assistive ______

A

Figure 13-2 Activities of home management. (Modified from Activities of Home Management Form, Occupational Therapy Department, University Hospital, Ohio State University, Columbus, Ohio.)

the activity, range of skills involved in performance, and various cultural meanings ascribed to it. For example, the patient may initially require assistance for retrieving items to make a sandwich but then would be able to assemble the sandwich independently. The practitioner should make evaluations and treatments meaningful to patients by involving them in the planning process for treatment sessions. Physical assistance to help the client complete the entire task (and not just a few steps) may be necessary to keep training sessions as functional and meaningful as possible.

Home management skills apply to women, men, and sometimes adolescents and children. Individuals may live independently or share home management responsibilities with their partners or families. In some homes, roles

Grading key:
I = Independent
MiA = Minimal assistance
MoA = Moderate assistance
MaA = Maximal assistance
D = Dependent
NA = Not applicable
0 = Not evaluated

CLEANING ACTIVITIES Date	8/25 Grade				REMARKS
Pick up object from floor	D				
Wipe up spills	D				
Make bed (daily)	D				
Use dust mop	I				
Shake dust mop	D				
Dust low surfaces	I				
Dust high surfaces	D				
Mop kitchen floor	D				
Sweep with broom	I				
Use dust pan and broom	MiA				
Use vacuum cleaner	D				
Use vacuum cleaner attachments	D				
Carry light cleaning tools	I				
Use carpet sweeper	I				
Clean bathtub	D				
Change sheets on bed	D				
Carry pail of water	D				

MEAL PREPARATION Date	8/25				REMARKS
Turn off water	I				
Turn off gas or electric range	I				
Light gas with match	D				
Pour hot water from pan to cup	D				
Open packaged goods	I				
Carry pan from sink to range	D				
Use can opener	D				
Handle milk bottle	I				
Dispose of garbage	D				
Remove things from refrigerator	D				
Bend to low cupboards	D				
Peel vegetables	D				
Cut up vegetables	D				
Handle sharp tools safely	D				
Break eggs	D				
Stir against resistance	D				
Measure flour	D				
Use eggbeater	D				
Use electric mixer	D				
Remove batter to pan	D				
Open oven door	I				
Carry pan to oven and put in	D				
Remove hot pan from oven to table	0				
Roll cookie dough or piecrust	D				

B

Figure 13-2, cont'd

may have to be reversed after the onset of a physical disability, with the partner who usually stays at home seeking outside employment and the disabled individual remaining at home.

If a client is going to be home alone, several basic ADL and IADL skills are necessary for safety and independence. ADL skills include independence with toileting, transfers, or alternative plans to allow for rest periods and the telephone or special call system for emergencies. Minimal IADL skills required to stay at home alone include abilities to (1) prepare or retrieve a simple meal; (2) employ safety precautions and exhibit good judgment; (3) take medication; and (4) obtain emergency aid. The practitioner can evaluate potential for remaining at home alone through the activities of home management evaluation. Safety management is also included in the home management evaluation.

MEAL SERVICE	Date 8/25 Grade				REMARKS
Set table for four	I				
Carry four glasses of water to table	D				
Carry hot casserole to table	D				
Clear table	I				
Scrape and stack dishes	I				
Wash dishes (light soil)	I				
Wipe silver	I				
Wash pots and pans	MiA				
Wipe up range and work areas	MoA				
Wring out dishcloth	I				

LAUNDRY	Date 8/25				REMARKS
Wash lingerie (by hand)	D				
Wring out, squeeze dry	D				
Hang on rack to dry	I				
Sprinkle clothes	I				
Iron blouse or slip	D				
Fold blouse or slip					
Use washing machine					

SEWING	Date 8/25				REMARKS
Thread needle and make knot					
Sew on buttons					
Mend rip					
Darn socks					
Use sewing machine					
Crochet					
Knit					
Embroider					
Cut with shears					

HEAVY HOUSEHOLD ACTIVITIES. WHO WILL DO THESE?

	Date 8/25				REMARKS
Wash household laundry					
Hang clothes					
Clean range					
Clean refrigerator					
Wax floors					
Marketing					
Turn mattresses					
Wash windows					
Put up curtains					

WORK HEIGHTS

SITTING/STANDING

Wheelchair ______ Chair X Stool X

Best height for
- Ironing: 17 1/2" seated
- Mixing: 26" on high stool at counter
- Dish washing: 26" on high stool at counter
- General work: ______

Maximal depth of counter area (normal reach): 25"

Maximal useful height above work surface: 33" if standing

Maximal useful height without counter surface: 68" if standing

Maximal reach below counter area: 20" if standing

Best height for chair: 17 1/2" - can be used at adjustable ironing board

Best height for stool with back support: 24" - can be used at sink or food preparation counter

SUGGESTIONS FOR HOME MODIFICATION

Remove scatter rugs in bedroom

Install guard rail on both sides of toilet

Install grab bars on wall next to bathtub

Place nonskid strips on bottom of bathtub

C

Figure 13-2, cont'd

Home Evaluation

When discharge from the treatment facility is anticipated, a home evaluation should be performed to facilitate the client's maximal independence in the living environment. Home evaluations help bridge the gap between inpatient care and life at home after discharge.[40] Ideally, physical therapy (PT) and OT practitioners should perform the evaluation together on a visit to the client's home. The client and family members or roommates should be present. However, time and budget limitations may not allow two clinicians to go to the client's home. Therefore one rehabilitation professional may perform the evaluation, or the evaluation may be referred to the home health agency that will provide home care services to the client. A home health agency is an agency that provides skilled therapy and nursing in the home environment. The client and a family member should be interviewed to determine the client's and family's expectations and the roles the client will assume in the home and community. The cultural or family values regarding a disabled member may influence role expectations and whether independence will be encouraged. Willingness and financial ability to make modifications in the home can also be determined.[54]

The OT practitioner with a large caseload needs to prioritize patients in need of home evaluations. More active patients take greater risks and have an increased risk of falling.[41] These patients should be given a high priority. The home session can be also be used to allow the patient and therapist to adapt therapeutic recommendations in the real conditions of life. For less active or wheelchair-dependent individuals, taking a wheelchair and other equipment into the home to ensure adequate space before bringing the patient into the home may be sufficient. Basic safety recommendations can be provided to the family in a time-efficient manner.

Sufficient time to allow the active client to demonstrate the required transfer and mobility skills should be scheduled for the home visit. The clinician may also ask the client to demonstrate selected self-care and home management tasks at home. During the evaluation the client should demonstrate the use of any ambulation aids and assistive devices. The clinician should bring a tape measure to measure width of doorways, height of stairs, height of bed, and other necessary dimensions.

The evaluator should begin by explaining the purposes and procedures of the home evaluation to the client and others present, if this explanation did not precede the visit. If the patient will rely on a walker or wheelchair for home mobility, the occupational therapist or OTA should take the mobility aid through the house to ensure that it fits in key areas. The evaluator can take the required measurements while surveying the general arrangement of rooms, furniture, and appliances. It may be helpful to sketch the size and arrangement of rooms for later reference and to attach the sketch to the home visit checklist (Figure 13-3). For more information on a variety of checklists, see Letts and colleagues' research.[29]

When the record of the home arrangement and dimensions is completed, the client should demonstrate mobility and transfer and essential self-care and home management skills. If relevant, the client's ability to use the entrance to the home and transfer to and from an automobile should be included in the home evaluation.

During the performance evaluation the clinician should observe safety factors, ease of mobility and performance, and limitations imposed by the environment. If the patient requires assistance for transfers and other activities, the caregiver should be instructed in appropriate methods. The patient may also be instructed in methods to improve maneuverability and simplify performance of tasks in a small space.

Before mentioning possible home modifications, educating the patient on legal rights of a tenant or renter with a disability is important.[56] Federal and state fair housing laws require the property owner to make **reasonable modifications** to the housing unit at their expense. Examples of these modifications include the installation of an access ramp and grab bars and widening the interior doorways. The person with a disability can also request a handicapped parking space be placed in a convenient location. If the client is planning to move to a new rental unit, the law grants disabled applicants the right to be judged on the same basis as all other tenants. Additionally, even if the building does not allow pets, the law requires a property owner to allow service animals for residents with a disability.[55] Basic education on these rights can help ease the transition from hospital to home.

At the end of the home evaluation the clinician can list problems, recommended modifications, and additional safety equipment and assistive devices. The most commonly needed changes are the following[54]:

- Addition of a ramp or railings at the entrance to the home
- Addition of safety grab bars around the toilet and bathtub (caution: it is not safe to rely on a towel rack for balance)
- Removal of scatter rugs, door sills, and extra furniture
- Securing of electrical cords away from walkways
- Rearrangement of kitchen storage and of furniture to accommodate a wheelchair
- Lowering of the clothes rod in the closet

For clients with balance impairments, an area for small children's toys must be designated so that walkways are free of obstacles. A bell on the collar of a cat or small dog is also recommended. Fold-away hinges increase the doorway capacity by two inches and allow wheelchair access to the room without reframing the opening.

The client may have trouble accessing and maneuvering in the bathroom with a wheelchair or walker. The clinician may recommend a **bedside commode** until a bathroom can be made accessible or modified to allow for independence with toileting (Figure 13-4). Shower seats can be used in the tub (if the client can transfer safely over the edge of the tub) and can also be used in a shower. A **transfer tub bench** (Figure 13-5) is recommended for individuals who cannot step over the edge of the tub safely or independently. A hand-held shower increases access to the water and also eliminates the need for standing or risky turns while bathing. Consider installing a clamp to secure the shower head in a location within reach when seated. Clamps can secure the shower head to the shower chair arm or the grab bar for convenience. A removable rubber threshold

HOME EVALUATION CHECKLIST

Name ______________________ Date ______________

Address ______________________________________

Diagnosis ____________________________________

Mobility status ☐ Ambulatory, no device ☐ Cane ☐ Walker ☐ Wheelchair

Exterior

Home located on ☐ Level surface ☐ Hill

Type of house ☐ Owns house ☐ Apartment ☐ Mobile home ☐ Board and care

Number of floors ☐ One story ☐ Two story ☐ Split level

Driveway surface ☐ Inclined ☐ Level ☐ Smooth ☐ Rough

Is the DRIVEWAY negotiable? ☐ Yes ☐ No

Is the GARAGE accessible? ☐ Yes ☐ No

Entrance

Accesible entrances ☐ Front ☐ Back ☐ Side

Steps
Number ________
Height of each ________
Width ________
Depth ________

Are there HANDRAILS? ☐ Yes ☐ No

If yes, where are they located? ☐ Left ☐ Right

HANDRAIL height from step surface? ________

If no how much room is avaliable for HANDRAILS? ________

Are landings negotiable? ☐ Yes ☐ No

Briefly describe any problems with LANDINGS: ______________________

Ramps ☐ Yes ☐ No
☐ Front ☐ Back
Height ________
Width ________
Length ________

Are there HANDRAILS? ☐ Yes ☐ No

If yes, where are they located? ☐ Left ☐ Right Height ________

If no ramp, how much room is avaliable for one? ______________________

Porch
Width ________
Length ________
Level at threshold? ☐ Yes ☐ No

Door
Width ________
Threshold height ________ Negotiable? ☐ Yes ☐ No
☐ Swing in
☐ Swing out
☐ Sliding

Interior

Living room

Is furniture arranged for easy maneuverability? ☐ Yes ☐ No

Is frequently used furniture accessible? ☐ Yes ☐ No

Type of floor covering: ______________________

Comments ______________________

Hallways

Can wheelchair or walking aid be maneuvered in hallway? ☐ Yes ☐ No
Hall width ________
Door width ________
Sharp turns ☐ Yes ☐ No

Steps? ☐ Yes ☐ No Number ________

Are there HANDRAILS? ☐ Yes ☐ No

If yes, where are they located? ☐ Left ☐ Right Height ________

Bedroom ☐ Single ☐ Shared

Is there room for a W/C? ☐ Yes ☐ No

Door:
Width ________
Threshold height ________ Negotiable? ☐ Yes ☐ No
☐ Swing in
☐ Swing out

A

Figure 13-3 Home visit checklist. (Modified from Occupational/Physical Therapy Home Evaluation Form, San Francisco, Ralph K. Davies Medical Center, and Occupational Therapy Home Evaluation Form, Berkeley and Oakland, Calif., 1993, Alta Bates Summit Medical Center.)

Bed:
- ☐ Twin
- ☐ Double
- ☐ Queen
- ☐ King
- ☐ Hospital bed

Overall height ________ Accessible? ☐ Yes ☐ No

Would hospital bed fit into room if needed? ☐ Yes ☐ No

Clothing:

Are drawers accessible? ☐ Yes ☐ No ☐ On right ☐ On left

Is closet accessible? ☐ Yes ☐ No ☐ On right ☐ On left

Comments: ________

Bathroom

Door: Width ________
Threshold height ________ Negotiable? ☐ Yes ☐ No

Tub: Height, floor-rim ________
Height, tub bottom rim ________
Tub width inside ________
Glass doors? ☐ Yes ☐ No
Width of tub doors ________
Overhead shower? ☐ Yes ☐ No
Is tub accessible? ☐ Yes ☐ No

Stall shower: ☐ Yes ☐ No
Door width ________
Height of bottom rim ________
Accessible? ☐ Yes ☐ No

Sink: Height ________
Faucet type ________
☐ Open
☐ Closed
Accessible? ☐ Yes ☐ No

Toilet: Height from floor ________
Location of toilet paper ________
Distance from toilet to side wall L ________ R ________

Grab bars: ☐ Yes ☐ No
Location ________

Comments: ________

Kitchen

Door: Width ________
Threshold height ________ Negotiable? ☐ Yes ☐ No

Stove: Height ________
Location of controls ☐ Front ☐ Back
Is stove accessible for use? ☐ Yes ☐ No

Oven: Height from floor to door hinge and door handle ________
Location of oven ________

Sink: Will w/c fit underneath? ☐ Yes ☐ No
Type of faucets ________

Cupboards:
Accessible from w/c? ☐ Yes ☐ No

Refrigerator:
Hinges on ☐ Left ☐ Right
Accessible from w/c? ☐ Yes ☐ No

Switches/outlets:
Accessible? ☐ Yes ☐ No

Kitchen table:
Height from floor ________
Accessible ☐ Yes ☐ No

Comments: ________

Laundry

Door: Width ________
Threshold height ________ Negotiable? ☐ Yes ☐ No

Steps: ☐ Yes ☐ No
Number ________
Height ________
Width ________
Are there HANDRAILS? ☐ Yes ☐ No
If yes, where are they located? ☐ Left ☐ Right Height ________

B

Figure 13-3, cont'd

Washer:
☐ Topload
☐ Front load
Accessible? ☐ Yes ☐ No
Dryer:
☐ Topload
☐ Front load
Accessible? ☐ Yes ☐ No

Safety

Throw rugs
☐ Yes ☐ No
Location ______
Phone
Accessible? ☐ Yes ☐ No
Location ______
Emergency phone numbers
☐ Yes ☐ No
Location ______
Mailbox
Accessible? ☐ Yes ☐ No
Location ______
Thermostat
Accessible? ☐ Yes ☐ No
Location ______
Electric outlets/switches
Accessible? ☐ Yes ☐ No
Imperfect floor?
☐ Yes ☐ No
Location ______

C

Sharp edged furniture?
☐ Yes ☐ No
Location ______
Insulated hot water pipes:
☐ Yes ☐ No
Location ______
Cluttered areas?
☐ Yes ☐ No
Location ______
Fire extinguisher?
☐ Yes ☐ No
Location ______

Equipment present: ______

Problem list: ______

Recommendations for modifications: ______

Equipment recommendations: ______

D

Figure 13-3, cont'd

ramp allows a wheelchair to glide over high thresholds for exterior doors or sliding glass doorways.[25]

For patients with severe physical impairments or who have progressive diseases, major home modifications may be necessary. For example, an automatic door opener allows the client to open locked interior or exterior doors from a remote location. Electronic stair lifts allow the client to ascend or descend stairs while seated, thus providing access to another floor of the home. A platform lift may be more economical and aesthetic than a large ramp extending into the street for front entry. Overhead lift tracking systems lift and transfer a person from a wheelchair to various locations in the home

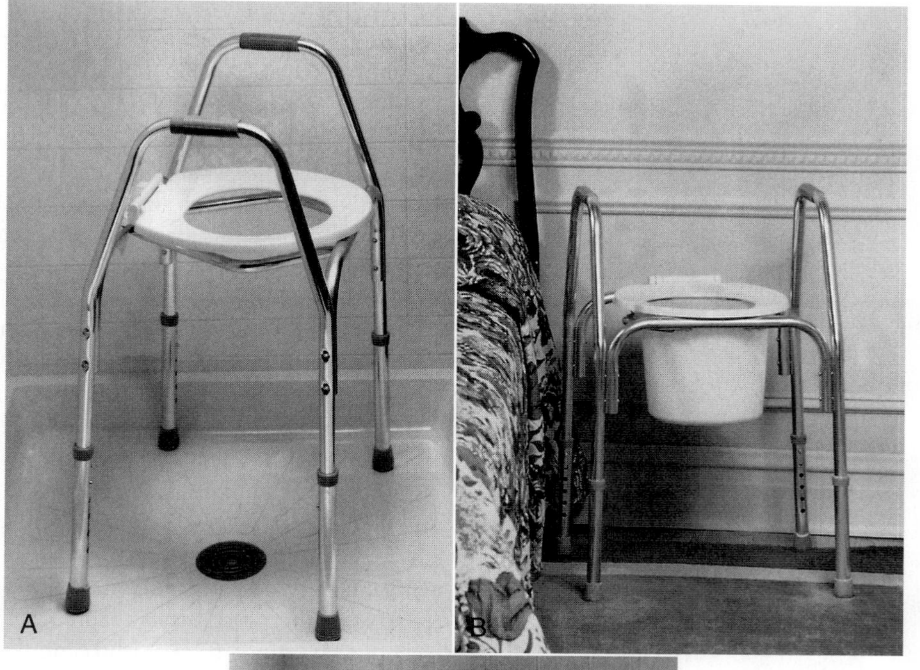

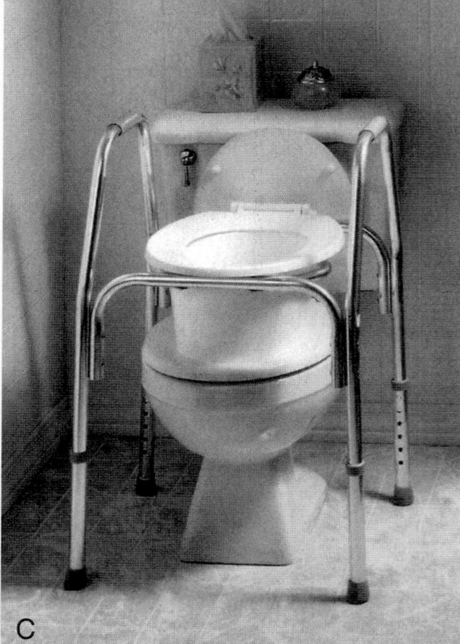

Figure 13-4 All-purpose commode. **A,** In shower; **B,** bedside; **C,** over toilet. (Courtesy Sammons, a BISSELL Co.)

while he or she is seated in a sling. If a client spends most of the time in a wheelchair, the walls and door jambs will most likely be scuffed and scratched. Installation of scratch-resistant plastic surfaces on the walls and door jambs can prevent such structural and cosmetic damage.[25]

Some additional safety measures should be considered. It is helpful to notify the local fire and police department that an individual with a disability resides in the home. An emergency exit plan should be established with two accessible exits, if possible. The evaluator should check whether smoke detectors work properly and that a fire extinguisher is within reach. The patient should keep important phone numbers on display near the phone or on a speed-dial function on the phone itself. The list should include family, neighbors, doctors, police and fire department, and the poison control center.[23]

When the home evaluation is completed, the evaluator should write a report summarizing the information on the form and describing the client's performance in the home. The report should conclude with a summary of the environmental barriers and the client's functional limitations. Recommendations should include equipment or alterations, with specifics in terms of size, building specifications, costs, sources, and specialized training required. Recommendations

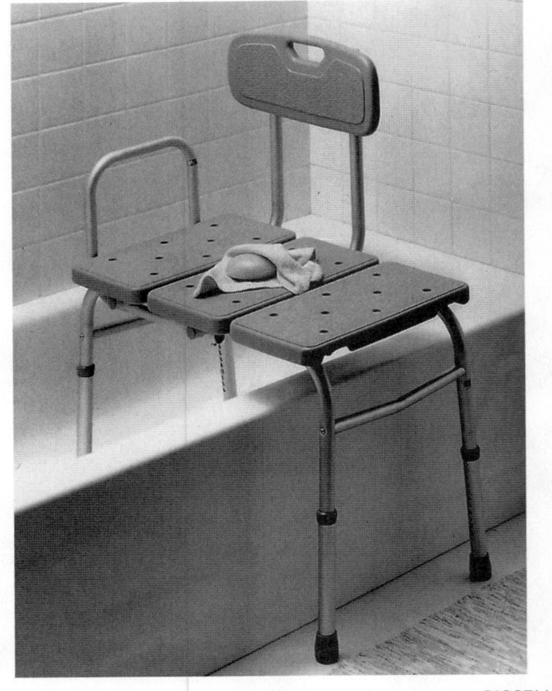

Figure 13-5 Transfer tub bench. (Courtesy Sammons, a BISSELL Co.)

may also include further functional goals to improve independence at home.

Home evaluation recommendations must be reviewed carefully with the client and family. The OT practitioner must use tact and diplomacy to present options and involve the client in a frank discussion of the recommendations. The client is free to refuse or consider alternative possibilities, and the therapist should facilitate client choice. Cultural values, aesthetic preferences, and family finances may be limiting factors in implementing needed changes. A social worker may help with handling funding for equipment and modifications, and the client should be made aware of this service when cost is discussed.[54]

The evaluator should include recommendations regarding the feasibility of the client remaining in or managing the home alone or being discharged to the home environment, as applicable. If any question regarding the client's ability to return home safely and independently exists, the home evaluation summary should include the functional skills the client needs to return home. The occupational therapist must remember to focus on preservation of autonomy and safety. Patients who do not receive home evaluations as a treatment intervention are more likely to lose autonomy after discharge than similar patients who received the evaluations.[41]

If a home visit is not possible, some information can be obtained by interviewing the client and family member after a trial home visit. The family member or caregiver may be instructed to complete the home visit checklist and to provide photographs or sketches of the rooms and their arrangements. Problems identified during the home visit should be discussed, and the necessary recommendations for their solution made, as described earlier.[54]

Community Living Skills

Money and Financial Management

If the client is to resume management of money and financial matters independently, the skills required for these tasks must be assessed. The evaluator must consider the effects of any cognitive, perceptual, or judgment problems on performance. The client may be capable of handling only small amounts of money or may need retraining with activities that require money management such as shopping, balancing a checkbook, paying bills, or making a budget. Adaptive writing devices or computer software can allow the client with a physical limitation to handle the paperwork aspects of money management with ease. An example is online banking. Caregivers who are new to the role of financial manager may require training and support with the unfamiliar role.

Community Mobility

Some clients can drive and can afford to have their own vehicle adapted or to purchase an adapted van (see Chapter 15). The client who cannot drive or who cannot afford an adapted vehicle must learn to use public transportation or travel on foot or in a wheelchair. The OT practitioner must then consider the client's physical, perceptual, cognitive, and social capabilities to be independent and safe with community mobility.

Physical capabilities to be considered are (1) whether the client has the endurance to be mobile in the community without fatigue and (2) whether the client is adequately independent with walker, cane, crutch, or wheelchair skills and transfers to go beyond the home environment. Necessary skills include managing uneven pavements, curbs, steps, ramps, and inclines and crossing streets. Using accessible transportation such as buses with lifts may also be included. Other skills to be evaluated before considering community mobility are how to (1) handle money; (2) carry objects in a wheelchair or with a walker; and (3) manage toileting in a public restroom.

Cognitive skills needed for community mobility include having basic topographic orientation, knowing where and how to obtain directions, and solving problems should they occur. If he or she is taking a bus, the client must know how to read a schedule and map. If the disability is new, the client may be developing new social skills, which initially will be stretched to the limit by community situations. Social skills include being assertive enough to obtain an accessible table at a restaurant, obtaining assistance with items that cannot be reached in the grocery store, and becoming comfortable with a new body image within the able-bodied community.

The client's community environment also needs to be assessed. Considerations include the following:

1. How safe is the neighborhood for a person vulnerable because of physical limitations?
2. What is the terrain like?
3. Are curb cutouts available?
4. Are the sidewalks smooth and even?
5. How far away is the nearest store or bus stop?

Accessibility of community transportation should also be considered. Some communities have door-to-door cab and van service, provided the client meets certain requirements, which may include arranging transportation up to 1 week in advance; going out to the front door and to the curb independently; and transferring independently into the vehicle. The client using a public bus must learn how to manage the electric lifts and how to strap a wheelchair into place on the bus. Neighboring bus stops must be evaluated because not all are wheelchair-accessible.

Community mobility requires preplanning by the OT practitioner and client; accurate assessment of the client's abilities; and awareness of potential physical, cognitive, and social barriers. A valuable resource by Armstrong and Lauzen, the *Community Integration Program*,[3] provides practical treatment protocols for a community living skills program. Efforts toward independence in community mobility are worth the investment because the client can expand life tasks beyond the home and interact with the community. A recreation therapist may take inpatients on outings and assess mobility while the client is out in the community. This information can be a good resource for problem solving and planning for a safe discharge.

Health Management

Health management includes the client's ability to understand the medical condition and to make reasonable decisions to maintain good health. Some practical aspects of health management include the client's abilities to handle medications and to know when to call a physician and how to make medical appointments. The evaluation of the client's ability to perform these activities will probably include other team members (e.g., nurse, physician).

The occupational therapist or OTA must assess each health management task separately and consider the performance skills and body functions required. The OT assessment can be helpful in determining which specific aspects of the task need to be modified for the client to be independent. For example, the OT practitioner may work jointly with a nurse to ensure that a client with hemiplegia and diabetes is able to manage insulin shots. The OT evaluation considers the client's cognitive and perceptual abilities to make judgments and physical abilities to draw the insulin out of the bottle, measure the insulin, and inject the insulin. If the client cannot safely manage the task, the OT practitioner may consider prefilled syringes. Different strategies for opening the medication bottles and measuring liquids may be necessary. Requesting prescriptions to be filled without childproof bottle tops may be helpful. Pill boxes equipped with alarms can help increase the patient's independence with heath management. Adaptive devices are available to allow easy application of eye drops for individuals with poor fine motor coordination or use of only one hand.

The OT practitioner may also evaluate and train the client in sub-skills needed to make a medical appointment such as using the phone, finding the appropriate phone numbers, and providing the needed information.

Patients with significant physical limitations such as an individual with high quadriplegia may have a number of caregivers to assist with ADL and health management. These patients must be educated on how to direct care to others to make sure medications are administered as prescribed and to prevent health risks such as urinary tract infections, skin ulcers, or autonomic dysreflexia (see Chapter 27).

Training in Activities of Daily Living/ Instrumental Activities of Daily Living

When ADL/IADL training is indicated, appropriate short-term and long-term objectives must be established based on the evaluation and the client's priorities and potential for independence. The Occupational Therapy Code of Ethics states that the OT practitioner should collaborate with service recipients in setting goals and priorities throughout the intervention process. Collaboration promotes awareness, compliance, and ability to apply OT to life situations. The more collaborative and goal focused the OT intervention is, the more likely a high level of achievement in desired outcomes in self-care activities will occur.[18]

The OT practitioner should estimate which ADL/IADL tasks are possible and which are impossible for the client to achieve. The clinician should explore with the client the possibility of alternate methods of performing the activities and using assistive devices. The level of assistance needed for each task should be determined. It may not be possible to estimate these factors until training is under way.

The ADL/IADL training program may be graded by beginning with a few simple tasks, which are gradually increased in number and complexity. Training should progress from dependent, to assisted, to supervised, to independent, with or without assistive devices.[54] The rate at which grading can occur depends on the client's potential for recovery, endurance, skills, and motivation.

Methods of Teaching Activities of Daily Living

The methods of teaching the client to perform ADL must be tailored to suit each client's learning style and ability. Clients who are alert and grasp instructions quickly may be able to perform an entire process after a brief demonstration and verbal instruction. Clients who have perceptual problems, poor memory, or difficulty following instructions require a more concrete, step-by-step approach in which assistance is reduced gradually as success is achieved. First, the clinician must prepare the environment by reducing extraneous stimuli. For such individuals, it is important to break down the activity into small steps and to progress through them slowly, one at a time. The clinician's slow demonstration of the task or step in the same place and in the same manner in which the client is expected to perform is helpful. Verbal instructions to accompany the demonstration may or may not be helpful, depending on the client's receptive language skills and ability to process and integrate two modes of sensory information simultaneously.

Helpful tactile and kinesthetic modes of instruction include (1) touching body parts to be moved, dressed, bathed, or positioned; (2) passively moving the part through the desired pattern to achieve a step or task; and (3) gently guiding the part manually through the task (see Chapters 10 and 21). Such techniques can augment or replace demonstration and verbal instruction, depending on the client's best avenues of learning. Skill, speed, and retention of learning require repeated task performance. Tasks may be repeated several times during the same training session, if time and the client's physical and emotional tolerance allow, or they may be repeated daily until desired retention or level of skill is achieved.

ADL training sessions allow a patient to experience and practice normal movement patterns with the therapist guiding the patient at key points of the body. This idea is a leading principle of neurodevelopmental technique (NDT). ADL training with NDT patterns can be a meaningful way for a patient to gain strength, balance, and endurance. If the patient is not expected to make physical improvements because of the nature of the physical dysfunction, the ADL training sessions should focus primarily on teaching compensatory strategies.

The process of *backward chaining* can be used in teaching ADL skills (see Chapter 10). This method is particularly useful in training clients with brain damage.[54]

Before beginning training in any ADL, the clinician must prepare by providing adequate space and arranging equipment, materials, and furniture for maximal convenience and safety. The clinician should be thoroughly familiar with the task to be performed and any special methods or assistive devices that will be used. The OT practitioner should be able to perform the task because the client is expected to perform it skillfully. This may include, for example, performance with the practitioner's nondominant hand.

Next the activity is presented to the client, usually in one or more modes of guidance, demonstration, and verbal instruction described earlier. The client then performs the activity—either along with the clinician or immediately after being shown, with supervision and assistance as required. Performance is modified and corrected as needed, and the process is repeated to ensure learning. Because other staff or family members often will help to reinforce the newly learned skills, family training is critical to ensure that the client carries over the skills from previous treatment sessions.

In the final phase of instruction, after mastering the task or several tasks, the client attempts to perform them independently. The OT practitioner should follow up by checking on performance in progress. Finally, the practitioner must check on adequacy of performance and carry-over of learning with nursing personnel, the caregiver, or the supervising family members.[24]

Recording Progress in Performance of Activities of Daily Living

The ADL checklists used to record performance on the initial evaluation usually have one or more spaces for recording changes in abilities and results of reevaluation during the training process. The sample checklist described earlier is designed and completed in this way (see Figure 13-1). Progress is usually summarized for inclusion in the medical record. The progress record should summarize changes in the client's abilities and current level of independence and estimate the client's potential for further independence, attitude, motivation for ADL training, and future goals for the ADL program. The progress record should also reflect how the client's current level of independence or assistance may affect discharge plans. For example, the client who continues to require moderate assistance with self-care may need to hire an attendant. Alternatively, the OT practitioner may justify a need for ongoing treatment when the client has potential for further independence.

Specific Techniques for Activities of Daily Living

Standard techniques to solve specific ADL problems are not practical in every situation. The OT practitioner, in collaboration with the patient, may need to explore a variety of methods or assistive devices to reach a solution. The OT practitioner sometimes needs to design a special device, method, splint, or piece of equipment to allow the client to perform a particular activity. Many assistive devices available today through rehabilitation equipment companies were originally created by OT practitioners and clients. Many special methods used to perform specific activities also evolved through trial-and-error approaches of clinicians and their clients. Clients often have good suggestions because they live with the limitation and are confronted regularly with the need to adapt the performance of daily tasks. Occasionally a solution is found but is unacceptable to the client because it involves excessive adaptive equipment, gadgets, or time. It is important to respect the patient's opinions throughout the entire training process to help him or her obtain personal goals.

The techniques and equipment specified in this chapter provide the OT student with basic skills to approach the patient with confidence but may not be appropriate for certain patients. The student should keep in mind that all adaptive equipment must be close at hand during the task. However, this stipulation may not be feasible if the patient is in a public place. A patient may resist adaptive equipment because of its aesthetic qualities or because of his or her cognitive impairments or resistance to change. Therefore alternative strategies to adaptive equipment must be explored. The patient's opinion of an adaptive device may change after he or she experiences the difficulty of trying the activity without the device.

The purpose of the following summary of techniques is to provide some general ideas about how to solve ADL problems for specific classifications of dysfunctions. (See References later for more detailed instruction in ADL methods.)

Limited Range of Motion and Strength

The major problem for clients with limited joint ROM is the lack of reach and joint excursion. Environmental adaptation and assistive devices are used to compensate. Individuals who lack muscle strength may require some of the same devices or techniques to conserve energy and to compensate for weakness. Obese individuals often suffer from limited ROM or ability to reach body parts and lack of muscle strength. Patients

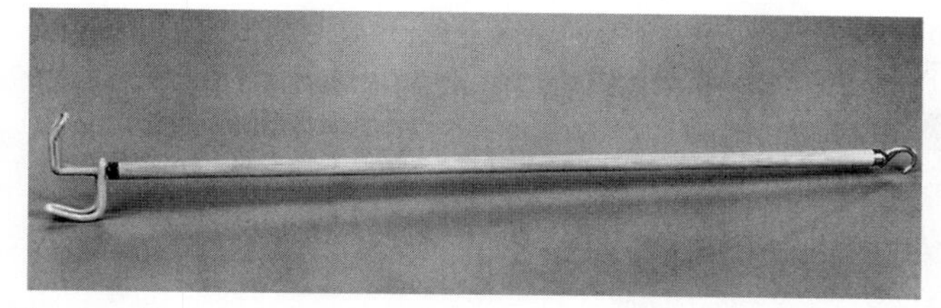

Figure 13-6 Dressing stick or reacher. (Courtesy Sammons, a BISSELL Co.)

recovering from a surgery may have postsurgical precautions that temporarily limit ROM. Some adaptations and devices are outlined in the following discussion.[30,34,46,54]

Dressing Activities

General suggestions for facilitating dressing include the following:

1. Use front-opening garments, one size larger than needed and made of fabrics with some stretch.
2. Use **dressing sticks** with a garter on one end and a neoprene-covered coat hook on the other for pushing and pulling garments off and on feet and legs (Figure 13-6) and to push a shirt or blouse over the head. Use a sock aid to pull on socks.
3. Use larger buttons or zippers with a loop on the pull tab.
4. Replace buttons, snaps, hooks, and eyes with Velcro or zippers (for those patients who cannot manage traditional fastenings). A cuff and collar extender installed in between the buttons of the shirt cuff widens the opening of the cuff without the need to unfasten. A small, barely visible spring helps extend the buttons' reach.
5. Eliminate the need to bend and tie shoelaces or to use finger joints in this fine motor activity by using elastic shoelaces, shoes with Velcro closures, or slip-on shoes.
6. Facilitate donning stockings without bending to the feet by using **stocking aids** from medical suppliers or homemade versions of garters attached to long webbing straps (Figure 13-7). Alternatively, kitchen rubber gloves with nodules help with grasp for donning stockings or TED (thromboembolic deterrent) hose.
7. Use one of several types of commercially available **buttonhooks** if finger coordination or ROM is limited (Figure 13-8).
8. Use **reachers** for picking up socks and shoes, arranging clothes, removing clothes from hangers, picking up objects on the floor (Figure 13-9), and donning pants.

Eating Activities

Assistive devices that can facilitate feeding include the following:

1. Built-up eating utensil handles can accommodate limited grasp or prehension (Figure 13-10). Utensils can be purchased with wide handles; alternatively, cylindrical foam, which is found at hardware stores in the pipe insulation section, can be added to regular utensils.
2. Elongated or specially curved handles on spoons and forks may be necessary to reach the mouth. A **swivel spoon** or spoon-fork combination can compensate for limited supination (Figure 13-11).
3. Long plastic straws and straw clips on glasses or cups can be used if neck, elbow, or shoulder ROM limits hand-to-mouth motion or if grasp is inadequate to hold the cup or glass.
4. **Universal cuffs** or utensil holders can be used if grasp is limited and built-up handles do not work (Figure 13-12). These cuffs wrap around the palm of the hand with an opening on the first web space. A variety of items can be placed in the opening, including eating utensils.
5. **Plate guards** or scoop dishes may be useful to prevent food from slipping off the plate if the patient lacks coordination when scooping the food with the utensil.

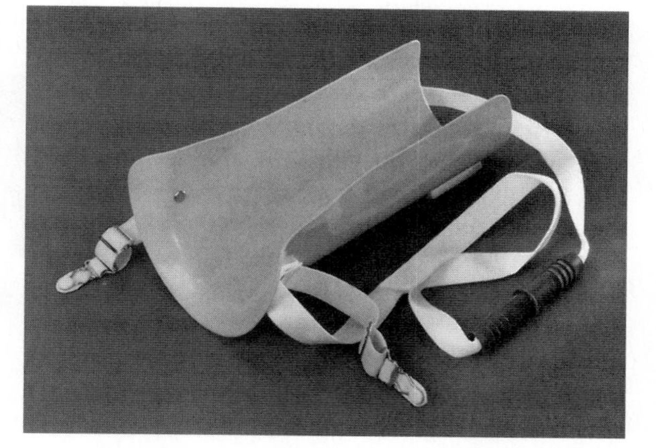

Figure 13-7 Sock aid. (Courtesy Sammons, a BISSELL Co.)

Hygiene and Grooming

Environmental adaptations that can facilitate bathing and grooming include the following:

1. A handheld showerhead on a flexible hose for bathing and shampooing hair facilitates showering while seated and allows the patient to control the direction of spray. Adding cylindrical foam to the showerhead is helpful for clients with limited grasp.
2. A long-handled bath brush or sponge with a soap holder (Figure 13-13) or long cloth scrubber can help the user to reach his or her legs, feet, and back. A wash mitt and soap on a rope can aid limited grasp. Putting a bar of soap in the foot of nylon pantyhose makes it easier to grasp.
3. A position-adjustable hair dryer may be helpful for those who prefer a hairstyle more elaborate than one that can be air-dried.[15] This device is useful for clients with limited ROM, upper extremity weakness, incoordination, and use of only one upper extremity. The dryer is adapted from a desk lamp with spring-balanced arms and a tension control knob at each joint. The lamp is removed and the hair dryer is fastened to the spring-balanced arms. The device is mounted on a table or countertop and can be adjusted for various heights and direction of airflow. This frees the client's hands to style his or her hair with brushes or combs. Specifications are available for constructing this device.[8] This product is also available commercially under the name Hands-Free Hair Dryer Pro Stand 2000

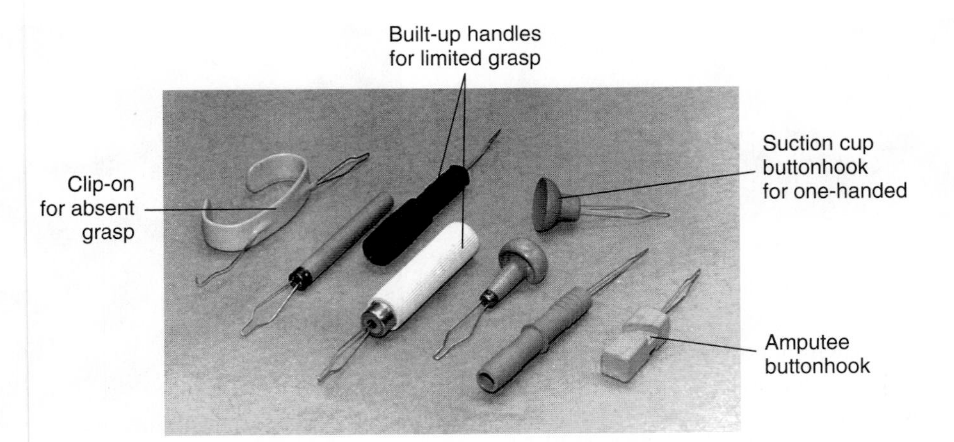

Figure 13-8 Buttonhooks to accommodate limited grasp, special types of grasp, or amputation.

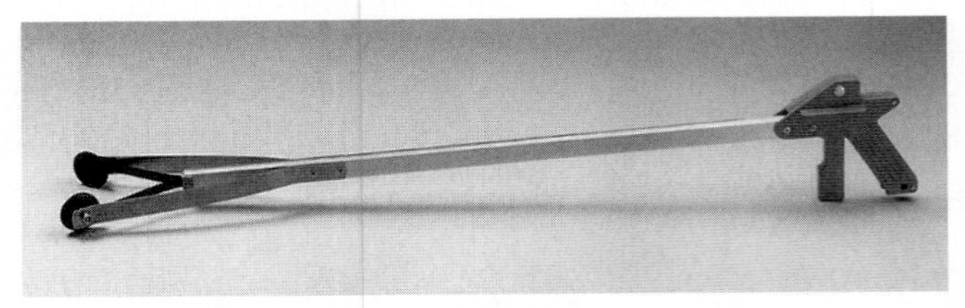

Figure 13-9 Extended-handle reacher.

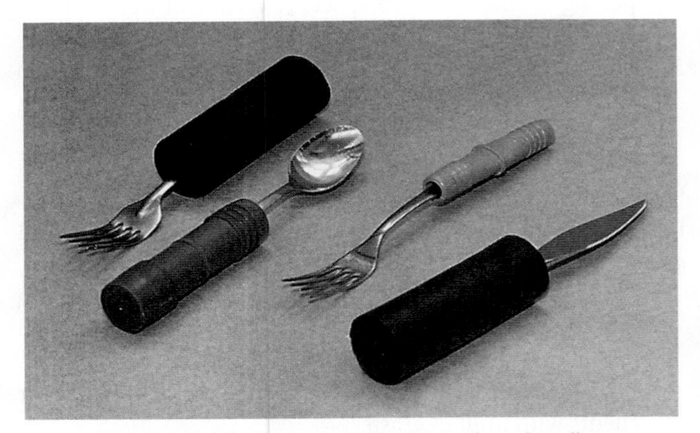

Figure 13-10 Eating utensils with built-up handles.

from rehabilitation product catalogs and infomercials on television.[37,49]

4. Long handles on a comb, brush, toothbrush, lipstick, mascara brush, and safety or electric razor may be useful for patients who have limited hand-to-head or hand-to-face movements. Extensions may be constructed from inexpensive wooden dowels or pieces of PVC pipe found in hardware stores.
5. Spray deodorant, hair spray, and spray powder or perfume can extend the reach by the distance the material sprays. Some persons may require special adaptations to operate the spray mechanism (Figure 13-14).
6. Electric toothbrushes and the Water-Pik system may be easier to manage than a standard toothbrush. Cylindrical foam to enlarge the toothbrush handle may help with grasp. Flossing aids decrease the need to directly handle and manipulate dental floss.[19]

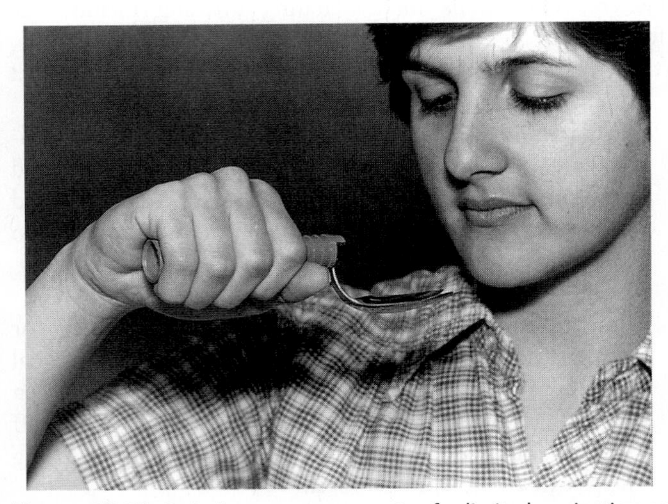

Figure 13-11 Swivel spoon compensates for limited supination or incoordination.

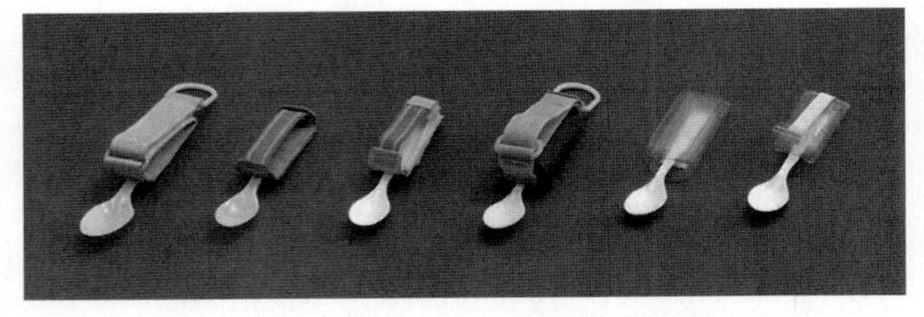

Figure 13-12 Utensil holders/universal cuffs. (Courtesy Sammons, a BISSELL Co.)

7. A short reacher can extend reach for using toilet paper. Several types of toilet tissue aids or tongs are available in catalogs of assistive devices.[5,17]
8. Dressing sticks can be used to pull garments up after using the toilet.
9. Safety rails (Figure 13-15) can be used for bathtub transfers, and safety mats or strips can be placed in the bathtub bottom to prevent slipping.
10. A transfer tub bench (see Figure 13-5), shower stool, or regular chair set in the bathtub or shower stall can eliminate the need to sit on the bathtub bottom or stand to shower, thus increasing safety.
11. Grab bars can be installed to prevent falls and to ease transfers.

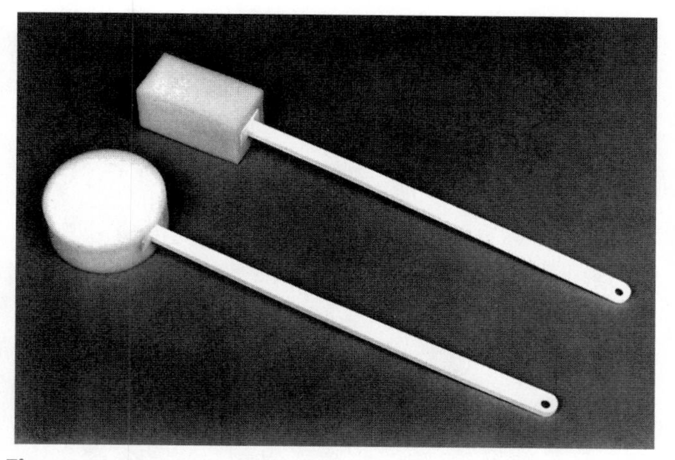

Figure 13-13 Long-handled bath sponges. (Courtesy Sammons, a BISSELL Co.)

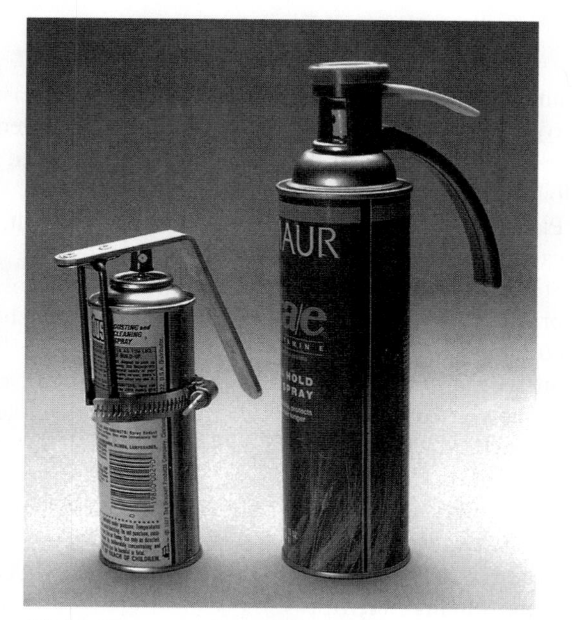

Figure 13-14 Spray can adapters. (Courtesy Sammons, a BISSELL Co.)

Communication and General Environment

Adaptations that can facilitate communication and use of common household fixtures include the following:

1. Telephones should be placed within easy reach. A clip-type receiver holder (Figure 13-16), extended receiver holder, large-button phone, speakerphone, or voice-activated phone may be necessary. Dialing sticks and push-button phones are other adaptations. Teach your patients how to store emergency contact and frequently dialed telephone numbers into the one-touch dialing feature. Use a blue tooth or wireless headset to allow for hands-free conversations. The Public Utilities Commission can often provide free telephones for landlines with adaptive features through the Deaf and Disabled Telecommunication Program.
2. Built-up pens and pencils with cylindrical foam to accommodate limited grasp and prehension can be used. A Wanchik writer and several other commercially available or custom-fabricated writing aids are helpful (Figure 13-17).

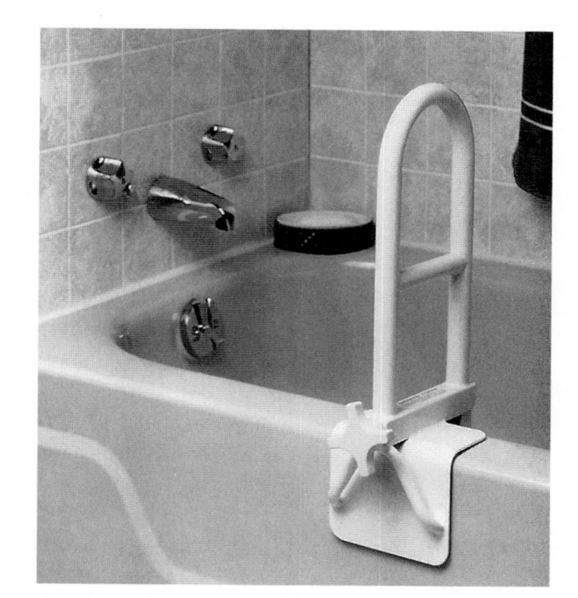

Figure 13-15 Bathtub safety rail. (Courtesy Sammons, a BISSELL Co.)

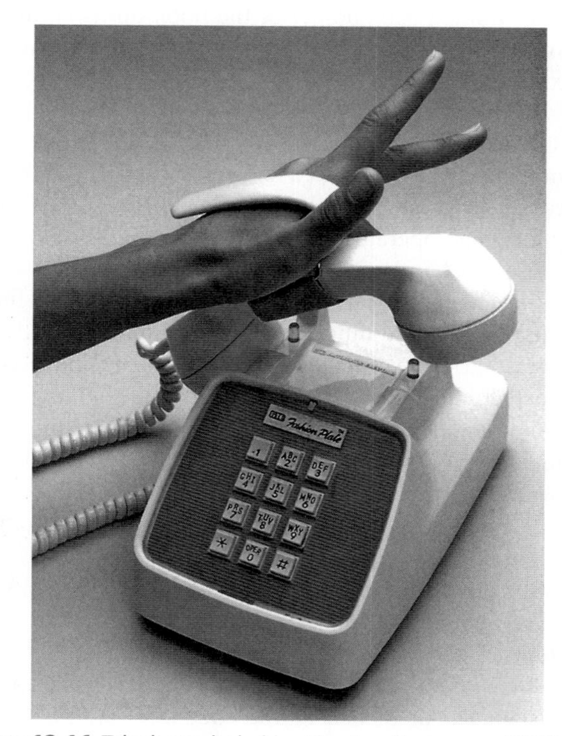

Figure 13-16 Telephone clip holder. (Courtesy Sammons, a BISSELL Co.)

3. Speech-recognition software such as Dragon Naturally Speaking from ScanSoft turns speech into text and can facilitate communication for those with limited or painful joints.[38]
4. A slip-on typing aid attached with a Velcro strip around the palm has a pointer under the index finger and requires minimal hand strength to use.
5. Lever-type doorknob extensions (Figure 13-18), car door openers, and adapted key holders can compensate for hand limitations.

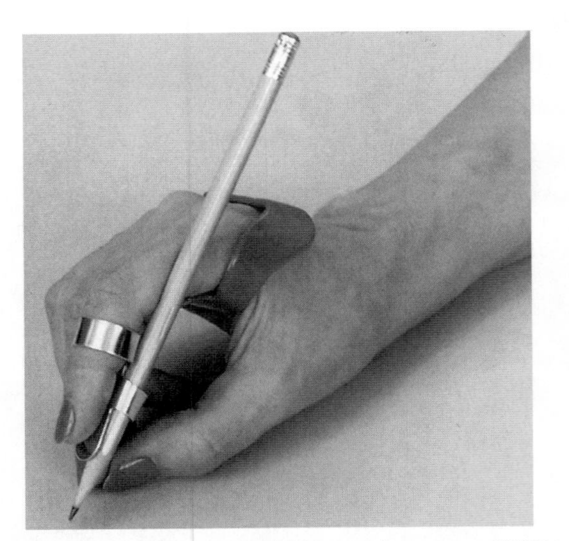

Figure 13-17 Wanchik writing aid. (Courtesy Sammons, a BISSELL Co.)

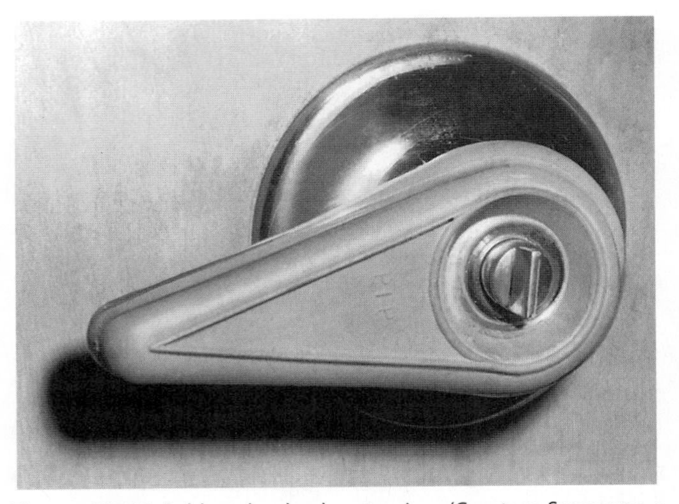

Figure 13-18 Rubber doorknob extension. (Courtesy Sammons, a BISSELL Co.)

6. Extended or built-up handles on faucets can accommodate limited grasp.
7. A wire-framed book holder or the Book Butler eliminates prolonged grasping of a book by holding the book open at a comfortable angle.[37,49]

Mobility and Transfers

The individual who has limited ROM *without* significant muscle weakness may benefit from the following assistive devices:

1. A glider chair operated by the feet can make transportation easier if hip, hand, and arm motions are limited.
2. Platform crutches can prevent stress on hand or finger joints and can accommodate limited grasp.
3. Enlarged grips on crutches, canes, and walkers can accommodate limited grasp.
4. A raised toilet seat can be used if hip and knee motion is limited.
5. A walker with padded grips and forearm troughs can be used if marked hand, forearm, or elbow joint limitations are a problem.
6. A walker or crutch bag and basket can carry objects. Some baskets include beverage holders.
7. A *transfer handle* at the side of the bed and a *couch-cane* allow clients to grasp onto the handles for leverage when transferring out of bed or the couch.[37,49] Adding furniture lifters or blocks to the legs of chairs, couches, or beds increases the height of the furniture and makes it easier to stand from or transfer to another surface.

Home Management Skills

Home management activities can be made easier by a variety of environmental adaptations, assistive devices, energy conservation methods, and work simplification techniques.[28,46] Persons with rheumatoid arthritis should use the principles of joint protection (see Chapter 29). Energy conservation allows patients to perform the same task while expending less energy. Using these principles, patients with weakness due to cardiac and/or pulmonary disorders can perform daily tasks while placing less demand on the body.[6] The demands on the body are measured by oxygen saturation levels and pulse rates. Home management for persons with limited ROM can be eased and improved with the following energy conservation principles:

1. Plan ahead. By managing time and pacing yourself, you can limit the need for excessive motions.
2. Store frequently used items on counters when possible or on the first shelves of cabinets (just above and below counters).
3. Sit whenever possible. Use a high stool to work comfortably at counter height. Alternatively, if a wheelchair is used, attach a drop-leaf table to the wall for meal preparation.
4. Use a utility cart of comfortable height to transport several items at once.
5. Use a reacher to pull down lightweight items (e.g., a cereal box) from high shelves.
6. Stabilize mixing bowls and dishes with nonslip mats.
7. Use lightweight utensils such as plastic or aluminum bowls and aluminum pots.
8. Use electric can openers and electric mixers.
9. The Black & Decker automatic jar opener opens jars of all sizes with the push of a button.[37,49]
10. Use adapted knives, electric scissors, or adapted loop scissors that are self-opening to open boxes or bags instead of tearing them open with your fingers (Figure 13-19).
11. Eliminate bending by using extended, flexible plastic handles on dust mops, brooms, and dustpans.
12. Use pull-out shelves to organize cupboards and eliminate bending.
13. Eliminate bending by using wall ovens, countertop broilers, and microwave ovens.
14. Eliminate leaning and bending by using a top-loading automatic washer and elevated dryer and a reacher. Wheelchair users can more easily operate front-loading appliances than other types.
15. Use an adjustable ironing board to make it possible to sit while ironing.

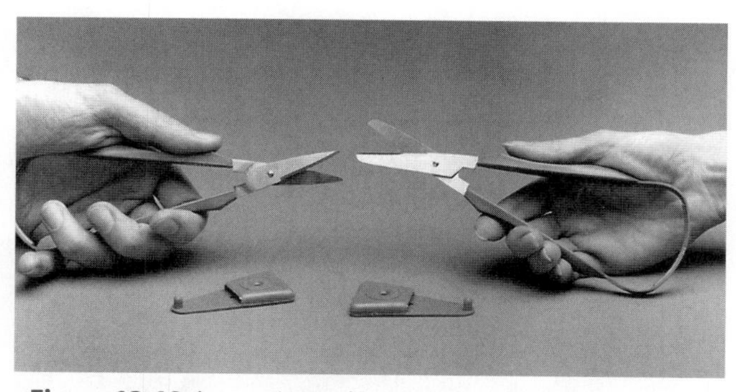

Figure 13-19 Loop scissors. (Courtesy Sammons, a BISSELL Co.)

16. For childcare by the ambulatory parent or caregiver, elevate the playpen and diaper table and use a bathinette or a plastic tub on the kitchen counter for bathing. These adaptations reduce the amount of bending and reaching. The crib mattress can be in a raised position until the child is 3 or 4 months old.
17. Use large, loose-fitting garments with hook and loop (Velcro) fastenings on children.
18. Use a reacher to pick up clothing and children's toys from the floor.

Problems of Incoordination

Incoordination can result from a variety of central nervous system (CNS) disorders such as Parkinson's disease, multiple sclerosis, cerebral palsy, and traumatic brain injuries (TBIs). Incoordination may take the form of tremors, ataxia, or athetoid or choreiform movements. Persons with incoordination may have difficulty maintaining safety and achieving adequate stability of gait, body parts, and objects to complete ADL.

Fatigue, emotional factors, and fears may increase the severity of incoordinated movement. The client must be taught appropriate energy conservation and work simplification techniques, along with appropriate work pacing and safety methods. The client who learns to avoid and reduce fatigue and fear will perform tasks better and with increased coordination.

The incoordinated individual with reasonable muscle strength can use weighted devices to help stabilize objects. A Velcro-fastened weight can be attached to the client's arm to decrease tremors and ataxia. Objects such as eating utensils, pens, and cups can be weighted.

Another technique that can be used throughout all ADL tasks is stabilizing the upper part of the involved upper extremity. This stabilization is accomplished by propping the elbow on a counter or tabletop, pivoting from the elbow and moving only the forearm, wrist, and hand in the activity. Stabilizing the arm reduces some of the incoordination and may allow the individual to accomplish gross and fine motor movements without assistive devices.[1,30,53] Stabilizing the trunk using seating positioning devices can greatly increase the fine coordination of the upper extremity (refer to Chapter 15).

Dressing Activities

Dressing difficulties encountered with incoordination can be reduced by using the following adaptations:

1. Front-opening garments that fit loosely can facilitate donning and removing garments.
2. Large buttons, Velcro, or zippers with loops on the tab can ease opening and closing fasteners. A buttonhook with a large, weighted handle may be helpful.
3. Elastic shoelaces, Velcro closures, other adapted shoe closures, and slip-on shoes eliminate the need for bow tying.
4. Trousers with elastic tops for women or Velcro closures for men are easier to manage than those with hooks, buttons, and zippers.
5. Brassieres with front openings or Velcro replacements for the usual hook and eye may be used with more ease. A slipover athletic-style elastic brassiere purchased one size larger may eliminate the need to manage brassiere fastenings. Regular (back-fastening) brassieres may be fastened in front at waist level and then slipped around to the back. Next the arms are put into the straps, which are worked up over the shoulders. Adaptive bras such as the "Sara bra" or the "Ability Bra" are easy to don for woman with poor coordination or limited hand and shoulder movement.
6. Men can wear clip-on ties. Alternatively, if the tie is stored loosely tied, it may be donned over the head and secured in place.
7. To compensate for balance problems and impaired fine motor control, dressing should be performed while sitting on or in the bed, in a wheelchair, or in a chair with arms.

Eating Activities

For clients with problems of incoordination, eating can be a challenge. Lack of control during eating is not only frustrating but also can cause embarrassment and social rejection. Therefore making eating safe, pleasurable, and as neat as possible is important. Some suggestions for achieving this goal include the following:

1. Use plate stabilizers such as nonskid mats, suction bases, Dycem, or damp dishtowels.
2. Use a plate guard or scoop dish to prevent food being pushed off the plate. The plate guard can be taken from home and clipped to any ordinary dinner plate (Figure 13-20).
3. Prevent spills during the plate-to-mouth movement by using weighted or swivel utensils to offer stability. Weighted cuffs may be placed on the forearm to decrease involuntary movements or tremors (Figure 13-21).
4. To eliminate the need to carry the glass or cup to the mouth (which may cause spills), use long plastic straws with a straw clip on a glass or cup with a weighted bottom. Plastic cups or hot beverage travel containers with covers and spouts can also reduce spills.
5. Use a resistance or friction-type arm brace similar to a mobile arm support to help control patterns of involuntary movement during feeding activities of adults with cerebral palsy and athetosis.[22] This brace may help many clients with severe incoordination to achieve some degree of independence in feeding.

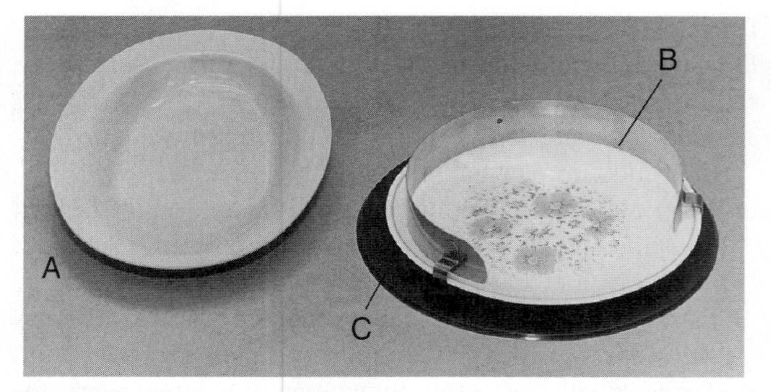

Figure 13-20 **A,** Scoop dish. **B,** Plate with plate guard. **C,** Nonskid mat.

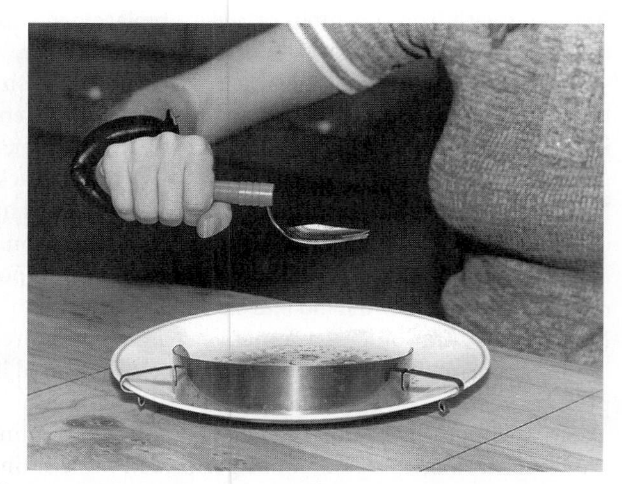

Figure 13-21 Weighted wrist cuff and swivel utensil can sometimes compensate for incoordination or involuntary motion.

Hygiene and Grooming

The following techniques can help a client stabilize and manipulate toilet articles:

1. If dropping is a problem, articles such as a razor, lipstick, and toothbrush can be attached to a cord. Small strips of rubber or friction tape placed around the objects help support the grasp. An electric toothbrush may be more easily managed than a regular one.
2. Weighted wrist cuffs may be helpful during hygiene activities requiring fine motor coordination such as applying makeup, shaving, and hair care.
3. The position-adjustable hair dryer described earlier for clients with limited ROM can be useful for those with incoordination as well.[15]
4. An electric razor rather than a blade razor offers stability and safety. A strap around the razor and the hand or neck can prevent dropping.
5. A suction nailbrush attached to the sink or counter can be used for nail or denture care (Figure 13-22).
6. Soap should be on a rope and can be worn around the neck (if safe for the particular client) or hung over bathtub or shower fixtures during the bath or shower to keep it within easy reach. A leg from a pair of pantyhose tied over a faucet, with a bar of soap in the toe, will stretch for use and keep soap within reach. Also, liquid soap bottles with a pump dispenser can be secured near the faucet. Consider securing these dispensers to the wall or having them built into the shower or vanity of the bathroom.

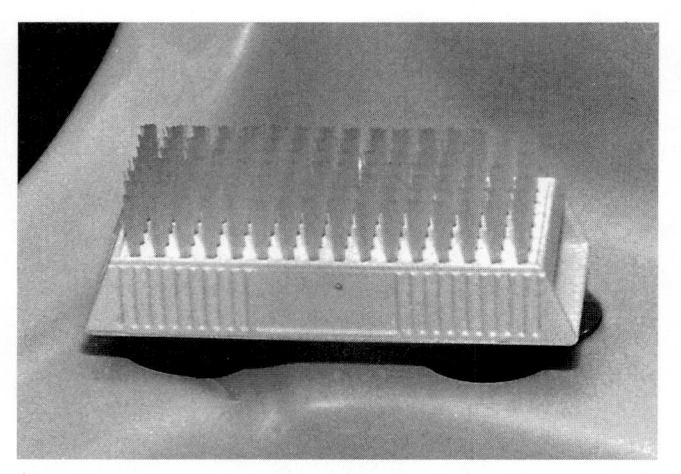

Figure 13-22 Suction brush attached to bathroom sink for dentures or fingernails. Brush can also be used in kitchen to wash vegetables and fruit.

7. An emery board or small piece of wood with fine sandpaper glued to it can be fastened to the tabletop for filing nails. A nail clipper can also be stabilized in the same manner.
8. Large-size roll-on or cream deodorants are controlled more easily than sprays.
9. Sanitary pads that stick to undergarments may be easier to manage than tampons.
10. A bath mitt with a pocket to hold the soap can be used for washing and eliminates the need for frequent soaping and for rinsing and wringing a washcloth.

The following recommendations can greatly increase safety during bathing. Nonskid mats should be used inside and outside the bathtub during bathing. Their suction bases should be fastened securely to the floor and bathtub before use. Safety grab bars should be installed on the wall next to the bathtub or fastened to the edge of the bathtub. Sitting on a bathtub seat or shower chair is safer than standing while showering or transferring to a bathtub bottom. Many uncoordinated clients require supervisory assistance during bathing. Sponge bathing while seated at a bathroom sink may substitute for bathing or showering several times a week.

Communication and General Environment

Adaptations that can facilitate communication and the use of common household fixtures by clients with incoordination include the following:

1. Doorknobs may be managed more easily if adapted with lever-type handles or covered with rubber or friction tape (see Figure 13-18).
2. A holder or headset for a telephone receiver, large-button phones, preprogrammed phone numbers, or speakerphones may be helpful. Voice-activated dialing is a convenient feature on most cellular phones.
3. Writing can be managed with a weighted, enlarged pencil or pen and securing the paper with a clipboard or tape. The

Wrist Hold-Down consists of a magnetized work surface and magnetized cups attached to the wrist to provide stability for writing or drawing.[49] Computer adaptations in software and types of keyboards and mice are discussed in Chapter 14.

4. Keys can be placed on an adapted rigid key holder that extends leverage for turning the key. However, inserting the key in the keyhole may be very difficult unless the incoordination is relatively mild. Changing the lock to require a combination or remote control button eliminates the need to retrieve and manipulate the keys.
5. Extended lever-type faucets are easier to manage than push-pull spigots and knobs. To prevent burns during bathing and kitchen activities, cold water should be turned on first and hot water added gradually. External temperature controls can be added directly to the water heater to prevent water from reaching scalding hot temperatures. These controls are considered environmentally friendly and are easy to install.
6. Lamps can be wired with switches that respond to light touch or to a remote signal. Wall switches can also eliminate the need to turn a small switch manually. Environmental control units or electronic aids to daily living (EADL) provide power to specific electronic devices throughout the home in one centralized and easily accessible area. Refer to Chapter 15 for more information.

Mobility and Transfers

Clients with problems of incoordination may use a variety of ambulation aids, depending on the type and severity of incoordination. Sometimes the OT practitioner must help the client with degenerative diseases to recognize the need for ambulation aids and accept their use. This may mean switching from a cane to crutches to a walker and finally to a wheelchair for some persons. Clients with incoordination can improve stability and mobility by using the following techniques:

1. Instead of lifting objects, slide them on counters or tabletops.
2. Use ambulation aids as appropriate.
3. Use a utility cart, preferably a custom-made cart that is heavy and has some friction on the wheels.
4. Remove door sills, throw rugs, and thick carpeting.
5. Install banisters on indoor and outdoor staircases with hand rails on both sides if possible.
6. Substitute ramps for stairs wherever possible.

Home Management Activities

The OT practitioner should make a careful assessment of homemaking activities performance to determine the following: (1) which activities can be done safely; (2) which activities can be done safely if modified or adapted; and (3) which activities cannot be done adequately or safely and therefore should be assigned to someone else. The major problem areas are stabilization of foods and equipment to prevent spilling and accidents and the safe handling of appliances, pots, pans, and household tools to prevent cuts, burns, bruises, electric shock, and falls. Suggestions for improving safety and function in home management tasks include the following[28,30,54]:

1. Use a wheelchair and wheelchair lapboard (even if ambulation is possible with devices). This saves energy and increases stability when balance and gait are unsteady.
2. If possible, use convenience and prepared foods to eliminate processes such as peeling, chopping, slicing, and mixing.
3. Use easy-open containers or store foods in plastic containers.
4. Use heavy utensils, mixing bowls, and pots and pans to increase stability.
5. Try using various types of jar openers including wall-mounted and portable.
6. Use nonskid mats on work surfaces. Line the kitchen sink with rubber mat cushions to prevent items from sliding or breaking.
7. Use electric appliances such as crockpots, electric fry pans, electric tea kettles, toaster ovens, and microwave ovens because they are safer to use than the range or oven.
8. Use a blender and countertop mixer because they are safer than handheld mixers and easier than mixing with a spoon or whisk.
9. If possible, adjust work heights of counters, sink, and range to minimize leaning, bending, reaching, and lifting, whether the client is standing or using a wheelchair. Use a stool at the counter to increase balance and stability.
10. Use long oven mitts, which give greater protection than potholders.
11. Use lightweight pots, pans, casserole dishes, and appliances with bilateral handles because they may be easier to hold and manage than those with one handle.
12. Use a cutting board with stainless steel nails (Figure 13-23) to stabilize meats, potatoes, and vegetables while cutting or peeling. When the cutting board is not in use, the nails should be covered with a large cork. To prevent slipping, the bottom of the board should have suction cups, be covered with stair tread, or be placed on a nonskid mat.
13. Use heavy dinnerware, which offers stability and control to the distal part of the upper extremity and may be easier to handle. If dropping and breaking are problems, durable plastic dinnerware may be more practical.
14. Cover the sink, utility cart, and countertops with protective rubber mats or mesh matting to stabilize items.
15. Use a serrated knife for cutting and chopping because it is easier to control.
16. To eliminate the need to carry and drain pots of hot liquids, use a steamer basket or deep-fry basket for preparing boiled foods.
17. Use tongs to turn foods during cooking and to serve foods because tongs offer more control and stability than a fork, spatula, or serving spoon.
18. Use a *bottle tipper* to safely pour liquids. Velcro straps hold the bottle into a wire frame while the client controls the tipping angle by pulling down on the wire frame until liquid slowly streams out of the bottle.[37,49]
19. Use blunt-ended loop scissors to open packages.

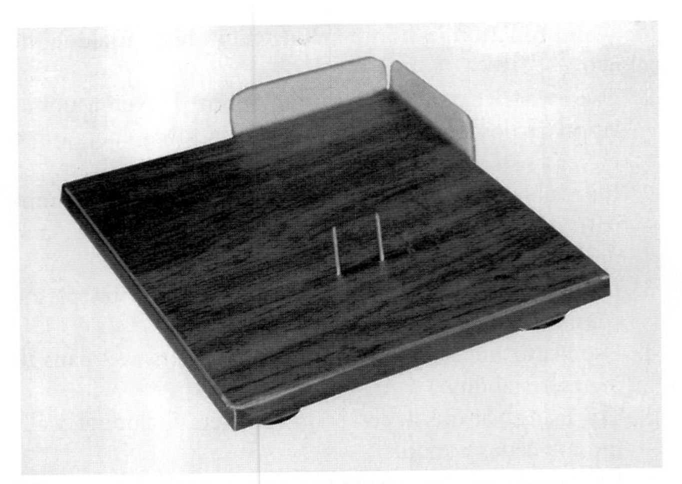

Figure 13-23 Cutting board with stainless-steel nails, suction-cup feet, and corner for stabilizing bread is useful for patients with incoordination or lacking use of one hand. (Courtesy Sammons, a BISSELL Co.)

20. The ambulatory client may find vacuuming easier with a heavy upright cleaner. The wheelchair user may be able to manage a lightweight tank-type vacuum cleaner or electric broom.
21. Use dust mitts or old athletic socks for dusting.
22. Avoid displaying objects that are easily broken or difficult to manage such as fragile knickknacks, unstable lamps, and dainty doilies.
23. Eliminate ironing by using no-iron fabrics, timed dryer, or spray-on Downy Wrinkle Releaser. Alternatively, assign this task to other members of the household.
24. Use front-loading washers, a laundry cart on wheels, and premeasured detergents, bleaches, and fabric softeners. Purex makes three-in-one laundry "sheets" that include detergent, fabric softener, and antistatic. This product is light and reduces the need for heavy lifting, pouring, and measuring.[45]
25. Sit while working with an infant. Use foam-rubber bath aids; an infant bath seat; and a wide, padded dressing table with safety straps with Velcro fastening to offer enough stability for bathing, dressing, and diapering an infant. Childcare may not be safe for individuals with significant incoordination difficulties.
26. Use disposable diapers with tape or Velcro fasteners because they are easier to manage than cloth diapers and pins.
27. Do not feed the infant with a spoon or fork unless the incoordination is mild or does not affect the upper extremities.
28. Dress the child in clothing that is large, loose, stretchy, nonslippery, and fastened with Velcro.

Hemiplegia or Use of Only One Upper Extremity

It is tempting but misleading to classify together all conditions that may result in the dysfunction of one upper extremity. Unilateral upper extremity amputations and temporary disorders such as fractures, burns, and peripheral neuropathy may lead to unilateral upper extremity dysfunction. Patients with unilateral upper extremity dysfunction resulting from such disorders are likely to learn compensatory techniques quickly and easily if they have normal functioning of sensory, perceptual, and cognitive systems. These patients may benefit from a few suggestions to help with ADL while they recover from the injury. However, hemiplegia is the most commonly seen diagnosis in which unilateral upper extremity dysfunction occurs, and this diagnosis requires a different approach.

Clients with hemiplegia require specialized methods of teaching; many have greater difficulty learning and performing one-handed skills than do persons with orthopedic or lower motor neuron dysfunction. The reason for this is that the head, trunk, and leg, as well as the arm, are involved; consequently, ambulation and balance difficulties may be impaired. Lack of trunk control reduces coordination of the distal upper extremity for ADL tasks. In addition, sensory, perceptual, cognitive, and speech disorders may affect the ability to learn and retain learning and performance. Finally, the presence of motor and ideational apraxia sometimes seen in this group of patients can limit their potential for learning new motor skills and remembering previous ones. The client with hemiplegia needs to be evaluated for sensory, perceptual, and cognitive deficits to determine potential for ADL performance and to establish appropriate teaching methods to facilitate learning.

The major problems for the one-handed worker are reduced work speed and dexterity and poor stabilization, a function usually assumed by the nondominant arm. The major problems for the client with hemiplegia are unsteady balance and the risk of injury because of sensory and perceptual loss.[1,28,30,32,33] *One-Handed in a Two-Handed World*[33] by Tommy K. Mayer is a good resource book for teaching ADL adaptations.

Dressing Activities

Individuals with hemiplegia may have difficulty donning and removing the clothing they wore before their disability. Suggestions for slight modifications of clothing are made throughout the following discussion on dressing. Exploring options in adaptive clothing can help individuals maintain independence and dignity, and the caregiver can assist with dressing without as much lifting and repositioning of the patient. A number of websites including www.easyaccessclothing.com sell adaptive clothing and provide ideas for patients to make modifications to their own clothing. Examples of adaptive clothing include button-down shirts that open or close with Velcro tabs, pants with extended Velcro flies to allow for easy access when using a urinal or catheter, seams sewn flat to help prevent pressure sores, wrist or finger loops to help individuals lift garments when dressing, and coats with cut-out backs to eliminate sitting on excess fabric that may get caught in the wheelchair spokes or cause pressure sores. The addition of a zipper opening at the side seams from ankle to waist allows the individual to wear fitted pants without struggling to don or doff them. This concept is helpful for fitted blazers, with a zipper forming a side opening down the length of the sleeves. These solutions can be introduced to a local tailor so that discrete modifications can be added to the individual's current wardrobe to help increase safety and dressing ease.

If balance is a problem, the client should dress while seated in a locked wheelchair or sturdy armchair. Clothing should be within easy reach. Reaching tongs may be helpful for securing articles and assisting in some dressing activities. Dressing and other ADL should be approached with a minimum of assistive devices.

One-Handed Dressing Techniques

Some dressing techniques for the client with hemiplegia employ neurodevelopmental (Bobath) treatment principles. The following one-handed dressing techniques can facilitate dressing for clients with use of one upper extremity. As a general rule, place the affected extremity in the garment first when dressing and remove last when undressing. This procedure allows more room to work with the garment when motor control is most impaired.

Shirts Front-opening shirts may be managed by any one of three methods. The first method can be used for jackets, robes, and front-opening dresses.

Method 1: Basic Over Head—Donning (Figure 13-24)

1. Grasp shirt collar with unaffected hand and shake out twists *(A)*.
2. Position shirt on lap with inside facing up and collar toward chest *(B)*.
3. Position sleeve opening on affected side so that it is as large as possible and close to the affected hand, which is resting on lap *(C)*.
4. Using unaffected hand, place affected hand in sleeve opening and work sleeve over elbow by pulling on garment *(D1, D2)*. Ensuring the sleeve is placed over the elbow will prevent shoulder injuries when placing the shirt over the head.
5. Put unaffected arm into its sleeve and raise up to slide or shake sleeve into position past elbow *(E)*.
6. With unaffected hand, gather shirt up middle of back from hem to collar and raise shirt overhead *(F)*.
7. Lean forward, duck head, and pass shirt over it *(G)*.
8. With unaffected hand, adjust shirt by leaning forward and working it down past both shoulders. Reach in back and pull shirttail down *(H)*.
9. Line shirt fronts up for buttoning and begin with bottom button *(I)*. Button sleeve cuff of affected arm. The sleeve cuff of unaffected arm may be prebuttoned if cuff opening is large.

A button may be sewn on with elastic thread or sewn onto a small tab of elastic and fastened inside shirt cuff. A small button attached to a crocheted loop of elastic thread is another alternative. Also, a cuff and collar extender can be added. Slip the button on loop through buttonhole in the garment so that the elastic loop is inside. Stretch the elastic loop to fit around original cuff button. This simple device can be transferred to each garment and positioned before the shirt is put on. The loop stretches to accommodate the width of the hand as it is pushed through the end of the sleeve.[50] Warning: Self-buttoning is a labor-intensive and frustrating task for patients with hemiplegia. Encourage these patients to wear a larger shirt and keep most buttons fastened before donning. Patients with hemiplegia may find it easier to button before donning or to have a caregiver arrange clothing fastened ahead of time.

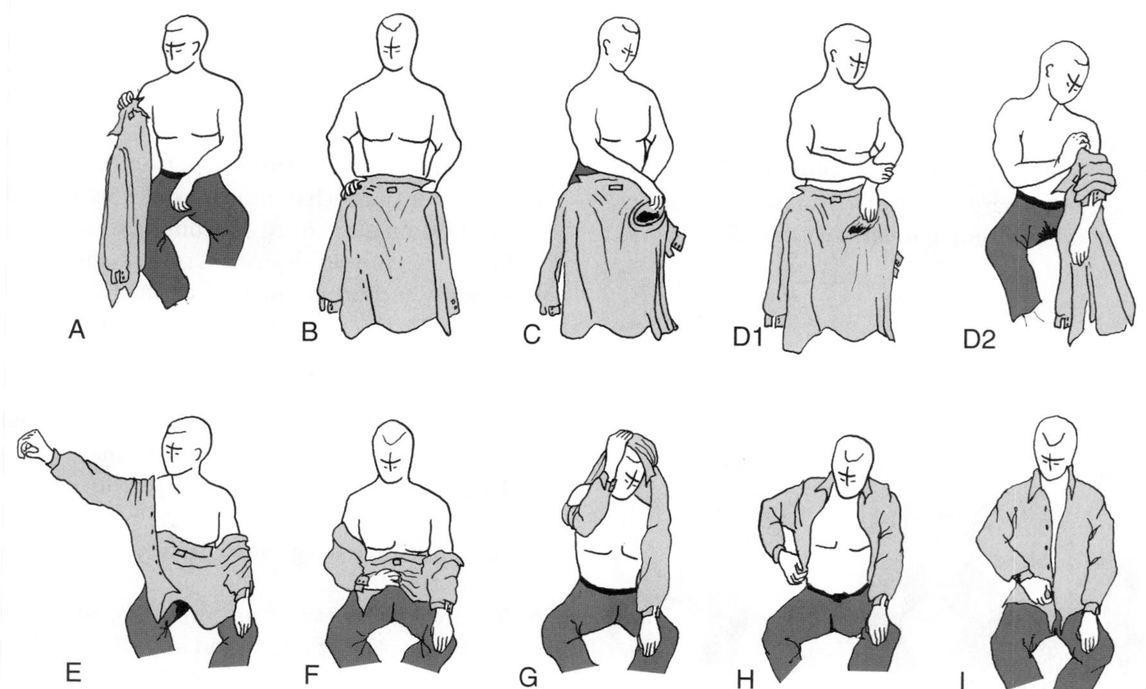

Figure 13-24 Steps in donning shirt: method 1 (basic over head). (Courtesy Christine Shaw, Metro Health Center for Rehabilitation, Metro Health Medical Center, Cleveland, Ohio.)

Method 1: Basic Over Head—Removing

1. Unbutton shirt.
2. Lean forward.
3. With unaffected hand, grasp collar or gather material up in back from collar to hem.
4. Lean forward, duck head, and pull shirt over head.
5. Remove sleeve from unaffected arm and then from affected arm.

Method 2: Over Head On/Shrug off—Donning. Method 2 may be used by clients who have shirt twisted or have trouble sliding the sleeve down onto unaffected arm.

1. Position shirt as described in method 1, steps 1 to 3.
2. With unaffected hand, place involved hand into shirt sleeve opening and work sleeve onto hand, but do *not* pull up over elbow.
3. Put unaffected arm into sleeve and bring arm out to 180 degrees of abduction. Tension of fabric from unaffected arm to wrist of affected arm will bring sleeve into position.
4. Lower arm and work sleeve on affected arm up over elbow.
5. Continue as in steps 6 to 9 of method 1 on p. 257.

Method 2: Over Head/Shrug off—Removing

1. Unbutton shirt.
2. With unaffected hand, push shirt off shoulders, first on affected side, then on unaffected side.
3. Pull on cuff of unaffected side with unaffected hand.
4. Work sleeve off by alternately shrugging shoulder and pulling down on cuff.
5. Lean forward, bring shirt around back, and pull sleeve off affected arm.

Method 3: Over Shoulder—Donning (Figure 13-25)

1. Position shirt and work onto arm as described in method 1, steps 1 to 4.
2. Pull sleeve on affected arm up to shoulder *(A)*.
3. With unaffected hand, grasp tip of collar that is on unaffected side, lean forward, and bring arm over and behind head to carry shirt around to unaffected side *(B)*.
4. Put unaffected arm into sleeve opening, directing it up and out *(C)*.
5. Adjust and button as described in method 1, steps 8 and 9.

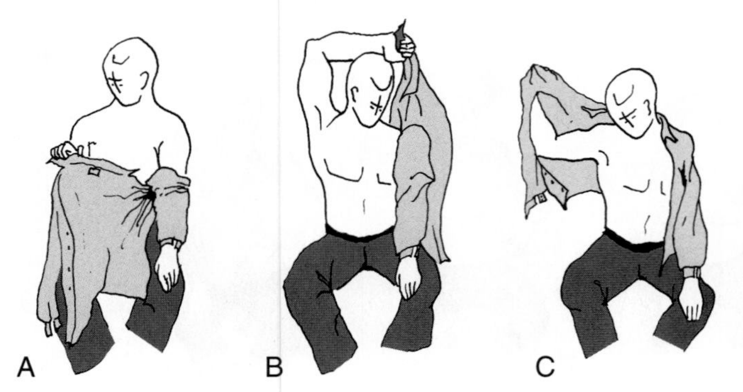

Figure 13-25 Steps in donning shirt: method 3 (over shoulder). (Courtesy Christine Shaw, Metro Health Center for Rehabilitation, Metro Health Medical Center, Cleveland, Ohio.)

Method 3: Over Shoulder—Removing. The shirt may be removed using the same procedure described for method 2.

Method 4: Donning Pullover Shirt (Over Head)

1. Position shirt on lap, with bottom toward chest and label facing down.
2. With unaffected hand, roll up bottom edge of shirt back up to sleeve on affected side.
3. Position sleeve opening so that it is as large as possible, and use unaffected hand to place affected hand into sleeve opening. Pull shirt up onto arm past elbow.
4. Insert unaffected arm into sleeve.
5. Adjust shirt on affected side up and onto shoulder.
6. Gather shirt back with unaffected hand, lean forward, duck head, and pass shirt over head.
7. Adjust shirt.

Method 4: Removing Pullover Shirt (Over Head)

1. Gather shirt up with unaffected hand, starting at top back.
2. Lean forward, duck head, and pull gathered fabric in back over head.
3. Remove from unaffected arm and then affected arm.

Trousers. Trousers may be managed by one of the following methods, which can be adapted for shorts and women's panties as well. Velcro or elastic may replace buttons and zippers. Trousers should be worn in a size slightly larger than worn previously and should have a wide opening at the ankles. They should be put on before the socks and shoes. Feet can slip forward when attempting to stand if the person is wearing socks; a bare foot has better traction. The client who is dressing in a wheelchair should place feet flat on the floor, not on the footrests of the wheelchair.

Method 1: Partial Standing—Donning (Figure 13-26)

1. Sit in sturdy armchair or in locked wheelchair *(A)*.
2. Position unaffected leg in front of midline of body with knee flexed to 90 degrees. Using unaffected hand, reach forward and grasp ankle of affected leg or sock around ankle *(B1)*. Lift affected leg over unaffected leg to crossed position *(B2)*.
3. Slip trousers onto affected leg up to position where foot is completely inside of trouser leg *(C)*. Do not pull up above knee, or it will be difficult inserting unaffected leg.
4. Uncross affected leg by grasping ankle or portion of sock around ankle *(D)*.
5. Insert unaffected leg and work trousers up onto hips as far as possible *(E1, E2)*.
6. To prevent trousers from dropping when pulling pants over hips, place affected hand in pocket or place one finger of affected hand into belt loop. If able to do so safely, stand and pull trousers over hips *(F1, F2)*.
7. If standing balance is good, remain standing to pull up zipper or button *(F3)*. Sit down to button front *(G)*.

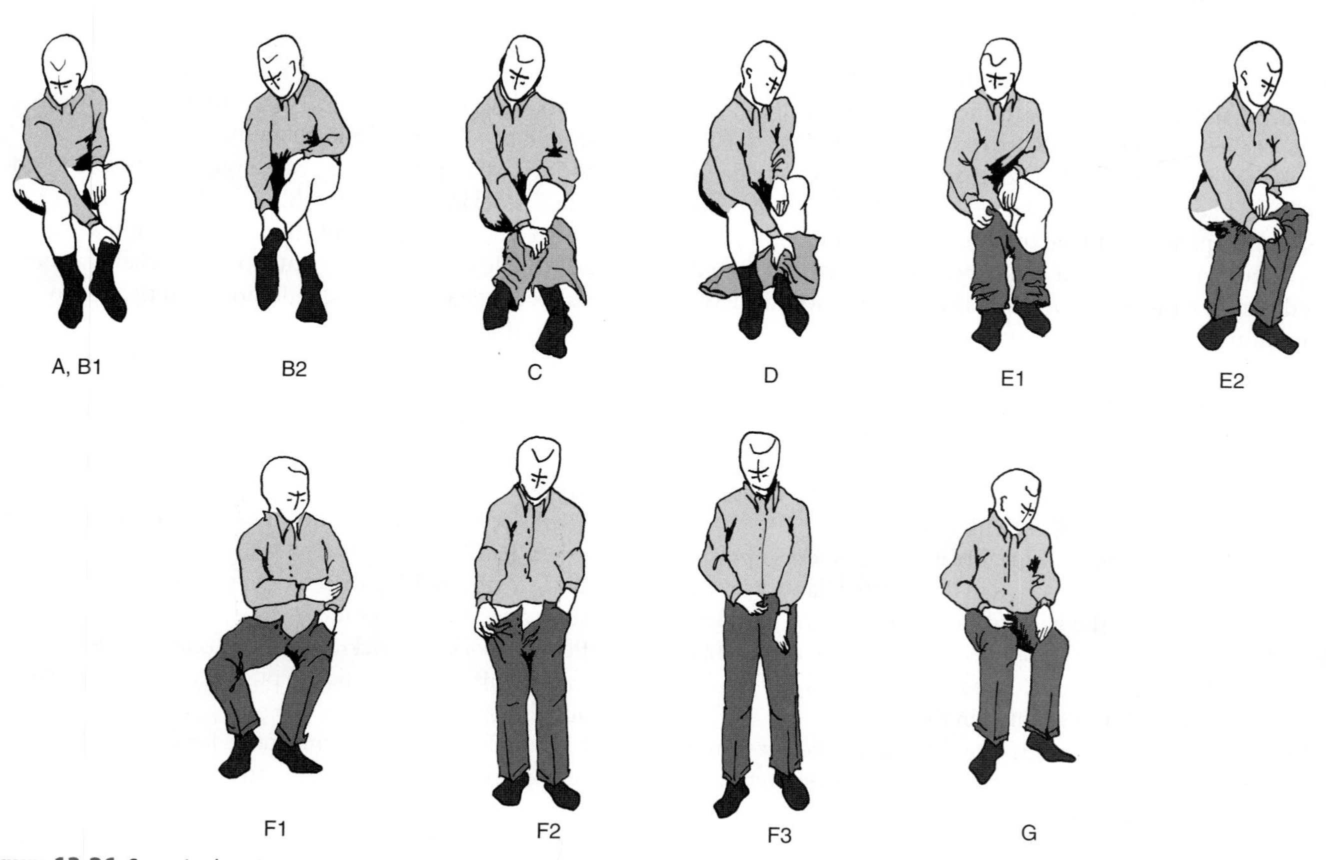

Figure 13-26 Steps in donning trousers: method 1 (partial standing). (Courtesy Christine Shaw, Metro Health Medical Center, Cleveland, Ohio.)

Method 1: Partial Standing—Removing

1. Unfasten trousers and work down on hips as far as possible while seated.
2. Stand, letting trousers drop past hips or work them down past hips.
3. Sit and remove trousers from unaffected leg.
4. Cross affected leg over unaffected leg, remove trousers, and uncross leg.

Method 2: Seated Bridging—Donning. Method 2 is used for clients who are in wheelchairs (brakes locked, footrests swung away) or in sturdy, straight armchairs (back against wall) and for patients who cannot stand independently.

1. Position trousers on legs as in method 1, steps 1 to 5.
2. Elevate hips by leaning back against chair and pushing down against floor with unaffected leg; this is called bridging. As hips are raised, work trousers over hips with unaffected hand. Again, the person's feet should be able to grip the floor (do not attempt when wearing only standard socks on feet).
3. Lower hips back into chair and fasten trousers.

Method 2: Seated Bridging—Removing

1. Unfasten trousers and work down on hips as far as possible while sitting.
2. Ensure that feet are positioned securely on the floor with no-slip socks or shoes to prevent hips from slipping forward and out of the chair.
3. Lean back against chair, push down against floor with unaffected leg to elevate hips, and with unaffected arm, work trousers down past hips.
4. Proceed as in method 1, steps 3 and 4.

Method 3: Recumbent Bridging—Donning. Method 3 is done in a recumbent position—that is, lying down or reclining in bed. It is more difficult to perform than methods done while sitting. If possible, the bed should be raised to a semireclining position for partial sitting. The firmer the mattress, the easier it is to maneuver.

1. Using unaffected hand, place affected knee in flexed position and cross over unaffected leg, which may be partially flexed to prevent affected leg from slipping.
2. Position trousers and pull onto affected leg first, up to knee. Then uncross leg.
3. Insert unaffected leg and work trousers up onto hips as far as possible.
4. With unaffected leg flexed, press down with foot and shoulder to elevate hips from bed. While in this bridged position, with unaffected arm, pull trousers over hips or work trousers up over hips by rolling from side to side.
5. Fasten trousers.

Method 3: Recumbent Bridging—Removing

1. Bridge hips as in putting trousers on in method 3, step 4.
2. Work trousers down past hips, remove unaffected leg, and then remove affected leg.

Brassiere (Back Opening)

DONNING. Clothing items such as brassieres, neckties, socks, stockings, and braces may be difficult to manage with one hand. The following methods are recommended.

1. Position brassiere on lap so that shoulder strap side is toward knees and inside is facing up. Tuck one end of brassiere into pants waistband or fasten it with a clothespin, and wrap other end around waist (wrapping toward affected side may be easiest). Hook brassiere in front at waist level and slip fastener around to back (at waistline level).
2. Place affected arm through shoulder strap, then place unaffected arm through other strap.
3. Work straps up over shoulders. Pull strap on affected side up over shoulder with unaffected arm. Put unaffected arm through its strap and work up over shoulder by directing arm up and out and pulling with hand.
4. Use unaffected hand to adjust breasts in brassiere cups.

If the client has some function in the affected hand, a fabric loop may be sewn to the back of brassiere near the fastener. The affected thumb may be slipped through this to stabilize the brassiere while the unaffected hand fastens it. Front-opening bras may also be adapted in this way.

In all cases, it is helpful if the brassiere has elastic straps and is made of stretch fabric. All-elastic brassieres, prefastened or without fasteners, may be put on using method 1 described previously for shirts.

REMOVING

1. Slip straps down off shoulders, unaffected side first.
2. Work straps down over arms and off hands.
3. Slip brassiere around to front with unaffected arm.
4. Unfasten and remove.

Necktie

DONNING. Clip-on neckties are convenient. If a conventional tie is used, the following method is recommended:

1. Place collar of shirt in up position, bring necktie around neck, and adjust it so that smaller end is at length desired when tying is completed.
2. Fasten small end to shirt front with tie clasp or spring-clip clothespin.
3. Loop long end around short end (one complete loop) and bring up between V at neck. Then bring tip down through loop at front and adjust tie, using ring and little fingers to hold tie end and thumb and forefingers to slide knot up tightly.

REMOVING. Pull knot at front of neck until small end slips up enough for tie to be slipped over head. Tie may be hung up in this state and replaced by slipping it over head, around upturned collar, with knot tightened as described in step 3 of donning.

Socks or Stockings

DONNING

1. Sit in straight armchair or in wheelchair with brakes locked, feet on floor, and footrest swung away.
2. With unaffected leg directly in front of midline of body, cross affected leg over it.
3. Open top of stocking by inserting thumb and first two fingers near cuff and spreading fingers apart.
4. Work stocking onto foot before pulling over heel. Care should be taken to eliminate wrinkles.
5. Work stocking up over leg. Shift weight from side to side to adjust stocking around thigh.
6. Thigh-high stockings with elastic band at top are often an acceptable substitute for pantyhose, especially for nonambulatory clients. Elastic should not be so tight as to impair circulation.
7. Pantyhose may be donned and doffed as a pair of slacks, except legs would be gathered up, one at a time, before placing feet into leg holes.

REMOVING

1. Work socks or stockings down as far as possible with unaffected arm.
2. With unaffected leg directly in front of midline of body, cross affected leg over it.
3. Remove sock or stocking from affected leg. Some clients may require dressing stick to push sock or stocking off heel and foot.
4. Lift unaffected leg to comfortable height or seat level and remove sock or stocking from foot.

Shoes. If possible, select slip-on shoes to eliminate lacing and tying. The client who uses an ankle-foot orthosis (AFO) or short leg brace usually needs shoes with fasteners.

1. Use elastic laces and leave shoes tied.
2. Use one-handed shoe-tying techniques (Figure 13-27).
3. Client can learn to tie a standard bow with one hand, but this requires excellent visual perceptual and motor planning skills along with much repetition.

ANKLE-FOOT ORTHOSIS. A client with hemiplegia who lacks adequate ankle dorsiflexion to walk safely and efficiently often uses an ankle-foot orthosis (AFO). The custom AFO is often

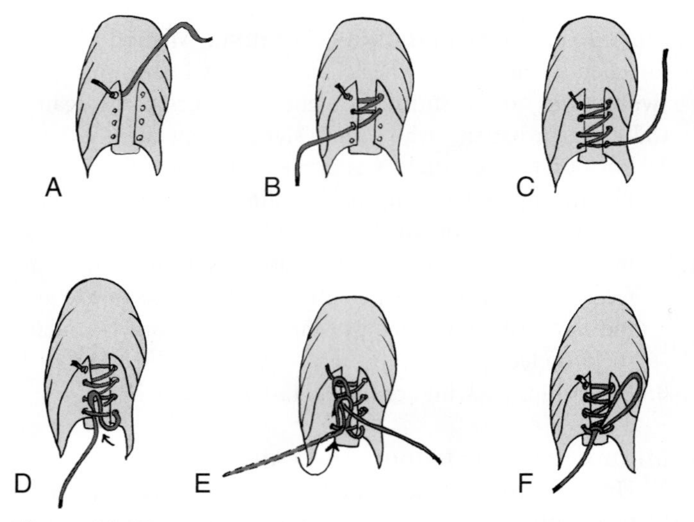

Figure 13-27 One-handed shoe-tying method. (Courtesy Christine Shaw, Metro Health Center for Rehabilitation, Metro Health Medical Center, Cleveland, Ohio.)

issued after the patient is discharged, so it may be necessary to practice this skill before the patient receives it.

Donning (Figure 13-28)

1. Sit in straight armchair or wheelchair with brakes locked and feet on floor *(A)*. Fasteners are loosened, and tongue of shoe is pulled back to allow AFO to fit into shoe *(B)*.
2. AFO and shoe are placed on floor between legs but closer to affected leg, facing up *(C)*.
3. With unaffected hand, lift affected leg behind knee and place toes into shoe *(D)*. It is important to keep or reposition affected leg, shoe, and AFO directly under affected knee, as much as possible.
4. Reach down with unaffected hand and lift AFO by the upright. Simultaneously, use unaffected foot against affected heel to keep shoe and AFO together *(E)*.
5. Heel is not pushed into shoe at this point. With unaffected hand, apply pressure directly downward on affected knee to force heel into shoe, if leg strength is not sufficient *(F)*.
6. Fasten Velcro calf strap and fasten shoes *(G)*. Affected leg may be placed on footstool to assist with reaching shoe fasteners.
7. To fasten shoes, one-handed bow tying may be used. Elastic shoelaces, Velcro-fastened shoes, or other commercially available shoe fasteners may be required if the client cannot tie his or her shoes.

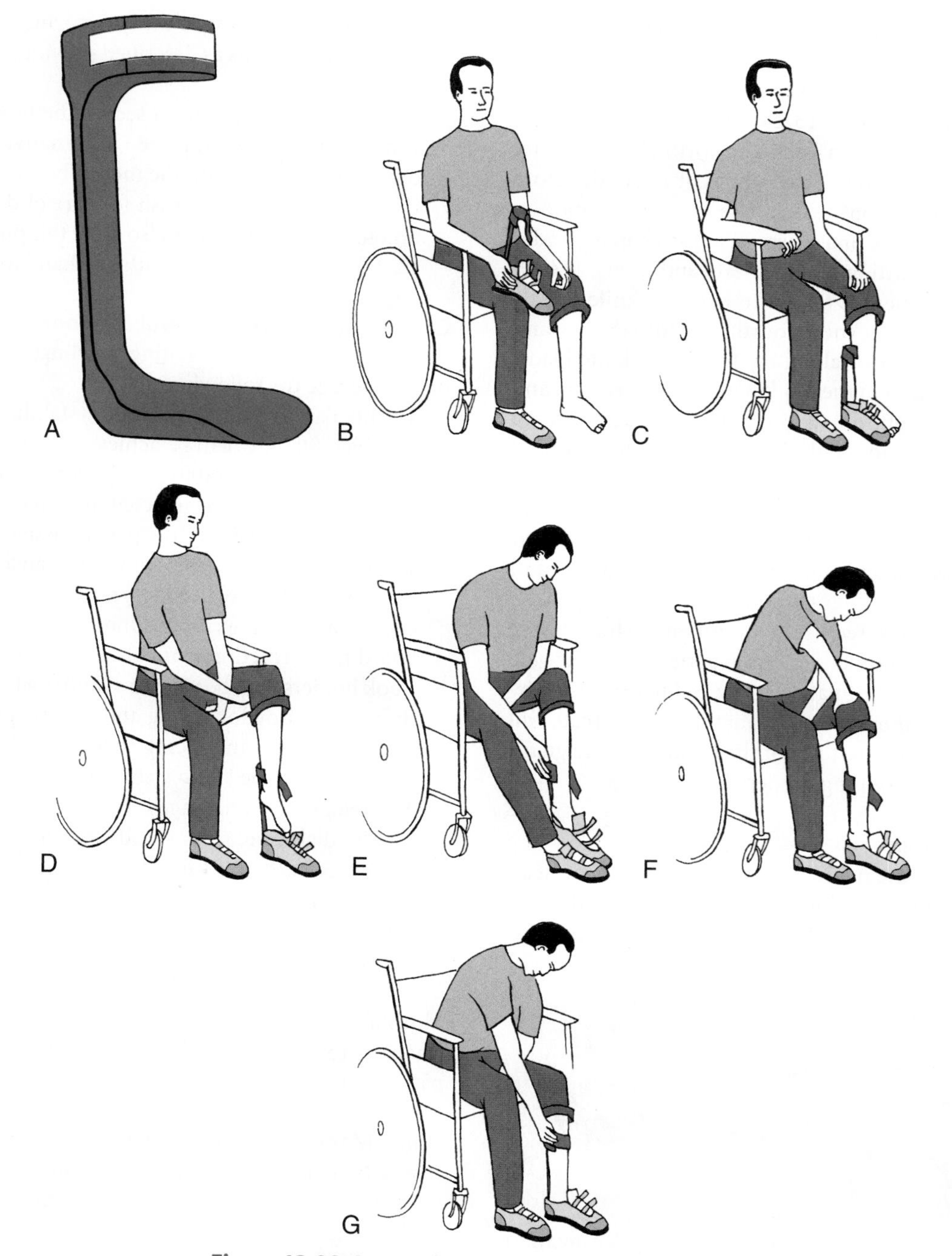

Figure 13-28 Steps in donning ankle-foot orthosis (AFO).

REMOVING: VARIATION 1

1. While seated as for donning an AFO, cross affected leg over unaffected leg.
2. Unfasten straps and laces with unaffected hand.
3. Using unaffected hand, push down on AFO upright until shoe is off foot.

REMOVING: VARIATION 2

1. Unfasten straps and laces.
2. Straighten affected leg by putting unaffected foot behind heel of shoe and pushing affected leg forward.
3. Push down on AFO upright with unaffected hand and at same time push forward on heel of AFO shoe with unaffected foot.

Eating Activities

A significant problem with using only one hand to eat is managing a knife and fork simultaneously for meat cutting. This problem can be solved by the use of a rocker knife for cutting meat and other foods (Figure 13-29). The knife cuts with a rocking motion rather than a back-and-forth slicing action. This motion holds the food in place while cutting it, therefore requiring only one hand for the task. Use of a rocking motion with a standard table knife or a sharp paring knife may be adequate to accomplish cutting tender meats and foods. If such a knife is used, the patient is taught to hold the knife handle between the thumb and the third, fourth, and fifth fingers, and the index finger is extended along the top of the knife blade. The knife point is placed in the food in a vertical position, and then the blade is brought down to cut the food. The rocking motion, using wrist flexion and extension, is continued until the food is cut.

The occupational therapist or OTA should keep in mind that one-handed meat cutting involves learning a new motor pattern and may be difficult for clients with hemiplegia and apraxia.

Eating activities may require a dominance shift. If the patient is right hand dominant and is experiencing right-side hemiplegia, left-hand coordination may need to be learned by practice. Using Dycem or a nonskid mat under the plate will keep the plate steady without use of the hands. A plate guard may be helpful when scooping slippery items.

Hygiene and Grooming

With the use of alternate methods and some assistive devices, hygiene and grooming activities can be accomplished using only one hand or one side of the body. Suggestions for achieving hygiene and grooming with one hand include the following:

1. Use an electric razor rather than a safety or disposable razor.
2. Use a bathtub seat or chair in the shower stall or bathtub. Use a suction-based bathmat, wash mitt, long-handled bath sponge, safety rails on the bathtub or wall, soap on a rope or suction soap holder, and suction brush for fingernail care.
3. Sponge-bathe while sitting at the toilet, using the wash mitt, suction brush, and suction soap holder.

The uninvolved forearm and hand can be washed by placing a soaped washcloth on the thigh and rubbing the hand and forearm on the cloth.

4. Use the position-adjustable hair dryer previously described. Such a device frees the unaffected upper extremity to hold a brush or comb to style the hair during blow-drying.[15]
5. Care for fingernails as described previously for clients with incoordination.
6. Use Dycem on the sink to secure the toothbrush in place while applying toothpaste. Alternatively, squeeze the toothpaste directly into the mouth before brushing teeth.
7. Use a suction denture brush for care of dentures. The suction fingernail brush may also serve this purpose (see Figure 13-22). Use a flossing aid with one hand for oral hygiene.

Communication and General Environment

Suggestions to facilitate writing, reading, and using the telephone include the following:

1. The primary problem in writing is stabilization of the paper or tablet. Stability can be achieved by using a clipboard or paperweight, or by taping the paper to the writing surface. In some instances the affected arm may be positioned on the tabletop to stabilize the paper passively.
2. The individual who must shift dominance to the nondominant extremity may need to practice to improve speed and coordination in writing. One-handed writing and keyboarding instruction manuals are available.
3. Book holders may be used to stabilize a book while reading or holding copy for typing and writing practice. For reading while seated in an easy chair, the client can position a soft pillow on the lap to stabilize a book.
4. The telephone is managed by lifting the receiver to listen for the dial tone, setting it down, dialing or pressing the buttons, and then lifting the receiver to the ear. To write while using the telephone, a telephone headset or earpiece can be used. A speakerphone can also leave hands free to take messages.

Mobility and Transfers

Chapter 15 describes principles of transfer techniques for patients with hemiplegia.

Home Management Activities

A variety of assistive devices make home management activities easier to perform.[28] The nature and severity of the disability determine how many home management activities realistically can be performed, which methods can be used,

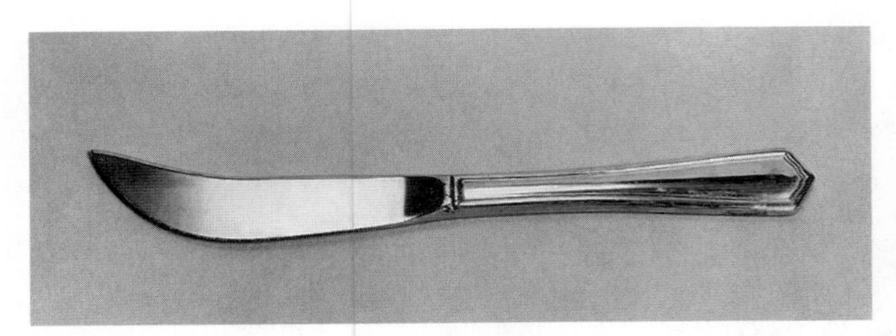

Figure 13-29 One-handed rocker knife. (Courtesy Sammons, a BISSELL Co.)

and how many assistive devices can be managed. Whether the client is disabled solely by the loss of function of one arm and hand (as in amputation or peripheral neuropathy) or whether both arm and leg are affected—along with possible visual, perceptual, and cognitive dysfunctions (as in hemiplegia)—makes a significant difference in planning treatment. Suggestions regarding home management for the client with use of one hand include the following (see References for further details)[28]:

1. Stabilization of items is a major problem for the homemaker who can use only one hand. Stabilize foods for cutting and peeling by using a board with two stainless steel or aluminum nails in it. A raised corner on the board stabilizes bread while making sandwiches or spreading butter. Suction cups or a rubber mat under the board will keep it from slipping. Rubber stair tread, shelf liner, or Dycem may be glued to the bottom of the board (see Figure 13-23).
2. Use sponge cloths, nonskid mats or pads, wet dishcloths, or suction devices to keep bowls and dishes from turning or sliding during food preparation. Use a pan holder—a steel rod frame with suction cups attached to the stove top—to keep the pot from spinning while the contents are being stirred or flipped.[37,49]
3. To open a jar, stabilize it between the knees or in a partially opened drawer while leaning against it. Break the air seal by sliding a bottle opener under the lid until the air is released; then use a wall-mounted opener like the Zim jar opener (Figure 13-30). When purchasing food items in jars, ask the grocer to open and gently reseal jars before bagging them.
4. Open boxes, sealed paper bags, and plastic bags by stabilizing between the knees or in a drawer, as just described, and cutting open with a household shears. Special box and bag openers are also available from ADL equipment vendors.[37,49]

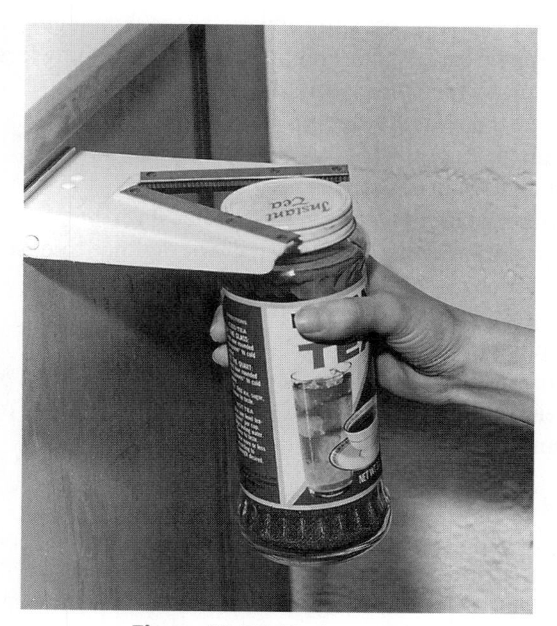

Figure 13-30 Zim jar opener.

5. Open an egg by holding it firmly in the palm of the hand, hitting it in the center against the edge of the bowl, and then using the thumb and index finger to push the top half of the shell up and the ring and little fingers to push the lower half down. Separate whites from yolks by using an egg separator or a funnel. Another solution is to use cholesterol-free eggs, such as Egg Beaters, from a carton.
6. Eliminate the need to stabilize the standard grater by using a grater with suction feet, or use an electric food processor.
7. Eliminate the need to use hand-cranked or electric can openers requiring two hands by using a one-handed electric can opener.
8. Use a utility cart to carry items from one place to another. A cart that is weighted or constructed of wood may be used as a minimal support during ambulation for some clients with mild balance or coordination impairments.
9. Transfer clothes to and from the washer or dryer by using a clothes carrier on wheels.
10. Use electrical appliances that can be managed with one hand to save time and energy. Some of these appliances include a lightweight electrical hand mixer, blender, and food processor. Safety factors and judgment need to be evaluated carefully for electrical appliances.
11. Floor care becomes a problem if ambulation and balance are affected in addition to the upper extremity. For clients with involvement of one arm only, a standard dust mop, carpet sweeper, or upright vacuum cleaner should present no problem. A self-wringing mop may be used if the mop handle is stabilized under the arm and the wringing lever operated with the unaffected arm. Floor cleaning systems such as Swiffer or Clorox Ready Mop dispense the cleanser through a pump, wipe up the floor with a disposable cleaning pad, and are easy to manage with one hand. Clients with balance and ambulation problems may manage some floor care from a sitting position. Dust mopping or using a carpet sweeper may be possible if gait and balance are adequate without the aid of a cane.
12. To easily push furniture aside and avoid scratching flooring while cleaning or rearranging, attach Magic Sliders to the bottoms of the feet or base of furniture. This product can be purchased at hardware stores.
13. Use a gas lighter with one hand (instead of a match requiring two hands) to light candles.

These suggestions are just a few of the possibilities to solve home management problems for clients with use of only one hand. The OT practitioner must evaluate each client to determine how the dysfunction affects performance of homemaking activities. One-handed techniques require more time and may be difficult for some clients to master. Activities should be paced to accommodate the client's physical endurance and tolerance for one-handed performance and use of special devices. Work simplification and energy conservation techniques should be employed.

New techniques and devices should be introduced on a graded basis as the client masters one technique and device and then another. Family members must be oriented to the client's skills, special methods, and work schedule. The clinician may help plan homemaking responsibilities with the family and client, focusing on which tasks will be shared with other family members and the procedures for supervising the client, if needed.

If special equipment and assistive devices are needed for ADL, obtaining them, if possible, while the person is receiving OT treatment is advisable. The OT practitioner can then train the client in their use and demonstrate to a family member before the items are used at home. After training, the clinician should provide the client with sources to replace items independently such as a consumer catalog or websites of adaptive equipment.[37,49]

Wheelchair-Dependent Clients with Good to Normal Arm Function (Paraplegia)

Clients who are confined to wheelchairs need to find ways to perform ADL from a seated position, to transport objects, and to adapt to an environment that is intended for standing and walking. Given normal upper extremity function, the wheelchair-dependent client can probably perform seated level activities independently. To do so, the client should have a stable spine and mobility precautions should be clearly identified. It is important to minimize transfers during self-care tasks because they require a lot of energy and can be a safety risk. Planning out the order of the self-care routine can reduce the number of transfers required.

Dressing Activities

Wheelchair-dependent clients should put clothing on in this order: stockings, undergarments, braces (if worn), trousers or slacks, shoes, shirt, or dress.[1]

Socks or Stockings

Donning

1. Put on socks or stockings while seated on bed or in wheelchair.
2. Pull one leg into flexion with one hand and cross over other leg.
3. Use other hand to slip sock or stocking over foot and pull it on.

Soft stretch socks or stockings are recommended. Pantyhose that are slightly large may be useful. Elastic garters or stockings with elastic tops may lead to skin breakdown and should be avoided. Dressing sticks or a stocking device may be helpful to some clients.

Removing. Remove socks or stockings by flexing leg as described for donning, then pushing sock or stocking down over heel. Dressing sticks may be needed to push sock or stocking off heel and toe and to retrieve it.

Trousers

Trousers and slacks are easier to fasten if they button or zip in front. If braces are worn, zippers in the side seams may be helpful. Wide-bottom slacks of stretch fabric are recommended. The following procedure is for putting on trousers, shorts, slacks, and underwear.

Donning

1. Long sit (thighs and calves on bed, knees extended) on bed with feet hanging off the foot of the bed and reach forward toward feet, or sit on bed and pull knees into flexed position.
2. While holding top of trousers, flip pants down to feet.
3. Work pant legs over feet and pull up to hips. Crossing ankles may help work pants on over heels.
4. In semireclining position, roll from hip to hip and pull up garment. When lying on the left hip, pull the trousers up over the right hip and vice versa.
5. Reaching tongs or fabric loops on the waistband may be helpful to pull garment up or position garment on feet if the client has impaired balance or limited ROM in the lower extremities or trunk.

Removing. Remove pants or underwear by reversing procedure for putting on. Dressing sticks may be helpful to push pants off feet.

Slips and Skirts

Donning

1. Sit on bed, slip garment over head, and let it drop to waist.
2. In semireclining position, roll from hip to hip and pull garment down over hips and thighs.

Slips and skirts slightly larger than usually worn are recommended. A-line, wraparound, and full skirts are easier to manage and lie more smoothly while the client is seated in a wheelchair than do narrow skirts. Long skirts and jackets may get caught in the wheel of the wheelchair during mobility and should be avoided for safety reasons.

Removing

1. In sitting or semireclining position, unfasten garment.
2. Roll from hip to hip, pulling garment up to waist level.
3. Pull garment off over head.

Shoes

Because of sensory loss and paralysis, shoes should be donned before any transfers to prevent the foot from slipping forward and to protect the foot from bruises.

Donning

1. Sit on edge of bed or in wheelchair.
2. Cross one leg over other and slip shoe on.
3. Put foot on footrest and push down on knee to push foot into shoe.

Removing

1. Cross leg as described earlier.
2. Remove shoe from crossed leg with one hand while maintaining balance with other hand, if necessary.

Shirts

Shirts, pajama jackets, robes, and dresses that open completely down the front may be put on while the client is seated in a wheelchair. If it is necessary to dress in bed, the following procedure can be used.

Donning

1. Balance body by putting palms of hands on mattress on either side of body. If balance is poor, assistance may be needed. Propping two pillows to support the back can leave both hands free.
2. If difficulty is encountered in customary methods of applying garment, open garment on lap with collar toward chest. Put arms into sleeves and pull up over elbows. Then hold on to shirttail or back of dress, pull garment over head, adjust, and button.

Fabrics should be wrinkle resistant, smooth, and durable.

Roomy sleeves and backs and full skirts are more suitable styles than more closely fitted garments.

Removing

1. While sitting in wheelchair or bed, open fastener.
2. Remove garment in usual manner.
3. If step 2 is not feasible, grasp collar with one hand while balancing with other hand. Gather material up from collar to hem.
4. Lean forward, duck head, and pull shirt over head.
5. Remove sleeve from supporting arm and then from the working arm.

Eating Activities

The wheelchair-dependent client with good to normal arm function generally can eat normally. Wheelchairs with removable desk arms and swing-away footrests are recommended so that the client can sit close to the table.

Hygiene and Grooming

Face and oral hygiene and arm and upper body care should present no problem. Reachers may be helpful to retrieve towels, washcloths, makeup, deodorant, and shaving supplies from storage areas, if necessary. Adjusting the sink height and removing the cabinetry below the sink may be necessary to allow the wheelchair to fit directly under the sink. A wall-mounted swivel-adjustable-arm mirror may be useful for makeup and face care. Tub baths or showers require some special equipment. Chapter 15 discusses transfer techniques for the toilet and bathtub. Suggestions to make bathing activities easier for the wheelchair-dependent client include the following:

1. Use a handheld showerhead, and keep a finger over the spray to determine sudden temperature changes in water. This method will help prevent burning the skin in areas with sensory loss.
2. Use long-handled bath brushes with soap insert for ease in reaching all parts of the body.
3. Use soap bars attached to a cord around the neck.
4. For sponge bath in a wheelchair, cover the chair with a sheet of plastic.
5. Use padded shower chairs or bathtub seats with cut-out bottom to allow for full body cleansing from a seated position.
6. Increase safety during transfers by installing grab bars on wall near the bathtub or shower and on the bathtub.
7. Fit bottom of the bathtub or shower with nonskid mat or adhesive material.
8. Remove doors on the bathtub and replace with a shower curtain to increase transfer space.

Communication and General Environment

With the exception of difficulty with reaching in some situations, wheelchair-dependent patients should have no problem using the telephone. Short-handled reachers may be used to grasp the receiver from the cradle. Numbers can be entered with a short, rubber-tipped, ¼-inch dowel stick (or the eraser end of a pencil). A cordless telephone eliminates reaching except when the phone needs recharging. These clients should be able to use writing implements, computers, and tape recorders with no difficulty, if the devices are placed on an easily accessible tabletop.

Managing doors may present some problems. If the door opens toward the client, opening it can be managed by the following procedure:

1. If doorknob is on the right, approach door from right and turn doorknob with left hand.
2. Open the door as far as possible and move wheelchair close enough so that it helps keep door open.
3. Holding door open with left hand, turn wheelchair with right hand and wheel through door.
4. Start closing door when halfway through.

If the door is heavy and opens out or away from the client, the following procedure is recommended[8]:

1. For a doorknob on the right, back up to door so that knob can be turned with right hand.
2. Open door and back through so that back wheels keep it open.
3. Also use left elbow to keep door open.
4. Wheel backward with right hand.

Mobility and Transfers

Chapter 15 discusses transfer techniques.

Home Management Activities

For a wheelchair-dependent person, the major home management problems are work heights; adequate space for maneuverability; access to storage areas; and transfer of supplies, equipment, and materials from place to place. If funds are available for kitchen remodeling, lowering counters and range to a comfortable height is recommended. However, such extensive adaptation is often not feasible. Suggestions for home management include the following[28]:

1. Remove lower cabinet doors to eliminate the need to maneuver around them for opening and closing. Commonly used items should be stored on counters or toward the front of easy-to-reach cabinets above and below the counter surfaces.
2. If entrance and inside doors are not wide enough, use a narrower wheelchair or make doors slightly wider by removing strips along the doorjambs. Offset hinges can replace standard door hinges and increase the doorjamb width by 2 inches (5 cm) (Figure 13-31).

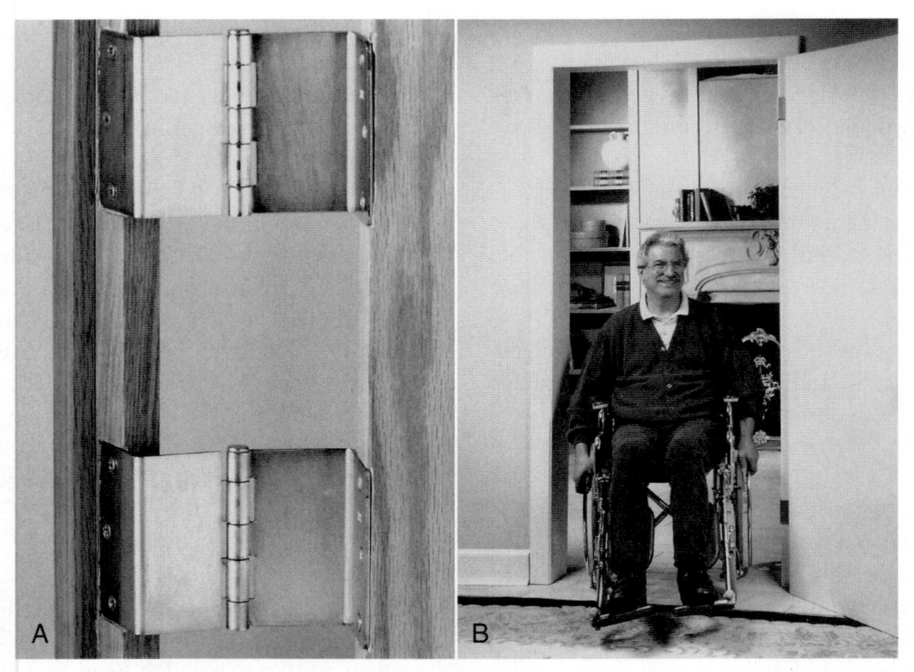

Figure 13-31 **A,** Offset hinges. **B,** Offset hinges widen doorway for wheelchair-dependent patient. (Courtesy Sammons, a BISSELL Co.)

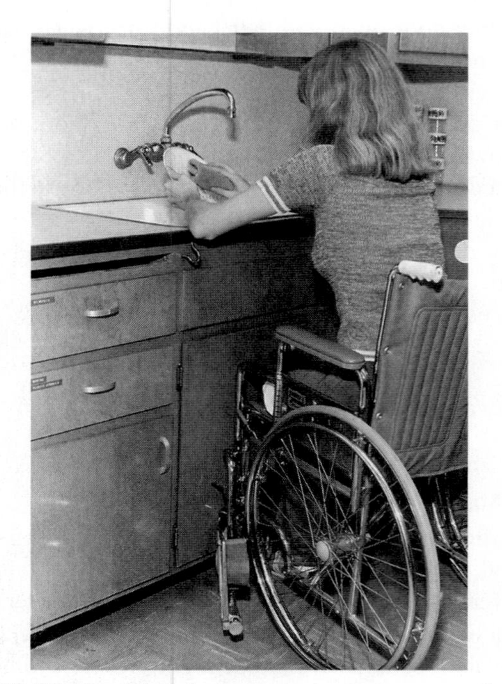

Figure 13-32 Wheelchair footrests are swung away to allow close access to sink.

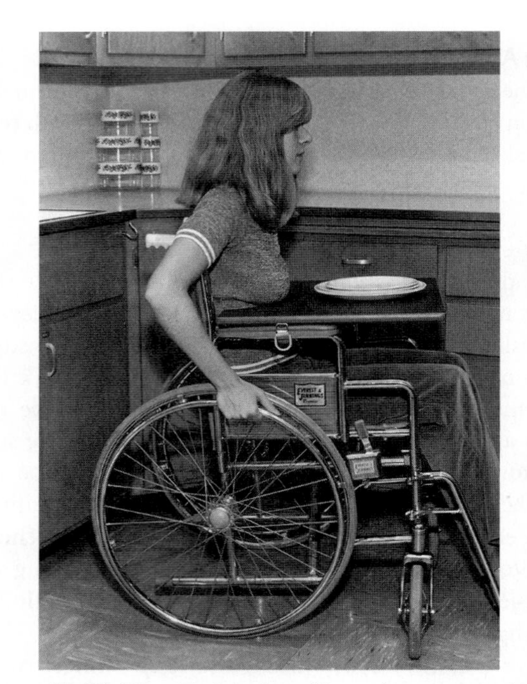

Figure 13-33 Wheelchair lapboard is used to transport items.

3. Increase the client's height with a wheelchair cushion so that standard countertops can be used.
4. Use detachable desk arms and swing-away detachable footrests to allow the client to roll close to counters and tables and also to stand at counters, if possible (Figure 13-32).
5. Transport items safely and easily by using a wheelchair lapboard. The lapboard can also serve as a work surface for preparing food and drying dishes. It also protects the lap from injury from hot pans and prevents utensils from falling into the lap (Figure 13-33).
6. Fasten a drop-leaf board to a bare wall or a slide-out board under a counter to provide the wheelchair-dependent cook with a work surface at a comfortable height in an otherwise standard kitchen.
7. Fit cabinets with custom-made or ready-made lazy Susans or pull-out shelves to eliminate the need to reach to the rear of the space (Figure 13-34).
8. Ideally, ranges should be at a lower level than standard height. If this is not possible, place controls at the front of the range and hang a mirror over the range, angled at such a degree that

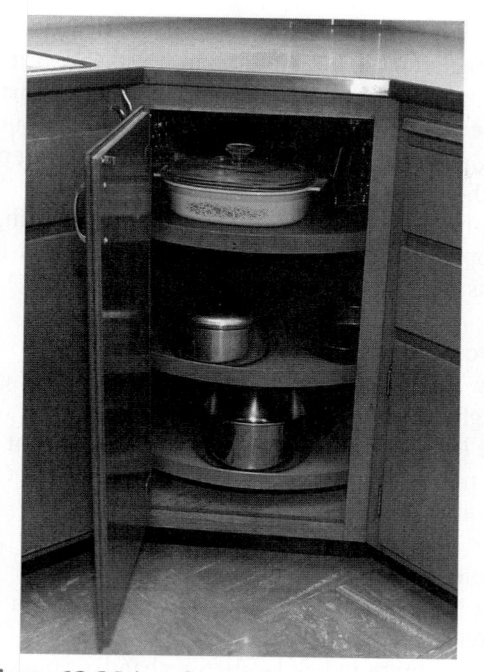

Figure 13-34 Lazy Susan in kitchen storage cabinet.

the client can see contents of pots. Oven-stove mirrors are commercially available from rehabilitation catalogs.[37,49]

9. Substitute small electric cooking units such as a portable electric range, toaster oven, and microwave ovens for the range if the patient cannot use the range safely.
10. Use front-loading washers and dryers.
11. Vacuum carpets with a carpet sweeper or tank-type cleaner that rolls easily and is lightweight or self- propelled. A retractable cord may be helpful to prevent tangling the cord in the wheels.

Wheelchair-Dependent Client with Upper Extremity Weakness (Quadriplegia)

In general, clients with muscle function from spinal cord levels C7 and C8 can follow the methods just described for paraplegia. Clients with muscle function from C6 can be relatively independent with adaptations and assistive devices. However, those with muscle function from C4 and C5 require considerable special equipment and assistance. Clients with muscle function from C6 may benefit from the use of a wrist-driven flexor hinge splint or tenodesis splint. Externally powered splints and arm braces or mobile arm supports are recommended for C3, C4, and C5 levels of muscle function.

Dressing Activities

Determining whether a patient meets the criteria for beginning dressing activities is a professional-level responsibility. However, the OTA can assist in the determination and should always closely observe patient appropriateness for this or any other activity.

Criteria

Training in dressing can begin once the spine is stable.[7,48] Before spinal stability is achieved, the client may require assistance donning a cervical or cervical thoracic orthosis as specified by doctor's orders. Minimal criteria for upper extremity dressing are the following: (1) fair to good muscle strength in deltoids, upper and middle trapezii, shoulder rotators, rhomboids, biceps, supinators, and radial wrist extensors; (2) ROM of 0 to 90 degrees in shoulder flexion and abduction, 0 to 80 degrees in shoulder internal rotation, 0 to 30 degrees in external rotation, and 15 to 140 degrees in elbow flexion; (3) sitting balance in bed or wheelchair, which may be achieved with the assistance of bed rails, an electric hospital bed, or a wheelchair safety belt; and (4) finger prehension, achieved with adequate tenodesis grasp or a wrist-hand orthosis.

Additional criteria for dressing the lower extremities are the following: (1) fair to good muscle strength in pectoralis major and minor, serratus anterior, and rhomboid major and minor; (2) ROM of 0 to 120 degrees in knee flexion, 0 to 110 degrees in hip flexion, and 0 to 80 degrees in hip external rotation; (3) body control for transfer from bed to wheelchair with minimal assistance; (4) ability to roll from side to side, balance in side lying, or turning from supine to prone position and back; and (5) vital capacity of 50% or greater.[48]

Contraindications

Dressing is contraindicated if any of the following factors are present: (1) unstable spine at site of injury; (2) unhealed pressure sores or tendency for skin breakdown during rolling, scooting, and transferring; (3) uncontrollable muscle spasms in legs; and (4) less than 50% vital capacity.[7,48]

Sequence of Dressing

The recommended sequence for training to dress is to put on underwear and trousers while still in bed, then transfer to a wheelchair to put on shirts, socks, and shoes.[48] Some patients may choose to put the socks on before the trousers because socks may help the feet slip through the trouser legs more easily.

Expected Proficiency

Clients with total spinal cord lesions at C7 and below can achieve total dressing, which includes both upper and lower extremity dressing skills. Although people with lesions at C6 can achieve total dressing, lower extremity dressing may be difficult or impracticable in terms of time and energy.

Clients with lesions at C5 to C6, with some exceptions, can independently achieve upper extremity dressing. However, these clients find it extremely difficult to put on a brassiere, tuck a shirt or blouse into a waistband, or fasten buttons on shirt fronts and cuffs. Factors such as age, physical proportions, coordination, coexistent medical problems, and motivation affect the client's degree of proficiency in dressing skills.[7]

Types of Clothing

Clothing should be loose and have front openings. Trousers need to be a size larger than usually worn to accommodate the urine collection device or leg braces, if worn. Avoid jeans or pants with thick seams during the first few months after onset of injury to avoid potential skin breakdown. The easiest fasteners to manage are zippers and Velcro closures. Because the quadriplegic client may use the thumb as a hook to manage clothing, loops attached to zipper pulls, underwear, and even the back of the shoes can be helpful. Belt loops on trousers are used for pulling and should be reinforced. Brassieres should have stretch straps and no underwires. Front-opening brassieres can be adapted by fastening loops and adding Velcro closures; back-opening styles can have loops added at each side of the fastening.

Shoes should be one-half to one size larger than normally worn to accommodate edema and spasticity and to avoid pressure sores. Shoe fasteners can be adapted with Velcro, elastic shoelaces, large buckles, or flip-back tongue closures. Loose woolen or cotton socks without elastic cuffs should be used initially. Ridgeless socks, available from ADL catalogs, can help protect the skin from breakdown and are easier to don. As skill is gained, nylon socks, which tend to stick to the skin, may be introduced. If neckties are used, the clip-on type or a regular tie that has been preknotted and can be slipped over the head may be manageable for some clients.[7,49]

The following techniques can make dressing easier for clients with upper extremity weakness.

Trousers and Undershorts

Donning

1. Sit on bed with bed rails up (long-sitting position). Trousers are positioned at foot of bed with trouser legs over end of bed and front side up.[48]
2. Sit up and lift one knee at a time by hooking right hand under right knee to pull leg into flexion; then put trousers over right foot. Return right leg to extended or semiextended position and repeat procedure with left hand and left knee.[7] It is important to maintain one leg at a time in flexion by holding it with one arm or by taking advantage of spasticity. If neither of these strategies works, a dressing band may be used to secure the leg. This is a piece of elasticized webbing sewn into a figure-eight pattern, with one small loop and one large loop. Small loop is hooked around foot and large hoop anchored over knee. Band is measured for each client so that its length is appropriate to maintain desired amount of knee flexion. Once trousers are in place, knee loop is pushed off knee and dressing band removed from foot with dressing stick.[13]
3. Work trousers up legs, using patting and sliding motions with palms of hands. Secure a piece of nonslip material such as Dycem to the palms of hands or wear push gloves to help grip and pull the material into place.
4. While still sitting with pants at midcalf height, insert dressing stick in front belt loop. Dressing stick is gripped by slipping its loop over wrist. Pull on dressing stick while extending trunk, returning to supine position. Return to sitting position and repeat this procedure, pulling on dressing sticks and maneuvering trousers up to thigh level.[48] If balance and flexibility are adequate, an alternative is for client to remain seated and lean on left elbow and pull trousers over right buttock, then reverse process for other side. Another alternative is for client to remain in supine position and roll to one side; throw opposite arm behind back; hook thumb in waistband, belt loop, or pocket; and pull trousers up over hips. These maneuvers can be repeated as needed to pull trousers over buttocks.[7]
5. Using palms of hands in pushing and smoothing motions, straighten trouser legs.
6. In supine position, fasten trouser placket by hooking thumb in loop on zipper pull, patting Velcro closed, or using hand splints and buttonhooks if buttons are present.[7,48]

Donning: Variation. For step 2, substitute the following:

Sit up and lift one knee at a time by hooking right hand under right knee to pull leg into flexion, then cross foot over opposite leg above knee. This position frees up foot to place trousers more easily and requires less trunk balance. Continue with all other steps.

Removing

1. Lying supine in bed with bed rails up, unfasten belt and placket fasteners.
2. Placing thumbs in belt loops, waistband, or pockets, work trousers past hips by stabilizing arms in shoulder extension and scooting body toward head of bed.
3. Use arms as described in step 2, and roll from side to side to slide trousers past buttocks.
4. Coming to sitting position and alternately pulling legs into flexion, push trousers down legs.[48]
5. Trousers can be pushed off over feet with dressing stick or by hooking thumbs in waistband.

Cardigans or Pullover Garments. Cardigan and pull-over garments include blouses, vests, sweaters, skirts, and front-opening dresses.[7,48] Upper extremity dressing is often performed in the wheelchair for greater trunk stability.

Donning

1. Position garment across thighs with back facing up and neck toward knees.
2. Place both arms under back of garment and in armholes.
3. Push sleeves up onto arms past elbows.
4. Using a wrist extension grip, hook thumbs under garment back and gather material up from neck to hem.
5. To pass garment over head, adduct and externally rotate shoulders and flex elbows while flexing head forward.
6. When garment is over head, relax shoulders and wrists and remove hands from back of garment. Most material will be gathered up at neck, across shoulders, and under arms.
7. To work garment down over body, shrug shoulders, lean forward, and use elbow flexion and wrist extension. Use wheelchair arms for balance if necessary. Additional maneuvers to accomplish task are to hook wrists into sleeves and pull material free from underarms or lean forward, reach back, and slide hand against material to aid in pulling garment down.
8. Garment can be buttoned from bottom to top with aid of buttonhook and wrist-hand orthosis if hand function is inadequate.

REMOVING

1. Sit in wheelchair and wear wrist-hand orthosis. Unfasten buttons (if any) while wearing splints and using button-hook. Remove splints for remaining steps.
2. For pullover garments, hook thumb in back of neckline, extend wrist, and pull garment over head while turning head toward side of raised arm. Maintain balance by resting against opposite wheelchair armrest or pushing on thigh with extended arm.
3. For cardigan garments, hook thumb in opposite armhole and push sleeve down arm. Elevation and depression of shoulders with trunk rotation can be used to have garment slip down arms as far as possible.
4. Hold one cuff with opposite thumb while elbow is flexed to pull arm out of sleeve.

Brassiere (Back Opening)

DONNING

1. Place brassiere across lap with straps toward knees and inside facing up.
2. Using a right-to-left procedure, hold end of brassiere closest to right side with hand or reacher and pass brassiere around back from right to left. Lean against brassiere at back to hold it in place while hooking thumb of left hand in a loop that has been attached near brassiere fastener. Hook right thumb in a similar loop on right side, and fasten brassiere in front at waist level.
3. Hook right thumb in edge of brassiere. Using wrist extension, elbow flexion, shoulder adduction, and internal rotation, rotate brassiere around body so that front of brassiere is in front of body.
4. While leaning on one forearm, hook opposite thumb in front end of strap and pull strap over shoulder, then repeat procedure on other side.[7,48]

REMOVING

1. Hook thumb under opposite brassiere strap and push down over shoulder while elevating shoulder.
2. Pull arm out of strap and repeat procedure for other arm.
3. Push brassiere down to waist level and turn around as described previously to bring fasteners to front.
4. Unfasten brassiere.

Alternatives to a back-opening bra are (1) a front-opening bra with loops to use a wrist extension grip or (2) a fully elastic bra, one size larger, with no fasteners. The larger bra can be donned like a pullover sweater.

Socks

DONNING

1. Sit in wheelchair (or on bed if balance is adequate) in cross-legged position with one ankle crossed over opposite knee.
2. Pull sock over foot with wrist extension grip and patting movements with palm of hand.[7,48]
3. If trunk balance is inadequate and cross-legged position cannot be maintained, prop foot on stool, chair, open drawer, or edge of bed, keeping opposite arm around upright of wheelchair for balance. Fastening wheelchair safety belt or leaning against wheelchair armrest on one side are alternatives to maintain balance.
4. Use stocking aid (see Figure 13-7) or soft sock aid to assist in putting on socks while in this position. Apply sock-to-sock aid by using thumbs and palms of hands to smooth sock out on cone.
5. Place cord loops of sock cone around wrist or thumb and throw cone beyond foot.
6. Maneuver sock aid over toes by pulling cords using elbow flexion. Insert foot as far as possible into cone.
7. To remove aid from sock after foot has been inserted, move heel forward off wheelchair footrest. Use wrist extension of one hand behind knee, and with other hand continue pulling cords of cone until it is removed and sock is in place on foot. Use palms to smooth sock with patting and stroking motion.[48]
8. Two loops can also be sewn on either side of top of sock so that thumbs can be hooked into loops and socks pulled on.

REMOVING

1. While sitting in wheelchair or lying in bed, use dressing stick or long-handled shoehorn to push sock down over heel. Cross legs if possible.
2. Use dressing stick with cup-hook on end to pull sock off toes.[8]

Shoes

DONNING

1. For putting on shoes, use same position as for donning socks.
2. Use extended-handle dressing aid and insert it into tongue of shoe; then place shoe opening over toes. Remove dressing aid from shoe and dangle shoe on toes.
3. Using palm of hand on sole of shoe, pull shoe toward heel of foot. Use one hand to stabilize leg while pushing other against sole of shoe to work shoe onto foot. Use thenar eminence and sides of hand for pushing motion.
4. With feet flat on floor or on wheelchair footrest and knees flexed 90 degrees, place long-handled shoehorn in heel of shoe and press down on flexed knee.
5. Fasten shoes.[48]

REMOVING

1. Sitting in wheelchair as described for donning socks, unfasten shoes.
2. Use shoehorn or dressing stick to push on heel counter of shoe, dislodging it from heel; then shoe will drop or can be pushed to floor with dressing stick.

Eating Activities

Eating may be assisted by a variety of devices, depending on the quadriplegic client's level of muscle function.[1] Levels C5 and above require mobile arm supports or externally powered splints and braces. A wrist splint and universal cuff may be used together if a wrist-hand orthosis (flexor hinge splint) is not used. The universal cuff holds the eating utensil, and the splint stabilizes the wrist. A nonskid mat and a plate with plate guard may provide adequate stability of the plate for pushing and picking up food (Figure 13-35).

The spoon-plate is an option for independent feeding for clients with high spinal cord injuries.[56] It is a portable device that can be adjusted in height to the level of the client's mouth. The plate is made of a high-temperature thermoplastic and is formed over a mold that has a cupped rim shaped to the approximate depth and length of a spoon. The client rotates the device with mouth and neck control. Food is removed from the rim of the plate with the mouth. Successful use of the device depends on adequate oral control, head and trunk control, and motivation. Wykoff and Mitani[56] provide further information on making or obtaining this device.

Also available for clients who have no use of their upper extremities is an electric self-feeder that requires only slight head motion and is activated by a chin switch (Figure 13-36). The Winsford Feeder uses a motorized pusher to fill a spoon and automatically moves the food to the client's mouth. A chin switch or a rocker switch activates it. Another assistive device to help with self-feeding is the assistive robotic arm (Assistant Robot Manipulator) mentioned in the assistive technology section later in this chapter.[14]

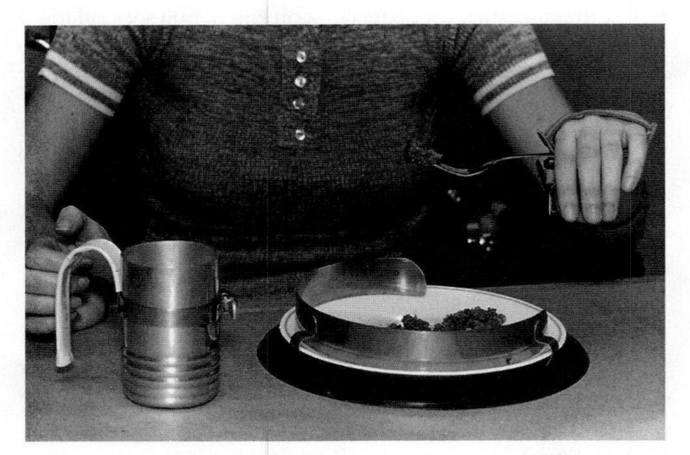

Figure 13-35 Self-feeding with aid of universal cuff, plate guard, nonskid mat, and clip cup holder to compensate for absent grasp.

A regular or swivel spoon-fork combination can be used when the client has minimal muscle function (C4 to C5). A long plastic straw with a straw clip to stabilize it in the cup or glass eliminates the need for picking up these drinking vessels. A bilateral or unilateral clip holder on a glass or cup allows many clients with hand and arm weakness to manage liquids without a straw.

Built-up utensils may be useful for clients with some functional grasp or tenodesis grasp. Cutting food may be managed with a Quad-Quip knife if arm strength is adequate to manage the device (Figure 13-37). When ordering a meal at a restaurant, the person can request that the server or cook cut the food into bite-size pieces.

Hygiene and Grooming

General suggestions to facilitate hygiene and grooming are the following[1]:

1. Use a shower or bathtub seat and transfer board for transfers.
2. Extend reach by using long-handled bath sponges with loop handle or built-up handle.
3. Eliminate need to grasp washcloth by using terry cloth or sponge bath mitts.
4. Hold comb and toothbrush with a universal cuff.[1]
5. Use the position-adjustable hair dryer described previously.[15] Use a universal cuff to hold brush or comb for hair styling while using this mounted hair dryer.
6. Use a clip holder for electric razor.
7. Use a suppository inserter for bowel program.
8. Use skin inspection mirror with long stem and looped handle for independent skin inspection (Figure 13-38). The degree of weakness must be considered for each client when selecting devices and when selecting and adapting methods.
9. Adapted leg-bag clamps to empty catheter leg bags are also available for patients with limited hand function. Velcro straps may substitute for elastic leg-bag straps. Use a clothespin with a bungee cord to help manage clothing during self-catheterization.

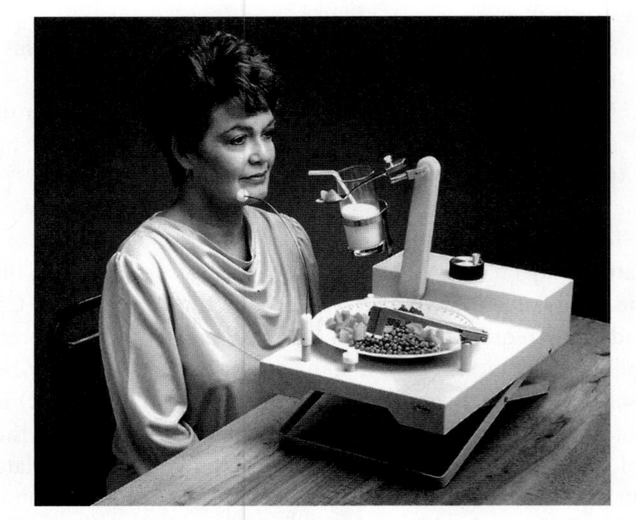

Figure 13-36 Electric self-feeder. (Courtesy Sammons, a BISSELL Co.)

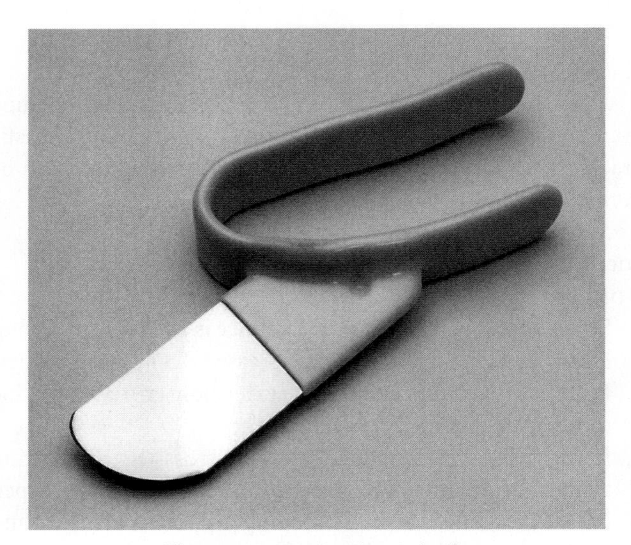

Figure 13-37 Quad-quip knife.

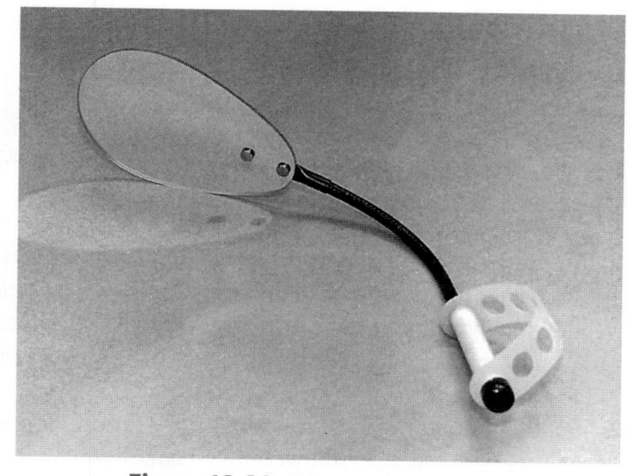

Figure 13-38 Skin inspection mirror.

Figure 13-39 Wand mouthstick. (Courtesy Sammons, a BISSELL Co.)

Communication and General Environment

Suggestions for facilitating communication include the following:

1. Turn pages with an electric page turner, mouthstick, or head wand if hand and arm function is inadequate (Figure 13-39).
2. For keyboarding, writing, operating a tape recorder, and painting, insert a pen, pencil, typing stick, or paintbrush in a universal cuff that has been positioned with the opening on the ulnar side of the palm (Figure 13-40).
3. Enter telephone numbers with the universal cuff and a pencil positioned with the eraser down. The receiver may need to be stationed in a telephone arm and positioned for listening or adapted with a telephone clip holder (see Figure 13-16). Special adaptations are available to substitute for the need to replace the receiver in the cradle. Set up and use speed dial options on the telephone. For patients with no arm function, a speakerphone can be used with a mouthstick to push the button to initiate a call; the operator assists with dialing. A voice-activated phone is also available for clients with little to no upper extremity function. If possible, add the telephone to a voice-activated environmental control unit (ECU).
4. Use personal computers with voice activation software, head pointers, or adaptive switches.
5. Built-up pencils and pens or special pencil holders are necessary for clients with hand weakness. The Wanchik writer is an effective adaptive writing device (see Figure 13-17). The slip-on writing aid holds the pen at an adjustable angle in the first web space and with a heat gun can be custom-fit to contour to the hand.

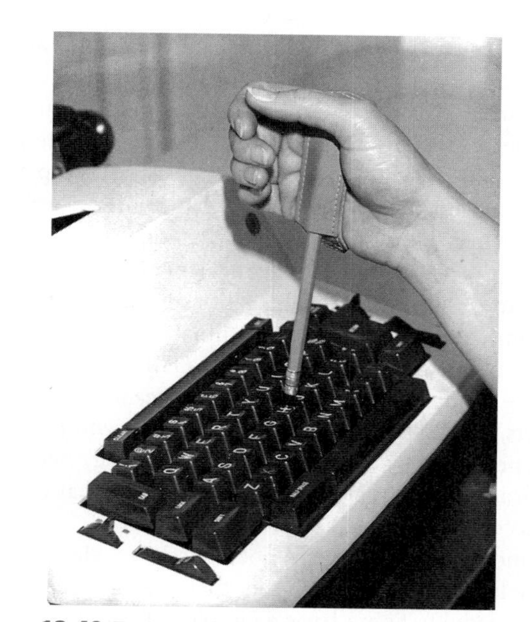

Figure 13-40 Typing with aid of utensil holder and typing stick.

6. Sophisticated augmented communication devices operated by mouth, pneumatic controls, and head control are available for clients with no upper extremity function.[54] (See Chapter 14.)
7. Audiocassettes may still be used by some clients. Kelly[26] described two mouthsticks and a cassette tape holder that allow persons with C3, C4, or C5 quadriplegia to operate a tape recorder or radio independently. The first mouthstick, a rod about 20 inches (50 cm) long with a friction tip, is used to depress the operating buttons and adjust the radio's volume and selector dials. The second mouthstick is a metal rod that separates into two prongs at its end. These prongs are 4 inches (10 cm) apart, and the mouthstick is used to insert cassettes from the cassette holder into the tape recorder and to remove cassettes from the recorder. The vertical cassette tape stand is made of metal, tilted backward at a 70-degree angle, and designed to hold eight tapes at its eight levels. Kelly[26] offers specifications on construction of these devices.
8. For managing knobs or controls that require a strong lateral pinch, the person can use a potato masher to interlace around the knob and use his or her entire hand to twist the knob.
9. Place a terry cloth wristband around a glass or mug to protect the hand from excessive hot or cold and to provide friction to require less force to hold.

Assistive Technology

For clients with severe physical impairments, options in assistive technology can help improve independence with ADL. According to the Human Activity Assistance Technology (HAAT) model, a person choosing the best system for his or her client must consider the person using the technology, the activity the technology will be used to perform, and the environment in which the technology will be used in order to set up the best system for the client.[47] The client's tolerance of technology and adaptive devices and his or her ability to learn complex commands should be considered. A complete discussion of assistive technology is provided in Chapter 14. Technology rapidly introduces new products to the general public. The OT practitioner should always stay up to date with the newest opportunities to enhance his or her clients' independence. Subscribing to product catalogs such as the *Disabled Dealer* (www.disableddealer.com) or attending yearly expositions such as the Abilities Expo (www.abilities-expo.com), the American Occupational Therapy Association (AOTA) national conference, or state OT association conferences are some ways to remain knowledgeable about current products. The *Computer Resource for People with Disabilities*, a book presented by the Alliance for Technology Access, provides product information on making a personal computer more accessible.

All individuals in modern society rely on electronic aids to daily living (EADL), products that use electricity to perform an activity. Some basic examples of EADLs are radios or lamps. Some EADLs require mobility and physical abilities to control.[46] By setting up a central unit, the therapist enables the client to control a number of appliances around the home from a centralized area.

Quartet Technology's Simplicity line is an example of a unit that can control a vast number of EADLs in the environment.[47] This device can perform tasks such as operating a personal computer; activating the controls normally performed by a remote control on a television, DVD player, or stereo; dialing and receiving options on a telephone; controlling the lighting and temperature in the room or house; and adjusting the exact position of a hospital bed. The therapist can work with his or her patient to find the easiest way to operate the system. This product responds to voice, sip and puff, switches, and radio remote.

A control device can be linked to all adaptive devices in the house, thus allowing a patient to independently perform detailed tasks such as turning a page in a book, dialing a friend on the telephone, opening a door, listening to a favorite song on a CD, and checking e-mail.[46]

A unique product for increasing independence for clients with significant physical impairments is the Assistant Robot Manipulator (ARM).[14] This robotic arm is attached to the power wheelchair and can be controlled with a joystick or switch to perform a wide variety of ADL. It can be used to assist with self-feeding, brushing teeth, picking up objects from the floor or overhead, opening the door to a microwave, inserting a DVD into the player, and scratching an itch. If a patient is cognitively capable of performing tasks but cannot physically participate, the ARM helps bridge this gap. With precise training, the patient can learn to perform enough tasks to rely less on caregiver assistance.[14]

An important factor to consider when recommending assistive technology is cost. Many new products are not covered by insurance. The therapist should consider whether the cost of the product can be justified if it will cut back on personal assistant or home modification needs. He or she should be realistic about the patient's training abilities. If the patient will be unable to use the full capabilities of the product, a more basic option should be considered.

Mobility and Transfers

Chapter 15 discusses principles of wheelchair transfer techniques for the quadriplegic client. Mobility depends on degree of weakness. Power wheelchairs operated by hand, chin, or pneumatic (sip and puff) controls have greatly increased the mobility of clients with severe upper and lower extremity weakness. Vans and public buses fitted with wheelchair lifts and stabilizing devices have provided such clients with transport to pursue community, vocational, educational, and avocational activities with an assistant. In addition, adaptations for hand controls have allowed many clients with at least C6-level function to drive independently.

Home Management Activities

Many wheelchair-dependent clients with upper extremity weakness are dependent or partly dependent for homemaking activities. Clients with muscle function of C6 or better may be independent for light homemaking with appropriate devices, adaptations, and safety awareness. Many of the suggestions for wheelchair maneuverability and environmental adaptation outlined for the paraplegic client apply to these clients as well. In addition, the patient with upper extremity weakness needs to use lightweight equipment and special devices. The *Mealtime Manual for People with Disability and the Aging* contains many excellent and specific suggestions that apply to the cook with weak upper extremities.[28]

Parenting with a Disability

The need for OT practitioners to address the ADL of parenting or caregiving is growing. An increasing number of people with disabilities are choosing to raise their own families. Some patients may already be parents at the time of injury or diagnosis of a disorder. Familiarizing such patients with helpful childcare products available for the general public (universal design) may be especially advantageous for a parent with a disability.[42] The practitioner may need to assist the patient in customizing products to meet more specific needs.

Funding for services and products may be available in the form of direct government financial assistance. The United States federal government allots funds specifically for parents with disabilities. Rehabilitative engineering departments at local hospitals often offer assistance in fabrication of custom products. The Rehabilitation Institute of Chicago and the National Rehabilitation Hospital in Washington D.C. have renowned rehabilitation engineering departments and are worth consulting. Volunteers for Medical Engineering is a philanthropic organization that helps create custom products.

Through the Looking Glass is a research, training, and service center devoted to families in which a parent or child has a disability.[43] This center, located in Berkeley, Calif., publishes a number of resources to help parents with disabilities perform childcare tasks independently. These resources discuss caregiving techniques, adaptive aids, and current research. The website, www.lookingglass.org, shows inspiring photos, information on obtaining publications, and updates on nationwide conferences, workshops, and support groups. Parents can also be referred to the Parent Empowerment Network to connect with other parents and find commercially available childcare products and tips.

Adapting the environment and introducing the client to a variety of parenting assistive devices can increase the client's independence with childcare activities. A client may have a physical disability too severe to allow him or her to care for the child safely. Nurturing assistance involves a hired aide who provides physical assistance to parents with young children.[39] The parent directs the nurturing assistant through the tasks. This process facilitates parental involvement to fulfill the emotional need for the parent and can help strengthen the parent-child bond.[39]

The following discussion lists ready-made or custom-made products to help assist with childcare activities for parents with a variety of disabilities. A full evaluation of the parent's abilities to physically and cognitively perform all childcare tasks is necessary to determine the safety of the parent and child.

The Babee Tenda Safety Convertible Crib is a crib with a toddler gate that allows a parent to retrieve the baby from the crib at wheelchair level. It reduces risks that may occur when parents with upper extremity weakness or pain attempt to reach over a standard, drop-down crib.

Velcro disposable diapers allow the parent to position and reposition closures without ripping the diaper.

This product helps those with dexterity impairments change diapers with ease.

Childproofing the home can be a difficult feat when the parent has strength or dexterity problems. Standard safety locks and gates block access to the parent with a disability, as well as the child. Tot-loks is a safety lock for cabinets that is released when a strong magnet is held up to the exact location of the latch. The magnet must be kept out of reach of the child to ensure safety.

Holding the child when the parent uses a wheelchair poses a safety problem. The Baby B'Air Airline Safety Harness was created for babies seated in the parent's lap during an airplane flight. It is threaded through the airline safety belt; however, it can also be used to secure the baby onto a parent in a wheelchair by threading it through the wheelchair safety belt.

A variety of baby holders that may be helpful for a parent who requires use of an assistive device when ambulating are commercially available. Some examples include the Baby Bjorn, the Over the Shoulder Baby Holder, and the Sling Rider. Depending on the temperament of the baby and the physical needs of the parent, one product might work better than others.

Positioning for breast-feeding may be problematic for patients with upper extremity weakness. "Meals on Wheels" was created specifically for a mother with cerebral palsy who was struggling with positioning her baby for breast-feeding while seated in her wheelchair. A rehabilitation engineer modified a wheelchair lap tray that was secured on the armrests of the chair to hold a baby positioning device on top.

Helping the parent with a disability maintain independence for childcare tasks is a dynamic activity. The OT practitioner must consider the ever-changing needs of a growing child and potential changes in the physical or cognitive status of the parent. Continual reassessment of childcare tasks is necessary to ensure the safest and easiest solutions.

Traveling with a Disability

The prospect of traveling can bring up numerous issues and concerns for individuals with disabilities. The practitioner should encourage clients to plan ahead for trips and provide them with the resources needed to help with planning. Travelers with a disability need to be educated about their rights and the resources available to them.

During airline travel, clients may encounter a variety of obstacles. The Air Carrier Access Act, passed in 1986, ensures that people with disabilities receive consistent and nondiscriminatory treatment when traveling by air.[44] The client is required to provide the airline with at least 48 hours notice to allow accommodations to be made. Most wheelchairs do not fit in the aisle of the plane, so the client needs to transfer to an aisle chair to get to his or her seat (see www.casa.gov.au/airsafe/disable/wheeltips.htm).[51] If the flight is long, the client should request that the aisle chair be available during the flight to allow him or her access to the bathroom.

All power wheelchairs must be stowed as checked luggage. Removing seat cushions or any other loose parts that could get lost during the flight is helpful. Attaching instructions on how to assemble or disassemble the chair for storage can help the flight crew properly handle the chair. For international travel, including illustrations or pictures on the instruction sheet may be wise.[52] If the client is traveling with a manual wheelchair that can be folded, he or she can request that it be stowed in the onboard coat closet. Traveling with basic wheelchair maintenance tools is helpful if problems occur during the flight. Clients should be advised to research ahead to have a list of wheelchair vendors at the destination in case repairs are needed.

Transferring while on the airplane can be difficult. The disabled person should ask the airline representative during the reservation process for as much information about the facilities on the type of plane for the specific flight. Any aircraft with 30 or more passengers built after 1990 is required to have movable armrests on some aisle seats to allow more room for the transfer.[44] If requested, the airline may provide a free upgrade to first class to clients traveling with wheelchairs to allow for a safer and more efficient boarding process. Some of the larger and newer aircraft have an accessible restroom with outward swinging doors and handrails; they are large enough to fit the aisle chair inside. Alternatively, it may be possible to swing and clip the doors to increase the space. If no accessible restrooms are available, there may be an area of the plane with a privacy curtain to allow a companion to assist with toileting activities or changing clothing.

It is important to know about the environment where the disabled person will be staying. If booking a hotel room, the disabled person should request an accessible room and specify what he or she needs. The person should ensure that the room and restroom have ample space for a wheelchair, if necessary, and should learn what bathroom equipment such as a shower chair or commode can be requested. If the person calling is not specific about needs, the hotel representative may claim that a room is accessible simply because grab bars are installed in the restroom.

The travel industry has recently become involved in making traveling easier for individuals with varying degrees of disabilities. Accessible bus tours, trains, and cruises are available.[44] One can rent an accessible van or arrange for basic hand controls to be installed into a rental car if needed. Providing clients with information on all the available resources may encourage them to travel.

Service Animals and Skilled Companions

Service animals can help to enhance independence in occupational performance for individuals with physical disabilities. Service animals can do much more than guide individuals with vision impairments. They can reduce the reliance on other people to perform tasks disabled individuals have difficulty performing on their own. Service animals are also known to help increase community participation, social contact, personal skill development, adjustment to challenges, and sense of responsibility.[9] Service animals often evoke feelings of "always having someone to watch over" and being "like an able-bodied person again."[9]

Some occupational therapists work with these animals during rehabilitation treatment sessions. These animals can provide the added mental, physical, and emotional support when patients are trying to learn or relearn living skills. These sessions can also screen patients for the need and appropriateness of a skilled companion or service animal of their own. Rehabilitation professionals can become advocates for their clients in obtaining, training, and adjusting to living with a service dog.[35] The Assistance Dog Institute provides coursework and advanced degrees for health care professionals to better understand training strategies and the complex relationship between dogs and humans in society.[4]

Numerous organizations throughout the United States train animals to become assistance dogs. Canine Companions for Independence pairs the participant and dog together and establishes a training team.[10] The team consists of the student, the service dog or skilled companion, and a facilitator to teach the handling process and help extend the abilities of the dog. The goal is to help develop the maximum amount of independence that a team can achieve with an assistance dog. This organization also trains animals to work directly with the health care professional as facility-based service animals and prepares dogs to work with hearing-impaired people.[10]

Helping Hands is an organization that trains Capuchin monkeys to assist individuals with quadriplegia with daily activities.[21] Their intelligence and fine motor dexterity allow these monkeys to perform a wide variety of tasks such as assisting with feeding or retrieving and placing a tissue on the nose after a sneeze. These monkeys have small hands, but they can be trained to don splints to allow them to expand their reach and allow them to open a large jar lid or respiration equipment valve. The affectionate and responsive nature of these animals allows them to become companions and improve mental and emotional quality of life.[21]

During the evaluation of occupational performance, the occupational therapist can screen patients for the appropriateness of introducing an assistance dog or skilled companion. Providing patients with knowledge and resources about service animals early after onset of a disability can inspire them to readjust their expectations for independence.

Summary

ADL and IADL are tasks of self-maintenance, mobility, communication, home management, and community living skills that allow a client to function independently and assume important occupational roles.

ADL and IADL are major life activities that consume significant time even for persons without disabilities. OT practitioners routinely evaluate performance in ADL to assess clients' level of functional independence. The OTA may establish service competency and special expertise in this practice area. Evaluation is performed through the interview and observation of performance. Evaluation results and ongoing progress are recorded on one of many available ADL checklists, and the content is summarized for the permanent medical record.

Treatment is directed toward training in independent living skills using methods in such activity areas as eating, dressing, mobility, home management, communication, and community living. The OTA practicing in this area should be familiar with the special equipment and methods for performing ADL needed by the client with specific functional problems.

Selected Reading Guide Questions

1. Define and differentiate between ADL and IADL. List three subcategories in both ADL and IADL.
2. Describe the role of OT in restoring ADL and IADL independence.
3. List at least three activities for each of the following subcategories of skills: self-care, mobility, communication, home management, and community living.
4. List three factors that the OT practitioner must consider before commencing ADL performance evaluation and training. Describe how each could limit or affect the client's ADL performance.
5. Discuss the concept of *maximal independence,* as defined in the text.
6. List the general steps in the procedure for ADL evaluation.
7. What is the purpose of the home evaluation?
8. List the steps in the home evaluation.
9. Who should be involved in a comprehensive home evaluation?
10. What other areas or factors are assessed in a home evaluation?

11. How does the OT practitioner record and report results of the home evaluation and make the necessary recommendations?
12. How does the OT practitioner, with the client, select ADL and IADL training objectives after an evaluation?
13. Describe three approaches to teaching ADL skills to a client with perception or memory deficits.
14. List the important factors to include in an ADL progress report.
15. Give an example of a health and safety management issue.
16. Explain how an OTA would establish service competency and maximal independence in providing ADL services within the legal guidelines of his or her state or other local jurisdiction.

Exercises

1. Demonstrate the use of at least three assistive devices mentioned in the text.
2. Teach a person to don a shirt, using one hand.
3. Teach another person how to don and remove trousers, as if the person had hemiplegia.
4. Teach a person how to make a sandwich with only one hand.
5. Teach a different person how to don and remove trousers, as if his or her legs were paralyzed.

References

1. Activities of daily living for patients with incoordination, limited range of motion, paraplegia, quadriplegia, and hemiplegia, Cleveland, 1968, Division of Occupational therapy, Highland View Hospital, Cuyahoga County Hospitals (unpublished).
2. Occupational Therapy Practice Framework: Domain and process, ed 2, *Am J Occup Ther* 62(6):625–683, 2008.
3. Armstrong M, Lauzen S: *Community integration program*, ed 2, Washington, 1994, Idyll Arbor.
4. ADI Degree Programs: http://www.assistancedog.org/college/degree_programs.html, Accessed October 7, 2004.
5. Bottom Buddy Toilet Aid. http://www.activeforever.com/p-1272-bottom-buddy-toilet-aid.aspx.
6. Branick L: Integrating the principles of energy conservation during everyday activities, *Caring* 22(1):30–31, 2004.
7. Bromley I: *Tetraplegia and paraplegia: a guide for physiotherapists*, ed 2, London, 1981, Churchill Livingstone.
8. Buchwald E: *Physical rehabilitation for daily living*, New York, 1952, McGraw-Hill.
9. Camp MM: The use of service dogs as an adaptive strategy: a qualitative study, *Am J Occup Ther* 55(5):509–517, 2001.
10. Canine Companion service. http://www.caninecompanions.org/-our_services.html Accessed October 2, 2004.
11. Christiansen C: Occupational performance assessment. In Christiansen C, Baum C, editors: *Occupational therapy: overcoming human performance deficits*, Thorofare, NJ, 1991, Slack.
12. Cynkin S, Robinson AM: *Occupational therapy and activities health: toward health through activities*, Boston, 1990, Little, Brown.
13. Easton LW, Horan AL: Dressing band, *Am J Occup Ther* 33:656, 1979.
14. Exact Dynamics BV: *Edisonstraat 96, NL-6942 PZ, Didam, the Netherlands Assistive Robotic Manipulator product information.* http://www.exactdynamics.nl/ retrieved from the web, November 3, 2004.
15. Feldmeier DM, Poole JL: The position-adjustable hair dryer, *Am J Occup Ther* 41:246, 1987.
16. Florey LL, Michelman SM: Occupational role history: a screening tool for psychiatric occupational therapy, *Am J Occup Ther* 36:301, 1982.
17. Freedom Wand Toilet Aid: *self-wipe, sanitary, wiping aid.* http://www.freedomwand.com Accessed September 16, 2010.
18. Gagne DE, Hoppes S: The effects of collaborative goal-focused occupational therapy on self-care skills: a pilot study, *Am J Occup Ther* 57(2):215–219, 2003.
19. Gripit Floss Holder. http://sale.dentist.net/products/gripit-floss-holder. Accessed September 19, 2010
20. Guerette P, Moran W: ADL awareness, *Team Rehabil Rep* June 1994.
21. *Helping Hands—Monkey Helpers for the Disabled.* http://www.helpinghandsmonkeys.org. Accessed October 8, 2010.
22. Holser P, Jones M, Ilanit T: A study of the upper extremity control brace, *Am J Occup Ther* 16:170, 1962.
23. *Home Safety Checklist*, San Francisco, 1995, California Department of Aging, Senior Housing Information and Support Center.
24. Hopkins HL, Smith HD, Tiffany EG: Therapeutic application of activity. In Hopkins HL, Smith HD, editors: *Willard and Spackman's occupational therapy*, ed 6, Philadelphia, 1983, Lippincott.
25. Jonathan's Son, Handcrafted solutions to your accessibility and mobility needs, Santa Rosa, CA.
26. Kelly SN: Adaptations for independent use of cassette tape recorder/radio by high-level quadriplegic patients, *Am J Occup Ther* 37:766, 1983.
27. Kemp BJ, Mitchell JM: Functional assessment in geriatric mental health. In Birren JE, et al: *Handbook of mental health and aging*, ed 2, San Diego, 1993, Academic Press.
28. Klinger JL: *Mealtime manual for people with disabilities and the aging*, Camden, NJ, 1978, Campbell Soup.
29. Letts L, et al: Person-environment assessments in occupational therapy, *Am J Occup Ther* 48:608–618, 1994.
30. Malick MH, Almasy BS: Activities of daily living and homemaking. In Hopkins HL, Smith HD, editors: *Willard and Spackman's occupational therapy*, ed 7, Philadelphia, 1988, Lippincott.
31. Malick MH, Almasy BS: Assessment and evaluation: life work tasks. In Hopkins HL, Smith HD, editors: *Willard and Spackman's occupational therapy*, ed 6, Philadelphia, 1983, Lippincott.
32. Matsusuyu J: The interest checklist, *Am J Occup Ther* 23:323, 1969.
33. Mayer TK: *One-handed in a two-handed world*, ed 2, Boston, 2000, Prince-Gallison Press.
34. Melvin JL: *Rheumatic disease: occupational therapy and rehabilitation*, ed 2, Philadelphia, 1982, Davis.
35. Madlin S: From puppy to service dog: raising service dogs for the rehabilitation team, *Rehabil Nurs* 26(1):12–17, 2001.
36. Moorhead L: The occupational history, *Am J Occup Ther* 23:329, 1969.
37. *North Coast Medical Rehabilitation Catalog 2004/ 2005*, Morgan Hill, 2004. http://www.ncmedical.com2004. Accessed October 3, 2010.
38. Nuance-Dragon Naturally Speaking. http://www.nuance.com/. Accessed October 8, 2010.

39. Nurturing Assistance: *Physical support for parents with disabilities.* http://www.enablelink.org/nurturing.html. Accessed October 3, 2010.
40. Nygard L, Grahn U, Rudenhammer A, et al: Reflecting on practice: are home visits prior to discharge worthwhile in geriatric inpatient care? Clients' and occupational therapists' perceptions, *Scand J Caring Sci* 18:193–203, 2004.
41. Pardessus V, et al: Benefits of home visits for falls and autonomy in the elderly: a randomized trial study, *Am J Phys Med Rehabil* 81(4):247–252, 2002.
42. Parent Empowerment Network, http://www.disabledparent.net Accessed October 8, 2010
43. Parents with Disabilities, http://lookingglass.org/index.php September 8, 2004, October 16, 2004, September 19, 2010. www.enablelink.org.
44. *Planet Mobility accessible air travel & airline tickets*http://www.planetmobility.com/go/travel/air. Accessed October 29, 2004.
45. Purex Complete 3-in-1 Laundry Dispenser. http://www.amazon.com/Complete-Dispenser-Detergent-Softener-Anti-static/dp Accessed September 16, 2010.
46. Public Utilities Commission: *Deaf & Disabled Telecommunication Program.* www.ddtp.org. Accessed September 16, 2010.
47. Quartet Technology, Inc: *Extraordinary technology that lets you get back to everyday living,* Tyngsboro, MA, www.enablelink.org.
48. Runge M: Self-dressing techniques for clients with spinal cord injury, *Am J Occup Ther* 21:367, 1967.
49. *Sammons Preston Rolyan 2004 Professional Rehabilitation Catalog*:Bolingbrook IL, 2004, http://www.sammonspreston-rolyan.com.
50. Sokaler R: A buttoning aid, *Am J Occup Ther* 35:737, 1981.
51. *Travel tips for wheelchair users*http://www.casa.gov.au/airsafe/disable/wheeltips.htm:Accessed October 29, 2004.
52. *Traveling with a disability*http://e-bility.com/articles/accessible_travels.shtml:January 2004, October 29, 2004.
53. Trombly CA: Activities of daily living. In Trombly CA, editor: *Occupational therapy for physical dysfunction,* ed 2, Baltimore, 1983, Williams & Wilkins.
54. Trombly CA: Retraining basic and instrumental activities of daily living. In Trombly CA, editor: *Occupational therapy for physical dysfunction,* ed 4, Baltimore, 1995, Williams & Wilkins.
55. *What are our rights as tenants with disabilities?* Palo Alto, 2004, Midpeninsula Citizens for Fair Housing (unpublished).
56. Wykoff E, Mitani M: The spoon plate: a self-feeding device, *Am J Occup Ther* 36:333, 1982.

Recommended Reading

Pendleton HM, Schultz-Krohn, Winifred: *Pedretti's occupational therapy practice skills for physical dysfunction,* ed 7, St. Louis, 2013, Elsevier, Inc.

Sine RD, et al: *Basic rehabilitation techniques: a self-instructional guide,* ed 3, Gaithersburg, Md, 1988, Aspen.

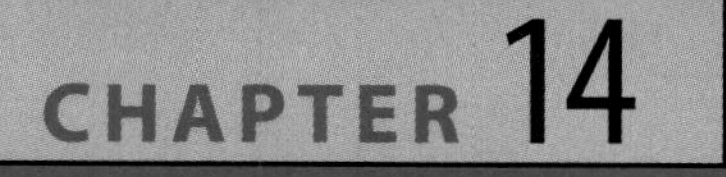

Assistive Technology

DENIS ANSON

Key Terms

Rehabilitation technology
Assistive technologies
Universal design
Human interface assessment (HIA) model
Electronic aids to daily living (EADL)
Power switching
Subsumed devices
X-10 system
Feature control
Augmentative and alternative communication
Message composition
Message transmission
Graphical communication
Physical keyboard
Virtual keyboard
Pointing systems
Eye tracking
Switch encoding
Speech input
Scanning input
Rate enhancement
Semantic compaction
Integrated controls
Compression/expansion
Speech output
Tactile output

Chapter Objectives

After studying this chapter, the student or practitioner will be able to:

1. Define assistive technology and contrast it with rehabilitative technologies.
2. Explain why universal design is not considered assistive technology.
3. Describe the Human Interface Assessment model.
4. Discuss the pros and cons of electronic aids to daily living for different populations.
5. Consider augmentative and alternative communications used both for augmentative and for alternative communication, and explain considerations for each use.
6. Discuss the pros and cons of different technologies for keyboarding for persons with disabilities.
7. Discuss the advantages and disadvantages of current speech input and voice output technologies.
8. Explain why Braille is mandated by the Individuals with Disabilities Education Act of 1997.

CASE STUDY

Mary, Part 1

Mary is a 26-year-old, would-be lawyer. Her path to the legal profession is obstructed by her C4 level, complete spinal cord injury, which she sustained 12 years previously in the automobile accident that killed her parents. Mary is bright, articulate, and exceptionally popular in her rural community. She recently received a new wheelchair with sip-and-puff controls, which allows her mobility in her home and community, and now she would like to attend law school. Ultimately, Mary would like to specialize in disability rights, to support the civil rights of others with profound disabilities. She feels that her "insider" perspective on the issues might make her arguments more compelling when disabled workers are seeking reasonable accommodations.

The admissions office at the nearby university—which includes a law program—suggests that Mary may have a difficult time completing the required work. As a law student, Mary will have to research legal precedence in case law and write briefs. She can get into the library, which meets many of the requirements of the Americans with Disabilities Act, but will need to be able to navigate the legal record, take notes of her findings, and write formal responses to legal challenges. The counselor feels that Mary, who has no movement below her neck, may find the challenges of the legal profession to exceed her capabilities.

Mary does have full-time attendant care, and the attendant would be allowed to sit with Mary in the classroom and take notes for her. (The school also provides lecture notes to disabled students within 3 days of a class session, if requested.) However, because Mary's attendant must constantly monitor Mary, her ability to focus on the lecture may be impaired. Also, because the attendant does not have the interest or background to study law, her ability to tell what is important is limited. Finally, because Mary generally changes attendants every 6 months or so, the attendant will not have a complete background to help with interpretation of the material Mary is studying. In her home life, Mary would very much like to be able to adjust the lights, the room temperature, and radio station (she prefers to study with music in the background) that is playing without interrupting her attendant. She knows that she will always be dependent on others for bathing, dressing, meal preparation, and many other aspects of her activities of daily living. However, she feels that her attendants might be able to remain in her employ longer if she were able to do more for herself and make fewer demands on them.

Mary has had an assistive technology consult and has obtained some of the recommended adaptations to allow her to attend law school.

1. What training strategies might help Mary learn to use her assistive technologies?
2. How would a clinician know that the assistive technology is performing as intended?
3. Now that Mary has assistive technology, would it be reasonable to expect her to perform like her able-bodied peers?
4. Now that Mary has assistive technology, is it reasonable to expect her to succeed in her goal of becoming a lawyer?

What Is Assistive Technology?

A discussion of assistive technology (AT) should begin with a description of the general limits of the topic. This is made difficult because the legal definitions of AT are not uniform. Assistive technologies are sometimes included in the category of rehabilitation technology.[20] In other cases, rehabilitation technology is considered an aspect of assistive technologies.[12,13] A third category of "universal designed technologies" does not seem to fit into either category.[19] For purposes of this discussion, the author presents a set of definitions that are within current practice, but not necessarily congruent with any particular statute.

Rehabilitative/Assistive/Universal Technologies

The category into which an enabling technology falls depends largely on its application, not on the nature of the device. What is for some people a convenience may for another be an AT.

Rehabilitation Technology

To rehabilitate is to restore to a prior level of function. To be consistent with general usage, therefore, the term **rehabilitation technology** should be used to describe those technologies that are intended to restore an individual to a previous level of function following the onset of pathology. When an occupational therapist uses a technological device to establish, restore, or modify functioning in the client, he or she is using a rehabilitative technology. Rehabilitative technologies are generally intended to be used within a therapy setting, by trained professionals, and over a short period of time. The expectation is that the professional may have significant training before applying the technology. The professional guiding the use of such technologies is expected to ensure the correct application of the technology and to protect the safety of the individual using the device. Physical agent modalities such as ultrasound, diathermy, paraffin, and functional electric stimulation, which may be used in OT as preparation for participation in meaningful activity, are examples of rehabilitative technologies. When these technologies have done their job, the client will have improved intrinsic function and the technology will be removed.

Assistive Technology

Central to occupational therapy is the belief that active engagement in meaningful activity supports the health and well-being of the individual. An individual who has functional limitations secondary to some pathology may not have the cognitive, motor, or psychological skills demanded by a desired meaningful activity and may require assistance to participate.

To assist is to help, aid, or support. There is no implication of restoration in assistance. Assistive technologies, therefore, are those technologies that assist a person with a disability in performing tasks. More specifically, assistive technologies are those technologies, whether designed for a person with a disability or designed for mass market and used by a person with a disability, which allow that person to perform tasks that an able-bodied person can do without technological assistance. It may be that an able-bodied person would prefer to use a technology to perform a task (e.g., using a television remote control), but it does not rise to the level of AT so long as it is possible for the able-bodied person to perform the task without the technology.

Assistive technologies replace or support an impaired function of the user without being expected to change the native functioning of the individual. A wheelchair, for example, replaces the function of walking but is not expected to teach the user to walk. Similarly, forearm crutches support independent standing but do not, of themselves, improve strength or bony integrity, so they will not change the ability of the user to stand without them.

Because they are not expected to change the native ability of the user, assistive technologies have different design considerations. They are expected to be used over prolonged periods of time, by individuals with limited training, and possibly with limited cognitive skills. The controls of the device must be readily understood so that constant retraining will not be required, although some training may be required to use the device. The device should not require deep understanding of its principles and functions to be useful.

One significant difference between rehabilitation technology and AT occurs at the end of the rehabilitation process. At this point, the client no longer uses rehabilitation technologies but may have just completed training in the use of assistive technologies. The assistive technologies go home with the client; the rehabilitation technologies generally remain in a clinic. Some technologies do not fit neatly into these categories because they may be used differently with different clients. Some clinicians use assisted communication as a tool to train unassisted speech for their clients. For other clients, assisted communication may be used to support or replace speech. In the first case, the technology is rehabilitative. In the second, the same technology may be assistive.

Universal Design

Universal design is a relatively new category of technology. The principles of universal design were published by The Center for Universal Design at North Carolina State University in 1997, and their application is still limited. The concept of universal design is simple: If devices are designed to meet the needs of people with a wide range of abilities, they will be more usable for all users, with and without disabilities.

This design philosophy could, in some cases, make AT unnecessary. A can-opener that has been designed for one-handed use by a busy housewife will also be usable by the cook who has had a CVA and now only has use of one hand. Because both individuals are using the same product for the same purpose, it is just technology, not AT. Some eBook readers include a feature to allow them to be used as "talking books." In an interesting reversal of the typical relationship, the Apple iPad includes this ability to allow blind users to access onscreen content, but the same feature can be used by commuters while driving. No adaptation is necessary because accommodations for the special needs of the person with a disability have already been designed into the product.

Role of Assistive Technology in Occupational Participation

The *Occupational Therapy Practice Framework*, 2nd Edition[1] defines the appropriate domain of occupational therapy as including the analysis of the performance skills and patterns of the individual and the activity demands of the occupation the individual is attempting to perform.

Human Interface Assessment

Anson's Human Interface Assessment (HIA) model provides a detailed look at the skills and abilities of the human in the skill areas of motor, process, and communication/interaction, as well as the demands of an activity (Figure 14-1, *A*). The HIA model suggests that when the demands of a task do not exceed the skills and abilities of an individual, no AT is required, even when a functional limitation exists (Figure 14-1, *B*). On the other hand, when a task makes demands that exceed the native abilities of the individual, the individual will not be able to perform the task in the prescribed manner (Figure 14-1, *C*). In these cases, an AT device may be used to bridge the gap between the demands and abilities (Figure 14-1, *D*).

Although an AT must be able to assist in performing the desired task, it also presents an interface that must match the needs of the client. A careful match among the sensory, cognitive, and motor abilities of the human and the input and output capabilities of assistive technologies is necessary.

When assisting a client to learn to use an AT, the attention of the OTA should first focus on whether the individual can control the technology. (Does the AT make demands beyond the ability of the client?). Once it is determined that the client can control the device, the focus should shift to the ability of the client to perform the tasks for which the AT was recommended. Unless the client's ability to perform the task has improved, the AT is not effective. A great risk in providing AT is the tendency to focus on the ability of the person to use the technology, while overlooking the tasks for which it should be used. If a man with a spinal cord injury is provided with an EADL, for example, is he able to independently control the temperature of the environment to avoid overheating?

Types of Electronic Enabling Technologies

Although modern technology can blur some of the distinctions presented as follows, it is useful to consider assistive technologies in categories for which they are applied. This chapter

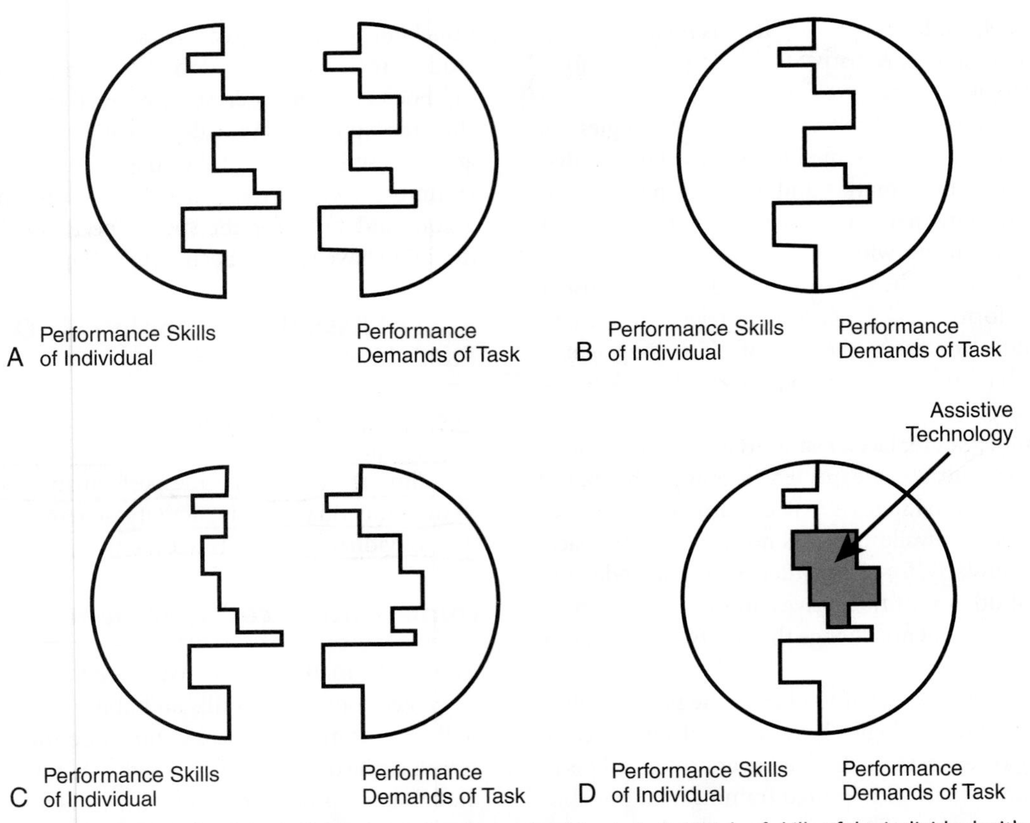

Figure 14-1 **A,** Skills of the individual and the demands of the task. **B,** Match of skills of the individual with the demands of the task. **C,** Skills of the individual and demands of the task mismatch. **D,** Assistive technology used to bridge gap between the skills of the individual and the demands of the task.

deals only with electronic assistive technologies, which, in terms of their primary application, may be considered to fall into three categories: electronic aids to daily living (EADL), alternative and augmentative communications (AACs), and general computer applications.

Electronic Aids to Daily Living

Electronic aids to daily living (EADL) are devices that can be used to control electrical devices in the client's environment. Before 1998,[41] this category of device was generally known as an *environmental control unit* (ECU) (though technically, this terminology should be reserved for furnace thermostats and similar controls). The more generic EADL applies to control of lighting and temperature but may also extend to control of radios, televisions, telephones, and other electrical and electronic devices in the environment of the client (Figure 14-2).[5,14-16,18,22,26,43]

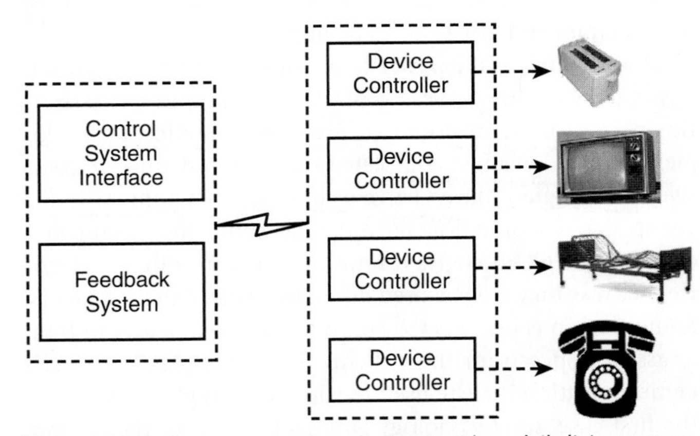

Figure 14-2 Components of an electronic aids to daily living system.

EADL systems may be characterized by the degree and types of control that they provide to the user. These levels of control are simple power switching, control of device features, and subsumed devices (Figure 14-3).

Power Switching

The simplest EADL provide simple switching of the electrical supply for devices in a room. Although not typically classified as EADL, the switch adaptations for switch-adapted toys provided to severely disabled children would, formally, be included in this category of device. Primitive EADL systems consisted of little more than a set of electrical switches and outlets in a box that is connected to devices within a room via extension cords. Second-generation EADL systems use various remote control technologies to switch power to electrical devices in the environment.

Regardless of the means used to communicate between the device and the controller, the user must know which control operates which device. Some systems, such as the TASH Ultra 4,[59] use colored markers on the control device and switch box to make this connection. Other systems, such as the X-10 system,[54] use encoding switches so that any control module can be controlled by any input of the controller. So long as the client is able to turn on the intended device reliably,

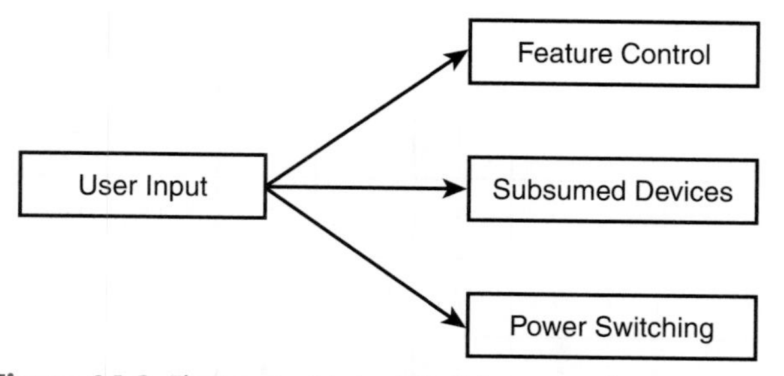

Figure 14-3 Electronic aids to daily living control components.

the coding is not relevant. However, systems like X-10 can offer more options than Ultra-4.

When working with a client on a power-switching EADL, it is important to ensure that the client can operate the controls of the device, to recognize which control operates which light or appliance, and to turn devices on and off at will. Ability to control devices should be evaluated when the client is relaxed and rested, as well as when fatigued. Unless the client can control his or her environment all through the day, the EADL will not be effective.

Feature Control

As electronic systems became more common in the home, devices that simply switched lights and coffee pots on and off failed to meet the needs of the individual with a disability who wanted to control the immediate environment. With wall current control, a person with a disability might be able to turn radios and televisions on and off but would have no control beyond that. A person with a disability might want to be able to surf cable channels as much as an able-bodied person with a television remote control. When advertisements are blaring from the speakers, a person with a disability might want to be able to turn down the sound or tune to another radio station. Nearly all home electronic devices are now delivered with a remote control, generally using infrared signals. Most of these remote controls are not usable by a person with a disability, due to demands for fine motor control and good sensory discrimination.

EADL systems designed to provide access to the home environment of a person with a disability must provide more than on/off control of home electronics. They must also provide control of the features of home electronic devices. Because of this need, EADL systems frequently have hybrid capabilities and incorporate a means of switching power directly to remote devices, often using X-10 technology. This allows operation of devices such as lights, fans, and coffee pots, as well as electrical door openers and other specialty devices.[50,51] These EADL systems typically also incorporate some form of infrared remote control, allowing them to mimic the signals of standard remote control devices. This control is provided either by programming in the standard sequences for all commercially available VCRs, televisions, and satellite decoders or through teaching systems, in which the EADL learns the codes beamed at it by the conventional remote. The advantage of the latter approach is that the EADL can learn any codes, even those that have not yet been invented. The disadvantage is that the controls must be taught, requiring more setup and configuration time for the user and caregivers.

Infrared remote control, as adopted by most entertainment systems controllers, is limited to approximate line of sight control. Unless the controller is aimed in the general direction of the device to be controlled (most have wide dispersion patterns), the signals will not be received. This means that an EADL cannot directly control, via infrared, any device located in another room. However, infrared repeaters, such as the X-10 Powermid[11] can overcome this limitation by using radio signals to send the control signals received in one room to a transmitter in the room of the device to be controlled. With a collection of repeaters, a person would be able to control any infrared device in the home from anywhere else in the home.

The proliferation of remote control devices is a problem shared by EADL users and able-bodied consumers alike. Many homes now are cluttered with separate remote controls for the television, the cable/satellite receiver, the DVD player/VHS recorder (either one or two devices), the home stereo/multimedia center, and other devices, all in the same room. Universal remote controls allow switching control from one device to another but are often cumbersome to operate and do not provide the full features of the controlled devices. As the number of devices to be controlled by an EADL increases, the complexity of the device does also. It is important to make sure, as the number of devices and options grow, that the client remains able to control the environment easily.

One interesting aspect of feature control by EADL is the relationship between EADL and computers. Some EADL systems, such as the Quartet Simplicity,[49] include features to allow the user to control a personal computer through the EADL. In general, this is little more than a pass-through of the control system of the EADL to a computer access system. Other EADL such as the PROXi[42] are designed to accept control inputs from a personal computer. The goal in both cases is to use the same input method to control a personal computer as to control the EADL. In general, the control demands of an EADL system are much less stringent than those for a computer. An input method that is adequate for EADL control may be tedious for general computer controls (see later). On the other hand, any system that allows fluid control of a computer will not be strained by the need to also control an EADL. The "proper" source of control will probably have to be decided on a case-by-case basis, as is illustrated later in this chapter in the section about augmentative communication systems.

Subsumed Devices

Finally, modern EADL frequently incorporate some common devices that are more easily replicated than controlled remotely. Some devices such as the telephone are so pervasive that any EADL system assumes that a telephone will be required. Incorporating telephone electronics into the EADL is actually less expensive, due to the standardization of telephone electronics, than inventing special systems to control a conventional telephone. Other systems designed for individuals with disabilities are so difficult to control remotely that the

EADL must incorporate an entire control system. Hospital beds, for example, have no provisions for remote control but need to be usable by a person with a disability.

Many EADL systems include a speakerphone that allows the user to originate and answer telephone calls using the EADL electronics to serve as a telephone. Because of existing standards, EADL phone systems are generally analog, single-line telephones, electronically similar to those found in the typical home. Many business settings now use multiline sets that are not compatible with home telephones. Some businesses are converting to digital interchanges; these are also not compatible with conventional telephones. Because of these compatibility issues, the telephone built into a standard EADL may not meet the needs of a disabled client in an office setting. Before recommending an EADL as an access solution for a client's office, therapists should check that the system is compatible with the telecommunications systems in place in that office. With the increasing popularity of "voice over Internet protocol" (VOIP), telephone operations may soon become part of the computer interface for many users. The relative ease of controlling a telephone from a computer is likely to make this the approach most often used by individuals with disabilities.

Because the target consumer for an EADL will have severe restrictions in mobility, the manufacturers of many of these systems assume that a significant portion of the customer's day will be spent in bed, so they include some sort of control system for standard hospital beds. These systems commonly allow the user to adjust head and foot height independently, extending the time the individual can be independent of assistance for positioning. As with telephone systems, different brands of hospital beds use different methods of control. It is essential that the clinician match the controls provided by the EADL with the inputs required for the bed to be controlled.

Controlling Electronic Aids to Daily Living

EADL systems are designed to allow the individual with limited physical capability to control devices in the immediate environment. As such, the method used to control the EADL must be within the capability of the client. Because these controls for EADL have features in common with other forms of electronic devices, the control strategies are discussed next.

Augmentative and Alternative Communication

The term augmentative and alternative communication (AAC) is used to describe systems that supplement (augment) or replace (alternative) communication by voice or gestures between people.[39] As used in AT, AAC may be defined as the use of technology to allow communication in ways that an able-bodied individual would be able to accomplish without assistance. Thus using a pencil to write a letter to Aunt May would not be an example of AAC for a person who is unable to speak because an able-bodied correspondent would be using the same technology (pencil and paper) for the same purpose (social communication). However, when a woman who is nonvocal uses the same pencil to explain to the doctor that she has sharp pains in her right leg, it becomes an AAC device because an able-bodied person would communicate this by voice.

A	B	C	D	E	F	I Hurt
G	H	I	J	K	L	I'm thirsty
M	N	O	P	Q	R	Head/Neck
S	T	U	V	W	X	Trunk
Y	Z	1	2	3	4	Arms
5	6	7	8	9	0	Legs

Figure 14-4 Low-technology alternative and augmentative communications system.

There are two different reasons that an individual might have a communication disorder. In a language disorder, the individual has difficulty in understanding and/or formulating messages, regardless of means of production. A person with a language disorder, in most cases, will not benefit from AAC. On the other hand, an individual with difficulty in motor control or muscle tone may be perfectly able to understand and formulate messages but not be able to speak intelligibly because of difficulty in controlling the oral musculature. Such a person has no difficulty with language composition, only with language transmission. This person may well benefit from an AAC device.

AAC devices range from extremely low technology to extremely high technology in design. In hospital intensive care units, low-tech communication boards can allow a person on a respirator to communicate basic needs (Figure 14-4). A low-tech communication board can allow a client to deliver basic messages or spell out more involved messages in a fashion that can be learned quickly. For a person capable only of yes/no responses, the communication partner can indicate the rows of the aid one at a time, asking if the desired letter is in the row. When the correct row is selected, the partner can move across a row until the communicator indicates the correct letter. This type of communication is inexpensive, quick to teach, and slow to use. In settings where there are limited communication needs, this type of AAC is adequate but will not serve for long-term or fluent communication needs.

To meet the communication needs of a person who will be nonvocal over a longer period of time, clinicians frequently recommend electronic AAC devices (Figure 14-5).

An AAC system used solely for expression of needs and wants can be fairly basic. The vocabulary used in this type of communication is limited, and because the expressions tend to be fairly short the communication rate is not of paramount importance. In some cases the communication system may consist only of an alerting buzzer, indicating that the individual is in need, to summon a caregiver. Low-tech communication systems such as that described earlier can meet basic communication needs for individuals whose physical skills are limited to eye blinks or directed eye movement.

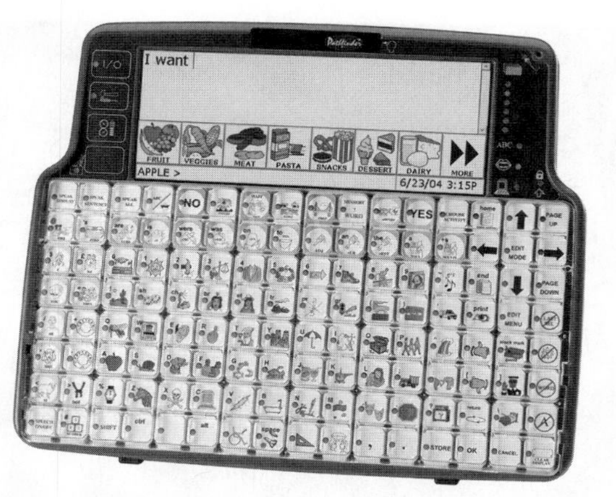

Figure 14-5 High-technology alternative and augmentative communications system (Pathfinder).

Most development in AAC seems to be focused around communicating basic needs and information transfer. Information transfer presents some of the most difficult technological problems because the content of information to be communicated cannot be predicted. Making these unpredictable bits of information available for fluent communication is the ongoing challenge of AAC development.

Social communication and social etiquette present significant challenges for users of AAC devices. Although the information content of these messages tends to be low, because the communication is based on convention, the dialogue should be both varied and spontaneous. AAC systems such as the Dynavox[25] have provisions for preprogrammed messages that can be retrieved for social conversation, but providing both fluency and variability of social discourse through AAC remains a challenge. Devices currently available allow moderately effective communication of wants. They are not nearly so effective in discussing dreams.

Message Composition

Most of the time, able-bodied people and individuals with disabilities plan their messages before speaking. (Many of us can remember the taste of foot when we have neglected this process.) An AAC device should allow the user to construct, preview, and edit communication utterances before they become apparent to the communication partner. This gives the user of an AAC device the ability to think before speaking. It also allows compensation for the rate difference between message composition via AAC and communication between able-bodied individuals.

Able-bodied individuals typically speak between 150 and 175 words per minute.[46] Augmentative communication rates are more typically on the order of 10 to 15 words per minute, resulting in a severe disparity between the rate of communication construction and expected rate of reception. Although input techniques (discussed later) offer some improvement in message construction rates, the rate of message assembly using AAC is such that many listeners will lose interest before an utterance can be delivered. If words are spaced too far apart, an able-bodied listener may not even be able to assemble them into a coherent message!

Perhaps the most difficult challenge when working with a new AAC user is convincing the client to use the device. Initially, the process of message composition and message transmission is so slow and difficult that the client may wish to continue to use his or her poorly understood natural voice. Indeed, in the early stages, such communication may be faster and allow easier communication. (In order to understand a person with a severely distorted voice, the communication partner must pay close attention. This close attention may also be sought by the communicator because this ensures continued attention.) In order to teach an individual to use an AAC device, it may be important for the clinician to be "unable" to understand the communicator's voice and to encourage him or her to use the AAC device to continue the conversation. Over time, using the AAC device will become more automatic for the client, both with the clinician and with others.

General Computer Access

The third category of electronic enabler is general computer access. Although computer use is ubiquitous among able-bodied individuals, it is an AT for individuals with a wide range of disabilities because the computer allows them to perform tasks for which they have no alternative method. Computers can be used to write messages or to research school subjects. For the person with a print impairment, the computer can provide access to printed information either through electronic documents, or through optical character recognition of printed documents, which can convert the printed page into an electronic document. Once a document is stored electronically, it can be presented as large text for the person with a visual acuity limitation or read aloud for the person who is blind or profoundly learning disabled. Computers can allow the manipulation of "virtual objects" to teach mathematical concepts, form constancy, and develop spatial relations skills that are commonly learned by manipulation of physical objects.[31] Smart phones and small personal electronics may be useful for the busy executive but may be the only means available for a person with attention deficit hyperactivity disorder (ADHD) to get to meetings on time.[60] For the executive, they are conveniences, but for the person with ADHD, they can be assistive technologies.

Individuals using computers can locate, organize, and present information at levels of complexity that are not possible without electronic aids. Through the emerging area of cognitive prosthetics, computers can be used to augment attention and thinking skills in people with cognitive limitations. Computer-based biofeedback can monitor and enhance attention to task. Research in temporal processing deficits has led to the development of computer-modified speech programs that can be used to enhance language learning and temporal processing skills.[45,57]

Beyond such rehabilitative applications, the performance-enhancing characteristics of the conventional computer can allow a person with physical or performance limitations to participate in activities that would be too demanding without the assistance of the computer. An able-bodied person would be able to write a note by hand.

A person with a disability may lack the physical capacities to hand-write a note, and would rely on the abilities of the computer. For the able-bodied person, the computer is a convenience. For the person with a disability, it is an AT because the task cannot be accomplished without it. The computer applications appropriate for a person with a disability include all the computer applications available to an able-bodied person.

Control Technologies

All electronic enabling technologies depend on the ability of the individual to control them. Although the functions of the various devices differ, the control strategies share common characteristics. Because the majority of electronic devices were designed for use by able-bodied persons, the controls of assistive technologies may be categorized in the ways that they are adapted from the standard controls. Electronic control may be divided into three broad categories: input adaptations, output adaptations, and performance enhancements.

Input to Assistive Technologies

A wide range of input strategies is available to control electronic enablers; these can be more easily considered in subcategories. Different authors have created different taxonomies for the categorization of input strategies, and some techniques are classified differently in these taxonomies. The categorization presented here should not be considered as uniquely correct, but merely as a convenience. Input strategies may be classified as those using physical keyboards, those using virtual keyboards, and those using scanning techniques.

Physical Keyboards

Physical keyboards generally supply an array of switches with each switch having a unique function. On more complex keyboards, modifier keys may change the function of a key, usually to a related function.[3,4] Physical keyboards appear on a wide range of electronic technologies including computers, calculators, telephones, and microwave ovens. In these applications, sequences of keys are used to generate meaningful units such as words, checkbook balances, telephone numbers, and the cooking time for a baked potato. Other keyboards may have immediate action when a key is pressed. The television remote control has keys that switch power or raise volume when pressed, for example.

Physical keyboards can be adapted to the needs of the individual with a disability in a number of ways (Figure 14-6). Most alphanumeric keyboards, for example, are arranged in the pattern of the conventional typewriter. This pattern was intentionally designed, for reasons relating to mechanical limitations, to slow down the user. Modern computers can accommodate higher speeds of keyboarding, and the QWERTY layout of the standard[7] keyboard is no longer required for anyone, but it is what most people have learned.

The QWERTY pattern of keys is seldom optimum for assistive technologies. Alternative keyboard patterns include the Dvorak Two Handed, Dvorak One Handed, and Chubon

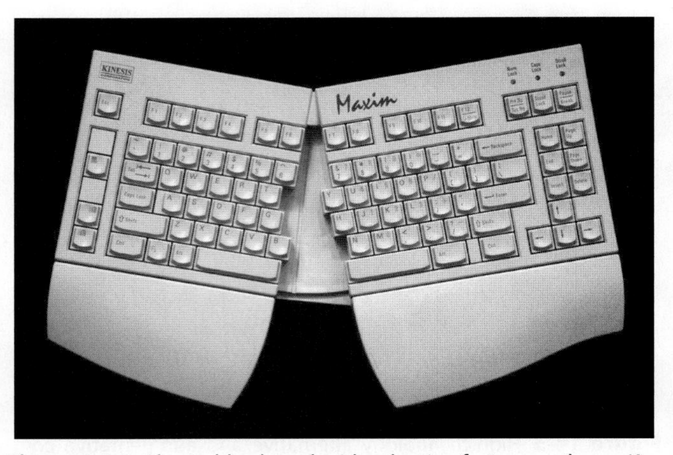

Figure 14-6 Physical keyboard with adaptive features—the myKey keyboard.

(Figure 14-7).[3] These patterns offer improvements in efficiency of typing that may allow a person with a disability to perform for functional periods of time.[7,8,27,32,34,52,53,55,56,62,65]

Initially, the process of using an alternative keyboard layout will be frustrating to users of standard keyboards because the keys are "in the wrong places." In assisting a client to learn to use the new keyboard layout, the clinician may need to employ highly engaging activities where speed is relatively unimportant. E-mail would be more effective than chat rooms, for example, because chat occurs quickly, and a slow typist can be left behind, whereas an e-mail exchange can be conducted at the speed of the typist. Word games depend more on the quality of typing than the speed of typing. Careful documentation of typing speed and accuracy can also be helpful because it allows the client to see progress from day to day.

The scale of the standard keyboard is designed to fit the fine-motor control and range of motion (ROM) of an able-bodied individual. The client with limitations in either ROM or motor control may find the conventional keyboard difficult to use. If the client has limitations in motor control, a keyboard with larger keys and/or additional space between keys may allow independent control of the device. This adaptation may also assist the person with a vision limitation. However, providing an equivalent number of options on larger keys increases the size of the keyboard, which may make it unusable for the person with limitations in ROM.

To accommodate limitations in ROM, the keyboard controls can be reduced in size. Smaller controls, placed closer together, will allow the selection of the full range of options with less demand for joint movement. However, the smaller controls will be more difficult to target for the person with limited motor control. A mini-keyboard is usable only by a person with good fine motor control and may be the only scale of keyboard usable by a person with limited ROM.

To accommodate both limited ROM and limited fine motor control, a keyboard can be designed with fewer options. Many augmentative communication devices can be configured with 4, 8, 32, or 64 keys on a keyboard of a single size. Modifier or "paging" keys can allow access to the full range of options for

~ ` { [}] # 3 @ 2 ! 1 V U P ^ 6 & 7 * 8 + = ←
TAB _ - $ 4 Q M I T S C K Z (9 : ; | \
CAPS LOCK % 5 J G N R E H B Y X) 0 ENTER
SHIFT ? / " ' F O A D L W < , > . SHIFT
CTRL ALT SPACE ALT CTRL

The Chubon Keyboard Layout

~ ` ! 1 @ 2 # 3 $ 4 J L M F P ? / { [}] ←
TAB % 5 ^ 6 Q > . O R S U Y B : ; + = | \
CAPS LOCK & 7 * 8 Z A E H T D C K _ - ENTER
SHIFT (9) 0 X < , I N W V G " ' SHIFT
CTRL ALT SPACE ALT CTRL

The Right-Handed Dvorak Layout

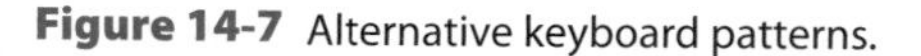

Figure 14-7 Alternative keyboard patterns.

the keyboard, but with reduced efficiency. In this approach, the person uses one or more keys of the keyboard to shift the meanings of all of the other keys of the keyboard. Unless this approach is combined with a dynamic display, the user must remember the meanings of the keys.

When the client is using either an expanded or a minikeyboard, the clinician must monitor whether task performance is actually better. Does typing speed measurably improve? Can the client complete a homework assignment in a reasonable amount of time? What kinds of errors are being made with the keyboard? Does the client strike elsewhere than the intended key? Does he or she drag across keys in the middle of the keyboard? The type of mistake can indicate what modifications are necessary.

Virtual Input Techniques

When an individual lacks the motor control to use an array of physical switches, a virtual keyboard may be used in its place. Virtual keyboards provide the functionality of a physical keyboard system, allowing the user to select directly from the array of options by performing a specified action. Instead of using physical switches for the actions to be performed, the meaning of the "selection" action may be encoded spatially (via pointing) or temporally (via sequenced actions).

Pointing Systems

Pointing systems are analogous to using a physical keyboard with a physical pointer such as a head or mouth-stick.[23] In these systems a graphical representation of a keyboard is presented to the user, and the user makes selections from it by pointing to a region of the virtual "keyboard" and performing a selection action. The selection action is typically either the operation of a single switch (e.g., clicking the mouse) or the act of holding the pointer steady for a period of time.

Several augmentative communication systems now use a "dynamic display" on which the graphical keyboard can be changed as the user makes selections so that the meaning of each location of the keyboard changes as a message is composed. Dynamic displays free the user from having to remember the current meaning of a key or having to decode a key with multiple images on it.

Pointing systems behave much like physical keyboard systems, and many of the considerations of physical keyboards apply. The key size must balance the demands for fine-motor

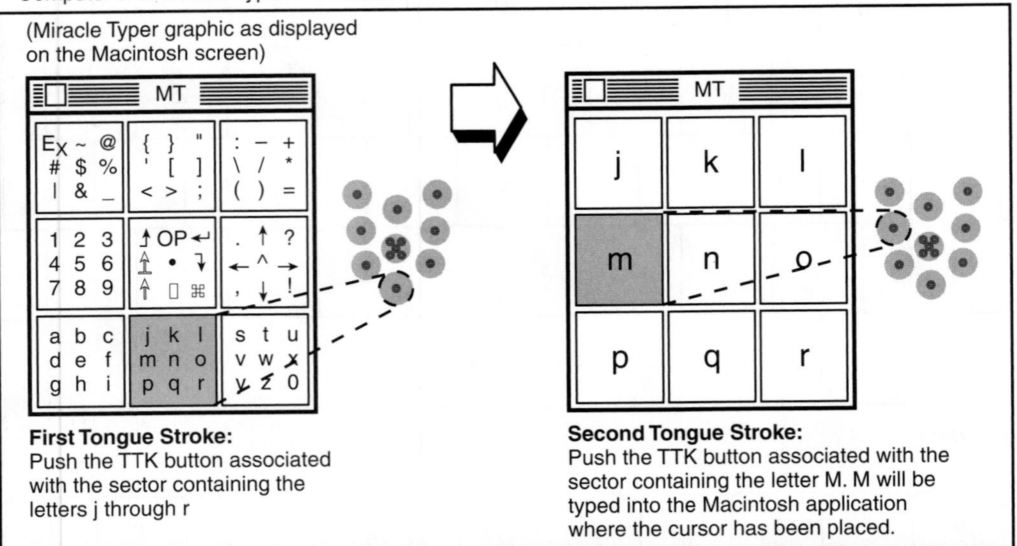

Figure 14-8 MiracleTyper enabling character selection by selection history.

control with the ROM available to the client. The keyboard pattern should be selected to enhance, not hinder, function. The selection technique should facilitate intentional selections while minimizing accidental actions.

Switch Encoding Inputs

The individual who lacks the ROM or fine-motor control necessary to use a physical or graphical keyboard may be able to use a switch encoding input method. In switch encoding, a small set of switches (from one to nine) is used to directly access the functionality of the device. The meaning of the switch may depend on the length of time it is held closed, as in Morse code,[6,9,33,35,44] or on the immediate history of the switch set, as in the Tongue Touch Keypad (see later for more extended discussion of this device).

In Morse code, a small set of switches is used to type. In single-switch Morse, a short switch closure produces an element called a "dit," which is typically written as an "*." A long switch closure produces the "dah" element, which is transcribed as "–." Patterns of switch closures produce the letters of the alphabet, numbers, and punctuation. Pauses longer than five times the short switch closure indicate the end of a character. Two-switch Morse is similar, except two switches are used: one to produce the "dit" element and a second to produce the "dah." Because the meaning of the switches is unambiguous, it is possible for the input time of the dit and dah to be the same length, potentially doubling typing speed. Three-switch Morse breaks the time dependence of Morse by using a third switch to indicate that the generated set of dits and dahs constitute a single letter.

Morse code is a highly efficient method of typing for a person with severe motor control limitations and, unlike other virtual keyboard techniques, can eventually become completely automatic.[9,44] Many Morse code users indicate that they do not "know" Morse code. They think in words, and the words appear on the screen, just as happens in touch-typing. Many Morse code users type at speeds approaching 25 words per minute, making this a means of functional writing.

Many therapists shy away from Morse because they do not know it themselves, and they are unwilling to ask a client to perform a task that they cannot. However, it is clear from clinical experience that Morse code is like touch-typing. When it is first being learned, it is difficult and frustrating; once learned, it becomes automatic and users are reluctant to go back to slower methods. The role of the therapist, therefore, is to provide the encouragement necessary for the client to get beyond the difficult and frustrating stage.

Another type of switch encoding uses immediate history (recent use) for selection. The Tongue Touch Keypad (TTK) from newAbilities[47] uses a set of nine switches on a keypad built into a mouthpiece resembling a dental orthotic.

Early versions of the product used an "onscreen keyboard" called Miracle Typer (Figure 14-8). When using this input method, the first switch selection chose a group of nine possible characters and the second switch action selected a specific character. This approach to typing was somewhat more efficient than Morse physically but did require the user to observe the screen to monitor the current switch meaning. Later versions of the TTK used the keypad only as a mouse emulator, allowing the user to select any onscreen keyboard desired for text entry.

A different approach to switch encoding is provided by the T9 keyboard (Figure 14-9).[61] In this novel interface, each key of the keyboard has several letters on it but the user types as if only the desired character were present. The keyboard software determines from the user's input what word might have been intended. The "disambiguation process" used in the T9 keyboard allows a high degree of accuracy in determining which character the user intended and also allows rapid learning of the keyboard. The T-9 keyboard is provided as an input

BRZ?	CLOJ	MEG.
ADFX	.-/	ISVY
QUNW	BkSpace	THKP

Figure 14-9 T9 Keyboard on a Palm V.

method for text messaging in many cell phones. For those with physical disabilities, this input technology is potentially compatible with pointing systems, described earlier, providing an excellent balance of target size and available options. However, because it depends on the user striking all the correct keys, it does not work accurately for a person who cannot spell.

The developers of the T9 keyboard are currently introducing a new input method that looks like a traditional onscreen keyboard but adds the disambiguation of the T9. The Swype input method, as this new technique is called, does not require the user to tap each key of a word. Instead, the user touches the first letter, then moves over each letter of the desired word, releasing at the last letter. Because of the disambiguation, the system does not require a high degree of precision in dragging over the letters. This input method is currently being tested for individuals with disabilities and is already available on some cell phones.

Speech Input

For many, speech input has a magical allure. What could be more natural than to speak to an EADL or computer and have one's wishes carried out? When first introduced by Dragon Systems[24] in 1990, large vocabulary speech input systems were enormously expensive and, for most, of limited utility. Although highly dedicated users were able to type using voice in 1990, almost no one with the option of the keyboard would choose to use voice for their daily work. These early systems required the user to pause between each word so that the input system could recognize the units of speech. Today (2011), the technology has evolved to allow continuous speech, with recognition accuracy greater than 90%.[37] (The companies producing speech products claim accuracy of greater than 95%.) Although this advance in speech technology is remarkable, it does not mean that speech input is the input method of choice for people with disabilities, for a number of reasons.

Speech recognition requires consistent speech. Although it is not necessary that the speech be absolutely clear, the user must say words the same way each time for an input system to recognize them. Because of this, the majority of people with speech impairments cannot use a speech input system. Slurring and variability of pronunciation will result in a low recognition rate.

Speech input requires a high degree of vigilance during training and use. To provide the highest initial accuracy, current speech technology must be trained to understand the voice of the intended user. To do this, the system presents onscreen text, which the potential user must read into the microphone of the recognition system. If the user lacks the cognitive skills to respond appropriately to the presented cues, the training process will be difficult. A few clinicians have reported success in training students with learning disabilities or other cognitive limitations to use speech input systems, but in general the success rate is poor. Even after training, the user must watch carefully for misrecognized words and correct them at the time the error is made. Modern speech recognition systems depend on context for their recognition. Each uncorrected error slightly changes the context, until the system can no longer recognize the words being spoken. Spell checking a document will not find misrecognized words because each word on the screen is a correctly spelled word. It just may not be the word the user intended!

Speech input is intrusive. One person in a shared office space talking to a computer will reduce the productivity of every other person in the office. If everyone in the office were talking to their computers, the resulting noise would be intolerable to many. Speech input may be acceptable for a person who works or lives alone but is not a good input method for most office or classroom settings.[37]

The type of speech system used depends on the device being controlled. For EADL systems, discrete speech ("lights—on") provides an acceptable level of control. The number of options is relatively small, and there is seldom a need for split-second control. Misrecognized words are unlikely to cause difficulty. Text generation for narrative description, however, places higher demands for input speed and transparency, and it may call for a continuous input method. Other computer applications, however, may work better with discrete rather than continuous input methods. Databases and spreadsheets typically have many small input areas, with limited information in each. These applications are much better suited to discrete speech than continuous.

Current research suggests that the most limiting and frustrating aspect of speech recognition is error correction. When teaching a client to use speech recognition, the methods used to correct errors should be a major focus of training. Where a speech system may offer a large number of correction methods, the clinician should focus on teaching the client to use one method consistently and accurately. Only after one method of error correction is mastered should other options be introduced.

Scanning Input Methods

For the individual with limited cognition and/or motor control, some variation in row-column scanning is sometimes used.[3,22,29] In scanning input, the system to be controlled sequentially offers choices to the user, and the user indicates assent when the correct choice is offered. Typically, such systems first offer groups of choices and, when a group is selected, offer the items of the group sequentially. Because the items were, in early systems, presented as a grid being offered a row at a time, such systems are commonly referred to as "row-column" scanning, even when no rows or columns are present.

Scanning input allows selection of specific choices with limited physical effort. Generally, the majority of the user's time is spent waiting for the desired choice to be offered, so the energy expenditure is relatively small. Unfortunately, the overall time expenditure is generally relatively large. When the system has only a few choices from which to select, as in most EADL systems, scanning is a viable input method. The time spent waiting while the system scans may be a minor annoyance, but the difference between turning on a light now versus a few moments later is relatively small. EADL systems are used intermittently throughout the day, rather than continuously, so the delays over the course of the day are acceptable in most cases.

For AAC or computer systems, however, the situation is different. In either application, the process of composing thoughts may require making hundreds or thousands of selections in sequence. The cumulative effect of the pauses in row-column scanning will slow productivity to the point that functional communication is tedious and may be impossible. Certainly, when productivity levels are mandated, the communication rate available via scanning input will not be adequate.

Rate Enhancement Options

For EADL systems, rate of control input is relatively unimportant. As noted earlier, the number of control options is relatively limited, and selections are rarely severely time constrained. However, for AAC and computer control systems, the number of selections to be made in sequence is high and rate can be critical. Rate enhancement technologies may increase the information transmitted by each selection when a person with a disability is unable to make selections as quickly as an able-bodied person.

To understand how rate enhancement works, one must appreciate how language production works. In general, language can be expressed in one of three ways: letter-by-letter spelling, prediction, and compaction/expansion. The latter two options allow enhancement of language generation rates.

Letter-by-Letter Spelling

Typical typing is an example of letter-by-letter representation and is relatively inefficient. In all languages and alphabets, there is a balance between the number of characters used to represent a language and the number of elements in a message. English, using the conventional alphabet, averages about 6 letters (selections) per word (including the spaces between words). When represented in Morse code, the same text will require roughly 18 selections per word. By comparison, the basic vocabulary of a person speaking Chinese can be produced by selecting a single ideogram per word. However, each ideogram must be selected from an array of thousands of choices. In general, having a larger number of characters in an alphabet allows each character to convey more meaning but may make the selection of each specific character more difficult.

Many AAC systems use an expanded set of "characters" in the form of pictograms or icons to represent entire words that may be selected by the user. Such semantic compaction allows a large vocabulary to be used within a device but requires a system of selection that may add complexity to the device.[21] For example, a device may require the user to select a word group (e.g., food) before selecting a specific word (e.g., hamburger) from the group. Using subcategories, it is theoretically possible to represent a vocabulary of more than 2 million words on a 128-key keypad with just three selections.

Prediction

Because messages in a language tend to follow similar patterns, it is possible to produce significant savings of effort using prediction technology. There are two types of prediction used in language production: word completion and word/phrase prediction.

In word completion, a communication system (AAC or computer based) will, after each keystroke, present a number of options to the user representing possible words that begin with these keystrokes. When the appropriate word is presented by the prediction system, the user may select that word directly rather than continuing to spell out the word. Overall, this strategy may reduce the number of selections required to complete a message.[10,30,36,38,40,48,58] However, it may not improve typing speed.[2,10,36,38,64,66] Anson[2] demonstrated that when typing from copy using the keyboard, typing speed was slowed in direct proportion to the frequency of using the prediction list. The burden of constantly scanning the prediction list overwhelms the potential speed savings of word completion systems under these conditions. However, when typing using an onscreen keyboard or scanning system, in which the user must scan the input array in any case, word completion does appear to increase typing speed and reduce the number of selections made.

Because most language is similar in structure, it is also possible, in some cases, to predict the word that will be used following a specific word. For example, after a person's first name is typed, the surname is often the next item typed. When this prediction is possible, the next word may be generated with a single selection. When combined with word completion, next-word prediction has the potential to decrease the effort of typing substantially. However, in many cases, this potential is unrealized. Many users, even when provided with next-word prediction, become so involved in spelling words that they ignore the predictions even when they are accurate. The cognitive effort of switching between "typing mode" and "list scanning" mode may be greater than the cognitive benefit of not having to spell a word out.[28]

Compression/Expansion

Compression/expansion strategies allow limited sets of commonly used words to be stored in unambiguous abbreviations. When these abbreviations are selected, either letter by letter or through word completion, the abbreviation is replaced by the expanded form of the word or phrase.[3,22]

Because the expansion can be many selections long, this technology offers an enormous potential for saving energy and time. However, the potential savings are available only when the user remembers to use the abbreviation rather than the expanded form of a word. Because of this limitation, abbreviations must be carefully selected. Many abbreviations are already in common use and can be stored conveniently. Most people will refer to the television by the abbreviation TV, which requires just 20% of the selections to represent. With an expansion system, each use of TV can automatically be converted to "television" with no additional effort of the user. Similarly, TTFN might be used to store the social message, "Ta-ta for now."

Effective abbreviations will be unique to the user, rather than general. An example of an effective form of abbreviation is found in the language shortcuts commonly used in note taking. These abbreviations form a shorthand generally unique to the individual that allows complex thoughts to be represented on the page quickly in the course of a lecture. A clinician should work carefully with the client to develop abbreviations that will be useful and easily remembered.

Another form of "abbreviations" that is less demanding to create is common spelling errors. For persons, either students or adult writers, who have cognitive deficits that influence spelling skills, expansions can be created to automatically correct misspelled words. In these cases the "abbreviation" is the way that the client generally misspells the word, and the "expansion" is the correct spelling of the word. Once a library of misspelled words is created, the individual is relieved of the need to worry about the correct spelling. There are those who will maintain that this form of adaptation will prevent the individual from ever learning the correct spelling. In cases where the client is still developing spelling skills, this is probably a valid concern, and the adaptation should not be used. But for the individual with a cognitive deficit, normal spelling skills may not be a priority. In cases where remediation is not possible, accommodation through compression/expansion technology is a desirable choice.

None of these technologies will allow a person with a disability to produce messages at the same rate as an able-bodied person. However, individually and collectively, these technologies can make message generation significantly more efficient than it would be without them. The techniques are not mutually exclusive. Icons can be predicted using "next word" techniques. Abbreviations can be used in conjunction with word completion and word prediction technologies.

Output Options

The control of assistive technologies involves a cycle of both human output and human input, matched to technology input and technology output. Individuals who have sensory limitations may have difficulty controlling assistive technologies (or common technologies) because they are unable to perceive the messages that are being sent to them by the technology. For these individuals, adaptations of the output of the technology may be required. These adaptations generally depend on one of three sensory modalities: vision, hearing, or tactile sensation.

Visual Output

The default output of many types of electronic technology is visual. Computer screens are designed to resemble the printed page. AAC systems have input that "looks" like a keyboard and, generally, a graphical message composition area. EADL use display panels and lighted icons to show current status of controlled devices. The perception of all these controls depends on the user having visual acuity at nearly normal levels. When the client has some vision, but that vision is limited, adaptations may be required.

Colors and Contrast

Many types of visual impairment affect the ability to separate foreground and background colors. In addition, bright background colors can produce a visual glare that makes the foreground difficult to perceive. In accommodating visual deficits, the clinician should explore the colors that are easily perceived by the individual and those that are difficult. Background colors, for most people, should be muted soft colors that do not produce a strong visual response. Icons and letters, on the other hand, may be represented in colors that provide visual contrast with the background. Very bright or strident colors should be avoided in both cases, and the specific colors and contrast levels required by the user must be selected on an individual basis.

Image Size

Visual acuity and display size present difficulties in output displays that closely mirror the issues that ROM and fine motor skills present in keyboard design. In most cases, a person with 20/20 vision can easily read text that is presented in letters about ⅙ of an inch high. (This is equivalent to a page printed in a 12-point font.) On a typical display, this allows the presentation of between 100 and 150 words of text at a time or a similar number of icons for selection. If the user has lower visual acuity or limited ability to process visual stimuli, the letter/icon size must be increased to accommodate that loss of acuity. Larger icons, however, require either fewer letters shown at a time or increased display size. For people with severe vision limitations, as with individuals with severe fine motor limitations, it would be impractical to display all choices at once.

Screen enlargement programs[3] typically overcome this limitation by enlarging only a part of the screen at a time and moving the portion that is expanded to the area most likely of interest to the user. The visual effect is similar to viewing the screen through a magnifying glass that the user moves over the display. Most programs can be configured to follow the text insertion point, the mouse pointer, or other changes on the display. With all such programs, a serious weakness is navigation. When the user can see only a small portion of the screen at a time, the landmarks that are normally available to indicate the layout of the text on a page may be invisible because they are not in the field of view. To be usable by the client, a screen enlargement program must provide a means of orienting to the location on the screen.

AAC systems can accommodate the needs of a user with low visual acuity using precisely the same techniques used for the person with limited fine motor control. The keyboard of the device can be configured with fewer, larger keys, each of which has a larger symbol to represent its meaning. However, as with keyboards for those with physical limitations, the result is either fewer communication options or a more complex interface for the user. Also, these accommodations do not adapt the size of the message composition display, which may be inaccessible to the user with vision limitations.

Speech Output

Speech output is a useful tool in two cases: (1) when it replaces voice for a person with a disability and (2) when the user is not able to use vision to access the technology. AAC devices using voice provide the most "normal" face-to-face communication available. Able-bodied people, in most conditions, communicate by voice.

People with disabilities generally want to communicate in similar fashion. In voice output, the device communicates with the user auditorially, converting printed words or commands into voice. Voice output technology has been in existence for much longer than voice input and is a more mature technology—not perfect, but more mature. The demands of voice output are different depending on the application and the intended listener. It is helpful to consider separately the systems where a second person is the listener and the systems where the user is the listener.

Second Person as Listener

"Second person as listener" systems substitute for speech when the user cannot be understood using normal speech. When used in AAC applications, voice output is almost always intended to be understood by a second person who may have little experience with synthetic voices. For example, if an AAC user is at the corner market, buying 2 lb of hamburger for dinner, the butcher is unlikely to have had much experience with a synthetic voice. When the AAC user is asking for directions on the street corner, the listener will face the additional challenge of hearing the AAC's voice over the sounds of trucks and buses.

To be understandable by novice listeners in real-world environments, a synthetic voice should be clear and as "human sounding" as possible. The voice will be easily understood to the extent that it sounds like what the listener expects to hear. Ideally, the voice should provide appropriate inflection in the spoken material and should be able to convey emotional content. Current AAC systems do not convey emotional content well, but high-end voices do sound much like a human speaker. Under adverse conditions, they will remain less understandable than a human speaker because facial and lip movements (which provide additional cues as to the sounds being produced) do not accompany synthetic voices.

User as Listener

When used for computer access or EADL, voice quality need not be as "human sounding." In either case, the user has the opportunity to learn to understand the voice in training. In EADL applications, there will be relatively few utterances that must be produced, and they can be designed to sound as different from each other as possible so that there is little chance of confusion. General voice output for an entire language is somewhat more difficult, however, because many words sound similar and are easily confused.

For general text reading, however, the primary issue is voicing speed. As noted earlier, humans generally produce between 150 and 175 words per minute. However, most humans also read between 300 and 400 words per minute. A person who depends on a human-sounding voice for reading printed material will be limited to reading at less than half the speed of able-bodied readers. To be an effective text access method, synthetic voice must be understandable at speeds in excess of 400 words per minute. This will obviously require significant training because untrained people without disabilities cannot understand speech at such speeds. However, with training, speech output is a useful way for a person with a vision limitation to access printed material.

Another application of voice output is "eyes-free" control. In the mass market for able-bodied consumers, these applications include presenting information over the telephone while driving or in other settings where a visual display might be difficult to use. All these situations are important for people with disabilities as well. In addition, assistive technologies using voice output may be intended for use by people with print impairments. The category of print impairments includes conditions that result in low vision and/or blindness, as well as conditions that result in the inability to translate visual stimuli to language and those that make manipulation of printed materials difficult.

Voice output technologies are problematic for people who are developing language skills. Because English is an irregular language, with many letter combinations making similar sounds, it is almost impossible to learn spelling by listening to the sound of words. Children who are blind from birth may not be good candidates for speech output as the primary language access method because the structure of words is lost when converted to speech. For these children, and for many others, tactile access is a better tool and is, in fact, mandated under the Individuals with Disabilities Education Act (IDEA).[61]

Tactile Output

The oldest method for individuals with vision deficits to access printed material is Braille. In 1829, Louis Braille developed the idea of adapting a military system that allowed writing secret messages and aiming artillery in darkness to provide a method of reading for students at the National Institute for the Young Blind in Paris.[17] Over time, this original system has been extended to allow communication of music, mathematics, and computer code to readers without vision. Basic Braille uses an array of six dots to represent letters and numbers. Traditional Braille, however, is usable only for static text such as printed books. Dynamic information cannot be represented by raised dots on a sheet of paper.

Technology access requires the use of refreshable Braille. Refreshable Braille displays use a set of piezoelectric pins to represent Braille letters. Changing electrical signals to the display moves the pins up and down, allowing a single display to represent different portions of a longer document.

Braille is not widely used among individuals who are blind.[17] By some estimates, only 10% of the blind population know and use Braille. It is not usable by those who have limited tactile sensation in addition to blindness. However, Braille is a skill that probably should be taught to a person who is blind and has good tactile discrimination. Most Braille readers are employed. Most people who are blind but do not read Braille are not employed. Although Braille may not be an essential skill for employment, the ability to learn Braille certainly correlates with the ability to hold a job.[17]

CASE STUDY

Mary, Part 2

Now that Mary, from the beginning of the chapter, has her AT, she must be trained to use it. As with all aspects of occupational therapy, her training should focus on meaningful activities. When Mary is using aids that are intended to allow her to write, she should use them to write. Initially, sending e-mail to friends is a good activity because it is highly engaging, is not rate dependent, and because friends are likely to be forgiving of misspellings. When Mary is using her EADL device, she should use it to control lights as it gets dark, to turn the television to her preferred channel, and to adjust the volume as needed. The hardest task for the clinician training Mary is to refrain from helping when the client is able to perform the task, although with difficulty.

1. Success in an AT intervention is determined by Mary's ability to perform tasks independently. Can she write a paper for her professor within the allotted time? Can she control the lights, furnace, and entertainment devices in her home? Can she communicate with friends? One of the best indicators of success is when Mary expands her ambitions. This tells the clinician that, for Mary, the range of what is possible has expanded.
2. The AT will not make tasks as easy as they are for her able-bodied peers. Tasks will still be more difficult but not impossible. AT does not guarantee success. It can, and does, give Mary the chance to succeed. Whether or not she does succeed depends on her drive, her innate capabilities, and her belief in herself. Once AT has made it possible for Mary to succeed, it is the job of the therapist to help her believe that she can.

Summary

The occupational therapy practitioner must remember that although disability makes few things impossible, it does make many things harder, and some sufficiently hard that they are "not worth it." AT can make many things easier for the person with a disability. Because AT makes them easier, many activities that were previously not worth the effort can become reasonable for a person with a disability. AT will never, in the terminology of the model of disability, remove the functional limitation. It can, however, allow engagement in occupation despite the functional limitation.

The key issue in all ATs is whether the individual is more able to perform desired tasks using the AT than without it. In many cases, an AT device that is provided for a specific task will have little utility in other tasks. This is not a new concept for occupational therapists. A built-up handle toothbrush makes brushing teeth easier, but a different device is necessary for brushing hair. In the same manner, an AT that is intended to allow a student to keep up on homework assignments may not be appropriate or adequate for chatting with friends online. The technology must match the task and must allow the individual to perform the task at a higher level with it than without it. At the current state of the art, however, AT cannot fully compensate for disability. Most tasks will still be hard, and some small number may be "not worth it." The occupational therapy practitioner who uses an interactive, collaborative, client-centered approach to consider AT solutions is likely to achieve the optimum result in terms of engagement in occupation.

Selected Reading Guide Questions

1. Compare and contrast rehabilitative and assistive technologies.
2. In what way do devices using universal design assist individuals with disabilities? Why are they not considered to be ATs?
3. According to the Human Interface Assessment model, why might a person with a disability not require any AT in the completion of some tasks?
4. In pediatric applications, complex EADL devices might not be considered appropriate. What sort of EADL might be used with a very young child?
5. Some EADL devices allow control of the features of devices in the environment. Discuss the benefit of providing such control. What additional load does this place on the user?
6. AAC devices can be used to provide alternative or augmentative communication. Discuss the difference between these two strategies. Might an AAC device be a rehabilitation technology in some applications?
7. What is the value of having a message composition area that is independent from the message transmission feature of an AAC device? Discuss the value for the communicator and for the communication partner.
8. How does a language disorder differ from a communication disorder? What sort of AAC device would help a person with a language disorder?
9. Consider the keypad providing control to a microwave oven. How might the keypad present difficulty to an individual who is blind? How might it be modified by an occupational therapist to improve its usability?
10. Word prediction and word completion are often touted as means to improve typing speed, yet the research suggests that they does not. What advantage might these technologies offer to improve productivity for a person with a disability?

11. Abbreviation expansion is generally considered as a means to type long words and phrases with only a few keystrokes, though this requires the user to remember the abbreviation. How else can this technology be used for individuals with learning disabilities, in ways that do not require memorization of keystroke sequences?
12. Refreshable Braille is expensive, whereas text to speech is inexpensive. Yet Braille training is mandated by IDEA. What factors support the learning of this old technology for individuals who are blind?

References

1. American Occupational Therapy Association Inc: *Occupational Therapy Practice Framework: Domain and Process,* ed 2, Bethesda, Maryland, 2008, AOTA Press.
2. Anson D: The Effect of Word Prediction on Typing Speed, *Am J Occup Ther* 47(11):1039–1042, 1993.
3. Anson D: *Alternative Computer Access: A Guide to Selection,* Philadelphia, 1997, F.A. Davis.
4. Anson D: The Future of Computer Access, *Am J Occup Ther* 55:106–108, 2001.
5. Anson D: Environmental Control. In Webster JG, editor: *Encyclopedia of Medical Devices and Instrumentation,* Vol 3, Hoboken, NJ, 2006, John Wiley & Sons, pp 211–215.
6. Anson D, Ames C, Fulton L, Margolis M, Miller M: Patterns For Life: A Study of Young Children's Ability to Use Patterned Switch Closures for Environmental Control. (2004) Retrieved Oct. 4, 2004, from http://atri.misericordia.edu/Papers/Patterns.php.
7. Anson D, Eck C, King J, Mooney R, Sansom C, Wilkerson B, Cychulis D: Efficacy of Alternate Keyboard Configurations: Dvorak vs. Reverse-QWERTY. (2001) Retrieved April 9, 2005, from http://atri.misericordia.edu/Papers/Dvorak.php.
8. Anson D, George S, Galup R, Shea B, Vetter R: Efficiency of the Chubon versus the QWERTY keyboard, *Assist Technol* 13(1): 40–45, 2001.
9. Anson D, Glodek M, Peiffer RM, Rubino CG, Schwartz PT: Long-term Speed and Accuracy of Morse code vs. Head-pointer Interface for Text Generation. Paper presented at the RESNA 2004 Annual Conference, Orlando, FL, 2004.
10. Anson D, Moist P, Przywara M, Wells H, Saylor H, Maxime H: The Effects of Word Completion and Word Prediction on Typing Rates Using On-screen Keyboards Assistive Technology (In-Press).
11. asiHome 36 Gumbletown Rd CS1, Paupack PA 18451, Phone: 800-263-8608, http://www.asihome.com/cgi-bin/ASIstore.pl?user_action=detail&catalogno=X10PEX01.
12. Assistive Technology Act of 1998, Pub. L. No. S. 2432 (1998).
13. Assistive Technology Act of 2004, Pub. L. No. HR 4278 (2004 Oct. 25, 2004).
14. Assistive Technology Partners: Direct Access Electronic Aids. (2002, 03/27/2002) Retrieved July 26, 2004, from http://www.uchsc.edu/atp/library/fastfacts/Direct%20Access%20Electronic%20Aids.htm.
15. Barnes MP: Environmental Control Systems—an Audit and Review, *Clin Rehabil* 8:326–366, 1994.
16. Butterfield T: Environmental Control Units. (2004, 7/26/2004) Retrieved July 26, 2004, from http://www.birf.info/artman/publish/article_418.shtml.
17. Canadian National Institute for the Blind: Braille Information Center. (2004, 2004) Retrieved July 29, 2004, from http://www.cnib.ca/eng/braille_information/
18. Center for Assistive Technology: Environmental Control Units. (2004, 7/26/2004) Retrieved July 26, 2004, from http://cat.buffalo.edu/newsletters/ecu.php.
19. Center for Universal Design: What is Universal Design? Principles of UD. (1997, 06/25/2004) Retrieved July 29, 2004, from http://www.design.ncsu.edu:8120/cud/univ_design/princ_overview.htm
20. Commission for the Blind and Visually Handicapped: CBVH Manual, REHABILITATION TECHNOLOGY - 8.20. (2002, 03/31/2000) Retrieved July 29, 2004, from http://www.nls.org/cbvh/8.20.htm.
21. Conti B: Semantic Compaction Systems—the home of Minspeak. (2004, 07/29/2004) Retrieved July 30, 2004, from http://www.minspeak.com/about1.html.
22. Cook AM, Hussey SM: *Assistive technologies: Principles and practice,* ed 2, Philadelphia, 2002, Mosby International.
23. DeVries RC, Deitz J, Anson D: et al 1998. A comparison of two computer access systems for functional text entry. 52:656–665.
24. Dragon Systems, Inc., 320 Nevada Street, Newton, Mass. 02460, USA, Phone: +1-617-965-5200, FAX: +1-617-965-2374.
25. DynaVox Systems LLC., 2100 Wharton Street, Suite 400, Pittsburgh, Penn. 15203 Phone: 1-800-344-1778, http://www.dynavoxsys.com.
26. Efthimiou J, Gordon WA, Sell GH, Stratford C: Electronic Assistive Devices: Their Impact on the Quality of Life of High-Level Quadriplegic Persons, *Archives of Physical Medicine and Rehabilitation* 62:131–134, 1981.
27. Fong Lee D: Alternative Keyboards, *Canad J Occup Ther* 62:175, 1995.
28. Gibler CD, Childress DS: Language anticipation with a computer-based scanning communication aid. Paper presented at the IEEE Computer Society Workshop on Computing to the Handicapped, Charlottesville, Va, 1982.
29. Glennen SL, DeCoste DC: *The Handbook of Augmentative and Alternative Communication,* San Diego, 1997, Singular Publishing Group.
30. Hunnicutt S, Carlberger J: Improving Word Prediction Using Markov Models and Heuristic Methods, *Augmentative and Alternative Communication* 17:255–264, 2001.
31. Intellitools: Number Concepts 2. (2004, 6/23/2004) Retrieved July 30, 2004, from http://intellitools.com/
32. Interactive MaM: The Dvorak keyboard. (1998) Retrieved Feb. 28, 2003, from http://www.maxmon.com/1936ad.htm.
33. Jarus T: Learning Morse code in rehabilitation: Visual, auditory, or combined method? *Br J Occup Ther* 57:127–130, 1994.
34. Kincaid C: Alternative Keyboards, *Exceptional Parent* 2:34–35, 1999.
35. King TW: *Modern Morse Code in Rehabilitation and Education: New Applications in Assistive Technology,* Boston, 2000, Allyn and Bacon.
36. Koester HH: *Word Prediction—When does it enhance text entry rate? Paper presented at the RESNA 2002,* Minneapolis, 2002, Minn.
37. Koester HH: Abandonment of Speech Recognition by New Users. Paper presented at the RESNA 26th International Annual Conference, Atlanta Georgia, 2003.
38. Koester HH, Levine SP: Effect of a Word Prediction Feature on User Performance, *Augmentative and Alternative Communication* 12:155–168, 1996.
39. Lloyd LL, Fuller DR, et al: *Augmentative and alternative communication: a handbook of principles and practices,* Boston, 1997, Allyn and Bacon.

40. MacArthur CA: Word processing with speech synthesis and word prediction: Effects on the dialogue journal writing of students with learning disabilities, *Learn Disabil Q* 21:1–16, 1998.
41. MacNeil V: Electronic Aids to Daily Living, *Team Rehabilitation Report* 9(3):53–56, 1998.
42. Madentec, Ltd., 4664 99 St., Edmonton, Alberta, Canada T6E 5H5, phone: (877) 623-3682, http://madentec.com.
43. McDonald DW, Boyle MA, Schumann TL: Environmental Control Unit Utilization by High-Level Spinal Cord Injured Patients, *Arch Phys Med Rehabil* 70:621–623, 1989.
44. McDonald JB, Schwejda P, Marriner NA, Wilson WR, Ross AM: *Advantages of Morse code as a computer input for school aged children with physical disabilities. Computers and the Handicapped*, Ottawa, 1982, National Research Council of Canada.
45. Merzenich M, Jenkins W, Johnston P, Schreiner C, Miller S, Tallal P: Temporal processing deficits of language-learning impaired children ameliorated by training, *Science* 271:77–81, 1996.
46. Miller GA: *Language and Speech*, San Francisco, 1981, Freeman.
47. newAbilities System Inc., 2938 Scott Blvd., Santa Clara, CA 95054. http://www.newabilities.com/
48. Newell AF, Arnott J, Booth L, Beattie W, Brophy B, Ricketts IW: Effect of "PAL" word prediction system on the quality and quantity of text generation, *Augment Altern Commun* 8:304–311, 1992.
49. Quartet Technology, Inc., 87 Progress Avenue, Tyngsboro, Mass. 01879, phone: 1.978.649.4328.
50. Quartet Technol: Frequently Asked Questions. (2004a) Retrieved Oct. 24, 2005, from http://www.qtiusa.com/faq.asp.
51. Quartet Technol: Quartet Technology, Inc. News. (2004b) Retrieved July 29, 2004, from http://www.qtiusa.com/ProdOverview.asp?ProdTypeID=1.
52. Quinn E: Keyboard ideology. (1998) Retrieved Sept. 6, 2000, from http://www.gontier.org/Quinn/WWW/ideology/Dvorak.html.
53. Rehr, D: Consider qwerty. Retrieved Feb. 28, 2003, from http://home.earthlink.net/~dcrehr/whyqwert.html.
54. Smarthome, Inc., 16542 Millikan Avenue, Irvine, Calif. 92606-5027, Phone: (949) 221-9200 x109.
55. Struck M: Focus on. One handed keyboarding options, *OT Practice* 4:55–56, 1999a.
56. Struck M: One-handed keyboarding options, *OT Practice* 4: 55–56, 1999b.
57. Tallal P, Miller S, Bedi G, Byma G, Wang X, Nagarajan S, Merzenich M: Language comprehension in language-learning impaired children improved with acoustically modified speech, *Science* 271:81–84, 1996.
58. Tam C, Reid D, Naumann S, O'Keefe B: Effects of Word Prediction and Location of Word Prediction Lists on Text Entry with Children with Spina Bifida and Hydrocephalus, *Augment Altern Commun* 18:147–162, 2002:(September).
59. Tash Inc., 3512 Mayland Ct., Richmond, Va, 23233 http://www.tashinc.com, phone: 1-800-463-5685 or (905) 686-4129.
60. TechDis Accessibility Database Team: TechDis PDA Project—Time Management and Organisation. (2002) Retrieved July 30, 2004, from http://www.techdis.ac.uk/PDA/time.htm.
61. Tegic Communications, 2001 Western Avenue, Suite 250, Seattle, Wash. 98121 http://www.tegic.com.
62. Trumbull M: Dvorak keyboard layout makes comeback 60 years later, *Christ Sci Monitor* 87:9, 1995.
63. Warger C: New IDEA '97 Requirements: Factors to Consider in Developing an IEP. (1999, 05/06/2004) Retrieved July 30, 2004, from http://www.hoagiesgifted.org/eric/e578.html.
64. Williams SC: How Speech Feedback and Word Prediction Software Can Help Students Write, *Teaching Exceptional Children* 34(3):72–78, 2002.
65. Zecevic A, Miller D, Harburn K: An evaluation of the ergonomics of three computer keyboards, *Ergonomics* 43:18–22, 2000.
66. Zordell J: The use of word prediction and spelling correction software with mildly handicapped students, *Closing Gap* 9(1):10–11, 1990.

CHAPTER 15

Moving in the Environment

TERU CREEL, MAUREEN MATTHEWS, CAROLE ADLER, AND MIRIAM MONAHAN

Key Terms

Durable medical equipment (DME)
Functional ambulation
Gait training
Pathological gait
Ambulation aids
Mobility assistive equipment (MAE)
Mobility-related activities of daily living (MRADL)
Power-operated vehicle (POV)
Rehabilitation technology supplier (RTS)
Skin breakdown
Spasticity
Contractures
Medical necessity
Vital capacity
Body mechanics
Positioning mass
Pelvic tilt
Clinical evaluation
Pre-driving tasks

Chapter Objectives

After studying this chapter, the student or practitioner will be able to do the following:

1. Define functional ambulation.
2. Discuss the role of the occupational therapy practitioner in functional ambulation.
3. Identify appropriate interventions to promote functional ambulation within occupational therapy treatment.
4. Identify safety issues in functional ambulation.
5. Recognize basic lower extremity orthotics and ambulation aids.
6. Understand the factors the occupational therapist considers in wheelchair evaluation, wheelchair measurement, and prescription completion.
7. Identify wheelchair safety considerations.
8. Follow guidelines for proper body mechanics.
9. Apply principles of proper body positioning.
10. Identify the steps necessary in performing various transfer techniques.
11. Identify considerations necessary to determine the appropriate transfer method based on the patient's clinical presentation.
12. List the 10 elements of a driving evaluation.
13. Describe the contribution of occupational therapy to the assessment of the disabled individual's driving.

Walking, climbing stairs, traveling within one's neighborhood, and driving a car are so universal and customary that most people would not consider these to be complex activities. The basic capacities to move within the environment, to reach objects of interest, to explore one's surroundings, and to come and go at will appear natural and easy. For persons with disabilities, however, mobility is rarely taken for granted or considered automatic. A disability may prevent a person from using his or her legs to walk or using hands to operate controls of motor vehicles. Cardiopulmonary and medical conditions may limit aerobic capacity or endurance, requiring the person to take frequent rests and to curtail walking to cover only the most basic of needs such as toileting. Deficits in motor coordination, flexibility, and strength may seriously impair movement and may make difficult any activities that require a combination of mobility (e.g., walking or moving in the environment) and stability (e.g., holding the hands steady as one must when carrying a cup of coffee or a watering can).

Visual, perceptual, and cognitive limitations can also impede free movement in one's environment. Lack of depth perception and visual acuity impairments can slow mobility even in individuals with conscious awareness of deficits. Visual field deficits and visual processing deficits can impose safety risks when one is moving or walking in congested or unfamiliar environments. Safe sequencing of transfers requires the ability to learn and retain new information. Generally speaking, the more complex the environment, the greater the demand is on all performance components.

Occupational therapy (OT) practitioners help persons with mobility restrictions to achieve maximum access to environments and objects of interest to them. Typically, occupational therapists provide remediation and compensatory training, and occupational therapy assistants (OTAs) assist in both areas. Clinicians at both levels must analyze the activities most valued and environments most used by their clients and must consider any future changes that can be predicted from an individual's medical history, prognosis, and developmental status.

This chapter guides the OTA in working with persons with mobility restrictions. Three main topics are explored. The first section addresses functional ambulation, which combines the act of walking within one's immediate environment (i.e., home or workplace) with other activities chosen by the individual. Feeding pets, preparing a meal and carrying it to a table, and doing simple housework are tasks that may involve functional ambulation. Functional ambulation may be conducted with aids such as walkers, canes, or crutches.

The second section concerns wheelchairs and their selection, measurement, fitting, and use. For many persons with disabilities, mobility becomes possible only with a wheelchair and specific positioning devices. Consequently, individual evaluation is necessary to select and fit this essential piece of personal medical equipment. Proper training in ergonomic use will allow the wheelchair-dependent individual many years of safe and comfortable mobility. Safe and efficient transfer techniques based on the individual's clinical status are introduced in this chapter. Attention is also given to the body mechanics required to safely assist an individual.

The third section covers community mobility, which for many in the United States of America is synonymous with driving. Increased advocacy by and for persons with disabilities has improved access and has yielded an increasing range of options for adapting motor vehicles for individual needs. Public transportation has also become increasingly accessible. Driving is a complex activity that requires multiple cognitive and perceptual skills. Evaluation of individuals with medical conditions and physical limitations is thus important for the safety of the disabled person and the public at large.

Mobility is an aspect of OT practice that requires close coordination with other health care providers, particularly physical therapists and providers of durable medical equipment (DME). Improving and maintaining the functional mobility of persons with disabilities can be one of the most gratifying practice areas. Consumers experience tremendous energy and empowerment when they can access and explore wider and more interesting environments.

SECTION I FUNCTIONAL AMBULATION

Teru Creel and Maureen Matthews

Functional Ambulation

Functional ambulation is a goal for many OT clients. Functional ambulation, a subcomponent of functional mobility, is the purposeful application of the mobility training taught to the client to enable movement from one position or place to another. Functional ambulation involves achieving a goal such as carrying a plate to the table or carrying groceries from the car to the house. If the individual is using an assistive aid to ambulate and simultaneously has a need to carry an object, solving the problem is more complex. Functional ambulation is applicable for individuals with a variety of diagnoses such as lower extremity amputation, cerebrovascular accident, acquired brain injury, or total hip replacement.

Functional mobility allows collaboration between the occupational therapist and the physical therapist. Together, the OT practitioner and the physical therapy practitioner provide the most appropriate technique and ambulation aid for use during functional ambulation. The physical therapist performs gait training (the treatments used to improve walking and ameliorate deviations from normal gait) and makes recommendations for ambulation aids. The occupational therapist applies these recommendations during functional activities and provides feedback to the physical therapy practitioner regarding functional outcomes using the recommended techniques and devices. The OTA carries out functional activities training as directed by the occupational therapist.

Basics of Ambulation

Ambulation or bipedal locomotion is a complex function. Locomotion is the act of getting from one place to another. For two-legged and four-legged animals, gait is the means of achieving locomotion.

The OT practitioner should have a basic understanding of ambulation terminology and techniques and of assistive aids commonly used during functional ambulation.

Gait is the means of achieving this action. Gait training is treatment used to improve gait.

The individuals seen by the OT-physical therapy team may exhibit pathological gait because of biomechanical or neurophysiological deficits. Problems noted may include decreased walking velocity, decreased weight bearing, increased swing time of the affected lower extremity, or an abnormal base of support. Functional deficits may include unsafe ambulation and insufficient energy. As the physical therapist evaluates the causes of the gait problems, orthotics and ambulation aids may be recommended. It is important that the OT practitioner reinforce the gait training by following the appropriate recommendations.

The OT practitioner should be familiar with basic lower extremity orthotics. Should it be determined that the individual has abnormal posture of the ankle, an ankle-foot orthosis (AFO) may be recommended. An AFO is a protective external device, commonly made of lightweight thermoplastic splinting material and applied to the ankle area to protect or compensate for joint instability.[6] Should it be determined that the individual has knee collapse or hyperextension, an external means of knee control such as a knee-ankle-foot orthosis (KAFO) may be recommended. A KAFO includes offset knee joints and a rigid AFO.[14]

An ambulation aid may be recommended for use during ambulation to compensate for impaired balance, decreased strength, pain during weight bearing on one or both lower extremities, or absence of a lower extremity. An ambulation aid may be necessary to help with fracture healing, to enhance body functions, or to improve functional mobility.[23]

Ambulation aids are numerous. Basic ambulation aids, from those providing the most support to the least, are a walker, crutches, a single crutch, bilateral canes, and a single cane.[23]

Table 15-1 Funtional Mobility Analysis

SITUATION: 53-YEAR-OLD HOMEMAKER WITH ANKLE AMPUTATION AMBULATING WITH A CANE	
Task Analysis Approach	**Example**
1. Identify the task(s) and specify the long- and short-term goals.	Task: Meal preparation; LTG: To prepare meal for family; STG: To prepare muffins from a mix
2. Gather necessary information concerning the following:	Necessary information specific to this client includes the following:
a. The action, including classification of the action and the movement	What motor skills are needed for this activity? What is the client's endurance level?
b. The environment, including the influence of both direct and indirect conditions	What are the environmental conditions for conducting this task? What supplies, people, and setting are required?
c. The client, including his or her interests and abilities and whether the minimal prerequisite skills for success are present	What information is known about the client? Interests and activities? What are the strengths and weaknesses from the OT assessment?
d. The prerequisite skills or performance components required of the client	What performance components are needed for functional ambulation to successfully bake muffins?
e. The expectations of outcome and movement	*Client successfully will bake muffins while ambulating with cane.*
3. Develop a strategy to make up for any deficits identified in #2.	Strategy: What adaptations will be necessary to accommodate availability of unilateral upper extremity to carry supplies because of use of an ambulation aid?
4. Plan the intervention strategy based on the preceding information concerning the individual-activity-environment interaction.	*Arrange supplies on countertop near oven to limit need for long distances of ambulation while carrying objects; use countertop or wheeled cart to transport bowls, pans, and other items.*
5. Effect the strategy.	Implement the task with the client.
a. Observe task and performance of the patients.	Observe and record outcomes.
b. Record what happened: What was the outcome and what was the approach and effect of the movement solution?	
6. Evaluate the observation.	*Evaluate whether the client was successful in baking muffins.*
a. Compare expectations and what happened.	Provide feedback to the client.
b. Provide feedback based on the comparison above and assist the patient in making decisions about the next attempt.	Plan next activity with client.
c. With the client, plan the next activity.	

Data from Higgins JR, Higgins S: The acquisition of locomotor skill. In Craik RL, Oatis CA, editors: *Gait analysis: theory and application*, St. Louis, 1995, Mosby.

The individual may begin ambulation with an aid that provides maximal support or stability and then may be progressed to an aid that provides less support or stability. Once again, the OT practitioner's communication with the physical therapist is essential to keeping abreast of any changes in the individual's ambulation aids and the use of such aids.

The basic ambulation techniques recommended by the physical therapist will vary from client to client, depending on the individual's goals, strengths, and weaknesses. General techniques may be applied to various clients based on the clinical judgment of the physical therapist. The OT practitioner reinforces the physical therapist's recommendations, incorporating these general techniques into functional ambulation activities.

During functional ambulation on a level surface, the OT practitioner is positioned slightly behind and to one side of the client. The therapist may position himself or herself to the stronger or weaker side of the client based on the recommendations and preference of the physical therapist. The therapist maintains contact with the client by using the gait belt. During ambulation, the therapist moves with (in the same direction as) the client. The therapist's outermost lower extremity moves with the ambulation aid, and the therapist's inside foot moves forward with the client's lower extremity.

Functional ambulation integrates ambulation into activities of daily living (ADL) and instrumental activities of daily living (IADL). Using an occupation-based approach, the OT practitioner considers the client's abilities within the performance context. What role(s) does the client desire to perform? What tasks does this role require of the client? Based on the answers to these questions, the OT plans for functional mobility activities with the goal of confident and safe functional ambulation in valued occupational roles and tasks; the OTA may carry out these functional ambulation activities.

When assessing the individual's needs based on roles and desired tasks, the OT practitioner performs a task analysis, analyzing the relationship between the client and his or her occupations and environment.[31] A task analysis serves the purpose of determining goals and targeting health outcomes. The task analysis identifies and examines meaningful and purposeful occupations.[20] Table 15-1 provides guidelines for such an analysis as it relates to functional ambulation.

Practical Instruction and Safety

Before beginning functional ambulation training, the OT practitioner should know basic client information. The occupational therapist reviews the medical record or pertinent notes reporting the client's current status and precautions. As part of this review, the occupational therapist confers with the physical therapy team member regarding the client's current ambulatory status, gait techniques, and ambulation aids or orthosis to be used. Throughout any functional ambulation activity, the occupational therapist or OTA reinforces the prescribed ambulation techniques and aids.

Another key to safe and successful functional ambulation is awareness of the client's endurance level. How easily does the client fatigue? What distance can the client ambulate? With this information in mind, the therapist can plan ahead for the functional ambulation activity. If the client may fatigue easily, the OT practitioner may have a wheelchair, chair, or stool readily available for use at appropriate intervals or in case of need.

To prepare the client for functional ambulation, the therapist begins with safe and appropriate footwear. The client should don nonskid shoes that fit well to avoid slipping. To increase the client's sense of security and to prevent a loss of balance or falls, the client should be instructed to avoid slippers or ill-fitting shoes or stocking feet.

The client's physiological responses should be monitored during the functional ambulation activity. The therapist should be aware of the client's precautions and respond appropriately. Physiological responses may include a change in breathing patterns, perspiration, reddened skin, a change in mental status, and decreased responsiveness.

During functional ambulation, the OT practitioner should be positioned slightly behind and to one side of the individual. Rather than grasping the individual's clothing, the OTA should maintain contact with the individual by using a gait belt to grasp with one hand, leaving the other hand free to assist with the functional activity.

The OTA should think ahead to be prepared for the unexpected. As with monitoring for fatigue level, the OTA must be prepared in case the unplanned occurs. Preparation includes having a wheelchair, walker, chair, or stool available should the activity need to be adjusted to a lower level of difficulty. Being prepared for the unexpected also involves watching for any obstacles or moving objects (e.g., individuals, therapists) that may come into the path of the client.

The OTA must not leave the client unattended during functional ambulation because the client may be unstable and a fall could result. The OTA should be certain that the area to be used for functional ambulation is free of any potential risks or safety hazards such as obstacles and that the floor is dry. Box 15-1 provides a summary of these important points.

Box 15-1

Safety for Functional Ambulation

1. Know the client (e.g., status, orthotics and aids, precautions).
2. Use appropriate footwear.
3. Clear potential hazards.
4. Monitor physiological responses.
5. Use a gait belt to guide the client. Do not use the client's clothes or upper extremity to guide the client.
6. Think ahead for the unexpected.
7. Do not leave the client unattended.

Functional Ambulation Application

Numerous opportunities for functional ambulation exist and are based on the individual and the specific requirements of the client's roles and desired tasks to be performed. Several typical functional ambulation activities follow. The activities may be modified for the individual clients. Functional ambulation may be incorporated during ADL, work and productive activities, and play or leisure activities.

Kitchen Ambulation

Functional ambulation may occur during meal preparation and cleanup within a kitchen. The OT practitioner must apply the gait-training techniques established by the physical therapist in combination with the treatment plan to accomplish meal preparation and cleanup tasks. For example, if the client has left hemiplegia and is ambulating with a quad-cane, the OT practitioner must solve problem to determine how the client will successfully accomplish the meal preparation activity. In this example, the OTA may guide the individual to ambulate to the left of the oven door in order to be able to open it with the unaffected right upper extremity. The same concept should be kept in mind for opening cabinet doors or drawers or refrigerator doors.

Transporting items such as food, plates, and eating utensils during functional ambulation invites creative problem solving on the part of the OT practitioner, particularly when the client is using an ambulation aid (Figures 15-1 and 15-2). Walker baskets, rolling carts, or countertops may be appropriate in these situations. Any such adaptation should be discussed to determine whether the client finds it acceptable.

Bathroom Ambulation

Functional ambulation to the sink, toilet, or edge of the bathtub or shower is an important concern for the occupational therapist. Great care should be taken during functional ambulation within the bathroom because of the many risks associated with water and hard surfaces. Spills on the floor and loose bath mats present tripping hazards. Educating clients about these dangers is essential.

Functional ambulation to the sink, using a walker in this example, may be performed in the following manner. First, approach as close to the sink as possible to enable the client to perform grooming and hygiene activities. If the walker has a walker basket or if a countertop or cabinets prohibit the client from positioning himself or herself close enough to use the sink safely, the client may need to cautiously maneuver the walker to one side and then carefully move forward toward the sink.

Ambulation to the toilet is another opportunity for OT intervention. The transfer to the toilet should be anticipated on entering the bathroom, and the client should be guided toward the toilet. Upon parallel alignment in front of the toilet, guide the client to maneuver himself or herself and

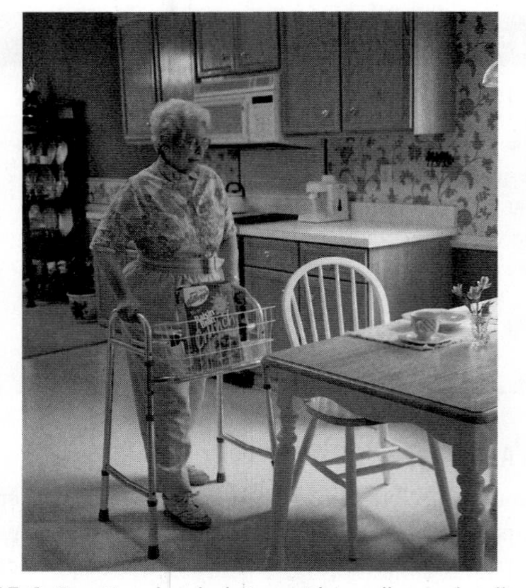

Figure 15-1 Functional ambulation with a walker and walker basket.

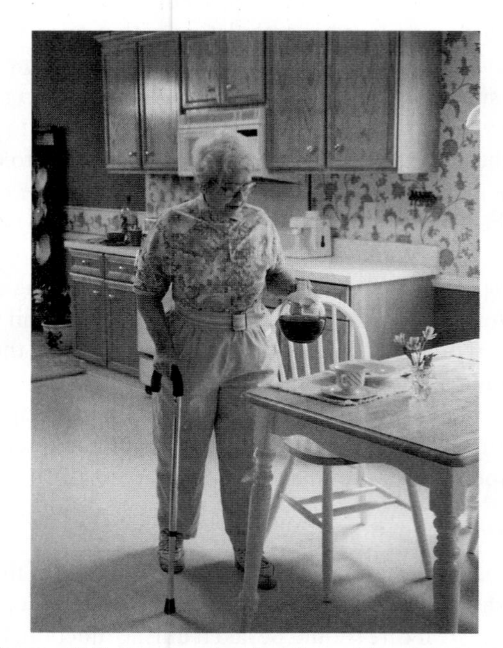

Figure 15-2 Functional ambulation with a straight cane.

the ambulation aid by pivoting to position him or her on the toilet. Guide the client to pivot the least distance possible, to prevent losing balance. If the toilet is to the left of the client, pivot clockwise approximately 90 degrees. If the toilet is on the right, pivot counterclockwise.

With ambulation to the edge of the bathtub or shower, the use of the bathtub or shower should be anticipated on entering the bathroom. The client should be guided toward the tub edge. Whether the client is ambulating with a walker, crutches, or cane or with no ambulation aid, the client should be aligned to prepare for a safe transfer as the client nears the edge. If a transfer tub bench, shower chair, or other equipment is necessary for the client, the client should be guided to position himself or herself before the transfer, thus limiting the risk of losing balance by using a technique requiring the least distance or extraneous movement.

Home Management Ambulation

Functional ambulation within the house during home management activities such as clothing care, cleaning, and household maintenance is another area for OT intervention. With clothing care, functional ambulation may be necessary during sorting, laundering, and storing of clothing. Cleaning including picking up, vacuuming, sweeping and mopping floors, dusting, and making beds is an ideal activity for including ambulation where appropriate. Household maintenance, which includes maintaining the home, yard, garden, appliances, and vehicles, may also incorporate functional ambulation. As with any OT intervention, the client should be consulted before the functional activity is begun in order to determine the home management activity that he or she most values.

Making the bed is an example of a homemaking activity. If the client uses a cane during ambulation, the client may stabilize himself or herself with the cane while using the other arm to straighten and pull up sheets and bedcovers. The client then moves around the bed to the other side to repeat the process. The client should be careful because he or she may lose balance while bending and straightening from bed height to a standing position throughout the activity.

Adaptations may be made to perform functional ambulation activities during household maintenance tasks such as yard work. For example, a client using a walker, crutches, or a cane may carefully ambulate, with assistance as needed, to the location in the yard needing weeding or pruning. Small yard tools may be carried in a walker basket or in a plastic shopping bag hung over the arm. During stationary activities such as weeding or pruning, the client may use a gardening stool. A stool may be used and moved to the next location as the yard work progresses.

Summary

Functional ambulation is the purposeful application of the mobility training taught to the client to enable movement from one position or place to another. It is applicable for clients with a variety of diagnoses, both biomechanical and neurologic, and across the age span.

Functional ambulation is an area in which the OT and physical therapy practitioners have an opportunity to collaborate. The physical therapist provides the gait training and ambulation aid recommendations; the occupational therapist and OTA reinforce and integrate these recommendations during purposeful activities.

Functional ambulation may be incorporated during ADL, work and productive activities, and play or leisure activities. The OT practitioner may often have an opportunity to incorporate functional ambulation into IADL.

SECTION II WHEELCHAIR ASSESSMENT AND TRANSFERS

Maureen Matthews and Carole Adler

For the person with a disability that makes ambulation impossible or impractical, a wheelchair provides access to environments and occupations. The case study of Kevin will illustrate this point. Throughout this section, consider Kevin's functionally relevant muscles, possible movements, and patterns of weakness. The occupational therapist weighed these and other factors in selecting an appropriate wheelchair and seating system and in determining the most efficient transfer techniques for him and his caregiver. The OTA's role is to assist in transfer training, wheelchair positioning and safety, and wheelchair adjustments, within the limits of service competency and local practice guidelines.

CASE STUDY

Kevin

Kevin is a 22-year-old male who sustained a C6 Asia A (sensory and motor complete) spinal cord injury after diving into shallow water. He was transferred to acute rehab from a hospital in the town where he was injured. He remained in acute rehab for 2½ months and received a minimum of 3 hours of occupational and physical therapy 6 days a week. In addition, he received psychology services, participated in multidisciplinary education classes and peer support groups, and avidly in therapeutic recreation activities.

Kevin was paralyzed in his hands, trunk, and lower extremities. He had a symmetrical C6 muscle picture with grade 4 muscle strength bilaterally in his trapezius, deltoids, biceps, and wrist extensors. Muscle strength was absent in triceps, hands, trunk, and lower extremities. Sensation was absent from the C7 dermatome throughout the rest of his body. Kevin's neck was immobilized in a cervical orthosis throughout his inpatient rehabilitation.

Kevin had been an athlete before his injury; he was active in water sports, particularly surfing. Now he is 5′9″ in height and weighs 150 lb. His normal weight before his injury was 175 lb.

Kevin required the physical assist of one caregiver for all of his personal care and mobility activities while he was out of his wheelchair including lower extremity dressing, bed mobility (primarily supine to sit and lower-extremity management because of significant spasticity), transfers, toileting, and bathing. Once in his wheelchair and in a wheelchair-accessible environment, he was modified independent (independent with the use of adaptive equipment and/or additional time) for feeding, sink-side grooming, upper-extremity dressing, and most tabletop activities. Absence of active trunk control made sitting balance a major challenge; however, he could independently perform weight shifts and position changes while sitting in his chair by using the wheelchair push handles.

Mobility Assistive Equipment

Mobility assistive equipment[12] (MAE) covers a range of equipment that assist disabled individuals in moving from place to place. Canes and walkers sit at the front end of this continuum, followed by manual wheelchairs, power-operated vehicles, and power wheelchairs. MAE must be medically necessary in order to be reimbursed by insurance. The type and complexity of the equipment recommended must restore the individual's ability to participate in mobility-related activities of daily living (MRADL) such as dressing, bathing, toileting, feeding, and grooming. A sequence of decisions will guide the clinician in selecting the most appropriate, medically justifiable MAE:

- Do specific mobility limitations prevent the client from participating in MRADL? This limitation could prevent the individual from completing an ADL, require an unreasonable amount of time for task completion, or place the individual at an increased risk of injury in attempting to perform the MRADL.
- What other conditions impede the individual's ability to complete MRADL tasks? Visual deficits, cognitive impairments, memory deficits, and other impairments should be identified. Secondary diagnoses, which may affect endurance, improvement, and safety, need to be considered.
- The client who is unable to participate actively in the MRADL may still require an MAE, provided there is a caregiver who will be able to use the device to better provide assistance in the MRADL.
- Safe operation of the MAE must be considered.
- What is the least expensive option to promote MRADL performance? Canes and walkers are least expensive, with custom power wheelchairs at the most costly end of the continuum.
- Does the home environment support the use of a wheeled mobility device? Consider obstacles, surfaces, stairs, and door widths. The device must be able to go through the bathroom door, for example, in order for the patient to shower or bathe in the tub.
- How will the device be propelled? How much upper body strength, range of motion, and endurance are required? Will one or both feet also assist with propulsion? Can the client safely and effectively maneuver the device in the MRADL home areas?
- If the client does not have sufficient strength and ability for a manual wheelchair, is the individual's strength and posture such that a power-operated vehicle (POV) or scooter may be of benefit? A POV/scooter has limited seating configuration, and a tiller is used to drive the vehicle. From a seated position, with legs in a dependent position and arms in front on the steering mechanism, is the client's endurance sufficient to benefit in MRADL performance?
- If not, will a power wheelchair allow the client to participate in MRADL?

A wheelchair can be the primary means of mobility for someone with a permanent or progressive disability such as cerebral palsy, brain injury, spinal cord injury, multiple sclerosis, or muscular dystrophy. It may be necessary as a temporary means of mobility by someone with a short-term illness or orthopedic problem. In addition to mobility, the wheelchair can substantially influence the total body positioning, skin integrity, overall function, and general well-being of the patient. Regardless of the diagnosis or condition of the patient, the OTA must appreciate and understand the complexity of wheelchair technology, available options and modifications, and the use, care, and cost of the wheelchair. The occupational therapist is responsible for the evaluation and measuring process; both occupational therapist and OTA may work together in the process by which equipment is funded.

Occupational therapists and physical therapists, depending on their respective roles at their treatment facilities, are usually responsible for evaluating, measuring, and selecting a wheelchair and seating system for the patient. Rehabilitation professionals including occupational therapists, physical therapists, OTAs, and physical therapy assistants also teach wheelchair safety and mobility skills to patients and their caregivers. The constant evolution of technology and variety of manufacturers' products make it helpful to have an experienced, knowledgeable, and certified rehabilitation technology supplier (RTS) on the ordering team. The RTS is a DME supplier who is proficient in ordering custom items and can offer an objective and broad mechanical perspective on the availability and appropriateness of the options being considered. The RTS is the patient's resource for insurance billing, repairs, and reordering when returning to the community.

Whether the patient requires a noncustom rental wheelchair for temporary use or a custom wheelchair for use over many years, an individualized prescription clearly outlining the specific features of the chair is necessary to ensure optimal performance, mobility, and enhancement of function. A wheelchair that has been prescribed by an inexperienced or untrained person is potentially hazardous and costly to the patient. An ill-fitting wheelchair can, in fact, contribute to unnecessary fatigue, skin breakdown, and trunk or extremity deformity and can inhibit function.[22] A wheelchair is an extension of the patient's body and should act to facilitate rather than inhibit good alignment, mobility, and function. For these reasons, the occupational therapist or the physical therapist must perform the evaluation and measurements and provide the prescription; OTAs with clinical experience and advanced training may assume some of the evaluation and measurement responsibilities in some settings, under local guidelines.

Box 15-2

Considerations in Recommendations for a Wheelchair

- Who will pay for the wheelchair?
- Who will determine the preferred durable medical equipment provider—the insurance company, the patient, or the therapist?
- What is the specific disability?
- What is the prognosis?
- Is ROM limited?
- Is strength or endurance limited?
- How will the patient propel the chair?
- How old is the patient?
- How long is the patient expected to use the wheelchair?
- What was the patient's lifestyle, and how has it changed?
- Is the patient active or sedentary?
- How will the dimensions of the chair affect the patient's ability to transfer to various surfaces?
- What is the maneuverability of the wheelchair in the patient's home or in the community (e.g., entrances and egress, door width, turning radius in bathroom and hallways, floor surfaces)?
- What is the ratio of indoor to outdoor activities?
- Where will the wheelchair be primarily used—in the home, at school, at work, or in the community?
- Which mode of transportation will be used? Will the patient be driving a van from the wheelchair? How will it be loaded and unloaded from the car?
- Which special needs (e.g., work heights, available assistance, accessibility of toilet facilities, and parking facilities) are recognized in the work or school environment?
- Does the patient participate in indoor or outdoor sports activities?
- How will the wheelchair affect the patient psychologically?
- Can accessories and custom modifications be medically justified, or are they luxury items?
- What resources does the patient have for equipment maintenance (e.g., self, family, caregivers)?

Wheelchair Evaluation

The therapist recommends a wheelchair that will be appropriate to meet not only immediate needs but also long-term needs. When evaluating for a wheelchair, the therapist must know the patient and have a broad perspective of the patient's clinical, functional, and environmental needs. The specific diagnosis, prognosis, and current and future problems (e.g., age, spasticity, loss of range of motion [ROM], muscle weakness, reduced endurance) may affect wheelchair use. The wheelchair will be used in a variety of environments. Box 15-2 lists questions to consider before making specific recommendations.

Before preparing the final prescription, the occupational therapist analyzes collected information to identify advantages and disadvantages of recommendations based on the patient's condition and how all specifics will integrate to provide an optimally effective mobility system. The occupational therapist works with the equipment supplier (RTS) and the reimbursement sources to facilitate payment for the most appropriate mobility system for the patient. The occupational therapist considers the patient's insurance benefits and provides documentation with thorough justification of the medical necessity of the wheelchair and any additional modifications. Therapists must explain clearly why particular features of a wheelchair are being recommended and must be aware of standard versus "up charge" items, the cost of each item, and how these items will affect the end product.

Wheelchair Ordering Considerations

Before selecting a specific brand and wheelchair specifications, the therapist should consider the following assessment sequence.[1,22,33]

Propelling the Wheelchair

The wheelchair may be propelled in a variety of ways, depending on the physical capacities of the user. The patient who is capable of self-propulsion with his or her arms on the rear wheels of the wheelchair must have sufficient and symmetrical grasp, arm strength, and physical endurance to maneuver the chair independently over varied terrain throughout the day.[33] An assortment of push rims is available to facilitate self-propelling, depending on the user's arm and grip strength. A patient with hemiplegia may propel a wheelchair using the unaffected arm and the ipsilateral leg to maneuver the wheelchair. A patient with tetraplegia may only have functional use of one arm and may be able to propel a one-arm drive wheelchair; however, a power chair may be more appropriate.

The surface that a chair is propelled over will influence the amount of strength and endurance required to move the chair. Hard, firm surfaces found in nursing homes and hospitals seldom replicate the challenges of a carpeted home environment. Propelling a wheelchair over a carpet requires much more exertion than does the same action over a hard tile or smooth wood surface.

Manual assist propulsion technology provides supplemental power to a manual wheelchair. By adding on to the manual frame, a battery-powered system assists the user in propelling the chair, literally minimizing the user's efforts while pushing the chair.

A power wheelchair is considered for those who have minimal or no use of the upper extremities, limited endurance, or shoulder dysfunction due to aging or pain. Power chairs are also preferred for inaccessible outdoor terrain.[9] Power wheelchairs have a wide variety of features and can be programmed; driven by foot, arm, head, or neck; or pneumatically controlled. Given today's sophisticated technology, assuming intact cognition and perception, even a person with the most severe physical limitations is capable of independently driving a power wheelchair.

For a chair that is to be propelled by the caregiver, the therapist considers ease of maneuverability and handling, as well as the positioning and mobility needs of the patient.

The therapist also analyzes the effect of the chair on the patient's current and future mobility and positioning needs. Lifestyle and environment, available resources such as ability to maintain the chair, transportation options, and available reimbursement sources are major determining factors.

Rental versus Purchase

The therapist estimates how long the patient will need the chair and whether the chair should be rented or purchased because these questions will affect the type of chair being considered. This decision is based on several clinical and functional issues. A rental chair is appropriate for short-term or temporary use such as when the patient's clinical picture, functional status, or body size is changing. Rental chairs may be necessary when the permanent wheelchair is being repaired. A rental wheelchair may also be useful when prognosis and expected outcome are unclear or when the patient has difficulty accepting the idea of using a wheelchair and needs to experience it initially as a temporary piece of equipment. Often the eventual functional outcome is unknown. In that case a chair can be rented for several months until a reevaluation determines whether a permanent chair will be necessary.[1] Medicare has defined capped periods for rental of wheelchairs. From 1 to 3 months, 80% of the charge is covered. From 4 to 10 months, 25% is covered. There are two options for funding after the eleventh month. In the first the Medicare wheelchair will convert to purchase after the thirteenth month, with the client responsible for all ongoing maintenance. In the second option, the client continues to rent for 5 more months. After that time, the vendor owns and maintains the chair, while the client uses it. The chair must be returned to the vendor when it is no longer necessary.[8]

A permanent wheelchair is indicated for the full-time user and for the patient with a progressive need for a wheelchair over a long period. It may be indicated when custom features are required and also when body size is changing, such as in the growing child.[1] Medicare funding guidelines require that a purchased wheelchair meet the client's needs for a 5-year period.[21] The clinician must project the disease progression over the next 5 years to determine the most appropriate device. This is most critical when degenerative disease processes are present or in the case of a growing child.

Frame Style

Once the method of propulsion and the permanence of the chair have been determined, the therapist considers wheelchair frame style. The frame style must be selected before specific dimensions and brand names can be determined. Wheelchair frames are now fabricated in titanium and aluminum materials. Frames differ in materials, durability, weight, and cost. A lighter-weight wheelchair requires less force to propel, is usually made with more durable components, and offers more adjustability. Frame weight, material, style, and custom options will significantly affect the patient's physical, functional, and mobility status—increasingly so over the long term.

Wheelchair Selection

The following decisions regarding patient needs are considered before the specific type of chair is determined[1]:

Manual versus Electric versus Manual Assist Wheelchair

Manual Wheelchair

Figure 15-3, *A* depicts a manual wheelchair. Individuals benefiting from a manual wheelchair should have sufficient strength and endurance to propel the chair at home and in the community over varied terrain. The effects of manual propulsion on upper-extremity joint health should be considered when recommending a manual chair. Standard manual wheelchairs exceed 35 lb. They can be difficult to maneuver and transport due to weight. A lighter-weight manual wheelchair is recommended for longer-term use.[8] Heavy-duty wheelchairs are available for individuals in excess of 250 lb, and extra-heavy duty wheelchairs can support clients weighing more than 300 lb. A heavy individual must be able to propel the chair or be pushed by others and may require a power chair as a result.

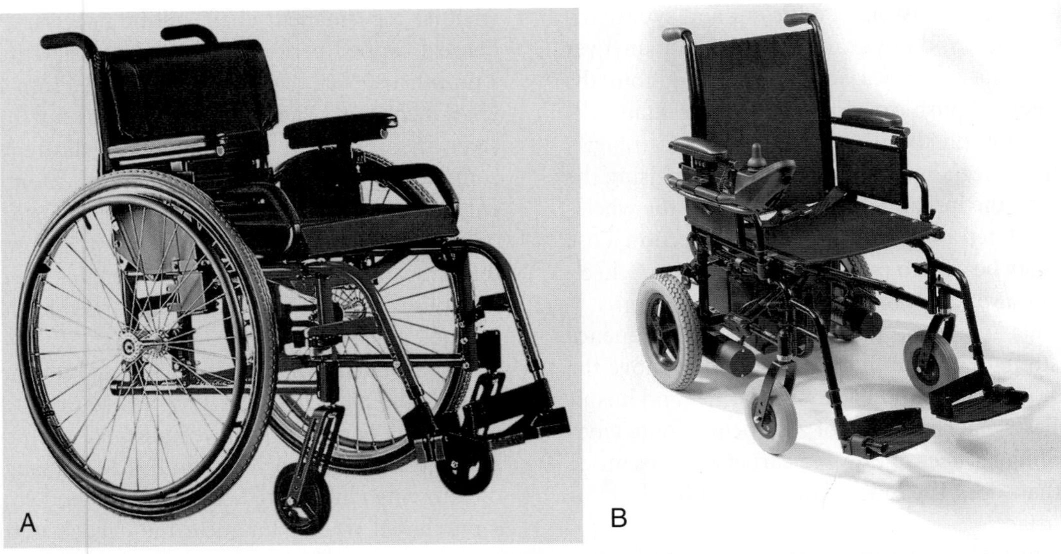

Figure 15-3 Manual versus electric wheelchair. **A,** Rigid frame chair with swing-away footrests. **B,** Power-driven wheelchair with hand control. (**A** courtesy Quickie Designs; **B** courtesy Invacare Corporation.)

POV/Scooter and Electric Wheelchair

Figure 15-3, *B* depicts an electric wheelchair. Questions to consider in the decision to recommend an electric wheelchair include the following:

- Does the user demonstrate insufficient endurance and functional ability to propel a manual wheelchair independently?
- Does the user demonstrate progressive functional loss that makes powered mobility an energy-conserving option?
- Is powered mobility needed to increase independence at school, at work, and in the community?
- Does the user demonstrate cognitive and perceptual ability to operate a power-driven system safely?
- Does the user or caregiver demonstrate responsibility for care and maintenance of equipment?
- Is a van available for transportation?
- Is the user's home accessible for use of a scooter or power wheelchair?
- What is the optimal driving control and seated posture for the client?
- Has the user been educated regarding the rear-, mid-, and front-wheel drive systems and been guided objectively in making the appropriate selection?

Manual Assist

Questions to consider in the decision to recommend manual assist include the following:

- Does the user have insufficient strength and endurance to propel the chair at home and in the community over varied terrain?
- Does the user desire and have the ability to provide some effort in propelling the chair?
- Does manual mobility enhance functional independence and cardiovascular conditioning of the wheelchair user?
- Will the caregiver be propelling the chair at any time? (A manual assist system is considerably heavier to "free-wheel.")
- What will be the long-term effects of the propulsion choice?
- Has the user been educated regarding the benefits and disadvantages of power assist versus straight power and been guided objectively in making the appropriate selection?

Manual Recline versus Power Recline versus Tilt Wheelchairs

Manual Recline Wheelchair

Figure 15-4, *A* depicts a manual recline wheelchair. Questions to consider in the decision to recommend a manual recline wheelchair include the following:

- Is the patient unable to sit upright because of hip contractures, poor balance, or fatigue?
- Is a caregiver available to assist with weight shifts and position changes?
- Is relative ease of maintenance a concern?
- Is cost a consideration?

Power Recline versus Tilt

Figure 15-4, *B* and *C* depict power recline and tilt. Questions to consider in deciding between power recline and tilt include the following:

- Does the patient have the potential to operate independently?
- Are independent weight shifts and position changes indicated for skin care and increased sitting tolerance?
- Does the user demonstrate safe and independent use of controls?
- Are there resources for care and maintenance of the equipment?
- Does the user have significant spasticity that is facilitated by hip and knee extension during the recline phase?
- Does the user have hip or knee contractures that prohibit his or her ability to recline fully?
- Will a power recline or tilt decrease or make more efficient use of caregiver time?

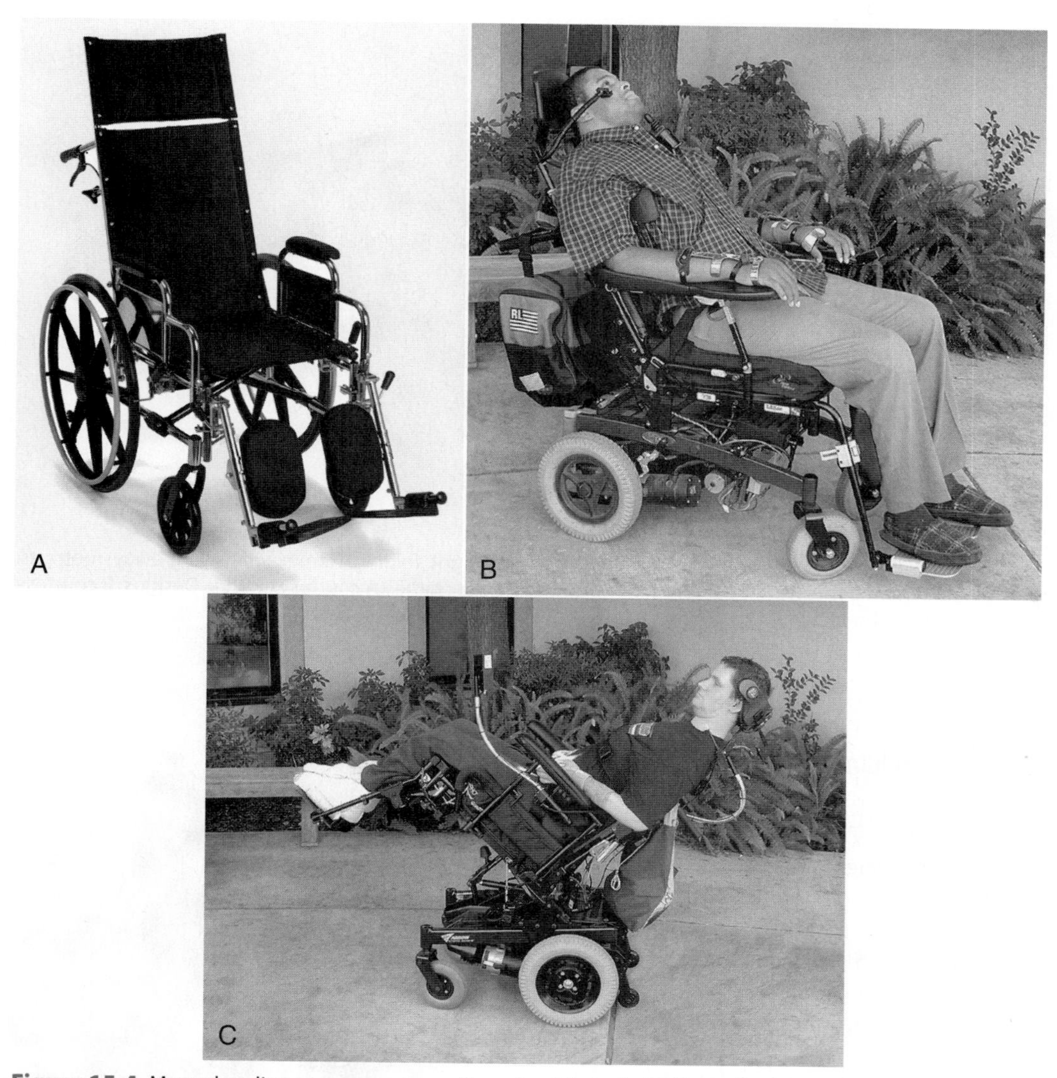

Figure 15-4 Manual recline versus power recline wheelchair. **A,** Reclining back on folding frame. **B,** Low-shear power recline with collar mount chin control on electric wheelchair. **C,** Tilt system with head control on electric wheelchair. (**A** courtesy Quickie Designs; **B** and **C** courtesy Luis Gonzalez, SCVMC.)

- Will a power recline or tilt reduce the need for transfers to the bed for catheterizations and rest periods throughout the day?
- Will the patient require quick position changes in the event of hypotension and/or autonomic dysreflexia?
- Has a reimbursement source been identified for this add-on feature?

Folding versus Rigid Manual Wheelchairs

Folding Wheelchairs

Figure 15-5, *A* depicts folding wheelchairs. In choosing a folding wheelchair, one should consider the following questions:

- Does the patient prefer a traditional-looking chair?
- Is the folding frame needed for transport, storage, or home accessibility?
- Which footrest style is necessary for transfers, desk clearance, and other daily living skills? (Elevating footrests are available only on folding frames.)
- Can the patient or caregiver load and fit the chair into necessary vehicles?

Equipment suppliers will have knowledge and a variety of brands available. Frame weight can range between approximately 28 and 50 lb depending on size and accessories. Frame adjustments and custom options depend on the model.

Rigid Wheelchair

Figure 15-5, *B* depicts a rigid wheelchair. In choosing a rigid wheelchair, one should consider the following questions:

- Does the user or caregiver have the upper extremity function and balance to load and unload the nonfolding frame from a vehicle if driving independently?
- Will the user benefit from the improved energy efficiency, decrease in weight, and performance of a rigid frame?

Footrest options are limited, and the frame is lighter (20 to 35 lb). Features include an adjustable seat angle, rear axle, caster mount, and back height. Efficient frame design maximizes performance. Options exist in frame material composition, frame colors, and aesthetics. These chairs are usually custom ordered through custom rehabilitation technology suppliers.

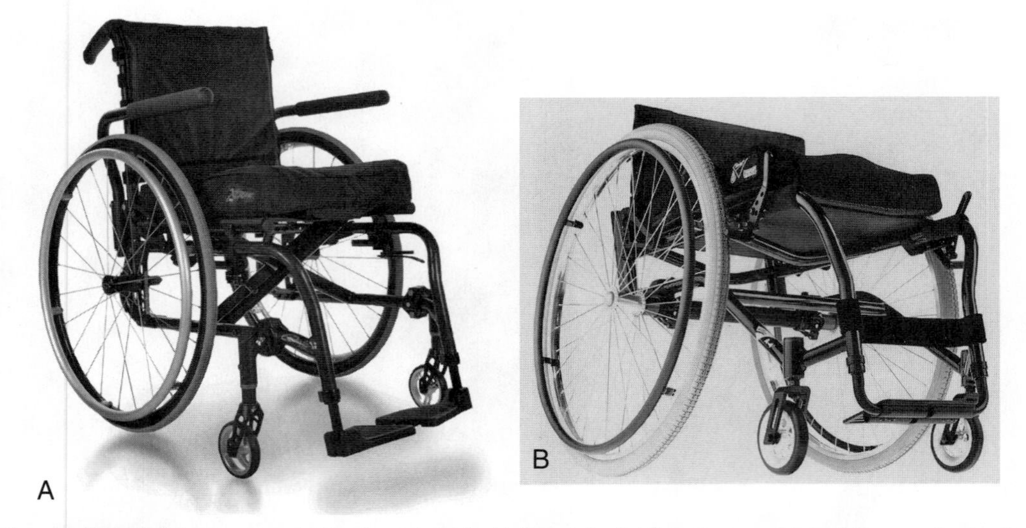

Figure 15-5 Folding versus rigid wheelchair. **A,** Lightweight folding frame with swing-away footrests. **B,** Rigid aluminum frame with tapered front end and solid foot cradle. (**A** courtesy Quickie Designs; **B** courtesy Invacare Corporation.)

Lightweight (Folding or Nonfolding) versus Standard-Weight (Folding) Wheelchairs

Lightweight Wheelchairs: Less Than 35 lb

Figure 15-5, *A* depicts a lightweight wheelchair. In choosing a lightweight wheelchair, one should consider the following questions:

- Does the user have the trunk balance and equilibrium necessary to handle a lighter frame weight?
- Does the lighter weight enhance mobility by reducing the user's fatigue?
- Will the user's ability to propel the chair or handle parts be enhanced by a lighter-weight frame?
- Are custom features (e.g., adjustable height back, seat angle, axle mount) necessary?

Standard-Weight Wheelchairs: More Than 35 lb

Figure 15-6 depicts standard-weight wheelchairs. In choosing a standard-weight wheelchair, one should consider the following questions:

- Does the user need the stability of a standard-weight chair?
- Does the user have the ability to propel a standard- weight chair?
- Can the caregiver manage the increased weight when loading the wheelchair and fitting into a vehicle?
- Will the increased weight of parts be unimportant during daily living skills?

Custom options are limited, and these wheelchairs are usually less expensive (except heavy-duty models required for users who weigh more than 250 lb).

Standard Available Features versus Custom Models

The price range, durability, and warranty within a specific manufacturer's model line are considered.

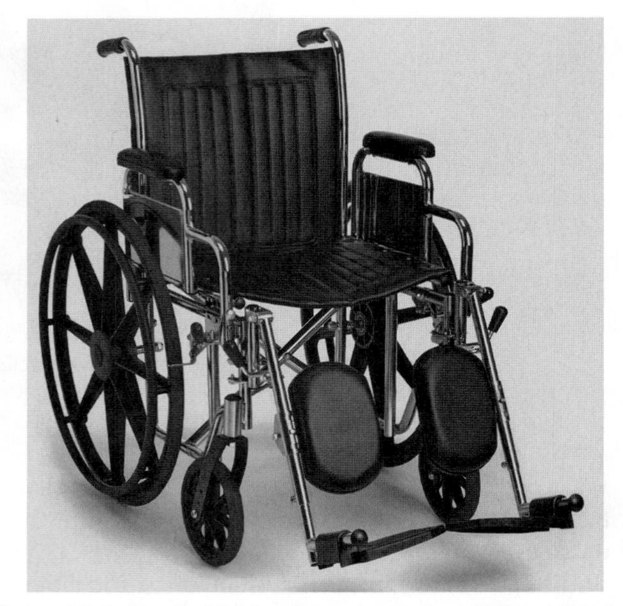

Figure 15-6 Standard folding frame (more than 35 lb) with swing-away footrests. (Courtesy Quickie Designs.)

Standard Available Features

When choosing from standard available features, one should consider the following questions:

- Is the chair required only for part-time use?
- Does the user have a limited life expectancy?
- Is the chair needed as a second or transportation chair, used only 10% to 20% of the time?
- Will the chair be primarily for indoor or sedentary use?
- Does the user depend on caregivers for propulsion?
- Will the chair be propelled only by the caregiver?
- Are custom features or specifications not necessary?
- Is substantial durability unimportant?

For standard wheelchairs, a limited warranty is available on the frame. Reimbursement limitations may restrict options. Limited sizes and options and adjustability are available. Standard chairs cost considerably less than custom wheelchairs.

Custom Models

- Will the patient be a full-time user?
- Is there a likely prognosis for long-term use of the wheelchair?
- Will this be the primary wheelchair?
- Is the user active both indoors and outdoors?
- Will this frame style improve potential for independent mobility?
- Is the user a growing adolescent, or does he or she have a progressive disorder requiring later modification of the chair?
- Are custom features, specifications, or positioning devices required?

Custom wheelchair frames usually have a lifetime warranty on the frame. A variety of specifications, options, and adjustments are available. Manufacturers often work with therapists and providers to solve a specific fitting problem. Experience is essential in ordering top-of-the-line and custom equipment.

Wheelchair Measurement Procedures

The patient is measured in the style of chair and with the seat cushion that most closely resembles those being ordered. If the patient will wear a brace or body jacket or need any additional devices in the chair, these should be in place during the measurement. Observation skills are important during this process. Measurements alone should not be used. The therapist "eyeballs" the entire body position every step of the way.[1,32] The procedures are given here as an aid for the OTA in understanding the process; again, only service-competent practitioners should engage in wheelchair measurement and prescription.

Seat Width

Figure 15-7, *A* addresses seat width.

- Objectives

1. Distributing the patient's weight over the widest possible surface
2. Keeping the overall width of the chair as narrow as possible

- Measurement

Measure across the widest part of either the thighs or hips while the patient is sitting in a chair comparable to that expected.

- Wheelchair Clearance

Add ½ to 1 inch on each side of the hip or thigh measurement taken. Consider how increasing the overall width of the chair will affect accessibility.

- Checking

Place the flat palm of the hand between the patient's hip or thigh and the wheelchair skirt and armrest.

- Considerations

1. User's potential weight gain or loss
2. Accessibility of varied environments

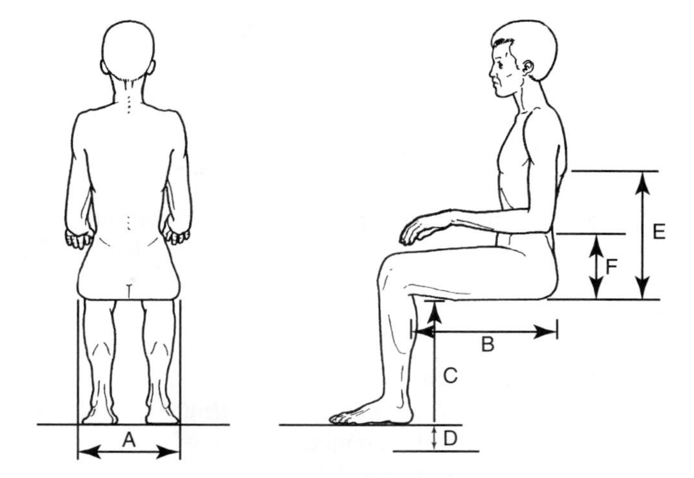

Figure 15-7 What and where to measure. **A,** Seat width. **B,** Seat depth. **C,** Seat height from floor. **D,** Footrest clearance. **E,** Back height. **F,** Armrest height. (Modified from Wilson A, McFarland SR: *Wheelchairs: a prescription guide,* Charlottesville, Va, 1986, Rehabilitation Press.)

3. Overall width of wheelchair; camber and axle mounting position, rim style, and wheel style can affect overall wheelchair width

Seat Depth

Figure 15-7, *B* addresses seat depth.

- Objective

The objective is to distribute the body weight along the sitting surface by bearing weight along the entire length of the thigh to just behind the knee. This approach is necessary to help prevent pressure sores on the buttocks and lower back and for optimal muscle tone normalization to assist in the prevention of pressure sores throughout the body.

- Measurement

Measure from the base of the back post to the inside of the bent knee; the seat edge clearance needs to be 1 to 2 inches less than this measurement.

- Checking

Check clearance behind the knees to prevent contact of the front edge of the seat upholstery with the popliteal space. Consider front angle of leg-rest or foot cradle.

- Considerations

1. Braces or back inserts that may be pushing the patient forward.
2. Postural changes throughout the day from fatigue or spasticity.
3. Thigh length discrepancy; the depth of the seat may be different for each leg.
4. If considering a power recliner, one should assume the patient will slide forward slightly throughout the day and should make depth adjustments accordingly.
5. Seat depth may need to be shortened to allow independent propulsion with the lower extremities.

Seat Height from Floor and Foot Adjustment

- Objectives

1. Supporting the patient's body while maintaining the thighs parallel to the floor (Figure 15-5, *C*)

2. Elevating the foot plates to provide ground clearance over varied surfaces and curb cuts (Figure 15-7, *D*)

- Measurements

Measure the top of the seat post to the floor and the popliteal fossa to the bottom of the heel.

- Wheelchair Clearance

The patient's thighs are kept parallel to the floor so that the body weight is distributed evenly along the entire depth of the seat. The lowest point of the footplates must clear the floor by at least 2 inches.

- Checking

Slip fingers under the patient's thighs at the front edge of the seat upholstery. Note: A custom seat height may be necessary to obtain footrest clearance. An inch of increased seat height raises the footplate 1 inch.

- Considerations

1. If the knees are too high, increased pressure at the ischial tuberosities puts the patient at risk for skin breakdown and pelvic deformity.
2. Sitting too high off the ground raises the patient's center of gravity, potentially a safety and stability problem. Sitting too high may interfere with visibility and seat height for transfers if the patient is driving a van from the wheelchair.

Back Height

Figure 15-7, *E* addresses back height.

- Objective

Providing back support consistent with physical and functional needs. The chair back should be low enough for maximal function and high enough for maximal support.

- Measurements

For full trunk support, measure from the top of the seat post to the top of the shoulders. For minimum trunk support, the top of the back upholstery should permit free arm movement, not irritate the skin or scapulae, and provide good total body alignment.

- Checking

Ensure that the patient is not being pushed forward because the back of the chair is too high or leaning backward over the top of the upholstery because the back is too low.

- Considerations

1. Adjustable-height backs (usually offer a 4-inch range)
2. Adjustable upholstery
3. Lumbar support or another commercially available or custom back insert to prevent kyphosis, scoliosis, or other long-term trunk deformity

Arm Height

Figure 15-7, *F* addresses arm height.

- Objectives

1. Maintaining posture and balance
2. Providing support and alignment for upper extremities
3. Allowing change in position by pushing down on armrests

- Measurements

With the patient in a comfortable position, measure from the seat post to the bottom of a bent elbow.

- Wheelchair Clearance

The height of the top of the armrest should be 1 inch higher than the height from the seat post to the patient's elbow.

- Checking

The patient's posture should look correct. The shoulders should not slouch forward or be subluxated or forced into elevation when the patient is in a normal sitting posture, with flexed elbows slightly forward on armrests.

- Considerations

1. Other uses of armrests such as increasing functional reach or holding a cushion in place.
2. Certain styles of armrests can increase the overall width of the chair.
3. Whether armrests are necessary at all.
4. The patient's ability to remove and replace the armrest from the chair independently.
5. Review all measurements against standards for a particular model of chair. Manufacturers have lists of the standard dimensions available and the cost for custom modifications.

Pediatric Wheelchair Considerations

Rarely does a standard wheelchair meet the fitting requirements of a child. The selection of size is variable; therefore custom seating systems specific to the pediatric population are available. A secondary goal is to consider a chair that will accommodate the child's growth.

For children younger than 5 years of age, a decision about whether to use a stroller base or a standard wheelchair base must be made. Considerations are the child's ability to propel the chair relative to the developmental level and the parent's preference for a stroller or a wheelchair.

Many variables must be considered when customizing a wheelchair frame. An experienced RTS or the wheelchair manufacturer should be consulted to ensure that a custom request will be successful.

Additional Seating and Positioning Considerations

A wheelchair evaluation is not complete until the seat cushion, back support, and any other positioning devices and the integration of those parts are carefully thought out, regardless of the diagnosis. Optimal body alignment has a profound effect on skin integrity, tone normalization, overall functional ability, and general well-being (Figure 15-8).[1]

The following are the goals of a comprehensive seating and positioning assessment.

Prevention of Deformity

Providing a symmetrical base of support preserves proper skeletal alignment and discourages spinal curvature and other body deformities.

Tone Normalization

By providing proper body alignment, as well as bilateral weight bearing and adaptive devices as needed, tone normalization can be maximized.

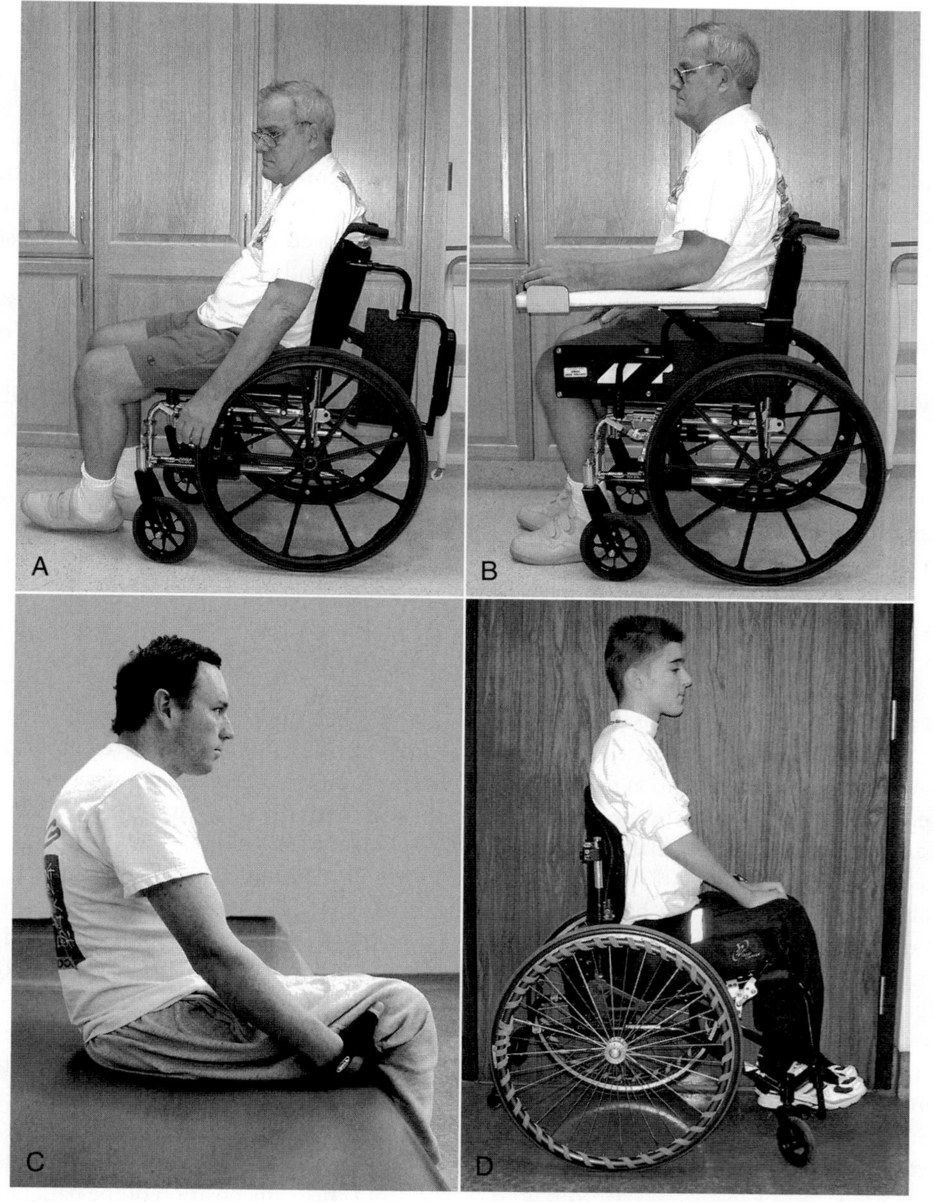

Figure 15-8 **A,** Stroke patient seated in wheelchair. Poor positioning results in kyphotic thoracic spine, posterior pelvic tilt, and unsupported affected side. **B,** Stroke patient seated in wheelchair with appropriate positioning devices. Seat and back insert support upright midline position with neutral pelvic tilt and equal weight bearing throughout. **C,** Spinal cord-injured patient sitting with back poorly supported results in posterior pelvic tilt, kyphotic thoracic spine, and absence of lumbar curve. **D,** Spinal cord–injured patient with rigid back support and pressure-relief seat cushion, resulting in erect thoracic spine, lumbar curve, and anterior tilted pelvis.

Pressure Management

The proper seat cushion can provide comfort; assist in trunk and pelvic alignment; and create a surface that minimizes pressure, heat, moisture, and shearing, the primary causes of skin breakdown. Pressure sores can be caused by improper alignment and an inappropriate sitting surface.

Promotion of Function

Pelvic and trunk stability is necessary to free the upper extremity for participation in all functional activities including wheelchair mobility and daily living skills.

Maximum Sitting Tolerance

Wheelchair sitting tolerance will increase as support, comfort, and symmetrical weight bearing are provided.

Optimal Respiratory Function

Support in an erect, well-aligned position can decrease compression of the diaphragm and thus increase vital capacity.

Provision for Proper Body Alignment

Good body alignment is necessary for prevention of deformity, normalization of tone, and promotion of movement.

The patient should be able not only to propel the wheelchair but also to move around within the wheelchair.

A wide variety of seating and positioning equipment is available for all levels of disability. New custom modifications regularly come on the market and are designed to meet a variety of patient needs. In addition, technology in this area is ever growing, and interest in wheelchair technology as a professional specialty is also growing. However, the skill of clinicians in this field ranges from extensive to negligible. Although it is an integral aspect of any wheelchair evaluation, the scope of seating and positioning equipment is much greater than can be addressed in this chapter. The suggested reading list at the end of this chapter gives additional resources.

Accessories

Once the measurements and the need for additional positioning devices have been determined, accessories are considered. A wide variety of accessories is available to meet individual needs. It is extremely important to understand the function of each accessory and how an accessory interacts with the rest of the chair and with seating and positioning equipment.[1,33]

Armrests come in fixed, flip-back, detachable, desk, standard, reclining, adjustable height, and tubular styles. The fixed armrest is a continuous part of the frame and is not detachable. It limits proximity to table, counter, and desk surfaces and prohibits side transfers. Flip-back, detachable desk, and standard-length arms are removable and allow side-approach transfers. Reclining arms are attached to the back post and recline with the back of the chair. Tubular arms are available on lightweight frames.

Footrests may be fixed, swing-away detachable, solid cradle, and elevating. The fixed footrests are attached to the wheelchair frame and are not removable. These footrests prevent the person from getting close to counters and may make some types of transfers more difficult. The swing-away detachable footrests can be moved to the side of the chair or removed entirely. This allows a closer approach to bed, bathtub, and counters and, when the footrests are removed, reduces the overall wheelchair length and weight for easy loading into a car. Detachable footrests lock into place on the chair with a locking device.[33] A solid cradle footrest is found on rigid, lightweight chairs and is not removable. Elevating leg rests are available for patients with such conditions as lower-extremity edema, blood pressure changes, and orthopedic problems.

The footplates may have heel loops and toe straps to aid in securing the foot on the footplate.[33] A calf strap can be used on a solid cradle or when additional support behind the calf is necessary. Other accessories can include seat belts, various brake styles, brake extensions, antitip devices, caster locks, arm supports, and head supports.

Preparing the Prescription

Once specific measurements and the need for modifications and accessories have been determined, the wheelchair prescription is completed. It should be concise and specific so that everything requested can be accurately interpreted by the DME supplier, who will submit a sales contract for payment authorization. Before-and-after pictures can be helpful in illustrating medical necessity. It is important that the requirements for payment authorization from a particular reimbursement source are known so that medical necessity can be demonstrated. The therapy practitioner who is documenting need must be aware of the cost of everything being requested and of the reason each item is necessary. Payment may be denied if clear reasons are not given to substantiate the need for every item and modification requested.

Before the wheelchair is delivered to the patient, the therapy provider should check the chair against the specific prescription and ensure that all specifications and accessories are correct. When a custom chair has been ordered, it is strongly recommended that the patient be fitted by the ordering therapist to ensure that the chair fits and that it provides all the elements that were expected when the prescription was generated.

Wheelchair Safety

Wheelchair parts tend to loosen over time and should be inspected and tightened on a regular basis. The OTA may have significant responsibility in this area.

Elements of safety for the wheelchair user and the caregiver include the following:

1. Brakes should be locked during all transfers.
2. The patient should never stand on the foot plates, which are placed in the "up" position during most transfers.
3. In most transfers, it is an advantage to have footrests swung away if possible.
4. If a caregiver is pushing the chair, he or she should be sure that the patient's elbows are not protruding from the armrests and that the patient's hands are not on the hand rims. If approaching from behind to assist in moving the wheelchair, the caregiver should inform the patient of this intent and check the position of the patient's feet and arms before proceeding.
5. To push the patient up a ramp, the person pushing should move in a normal, forward direction. If the ramp is negotiated independently, the patient should lean slightly forward while propelling the wheelchair up the incline.[34]
6. To push the patient down a ramp, the caretaker should tilt the wheelchair backward by pushing the foot down on the tipping levers to its balance position, which is a tilt of approximately 30 degrees. Then the caregiver should ease the wheelchair down the ramp in a forward direction, while maintaining the chair in its balance position. The caregiver should keep his or her knees slightly bent and back straight.[34] The caregiver may also move down the ramp backward while the patient maintains some control of the large wheels to prevent rapid backward motion. This approach is useful if the grade is relatively steep. Ramps with only a slight grade can also be managed in a forward direction if the caregiver maintains grasp and pull on the hand grips and the patient again maintains some control

of the big wheels to prevent rapid forward motion. If the ramp is negotiated independently, the patient should move down the ramp facing forward while leaning backward slightly and maintaining control of speed by grasping the hand rims. The patient can descend a steep grade by traversing the ramp to slow the chair. Gloves may be helpful to reduce the effect of friction.[34]
7. A caregiver can manage ascending curbs by approaching them forward, tipping the wheelchair back, and pushing the foot down on the tipping levers, thus lifting the front casters onto the curb and pushing forward. The large wheels are then in contact with the curb and roll on with ease as the chair is lifted slightly onto the curb.
8. A curb should be descended using a backward approach. A caregiver can move himself or herself and the chair around and pull the wheelchair to the edge of the curb. Standing below the curb, the caregiver can guide the large wheels off the curb by slowly pulling the wheelchair backward until it begins to descend. After the large wheels are safely on the street surface, the assistant can tilt the chair back to clear the casters, move backward, lower the casters to the street surface, and then turn around.[34]

With good strength and coordination, many patients can be trained to manage curbs independently. To mount and descend a curb, the patient must have a good bilateral grip, arm strength, and balance. To mount the curb, the patient tilts the chair onto the rear wheels and pushes forward until the front wheels hang over the curb, then lowers them gently. The patient then leans forward and forcefully pushes forward on the hand rims to bring the rear wheels up on the pavement. To descend a curb, the patient should lean forward and push slowly backward until the rear and then the front wheels roll down the curb.[10]

Transfer Techniques

Transferring is the process of moving a patient's body from one surface to another. Transfer may be done by the patient unaided, by the patient with the aid of caregivers, or by caregivers. Transfer includes the sequence of events that must occur both before and after the move, such as the pretransfer sequence of bed mobility and the posttransfer phase of wheelchair positioning. Assuming that a patient has some physical or cognitive limitations, it will be necessary for the OTA to assist in or supervise a transfer. Many clinicians are unsure of the transfer type and technique to employ or feel perplexed when a particular technique does not succeed with a given patient. It is important to remember that each patient, practitioner, and situation is different. This chapter does not include an outline of all techniques but presents the basic techniques with generalized principles. Each transfer must be adapted for the particular patient and his or her needs. The discussion in this chapter includes directions for some transfer techniques that are most commonly employed in practice. These techniques are the stand pivot, bent pivot, and one-person and two-person dependent transfers.

Preliminary Concepts

Clinicians must consider the following when selecting and carrying out transfer techniques to ensure safety for both the patient and self:

1. The patient's assets and limitations, especially the patient's physical, cognitive, perceptual, and behavioral abilities and deficits.
2. The clinician's own physical abilities and limitations, as well as ability to communicate clear, sequential instructions to the patient (and if necessary to the long-term caregiver of the patient).
3. The clinician's knowledge of correct moving and lifting techniques.

Guidelines for Using Proper Mechanics

The following are the basic principles of body mechanics[2]:

1. Get close to the patient or move the patient closer to you.
2. Square off with the patient (face head on).
3. Bend knees; use the legs, not the back.
4. Keep a neutral spine (not bent or arched back).
5. Keep a wide base of support.
6. Keep your heels down.
7. Do not tackle more than you can handle; ask for help.
8. Do not combine movements. Avoid rotating at the same time as bending forward or backward.
9. The clinician should consider the following questions before performing a transfer:

- What medical precautions affect the patient's mobility or method of transfer?
- Can the transfer be performed safely by one person, or is assistance required?
- Has enough time been allotted for safe execution of a transfer? Are you in a hurry?
- Does the patient understand what is going to happen? If not, does he or she demonstrate fear or confusion? Is the practitioner prepared for this limitation?
- Is the equipment that the patient is being transferred to and from in good working order and in a locked position?
- What is the height of the bed (or surface) in relation to the wheelchair? Can the heights be adjusted?
- Is all equipment placed in the correct position?
- Is all unnecessary bedding and equipment moved out of the way to work without obstructions?
- Is the patient dressed properly in case you need to use a waistband to assist? If not, do you need a transfer belt or other assistance?
- What are the other components of the transfer such as leg management and bed mobility?
- It is important for the OTA to be familiar with as many types of transfers as possible so that each situation can be resolved as it arises.

Many classifications of transfers exist and are based on the amount of clinician participation. Classifications range from *dependent,* in which the patient cannot participate and the therapist moves the patient, to *independent,* in which the patient moves independently while the clinician merely supervises, observes, or provides input for appropriate technique as related to the patient's disability.

Before attempting to move a patient, the OTA must understand the biomechanics of movement and the effect of the patient's center of positioning mass on transfers.

Principles of Body Positioning

Pelvic Tilt

Generally, after the acute onset of a disability or prolonged time spent in bed, patients assume a posterior pelvic tilt (i.e., a slouched position with lumbar flexion). In turn, this posture moves the center of mass back toward the buttocks. The therapist may need to verbally cue or assist the patient into a neutral or slightly anterior pelvic tilt position to move the center of mass forward over the center of the patient's body.[25]

Trunk Alignment

One may observe that the patient's trunk alignment is shifted to either the right or the left side. If the clinician assists in moving the patient while the patient's weight is shifted to one side, the movement could throw both the patient and the OTA off balance. The patient may need verbal cues or physical assistance to come to and maintain a midline trunk position before and during the transfer.

Weight Shifting

The transfer is initiated by shifting the patient's weight forward, removing weight from the buttocks. This movement allows the patient to stand, partially stand, or be pivoted by the clinician. This step must be performed regardless of the type of transfer.

Lower Extremity Positioning

The patient's feet must be placed firmly on the floor with ankles stabilized and with knees aligned at 90 degrees of flexion over the feet. This position allows the weight to be shifted easily onto and over the feet. Heels should be pointing toward the surface to which the patient is transferring. The patient should either wear shoes or be barefoot to prevent slipping out of position. The feet can easily pivot in this position, and the risk of twisting or injuring an ankle or knee is minimized.

Upper Extremity Positioning

The patient's arms must be in a safe position or in a position in which he or she can assist in the transfer. If one or both of the upper extremities is nonfunctional, the arms should be placed in a safe position that will not be in the way during the transfer (e.g., in the patient's lap). If the patient has partial or full movement, motor control, or strength, he or she can assist in the transfer either by reaching toward the surface to be reached or by pushing off from the surface to be left. The clinician's decision is based on prior knowledge of the patient's motor function.

Preparing Equipment and Patient for Transfer

The transfer process includes setting up the environment, positioning the wheelchair, and helping the patient into a pretransfer position. The following is a general overview of these steps.

Positioning the Wheelchair

1. Place the wheelchair at approximately a 30-degree angle to the surface to which the patient is transferring.
2. Lock the brakes on the wheelchair and the bed.
3. Place both of the patient's feet firmly on the floor, hip width apart and with knees over the feet.
4. Remove the armrest closer to the bed.
5. Remove the pelvic seatbelt.
6. Remove the chest belt and trunk or lateral supports.

Bed Mobility in Preparation for Transfer

Rolling the Hemiplegic Patient

Before rolling the patient, the practitioner may need to put his or her hand under the patient's scapula on the weak side and gently mobilize it forward to prevent the patient from rolling onto the shoulder, potentially causing pain and injury.

1. Assist the patient in clasping the strong hand around the wrist of the weak arm, and lift upper extremities toward the ceiling.
2. Flex the patient's knees.
3. The practitioner may assist the patient to roll onto his or her side by moving the arms, then the legs, and by holding one hand at the scapula area and the other at the hip, guiding the roll.

Side-Lying to Sit Up at the Edge of Bed

- Bring the patient's feet off the edge of the bed.
- Stabilize the patient's lower extremities.
- Shift the patient's body to an upright sitting position.
- Place the patient's hands on the bed at the sides of his or her body to help maintain balance.

Scooting to the Edge of the Bed

When working with a patient who has had a stroke or traumatic brain injury, walk the patient's hips toward the edge of the bed. Shift the patient's weight to the unaffected side, position your hand behind the opposite buttock, and guide the patient forward. Shift the patient's weight to the affected side and repeat the procedure if necessary. Move forward until the patient's feet are flat on the floor.

In the case of an individual with spinal cord injury, grasp the patient's legs from behind the knees and pull the patient forward, placing the patient's feet firmly on the floor and being sure that the ankles are in a neutral position.

Stand Pivot Transfers

The standing pivot transfer requires the patient to be able to come to a standing position and pivot on one or both feet. It is most commonly used with patients who have hemiplegia, hemiparesis, or a general loss of strength or balance.

Wheelchair to Bed or Mat Transfer

1. Help the patient scoot to the edge of the surface and put his or her feet flat on the floor. The patient's ankles should be pointed toward the surface to which the patient is transferring.
2. Stand on the patient's affected side with hands either on the patient's scapulae or around the patient's waist or hips.

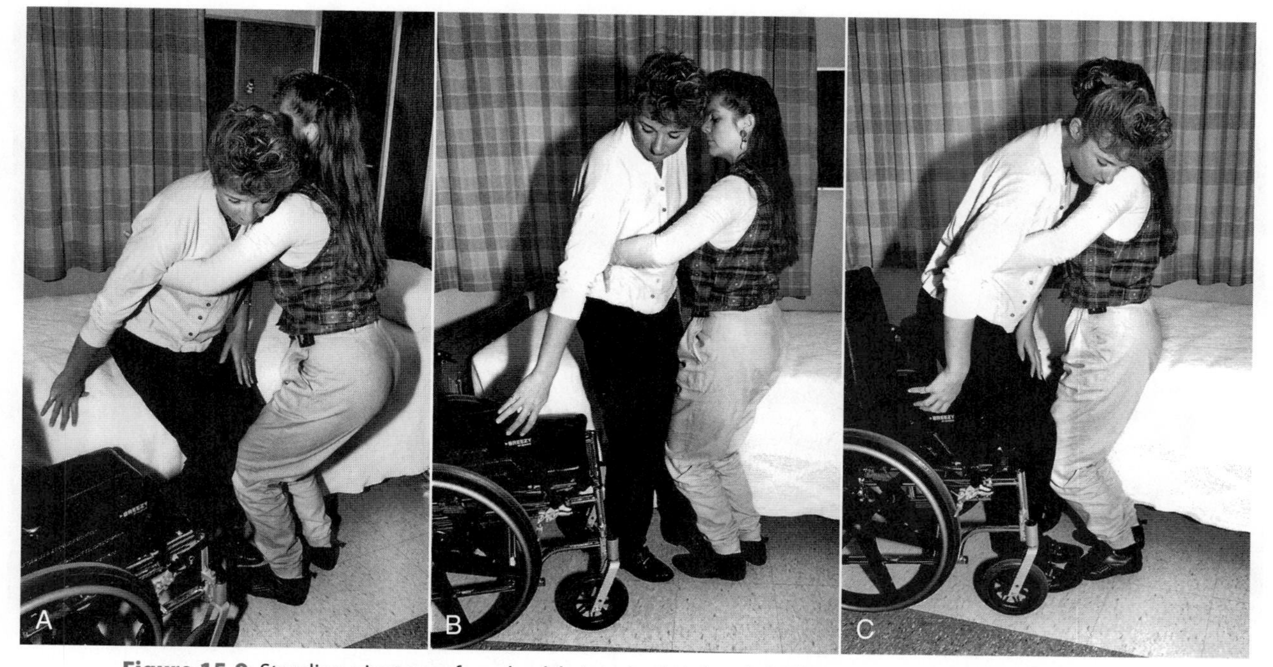

Figure 15-9 Standing pivot transfer; wheelchair to bed, assisted. **A,** Therapist stands on patient's affected side and stabilizes patient's foot and knee. She assists by guiding patient forward and initiates lifting buttocks up. **B,** Patient reaches toward transfer surface. **C,** Therapist guides the patient toward transfer surface. (Courtesy Luis Gonzalez, SCVMC.)

Stabilize the patient's foot and knee with your own foot and knee. Provide assistance by guiding the patient forward as the buttocks are lifted up and toward the transfer surface (Figure 15-9, *A*).
3. The patient either reaches toward the surface to which he or she is transferring or pushes off the surface from which he or she is transferring (Figure 15-9, *B*).
4. Guide the patient toward the transfer surface and gently help him or her down to a sitting position (Figure 15-9, *C*).

Variations: Stand Pivot and/or Stand/Step Transfer

A stand pivot and/or stand/step transfer is generally used when a patient can take small steps toward the surface goal and not just pivot toward the goal. The clinician's intervention may range from physical assistance to accommodate for potential loss of balance to facilitation of near normal movement, equal weight bearing, and maintenance of appropriate posture for patients with hemiplegia or hemiparesis. If a patient demonstrates impaired cognition or a behavior deficit including impulsiveness and poor safety judgment, the clinician may need to provide verbal cues or physical guidance.

Sliding Board Transfers

Sliding board transfers are best used with those who cannot bear weight on the lower extremities and who have paralysis, weakness, or poor endurance in their upper extremities. The patient who is going to assist the caregiver in this transfer should have good upper extremity strength. Sliding board transfer is most often employed with persons who have lower extremity amputations or individuals with spinal cord injuries.

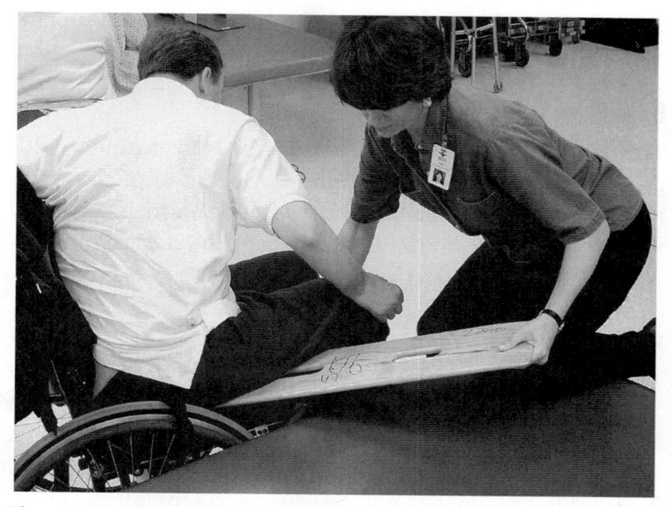

Figure 15-10 Positioning sliding board. Lift leg closest to transfer surface. Place board midthigh between buttocks and knee, angled toward opposite hip. (Courtesy Luis Gonzalez, SCVMC.)

Method

1. Position and set up the wheelchair as previously outlined.
2. Lift the leg closer to the transfer surface. Place the board midthigh between the buttocks and knee, angled toward the opposite hip. The board must be firmly under the thigh and firmly on the surface to which the patient is transferring (Figure 15-10).
3. Block the patient's knees with the practitioner's knees.
4. Instruct the patient to place one hand on the edge of the board and the other hand on the wheelchair seat.
5. Instruct the patient to lean forward.

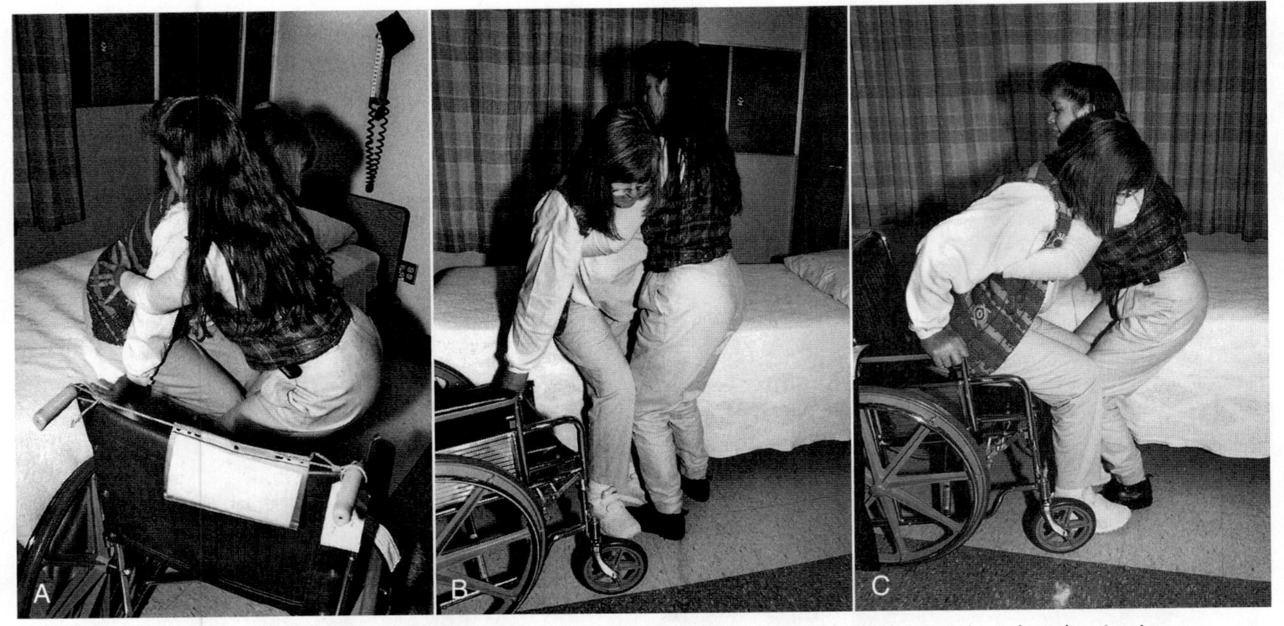

Figure 15-11 Bent pivot transfer; bed to wheelchair. **A,** Therapist grasps patient around trunk and assists in shifting patient's weight forward over feet. **B,** Patient reaches toward wheelchair. **C,** Therapist assists patient down toward sitting position. (Courtesy Luis Gonzalez, SCVMC.)

6. The patient should transfer his or her upper body weight in the direction opposite to which he or she is going. The patient uses both arms to lift or slide buttocks along the board.
7. Assist the patient where needed to shift weight and support the trunk while moving to the intended surface.

Bent Pivot Transfer: Bed to Wheelchair

The bent pivot transfer is used when the patient cannot initiate or maintain a standing position. A clinician often prefers to keep a patient in the bent knee position to maintain equal weight bearing, provide optimal trunk and lower extremity support, and perform a safer and easier clinician-assisted transfer.

Procedure

1. Assist the patient to scoot to the edge of the bed until both of the patient's feet are flat on the floor. Grasp the patient around the waist or hips or even under the buttocks if a moderate or maximal amount of assistance is required.
2. Assist the patient to align the trunk into a midline position.
3. Shift the weight forward from the buttocks toward and over the patient's feet (Figure 15-11, *A*).
4. Have the patient either reach toward the surface he or she is transferring to or push from the surface from which he or she is transferring (Figure 15-11, *B*).
5. Assist the patient by guiding and pivoting the patient around toward the transfer surface (Figure 15-11, *C*).

Depending on the amount of assistance required, the pivoting portion can be done in two or three steps, with the clinician repositioning himself or herself and the patient's lower extremities between steps. The clinician has a variety of choices of where to hold or grasp the patient during the bent pivot transfer, depending on the weight and height of the patient in relation to the clinician and the patient's ability to assist in the transfer. Variations include using both hands and arms at the waist, or trunk, or one or both hands under the buttocks. The clinician never grasps under the patient's weak arm or grasps the weak arm, an action that could cause significant injury because of weak musculature and poor stability around the shoulder girdle. The choice is made with consideration to proper body mechanics. Trial and error of technique is advised to allow for optimal facilitation of patient independence, safety, and the clinician's proper body mechanics.

Dependent Transfers

The dependent transfer is designed for use with the patient who has minimal to no functional ability. If this transfer is performed incorrectly, it is potentially hazardous for both clinician and patient. This transfer should be practiced with able-bodied persons and initially used with the patient only when another person is available to assist.[2]

The purpose of the dependent transfer is to move the patient from surface to surface. The requirements are that the patient be cooperative and willing to follow instructions. The clinician should be keenly aware of correct body mechanics, as well as his or her own physical limitations. With heavy patients, it is always best to use the two-person transfer or at least to have a second person available to spot the transfer.

One-Person Dependent Sliding Board Transfer

The procedure for transferring the patient from wheelchair to bed is the following:

1. Set up the wheelchair and bed as described previously.
2. Position the patient's feet together on the floor, directly under the knees, and swing the outside footrest away. Grasp the patient's legs from behind the knees, and pull the patient slightly forward in the wheelchair so that the buttocks will clear the big wheel when the transfer is made (Figure 15-12, *A*).

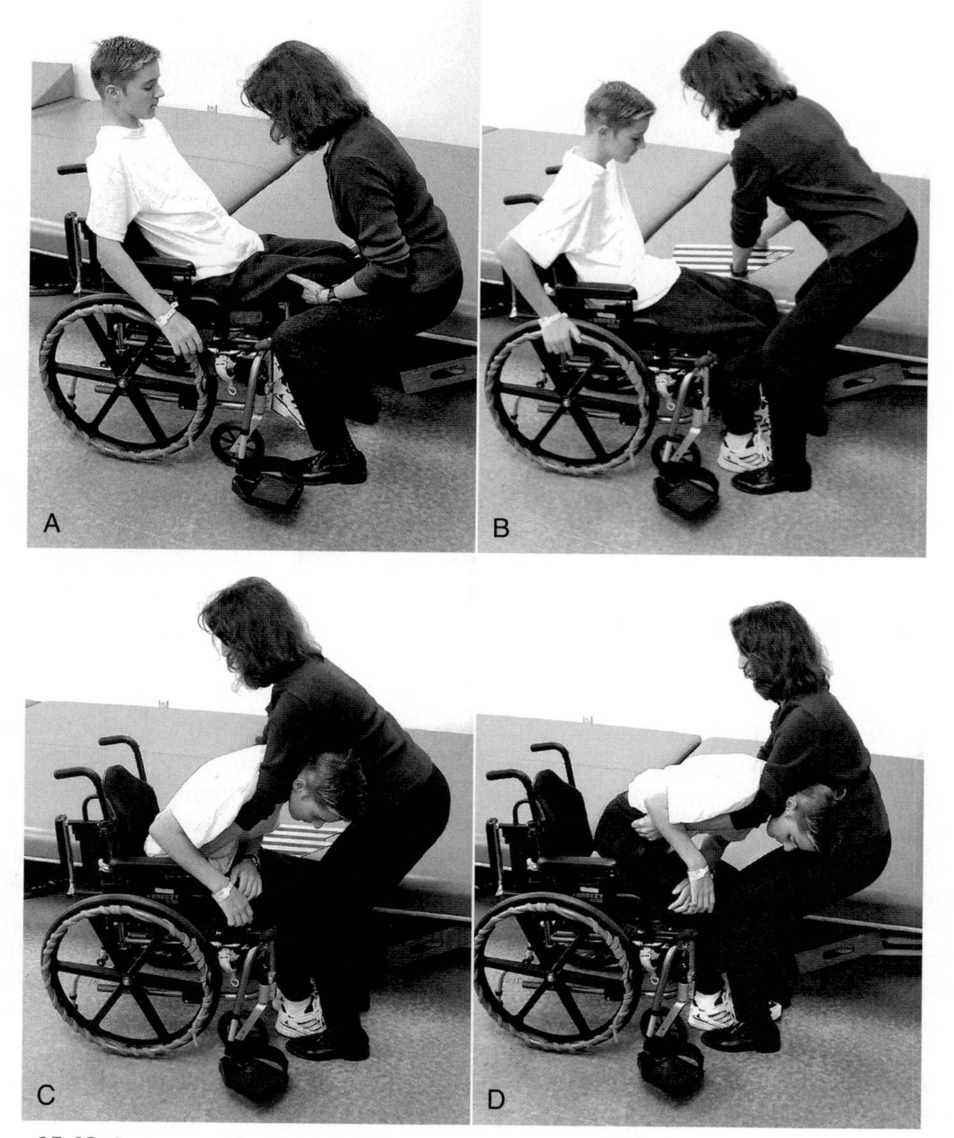

Figure 15-12 One-person dependent sliding board transfer. **A,** Therapist positions wheelchair and patient and pulls patient forward in chair. **B,** Therapist stabilizes patient's knees and feet after placing sliding board. **C,** Therapist grasps patient's pants at lowest point of buttocks. **D,** Therapist rocks with patient and shifts patient's weight over patient's feet, making sure patient's back remains straight.

3. Place a sliding board under the patient's inside thigh, midway between the buttocks and the knee, to form a bridge from the bed to the wheelchair. The sliding board is angled toward the patient's opposite hip.
4. Stabilize the patient's feet by placing your own feet laterally around the patient's feet.
5. Stabilize the patient's knees by placing your own knees firmly against the anterolateral aspect of the patient's knees (Figure 15-12, *B*).
6. Help the patient lean over the knees by pulling him or her forward from the shoulders. The patient's head and trunk should lean opposite the direction of the transfer. The patient's hands can rest on the lap.
7. Reach under the patient's outside arm and grasp the waistband of the trousers or under the buttock. On the other side, reach over the patient's back and grasp the waistband or under the buttock (Figure 15-12, *C*).
8. After your arms are positioned correctly, lock them to stabilize the patient's trunk. Keep your knees slightly bent and brace them firmly against the patient's knees.
9. Gently rock with the patient to gain some momentum, and prepare to move after the count of three. Count to three aloud, with the patient. On three, holding your knees tightly against the patient's knees, transfer the patient's weight over his or her feet. Keep your back straight to maintain good body mechanics (Figure 15-12, *D*).
10. Pivot with the patient and move him or her onto the sliding board (Figure 15-12, *E*). Reposition yourself and the patient's feet and repeat the pivot until the patient is firmly

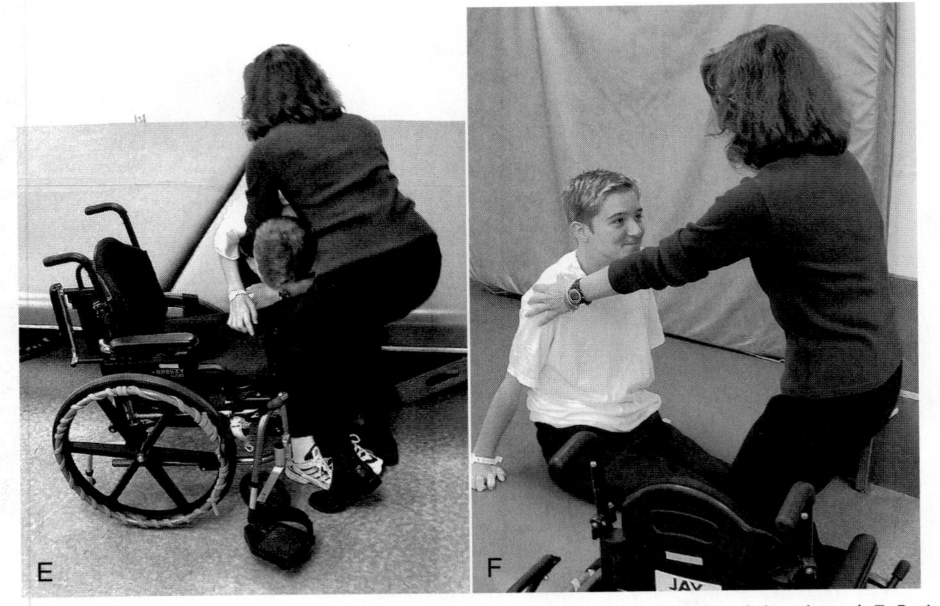

Figure 15-12, cont'd **E,** Therapist pivots with patient and moves patient onto sliding board. **F,** Patient is stabilized on bed. (Courtesy Luis Gonzales, SCVMC.)

seated on the bed surface, perpendicular to the edge of the mattress and as far back as possible. This step can usually be achieved in two or three stages (Figure 15-12, *F*).

11. Secure the patient on the bed by easing him or her against the back of an elevated bed or on the mattress in a side-lying position, then by lifting the legs onto the bed.
12. The one-person dependent sliding board transfer can be adapted to move the patient to other surfaces. It should be attempted only when clinician and patient feel secure with the wheelchair-to-bed transfer.

Two-Person Dependent Transfers

Bent Pivot: with or without a Sliding Board Bed to Wheelchair

A bent pivot transfer is used to allow increased clinician interaction and support. It allows the clinician greater control of the patient's trunk and buttocks during the transfer. This technique can also be employed during a two-person dependent transfer. It is often used with neurologically involved patients because trunk flexion and equal weight bearing are often desirable with this diagnosis. The steps in this two-person procedure are the following:

1. Set up the wheelchair and bed as described previously.
2. One clinician assumes a position in front of the patient and the other in back.
3. The clinician in front assists in walking the patient's hips forward until the feet are flat on the floor.
4. The same clinician stabilizes the patient's knees and feet by placing his or her knees and feet lateral to each of the patient's.
5. The clinician in back positions himself or herself squarely behind the patient's buttocks, grasping either the patient's waistband or the sides of the patient's pants, creating a slinging effect or placing his or her hands under the buttocks. Maintain proper body mechanics (Figure 15-13, *A*).
6. The clinician in front moves the patient's trunk into a midline position; grasps the patient around the back of the shoulders, waist, or hips; and guides the patient to lean forward and shift his or her weight forward, over the feet and off the buttocks. The patient's head and trunk should lean in the direction opposite the transfer. The patient's hands can rest on the lap (Figure 15-13, *B*).
7. As the clinician in front shifts the patient's weight forward, the clinician in back shifts the patient's buttocks in the direction of the transfer. This process can be done in two or three steps, making sure the patient's buttocks land on a safe, solid surface. The clinicians reposition themselves and the patient to maintain safe and proper body mechanics (Figure 15-13, *C*).
8. The clinicians should be sure they coordinate the time of the transfer with the patient and one another by counting to three aloud and instructing the team to initiate the transfer on three.
9. Transfer or gait belts may be employed to offer a place to grasp while one is assisting the patient in a transfer. The belt is placed securely around the waist and often used instead of the patient's waistband. The belt should not be allowed to slide up the patient's trunk.

Mechanical Lift Transfer

Some patients, because of body size, extent of disability, or the health and well-being of the caregiver, require the use of a mechanical lift. A variety of manual and electric lifting devices can be used to transfer patients of any weight (Figure 15-14). A properly trained caregiver, even one who is considerably smaller than the patient, can learn to use the mechanical lift safely and independently.[34] The patient's physical size, the environment in which the lift will be used, and the uses to which the lift will be put must be considered to order the appropriate

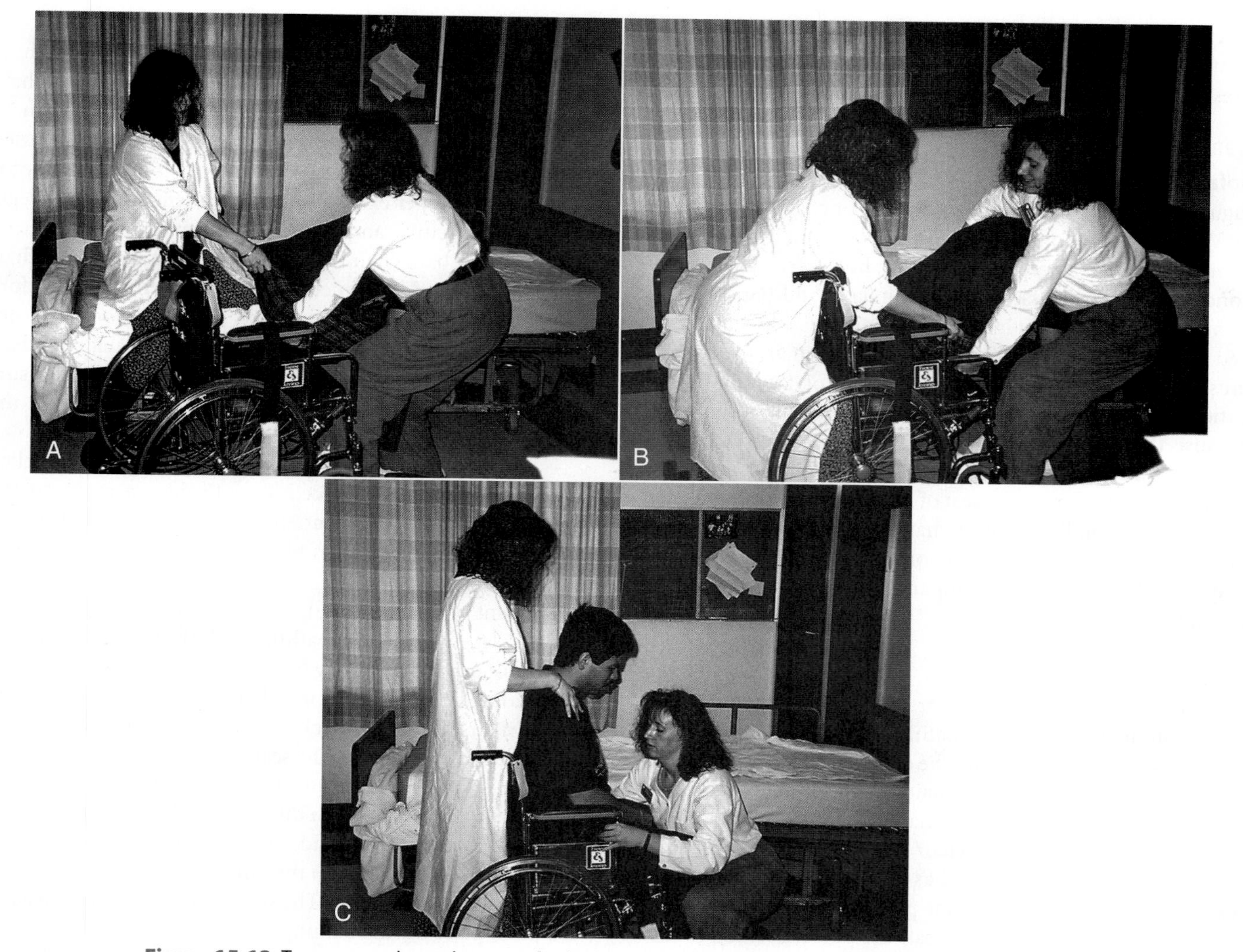

Figure 15-13 Two-person dependent transfer, bed to wheelchair. **A,** One therapist positions self in front of patient, blocking feet and knees. The therapist in back positions self behind patient's buttocks and assists by lifting. **B,** Person in front rocks patient forward and unweights buttocks as the back therapist shifts buttocks toward wheelchair. **C,** Both therapists position patient in upright, midline position in wheelchair. Seat belt is secured and positioning devices are added. (Courtesy Luis Gonzales, SCVMC.)

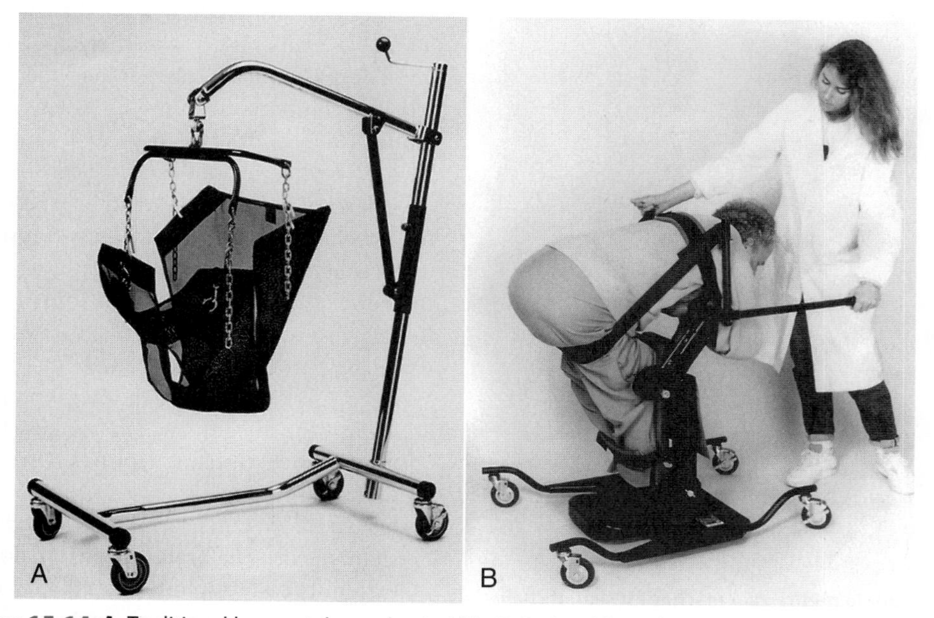

Figure 15-14 **A,** Traditional boom-style mechanical lift. **B,** Patient lift useful in transferring individuals with spinal cord injury. (**A** courtesy Trans-Aid Lifts, Sunrise Medical; **B** courtesy EZ-Pivot, Rand-Scott.)

mechanical lift. The patient and caregiver should demonstrate safe use of the lift to the clinician before the clinician prescribes it.

Transfers to Household Surfaces

Sofa or Chair

Figure 15-15 addresses transfers to sofas or chairs.

Wheelchair-to-sofa and wheelchair-to-chair transfers are similar to wheelchair-to-bed transfers; however, a few unique concerns should be assessed. The clinician and patient need to be aware that the chair may be light and not as stable as a bed or wheelchair. When transferring to the chair, the patient must be instructed to reach for the seat of the chair. The patient should not reach for the armrest or back of the chair because this action may cause the chair to tip over. When moving from a chair to the wheelchair, the patient should use a hand to push off from the seat of the chair as he or she comes to standing. Standing from a chair is often more difficult if the chair is low or the seat cushions are soft. Dense cushions may be added to increase height and provide a firm surface to which to transfer.

Toilet

In general, wheelchair-to-toilet transfers are difficult because of the confined space in most bathrooms and the inability and lack of support of a toilet seat. The clinician and patient should attempt to position the wheelchair next to or at an appropriate angle to the toilet. The clinician should analyze the space around the toilet and wheelchair to ensure no obstacles are present. Adaptive devices such as grab bars and raised toilet seats can be added to increase the patient's independence during this transfer. (Raised toilet seats are poorly secured to toilets and may be unsafe for some patients.) The patient can use these devices to support himself or herself during transfers and maintain a level surface to which to transfer.

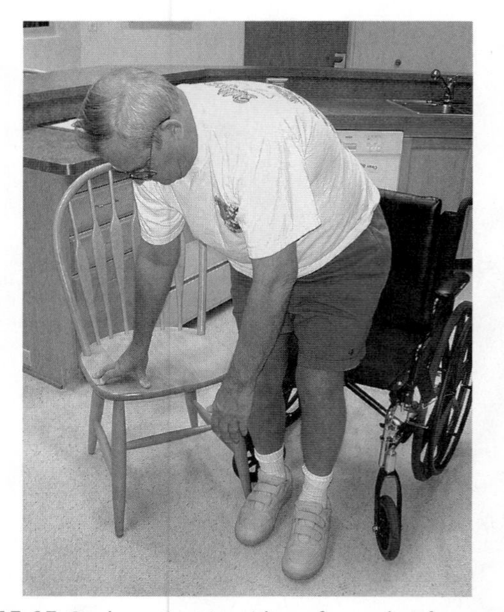

Figure 15-15 Stroke patient in midtransfer reaches for seat of chair, pivots, and lowers body to sitting. (Courtesy Luis Gonzales, SCVMC.)

Bathtub

The clinician should be cautious when assessing or teaching bathtub transfers because the bathtub is one of the most hazardous areas of the home. Transfers from the wheelchair to the bottom of the bathtub are extremely difficult and used only with patients who have good bilateral strength and motor control of the upper extremities (e.g., patients with paraplegia and lower extremity amputation). A commercially produced bath bench or bath chair or a well-secured straight-back chair is commonly used by clinicians for seated bathing. Therefore whether a standing pivot, bent pivot, or sliding board transfer is performed, the technique is similar to a wheelchair-to-chair transfer. However, the confined space, the slick bathtub surfaces, and the bathtub wall between the wheelchair and the bathtub seat may complicate the transfer.

If a standing pivot transfer is employed, the locked wheelchair should be placed at a 45-degree angle to the bathtub if possible. The patient should stand, pivot, sit on the bathtub chair, and then place the lower extremities into the bathtub.

If a bent pivot or sliding board transfer is used, the wheelchair is placed next to the bathtub with the armrest removed. The transfer tub bench may be used, which removes the need for a sliding board. This approach allows the wheelchair to be placed right next to the bench, thus allowing a safe and easy transfer of the buttocks to the seat.

If the transfer requires the assist of a caregiver, a transfer sling is an additional option during a "bare bottom" transfer. The cloth sling is placed under the patient's trochanters, and the sling handles are used in the same manner as grabbing the sides of the patient's pants. The sling can either be removed or remain in place during bathing.

The patient may exit by first placing one foot securely outside the bathtub on a nonskid floor surface and then performing a standing or seated transfer back to the wheelchair.

Car Transfers

A car transfer is often the most challenging for clinicians because it involves trial-and-error methods to develop a technique that is not only safe but also easy for the patient and caregiver to carry out. The clinician often uses the patient's existing transfer technique. The patient's size, degree of disability, and vehicle style (two-door vs. four-door) must be considered. These factors will affect level of independence and may necessitate a change in the usual technique to allow a safe, easy transfer.

In general, it is difficult to get a wheelchair close enough to the car seat, especially with four-door vehicles. The following are some additional considerations when making wheelchair-to-car transfers:

1. Car seats are often much lower than the standard wheelchair seat height, which makes the uneven transfer much more difficult, especially from the car seat to the wheelchair.
2. Occasionally, patients have orthopedic injuries that necessitate the use of a brace such as a halo body jacket or lower extremity cast or splint. The clinician often must alter technique to accommodate these devices.

3. The clinician may suggest use of an extra long sliding board for this transfer, to compensate for the large gap between transfer surfaces.
4. Because uphill transfers are difficult and the level of assistance may increase for this transfer, the clinician may choose a two-person assist instead of a one-person assist transfer to ensure a safe and smooth technique.

Summary

A wheelchair that fits well and can be managed safely and easily by its user and caregiver is one of the most important factors in the patient's ability to perform ADL with maximal independence.[7] Wheelchair users must learn the capabilities and limitations of the wheelchair and safe methods of performing all self-care and mobility skills. If there is a caregiver, he or she needs to be thoroughly familiar with safe and correct techniques of handling the wheelchair, positioning equipment, and the patient.

Transfer skills are among the most important activities that the wheelchair user must master. The ability to transfer increases the possibility of mobility and travel. However, transfers can be hazardous. Safe methods must be learned and followed.[34] Several basic transfer techniques are outlined in this chapter. Additional methods and more detailed training and instructions are available, as cited previously.

It should be recognized that many wheelchair users with exceptional abilities have developed unique methods of wheelchair management. Although such innovative approaches may work well for the person who has devised and mastered them, they cannot be considered basic procedures that everyone can learn.[34]

SECTION III IMPORTANCE OF DRIVING AND COMMUNITY MOBILITY

Miriam Monahan

Driving and community mobility are key IADL that play a pivotal role in community independence and social interactions. A driver's license symbolizes a rite of passage to adulthood for the teenager. Driving is the primary means of transportation in any area that lacks or has only limited mass transit options. Most adults rely on driving to access employment, medical care, and leisure activities; maintain relationships with friends and family; and carry out responsibilities such as shopping and transporting others. The ability to drive is instrumental in obtaining and maintaining an independent lifestyle. Depending on the client and his or her living environment, public transportation and walking may be just as critical to accessing the community as driving is in another environment. Community mobility can include walking, biking, using a scooter or wheelchair in the community, and riding as a passenger in a motor vehicle or on mass transit. Occupational therapists and OTAs address driving and other aspects of community mobility with clients of all ages.[5] OTs' and OTAs' interventions may include addressing their client's ability to be safe as a pedestrian or cyclist. Interventions may include addressing their client's ability to safely access mass transportation or ride as a passenger in a motor vehicle. Interventions may include addressing the needs of clients who are first-time drivers with special needs or experienced drivers after an injury or illness.[5]

Occupational Therapy and Driving

Driving requires continuous integration of visual, perceptual, cognitive, and motor skills. For example, every action a driver takes begins with searching the environment for critical information while ignoring unnecessary information, processing what is seen, making a decision, making a plan to respond, and then physically reacting to the situation, all in a timely manner. A complex task, driving carries more risk of harm than most other IADL or ADL. Consequently, evaluation of the ability to drive is critical for individuals whose medical condition or disability may impair any of the skills involved. All OT practitioners have the expertise to address driving as an IADL.[5] In this capacity OT practitioners can identify patients or clients who may be at risk if they begin to learn to drive, resume driving, or continue to drive. Where concerns exist, the OT practitioner can refer the patient to an OT practitioner (either a therapist or an assistant) who specializes in driver rehabilitation. These practitioners typically work within a driver rehabilitation program. They often have additional training to be a driving school instructor or work with a driving school instructor. In addition, these practitioners often have specialized training to address the specific needs of drivers. For example, they may provide low-vision driver training techniques, prescribe adaptive equipment, teach a driver to use adaptive driving equipment, and be able to identify strategies to compensate for cognitive limitations in the driving task. The driver rehabilitation program can be a resource to identify whether a person is appropriate to learn to drive, resume driving, or should stop driving. The occupational therapist is responsible for the overall driving evaluation but may delegate specific assessments and aspects of the treatment plan to the OTA.

Driving across the Span of OT Practice

Driving assessment and intervention are relevant across all practice areas in OT. All OT practitioners should consider assessing driving when assessing other activities of daily living. The occupational therapist should decide whether the patient's need can be managed within their expertise or whether the need requires the intervention of an OT specializing in driving. Occupational therapists and OTAs working in the school system with students with learning disabilities can begin addressing pre-driving skills. Pre-driving skills include community independence such as crossing streets, financial management, and appropriate social interactions. Children who use wheelchairs may require OT services to address safe transfers and vehicle transportation options. When these students approach driving age the student and family may need resources for a driver rehabilitation program. The patient seen primarily for hand therapy who is using a splint or sling needs

OT to address how to steer safely, use a turn signal, or turn on the defrost control. The OT practitioner involved in work hardening may need to address seating and positioning in the car for the chronic back pain patient. The OT practitioner practicing in geriatrics often addresses whether it is safe for a client to continue current driving patterns. The practitioner working in adult rehabilitation with patients who have had strokes, spinal cord injuries, or traumatic brain injuries must identify when a referral to driver rehabilitation services is appropriate. Those working in adult rehabilitation may be working with patients with progressive neurological conditions such as lower extremity neuropathy, muscular dystrophy, multiple sclerosis, and Parkinson's disease. These patients may be able to maintain driving with modifications or may require counseling for driving cessation and alternative transportation. The practitioner would identify when a referral to driver rehabilitation is appropriate. The occupational therapist and OTA working in these practice areas do not need to be driving experts but should be knowledgeable about when to refer a client to a driver rehabilitation program. All OT practitioners should recognize driving as a critical IADL.

Purpose of the Driving Evaluation

An individual entering a driving rehabilitation program for the first time is initially seen for an evaluation to help establish a baseline of skills and appropriate goals. The outcome of the evaluation might be that:

- The individual is safe to drive without further intervention
- The individual needs further driver rehabilitation services in order to be safe to drive
- The individual is unsafe to continue driving and would not benefit from further driver rehabilitation

OT must address alternative transportation holistically when driving cessation is recommended, as discussed later in the chapter. If the individual requires further driver rehabilitation services in order to be safe to drive, driving skills may be retrained in the car or in the clinic. Interventions may address areas of cognitive, visual, visual-perceptual, and/or motor skills. Driver evaluations may form the basis for a plan of care to address driver training with adaptive equipment and may serve as a template for identifying vehicle modifications when appropriate.

Candidates for Driving Assessment

Health care professionals including physicians, therapists, and case managers play an important role in identifying individuals who require a driver evaluation. In December 1999 the American Medical Association made the following statement to physicians on impaired drivers: "Physicians have an ethical responsibility to assess patients' physical or mental impairments that might adversely affect driving abilities. A physician may suggest that the individual seek further assessments and evaluation in occupational therapy."[3] Driver rehabilitation services are generally not covered by insurance plans. By thoroughly screening referrals for appropriateness, therapists conserve patient resources and provide cost-effective treatment. For example, a patient with a cognitive impairment who is unsafe in the kitchen or in managing his medications or basic finances would not be a good candidate to return to driving until assessed as independent in these skill areas. In order to drive, a person must have the cognitive skills to be safe at home and in the community. Vision skills must meet the state's licensing requirements before the client can be referred to a driver rehabilitation program. A referral to a qualified driver evaluation program should be considered if any of the following conditions arise and the OT practitioner feels the person's cognitive skills may be at an appropriate level for driving:

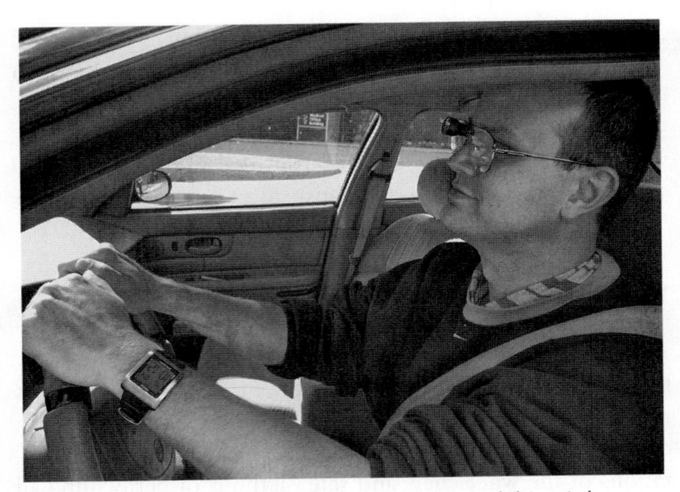

Figure 15-16 Driver with low vision driving with bioptic lenses.

1. The patient, family, or health care professional expresses concerns about the driver's safety or competence.
2. The patient has limitations that preclude use of the standard driving pattern of two-handed steering and right foot on the gas and brake.
3. The patient has a neurologic condition (e.g., traumatic brain injury, cerebrovascular accident, peripheral neuropathy, Parkinson's disease, dementia, multiple sclerosis, muscular dystrophy, polio).
4. The patient has impaired or low vision but meets the vision requirements for licensing in the state of residence. A variety of lenses that enable driving for persons with low vision (Figure 15-16) are available.
5. The patient is a student with learning impairments or physical disabilities (e.g., cerebral palsy, spina bifida, attention deficit disorder, autism spectrum disorder).

Driving Evaluation

Driver rehabilitation programs vary greatly in the types of services offered. Some programs offer clinical evaluations or simulator road tests. These programs are valuable in general problem identification, but research shows that performance during simulations does not predict road performance. A comprehensive driver evaluation program includes both a clinical and a driving component in a special evaluation vehicle.[16,17,19]

One of the important elements of a driving evaluation is direct observation of driving behavior. A driver who tailgates and speeds will be at a much greater risk than the individual who keeps a large following distance and stays at or below the speed limit. With a mild delay in cognitive processing speed, the risk as a tailgater or a speeder is magnified. What may seem insignificant in the clinic may actually take on large significance on the road because of driving behaviors. Conversely, what may seem to be a significant deficit in the clinic may be a minimal factor behind the wheel when a person has conservative driving behaviors. In general people are not good critics of their own driving behaviors, and therefore self-report is not always reliable.

Clinical Evaluation

The clinical evaluation, also referred to as a *prescreening evaluation* or *pre-driving evaluation,* aims to identify strengths and problem areas related to driving. This evaluation is conducted by the occupational therapist, who may delegate assessments to the OTA. The clinical evaluation begins with a review of medical information such as medical history, vision history, medication and side effects, episodes of seizure, or loss of consciousness. An interview concerning ADLs and IADLs is conducted to determine routines, supports, and independence levels at home and in the community. The interview should include driving history of crashes, violations, and license restrictions, as well as driving goals and routine driving environments. Driving environment includes questions such as (1) does the driver plan to drive in city traffic or only in a small local community? and (2) does the driver restrict driving to daytime hours and familiar routes?

Vision Screening

A comprehensive vision assessment includes acuity, ocular-motor skills, peripheral fields, and depth perception. Standards for distance acuity and peripheral field vary by state jurisdiction. Comprehensive vision screening is important because vision is the primary sense used to gather information required for driving-related decision making (see Chapter 22).

Motor and Sensory

Muscle strength, active range of motion (ROM), grip, and right foot reaction time are often cited as the basic required measurements.[11,13,16,24,30] In addition, muscle tone, dynamic sitting and standing balance, transfer status, ambulation status, type of ambulation device, and endurance are also important components to the evaluation.[27] Sensory awareness of the right lower extremity is critical, and for the upper extremities it is also important. Awareness of light touch, deep pressure, kinesthesia, and proprioception are critical for the right lower extremity to locate the pedals and apply appropriate pressure. Our upper extremities use sensory abilities to locate and operate the turn signals, air controls, and wipers/washer fluid controls while keeping our eyes on the road. Coordination is also important in order to control the steering wheel and move the foot accurately between the pedals. In addition, coordination is important for manipulation of other controls such as levers, dials, gear selectors, and seatbelt.[27] During the assessment of physical/sensory measurements, the evaluator should determine what equipment or modifications, if any, should be used during the road evaluation. Sensory and physical deficits may indicate the need for adaptive equipment. However, given intact cognitive skills, many persons with motor impairments can drive successfully with adaptive equipment (Figure 15-17).

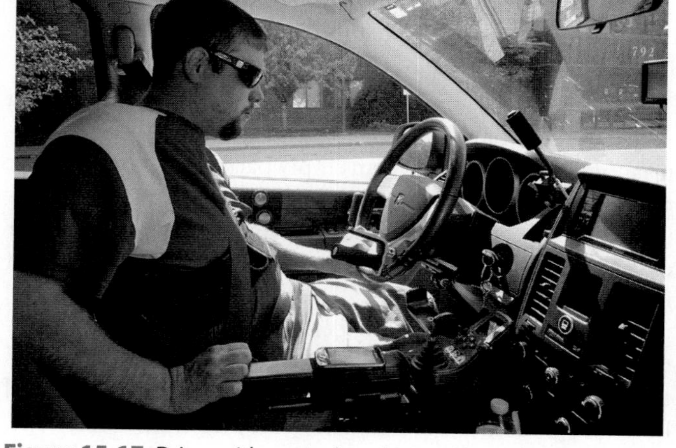

Figure 15-17 Driver with a spinal cord injury driving while seated in a wheelchair in a modified van.

Cognitive and Visual-Perceptual Skills

Driving requires adequate reliable perception of a rapidly changing environment, blending both cognitive and visual-perceptual skills. Specific mental functions that require assessment include processing speed, selective and divided attention, attention shift, problem solving, judgment, auditory and visual memory,[27] and, most importantly, self-awareness of how the disability affects the individual's driving skills. Visual perception determines how the driver interprets what he or she sees in the driving environment. Components of visual perception include visual organization, visual search and scanning, spatial relations, and visual processing speed.[13,16,19,24,30] Standardized tests that assess these skills and that have been studied for their correlation to driving performance are available. These tests should be used whenever possible to identify the driver's abilities.

Road Evaluation

Most driver rehabilitation programs use an evaluation vehicle. The vehicle may be a car or a specialized van. The vehicle is equipped with an instructor's brake and rearview mirror for the evaluator, similar to a driver education vehicle. Any adaptive equipment recommended in the clinical evaluation should be available in the evaluation vehicle.

Pre-driving Tasks

Pre-driving tasks include mobility to the vehicle, inserting and turning a key (or keyless entry operation), opening and closing the door, entering and exiting the vehicle, loading and unloading mobility devices (cane, walker, wheelchair), adjusting the driver seat, adjusting the mirrors, and fastening the seat belt.

Patients with physical, visual, or mental function limitations may have difficulty with some aspects of the pre-driving task.

Route Planning and Road Evaluation

The route for the driving evaluation is critical for assessing specific skills. A new driver should be evaluated in an appropriate environment such as an empty parking lot or low-traffic residential setting. Emphasis should be placed on maneuvering the vehicle for braking, accelerating, and turning. A driver education background or the assistance of a driver educator is helpful.

The environment for an experienced driver learning adaptive equipment should be similar to that for a new driver and should address the same skills. The experienced driver will likely progress more quickly into complex traffic situations. For example, an individual with paraplegia driving with hand controls to operate the accelerator and brake will need to master the controls in a controlled or low-traffic driving environment before progressing to more complex traffic. The patient who has had a stroke or traumatic brain injury and who is learning to drive with a steering device or a left foot accelerator (allows the driver to use their left foot to control the accelerator) should always begin in low-traffic environments. Eventually, such patients must be evaluated in a traffic environment that will test any cognitive and visual-perceptual deficits; this testing should include complex environments that require rapid visual scanning, quick decisions, visual perception, and divided attention.

An individual with memory deficits should be evaluated in *familiar* areas where they can be challenged with trip planning. For example, the OT practitioner may ask the driver to travel to three routine destinations such as the client's grocery store, post office, and church. Recalling of the driving route and destinations can distract an individual with memory deficits from the driving task, causing him or her to make a driving error. If the evaluator compensates by providing directions (such as "turn right at the next block"), getting an accurate assessment of the person's memory skills for driving is impossible. For individuals with memory deficits, the role of driver rehabilitation is often to identify when an individual needs to stop driving.

The older driver or any driver who limits driving to a few destinations in his or her local area may be appropriate to evaluate from home to these destinations. This concept of modifying the driving environment for the road assessment is similar to that used in cooking. If the individual prepares only microwave meals, the therapist would not ask him to cook a Thanksgiving dinner as part of the evaluation. However, making certain the driver has the ability to manage detours and other unexpected driving situations is necessary even in a limited driving environment. Skills assessed in the road evaluation are shown in Box 15-3.

Box 15-3

Skills Assessed in Road Evaluations

1. Maneuvering the vehicle
   - Acceleration and braking
   - Turning
   - Speed control
   - Lane changes
   - Parking and backing
2. Skills at varying types of intersections and driving environments
   - Rural roads
   - Parking lots
   - Residential
   - Business traffic
   - Interstate
3. Executive functions
   - Route planning
   - Decision and problem solving
   - Judgment and insight

Interpretation of the Evaluation

The clinical evaluation helps to identify which deficits are affecting the driving performance. For example, missing a red light may result from decreased speed of the right foot moving between the gas and brake or from problems in visual scanning or cognitive processing speed. Rehabilitation approach and potential will vary depending on the deficit and the severity.

Careful evaluation of the benefit of recommended adaptive equipment used during the evaluation is critical for individuals who require modifications. The equipment can be costly and is often paid for out of pocket. Further evaluation and training may be necessary before any final recommendations are made.

As a result of the evaluation, the occupational therapist can recommend that the patient do the following:

1. Resume driving
2. Discontinue driving
3. Receive driving rehabilitation services before returning to drive

Rehabilitation

Rehabilitation of driving skills can take many forms and may occur in the clinic or while driving. The occupational therapist may delegate the rehabilitation to the OTA, a driving school instructor, or family members. Toglia identifies three areas that rehabilitation can address: the *person*, the *environment*, and the *task*.[15,30]

A *person* may be able to learn strategies to compensate for deficits or to improve visual skills, specific mental functions, or physical abilities. For example, the individual with disorganized visual scanning may be instructed on new search patterns while driving, riding as a passenger, or using tools such as a visual scanning board in the clinic. Driving simulators or computerized programs can be appropriate in some cases to develop cognitive and visual skills for driving.

The driving *environment* may need to be adjusted. For example, the elderly individual with decreased cognitive processing speed may benefit from limitations on driving conditions such as confining driving to daytime hours, avoiding rush hours, or revising driving routes to avoid complex intersections.

The driving *task* can be altered to make it simpler by adding a spinner knob for the individual with an upper extremity deficit or installing blind spot and rear view convex mirrors for the individual with limited neck rotation. Adaptive equipment such as hand controls, reduced effort steering, and electronic gas/brake systems may be recommended to reduce the physical demands of driving. The person should be trained with the adaptive equipment in a variety of traffic conditions.

Driving Cessation

Anyone practicing in the area of driver rehabilitation will at one time or another need to recommend driving cessation. It is critical that the therapist and assistant attend to the emotional impact on the individual who can no longer drive. Be aware that some individuals may threaten suicide. Having medical supports and community resources in place is critical. Working closely with the individual's physicians, other medical professionals, and family can help ease the transition. Driving is the link to many other roles and to community participation. OT practitioners should address plans for alternative transportation so that the individual can maintain as many community roles as possible. If a transition plan is not provided and implemented, isolation and depression often follow.

Studies have shown that many older Americans who do not drive stay home because transportation options are lacking. As a group they are less likely to use alternatives to the automobile.[17,28] Most rely on family and friends for transportation[16,29] and in doing so experience feelings of indebtedness that become burdensome and demeaning.[11,18] Resources such as the Area Agency on Aging (AAA) can provide information on transportation alternatives.

Modes of Community Mobility

Community mobility is defined by the *Occupational Therapy Practice Framework, 2nd ed,* as "moving [oneself] in the community and using private or public transportation."[4,15] Community mobility may be achieved by driving or using the bus, train, subway, taxi, volunteer drivers, friends, family, and special paratransit services. A holistic approach is crucial for addressing community mobility. This includes assessment of the individual's goals, his or her purposes for community access, and the individual's performance skills. Knowledge of transportation options for each locality as well as funding sources available to clients is necessary.

Task Demands

Environments

Urban areas often offer public transit systems by bus, rail, or both. However, many people live outside these areas.

In rural areas of the country, nondrivers have limited options for transportation. They depend on family and friends. Those who are physically capable may ride a bicycle or walk. In many areas of the country community transportation agencies offer door-to-door service for medical appointments. Walking can be an option but is not an appropriate mode of community transportation for everyone. One in three older nondrivers walks on a given day in denser areas, as compared with 1 in 14 in more spread-out areas.[3,7] Inclement weather affects conditions for walking.

Motor

Motor demands in the community may challenge endurance, functional balance, and use of a mobility device in public settings. For example, the individual may need to be assessed for the ability to climb the stairs of a bus. Poor sidewalk conditions or hills or wet or icy conditions may challenge an individual's balance for walking or may prevent efficient and effective propelling of a manual wheelchair. Assessment of vehicle transfers may be necessary. For the individual who requires physical assistance, the caregiver and the client need training together with the vehicle. Loading and unloading of the walker or wheelchair will also need to be addressed.

Mental Function

Mental function demands in community mobility are varied. Examples may include navigation, safety in public settings, and use of public transit systems. For example, an individual may have difficulty interpreting a bus system schedule. The individual with limited social skills may not know how to address strangers on the bus route. Individuals with cognitive limitations may need to develop the skills for arranging rides from volunteer drivers and taxi services. Other relevant tasks that may be limited due to cognitive impairments include time management, financial management, and trip planning.

Visual Functions

Vision limitations can affect individuals in a number of different ways. The individual with low acuity may find reading a bus schedule or a bus route sign challenging. The individual with a visual field cut walking in a parking lot may not be aware of cars backing up. An individual with visual-motor deficits may find it challenging to scan the environment accurately and efficiently to cross the street.

Intervention

Mass Transit

In urban areas the OTA can provide bus (or subway) training to assist the individual to develop the cognitive skills for using the transit system. The following progression could be used for a client with a learning disability, brain injury, or stroke who may otherwise have the capabilities to use mass transit.

- Stage 1 focuses on comprehension of the task. This involves working with the individual to read and understand the system schedule. To build skills gradually, the OTA would ask the individual to plan a route to get to a destination that does not involve transfers to another bus or subway line.
- Stage 2 consists of close supervision while the person performs the task. For example, this may mean riding with the individual in the same seat to accustom him or her to the idea of paying the fare, talking to the bus driver, or reading the schedule to ensure that the right train or bus is taken.

- Stage 3 provides distant supervision to ensure independence in the task. The OTA would ride with the individual but not next to him or her. This allows the OTA to observe whether the individual can carry out the steps in stage 1 and 2 without support.
- Stage 4 provides supervision at a further remove. For example, the OTA might follow in a car behind a bus or in the next train car if the individual is traveling by train. The goal in stage 4 is to be out of sight but available to "rescue" the client, if need be. If the individual can plan the route, manage the time responsibilities, and address the financial aspects, he or she may have reached independence in a simple route.

When the task is completed successfully to stage 4, increased complexity (i.e., bus or train transfers) can be added. Depending on the individual's skills and deficits, training for increased complexity may start at stage 1; for the more capable client, stage 3 may be an appropriate place to begin.

Transportation as a Passenger

The OTA can educate the caregiver who is providing transportation. Proper body mechanics, communication techniques to prevent agitation, and assistive devices are a few of the areas that can be taught.[24] Another role for OT professionals is to identify appropriate candidates for paratransit services.[26] Typically, these services provide wheelchair-accessible vehicles for those who cannot ride regular public transportation.

Pedestrian Safety

A pedestrian must habitually exercise a wide range of skills. In addition to the motor and visual components, the pedestrian uses topographical orientation, abstract thinking, problem solving, and reasoning skills to move in various environments. Once an occupational therapist has completed the evaluation of pedestrian safety, an OTA can train an individual with cognitive deficits to cross the street and ambulate safely in the community. If the individual has visual or motor limitations, additional training techniques would be necessary. For example, the individual may require techniques to move a mobility device such as a walker or wheelchair safely in the community. For the individual with a vision impairment, techniques in visual scanning may be necessary.

Box 15-4

Additional Resources

Websites for Pertinent Associations

AAA Foundation for Traffic Safety
Publishers of consumer pamphlets and products
http://www.aaafts.org

ADED, the Association for Driver Rehabilitation Specialists
CDRS information, disability fact sheets, bulletin board for driver evaluators
http://www.driver-ed.org

American Association of Retired Persons
Information and publication on older driver issues
http://www.aarp.org

National Mobility Equipment Dealers Association
Product manufacturers and equipment installers
http://www.nmeda.org

National Highway Traffic Safety Administration
Airbag on-off switch and consumer information
http://www.nhtsa.dot.gov

Summary

Driving and community mobility is essential for fulfilling many areas of human occupation: education, work, leisure, and social participation. The occupational therapist and OTA must consider the individual's community mobility needs in the context of desired occupations and desired participation.

All OT practitioners can address driving and/or community across all practice areas. The OT practitioner may identify when a person has developed appropriate skills for driving and refer him or her to an OT driver rehabilitation program. The OT practitioner may identify deficits in performance skills that may affect driving when evaluating an individual and make a referral to driver rehabilitation. Occupational therapists practicing outside of driver rehabilitation may need to advise the patient, physician, and family members that the patient should not drive if the practitioner identifies severe performance skills impairments that are not appropriate for rehabilitation.

In the United States the automobile has become the primary mode of community mobility. Driving is the IADL most likely to affect the safety of other people. All health care professionals need to anticipate which patients or clients may be at risk. The medical community views OT as a key resource for information and evaluation. The American Occupational Therapy Association (AOTA) has helpful information regarding community mobility and driving safety for the generalist OT and the OT specializing in driving and community mobility. Additional resources are offered through a number of organizations (Box 15-4).

Community mobility can be achieved by a variety of means, by walking or using public or private transportation. The individual's performance skills, goals for accessing the community, and community resources are important considerations when addressing community mobility. The OT practitioner can help identify the appropriate means for community mobility and provide a rehabilitation approach to help individuals reach a level of independence for routine and novel transportation situations.

Selected Reading Guide Questions

1. Define functional ambulation.
2. List three ADL or IADL in which functional ambulation may occur.
3. Who provides gait training?

4. What is the role of the OT practitioner in functional ambulation?
5. How do the OT and physical therapy practitioners collaborate in functional ambulation?
6. List and describe safety issues for functional ambulation.
7. Name five basic ambulation aids in order of most supportive to least supportive.
8. Discuss why great care should be taken during functional ambulation within the bathroom.
9. List at least three diagnoses for which functional ambulation may be appropriate as part of OT services.
10. What purpose does a task analysis serve in preparation for functional ambulation?
11. What suggestions could be made regarding carrying items during functional ambulation when an ambulation aid is used?
12. What is the objective in measuring seat width?
13. What is the danger of having a wheelchair seat that is too deep?
14. What is the minimal distance for safety from the floor to the bottom of the wheelchair step plate?
15. List three types of wheelchair frames and the general uses of each.
16. Describe three types of wheelchair propulsion systems and tell when each would be used.
17. What are the advantages of detachable desk arms and swing-away footrests?
18. Discuss the factors for consideration before wheelchair selection.
19. Name and discuss the rationale for at least three general wheelchair safety principles.
20. Describe or demonstrate how to descend a curb in a wheelchair with the help of an assistant.
21. Describe or demonstrate how to descend a ramp in a wheelchair with the help of an assistant.
22. List four safety principles for correct moving and lifting technique during wheelchair transfers.
23. Describe or demonstrate the basic standing-pivot transfer from a bed to a wheelchair.
24. Describe or demonstrate the wheelchair-to-bed transfer, using a sliding board.
25. Describe the correct placement of a sliding board before a transfer.
26. In what circumstances would a sliding board transfer technique be used?
27. List the requirements for patient and clinician to perform the dependent transfer safely and correctly.
28. List two potential problems and solutions that can occur with the wheelchair-to-car transfer.
29. When is the mechanical lift transfer most appropriate?
30. Explain why driving is an important activity.
31. Describe some of the skills assessed during the driving evaluation.
32. What is meant by a pre-driving task? Give some examples.
33. Describe examples of community mobility.
34. What are some of the cognitive skills used in driving?
35. What are some of the physical skills used in driving?
36. Select a practice area of OT and a typical patient condition seen in that area, and describe how driving may be negatively affected by the condition.

References

1. Adler C: *Wheelchairs and seat cushions: a comprehensive guide for evaluation and ordering*, San Jose, Calif, 1987, Santa Clara Valley Medical Center, Occupational Therapy Department.
2. Adler C, Musik D, Tipton-Burton M: *Body mechanics and transfers: multidisciplinary cross-training manual*, San Jose, Calif, 1994, Santa Clara Valley Medical Center.
3. American Medical Association and the National Highway Traffic Safety Administration: *Physician's guide to assessing and counseling older drivers*, Chicago, 2003, American Medical Association.
4. American Occupational Therapy Association: *Occupational therapy practice framework: domain and process*, ed 2, Bethesda, Md, 2008, the Association.
5. American Occupational Therapy Association: Statements driving and community mobility, *Am J Occup Ther* 59(6):666–669, 2005.
6. Anderson KN, Anderson LE, Glanze WD, editors: *Mosby's medical, nursing and allied health dictionary*, ed 6, St. Louis, 2002, Mosby.
7. Bailey L: *Aging Americans: stranded without options, executive summary*, Surface Transportation Policy Project, 2004, Washington DC. www.transact.org.
8. Berner TF: Overview of manual wheelchairs and what to consider when making seating and positioning selections, *OT Pract* 12(19):CE1–CE8, 2007.
9. Breske S: The drive for independence, *Rehabilitation* 3:11–16, 1994.
10. Bromley I: *Tetraplegia and paraplegia: a guide for physiotherapists*, ed 3, London, 1985, Churchill Livingstone.
11. Carp FM: Retired people as automobile passengers, *Gerontologist* 12:73–78, 1972. Cited in Kostyniuk LP, Shope JT: Driving and alternatives: older drivers in Michigan, *J Safety Res* 34(4):407–414, 2003.
12. Center for Medicare & Medicaid Services: *Clinical criteria for MAE coverage*, Baltimore, Md, 2010, Author. Retrieved June 1, 2011 from http://www.cms.gov/CoverageGenInfo/Downloads/MAEAlgorithm.pdf. 2010-09-07.
13. Seals Easter: *Transportation solutions for caregivers: a starting point*, www.easterseals.com/transportation.
14. Esquenazi A, Hirai B: Gait analysis in stroke and head injury. In Craik RL, Oatis CA, editors: *Gait analysis: theory and application*, St. Louis, 1995, Mosby.
15. Gourley M: OT assessments save thousands for paratransit service, *OT Pract* 5(23):11, 2000.
16. Kostyniuk LP, Shope JT: *Reduction and cessation of driving among older drivers: focus groups* (Rep. No. UMTRI-98-26). Ann Arbor MI, 1998, The University of Michigan Transportation Research Institute. Cited in Kostyniuk LP, Shope JT: Driving and alternatives: older drivers in Michigan. *J Safety* Res 34(4):407–414, 2003.
17. Kostyniuk LP, Shope JT: Driving and alternatives: older drivers in Michigan, *J Safety Res* 34(4):407–414, 2003.
18. Latson LF: Overview of disabled drivers' evaluation process, *Phys Disabil Special Interest Sect Newslett* 10(4), 1987.
19. Lillie SM: Evaluation for driving. In Yoshikawa TT, Cobbs EL, Brummel-Smith K, editors: *Ambulatory geriatric care*, St. Louis, 1993, Mosby.
20. Moyers PA: The guide to occupational therapy practice, *Am J Occup Ther* 53(3):258–262, 1999.

21. National Government Services: *9/23/2010 Common Claim Completion Issues Act Teleconference—Questions and Answers Summary*, Indianapolis, Ind, Author. Retrieved June 1, 2011, from http://www.ngsmedicare.com/wps/portal/ngsmedicare/!ut.2010-09-23.
22. Pezenik D, Itoh M, Lee M: Wheelchair prescription. In Ruskin AP, editor: *Current therapy in physiatry*, Philadelphia, 1984, WB Saunders.
23. Pierson FM, Fairchild SL: *Principles and techniques of patient care*, ed 3, Philadelphia, 2002, WB Saunders.
24. Sabo S, Shipp M: *Disabilities and their implications for driving*, Ruston, LA, 1989, Center for Rehabilitation Sciences and Biomedical Engineering, Louisiana Tech University.
25. Santa Clara Valley Medical Center, Physical Therapy Department: *Lifting and moving techniques*, San Jose, Calif, 1985, Santa Clara Valley Medical Center.
26. *Statement of assurances for providers of driver evaluation services*, Downey, Calif, 1990, State of California Department of Rehabilitation Mobility Evaluation Program.
27. Stav, Wendy B: *Driving rehabilitation: a guide for assessment and intervention*, San Antonio, 2004, PsychCorp, p. 17, pp. 20–21.
28. Strano CM: Driver evaluation and training of the physically disabled driver: additional comments, *Phys Disabil Special Interest Sect Newslett* 10(4), 1987.
29. Taira ED, editor: *Assessing the driving ability of the elderly*, Binghamton, NY, 1989, Hayworth.
30. Toglia J: *The multicontextual approach to rehabilitation of awareness, memory and executive function impairments*, Chicago, 2001, workshop presented at the Rehabilitation Institute of Chicago.
31. Watson DE, Watson SA: *Task analysis: an occupational performance approach*, ed 2, Bethesda, Md, 2003, American Occupational Therapy Association.
32. *Wheelchair prescription: measuring the patient*, (Booklet no. 1), Camarillo, Calif, 1979, Everest & Jennings.
33. *Wheelchair prescription: safety and handling*, (Booklet no. 3), Camarillo, Calif, 1983, Everest & Jennings.
34. *Wheelchair prescription: wheelchair selection*, (Booklet no. 2), Camarillo, Calif, 1979, Everest & Jennings.

Suggested Readings

Bergen A, Presperin J, Tallman T: *Positioning for function*, Valhalla, NY, 1990, Valhalla Rehabilitation Publications.

Bonninger M: *Preservation of upper limb function following spinal cord injury: a clinical practice guideline for health-care professionals, consortium for spinal cord medicine*, Washington, DC, 2005, Paralyzed Veterans of America.

Davies PM: *Steps to follow: a guide to the treatment of adult hemiplegia*, New York, 1985, Springer-Verlag.

Ford JR, Duckworth B: *Physical management for the quadriplegic patient*, Philadelphia, 1974, FA Davis.

Gee ZL, Passarella PM: *Nursing care of the stroke patient: a therapeutic approach*, Pittsburgh, PA, 1985, AREN Publications.

Higgins JR, Higgins S: The acquisition of locomotor skill. In Craik RL, Oatis CA, editors: *Gait analysis: theory and application*, St. Louis, 1995, Mosby.

Hill JP, editor: *Spinal cord injury: a guide to functional outcomes in occupational therapy*, Rockville, MD, 1986, Aspen.

Leonard CT: The neurophysiology of human locomotion. In Craik RL, Oatis CA, editors: *Gait analysis: theory and application*, St. Louis, 1995, Mosby.

Whiteneck G: *Outcomes following traumatic spinal cord injury: clinical practice guidelines for health-care professionals, consortium for spinal cord medicine*, Washington, DC, 1999, Paralyzed Veterans of America.

Wilson AB, McFarland SR: *Wheelchairs: a prescription guide*, Charlottesville, Va, 1992, Rehabilitation Press.

CHAPTER 16

Sexuality: An Activity of Daily Living

JESSICA FARMAN AND GORDON UMPHRED BURTON

Key Terms

Disability
Sexual dysfunction
Sexual function
Sexual rehabilitation
Sexuality
Sexuality counseling

Chapter Objectives

After studying this chapter, the student or practitioner will be able to:

1. Define sexuality.
2. Describe the normal human sexual response cycle.
3. List the effects of aging on sexual function.
4. Identify the occupational therapy practitioner's role in sexuality intervention.
5. Understand and apply the levels of the permission, limited information, specific suggestions, and intensive therapy (PLISSIT) model that are appropriate for occupational therapy practitioners.
6. Identify sexual impairments and how they affect function.
7. Plan interventions for impairments affecting sexual function.

A discussion of sexuality includes not only specific sexual practices but also the attitudes, behaviors, thoughts, and feelings associated with sex and sexuality. These include an individual's perception of self as a sexual being, body image, self-esteem, participation and roles in relationships (sexual and other), sexual orientation (heterosexual, homosexual, or bisexual), and beliefs and attitudes toward a wide range of sexual behaviors including masturbation, coitus, oral-genital sex, cuddling, and sensuality. Romano[26] defines sexuality expertly: "Sexuality is more than the art of sexual intercourse. It involves for most … the whole business of relating to another person; the tenderness, the desire to give as well as take, the compliments, casual caresses, reciprocal concerns, tolerance, the forms of communication that both include and go beyond words … sexuality includes a range of behavior from smiling through orgasm; it is not just what happens between two people in bed."[15]

Why should the occupational therapy assistant (OTA) be concerned with issues of sensuality or sexuality when dealing with a patient? Sexuality is one aspect of activities of daily living (ADL) and is within occupational performance, the domain of occupational therapy. Everyone can enjoy sex. Health care professionals must be aware of their own attitudes toward sexuality. Our patients may be different from ourselves: they may be older, may be of a different sexual orientation, or may have permanent or temporary disabilities. And just as differences among human beings are inherent, therapists must consider and respect the variances in sexual behaviors, preferences, and beliefs among individuals.[15]

Normal Human Sexual Response

The OTA must have an understanding of the normal human sexual response cycle before one can explore the relationship between sexuality and disability. Masters and Johnson divided the human sexual response cycle into four segments: (1) excitement, (2) plateau, (3) orgasm, and (4) resolution. In each phase, definite physical changes occur in both sexes. During the excitement phase, physiologic reactions occur as a result of somatosensory or psychogenic stimulation. In females, the nipples become erect, the vagina swells and becomes lubricated, the clitoris and the labia minora and majora swell, and the uterus and cervix retract. In males, the penis grows erect and the testes rise. In both sexes blood pressure and heart rate increase.[15]

During the plateau phase, respiration increases and blood pressure and heart rate increase further. In females the areola surrounding the nipple swells, the orgasmic platform forms (vasocongestion of the outer two thirds of the vagina), and the color of the labia minora deepens from pink to red. In males a full erection is achieved as the testes elevate further and the Cowper gland secretes preejaculatory fluid.[15]

Orgasms differ between the sexes; some women can achieve multiple orgasms. In both sexes, peak pulse rate, blood pressure, and respiration increase, as does muscle tone. Rhythmic contractions of the orgasmic platform and the uterus occur in women, and rhythmic contractions of the penis project semen forward in males.[15]

The resolution phase is characterized by the return to preexcitement status including reductions in blood pressure, heart rate, and respiration. The genitals and breasts return to preexcitement size.[15]

Aging and the Human Sexual Response Cycle

In normal human development, changes occur during the aging process.

Women

Generally between the ages of 40 and 50, women experience menopause, the cessation of menstruation caused by a lack of production of estrogen that occurs over a period of several months to a few years. The major effects of menopause are as follows[15]:

- Vasomotor syndrome (hot flashes)
- Atrophic vaginitis (thinning of the vaginal walls)
- Osteoporosis
- A decrease in the rate, amount, and type of vaginal fluid, which can cause pain during intercourse and may lead to infection
- Loss of contractility of vaginal muscles, which can cause shorter orgasms
- Decreased size of the uterus and clitoris and atrophy of the clitoral hood
- Loss of elasticity in breast tissue, causing sagging

Men

As men grow older the following changes occur:

- Erections are often less full, take longer to achieve, and may require direct stimulation.
- Ejaculatory control increases, ejaculation may only occur every third sexual episode and is less forceful, and loss of erection after orgasm may occur faster.
- The man may not be able to achieve another erection for 12 to 24 hours after orgasm.
- Sperm volume decreases and the ejaculation may be less intense, which may affect the intensity of orgasm.
- The size and firmness of the testes diminish.
- The testosterone level decreases.

Many elderly persons continue to enjoy sexual activity; however, a decline in sexual activity among elderly persons is not uncommon. Older persons do not necessarily lose their desire for sex, but circumstances can make it difficult for them to engage in active sexual relationships. Leading causes of altered sexual activity in the older adult include difficulty finding partners, illness, medication effects, death of a partner, divorce, biases about masturbation, societal attitudes about sex and the elderly, and even their own biases and prejudices toward sexuality. Elderly persons may view sex as something that only young, attractive persons do.[15]

Sexuality and Neurologic Function

Sexual function is controlled by the brain, spinal cord, and peripheral nerves, whereas control of libido and sexual pleasure are mediated by several areas in the cortex, midbrain, and brainstem. Men experience reflexogenic and psychogenic erections, each of which has a different origin. Reflexogenic erections are caused by direct stimulation to the penis and may occur without conscious awareness, even in the absence of penile sensation. Psychogenic erections originate from mental activity such as sexual fantasies and stimulating visual input and do not require direct penile stimulation. Reflexogenic erections are controlled by the nervous system through the sacral roots, and psychogenic erections involve the sympathetic nerves. Female sexual function is similar to that of males regarding nerve innervation.

Neurologic disability can cause organic impotence by altering the blood flow needed for penile erection and can cause problems with emission and ejaculation in males and with lubrication, clitoral engorgement, and orgasm in females.[15]

Societal Attitudes

Attitudes on the part of the public or the patient's family members may affect the patient emotionally or psychologically. Although the Americans with Disabilities Act has resulted in some improvement in public attitude, the fact remains that many persons still harshly judge individuals who appear "different" from the rest of society and regard disabled individuals with fear and shame. Persons with disabilities perceive these attitudes and as a result avoid social or public situations. The media seldom depict persons with disabilities as full partners in sexual relationships. The patient and partner, family members, and others may share the view that persons with disabilities are sexless, "different," and undeserving of social and sexual fulfillment. These attitudes can affect patients' existing relationships and their willingness to pursue new relationships.[6,15,25]

Role of Occupational Therapy

When persons experience changes in sexual function, they may require professional intervention to cope with these changes. What is the role of occupational therapy in sexuality intervention for these patients, and what is required to fulfill this role?

Sexuality long has been considered an appropriate area for occupational therapy intervention. Recent literature further supports the role of occupational therapy in sexuality.[12,25,27] Andamo[2] states that "sexual function should be included in the occupational therapy evaluation as it relates to the identification of the patient's abilities and limitations in his daily living necessary for the resumption of his various roles." Neistadt[24] notes that as "holistic caregivers, dedicated to facilitating quality lives, OTs should be prepared to address sexuality issues with their adolescent and adult patients." Couldrick[12] argues that "with awareness and skill development, OTs can affirm sexual identity, they can listen, and, with sometimes simple measures, they can address issues that fall within their professional roles." The American Occupational Therapy Association has confirmed the role of occupational therapy by including sexual activity as an ADL within the areas of occupation in the *Occupational Therapy Practice Framework,* second edition.[4]

Occupational therapists (OTs) are well prepared to address sexuality problems with patients. The sensory, motor, cognitive, and psychosocial impairments that interfere with sexual function are the same ones that affect other areas of occupation addressed by occupational therapy, including other ADL and work and leisure activities. Occupational therapy practitioners' skills of activity analysis and adaptation, holistic orientation, and knowledge of biologic and behavioral sciences help them deal effectively with patients' sexual difficulties.[3,5,6,15] Research indicates that dependence in ADL is often associated with a reduction of sexual activity,[14,15,21,23,29] further supporting the role of occupational therapy in sexual rehabilitation.

Most OTs receive some training in sexuality intervention, but this training is less comprehensive in OTA education. Further study or in-service training is generally required, and for the OTA it must include supervised experience in association with an OT skilled in sexuality intervention.[15,16,20] The references at the end of the chapter can be used to further one's understanding of sexual function and disability. Numerous films, books, and articles can be helpful in deepening one's skill level in this area.[7,11,13,15]

Team Approach

Although occupational therapy practitioners must be involved in sexual health care, effective sexual rehabilitation, like all rehabilitation, requires a team approach. The rehabilitation team must address all the individual's problems in a holistic way, and all team members should be knowledgeable about sexual issues and treatment options. If each member of the treatment team is knowledgeable and skilled in this area, the patient can choose the team member with whom he or she is most comfortable to address sexual issues. In addition, each team member has different expertise from which the patient may benefit. The physician may best address problems related to erectile dysfunction; relationship changes may require social work intervention; and the speech and language pathologist may best address communication difficulties.[15]

In practice, it is more common for the health care team to ignore sexuality issues. In a study of 110 post myocardial infarction (MI) patients, only one third of patients received information about sexual function from health care staff.[1]

Rehabilitation professionals cite various reasons for not addressing sexuality with their patients, with the most common responses being that another team member is responsible for this intervention and that their knowledge is inadequate. In a pilot study of health care professionals who treat stroke patients, including occupational and physical therapists, lack of training was cited as the primary reason for failing to address sexuality. Lack of experience ranked second. More than half felt concern about offending or embarrassing the patient. Perceptions of which team member is most responsible for addressing sexual function varied. The physician, social worker, and psychologist are most often cited as responsible for sexuality intervention.[15]

In another study on sexuality counseling following spinal cord injury, patients indicated a preference to speak with their occupational or physical therapist or nurse about their sexual concerns. Participants reported a positive response to therapists who used an open and direct style of communicating; they reported feeling frustrated, embarrassed, or intimidated by therapists who did not. Although many of the subjects were not ready to discuss sexuality early in their rehabilitation, they concurred that knowing resources were available when they needed them was vital.[15]

Besides being neglected in the clinic, sexual rehabilitation has received little attention in research. However, a general positive correlation has been found between successful sexual rehabilitation and positive adjustment to disability. The literature shows that patients with disabilities are interested in the inclusion of sexuality in rehabilitation and give sexuality a high priority.[3,15]

In clinical rehabilitation, "a job title does not always define competencies," and "no job title ... excludes discussion of sexuality," according to Chipouras and colleagues.[8] The qualities necessary in a competent sexuality counselor for persons with disabilities have been described variously. Chipouras and colleagues[8] emphasize comfort with sexuality, including one's own; comfort with disability; empathy; nonprojection of one's own morals onto the patient; awareness of available resources; basic knowledge of human sexuality; and awareness of one's own competency and willingness to refer to others as needed. The foundation of sexuality counseling consists of awareness and knowledge, which one can gain through reading, in-service education, coursework, and workshops. Therapists must develop skill in sexuality counseling through practice, as for all clinical skills. Discomfort in dealing with sexuality need be no different than discomfort with other difficult disability issues. OTs and OTAs address many personal and sometimes painful issues with their patients. Increased competency, skill, and comfort come with practice. Practice of sexuality interventions through role play with other staff members may be helpful in achieving greater comfort in conducting sexuality interventions.

PLISSIT

The therapist may use various frameworks and models to address sexuality issues in health care. Among the earliest and most prevalent is the PLISSIT model, developed by psychologist Jack Annon.[5] PLISSIT is an acronym for four levels of intervention: permission, limited information, specific suggestions, and intensive therapy (Figure 16-1). Using this model, the practitioner can determine the type and extent of sexuality intervention needed, whether he or she has the skills to perform the intervention, and whether to refer to a more qualified counselor (Box 16-1).[15]

Permission

Permission is the most basic and most frequently required intervention. Permission consists of reassuring patients that their actions and feelings are normal and acceptable. All OTs and OTAs should strive to perform permission-level sexuality interventions. Recognizing that sexual behavior varies widely and not projecting one's own values or morals onto the patient is most important.

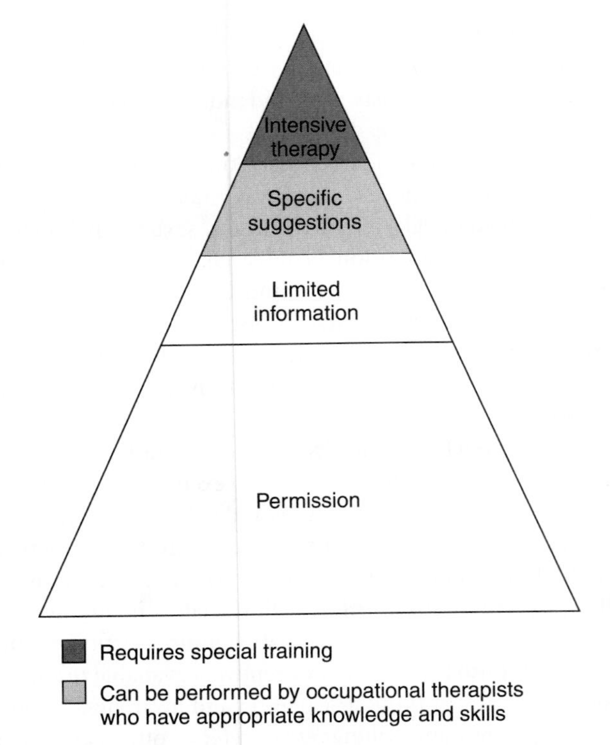

Figure 16-1 The permission, limited information, specific suggestions, and intensive therapy (PLISSIT) model. (From Gillen G: *Stroke rehabilitation: a function-based approach,* ed 3, St Louis, 2010, Elsevier.)

The practitioner must be proactive to provide patients with permission. Waiting for the patient to bring up sexual issues is not enough; the therapist must let the patient know that expressing sexual concerns is acceptable. The simplest way to do this is to ask, "People who have been diagnosed with Parkinson disease sometimes have concerns or questions about how they will be affected sexually. Do you have any concerns or questions in this area?" This line of questioning serves to normalize the concerns and gives patients the opportunity to say "no" if they are not comfortable discussing sexuality with that person at that time. Asking also lets patients know that sexual concerns are considered legitimate and gives them permission to bring up sexual issues again if their needs change. The therapist should ask questions in a language appropriate for the patient's understanding including the use of slang terms if necessary.[15]

The best time to bring up sexuality is at the initial evaluation, when other ADL issues are also being addressed. This should be done by the evaluating OT. If this is not feasible because of time constraints or because the evaluating therapist will not be treating the patient, sexuality should be brought up as soon as is comfortable, generally by the OT rather than the OTA. Sexual concerns should be explored before home visits and in the formulation of discharge plans because the patient's needs and concerns change throughout rehabilitation.[15]

Opportunities to give patients permission to express themselves as sexual beings often occur spontaneously. On one rehabilitation unit, a 38-year-old man with a diagnosis of right cerebrovascular accident was playing a getting-to-know-you game with the other patients, all of whom were older women. As part of the activity, each member of the group was asked to name something he or she liked. The women named things such as chocolate, flowers, and pets. The man said, "I like women." After a few seconds of silence, the OT running the group said, "Of course you do; what could be more natural?" The group members all nodded, and the activity continued.[15]

Box 16-1

Competencies for Sexuality Interventions at Each PLISSIT Level

Permission

To perform this level of sexuality intervention, the therapist should do the following:

- Acknowledge the sexuality of all persons.
- Be comfortable with his or her own sexuality.
- Believe that interest in sexuality is appropriate for everyone.
- Be comfortable speaking directly about sexual issues (or be willing to overcome discomfort).
- Refrain from projecting personal sexual morals and values onto others.

Limited Information

To provide this level of intervention, the therapist should fulfill the criteria listed for Permission and do the following:

- Have a basic understanding of human sexuality and its many variations.
- Understand the physiology of human sexual response.
- Be able to analyze the effects of physical disability on various sexual activities.
- Be willing to seek and provide accurate sexual information.
- Be aware of the limitations of his or her own knowledge base.

Specific Suggestions

To perform this level of intervention, the therapist should fulfill the criteria for Permission and Limited Information and do the following:

- Be familiar with various sexual activities.
- Be comfortable discussing specific sexual activities.
- Be able to conduct a sexual problem history.
- Be able to adapt various sexual activities to accommodate functional limitations.

Intensive Therapy

To perform this level of sexuality intervention, the therapist should fulfill the criteria for Permission, Limited Information, and Specific Suggestions and do the following:

- Have formal training in sex therapy, sexuality counseling, or psychotherapy.

From Gillen G: *Stroke rehabilitation: a function-based approach,* ed 3, St Louis, 2010, Elsevier.

Limited Information

Sometimes simply reassuring patients about sexuality is not enough. If patients do have concerns or questions, they may require specific information related to their stated concerns.[15] Some patients may need sex (sexuality) education because they may never have received the information even before the disability occurred.[17] Most OTs are qualified to provide patients with limited information. This level of intervention is often concerned with dispelling myths or misconceptions about sexuality. Limited information may be related to facts about the effect of disability on sexuality and sexual function. Handouts, pamphlets, and group education programs are good ways to provide limited information. Patients may read and absorb information on their own and ask the practitioner for clarification as needed. The important point is to limit the information to the patient's specific concerns. The accuracy of the information is also paramount. If the therapist does not have the information, he or she should help the patient get it before making a referral to another practitioner. For example, a patient with a complex cardiac history asks whether it is safe to have sex. Although the patient's physician can provide the answer, it is not enough for the therapist to say, "Ask your physician." By bringing up the concern to the therapist, the patient has chosen that person as an advocate. The therapist might respond, "Your physician is best equipped to answer that question. Would you feel comfortable asking her yourself, or would you like me to contact her for you?"[15]

Specific Suggestions

If a patient is experiencing a sexual problem, limited information may not be enough to solve it. The next level of intervention is specific suggestions aimed at solving the specific problem. This type of intervention requires more knowledge, time, and skill from the therapist but is appropriate for some OTs and occupational therapy assistants. The therapist should meet with the patient (and partner, if appropriate) in a comfortable, private setting and obtain a sexual problem history. This history should include the following:

- The patient's assessment of the problem and its cause, onset, and course
- The patient's attempts to solve the problem
- The patient's goals

Just as the OT would not initiate treatment of other problems without a full evaluation, the therapist must understand the sexual problem fully before making specific suggestions. After obtaining the sexual problem history, the therapist should develop goals in collaboration with the patient. If the patient's primary therapeutic relationship is with the OTA, the OTA and OT need to work in collaboration to establish methods to achieve stated goals. The goals may address learning the effects of the particular diagnosis on sexual function; adapting to changes in sensory, motor, or cognitive function; adapting to psychosocial and role changes; and improving sexual communication.[15]

One male paraplegic patient reported sexual problems after a weekend visit home. A sexual problem history revealed that he had always preferred the male-superior position for intercourse. Since his injury, lower extremity weakness had prevented adequate pelvic thrusting in this position. With the occupational therapy assistant, the patient discussed various new positions to increase mobility: sidelying or sitting in a chair with his partner seated facing him.[15]

Intensive Therapy

If the patient's problems are beyond the scope of goal-oriented specific suggestions, he or she may require intensive therapy. This level of intervention is based on specialized treatment skills and is beyond the scope of most OTs. Finding an appropriate referral for such patients such as a psychologist, social worker, or sex therapist is advisable. If the sexual problems predate or are not related to the onset of disability, the patient may require referral.[15]

The PLISSIT model enables the health care professional to adapt a sexuality program to the needs of the setting and the population served. Although permission to express sexual concern is universal, the need for limited information and specific suggestions varies. The best way to assess the need for sexuality intervention is to ask patients about their concerns. OT Evelyn Andamo's treatment model[2] uses a written problem checklist in which the patient is asked to identify problems in whatever role he or she fills including that of sexual partner. By addressing sexuality in a multiproblem context, this model helps normalize sexual concerns. The checklist includes two items related to sexual problems and concerns about sexual activity. Patients who check either item receive further intervention as needed including problem clarification, sexual history taking, and the development of treatment goals and treatment planning. The OT can adapt any evaluation to include questions about sexual concerns and collaborate with the occupational therapy assistant on such findings. Questions can be repeated before home visits or as discharge approaches because patients' concerns change over time.[15]

Underlying some health care workers' reluctance to address sexuality may be a fear of opening a Pandora's box of issues too difficult or intimate for them to handle. This is seldom the case. Most persons do not wish to disclose their sexual problems or to include strangers in their intimate relationships. They want and benefit from the least intervention possible to help them solve their sexual problems and deal with their concerns. Other therapists fear that providing permission to discuss sexual concerns will provoke inappropriate patient sexual behavior. The literature indicates that many health care workers are exposed to inappropriate sexual behavior on the part of patients during their careers, and they often lack training in dealing with these behaviors. Less experienced therapists and students tend to ignore the behaviors even when they are severe, which may result in high stress and difficult working conditions. Of course, any therapist who is exposed to sexual or other inappropriate behavior by anyone should address the problem immediately. Patient behaviors should be documented in the medical records; other staff members may also be affected. All new therapists and students should be encouraged to report harassment and seek help with difficult situations.

Providing permission to patients to address sexual issues directly actually decreases inappropriate behaviors. Flirting, sexual jokes, and innuendos are often a patient's way of indirectly expressing doubts and concerns about sexuality after disability. One spinal cord injured patient, B.L., overheard his OT inviting some coworkers to her home and asked, "When are you going to invite me over?" The therapist replied, "You know, B.L., that I'm your therapist, and although you're a really nice person, it would be unethical for us to have a social relationship. But tell me, are you interested in developing new social relationships?" This question led to a lively discussion about B.L.'s returning interest in women and sex. The therapist was understanding and supportive. The patient made no further advances to her. By refocusing attention on the patient, the therapist deflected the unwanted attention and responded to the patient's real need for permission to acknowledge his returning sexual feelings.[15]

Developing Competency

Competency in sexuality intervention comprises three elements (see Box 16-1): comfort, knowledge, and skill. These elements are interrelated; individuals are more comfortable with things they know well (knowledge) and do well (skill). Suggestions for improving these competencies can be found in Box 16-2.

Box 16-2

Improving Competency in Sexuality Intervention

Comfort

- Reading (See resources and references at end of chapter.)
- Films (e.g., *Sexuality Reborn,* Kessler Institute for Rehabilitation)
- Disability literature

Knowledge

- Readings (See resources and references at end of chapter.)
- Lectures
- In-service education

Skill

- Role-playing with other staff members
- Acquiring skill through practice
- Seeking a mentor who specializes in sexuality, for private supervision

Dealing with Physical Symptoms of Dysfunction

Activity Analysis

In order to provide specific suggestions, the OT practitioner must analyze the components of the activity. This process entails objectively examining the physical, social, and cultural contexts and communication/interaction skills and cognitive functions of the patient and partner. The clinician can approach this as just one more ADL that may need professional assistance and must be analyzed accordingly. The clinician needs to be sensitive to the individual's premorbid function including frequency of sexual activity, preferences, and sexual orientation. Suggestions need to be individualized, just as they would for any other ADL.

This section discusses specific symptoms that may create problems with sexual functioning for disabled persons and their partners (Table 16-1).

Endurance

Low endurance can create problems during sex because the individual may not be able to tolerate prolonged activity. Suggestions include the following: timing sex when energy is highest; wait 2 to 3 hours after meals before engaging in sex to allow for digestion; deemphasize intercourse through exploration of other sexual activities including oral-genital sex and mutual masturbation[15]; and assume positions that require less energy (Figures 16-2 and 16-3).

Loss of Mobility and Contractures

This can include mobility deficits due to impaired muscle tone, hemiplegia, and paralysis. Many movement patterns are restricted, and sexual positions will be limited by reduced range of motion.

Suggestions include positioning for comfort using pillows or bolsters and exploring positions that provide support and permit movement. An able-bodied partner may assume a superior position (Figures 16-4 to 16-6). Activity analysis can reveal positions that will allow for sexual activity focusing on

Table 16-1 Conditions and Possible Effects on Sexual Functioning

Diagnosis	Anxiety/ Fear	Contractures	Cultural Barriers	Decreased Libido	Depression	Impotence	Incontinence
Amputations	x	x	x		x		
Arthritis	x	x	x	x	x		
Burns	x	x	x		x		
Cardiac condition	x		x	x	x	x*	
Cerebral palsy	x	x	x		x		x
CVA	x	x	x	x	x	x	x
Diabetes	x		x	x	x	x	
Hand injury	x	x	x		x		
Head injury	x	x	x	x+	x	x	x
HIV	x		x	x	x		
Musculoskeletal injury	x	x	x		x		x
Pulmonary diseases	x		x	x	x	x	x
Spinal cord injury	x	x	x		x	x	x

CVA, cerebrovascular accident; ROM, range of motion; *, fear or medication as possible causes; x, Possible involvement; +, increased or decreased.

abilities, without focusing on the limitations. Creative problem solving is important (Figure 16-7).

Joint Degeneration

Conditions such as arthritis can cause pain, damage to the joints, and contractures. For the patient who has limited hip abduction, a side-lying position may be more advisable (see Figure 16-7).

Avoid situations that put stress and repetitive weight bearing on the joints (see Figure 16-4).

Pain

Pain limits the enjoyment of sexual activities.[19,24] Plan for sexual activities for a time of day when pain is diminished and energy is at its highest. Schedule pain medications in conjunction with sexual activity. Alternatives to intercourse may be suggested (i.e., mutual masturbation, oral sex). Encourage communication between partners; the unaffected partner may feel that her or his needs are not being considered or met, possibly because the partner does not understand the strong

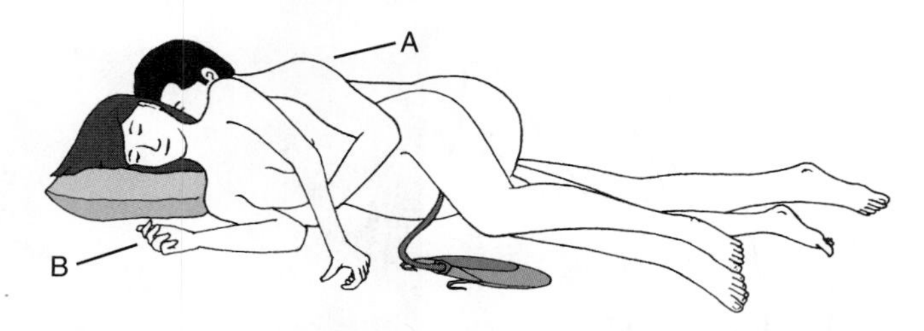

Figure 16-2 Partner B does not need to expend much energy in this position, and both partners can avoid swayback. Either person may have hemiparesis. Partner B does not need hip abduction, and pressure on stoma bag is avoided. (From Pendleton, HM: PEDRETTI'S OCCUPATIONAL THERAPY, 7th edition, St. Louis, Mosby, 2012.)

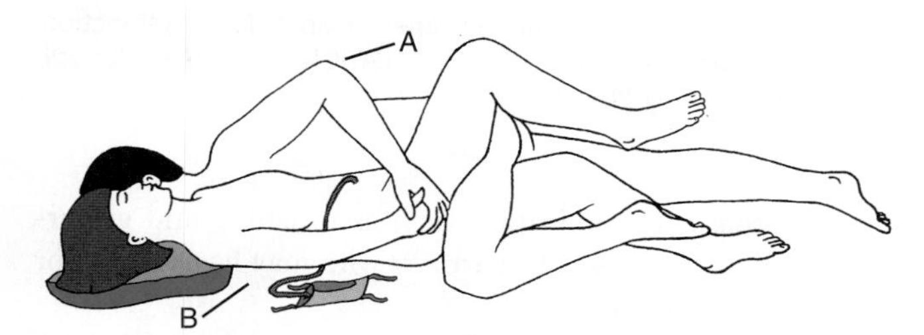

Figure 16-3 This position can be used if either partner has hemiparesis or if low endurance is a problem. Partner A can avoid swayback in this position. (From Pendleton, HM: PEDRETTI'S OCCUPATIONAL THERAPY, 7th edition, St. Louis, Mosby, 2012.)

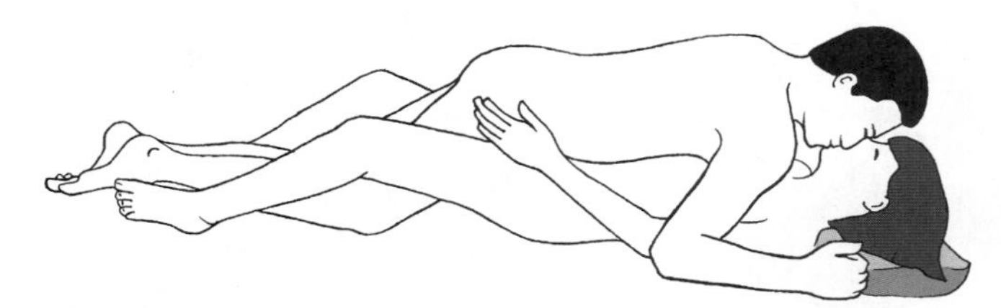

Figure 16-4 This position places pressure on the female's bladder and requires hip abduction but little energy expenditure for her. (From Pendleton, HM: PEDRETTI'S OCCUPATIONAL THERAPY, 7th edition, St. Louis, Mosby, 2012.)

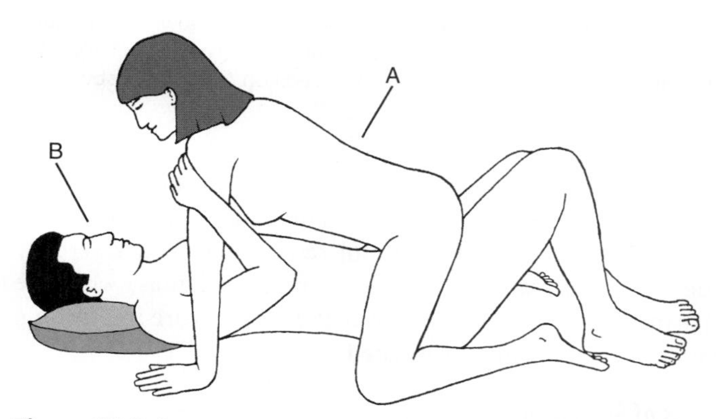

Figure 16-5 Partner A must have hip abduction, balance, and endurance, but there is no pressure on the bladder or stoma. If a catheter is used, it would be unrestricted. Back pain can be avoided by keeping the trunk vertical. Partner B's hip flexors could be contracted. If low back pain is a problem, legs should be flexed and a roll placed under the lower back. If stoma appliance is used, this position would avoid interference. This position is effective if low endurance is a problem for partner B. (From Pendleton, HM: PEDRETTI'S OCCUPATIONAL THERAPY, 7th edition, St. Louis, Mosby, 2012.)

Limited ROM	Loss of mobility	Loss of sensation	Low endurance	Medication	Paralysis/ spasticity	Poor body image	Tremor	Catheter/ostomy
	x	x				x		
x	x		x	x		x		
x	x	x	x		x	x		
	x		x	x		x		
x	x	x	x		x	x	x	x
x	x	x	x	x	x	x	x	x
	x	x	x			x	x	
x	x	x			x	x		
x	x	x	x	x	x	x	x	x
			x	x		x		
x	x	x	x	x	x	x	x	
	x	x	x	x		x		
x	x	x	x	x	x	x	x	x

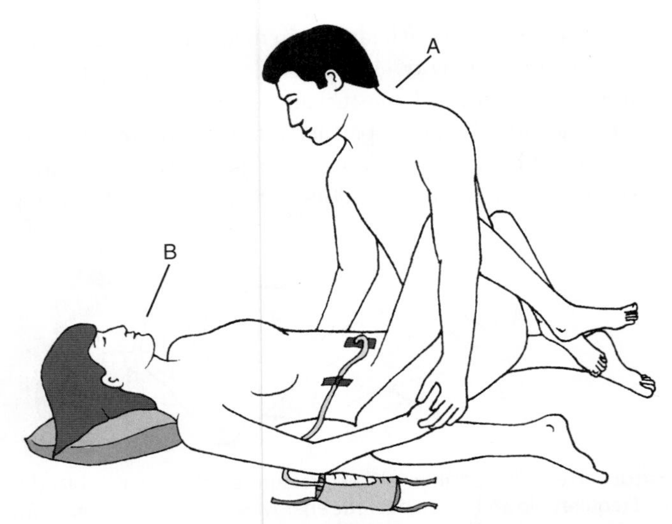

Figure 16-6 This position keeps pressure off the bladder, lessens the risk of tubing becoming bent, reduces pressure on back (especially if a small roll is used under the low back), and does not require partner B to use much energy. Legs do not need to be as high as shown. This position can be comfortable if hip flexors are contracted. (From Pendleton, HM: PEDRETTI'S OCCUPATIONAL THERAPY, 7th edition, St. Louis, Mosby, 2012.)

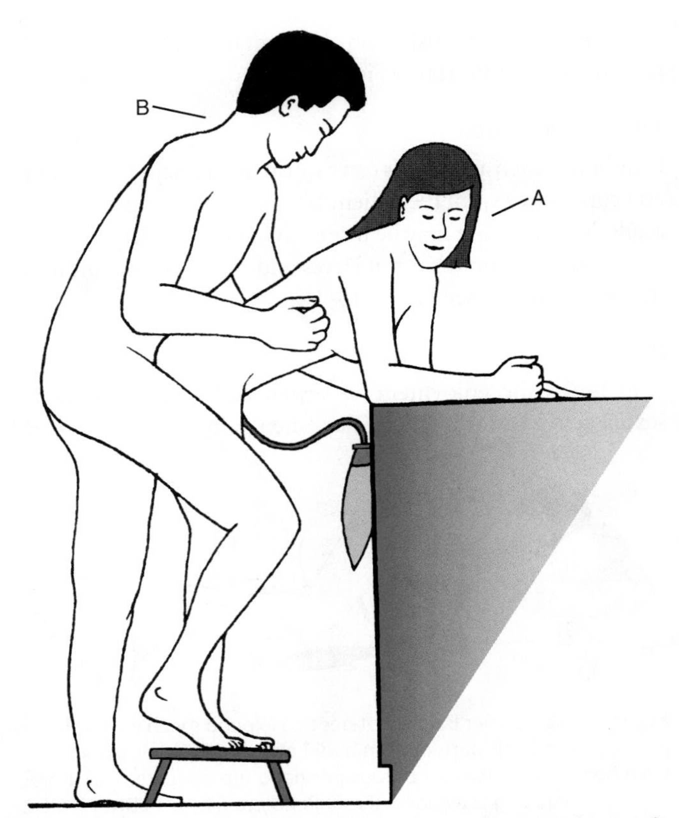

Figure 16-7 Partner A needs little hip abduction but good strength. Partner B may find decreased strain on his back. This position cannot be used if either partner has hip, knee, or ankle joint dysfunction. (From Pendleton, HM: PEDRETTI'S OCCUPATIONAL THERAPY, 7th edition, St. Louis, Mosby, 2012.)

negative effect of pain and cannot see a physical problem. The partner may perceive that the person in pain is just not interested. If touch creates a painful response, consider verbally describing or reading a sexually stimulating fantasy while the partner masturbates. In this way the partners are interacting, and neither person feels isolated.

Loss of Sensation

Loss of sensation can affect the sexual relationship through the lack of erogenous stimulation in the affected area. The loss can potentially block proper feedback so that an area is negatively affected through abrasion (e.g., vagina not being sufficiently lubricated). Lack of sensation may signify a break in the reflex loop, which may hamper reflexogenic erections (in the male) or lubrication (in the female); either of these issues can be addressed. Encourage good communication between partners so that the partner is aware of sensory losses. Encourage touch to unaffected areas. New erogenous zones can develop to compensate for the ones lost.[24]

Cognitive/Perceptual Impairments

Patients with cognitive/perceptual impairments and their partners may try the following suggestions:

- Simple positions are recommended (see Figures 16-4, 16-5, 16-8, and 16-9). Achieving a routine of sexual activity may be helpful if the person has difficulty moving spontaneously. When the brain becomes used to a routine, it does not have to work as hard to plan movements and the patient does not have to concentrate on how he or she is moving.[15]
- Perceptual deficits such as hemianopsia or unilateral neglect may cause a person to ignore parts of the partner's body or not respond when approached from the affected side. The unaffected partner must be sensitive to these deficits.
- Nonverbal communication such as touching and gesturing are encouraged with partners who may have speech or language disorders.[15]
- Distractions such as loud music should be kept to a minimum.[15]
- Individuals with memory impairment should keep a log of daily activities including sexual activities in an effort to remain oriented.[15]
- Sexual role changes such as increased sexual initiation by the nonaffected partner can help minimize the effects of cognitive changes on sexual function.

Inadequate Vaginal Lubrication

Lubricated condoms or water-based lubricants are recommended. Foreplay should be extended to ensure adequate lubrication of the vagina before intercourse. Partners need to be informed that impaired or delayed vaginal lubrication might be a normal age-related change, if the partner is older. A consultation with a gynecologist may be indicated.

Erectile Dysfunction

A ring placed on the base of the penis may help maintain blood flow into the penis and help maintain an erection.[15] Forms of sex that do not require an erect penis (such as using a vibrator or engaging in oral or manual sex) may meet the client's and the partner's needs. Medications for erectile dysfunction

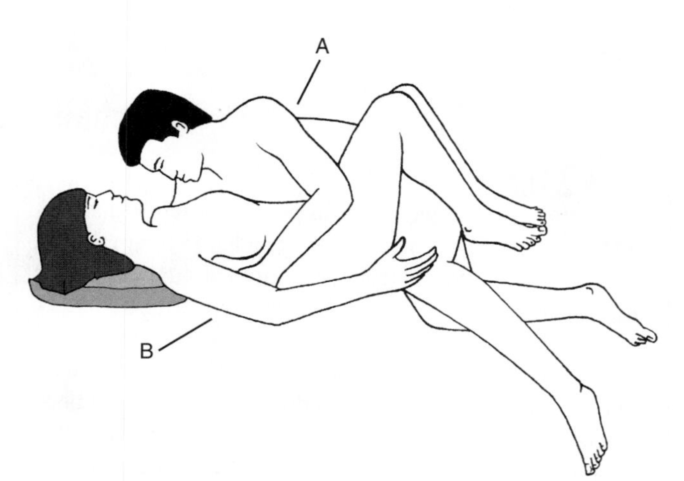

Figure 16-8 Vaginal entry of partner B requires no hip abduction, and hip flexion tightness would not impede performance. Energy requirements for both parties are minimal. Bladder pressure and safety of catheter and stoma appliance should not be concerns with this position for partner B. This position may be recommended if partner B has back pain or is paralyzed. A roll can be used to support the lumbar spine. (From Pendleton, HM: PEDRETTI'S OCCUPATIONAL THERAPY, 7th edition, St. Louis, Mosby, 2012.)

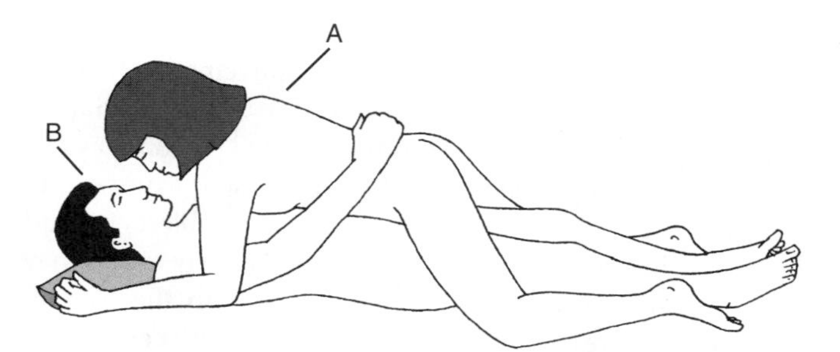

Figure 16-9 This position can be used if partner B is paralyzed or has limited range of motion. Partner B's back may need a roll for support, and he must be concerned about pressure on his bladder. (From Pendleton, HM: PEDRETTI'S OCCUPATIONAL THERAPY, 7th edition, St. Louis, Mosby, 2012.)

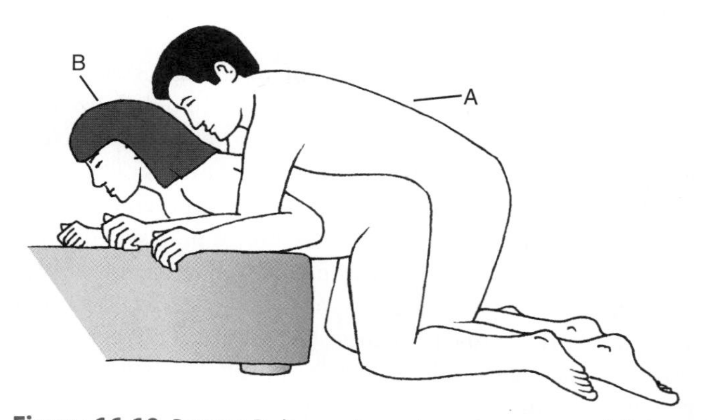

Figure 16-10 Partner B does not need much energy and little or no abduction of hips for this rear vaginal entry position. This position would not be good for persons with back, hip, or knee joint degeneration because of weight on the knees and inevitable movement at the hips. (From Pendleton, HM: PEDRETTI'S OCCUPATIONAL THERAPY, 7th edition, St. Louis, Mosby, 2012.)

may be indicated such as Viagra, Levitra, or Cialis. A referral to the physician would be warranted; the OT practitioner needs to consult with the doctor before even mentioning these possibilities. Other treatment options for erectile dysfunction require consultation with a urologist. These include vacuum constrictor devices, injection of vasoactive agents, and penile prosthesis implantion.[15] The patient should be encouraged to explore his body in an effort to stimulate a reflexogenic erection. Rubbing the penis, thighs, or anus may be effective. Some quadriplegic men have even reported that rubbing the big toe can stimulate an erection. If the reflex loop is impaired, an erection may be impossible without physical or chemical assistance, and alternative methods may need to be explored.

Dealing with Other Barriers to Sexuality

Incontinence

Patients with incontinence and their partners may try the following suggestions:

- The patient should avoid fluids before engaging in sexual activity.[15]
- Men may wear a condom to prevent leakage onto the partner.[15]
- Patients on a voiding schedule should be encouraged to adhere to the schedule to prevent accidents.
- Towels should be available in case of accidents, and the patient should discuss his or her situation before engaging in sexual activity, to prevent embarrassment.[15]
- The patient should empty his or her bladder before engaging in sexual activity.[15]

Catheter care should be addressed. If there is an indwelling catheter, pressure should not be placed on the bladder. The OT practitioner should have the nurse or the physician determine the length of time that flow of urine can safely be restricted. Similarly, the nurse or physician should issue safe guidelines for fluid restrictions before sexual activity. Sexual positions that avoid pressure on the bladder should be used (see Figures 16-3 to 16-10). Many of the same positions may be used if the patient has a stoma appliance.

Medications

The side effects of medications may cause erectile dysfunction or delayed sexual response and other problems. Diuretics, antihypertensives, and antidepressants may cause erectile dysfunction, decreased libido, and loss of orgasm. Side effects of medication should be discussed with the physician. The occupational therapy assistant can direct the patient to the physician.

Other Aspects of Sexuality

Isolation

The environment comprises objects, persons, and events that affect the individual and that the individual affects. Some of the objects with which disabled persons interact are wheelchairs, braces, canes, crutches, and splints. These objects are all hard, cold, and angular and generally communicate a "hard exterior" and a fragile interior, which is viewed as not "huggable" and soft or safe to hug. People may avoid embracing a person in a wheelchair, in braces, or on crutches for fear of hurting or knocking him or her down. Thus the disabled person may feel isolated because of appliances or, as one patient expressed it, "in a plastic bubble." People may relate to the objects around the patient in a nonsensual manner; thus everyday events may reinforce isolation and lack of sensuousness in the patient. Patients who have been discharged from the health care facility for a time feel more isolated than others. Even in the relatively acute phase of a disability, the clinician and patient may role-play how to deal with a new partner and how to explain the patient's equipment (e.g., catheters). Doing so may help ease the patient's anxieties and promote comfort with such issues.

Contraception

Disabled persons must be aware of many issues regarding birth control. The patient and partner first should realize that most disabling conditions do not impair fertility. Therefore the patient must consider contraception options. The functional abilities needed to use condoms, a diaphragm, or a cervical cap include fine motor abilities, motor praxis, and intact cognitive and perceptual function.[15] However, in some cases the nondisabled partner can assist with contraception and work it into the sexual repertoire. Oral contraceptives or contraceptive patches would require a consultation with a gynecologist; they may increase the risk of clotting, especially when the woman has impaired mobility or paralysis. A consultation with the physician would be required to determine the most appropriate birth control method. The patient should be educated about safe sex practices.

Adaptive Aids

Disabled patients may need to use adaptive aids, especially if they lack hand function. One aid is a vibrator for foreplay or masturbation.[22,24] Special vibrators have been adapted for men and women.[22,24] Pillows can be used for positioning, and other devices can be used for patients with special needs. The occupational therapy practitioner may prepare the patient for the concept of using sexual aids before asking the person to use such devices. For example, the OTA might ask the patient in private to explore the sensation that the vibrator produces in the lower extremities. When told about the potential functional benefits, the patient may discover the vibrator has practical application or at least will be more open to it as a sexual aid.

Pregnancy, Delivery, and Child Care

Pregnancy may result in complications that may affect the patient's function and mobility.[28] Increased weight impedes transfers and increases the possibility of dysreflexia (autonomic hyperreflexia) or increased bladder and bowel care.[9,10,28] The birth may present unique situations. For example, induction of labor may be contraindicated and present challenges to the medical team. After the birth, the disabled parent may require modifications to accommodate prenatal care and parenting; consultations may be necessary for the disabled patient to achieve an optimal level of functioning as a parent.[18,28]

CASE STUDY

"I Want to Get Out of the Wheelchair So That I Can Chase a Man"

W.A. is a 62-year-old woman who previously suffered a right middle cerebral artery stroke with resulting left hemiparesis. After her initial and rehabilitation hospitalizations, she was discharged home for continued occupational and physical therapy. She lived in a senior housing development, which had a social room on the premises. W.A. had been widowed for more than 15 years and reported that her husband had been an alcoholic and a "terrible man." During W.A.'s initial evaluation at home, the OT asked what her goals for rehabilitation were. W.A. was quick to reply, "I want to be able to get out of the wheelchair so that I can chase a man." Sexuality had not been addressed until this point in the evaluation. The therapist took the opportunity to ask W.A. whether she had a significant man in her life, to which W.A. replied "no." The therapist asked W.A. whether she had any concerns about resuming sexual activities after the stroke; again W.A. replied "no." She explained that she was not looking to marry again and simply wanted to be exposed to others so that she could flirt. During this conversation the therapist realized that further exploration of sexual function was geared toward getting W.A. out into the community again. W.A. had been limited in this endeavor because of poor mobility and wheelchair dependency.

In this example, the therapist used the permission level of the PLISSIT model. The patient brought up the topic herself, and it was discovered through further questioning that W.A. was really referring to a need to socialize, not so much as to act on her sexual desires. In subsequent conversations, W.A.'s OT reassessed this situation, particularly as W.A. made progress with ADL and functional mobility. After 6 months of treatment, W.A. was getting back out into the community, attending an adult day care center, and participating in bingo games in her building. She was taught how to transfer on and off the furniture in the social room to allow greater independence and a sense of normalcy. All areas of function including sexuality were reevaluated periodically during W.A.'s treatment program, and her goals remained unchanged from her initial evaluation.

In this example the issue of sexuality was related less directly to actual sexual activities than to socialization and flirting. Had the therapist neglected to pursue W.A.'s early statement about wanting to "chase a man," the patient's needs might never have been addressed.

Summary

For most people, sexuality is entwined with personal identity. Sexuality is classified as an ADL in the Occupational Therapy Practice Framework 2nd Edition. Thus the OTA should anticipate that disabled patients will require evaluation, assistance, information, and intervention in this area. The PLISSIT model helps the practitioner identify the type of sexuality intervention required. Communicating with patients about sexuality requires professional dignity and the greatest possible flexibility from the practitioner. Among the specific qualities and skills the practitioner should possess are knowledge of sexual theory and practices; tolerance; appreciation for the needs, views, and practices of others; excellent verbal and nonverbal communication skills; utmost discretion; and an understanding of the limitations of the OTA's role. The OTA is encouraged to seek additional training in this area and to obtain appropriate supervision when providing services to disabled patients related to issues of sexuality.

Selected Reading Guide Questions

1. Explain why the newly disabled patient might flirt with a staff member. Describe appropriate and helpful ways to respond.
2. Why might a patient ask the OTA, rather than the physician, about sexual aspects of a disability?
3. Describe the conditions (environment) in which a sexual history interview or other discussion of sexual matters is best conducted.
4. Give specific suggestions for addressing the following physical symptoms in sexual activities: low endurance, loss of mobility or contractures, joint degeneration, pain, loss of sensation, and incontinence.
5. List and discuss the effects of aging on sexuality for both men and women.
6. Discuss isolating aspects of the disabled patient's environment, and suggest methods to reduce isolation.
7. Describe effects of medications on sexuality.
8. Identify the acronym PLISSIT, and explain each component. Identify which components can be performed by the OTA and which require more education.

References

1. Akdolun N, Terakye G: Sexual problems before and after myocardial infarction: patients' need for information, *Rehabil Nurs* 26(4):152-158.
2. Andamo EM: Treatment model: occupational therapy for sexual dysfunction, *Sex Disabil* 4:26, 1980.
3. Andrews AB, Veronen LJ: Sexual assault and people with disabilities, *J Social Work Human Sexuality* 8(2):137–159, 1993.
4. American Occupational Therapy Association: *Occupational therapy practice framework: domain and process*, ed 2, Bethesda, MD, 2008, the Association.
5. Annon JS: *The behavioral treatment of sexual problems* (vols 1-2), Honolulu, 1974, Enabling Systems Inc.
6. Black K, Sipski ML, Strauss SS: Sexual satisfaction and sexual drive in spinal cord injured women, *J Spinal Cord Med* 21(3): 240–244, 1998.
7. Boyle PS: Training in sexuality and disability: preparing social workers to provide services to individuals with disabilities, *J Social Work Human Sexuality* 8(2):45–62, 1993.
8. Chipouras S, Cornelius DA, Makas E, et al: *Who cares? A handbook on sex education and counseling services for disabled people*, ed 2, Baltimore, 1982, University Park Press.
9. Cole SS, Cole TM: Sexuality, disability, and reproductive issues for persons with disabilities. In Haseltine FP, Cole SS, Gray DB, editors: *Reproductive issues for persons with physical disabilities*, Baltimore, 1993, Brookes.
10. Cole SS, Cole TM: Sexuality, disability, and reproductive issues through the life span, *Sexuality Disabil* 11(3):189–205, 1993.
11. Cornelius DA, Chipouras S, Makas E, et al: *Who cares? a handbook on sex education and counseling services for disabled people*, Baltimore, 1982, University Park Press.
12. Couldrick L: Sexual expression and occupational therapy, *Br J Occup Ther* 68(7):315–318, 2005.
13. Ducharme S, Gill KM: Sexual values, training, and professional roles, *J Head Trauma Rehabil* 5(2):38–45, 1991.
14. Edwards DF, Baum CM: Caregivers burden across stages of dementia, *Occup Ther Pract* 2(1):17–31, 1990.
15. Farman J, Dicker-Friedman J: Sexual function and intimacy. In Gillen G, editor: *Stroke Rehabilitation: A Function Based Approach*, 3rd edition, 2011.
16. Goldstein H, Runyon C: An occupational therapy education module to increase sensitivity about geriatric sexuality, *Phys Occup Ther Geriatr* 11(2):57, 1993.
17. Greydanus DE, Rimsza ME, Newhouse PA: Adolescent sexuality and disability, *Adolesc Med* 13(2):223–247, 2002.
18. Haseltine FP, Cole SS, Gray DB: *Reproductive issues for persons with physical disabilities*, Baltimore, 1993, Paul Brooks.
19. Hebert L: *Sex and back pain*, Bloomington, Minn, 1987, Educational Opportunities.
20. Johnson TC: Understanding the sexual behaviors of young children, *Sexuality Information and Education Council of the United States Report*, 1991.
21. Krause JS, Crewe NM: Chronological age, time since injury, and time of measurement: effect on adjustment after spinal cord injury, *Arch Phys Med Rehabil* 72:91–100, 1991.
22. Kroll K, Klein EL: *Enabling romance*, New York, 1992, Harmony.
23. McCabe MP, Taleporos G: Sexual esteem, sexual satisfaction, and sexual behavior among people with physical disability, *Arch Sexual Behav* 32(4):359–369, 2003.
24. Neistadt ME, Freda M: *Choices: a guide to sex counseling with physically disabled adults*, Malabar, FL, 1987, Krieger.
25. Pollard N: Sakellariou D: Sex and occupational therapy: contradictions or contraindications? *Br J Occup Ther* 70(8):162–165, 2007.
26. Romano MD: Sexuality and the disabled female, *Accent Living*, 1973:winter.
27. Sakellarious D: Algado SS: Sexuality and occupational therapy: exploring the link, *Br J Occup Ther* 69(8):150–156, 2006.
28. Sipski M, Alexander C: *Sexual function in people with disability and chronic illness*, Gaithersburg, Md, 1997, Aspen Publishing.
29. Verduyn WH: Spinal cord injured women, pregnancy, and delivery, *Sex Disabil* 11(3):29–43, 1993.

Recommended Reading/Resources

Alexander C, Sipski M: Sexuality Reborn; Kessler Institute for Rehabilitation (film).

Finger WW: Prevention, assessment and treatment of sexual dysfunction following stroke, *Sex Disabil* 11:1, 1993.

Gender AR: An overview of the nurse's role in dealing with sexuality, *Sexual Disabil* 10(2):70–71, 1992.

Gregory MF: *Sexual adjustment: a guide for the spinal cord injured*, Bloomington, Ill, 1993, Accent On Living.

Jackson AB, Wadley V: A multicenter study of women's self-reported reproductive health after spinal cord injury, *Arch Phys Med Rehabil* 80(11):1420–1428, 1999.

Kempton W, Caparulo F: *Sex education for persons with disabilities that hinder learning: a teacher's guide*, Santa Barbara, CA, 1989, James Stanfield.

Kettl P, Zarefoss S, Jacoby K, et al: Female sexuality after spinal cord injury, *Sex Disabil* 9:287–295, 1991.

Kroll K, Levy Klein E: *Enabling romance,* In Bethesda, Md., 1995, Woodbine House.

Leyson JF: *Sexual rehabilitation of the spinal-cord-injured patient,* Totowa, NJ, 1991, Humana Press.

Mackelprang R, Valentine D: *Sexuality and disabilities: a guide for human service practitioners,* Binghamton, NY, 1993, Haworth Press.

Neufeld JA, Klingbeil F, Bryen DN, et al: Adolescent sexuality and disability, *Phys Med Rehabil Clin N Am* 13(4):857–873, 2002.

Nosek MA, Walter LA: Community integration of women with spinal cord injuries: an examination of psychological, social, vocational, and environmental factors, *Topics Spinal Cord Inj Rehabil* 4(2): 41–55, 1998.

Novak PP, MM Mitchell MM: Professional involvement in sexuality counseling for patients with spinal cord injuries, *Am J Occup Ther* 42(2):105–112, 1988.

Sandowski C: *Sexual concern when illness or disability strikes,* Springfield, Ill, 1989, Charles C Thomas. In Resources for people with disabilities and chronic conditions, ed 2, Lexington, Ky, 1993, Resources for Rehabilitation.

Sandowski C: Responding to the sexual concerns of persons with disabilities, *J Soc Work Hum Sex* 8(2):29–43, 1993.

Sipski M, Alexander C: *Sexual function in people with disability and chronic illness,* Gaithersburg, Md, 1997, Aspen.

Sobsey D, Gray S, editors: *Disability, sexuality, and abuse,* Baltimore, 1991, Paul H. Brooks.

Resources-Agencies and Support Centers

American Association of Sex Education Counselors and Therapists
435 North Michigan Ave., Suite 1717
Chicago, IL 60611
(312) 644-0828
www.aasect.org

American Congress of Rehabilitation Medicine
6801 Lake Plaza Drive, Suite B-205
Indianapolis, IN 46220
(317) 915-2250
www.acrm.org

Planned Parenthood Federation of America
www.plannedparenthood.org
SEICUS (Sex Education and Information Council of the United States)
90 John St Suite 704
New York, NY 10038
(212) 819-9770
www.seicus.org

Sexuality and Disability Training Center
Boston University Medical Center
88 East Newton St.
Boston, MA 02118
(617) 638-7358
www.stanleyducharme.com

The Task Force on Sexuality and Disability of the American Congress of Rehabilitation Medicine
5700 Old Orchard Road
Skokie, IL 60077
(708) 966-0095
www.acrm.org

Specific Websites

Disability resources: www.menstuff.org
Institute on Independent Living: www.independentliving.org
Kessler Institute for Rehab: www.kessler-rehab.com
National Institute of Aging: www.nia.nih.gov
National Sexuality Resource Center: nsrc.sfsu.edu
Sexual Health Network: www.sexualhealth.org
Spinal cord injuries: www.spinalcord.org

CHAPTER 17 Work

DENISE HARUKO HA, JILL J. PAGE, AND CHRISTINE M. WIETLISBACH

Key Terms

Industrial therapy
Vocational Rehabilitation Act
Americans with Disabilities Act (ADA)
Occupational Safety and Health Administration (OSHA)
Musculoskeletal disorders (MSDs)
Industrial or occupational rehabilitation
Vocational evaluation
Functional capacity evaluation (FCE)
Validity
Work hardening
Work conditioning
Job demands analysis (JDA)
Pre-employment screening
Reasonable accommodation
Worksite evaluation
Ergonomics
Work readiness program

Chapter Objectives

After studying this chapter, the student or practitioner will be able to do the following:

1. Describe the history of occupational therapy's involvement with work rehabilitation and development.
2. Recognize names of assessments and evaluations used in general work evaluations.
3. Describe the purpose of a functional capacity evaluation.
4. Describe the services provided in work hardening programs.
5. Discuss the purpose of transitional work and modified duty programs.
6. Explain why and how pre-employment testing is conducted.
7. Discuss the concepts of "essential functions" and "reasonable accommodations."
8. Describe the process and requirements of a school-to-work transition program.
9. Explain how a work readiness program differs from other work programs.

Work is the major occupation of able-bodied adults and a cherished goal for many adults with disabilities. According to the Bureau of Labor Statistics (BLS), as of September 2010, the percentage of individuals without a disability in the labor force was 69.9. The unemployment rate for those with disabilities was 14.8%, compared with 9% for persons with no disability, not seasonally adjusted.[66] Occupational therapy (OT) practitioners are particularly suited to provide services to help individuals pursue their return to work goals throughout the lifespan, because of strong professional preparation in the nature of occupation, the analysis of activities, and the physical and mental factors that support engagement in occupation.

History of Occupational Therapy Involvement in Work Programs

OT has recognized and applied work as therapy since its founding.[23] Work programs for persons with mental illness began during the Moral Treatment movement, which started in Europe in the late eighteenth and early nineteenth centuries. The early leaders of OT identified the importance of work when they defined the profession's focus and purpose. Dr. Herbert Hall helped establish a medical workshop at Massachusetts General Hospital in Boston, where clients were involved in "work cure."[21] In this workshop, clients produced marketable goods and received a share of the profits. The focus of treatment in these curative workshops was to restore the impaired body part to as normal function as possible, with the goal of returning the client to work.

In the early 1900s the medical profession did not seem to consider vocational readiness programs important. The focus of care for persons with physical illnesses was primarily palliative, involving immobilization and bed rest. This attitude shifted after World War I with the need to rehabilitate large numbers of injured soldiers, to restore their functional capacities, and to help them gain employment.

The U.S. Federal Board for Vocational Education (FBVE) was created after the adoption of the Vocational Education Act of 1917.[29] In 1918 the Division of Orthopaedic Surgery in the Medical Department of the Army organized a reconstruction program for disabled soldiers, on which one of the founders of OT, Thomas Kidner, served as an advisor.[29] This program led to the development of a program to train reconstruction aides, precursors to occupational and physical therapists. Treatment involved both handicrafts and vocational education. The reconstruction aides used work activities to return as many as possible of the injured soldiers to military duty or civilian life.

In 1920 Congress passed the Civilian Rehabilitation Act of 1920 (Smith-Fess Act, Public Law 66-236). This law provided funds for vocational guidance and training, work adjustment, prostheses, and placement services.[29] If therapy was part of a medical treatment program, the law provided payment for OT services; however, it did not pay for physician services. Physicians either provided free services or received payment through state or volunteer contributions. This practice limited OT services in vocational rehabilitation to those states that supplemented federal program funds to support services such as the curative workshops. The Social Security Act of 1935 defined rehabilitation as "the rendering of a person disabled fit to engage in a renumerative occupation." This definition was the first attempt to provide vocational rehabilitation to the physically handicapped in the community.[36]

In 1937 industrial therapy (called "employment therapy") was born.[41] The occupational therapist used activities as treatment modalities. Patients commonly held work assignments in the hospital that matched their experience, aptitude, and interests. Sheltered work environments within the hospital including the hospital laundry, barber shop, and carpenter shop employed patients.

The term *prevocational* started appearing in the literature by the late 1930s. It referred to the use of "crafts to develop skills readily transferable to industry."[68] Prevocational therapy prepared patients for the work role. Occupational therapists worked as directors, work evaluators, and prevocational therapists within work programs. In the 1940s prevocational programs and work evaluation were accepted as part of OT practice. Patients in acute care facilities who were physically disabled were transferred to outpatient or rehabilitation prevocational and vocational programs.

World War II brought increased opportunity for OTs to become involved in work programs. With the advancement of medicine and pharmacology, many injured soldiers survived their wounds. Federal funding for rehabilitating the disabled veterans increased as the government discharged the disabled soldiers. Work programs were designed to evaluate and rehabilitate injured veterans.[13]

In 1943 the Barden-LaFollette Act (Public Law 78-113) modified the original provisions of the Civilian Rehabilitation Act of 1920.[29] This law, also known as the Vocational Rehabilitation Act, covered many medical services including OT and vocational guidance. Services were expanded to those with physical and mental limitations. The Barden-LaFollette Act also created the Office of Vocational Rehabilitation, a state and federally funded agency still in existence today. This agency provides disabled people with job training and placement services. Industrial therapy continued in various settings as a form of vocational rehabilitation.

During the 1950s many OTs believed that work evaluation belonged to the newly established profession of vocational rehabilitation rather than to OT.[41] OT involvement declined, and vocational counselors, vocational evaluators, and work adjusters became the leaders in this field. However, a few OTs remained active in work programming.

A high point in the development of prevocational exploration and training techniques in the field of OT occurred in 1960.[29] Thelma Wellerson and Bernard Rosenberg published an article on the development of the TOWER (*T*esting, *O*rientation, and *W*ork *E*valuation in *R*ehabilitation) system in New York.[29] The TOWER system was one of the first work sample programs to use real job samples in a simulated work environment.[29] Lilian S. Wegg gave the Eleanor Clarke Slagle Lecture on "Essentials of Work Evaluation," which was based on her experiences at the May T. Morrison Center for Rehabilitation in San Francisco. Wegg promoted OT involvement both in sound testing procedures and in training programs.[67] Florence S. Cromwell established norms for disabled populations on certain prevocational tests while evaluating the performance of adults with cerebral palsy at the United Cerebral Palsy Organization.[29] Cromwell continued to advocate for work-related therapy over the next few decades.

Occupational behavior theory, which emerged in the mid-1960s and early 1970s, offered a return to the profession's concern for occupation. Mary Reilly believed that productive activity as treatment was unique to OT.[29] Occupational behavior theory advocated that persons achieve healthy living only through a balance of work, rest, and play.

Increasing industrial development in the late 1970s and early 1980s opened up a whole new arena for occupational therapists and OT assistants (OTAs): industrial rehabilitation and work hardening.[29] Work hardening used actual work tasks in a simulated structured work environment, generally in community-based settings.[6] OT practitioners combined their knowledge of neuromuscular characteristics (including range of motion and endurance) with task analysis skills and knowledge of the psychosocial aspects of work. These foundation professional skills were invaluable in evaluating, planning, and implementing work hardening programs. In 1989 the Commission on Accreditation of Rehabilitation Facilities (CARF) developed work hardening standards that required an interdisciplinary approach, with a team comprising OTs, physical therapists, psychologists, and vocational specialists.[12]

The Americans with Disabilities Act of 1990 (ADA; Public Law 101-336) opened major markets for OTs.[29] Occupational therapists were involved with providing work training for persons with disabilities and provided assistance to employers with meeting the requirements of the ADA. This legislation continues to have important implications for work practice. The original law was revised in 2008 with the ADA Amendments Act (ADAAA, Public Law 110-325) to clarify and expand the meaning and application of the definition of disability.

In 1992 AOTA published a document called *Statement: Occupational Therapy Services in Work Practice,* which defined work as "all productive activities" and included life roles such as "homemaker, employee, volunteer, student, or hobbyist."[5] This document was replaced in 2000 by the AOTA's statement *Occupational Therapy Services in Facilitating Work*

Performance, which affirms that "occupational therapists and OTAs contribute to the delivery of services for the promotion and management of productive occupations, as well as the prevention and treatment of work-related disability."[4]A revision of *Occupational Therapy Services in Facilitating Work Performance* was issued by AOTA in 2005.[3]

In 2002 the Occupational Safety and Health Administration (OSHA) unveiled a comprehensive ergonomics approach aimed at reducing musculoskeletal disorders (MSDs) in the workplace. The four-pronged, comprehensive approach includes guidelines, enforcement, outreach and assistance, and a national advisory committee on ergonomics.[65] OT practitioners continue to consult employers and employees, making recommendations about equipment, posture, and body mechanics to prevent injuries. Ergonomic intervention continues to offer many opportunities for OT practitioners who have received additional training and education in this area.

Work and Industry has been identified as a key practice area in the twenty-first century by the American Occupational Therapy Association (AOTA) Centennial vision. The AOTA encourages OT practitioners to become involved in this practice area to help individuals participate in the worker role.

Role of the Occupational Therapy Assistant in Work Programs

OTAs play an important role in helping individuals participate in all aspects of work. According to the *Occupational Therapy Practice Framework: Domain and Process, 2nd ed,* work is defined by Mosey as "activities needed for engaging in renumerative employment or volunteer activities," which include the following: "employment interests and pursuits, employment seeking and acquisition, job performance, retirement preparation and adjustment, volunteer exploration, and volunteer participation."[2] The AOTA 2005 statement, *Occupational Therapy Services in Facilitating Work Performance,* documented that "occupational therapists and OT provide services to individuals or populations with deficits or problems in the area of work performance."[3] Whereas occupational therapists focus on identifying and analyzing problems, as well as selecting or designing appropriate assessments and interventions to address the problem, the OTA focuses on direct delivery of services and reporting and documenting client response and progress.[3,32] OTAs provide OT services under the supervision of and in collaboration with occupational therapists.[1]

OTAs provide work-related services in a variety of settings including, but not limited to, "acute care and rehabilitation facilities, industrial sites and office environments, psychiatric treatment centers, and in the community."[3]

Industrial Rehabilitation

The range of services provided to injured workers and industry is often described as industrial or occupational rehabilitation. The terms are used interchangeably in this chapter. Industrial rehabilitation includes vocational evaluation, functional capacity evaluation, job demands analysis, pre-employment screening, work hardening/conditioning, onsite rehabilitation, modified/transitional duty development, education, ergonomics, wellness, and preventive services. Occupational therapists and OTAs collaborate in providing these services, and this area of practice provides a tangible way for therapists to experience the tremendous reward of seeing lives changed through their efforts. The AOTA has developed a Work and Industry Special Interest Section (WISIS) for those who are involved with or who wish to know more about this area of specialization.

Vocational Evaluations

Work evaluations or vocational evaluations constitute "a comprehensive process that systematically uses work, real or simulated, as the focal point for vocational assessment and exploration to assist individuals in their vocational development."[18] According to CARF, the following factors are addressed in the traditional vocational evaluation model: physical and psychomotor capacities; intellectual capacities; emotional stability; interests, attitudes, and knowledge of occupational information; aptitudes and achievements (vocational and educational); work skills and work tolerances; work habits; work-related capabilities; and job-seeking skills.[25] This evaluation can take from 3 to 10 consecutive days to complete, depending on the goals of the assessment. Vocational evaluators generally conduct these types of assessments in private vocational agencies; however, some OTs (with OTAs) also conduct these evaluations in public and private medical or nonmedical settings. Vocational rehabilitation (VR), worker's compensation, and long-term disability carriers pay for these services, but most medical plans do not.

Standardized work samples are the primary tools used in a vocational evaluation. A work sample is a "well-defined work activity involving tasks, materials, and tools that are identical or similar to those in an actual job or cluster of jobs. Work samples are used to assess an individual's vocational aptitude, worker characteristics, and vocational interests."[26] Some of the more common work samples used by occupational therapists are the WEST system, Valpar Component Work Samples, and the Jewish Employment Vocational Services System (Figure 17-1). Dexterity tests such as the Bennett Hand Tool (Figure 17-2), Crawford Small Parts, and Purdue Pegboard evaluate motor skills.[25] When standardized work samples are not available to assess specific skills needed for a particular occupation, specially designed situational assessments are also used to create real-life work situations that are related to actual work tasks conducted on particular jobs. For example, a person who is interested in working as a floral arranger could be evaluated on his or her motor skills to determine the presence of the coordination, energy, and strength and effort to grip and manipulate tools to cut the stems of flowers and plants and arrange them in floral containers. Individuals can also be evaluated in real worksites and perform actual job tasks that one would perform on the job.

Two different types of vocational evaluations are common: *general* and *specific.* A general vocational evaluation is a comprehensive assessment of a person's potential to do any type of work. For an individual who has never worked, does not have a job to which to return, or cannot return to the previous job because of disability, this type of evaluation helps determine aptitudes, abilities, and interests. It yields a range of reasonable options for work. For example, the treating physician of a person who worked as a truck driver and suffered a traumatic brain injury that resulted in cognitive and physical limitations (including seizure precautions) advised the patient to pursue a different line of work. This patient could benefit from a general vocational evaluation to help identify other vocational interests and abilities by exploring cognitive and motor skills and physical and mental tolerances that could be applied to a different occupation.

A specific vocational evaluation assesses a person's readiness to return to a particular occupation. For a person who had a stroke and wants to return to work as a general office clerk, a specifically tailored vocational evaluation to assess the person's ability to return to this particular type of work is necessary. Clerical work samples and specially designed situational assessments that assess the person's ability to multitask, pay attention to detail, file, answer a telephone, and take messages can be incorporated into the vocational evaluation.

OTAs who have received additional training in standardized work samples and vocational assessments can assist in conducting portions of a vocational evaluation. The occupational therapist or vocational evaluator conducts the initial intake and writes the final report that analyzes and summarizes the test results and provides specific recommendations toward a work goal.

Functional Capacity Evaluation

A functional capacity evaluation (FCE) is an objective assessment of an individual's ability to perform work-related activity.[19,35] These functionally based tests have been used since the early 1970s for making decisions about returning to work. At that time, primarily occupational and physical therapists performed FCEs.[27] Today, the FCE can be used in many different ways and can be performed by practitioners from many disciplines. Occupational therapists are remarkably qualified to conduct FCEs due to their education and background in

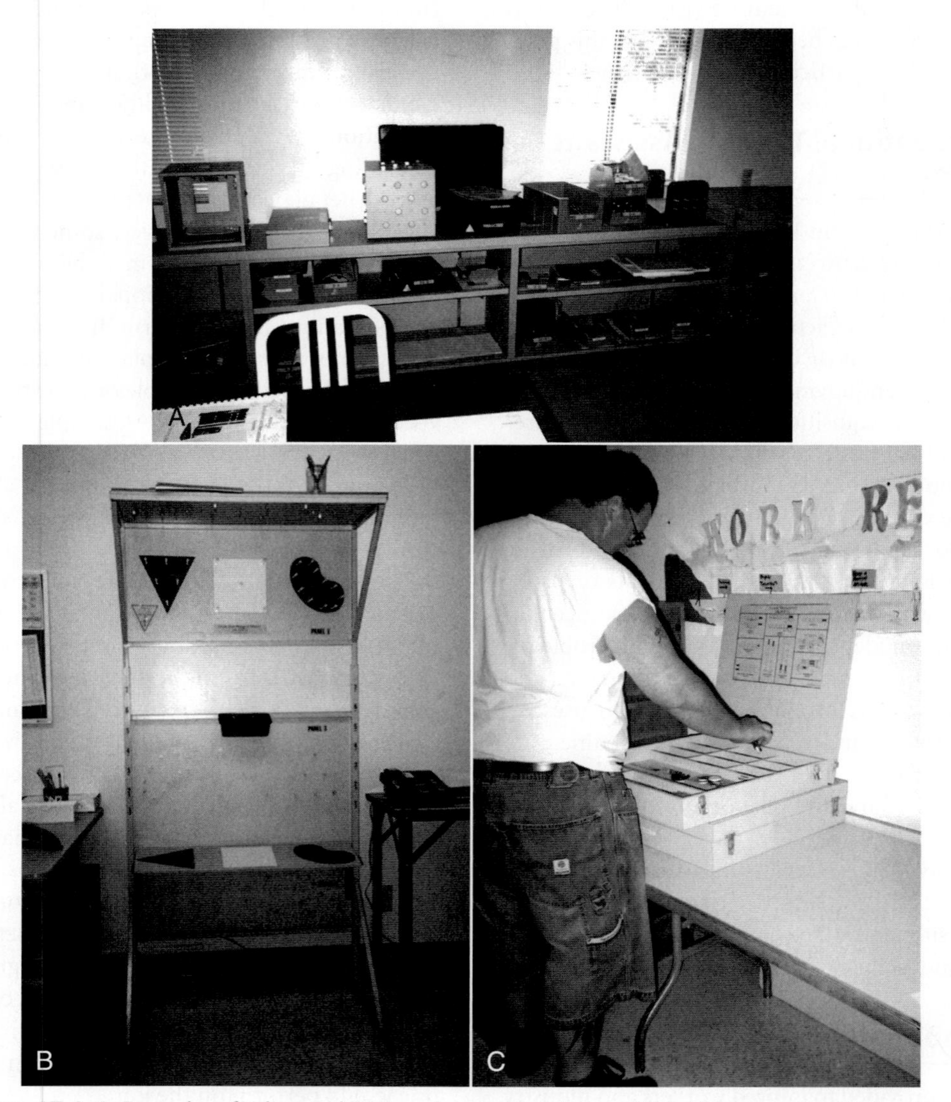

Figure 17-1 **A,** Examples of Valpar and JEVS work samples. **B,** Valpar 9 Total Body Range of Motion is used to evaluate functional abilities such as standing, bending, crouching, reaching, and gross manipulation and handling. **C,** Valpar 10 is used to evaluate a person's ability to follow a multistep sequence to inspect metal parts with various jigs and tools.

task analysis.[2,4] In many states, OTAs and physical therapy assistants can participate in the portions of the FCE that do not require interpretation. The FCE can be used to set goals for rehabilitation and readiness for returning to work, assess residual work capacity, determine disability status, screen for physical compatibility before hiring a new employee, and summarize the person's status for case closure.[50] An FCE usually comprises review of medical records, interview, musculoskeletal screening, evaluation of physical performance, formation of recommendations, and report generation.[31] The evaluation of physical performance may involve assessing the client's physiology including cardiovascular (i.e., blood pressure and heart rate response), biomechanics, and muscular endurance over the course of strength, position tolerance, and mobility tasks. The tested tasks reflect the physical demands required for the client's job, or the evaluation may be generic in terms of assessing physical performance. The report usually contains information regarding the overall level of work, tolerance for work over the course of a day, individual task scores, job match information, level of client participation (cooperative or self-limiting), and interventions for consideration.[31,33]

A wide variety of FCEs are currently used in practice including both commercially available systems and evaluations developed by individual therapists or clinics (Box 17-1, Figure 17-3). A well-designed FCE is comprehensive, standardized, practical, objective, reliable, and valid.[31,33,54]

A comprehensive FCE will include all the physical demands of work as defined by the *Dictionary of Occupational Titles*, published by the U.S. Department of Labor, last revised in 1991[64] (Box 17-2). The evaluation also needs to be practical in

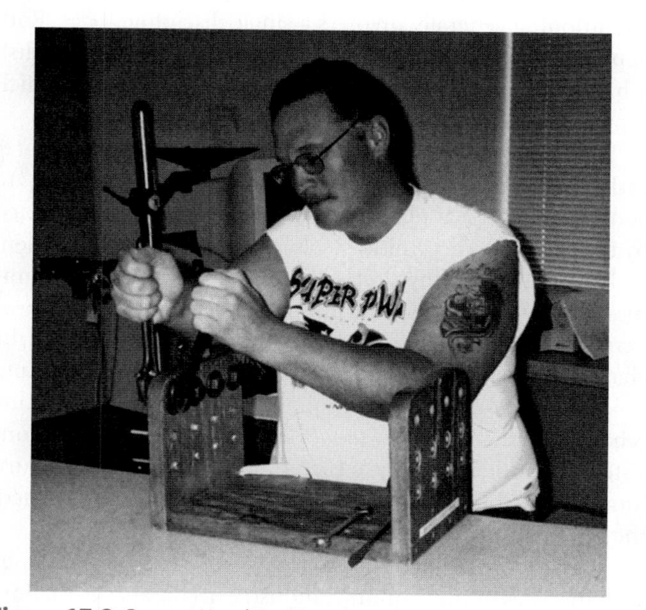

Figure 17-2 Bennet Hand Tool is a dexterity test to assess a person's ability to use hand tools.

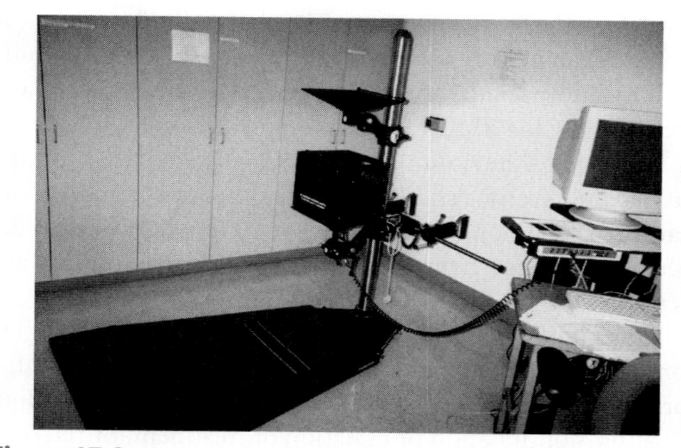

Figure 17-3 An example of a functional capacity evaluation system (BTE Technologies Focus System).

Box 17-1

Various Functional Capacity Evaluation Systems

- Blankenship
- BTE Technologies
- DSI
- Ergoscience
- Evaluwriter
- J-Tech
- Key
- Matheson
- Medigraph
- Occucare
- Procomp
- Valpar-Joule
- West/Epic
- Workhab
- Worksteps
- Workwell

Box 17-2

Twenty Physical Demands of Work

- Lifting
- Standing
- Walking
- Sitting
- Carrying
- Pushing
- Pulling
- Climbing
- Balancing
- Stooping
- Kneeling
- Crouching
- Crawling
- Reaching
- Handling
- Fingering
- Feeling
- Talking
- Hearing
- Seeing

From U.S. Department of Labor, Employment and Training Administration: *Revised dictionary of occupational titles*, vol 1 and 2, ed 4, Washington, DC, 1991, U.S. Government Printing Office.

length of testing, cost, space, and report generation.[33,50] Standardization results in having a procedure manual, task definitions and instructions, a scoring methodology, and equipment requirements and setup.[33,35,50] This structure ensures fair and consistent assessment and minimizes subjectivity. Objectivity during the course of the FCE does not preclude clinical judgment and decision making, but it does require client cooperation during testing, as well as a measure as free as possible of examiner bias for documenting physical performance.[54]

The most important aspects of FCE are reliability and validity of the testing protocol. Establishing reliability is the first step in determining validity, or accuracy of the results. Once reliability has been proven, validity can be assessed. The term **validity** has been used in many ways, often with a significance placed on issues surrounding sincerity of effort. In scientific terms, validity means accuracy. It asks the question "does the FCE provide results that truly describe how the client can perform at work?"[33,54] The first FCE to be studied for validity and published in peer-reviewed literature was developed by the occupational therapist Susan Smith. It was an important contribution to the knowledge base.[58] Without reliability and validity, a referral source cannot know that the results of the evaluation would not vary if the individual were tested by another therapist or if the results are accurate.[31,33,35]

The FCE is a tremendous tool in the course of rehabilitation. It provides a therapist with objective findings that support thoughtful and appropriate recommendations regarding initiation, continuation or cessation of treatment, or referrals to another service. Because of their enormous influence on a patient's life, valid results, carefully documented, must be ensured.[31,33]

Work Hardening and Work Conditioning

Work hardening refers to formal, multidisciplinary programs for rehabilitating the injured worker.[15,30,34,48] The idea of using work for rehabilitation is at the core of OT. Restoring function to all areas of life—work, leisure, and self-care—is the basic goal of the profession.[48] In the 1970s occupational rehabilitation was seen as a means for improving strategies to control work-related injuries.[15,30,34,48] Leonard Matheson was first to illustrate work hardening.[30,34,48] The goal then, as now, was to rehabilitate injured workers, maximize their function, and return them to work as quickly and safely as possible. The delivery system for this type of rehabilitation has evolved over time from a lengthy hospital-based program, to structured interdisciplinary programs in outpatient settings, to the more progressive partnership between outpatient intervention and transitional work. We now see rehabilitation occurring at the workplace in company-sponsored clinics. In the 1980s CARF developed guidelines for work-hardening programs and offered certification for a fee through adherence to their guidelines and periodic survey.[15,30,34,48] In 1991 a committee from the American Physical Therapy Association (APTA) developed another set of principles for clinics that wanted to follow recognized standards but did not adopt CARF's accreditation process.[15,30,34]

The disciplines represented on the work-hardening team may include occupational and physical therapists and assistants, psychologists, vocational evaluators and counselors, licensed practical counselors, addiction counselors, exercise physiologists, and dieticians.[15,30,34] The programs typically range from 4 to 8 weeks, with entry and exit evaluation (usually FCE or a derivative thereof), a job site evaluation, graded activity, work simulation, strength and cardiovascular conditioning, education, individualized goal setting, and program modification. The goal is return to work at either full or modified duty.[15,30,34] Actual equipment from the job is preferred during the work simulation in order to maximize the cooperation of the worker and more closely replicate the actual demands of the job.[30] **Work conditioning** is more often defined as physical conditioning alone. It covers strength, aerobic fitness, flexibility, coordination, and endurance. Work conditioning generally involves a single discipline.[15,30,34] Both approaches involve evaluation of the worker to establish a baseline from which to plan treatment and against which progress can be measured.

Ensuring positive outcomes for the injured worker requires early intervention and a customized plan of treatment to address the various physical and psychosocial areas affected by the injury.[57] The multidisciplinary team allows the patient to benefit from many areas of expertise that share a common goal. Intervening and initiating the rehabilitation program as soon as possible after injury dramatically increase the chances for a successful return to work. Transitional work and modified-duty programs combine or progress through acute rehabilitation and return to work; they move at a pace consistent with the individual's current ability and seek to return him or her to full work duty. If this goal cannot be reached, they strive to maximize the individual's work capacity.

Industrial rehabilitation programs will continue to change with the tides of the economy, industry needs, and legislation. Occupational therapists and OTAs are vital in shaping and directing the changes that await us.

Job Demands Analysis

Assessing the physical demands of a job often benefits rehabilitation because recommendations for initial evaluation or return to work require objective information about the client's abilities and the job itself. A well-written job description that includes the essential tasks of the job, physical requirements, cognitive aptitudes, educational requirements, equipment operated, and environmental exposures assists in selecting suitable candidates for employment, setting compensation packages, and making appropriate return-to-work decisions after an injury.[10]

Approaches to **job demands analysis** (JDA) include questionnaires, interview, observation, and formal measurement.[10] Interviewing incumbents (workers occupying the same or similar jobs) or supervisors about the job requirements is common,[49] yet however interesting the interviews, such an informal approach often leads to narrative descriptions with little functional information and questionable accuracy of demand estimates.[24,42,49] As with other types of assessment, an objective process for analyzing the demands of the job is important. A standardized classification system with consistent terminology is crucial to making the assessment understandable to a range of professionals. The *Dictionary of Occupational Titles* (DOT) defines the physical demands of work and defines occupations in the United States.[63] Tables 17-1 through 17-3 list some common terms and classifications from the DOT. The DOT provides definitions for the overall level of work, the strength demands, and the frequencies for the physical demands.[63,64]

Jobs comprise the tasks that are performed, the physical demands of those tasks, and the frequency of the physical demands including weights handled, forces exerted, and distances ambulated and reached.[10] The frequency of each physical demand must be weighted according to a common standard for the given duration of each task because there is often significant difference in the amount of time spent in each task during the workday. For example, the job of "loader" in ABC warehouse comprises two tasks: (1) loading crates with boxes and (2) wrapping the crate with packing tape after it is loaded. The "loader" completes 48 cycles of loading and taping in an 8-hour shift, and loading the crate takes approximately 80% of the work shift. The boxes weigh 10 lb each. To correctly assess the overall level of work, the occupational therapist must determine the amount of weight lifted and the frequency of the manual materials handling.

Task 1 presents the physical demands of lifting, carrying, stooping, walking, reaching, handling, and standing. Task 2 has the demands of walking, reaching, handling, fingering, and standing. To total the amount of the physical demands for the job of "loader," one must determine how much time is spent in each physical demand within each task and then account for the proportion of the time that the task is performed during the workday. This type of assessment can be

Table 17-1 Definitions for Overall Level of Work

Level of Work	Definition
Sedentary	Exerting up to 10 pounds of force occasionally or a negligible amount of force frequently to lift, carry, push, pull or otherwise move objects, including the human body. Sedentary work involves sitting most of the time but may involve walking or standing for brief periods of time. Jobs are sedentary if walking and standing are required only occasionally, but all other sedentary criteria are met.
Light	Exerting up to 20 pounds of force occasionally, or up to 10 pounds of force frequently, or a negligible amount of force constantly to move objects. Physical demand requirements are in excess of those for sedentary work. Although the weight lifted may be only a negligible amount, a job should be rated light work when it requires walking or standing to a significant degree, when it requires sitting most of the time but entails pushing or pulling of arm or leg controls, or when the job requires working at a production rate pace entailing the constant pushing or pulling of materials even though the weight of those materials is negligible. NOTE: The constant stress and strain of maintaining a production rate pace, especially in an industrial setting, can be physically demanding of a worker even if the amount of force exerted is negligible.
Medium	Exerting 20 to 50 pounds of force occasionally, 10 to 25 pounds of force frequently, or greater than negligible up to 10 pounds of force constantly to move objects. Physical demand requirements are in excess of those for light work.
Heavy	Exerting 50 to 100 pounds of force occasionally, 25 to 50 pounds of force frequently, or 10 to 20 pounds of force constantly to move objects. Physical demand requirements are in excess of those for medium work.
Very Heavy	Exerting force in excess of 100 pounds of force occasionally, more than 50 pounds of force frequently, or more than 20 pounds of force constantly to move objects. Physical demand requirements are in excess of those for heavy work.

Data compiled from US Department of Labor, Employment and Training Administration: *Revised dictionary of occupational titles*, Vol. I & II, ed 4, Washington, DC, 1991, US Government Printing Office; US Department of Labor, Employment and Training Administration: *The revised handbook for analyzing jobs*, Indianapolis, 1991, JIST Works.

Table 17-2 Definitions for Physical Demand Frequencies

Physical Demand Frequency	Definition
Never	Activity or condition does not exist
Occasionally	Up to 1/3 of the day
Frequently	1/3 to 2/3 of the day
Constantly	2/3 to full day

Data compiled from US Department of Labor, Employment and Training Administration: *Revised dictionary of occupational titles*, Vol. I & II, ed 4, Washington, DC, 1991, US Government Printing Office; US Department of Labor, Employment and Training Administration: *The revised handbook for analyzing jobs*, Indianapolis, 1991, JIST Works.

Table 17-3 Strength Demands of Work

	FREQUENCY OF FORCE EXERTION OR WEIGHT CARRIED		
Strength Rating	Occasional (up to 1/3 of the day)	Frequent (1/3 to 2/3 of the day)	Constant (over 2/3 of the day)
Sedentary	10 lbs.	Negligible	Negligible
Light	20 lbs.	10 lbs.	Negligible
Medium	20-50 lbs.	10-25 lbs.	10 lbs.
Heavy	50-100 lbs.	25-50 lbs.	10-20 lbs.
Very Heavy	Over 100 lbs.	50-100 lbs.	20-50 lbs.

Data from US Department of Labor, Employment and Training Administration: *Revised dictionary of occupational titles*, Vol. I & II, ed 4, Washington, DC, 1991, US Government Printing Office.

performed manually, as well as with the application of various software protocols available in the marketplace.

Whatever methods they use, clinicians should strive toward an accurate picture of the job and its requirements. An emphasis on functional demands makes for an easier application in the rehabilitation continuum.

Pre-Employment Testing

Functional testing commonly focuses on assessing a person's ability to meet certain physical requirements before he or she is hired for a job.[51] Pre-employment testing can consist of isometric testing, range-of-motion testing, or actual measurement of a person's ability to perform selected tasks from the job description. Pre-employment screening can be integral to a company's comprehensive injury prevention and management strategy.[51] Because of their task analysis training and holistic approach, OTs and OTAs are excellent candidates for assisting companies with the expansion of plans to more effectively manage employee injuries.

From a business perspective, a company must take the time to thoroughly develop its screening process and be able to defend the necessity of the screening. Company representatives should be prepared to explain and demonstrate the applicability of the screen to the job in question.[51] Pre-employment testing can also occur at several points in the hiring process; however, many health care providers and legal experts recommend such testing occur after an offer of employment.[22,37] A conditional offer is extended to the applicant based on the applicant's ability to meet a variety of conditions such as passing a drug screen, acceptable background check, and physical testing.

If the applicant passes the screening, then he or she is hired and begins working. If the applicant does not pass, the employer must assess whether the applicant has a disability, as defined under the Americans with Disabilities Amendments Act of 2008 (ADAAA).[7] If a disability exists, the employer must determine whether to offer reasonable accommodation to the applicant so that he or she can perform the job. "Reasonable" means that the accommodation does not place the employer under undue financial strain. If the company offers accommodation to the applicant, the hiring process is completed and employment begins. If the company cannot offer reasonable accommodation or if the applicant does not have a disability but fails the screening nonetheless, the employer can choose to rescind the offer of employment, examine opportunities for alternative placement elsewhere in the company, or offer remediation of some type. If certain criteria are met, the company may allow the applicant to retest.[51]

Once jobs are selected for testing, their respective physical demands must be evaluated. This evaluation can be done by survey, questionnaire, or observation—either directly or by video.[10] The job description must include information about physical demands and describe the essential tasks of the job. It must be written clearly so that one can test for an individual's ability to perform job tasks that are specific to this job.[10] The selection of a reliable and valid method for testing an individual's ability is crucial. Such a method may include a standardized battery of physical demand tests or job-specific tasks developed to improve the applicant's understanding of the relevance of the task and the company's defensibility about hiring decisions.[17,51] The clinician must encourage companies to have written policies regarding the screening process including screening failures.[51] Continuing documentation and follow-up help to develop a definitive paper trail that establishes the business necessity of a pre-employment screening process, the steps taken to select and analyze the job and tasks to be tested, the implementation phase, and ongoing quality assurance to monitor any changes in the job and reflect subsequent changes in the screen.[51]

Worksite Evaluations

Worksite evaluations are on-the-job assessments to determine whether an individual can return to work after onset of a disability or can benefit from reasonable accommodations to maintain employment.[28] Consider, for example, a man who worked at a manufacturing company as a machine operator before his stroke. The man's employer is willing to take him back as long as he can meet the physical and cognitive demands of the job. An OTA can go to the worksite with an occupational therapist or another member of the vocational rehabilitation team to help evaluate the person's ability to operate the machinery and carry out the essential functions of the job. Another example might be a woman who worked previously as an office clerk without any difficulties but whose postpolio syndrome now causes extreme fatigue, pain, and muscle weakness with repetitive tasks. She could benefit from a worksite evaluation to identify reasonable accommodations to allow her to continue her job while minimizing her symptoms. Along with the work, the occupational therapist assesses several factors at the worksite including the essential functions of the job, the functional assets and limitations of the worker, and the physical environment of the workplace.[39]

A worksite evaluation is usually conducted after a job analysis. Larger companies may already have specific job analyses. If no job analysis exists and if the employer is willing, the occupational therapist can conduct one; alternately, a job description could be obtained from the employer before the occupational therapist goes to the worksite. If no written job description exists, a phone interview with the worker's supervisor or manager should elicit information regarding the essential functions and physical and cognitive requirements of the job. After this information is obtained, the occupational therapist schedules a time to meet at the worksite with the employer and the worker.

Taking photographs or video recordings at the worksite can be useful; however, permission must be obtained from both the employer and the worker. The OTA should also bring a tape measure to measure heights of work surfaces, widths of doorways, and so on, depending on the person's needs. Drawing a layout of the work area, using graph paper to draw the room to scale, is also helpful, especially when the worker requires a wheelchair. Critical measurements can be recorded on the diagram.

The worksite evaluation determines whether the person can carry out the essential functions of the job safely and adequately with or without any reasonable accommodations. Ergonomic principles (addressed in the following section) should be considered and applied when the occupational therapist is recommending reasonable accommodations. Identifying reasonable accommodations requires cooperation between the person with the disability, the employer, and the occupational therapist or OTA.[52] Each person has valuable insights and information to contribute to the process of identifying the best accommodations. The Job Accommodation Network (JAN), a product of the President's Committee for the Employment of People with Disabilities, is the best resource for assisting employers and disabled workers with reasonable accommodations.[55] Their website (http://askjan.org/) points out that most job accommodations are not expensive. According to JAN, more than half of all accommodations cost under $500. They can involve any of the following: altering the job duties or work schedule, modifying the facility, purchasing adaptive equipment or providing assistive technology, or modifying or designing a new product. After the worksite evaluation is completed, the OTA helps prepare the report, which is then sent to the qualified employee, the referring party, and the employer. The problem areas that relate to the essential job functions should be clearly listed, as should the accommodations necessary to solve them. If training is necessary for use of a recommended accommodation, sources for the training should be identified. If commercially available equipment is recommended, exact model numbers, local sources, and approximate expenses should be provided.[61] If custom equipment needs to be fabricated, the report should include sources, cost estimates, and the amount of time required to fabricate the equipment. The report should summarize the evaluation findings and the recommended accommodations.

Ergonomic and Injury Prevention Consultation

The term ergonomics comes from the Greek words *ergos,* meaning "work," and *nomos,* meaning "laws." Thus the term represents the laws of work.[16] OT practitioners use the science of ergonomics to assist clients to fully engage in work. Ergonomics addresses human performance and well-being in relation to occupational tasks, equipment, tools, and the environment. The science of ergonomics seeks to improve the health, safety, and efficiency of both the worker and the workplace.[43] Corporate clients increasingly seek the assistance of professionals trained in ergonomics to improve the fit between workers and their jobs. OT practitioners are uniquely qualified to fulfill this role.[7]

Work settings and work processes are often designed to satisfy space and budget limitations and the demands of productivity and aesthetics. When designs fail to consider the people who will use the work settings and processes, musculoskeletal strain and inefficiency can result. Every worker brings his or her own unique set of performance skills, performance patterns, and client factors to the workplace. Matching individual employees' strengths and limitations with the context and activity demands of the job can improve both worker comfort and workplace productivity.[38,62]

The principles of ergonomics address a wide variety of work-related issues. Common issues include workplace and work process design, work-related stress, the disabled and aging workforces, tool and equipment design, and architectural design and accessibility. Ergonomic intervention can be applied proactively by preventing problems before they occur or reactively by addressing worker-job "fit" problems after an injury or other problem is identified.[20]

An example of an ergonomic intervention strategy is modifying the style of a tool handle to help a worker's wrist stay in a neutral, more comfortable position. The modification could occur before an employee's first day at work, in a proactive effort to prevent wrist injury. On the other hand, the tool might be modified only after a worker suffers a wrist injury. This step would be a reactive adjustment to the injury itself. Regardless of the timing, the tool modification helps to improve the fit between the worker and his or her job.

In 2004 the AOTA identified ergonomics consulting as one of the top six emerging practice areas for the profession of OT.[40] The OTA interested in the field of ergonomics will find that the holistic nature of OT training is an asset. The OT practitioner uses his or her knowledge of the human body, psychosocial issues, and creative problem solving to help make the work environment safer and more efficient.

OT practitioners are not, however, the only professionals suited to provide ergonomic consultation services. Ergonomics consultants come from a variety of academic fields. Backgrounds in engineering, business administration, computer science, industrial hygiene, psychology, or architecture are also good foundations for a career in ergonomics.[14] Regardless of one's academic degree, training beyond college graduation is generally required to begin working in the field. Box 17-3 outlines a variety of ways to gain advanced training in ergonomics.[59]

Many occupational therapists and OTAs provide ergonomic consultation as part of work hardening, traditional rehabilitation, or wellness and prevention programs. These OT practitioners may only require a few weekends of continuing education courses to master basic ergonomic intervention skills. A smaller number of OTs and OTAs actually specialize in ergonomics and, with a significant amount of advanced training, become professional ergonomists. These practitioners generally seek board certification as a Certified Professional Ergonomist.

OT practitioners might provide ergonomic consultation under the umbrella of OT services or as an independent ergonomic consultant or injury-prevention specialist. When ergonomic consultation is delivered as an OT service, OTAs act under the supervision of and in partnership with an occupational therapist. The OTA contributes to the ergonomic risk factor assessment process as delegated by the occupational therapist and also provides input into the intervention plan. The OTA will then assist the occupational therapist in implementing ergonomic intervention strategies and outcome measurements. The occupational therapist–OTA partnership can be especially rewarding in the area of ergonomic consultation services because of the tremendous need for detailed problem

Box 17-3

Education and Training Opportunities in Ergonomics

Education and training beyond occupational therapy entry-level practice is necessary for achieving advanced competence in ergonomics.

- University-sponsored graduate certificate programs in ergonomics are available through Texas Women's University, Cleveland State University, University of Central Florida, and the University of Massachusetts. These graduate-level courses typically require four to five courses for a total of 12 to 16 credit hours.
- Continuing education providers offer several-day courses that earn the occupational therapist eligibility for certifications such as the Ergonomics Evaluation Specialist available through Roy Matheson and Associates, Inc. (www.roymatheson.com) and the Certified Ergonomics Assessment Specialist available through the Back School of Atlanta (www.backschoolofatlanta.com).
- The Oxford Research Institute (www.oxfordresearch.org) offers the following advanced-level certifications: Certified Industrial Ergonomist, Certified Associate Ergonomist, and Certified Human Factors Engineering Professional.
- The Board of Certification in Professional Ergonomics (BCPE) (www.bcpe.org) offers the highest level of certification in the field of ergonomics: the Certified Professional Ergonomist. Other advanced-level certifications available through the BCPE include Associate Ergonomics Professional, Certified Ergonomics Associate, Certified Human Factors Professional, and Associate Human Factors Professional.

From Snodgrass J: Getting comfortable: developing a clinical specialty in ergonomics has its own challenges and rewards, *Rehab Manag* July:24-27, 2004.

solving. The team approach almost always heightens creativity and minimizes oversight.

OTAs with appropriate skills and aptitudes can also act as independent ergonomic consultants or injury-prevention specialists outside the arena of OT. The education of OTAs opens up new avenues of employment that are independent of the field of OT. The traditional occupational therapist–OTA supervision model does not apply when the services rendered are not called OT or billed as OT services.

An OTA could obtain advanced training in ergonomics, safety, and/or injury prevention and then offer his or her services to corporate clients as an independent contractor. Practitioners who pursue this avenue of independent practice should clarify with their state regulatory agencies and review their states' OT practice acts for specific guidelines regarding use of the OTA title while working in this area.[1]

One of the most common reasons that a corporate client seeks the services of an ergonomic specialist or injury prevention consultant is work-related musculoskeletal disorders. Work-related musculoskeletal disorders account for approximately one third of all occupational injuries and illnesses reported to the U.S. Bureau of Labor Statistics, and employers annually pay more than $45 billion in workers compensation and other associated expenses associated with these disorders.[9] These statistics indicate that work-related musculoskeletal disorders are at crisis level in the workplace. The financial losses to individuals, industry, and the economy are great. However, these monetary losses pale in comparison to the physical and emotional suffering endured by injured workers.

Work-related musculoskeletal disorders (MSDs) are a class of soft tissue injuries that affect the muscles, tendons, and nerves. These disorders come on slowly and develop over time as a result of repeated microtraumas to the body. They occur when the body is denied the opportunity to adequately rest and repair itself. The term *work-related musculoskeletal disorder* is the most current terminology. These same disorders have also been called *cumulative trauma disorders* (CTDs) or *repetitive strain injuries* (RSIs). Common diagnoses within this class of disorders are carpal tunnel syndrome, De Quervain's tendonitis, lateral epicondylitis (i.e., "tennis elbow"), and some back injuries.[53]

Research has identified specific physical activity demands that place people at risk for developing work-related musculoskeletal disorders. Risk factors include repetition, force, awkward or static posturing, prolonged direct pressure on soft tissue, vibration, exposure to cold, and inappropriate or inadequate hand tools.[44-47,53] Additionally, psychosocial stressors at work are thought to contribute to these disorders.[11] Stressors might include excessive volume or productivity expectations, work that is beyond the emotional or intellectual capacity of the employee, or working for a superior who does not express appropriate appreciation. The ergonomics consultant must address a combination of physical and psychosocial risk factors as part of a successful injury-prevention program.

The goal of ergonomic intervention is to reduce or eliminate risk factors for development of work-related musculoskeletal disorders as soon as they are identified—whether the ergonomic consultation occurs proactively or reactively after a worker's injury. The ergonomic consultant identifies risk factors and suggests possible strategies to control them. Risk-factor control strategies can be categorized as engineering controls, work practice controls, administrative controls, and personal protective equipment.[47]

Engineering controls include strategies for designing or modifying the workstation, work methods, and/or tools. The goal is to eliminate or reduce excessive exertion, awkward postures, and repetition. Workstations should be designed or modified to accommodate the actual worker at the workstation. If more than one person uses a workstation, elements of the workstation should be adjustable to each worker. Work methods should be designed or modified to minimize static and awkward posturing, repetitive motions, and excessive force. Tools and handles should be designed for a specific job to minimize contact stress, vibration, and forceful motion by the workers' hands.[47]

Work practice controls include policy and procedures for safe and proper task performance. Workers should receive training in proper body mechanics, tool maintenance, and workstation adjustability features. New workers and workers who have been away from their jobs for a while should be allowed adequate break-in periods to condition their bodies

Box 17-4

OSHA and NIOSH

The Occupational Safety and Health Act of 1970 created both the National Institute for Occupational Safety and Health (NIOSH) and the Occupational Safety and Health Administration (OSHA). Although NIOSH and OSHA were created by the same Act of Congress, they are two distinct agencies with separate responsibilities.

OSHA is under the U.S. Department of Labor and, as a regulatory agency, is responsible for developing and enforcing workplace safety and health regulations. OSHA developed the following publication guidelines to assist industries in developing in-house ergonomic programs:

- Ergonomic Program Management Guidelines for Meatpacking Plants (1993) (OSHA Publication 3123)
- Guidelines for Nursing Homes: Ergonomics for the Prevention of Musculoskeletal Disorders (Revised 2009) (OSHA Publication 3182)
- Guidelines for Retail Grocery Stores: Ergonomics for the Prevention of Musculoskeletal Disorders (2004) (OSHA Publication 3192-05N)
- Guidelines for Poultry Processing: Ergonomics for the Prevention of Musculoskeletal Disorders (2004) (OSHA Publication 3213-09N)
- Guidelines for Shipyards: Ergonomics for the Prevention of Musculoskeletal Disorders (2008) (OSHA Publication 3341-03N)

These publications can be ordered at www.osha.gov or by calling 1-800-321-OSHA.

NIOSH is part of the Centers for Disease Control and Prevention (CDC) within the U.S. Department of Health and Human Services. NIOSH is an agency established to conduct research and make recommendations for preventing work-related injury and illness. NIOSH and OSHA often work together toward the common goal of protecting worker safety and health.

NIOSH currently offers several publications to assist with ergonomic intervention efforts. The following may be of interest to OTAs wanting to get involved with ergonomics:

- Elements of Ergonomic Programs: A Primer Based on Workplace Evaluations of Musculoskeletal Disorders (1997) (NIOSH Publication 97-117)
- Simple Solutions: Ergonomics for Construction Workers (2007) (NIOSH Publication 2007-122)
- Ergonomic Guidelines for Manual Material Handling (2007) (NIOSH Publication 2007-131)
- Safe Lifting and Movement of Nursing Home Residents (2006) (NIOSH Publication 2006-117)
- Conference Proceedings: Prevention of Musculoskeletal Disorders for Children and Adolescents Working in Agriculture (2004) (NIOSH Publication 2004-119)
- Easy Ergonomics: A Guide to Selecting Non-Powered Hand Tools (2004) (NIOSH Publication 2004-164)
- Simple Solutions: Ergonomics for Farm Workers (2001) (NIOSH Publication 2001-111)
- Ergonomic Interventions for the Soft Drink Beverage Delivery Industry (1996) (NIOSH Publication 96-109)

These publications (and others) can be ordered from the CDC-NIOSH website: http://www.cdc.gov/niosh/ or by calling NIOSH at 1-800-CDC-INFO (1-800-232-4636); outside the United States, 513-533-8328.

to the physical demands of the work. Management should constantly monitor the use and effectiveness of work practice controls and adjust techniques, production rates, and staffing as needed to maintain a safe and healthy work environment.[47]

Selection and use of personal protective equipment should be specific to the task. Equipment should be available in a variety of sizes to accommodate the size difference between workers. Proper fit is especially important for gloves. Poorly fitting gloves can reduce blood flow and sensory feedback, leading to slippage and use of excessive grip and pinch forces. Protection against cold temperatures less than 40° F is required to protect joints and soft tissues. Back braces and upper extremity splints should not be considered personal protective equipment. These devices should be used only with the advice and under the supervision of employee health personnel.[47]

Finally, administrative controls are an option when musculoskeletal injury risk factors cannot be adequately reduced or eliminated via engineering controls, work practice controls, and personal protective equipment. Administrative controls reduce duration, frequency, and severity of exposure to risk factors. Methods include decreasing production rates, limiting overtime work, providing periodic rest breaks throughout the day, increasing staffing levels, and using job rotation/job enlargement to include other jobs and tasks that use different muscle-tendon groups.[47]

Many resources are available for the OTA interested in learning more about ergonomics and injury-prevention programs. The U.S. Occupational Safety and Health Administration (OSHA) and the National Institute for Occupational Safety and Health (NIOSH) serve as excellent starting points. In the 1990s and the early 2000s, these government agencies developed guidelines and recommendations for public and private sector organizations seeking assistance in establishing musculoskeletal injury prevention programs. Informational booklets available through OSHA and NIOSH are a good resource for OT practitioners who want to provide ergonomic and injury-prevention consultation services to industry. Box 17-4 offers information on OSHA and NIOSH and provides a partial listing of their ergonomic and injury-prevention program resource material.

Transition Services from School to Work

OTAs can make a valuable contribution to students with disabilities transitioning from school to the community. The 1997 amendments to the Individuals with Disabilities Education Act (IDEA) of 1990 specified that transition planning is to be part of the Individualized Education Program (IEP). Representatives from community agencies that provide post-school services such as state-sponsored vocational rehabilitation must join the education team. Related services such as OT must serve as formal contributors to transition planning for students who need these services.[60] IDEA defines transition services as "a coordinated set of activities for a student designed within an outcome-oriented process, which promotes movement from school to post-school activities, includes postsecondary education, vocational training, integrated employment (included supported employment), continuing and adult education, adult services, independent living, or community participation."[59] OT's unique focus on occupational performance can be a strong asset to the transition team.

The three main roles in which an OT practitioner participates are transition-related evaluation, service planning, and service implementation. The OTA is primarily involved in service implementation, whereas the occupational therapist is primarily responsible for the evaluation and service planning. The OT practitioner contributes vital information about students' performance abilities and needs in any of the transition domains: domestic, vocational, school, recreation, and community.

Transition-Related Evaluation

Effective transition-related evaluation primarily uses nonstandardized interviews, situational observation, and activity analysis approaches. These approaches are top-down, meaning that they first consider what the student wants or needs to do and secondarily identify the occupational performance issues that are causing difficulties.[8] The transition team helps the student identify a positive, shared vision for the future. This can include living alone or with others in the community, attending postsecondary schools or training programs, working in a paid or volunteer job, using community services, and participating in activities of interest. The occupational therapist and other members on the team work together to identify the student's present interests and abilities within the context in which performance is expected or required. The evaluation process also allows the team to identify areas in which the student is likely to need ongoing support and resources to achieve the vision and goals for the future.

Service Planning

In a collaborative transition team, the team members collectively share information and write the student's goals.[60] The team members do not write discipline-specific goals that focus on remediating the student's underlying deficits. The occupational therapist, for example, does not need to write specific goals addressing cognitive, motor, or psychosocial skills. Instead, two or more group members gather together to write the goals and collaborate with the student to accomplish the goals. A student with limited movement in his or her arms and hands may seek to complete written assignments. The occupational therapist may take the lead in evaluating the effectiveness of using alternative writing methods such as assistive technology. He or she makes recommendations to the student and the team. If the team supports the recommendations, the team would assign responsibility for obtaining the equipment, as well as providing training to the student and other team members.

Program Implementation

The occupational therapist and/or the OTA collaborates with the student and his or her teachers, parents, employers, coworkers, and others as needed to address the student's goals in the areas of domestic activities, vocational activities, school, recreation, and community. Transition services are delivered in the student's natural environments. Therefore, OTAs may work in the student's school, at the student's workplace, in the student's home, or in any other relevant setting in the community. Collaborative problem solving with others involved in the student's environment is essential to help the student use alternative methods to complete necessary activities. For example, an OTA may introduce and train the teacher in using assistive technology to help a student access the computer at school to do written assignments. The OTA may provide direct or consultative services to help maximize fit between the student's abilities and the demands of any environment. Evaluating whether the student reaches his or her goals should be the outcome measure to evaluate the effectiveness of OT services.

Work Readiness Programs

Some people who have survived a major accident or illness cannot return to their prior employment and need to explore other options for employment. For example, a person who previously worked as a roofer and has suffered a C4 complete spinal cord injury can no longer physically carry out the job demands of a roofer. This person may want to return to some type of meaningful work but will require guidance and direction to explore his or her present abilities and work skills to set realistic vocational goals.

A **work readiness program** is designed for individuals who desire to work. This program helps these people identify vocational options that match their interests, skills, and abilities. At Rancho Los Amigos National Rehabilitation Center in Downey, Calif., an occupational therapist designed and currently leads a work readiness program; however, an OTA could lead the groups as well. The 6-week program meets three times a week for 2 hours. It consists primarily of group sessions but offers a few individual sessions. Topics include the following: work habits, values, goals, interests, work skills, vocational exploration, job-hunting strategies, and community resources. Instruction, group discussion, and hands-on exploration of work skills using standardized work samples and situational assessments help people explore their readiness to work and discover their potential for pursuing training for a different occupation. Each person's program is individualized to address specific goals and interests. For example, a person who is interested in working with computers would try different work-related tasks that require a computer, to determine his or her aptitude for this work. If the person was not familiar with the types of jobs a person could do with a computer, he or she would be taught how to do vocational research, using reference books or the Internet.

A work readiness program can help people identify specific goals to pursue and develop a plan to help them work toward their goals. Such a program can help a person prepare to return to work but does not provide a job for the participant. At the completion of the program, if a person demonstrates readiness to work, he or she can be referred to the State Department of Rehabilitation for assistance with job training and job placement. After a client has completed a work readiness program, the occupational therapist can provide valuable information on the person's skills, aptitudes, and interests to assist the rehabilitation counselor with developing a feasible plan for the worker.

Older Workers

Baby boomers comprise the largest percentage of the working population.[56] As workers age, employers may need to be sensitive to those who develop multiple disabilities that affect their job performance. Changes in the workplace offer new opportunities for occupational therapists and OTAs to help aging workers stay employed despite the challenges of their functional limitations. As older workers retire, OTAs can help them plan for their retirement and explore ways to remain active in the community through participation in leisure pursuits or volunteer activities. OTs and OTAs can help older individuals identify their strengths and abilities and provide community resources to allow meaningful participation in valued occupations.

Summary

This chapter gives an overview of the range of work programs in which occupational therapists and OTAs currently practice. Little has been published specific to OTA involvement in work and industry. Opportunities for OTAs to expand their role and involvement in hospitals, schools, industrial settings, and in the community in the area of work practice are tremendous. OTAs must be proactive in communicating the need for and benefits of these programs in all communities to help restore the worker role in many people's lives.

Selected Study Guide Questions

1. How has OT involvement in work programs evolved over the years?
2. What is the role of the OTA in work programs?
3. Describe the difference between a functional capacity evaluation and a vocational evaluation.
4. Name the common applications of the results of a job demands analysis.
5. What are the possible outcomes of postoffer testing?
6. Describe the optimal sequence for postoffer screening.
7. Describe the difference between work hardening and work conditioning.
8. Why is having actual work equipment for use during simulation beneficial?
9. What is "ergonomics?"
10. Explain the circumstances under which an OTA may provide ergonomic services without the supervision of an occupational therapist.
11. What are work-related musculoskeletal disorders, and why would an ergonomic consultant be concerned with these disorders?
12. Name two excellent government resources for the OTA who is interested in practicing in the area of ergonomics and injury prevention.
13. What is the OTA's role in school-to-work transition programs?
14. What kind of client can benefit from participation in a work readiness program?

References

1. American Occupational Therapy Association: Guidelines for supervision, roles, and responsibilities during delivery of occupational therapy services, *Am J Occup Ther* 63(6):797–803, 2009.
2. American Occupational Therapy Association: Occupational therapy practice framework: domain and process, *Am J Occup Ther* 62(6):625–683, 2008.
3. American Occupational Therapy Association: Statement: occupational therapy services in facilitating work performance, *Am J Occup Ther* 59:676–679, 2005.
4. American Occupational Therapy Association: Statement: Occupational therapy services in facilitating work performance, *Am J Occup Ther* 54(6):626–628, 2000.
5. American Occupational Therapy Association: Statement: occupational therapy services in work practice, *Am J Occup Ther* 46:1086–1088, 1992.
6. American Occupational Therapy Association: Work hardening guidelines, *Am J Occup Ther* 40:841–843, 1986.
7. Bade S, Eckert J: Occupational therapists' critical value in work rehabilitation and ergonomics, *Work* 31:101–111, 2008.
8. Baum CM, Law M: Occupational therapy practice: focusing on occupational performance, *Am J Occup Ther* 51:277–288, 1997.
9. Biddle J, Roberts K: More evidence of the need for an ergonomic standard, *Am J Ind Med* 45:329, 2004.
10. Bohr PC: Work analysis. In King PM, editor: *Sourcebook of occupational rehabilitation*, New York, 1998, Plenum Press.
11. Cohen AL, et al: *Elements of ergonomics programs: a primer based on workplace evaluations of musculoskeletal disorders*, Washington DC, 1997, US Government Printing Office.
12. Commission on Accreditation of Rehabilitation Facilities: Standards manual for organizations serving people with disabilities, *Tuscon, Ariz*, 1989. CARF.
13. Cromwell FS: Work-related programming in occupational therapy: its roots, course, and prognosis, *Occup Ther Healthcare* 2(4):9–25, 1985.
14. Dahl R, Ergonomics: In Kornblau B, Jacobs K, editors: *Work: principles and practice*, Bethesda, Md, 2000, AOTA.
15. Darphin LE: Work-hardening and work-conditioning perspectives. In Isernhagen SJ, editor: *The comprehensive guide to work injury management*, Gaithersburg, Md, 1995, Aspen Publishers, Inc.
16. Davis H, Rodgers S: Using this book for ergonomics in industry: introduction. In Eggleton E, editor: *Ergonomic design for people at work*, 1, New York, 1983, Van Nostrand Reinhold.

17. Equal Employment Opportunity Commission: *Uniform guidelines on employee selection procedures*, Washington, DC, the Author.
18. Eser G: *Overview of vocational evaluation*, Las Vegas, 1983, Stout University Training Workshop.
19. Gibson L, Strong J: A conceptual framework of functional capacity evaluation for occupational therapy in work rehabilitation, *Austral Occup Ther J* 50(2):64–71, 2003.
20. Grayson D, Dale AM, Bohr P, Wolf L: Evanoff, B: Ergonomic evaluation: Part of a treatment protocol for musculoskeletal injuries, *AAOHN J* 53(10):450–457, 2005.
21. Hall H, Buck M: *The work of our hands*, New York, 1919, Moffat, Yard.
22. Harbin G, Olson J: Post-offer, pre-placement testing in industry, *Am J Industr Med* vol. 47, No. 4:296–307, 2005.
23. Harvey-Krefting L: The concept of work in occupational therapy: a historical review, *Am J Occup Ther* 39:301–307, 1985.
24. Homan NM, Armstrong TJ: Evaluation of three methodologies for assessing work activity during computer use, *Am Industr Hygiene Assoc J* vol. 64, No.1:48–55, 2003.
25. Holmes D: The role of the occupational therapist-work evaluator, *Am J Occup Ther* 39(5), 1985.
26. Hursh N, Kerns A: *Vocational assessment and evaluation systems: a comparison*, Boston, 1988, College-Hill Press.
27. Isernhagen SJ: Advancements in functional capacity evaluation. In D'Orazio BP, editor: *Back pain rehabilitation*, Boston, 1993, Butterworth.
28. Jacobs K: Preparing for return to work. In Trombly CA, editor: *Occupational therapy for physical dysfunction*, ed 4, Baltimore, 1995, Williams & Wilkins.
29. Jacobs K, Baker NA: The history of work-related therapy in occupational therapy. In Kornblau BL, Jacobs K, editors: *Work: principles and practice*, Bethesda, Md, 2000, AOTA.
30. King PM: Work hardening and work conditioning. In King PM, editor: *Sourcebook of occupational rehabilitation*, New York, 1998, Plenum Press.
31. King P, Tuckwell N, Barrett T: A critical review of functional capacity evaluations, *Phys Ther* 78(8):852–866, 1998.
32. Larson B: Work injury activities. In Ryan S, Sladyk K, editors: *Ryan's occupational therapy assistant*, ed 3, Thorofare, NJ, 2001, Slack.
33. Lechner DE: Functional capacity evaluation. In King PM, editor: *Sourcebook of occupational rehabilitation*, New York, 1998, Plenum Press.
34. Lechner DE: Work hardening and work conditioning interventions: do they affect disability? *Phys Ther* 74(5):102–124, 1994.
35. Lechner D, Roth D, Stratton K: Functional capacity evaluation in work disability, *Work* 1:37–47, 1991.
36. Legislative Committee: National Rehabilitation Association: Meeting the nation's needs by the expansion of the program of vocational rehabilitation of physically handicapped persons, *Occup Ther Rehab* 16(3):186, 1937.
37. Littleton M: Cost-effectiveness of prework screening program for the University of Illinois at Chicago physical plant, *Work 21*, No. 3:243–250, 2003.
38. Leyshon R, Chalova K, Gerson L, et al: Ergonomic interventions for office workers with musculoskeletal disorders: a systematic review, *Work* 35:335–348, 2010.
39. MacFarlane B: Job modification, *Work Special Int Section News* 2(1):1–2, 1988.
40. Malugani M: Emerging areas in OT, Monster Worldwide (http://content.monster.com) on the AOTA website 12/24/04 (http://www.otjoblink.org/links/link09.asp), 2004.
41. Marshall EM: Looking back, *Am J Occup Ther* 39(5), 1985.
42. Mikkelson S, Vilstrup I, Lassen CF, et al: Validity of questionnaire self-reports on computer, mouse and keyboard usage during a four-week period, *Occup Environ Med* 64(8):541–547, 2007.
43. O'Callaghan J: Primary prevention and ergonomics: the role of rehabilitation specialists in preventing occupational injury. In Rothman J, Levine R, editors: *Prevention practice: strategies for physical therapy and occupational therapy*, Philadelphia, 1992, WB Saunders.
44. Occupational Safety and Health Administration: *Ergonomics for the prevention of musculoskeletal disorders: guidelines for nursing homes*, Washington, DC, 2003, US Government Printing Office.
45. Occupational Safety and Health Administration: *Ergonomics for the prevention of musculoskeletal disorders: guidelines for poultry processing*, Washington, DC, 2004, US Government Printing Office.
46. Occupational Safety and Health Administration: *Ergonomics for the prevention of musculoskeletal disorders: guidelines for retail grocery stores*, Washington, DC, 2004, US Government Printing Office.
47. Occupational Safety and Health Administration: *Ergonomics program management guidelines for meatpacking plants*, Washington, DC, 1990, US Government Printing Office.
48. Ogden-Niemeyer L, Jacobs K: Definition and history of work hardening. In Ogden-Niemeyer L, Jacobs K, editors: *Work hardening state of the art*, Thorofare, NJ, 1989, lack.
49. Owens LA, Buchholz RL: Functional capacity assessment, worker evaluation strategies, and the disability management process. In Shrey DE, Lacerte M, editors: *Principals and practices of disability management in industry*, Winter Park, FL, 1995, GR Press, Inc.
50. Page J: Functional capacity evaluation-making the right decision, *RehabPro* 9(4):34–35, 2001.
51. Perry LL: Preemployment and preplacement testing. In King PM, editor: *Sourcebook of occupational rehabilitation*, New York, 1998, Plenum Press.
52. Pinel P: *A treatise on insanity*, New York, 1962, Hafner Publishing Co.
53. Putz-Anderson V, editor: *Cumulative trauma disorders: a manual for musculoskeletal diseases of the upper limbs*, Bristol, Pa, 1988, Taylor & Francis.
54. Rothstein J, Echternach J: *Primer on measurement: an introductory guide to measurement issues featuring the APTA's standards for tests and measurements in physical therapy practice*, Fairfax, Va, 1993, APTA.
55. Ryan DJ: *Job search handbook for people with disabilities*, Indianapolis, 2000, JIST Pub Inc.
56. Sabata D, Endicott S: *Workplace changes: seizing opportunities for persons with disabilities in the workplace*, 21, Bethesda, Md, 2007, Work Programs Special Interest Section Quarterly/American Occupational Therapy Association. 2.
57. Shrey DE: Worksite disability management and industrial rehabilitation: an overview. In Shrey DE, Lacerte M, editors: *Principals and practices of disability management in industry*, Winter Park, FL, 1995, CRC Press, Inc.
58. Smith SL, Cunningham S, Weinberg R: The predictive validity of the functional capacities evaluation, *Am J Occup Ther* 40: 564–567, 1986.
59. Snodgrass JE: Getting comfortable: developing a clinical specialty in ergonomics has its own challenges and rewards, *Rehab Manag*, 24–27 July 2004.

60. Spencer K: Transition from school to adult life. In Kornblau B, Jacobs K, editors: *Work: principles and practice*, Betheseda, Md, 2000, AOTA.
61. Symons J, Veran A: Conducting worksite evaluations to identify reasonable accommodations. In Hamil J, editor: *Integrating assistive technology into your practice, AOTA online course*, Bethesda, Md, 2000, AOTA.
62. Tompa E, Dolinschi R, deOliveira C, et al: A systematic review of workplace ergonomic interventions with economic analysis, *J Occup Rehabil* 20:220–234, 2010.
63. US Department of Labor: ed 4, *Employment and training administration: revised dictionary of occupational titles*, vol. I & II, Washington, DC, 1991, US Government Printing Office.
64. US Department of Labor: *Employment and Training Administration: The revised handbook for analyzing jobs*, Indianapolis, 1991, JIST Works.
65. US Department of Labor, Occupational Safety and Health Administration: *OSHA effective ergonomics: strategy for success*, www.osha.gov.
66. US Department of Labor: *Office of Disability Employment Policy (ODEP) website retrieved*, October 16, 2010. Available at www.dol.gov/odep/.
67. Wegg LS: The essentials of work evaluation, *Am J Occup Ther* 14:65–69, 1960. 79.
68. Young ES: Setting up an industrial program for the tuberculosis patient, *Occup Ther Rehab* 18(3):163, 1939.

CHAPTER 18

Promoting Engagement in Leisure and Social Participation

STEVE PARK AND SUE BYERS-CONNON

Key Terms

Leisure
Social participation
Life satisfaction
Well-being
Quality of life
Health
Client-centered

Chapter Objectives

After studying this chapter, the student or practitioner will be able to do the following:

1. Identify the characteristics that distinguish leisure and social participation from other areas of occupation.
2. Apply the *Occupational Therapy Practice Framework* to leisure and social participation with clients.
3. Explain the contribution of leisure and social participation to life satisfaction, quality of life, well-being, and health for all persons.
4. Appreciate the leisure and social challenges faced by some persons with physical disabilities.
5. Apply different client-centered methods to gather information about the importance and meaning of leisure and social participation.
6. Implement occupational therapy intervention that promotes the benefit of engaging in leisure and social activities.

"Because we freely choose them, our play and leisure activities may be some of the purest expressions of who we are as persons."
Anita C. Bundy[11]

CASE STUDY

Winnie, Part 1: Engaging in Valued Daily Life Activities*

Maintaining a healthy balance between work and leisure can be a challenge, as many people struggle to make time for activities they enjoy. Winnie, a 74-year-old woman, has never had this problem. Throughout her life, Winnie maintained a beneficial balance between work and leisure activities, enjoying the best of both. As a young woman, she enjoyed dance lessons, traveling, and attending the theater while also working various jobs as a model, bookkeeper, and secretary. She raised five children and volunteered at her children's school.

After her children left home, she worked full-time as an administrative secretary in the allied health division at a community college. Since her retirement, Winnie continues to maintain an active life. Her leisure pursuits are many; she particularly enjoys gardening, embroidery, cooking, and swimming. Winnie and her husband Bill often go out to dance, and she is a member of a tap dancing group that performs at various fundraising activities in association with the local Elks Club. Winnie is also an active volunteer at her church and is responsible each Sunday for the altar flower arrangements.

Family and friends are the center of Winnie's life. At regular family gatherings with children and grandchildren, everyone enjoys a good meal (particularly Winnie's cheesecake) and the friendly competition of a board game. Winnie attends her grandchildren's sporting events, rarely missing a game. Winnie hand-embroidered a unique Christmas stocking for each of her children and grandchildren. Her sense of humor, ready smiles, and bountiful laugh are familiar to many. She and several friends who were born in May are known as the "May Babies." Every year they celebrate their birthdays by going to the beach, where they enjoy playing cards, cooking their favorite seafood stew, and visiting the local casino.

Two and a half months before her 75th birthday, Winnie had a stroke.

*People generally use first names in leisure and social situations, so we refer to clients (including elders) in this chapter by their first names.

Leisure and Social Participation

"There are many ... rhythms ... the big four—work and play and rest and sleep, which our organism must be able to balance even under difficulty." Adolf Meyer[49]

From the beginning of the profession, occupational therapy (OT) practitioners emphasized the importance of a healthy balance in daily activities. This tradition continues as occupational therapists and occupational therapy assistants (OTAs) address the broad array of activities in which humans engage. Participation in life through engagement in a variety of daily activities (occupation) is the primary focus and outcome for clients receiving OT services. Leisure and social participation (also called leisure and social activities) are two of the areas of occupation, the others being activities of daily living (ADL), instrumental ADL (IADL), rest and sleep, education, work, and play (Box 18-1).[2]

Although the American Occupational Therapy Association (AOTA) defines each area of occupation, what specifically identifies a daily activity as leisure, social participation, or another area? One perspective identifies leisure as the time spent in activities left over after a person completes obligatory activities such as ADL, IADL, education, or work.[12,60] For example, Robin travels for work, meeting with clients during the day and often during mealtimes. These engagements take up much of her time on the road; she spends her free time in the hotel reading novels, relaxing in the bath, and phoning friends. The activities associated with work are considered obligatory; her free-time activities are considered discretionary. Thus from this perspective, if an activity is *not* identified as obligatory, by default it is designated as leisure.

Another perspective identifies leisure activities according to agreed-upon, recognizable features a specific society associates with leisure.[12,60] Common features among Western societies include pleasurable, creative, stimulating, physically or mentally challenging, relaxing, artistic, energetic, competitive, and social. If an activity typically embodies one these features, it is customarily identified as leisure. These features can be used to differentiate leisure activities such as active versus sedentary, relaxing versus energetic, or social versus solitary. For example, Brad likes to pursue more solitary and physically challenging activities such as running through the park and swimming laps. Geneva enjoys more social and mentally challenging activities such as playing chess and participating in a book club. Thus many activities are considered leisure by society, although they can take different forms and different societies may value different characteristics.[77] Categorizing leisure activities by their common features acknowledges the social nature commonly associated with leisure. This perspective, however, designates social activity a subcategory of leisure. Leisure activities should be differentiated from social activities because not all social activities involve leisure (and vice versa).[10] Interestingly, when older adults discuss the role of activities in their lives, they tend to refer to activities as social, physical, or mental[67] rather than self-care, productive, or play/leisure, the categories OT practitioners often use.

Box 18-1

Occupational Therapy Practice Framework: Leisure and Social Participation

Leisure

Leisure is "[a] nonobligatory activity that is intrinsically motivated and engaged in during discretionary time, that is, time not committed to obligatory occupations such as work, self-care, or sleep."[56]

- Exploration: Identifying interests, skills, opportunities, and appropriate leisure activities.
- Participation: Planning and participating in appropriate leisure activities; maintaining a balance of leisure activities with other areas of occupation; and obtaining, using, and maintaining equipment and supplies as appropriate.

Social Participation

Social participation is "organized patterns of behavior that are characteristic and expected of an individual or an individual interacting with others within a given social system."[52]

- Community: Engaging in activities that result in successful interaction at the community level (i.e., neighborhood, organizations, work, school).
- Family: Engaging in "[activities that result in] successful interaction in specific required and/or desired familial roles."[52]
- Peer, Friend: Engaging in activities at different levels of intimacy including engaging in desired sexual activity.

Modified from American Occupational Therapy Association: Occupational therapy practice framework: domain and process, ed 2, *Am J Occup Ther* 62(6):625, 2008.

A potential problem exists when conceptualizing leisure as free-time, discretionary activities or activities identified by society as leisure. For any one person, not all free time may be experienced as leisure (at times, free time can be boring) and activities identified by society as leisure may not be experienced by a person as leisure.[70,71] These conceptions of leisure do not account for a person's unique perspective of and meaning associated with his or her engagement in activities. For example, Tyrome attends a going-away party for a coworker and experiences the party as leisure. Scott attends the same party, considering it obligatory, and experiences it more as work. To confuse matters even more, it is a social activity for both. To account for each person's unique perspective and the fact that most activities could be experienced as leisure, professionals need to understand leisure as an experience, a state of mind unique to each person.[12,59,70,71,76]

Although different activities may be experienced as leisure, research highlights qualities that characterize an activity as more leisurely than work (Box 18-2).[6,59,65,69,76] For the person to consider an activity as leisure, he or she does not need to experience each and every quality. Rather, if the person experiences many of these qualities, the activity will more likely be experienced as leisure. More importantly, the greater the intensity of each characteristic experienced, the more the activity will be experienced as leisure.[11,12] Given the qualities associated with experiencing leisure, how are these related to life satisfaction, well-being, quality of life, and health?

Box 18-2

Characteristics of Leisure Activities

Freedom of choice: The person freely chooses the activity (nonobligatory).
Sense of control: The person feels in charge during the activity.
Sense of enjoyment: The activity evokes pleasurable feelings.
Timelessness: Time seems to fly by while engaged in the activity.
Sense of competence: The person feels a sense of proficiency and accomplishment.
Spontaneity: The person could participate in the activity on the spur of the moment.
Intrinsic satisfaction: The person feels a sense of doing something worthwhile.
Companionship: The person experiences a sense of camaraderie and friendship.
Lack of external judgment: The person's performance is not evaluated by others.
Relaxation: The person feels a sense of relief from physical effort and emotional tension.
Novelty: The person engages in something new and different.
Freedom: The activity provides an escape from the daily necessities of life.

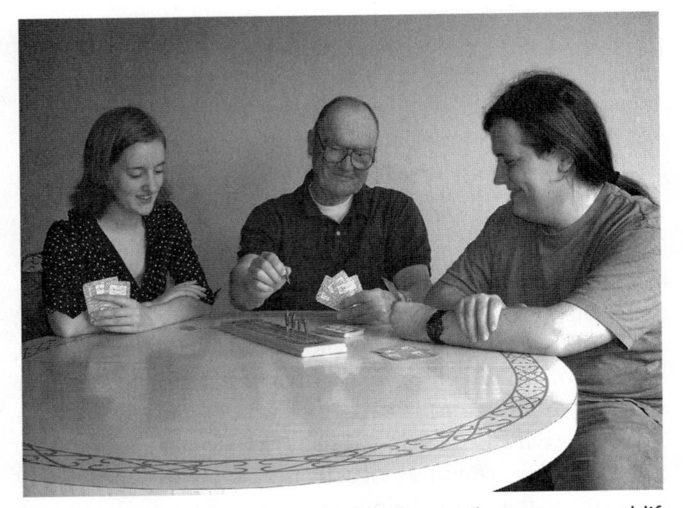

Figure 18-1 Spending time with family contributes to general life satisfaction.

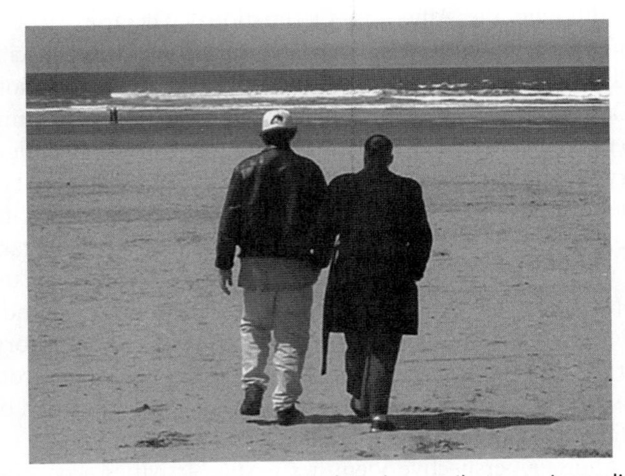

Figure 18-2 Spending time with friends contributes to immediate day-to-day happiness.

Importance of Leisure and Social Activities in Everyday Life

Considerable evidence suggests that participation in meaningful leisure and social activities is related to and significantly influences a person's well-being, life satisfaction, quality of life, or health, particularly for older adults.[13,17,21,25,31,33,40,58] Older adults who are more active tend to live longer, and evidence suggests that social and productive activities (which include leisure) can be as effective as physical fitness activities in reducing a person's risk of death and enhancing quality of life.[27] Moreover, greater social integration is linked to a greater likelihood of survival.[32]

Satisfaction with leisure activities and the quality of social interactions appears more important to quality of life and life satisfaction than frequency of leisure participation.[44,67] For older adults living independently in the community, less frequent participation in and decreased access to leisure activities do not automatically equate to diminished life satisfaction—rather, "even valued [leisure] activities, pursued infrequently, may add meaning and satisfaction to the lives of elderly people."[28] Moreover, whereas spending time with family contributes to a general sense of life satisfaction, spending time with friends engenders immediate day-to-day happiness and generates more positive feelings and is associated with greater quality of life, well-being, and morale than spending time with family (Figures 18-1 and 18-2).[26,39,43] Engagement in leisure pursuits helps develop social support networks,[40] and the prospect of establishing social connections is a primary reason why adults may choose to pursue an activity.[67] Most pointedly, when older adults discuss activities in their lives that have the most meaning, they rarely mention basic ADL tasks.[67] Rather, leisure and social activities are viewed as having the most meaning in their everyday lives.

Importance for People with Disabilities

Research also highlights the importance of leisure and social activities in the everyday lives of adults experiencing physical disabilities. For persons with severe multiple traumas, the most important contributors to overall life satisfaction are family life, a sufficient social network, satisfaction with leisure, and vocation.[4] A strong relationship appears to exist between well-being and involvement in leisure and social activities for persons with stroke, more so than other factors.[1,78] Adults with congenital disabilities report the importance of leisure in their lives, believing that leisure participation contributes to their physical and mental health.[73] They describe the pure joy of engaging in leisure activities and the sense of belonging and self-worth that leisure and social activities promote.

Diminished Participation for People with Disabilities

Although adults with physical disabilities can experience the benefits of leisure and social activities (similar to people without disabilities), considerable evidence suggests that many do not. Many adults with physical disabilities are unhappy with their reduced participation in leisure and social activities and experience a subsequent decline in well-being and quality of life. Research confirms that persons after a stroke do not participate in as many leisure and social activities, particularly outside the home, and they identify this as a significant concern.[1,29,54,64,83] Similarly, reduced leisure and social participation occur with adults experiencing arthritis,[63,74,84] cardiac conditions,[24] spinal cord injuries,[10] and traumatic brain injuries.[8,86] For older residents living in assisted living centers, concerns exist about their leisure and social participation: (1) engaging in center-sponsored activities because they are convenient and available, not because they are meaningful; (2) occupying their time with predominantly group activities designed to promote socialization; and (3) missing the opportunity to engage in activities more on their own.[20] These and other research studies demonstrate that participation in leisure and social activities is a significant concern for adults experiencing physical disabilities, indicating OT practitioners can provide a needed service in this area.

Facilitating Leisure and Social Participation

"Leisure is an occupational performance area, a state of mind, time to be filled, and a tangible activity through which therapeutic goals are met." Melinda Suto[76]

Adults experiencing physical disabilities advocate for leisure and social activities to be an integral part of their rehabilitation. Persons with stroke receiving inpatient rehabilitation services report that leisure activities are a means to their recovery and a lifeline to regain a sense of control over their situations.[19] They strongly desire more leisure and social activities during inpatient rehabilitation and believe this may speed their recovery, alleviate boredom, and ward off potential depression. However, OT and rehabilitation services (particularly inpatient services) place greater emphasis on physical independence in mobility, basic ADL, and household tasks and limited emphasis on leisure and social participation.[8,38,63,73,80] As Radomski so pointedly stated after reviewing the stroke rehabilitation literature, "we have succeeded in facilitating the recovery of patients' physical skills after stroke but not in advancing their resumption of the social, leisure, and productive activities that make life worth living.[61]

Although helping clients achieve greater ADL independence can be important, exclusive focus on this outcome ignores what is important to everyone—disability or not. Engagement in leisure and social activities brings greater life satisfaction, quality of life, and well-being than does independent performance of basic ADL tasks. Although people with disabilities recognize the significance of leisure and social activities, clients sometimes may not recognize this importance,[8,76] particularly if they were admitted to the hospital for a reason secondary to a health condition. Such clients often just want to get better; leisure and social activities may be the last thing on their minds. In these situations, OT practitioners should not force the issue. Rather, they should thoughtfully and considerately explore, in collaboration with the client, leisure and social activities of importance, gently advocating that leisure and social participation could be a significant aspect of recovery.

Overview of Occupational Therapy Process

OT practitioners begin the evaluation process by creating an occupational profile[2] that includes gathering information about the meaning of leisure and social activities in the client's life. The evaluation process includes an analysis of occupational performance and should examine the client's ability to engage in desired leisure and social activities including what supports and hinders his or her participation. Once this information is gathered, OT practitioners develop the intervention plan, collaborating with the client to develop realistic and achievable goals that focus on leisure and social participation, and selecting methods appropriate to the goals and the situation. The plan is then implemented; after a period of intervention, the client and OT practitioner(s) evaluate whether the desired outcome was achieved—that is, whether the client's leisure and social participation improved. The following sections illustrate this process.

Evaluation Process

"It is important that [OT practitioners] learn from each client what occupations are important for his or her health and well-being and how current problems are interfering with performance of those occupations." Mary Law, Sandy Steinwender, Leanne Leclair[42]

Following a client-centered approach, OT practitioners seek to understand the client's perspective on important and meaningful leisure and social activities, particularly those of current concern. The evaluation process is the same as for other areas of occupation; interviews, observations, and standardized assessments are used to gather needed information.[2] Although the occupational therapist begins and completes the initial evaluation, the OTA may perform specific evaluation procedures once service competency is established.[3] The OTA may conduct an interview, observe a client, or administer a standardized assessment and then share the information with the occupational therapist, who is responsible for its interpretation.

An important consideration during the information gathering process is the client's socio-cultural background and beliefs regarding leisure and social participation that influence his or her perceptions about the value, choice, and degree of desired engagement in specific leisure and social activities.[9,55] Through understanding the client's socio-cultural perspectives on leisure and social activities (which can be different from one's own), OT practitioners can ensure any proposed intervention is in accord with the client's socio-cultural background and preferences[82] (see Case Study: Gabriella). This often necessitates examining one's own socio-cultural background and beliefs in regard to leisure and social activities to ensure that one's own values and beliefs are not unintentionally imposed on a client.[5,55]

CASE STUDY

Gabriella

Gabriella, 79 years old and grandmother to 12, recently fell and broke her hip. Until she can return home, she is undergoing rehabilitation at a local skilled nursing facility (SNF). Her youngest grandson, Miguel, will be 8 years old in 3 weeks, and she wants to go on a weekend pass to join her family in the traditional birthday celebration. Gabriella always made her "famous" tamales for family celebrations, for which her extended family will travel miles. Recognizing the importance to Gabriella to retain her role in the family, the OTA broached the possibility of making tamales in the SNF kitchen. Gabriella told her, however, it would be difficult to make them in a kitchen that does not have all the cooking equipment that she has at home and cooking from a wheelchair seems like a lot of work. She also confided "it's time someone else stepped up and made the tamales," an acknowldgement that Gabriella's matriarchal role within the family was changing. However, the OTA continued to talk with Gabriella about what her family celebrations usually entailed and Gabriella mentioned that the highlight of the party is always the breaking of the piñata. The OTA proceeded to ask Gabriella if she might consider making a paper-mache piñata for the party, particularly as the SNF had the supplies and they could enlist the help of other residents if she desired. Gabriella thought it was a great idea and started to make plans to create a large sun, filled with candy for her grandson and birthday guests to enjoy.

Interviewing Clients

The purpose of interviewing is to gather essential information to begin intervention, but not all information need be gathered during one session. Working collaboratively, the occupational therapist and OTA may decide that the occupational therapist will briefly review leisure and social activities with a client at initiation of the evaluation and that the OTA will follow with a more in-depth interview. An informal, conversational style that prompts the client to tell stories about his or her leisure and social activities will better elicit the type of information desired—the meaning of leisure and social participation in the client's life (Figure 18-3). To ensure a client-centered approach, the OTA should begin by asking the client what he or she considers leisure and explore the client's thoughts and feelings about leisure and social participation.[60,76]

The OTA should not continue on to another question after receiving only a brief response to a previous one. The meaning of and benefits received from leisure and social activities cannot be communicated adequately, nor understood by the interviewer, with a one-word or one-sentence response. Follow-up questions can fully illuminate the meaning of activities (Table 18-1). A conversation with careful follow-up questions elicits rich narrative data useful to plan intervention.[12] By the end of the conversation, the OTA should understand (1) the meaning of leisure and social activities in the client's life; and (2) specific leisure and social activities of most importance and concern to the client that could be addressed during therapy. If a client has difficulty communicating, a similar conversation with family members should occur.

Information about leisure and social activities should be gathered throughout intervention, reflected upon, and used to modify the intervention plan.[2] The OTA should be sensitive to when a client might be ready to explore new pursuits. The client who cannot resume previous activities is confronted with a loss of self, a particularly distressing feeling. When a client shows readiness to consider new interests, the client and OTA can explore potential activities that have features similar to those in which the client previously engaged and in which the client may be successful and satisfied (see Case Study: Dimitri).[76]

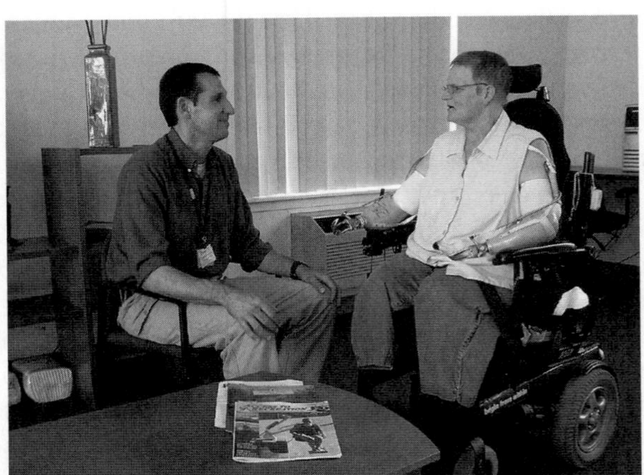

Figure 18-3 An informal conversation best elicits the meaning of leisure and social participation.

CASE STUDY

Dimitri

Dimitri, a 28-year-old carpet layer, experienced multiple physical traumas from an auto accident. He was admitted to inpatient rehabilitation for a short stay. Although leisure was mentioned during the initial evaluation, Dimitri's priority was to get stronger to manage his basic ADL tasks and return to work. Three days before discharge, Dimitri began to acknowledge that he could not return to work as soon as he hoped and that he would have a lot of free time on his hands. At this time, he and the OTA began exploring his interests and how he might occupy his time at home, focusing on those leisure and social activities of interest that were within his capabilities.

Table 18-1 Interview Questions Regarding Client's Leisure and Social Participation

General Questions	Follow-Up Questions
What do you consider leisure in your life?	What makes it leisure for you?
What do you like to do with friends? With family?	What is important about spending time with friends? With family?
What do you particularly enjoy doing?	What makes those things enjoyable?
What type of leisure activities do you prefer?	Creative? Intellectual? Physical? Relaxing? Competitive? Social? Solitary?
What do you like to do because you want to do it, not because you feel you have to do it?	What are those times like when you do things you don't necessarily have to do?
Are there times when you forget about everything else and time seems to fly?	What makes time fly? What is it that makes you forget about everything else?
Are there things you do that you feel you can do the way you want?	What allows you to do it the way you want? What is it that appeals to you about doing it the way you want?
What is (or has been) your routine of engaging in enjoyable activities? Getting together with friends? Family?	What is important about routinely engaging in enjoyable activities? Getting together regularly with friends? With family?
Are there leisure and social activities of concern to you right now?	What is of most concern? What is most important to you?

Modified from Bundy AC: Assessment of play and leisure: delineation of the problem, *Am J Occup Ther* 47(3):217-219.

Observing Clients

Whenever feasible, the OTA should observe a client engage in specific desired leisure and social activities, noting the effectiveness of the client's performance skills[2] (see Case Study: Stella). Turner and colleagues[80] note that OT practitioners, when gathering information about leisure, may be focusing primarily on general information about the client's leisure interests rather the actual performance of leisure activities, indicating a greater need to focus on the performance of leisure activities during the evaluation process.

CASE STUDY

Stella

Stella was recently diagnosed with Parkinson disease and began outpatient OT. The occupational therapist conducted the initial evaluation, during which she learned that Stella enjoyed creating greeting cards for friends and family on the computer but had stopped because of the difficulty and frustration she experienced as a result of the disease. The occupational therapist discussed the evaluation results and intervention plan with the OTA, who then assumed responsibility for intervention. The OTA began by asking Stella if she could observe her using the computer in the clinic, explaining this would provide her with a clearer understanding of Stella's performance skills that supported and hindered her ability to use the computer and to perform other activities in her daily life.

Administering Standardized Assessments

Standardized assessments that focus on leisure and social activities may complement the evaluation process, although usage reported by OT practitioners is low.[80] Standardized interest checklists such as the original Neuropsychiatric Institute (NPI) Interest Check List[47] and updated versions such as the Modified Interest Checklist[50] and Interest Checklist (UK)[34] provide an overview of a client's interest in specific leisure and social activities. These types of checklists list a variety of activities for which the client identifies those he or she pursued in the past, is currently participating in, or might want to pursue in the future, as well as his or her degree of interest (e.g., none, some, strong). These checklists typically do not ask the client to add to the list other activities he or she considers as leisure or social, nor do they explore the meaning of the activities to the client. A conversation is required to solicit this information. Moreover, interest checklists need to be updated periodically to reflect socio-cultural changes in how people typically occupy leisure and social time. A more interactive assessment than written interest checklists, the Activity Card Sort[7] uses a set of 89 photographs to help clients identify instrumental, low physical-demand leisure, high physical-demand leisure, and social activities in which the client participates. Lastly, recognizing the importance of distinguishing participating in leisure versus social activities and engaging with friends versus family, the Mastricht Social Participation Profile[46] assesses the frequency with which a person engages in 26 different activities, providing a profile of engagement over a 4-week period.

Other standardized assessments ask the client to identify activities that he or she considers leisure or social and identifies the client's performance pattern for those and other activities. The Occupational Questionnaire (OQ)[72] is a self-report assessment based on the Model of Human Occupation.[37] The OQ requires the client to document the main activity in which he or she engages for each half-hour throughout a morning, day, and evening and identify each activity as work, daily living task, recreation, or rest (Figure 18-4). For each activity, the client rates how well he or she does the activity, how important it is, and how much he or she enjoys it. Using the OQ allows the OTA to understand which activities the client considers leisure (if any) and to explore the meaning of leisure from the client's perspective. The Canadian Occupational Performance Measure (COPM)[41] is another standardized assessment that allows a client to identify activities that he or she considers leisure and social. During this interview-based assessment, the OT practitioner asks a client to identify self-care, productive, and leisure

Typical Activities For the half hour beginning at:	I consider this activity to be: 1= Work 2= Daily living task 3= Recreation 4= Rest	I think that I do this: 1= Very well 2= Well 3= Above average 4= Poorly 5= Very poorly	For me this activity is: 1= Extremely important 2= Important 3= Take it or leave it 4= Rather not do it 5= Total waste of time	How much do you enjoy this activity: 1= Like it very much 2= Like it 3= Neither like it nor dislike it 4= Dislike it 5= Strongly dislike it
5.00 a.m.	1 2 3 4	1 2 3 4 5	1 2 3 4 5	1 2 3 4 5
5.30	1 2 3 4	1 2 3 4 5	1 2 3 4 5	1 2 3 4 5
6.00	1 2 3 4	1 2 3 4 5	1 2 3 4 5	1 2 3 4 5
6.30	1 2 3 4	1 2 3 4 5	1 2 3 4 5	1 2 3 4 5
7.00	1 2 3 4	1 2 3 4 5	1 2 3 4 5	1 2 3 4 5
7.30	1 2 3 4	1 2 3 4 5	1 2 3 4 5	1 2 3 4 5
8.00 a.m.	1 2 3 4	1 2 3 4 5	1 2 3 4 5	1 2 3 4 5
8.30	1 2 3 4	1 2 3 4 5	1 2 3 4 5	1 2 3 4 5
9.00 a.m.	1 2 3 4	1 2 3 4 5	1 2 3 4 5	1 2 3 4 5
9.30	1 2 3 4	1 2 3 4 5	1 2 3 4 5	1 2 3 4 5

Figure 18-4 The Occupational Questionnaire: a sample selection. (From Smith NR, Kielhofner G, Watts J: *Occupational questionnaire,* Chicago, 1986, Model of Human Occupation Clearinghouse.)

Box 18-3

Sample Questions from the Leisure Interest Measure

Domain	Question	Answers
Physical	I like leisure activities that require physical challenge. _______	Never true
Outdoor	I like the fresh air of outdoor settings. _______	Seldom true
Mechanical	I like repairing or building things in my leisure time. _______	Somewhat true
Artistic	I like to be original in my leisure activities. _______	Often true
Service	I often participate in service activities in my leisure time. _______	Always true
Social	I prefer to engage in leisure activities that require social interaction. _______	
Cultural	I have a strong attraction to the cultural arts. _______	
Reading	I like to read in my free time. _______	

Modified from Ragheb MG, Beard JG: *Leisure interest measure,* Ravensdale, Wash, 1991, Idyll Arbor.

activities considered important and that the client needs, wants, or is expected to do. The COPM also prompts the interviewer to ask about quiet, active, and social activities. Interestingly, research indicates that use of the COPM identifies additional leisure concerns for people with physical disabilities beyond those identified in typical interview procedures.[22,48,81]

Other self-report standardized assessments focus on the meaning and experience of leisure and social activities. Instead of asking the client to identify specific activities in his or her daily life, the client rates his or her perspective on specific qualities associated with leisure (Box 18-3). The Idyll Arbor Leisure Battery,[62] a battery of assessments developed

CASE STUDY

Winnie, Part 2: Focusing on Valued Activities after Her Stroke

While in the hospital, Winnie also developed bronchitis. Because of her limited cardiopulmonary endurance, she was subsequently transferred to a skilled nursing facility (SNF) for extended (and less intensive) rehabilitation. On admission, she needed substantial assistance with getting in and out of bed, completing basic ADL tasks, and propelling her wheelchair. She could barely raise her affected right arm to shoulder level or grasp objects; she was frustrated that she could not write her name or use a fork properly. She experienced episodes of eyestrain, difficulty concentrating, and fatigue, particularly at the end of days when her family and friends visited.

Winnie currently struggles to accept her condition and is concerned she might not recover in time for the "May Babies" annual birthday celebration, which is 7 weeks away. The occupational therapist interviewed Winnie on admission and identified that leisure and social activities were particularly important. The occupational therapist and OTA decided Jodi (the OTA) would conduct a more extensive interview. Because Jodi had demonstrated competency with in-depth interviews, they considered this an efficient use of time.

Using client-centered questions as a guide (see Table 18-1), Jodi obtained more detail about the meaning of leisure and social activities in Winnie's life. Throughout their conversation, Winnie conveyed that leisure and social activities are an integral aspect of who she is, not just something she does for the sake of keeping busy. She related the importance of maintaining her long-time friendships with the "May Babies" and teared up while talking about their annual birthday celebration, a few months away. She mentioned that when she plays board games with her children and grandchildren the time seems to fly, and before they know it, her grandchildren's bedtime has passed. She commented on the raucous laughter that permeates the house during every family board game. Winnie shared that her daughter-in-law is involved in making quilts for families of soldiers who died in Iraq and Afghanistan and is disappointed she can't help because of her stroke. Maintaining her physical fitness is also important, with swimming being her top priority. Most of all, she is happy when she spends any time with her family, commenting she considers this time a blessing rather than a responsibility. As the conversation with Winnie progressed, Jodi realized she was gathering the information she needed, decided against incorporating an interest checklist, and continued the conversation.

When discussing her valued activities, Winnie repeatedly commented, "I don't see how I'm ever going to do them again." Jodi recognized the extent to which Winnie valued leisure and social activities and gently presented the possibility Winnie would again be able to engage in leisure and social pursuits. Jodi explained they could explore ways she could still be involved in valued leisure and social activities with her family and friends, perhaps engaging in old ones and also considering new ones. By being thoughtful and considerate of Winnie's perspective and gently advocating for Winnie to consider leisure and social activities at this stage of her recovery from stroke, Jodi set the stage for Winnie to begin reclaiming her well-being and quality of life. They were now ready to plan and begin intervention.

within the field of therapeutic recreation, contains the Leisure Attitude Measure, Leisure Interest Measure, Leisure Satisfaction Scale, and Leisure Motivation Scale—all self-report questionnaires that explore various leisure qualities. Although standardized assessments may appear to be a quick and easy method to gather information, the OTA should typically start with an interview and use a standardized assessment to supplement the information gathered during the interview.

Intervention

The intervention process for leisure and social participation is the same as for other areas of occupation—that is, an intervention plan is developed (including the establishment of goals), implemented, monitored, and reviewed.[2] Intervention should occur in collaboration with the client and should be tailored to each client, focusing on promoting, restoring, maintaining, and/or modifying a client's current and future participation in leisure and social activities, and/or preventing a loss of participation. Strategies to enhance a client's well-being, life satisfaction, and quality of life should not focus exclusively on engaging clients in just any leisure or social activities. Engaging in activities just to keep busy does not produce the same results as engaging in activities because they are personally meaningful.[20] Thus incorporating leisure and social activities into the therapy process should be client centered and unique to each client.

Because activities are both the means and end of OT, leisure and social activities could be the process by which a client regains performance skills to support his or her participation in daily life activities.[2] For example, by engaging in a favored woodworking project, a client could develop greater skill in grasping, manipulating, and using tools and materials—necessities for many daily activities. However, this approach accounts neither for the fact a client may experience therapy as work (even when engaged in favored leisure pursuits) nor for the inherent benefits of engaging in leisure and social activities. The greater good of leisure and social participation resides in its contribution to a client's quality of life, well-being, and life satisfaction rather than the performance skills he or she may be learning. For example, after a lower limb amputation, a young woman's achievement of going to the movies for the first time with her friends, thoroughly enjoying the time, and feeling great about it afterward far outweighs whether she can effectively and independently negotiate curbs and steps during a community outing. A client's sense of satisfaction, enjoyment, competence, camaraderie, and other qualities associated with engagement in leisure and social activities should be valued equally to the achievement of specific performance skills.

OT practitioners have raised concerns regarding payment, sometimes believing insurance will not reimburse for leisure or social activities.[68] Although each insurance plan is different, Medicare will reimburse for services when leisure or social activities are included.[14] As long as reimbursement criteria are complied with and documented accordingly, leisure and social activities may be incorporated into and become the focus of OT, particularly as a means to achieve greater "independent functioning." In doing so, OT practitioners communicate the contribution of all activities to a person's functioning and his or her well-being, life-satisfaction, quality of life, and health.

Familiarity with a variety of leisure and social activities and knowledge of how to adapt activities to improve a client's performance provide the OTA with the skills to promote a client's engagement in those activities. The OTA can assist a client's increased participation by helping him or her learn to engage in previous activities in new adapted manners and/or explore new activity interests. Additionally, the OTA can create a therapeutic context that capitalizes on the inherent joy and satisfaction of engagement in leisure and social activities.

Intervention Guidelines

An inability to resume a leisure or social activity is seldom attributable solely to physical factors.[51] Less obvious and more complex reasons are usually involved. OT practitioners will need to consider all elements that support and hinder a client's engagement (i.e., the client's performance skills, performance patterns, activity demands, client factors, and context and environment).[2] The following guidelines are based on research and reflect those issues particularly relevant to leisure and social activities for people with disabilities and older adults. To fully address clients' leisure and social concerns, OTAs will need to draw on the entire breadth of knowledge and skills they possess.

Consider Client's Previous Level of Engagement

If a client engaged in many leisure and social activities before the onset of a health condition, a wider range of options for intervention is possible. People who have a wide range of interests are more likely to continue engaging in a previous leisure activity than those with a narrow range.[36] This situation was certainly the case for Winnie. Given Winnie's wide range of leisure and social interests, the OTA can draw from more choices and thus is more likely to achieve engagement in some activities, although perhaps in an adapted manner.

Clients who previously participated in a limited range of leisure and social activities and who cannot perform or are not interested in previous activities are likely to need to develop new interests.[36] In these situations, the OTA may gently propose new leisure and social options that are within the person's capability (see Case Study: Edwin).

> **CASE STUDY**
>
> **Edwin**
>
> Edwin, 54 years old, is in inpatient rehabilitation after falling from his roof and sustaining a back injury and minor brain injury. Before his accident, according to his wife, he spent all his spare time restoring old cars with his two brothers, and playing golf. This information presented a dilemma for the OTA. She recognized that Edwin would not be able to return to these activities any time soon, yet she was unaware of any other leisure or social pursuits Edwin previously enjoyed. During one session learning bathroom transfers, the OTA asked Edwin whether there was anything that he ever dreamed of doing. Edwin recalled he once thought about becoming a pastry chef but did not think it a particularly masculine career. The OTA suggested he might want to explore this idea and bake something for his wife. Edwin agreed, and the OTA recommended he choose a recipe from among the easy ones in the department recipe file. During their next kitchen session that focused on safe mobility, Edwin made a banana cream pie for his wife. Edwin was pleased with how it turned out, despite dropping some of the filling on the floor. Edwin began to recognize that it was possible to replace his former interests with ones that were within his current capacity and that he enjoyed.

If leisure and/or social activities are not a top priority in the client's life, the OTA should not press a client to accept that such activities will be good for him or her. For example, if a client experiences a condition that prevents him or her from returning to work, the client is less likely to want to substitute leisure and social pursuits for previous productive activities.[51] In these situations, the OTA should acknowledge and work with the client's desire for productive—not leisure or social—activities. However, the OTA may want to share that engaging in leisure and social activities after a disability significantly contributes to life satisfaction, quality of life, and well-being. The choice to pursue leisure and social activities, however, is always the client's.

Consider Client's Personal Standards of Performance

The quality of performance considered acceptable by a client may determine whether he or she wants to pursue a leisure or social activity. Some clients are willing to resume activities at a lesser level of competence; others are not interested if they cannot perform to their previous standard,[36,68,86] particularly if they considered themselves proficient (see Case Study: Jean).

Encouraging a client to engage in previously enjoyed activities may have the undesired effect of making the client feel less than adequate.[51] In these situations, the OTA may prefer to introduce new activities for which the client–not having a previous standard–may be less likely to judge his or her performance negatively. Other clients choose not to engage in an activity because they cannot do it the way they did it

CASE STUDY

Jean

Jean, 68 years old, loved to play word games and took great pride in her skill. She was diagnosed with early-onset dementia and began attending an adult day program in which the OTA, learning from her family that Jean liked games, tried to involve her in simple word games. Jean refused. Only after carefully observing Jean's reluctance did the OTA realize Jean refused because she recognized she could not play to her previous skill level.

CASE STUDY

Catherine

Catherine, 82 years old, is receiving outpatient OT to learn more about joint protection techniques after a severe exacerbation of rheumatoid arthritis. She identified her favorite activity, which she feels free to do in her own way, as making her special chocolate chip cookies. She takes great joy in adding various surprise ingredients such as dried cranberries or crushed mints and looks forward to her great-granddaughter's reaction when she babysits her each weekend. The OTA suggested that instead of making cookies from scratch, Catherine could save energy by using prepackaged dough and preserve her joints by cutting the tube of dough with a rocker knife. Catherine immediately rejected the idea because it was not the way she makes cookies. The OTA needed to shift focus and collaborate with Catherine on ways to save energy and protect her joints while still engaging in valued activities in a manner acceptable to Catherine.

before their new health condition (see Case Study: Catherine). In other cases, clients might not want to engage in activities for fear of family members' (and others') disapproval (or the perception of disapproval) of less than perfect performance[36] (see Case Study: Marie). If a client is frustrated with his or her diminished ability to engage in a specific leisure or social activity, he or she is less likely to consider using adaptive equipment.[68] OTAs must respect client choices and rejection of activities, particularly if the client is frustrated. Collaboration with the client can identify other leisure and social activities in which he or she might feel more comfortable and competent.

Emphasize Choice and Control during Activities

When activities are chosen for them and they do not feel in control, clients are less likely to want to participate.[51] Results from the Well Elderly Program[17,35] and a wellness program based on the Model of Human Occupation (MOHO) for healthy older adults[87] indicate that life satisfaction, well-being, and quality of life are enhanced when older adults are given the opportunity to explore and choose what they would like to do and when opportunities are provided that are challenging yet within their capabilities (see Case Study: Community Residence).

CASE STUDY

Marie

Marie, 32 years old, was scheduled for an overnight home visit during her final week of rehabilitation after the onset of Guillain-Barré syndrome. Marie's husband wanted to surprise her with reservations at her favorite restaurant and consulted with the OTA. During their conversation, the OTA shared that Marie had mentioned several times she thought other people were embarrassed when she spilled food and drinks. The OTA carefully suggested that her husband consider a quiet dinner alone at home because some people are uncomfortable going out in public the first time; he agreed. She also suggested to Marie that she might consider discussing her feelings with her husband. On Monday, Marie reported she and her husband had enjoyed two nice dinners at home and had talked a lot over the weekend. She said she was relieved the OTA had addressed the issue of her embarrassment with handling food and utensils with both her husband and her.

CASE STUDY

Community Residence

An OTA working at a community residence for persons with HIV disease is responsible for assisting weekly activities with residents. During one session, the residents said they wanted a barbecue at the end of the month. The OTA helped them develop a plan and decide who would do what. The day of the barbecue, the OTA arrived a few hours early to help with preparations and was pleasantly surprised. Several residents had taken it upon themselves to ask neighbors for donations of flowers and plants and had decorated the residence. Other residents had already prepared their dishes and were helping others to make theirs. Two residents were busy rehearsing a funny poem they wrote for the invited volunteer staff, a spur-of-the-moment decision on their part. Through assisting self-choice and promoting self-control, the OTA contributed to increased enjoyment and satisfaction in the residents' daily lives.

Emphasize Exploration, not only Performance

For many clients, participating in structured leisure exploration programs may be of benefit to assist their eventual engagement in leisure and social activities.[23,53] These types of programs (similar to the previously mentioned programs but developed from a leisure perspective) help clients explore the importance of leisure, develop greater awareness of their perceptions in regard to leisure, identify leisure activities of interest, and develop competence to eventually engage in leisure activities.

Consider Attitudes of Family Members, Friends, and Others

Support from family, friends, and others is an important environmental factor with leisure and social activities.[36,73] Family members' positive attitudes and beliefs, particularly those of spouses and partners, can encourage and support a client to resume prior activities or begin new pursuits. The OTA should also be aware if family members provide only minimal encouragement or even actively discourage leisure and social endeavours.[36] The OTA could share with a client's family and friends that their support and encouragement are particularly important in regard to engagement in leisure and social activity. As seen later, this encouragement was a key factor during Winnie's OT. Moreover, when family and friends support the use of adaptive equipment, the client is more likely to accept and use it successfully.[68] The OTA should involve the client and appropriate family members and friends actively while identifying options for adaptive equipment and skills training (see Case Study: Velda).

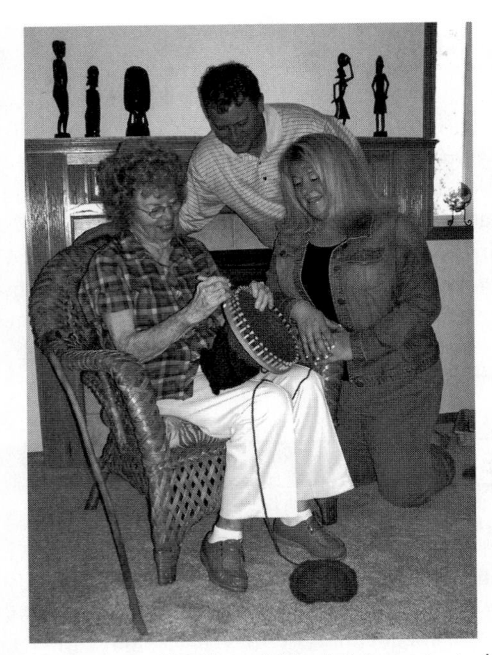

Figure 18-5 Support of family and friends is important when learning different ways to engage in leisure activities.

CASE STUDY

Velda

Velda is 69 years old. She had polio when she was 3 years old and now lives in an assisted living complex. The OTA is responsible for fostering the residents' participation in valued leisure and social activities. Once every 2 months, the OTA introduces a new handicraft for residents to try. Velda's "gaggle of friends" (as Velda refers to them) look forward to this activity, but Velda often says "if it involves a new-fangled device, I just won't learn it." One month, the OTA introduced rake-knitting and suggested to Velda's friends that they playfully tease Velda into trying this "new-fangled device." It worked; Velda liked it and purchased the required wooden frame so that she could make scarves whenever she wanted (Figure 18-5).

Suggest Activities That Appeal to a Client's Altruistic Nature

Because older adults particularly want to engage in responsible roles and feel depended on,[30] the OTA should explore options for leisure and social activities that appeal to a client's altruistic nature. Evidence suggests that when older adults are invited to participate in activities primarily for the benefit of others, such as decorating Valentine cookies for preschool children rather than just decorating Valentine cookies, they are more motivated and likely to participate.[15,16,30,85] When clients are reluctant to consider leisure activities during therapy because they believe it is not "real work" or "frivolous," they are more likely to agree and participate if the activity is presented as something that would benefit someone else. Most importantly, such reasons help a client believe he or she is worthwhile and doing something of value and help establish a sense of community and connectedness.[16] As seen later, this incentive was another key factor during Winnie's OT.

Identify Barriers to Transportation and Accessibility in the Community

One of the biggest barriers to engaging in leisure and social pursuits is difficulty with transportation and accessibility in the community.[73] Given the tendency for adults with physical disabilities to participate in substantially more home-based, sedentary, and solitary leisure and social activities,[1,8,83,86] OTAs should be familiar with community resources including feasible means of transportation that might support a client's engagement in activities, particularly social, outside the home. They can then help educate clients and families how best to access and use suitable community resources (see Case Study: Jason). Moreover, helping clients to engage in enjoyable and social activities outside the home may also provide needed respite for family members.[81] (See Case Study: Jason)

CASE STUDY

Jason

Before his T-8 spinal cord injury, Jason, who is 33 years old, enjoyed a wide variety of social and leisure activities in the community. He played music with friends once a week, coached his daughter's soccer team, and typically ended the workweek with a date with his partner. The OTA who worked with him at the outpatient clinic knew of community resources and was familiar with the accessibility challenges people using wheelchairs face. She supported Jason's desire to get out of the house and explored with him community options that would be interesting, practical, and accessible. Jason could participate in his community and was no longer a captive in his home.

Consider the Leisure and Social Participation Desires of Family Caregivers

Although the primary focus of intervention is the client, OTAs should also consider the leisure and social participation desires of family members who care for the client, particularly as many caregivers express diminished satisfaction with their own participation in leisure and social activities.[75] Some caregivers (particularly those with a strong family orientation) may find it hard to understand or accept that leisure is important simply because it is good for them. Here it is valuable to educate the caregiver and encourage reflection on results to help them see that taking the time to engage in chosen leisure and social activities (outside of their caregiving services) can enhance their own ability to take care of the client.[66]

Focus on Social Participation and Leisure

When identifying activities, the OTA should consider options beyond typical leisure pursuits such as arts, crafts, and hobbies. Because the primary motivation to engage in leisure activities may be to meet new people, establish friendships, and feel a sense of belonging,[73] social activities should be identified. Older adults report that relationships with others are important; one of their strategies to establish social relationships is attendance at more formal gatherings[18] such as civic groups or volunteer organizations. Thus the OTA should consider options within the community to meet a client's social needs, particularly those that may not involve family members. One innovative idea involved a group of older adults who could not leave their homes.[79] A local agency arranged, once a week, a conference call during which each adult sang a song with (and for) everyone else. Invariably, each performance was followed by applause and compliments. The agency also arranged other conference calls, tailored to their individual interests, for other clients. For older adults with Internet access, usage of social network sites is on the rise, for sharing photos, news, and other information among a network of contacts.[45] These and other innovations can provide valuable social engagement for many older adults and persons experiencing physical disabilities.

Focus on Developing a Routine of Leisure and Social Activities

The final guideline reinforces the importance of establishing and engaging in a routine of activities (the client's performance patterns). Older adults report that it is important to keep active in a variety of activities and to set aside time for quiet periods and rest.[18] Although pattern and routine are useful, a routine of leisure and social activities should be flexible to allow for spontaneity. For example, people with arthritis may reduce the expression of symptoms by pacing and planning of activities throughout the day and week. However, these strategies may constrain spontaneity because of less flexible scheduling.[74] Because spontaneity can be a key quality of leisure, the OTA should encourage clients to plan daily or weekly routines that allow room for spontaneous decisions.

Given the benefits of participating in leisure and social activities, all OT practitioners should recommend, particularly for those who are older and experiencing greater challenges resulting from physical impairments,[27] engagement in a broad range of relaxing, physical, and social activities.[24] If OT practitioners believe a balance of activities is important, a routine of activities should be promoted in which leisure and social participation is valued and balanced in relation to other activities in a client's life.

CASE STUDY

Winnie, Part 3: Engaging in Valued Activities after Her Stroke

In addition to targeting Winnie's ability to perform ADL tasks safely and more independently and setting goals to that effect, Jodi, Winnie, and the occupational therapist agreed that leisure and social participation should also be a primary focus and outcome during Winnie's anticipated 6-week rehabilitation stay. When asked, Winnie identified her activities of concern as the following:

1. Preparing food for her family
2. Attending the "May Babies" birthday celebration
3. Having fun with her children and grandchildren
4. Volunteering with her daughter-in-law to make quilts
5. Getting back to swimming

Jodi explained that although they would address all her concerns, only one would become an official goal and documented with her ADL and mobility goals. When asked which concern was most important, Winnie chose making quilts for families of soldiers. When asked for clarification, Winnie said she was feeling useless and would feel better if she was doing something for someone else. Thus a goal was documented: "By discharge, patient will satisfactorily engage in her valued leisure pursuit of making quilts for soldiers' families as a volunteer activity." Jodi assured Winnie that her other leisure and social concerns would be addressed and incorporated into therapy sessions that focused on improving Winnie's ability to perform ADL and IADL tasks such as preparing treats and meals for her family and learning to safely move about the community in order to attend the "May Babies" celebration and get back to swimming.

During Winnie's first week, intervention focused primarily on basic ADL and mobility tasks. However, as Winnie identified that spending time with her family was important, Jodi asked if it would be a good idea if some family members visited during lunch when Winnie was less fatigued. She agreed but felt uncomfortable about asking them and requested Jodi to do this. When Jodi discussed this with Winnie's son, he took charge and arranged a flexible schedule for family and friends to visit throughout the week. Jodi also mentioned to him the importance of Winnie maintaining her role as family matriarch, making choices and feeling a sense of control. Jodi emphasized that although family members were concerned about Winnie, they shouldn't be overprotective; instead, they could encourage her to be as active as she wanted. For example, they could ask Winnie if she preferred to visit in her room, in the lounge, or outside, even if this required her family's help with mobility. Further,

CASE STUDY—cont'd

knowing that Winnie's eyestrain and limited concentration were troubling, Jodi suggested short and simple board games that Winnie could choose to play with family members, particularly when her grandchildren visited.

Several "May Babies" visited Winnie. One dropped by at the end of a session when Winnie was working on safe transfers in the bathroom. Winnie's friend happened to mention that they were starting to plan the meals for their birthday beach celebration. Jodi immediately recognized Winnie might feel left out and skillfully steered the conversation such that by the end, Winnie and her friend planned to get all the "May Babies" together at the SNF that weekend so that Winnie could help plan the celebration, a role important to her.

As the weeks progressed, Jodi and Winnie considered Winnie's interests and leisure activities and incorporated them into her intervention sessions. They spent several sessions a week in the kitchen, developing her performance skills while preparing muffins for her husband, bread for her children, and cookies for her grandchildren. Jodi asked whether Winnie wanted to give anything special to the "May Babies" for their birthdays. Winnie mentioned that they all enjoyed cooking and thought potted fresh herbs would be a nice gift. To develop her performance skills for all daily life activities, Winnie transplanted several herbs into pots and began sponge painting each one. After Winnie completed the first one, Jodi made arrangements with staff so that Winnie and her grandchildren could complete these together on the weekend in the OT room.

During the latter part of her stay, Winnie was getting better at moving around the room and could walk with minimal support of her husband down the hallway, albeit a bit slowly and unsteadily. As discharge was getting closer, Jody and Winnie began to consider how she would spend her time once she returned home. Jodi ensured that all team members were aware that many of Winnie's leisure and social interests occurred outside the home and were working with Winnie to help her gain as much independence as possible. Taxis and public transportation were options for her. Although Winnie could see herself eventually returning to swimming, she was hesitant about being around others in public. She wasn't sure how accessible the pool might be and didn't know whether someone could help her if she got into trouble, both in the locker room and in the pool. Jodi gently suggested that it might be good for Winnie to advocate for herself. To do so, she suggested Winnie keep track of her concerns, develop a list of questions, and then call the swim center.

From the beginning, Winnie's official goal was to work together with her daughter-in-law to embroider quilts for soldiers' families and feel satisfied doing so. Jodi initially scheduled a time with Winnie and her daughter-in-law to discuss their original plans and explore ways in which Winnie could continue to participate. Listening to Winnie describe the process of quilt making, Jodi used activity analysis to identify aspects of the activity within Winnie's current ability and to note those for which she would need to further develop her skills or adapt the method. To begin, Jodi recommended that Winnie and her daughter-in-law plan which fabrics they wanted to use and that her daughter-in-law bring them to the SNF. Because this week was the second of rehabilitation, Jodi surmised that Winnie would be frustrated with using scissors because she was not using her right hand to feed herself. Instead, Jodie suggested Winnie solicit her grandchildren's help and direct them to cut the fabric squares. They could do it together during the evenings, thus giving Winnie a reason to be a bit active in the evening, spend time with her grandchildren, and improve her endurance. The original plan was for Winnie to embroider some of the quilt squares after they were cut. Because embroidering would be difficult with Winnie's continued eyestrain and diminished hand control, Jodi inquired whether she was willing to forego embroidery and focus on creating a simpler yet still beautiful quilt. Winnie concurred and began to plan the quilt's design.

By the third week, the last of the fabric squares was cut, and Jodi scheduled an afternoon session for Winnie to focus on improving her standing balance while using her right arm for balance as she ironed the squares with her left. This process took several sessions, and by the fourth week, the fabric squares were ready to be sewn together. Jodi showed Winnie a method whereby Winnie could pin the fabric with her left hand (which was awkward at first) while using her affected right hand to stabilize the fabric while she pinned. Jodi mentioned that this would foster better control and quality of movement. Jodi also knew that if Winnie made a mistake during the pinning, it could easily be corrected. After their first practice session, Winnie again took charge and solicited the help of her grandchildren during the evenings and weekends. She insisted, however, that she would do all the pinning; her grandchildren would serve only as assistants.

Pinning half of the squares took until the next week to complete, and Winnie mentioned to everyone that she did it all (perhaps "forgetting" that her grandchildren did help a bit!). At this point, discharge was 1 week away and Jodi made plans for Winnie and her daughter-in-law to begin sewing the squares together. Winnie was reluctant to use the sewing machine, fearing a mistake. Jodi and Winnie tried different methods and discovered an effective technique for Winnie to help her daughter-in-law with the performance skills Winnie had been developing. Although Winnie did not have time to complete the quilt before discharge, when she and Jodi reviewed her goal to engage in a favored leisure activity to her satisfaction, Winnie agreed the goal had been met and acknowledged that although it was not the way she used to do it, she felt good that she was doing something useful. When Winnie was discharged home, she still required slight assistance with some mobility and ADL tasks but reported more self-worth and joy in her daily life, in part from engaging in leisure and social activities again.

Summary

More professionals are advocating that rehabilitation and OT services increase the time devoted to leisure and social activities and decrease the time devoted to basic ADL tasks, particularly for clients living in the community.[8,19,57,83,88] Given the benefits of participating in leisure and social activities for all persons, OT practitioners need to address leisure and social participation throughout all phases of their practice. To relegate leisure and social activities to the back burner or consider leisure and social activities only as a means to regain performance skills diminishes the opportunity for clients to experience joy and satisfaction in their daily lives. By implementing intervention that promotes the benefits of leisure and social participation, OT practitioners can help their clients enjoy walking the family dog, laughing with a best friend, making a quilt for a first grandchild, and watching sunsets at the beach with a loved one. By engagement in these activities, clients and others can recognize that how one occupies one's daily life is truly related to one's health, well-being, life satisfaction, and quality of life.

"The experience of leisure neither cures nor removes the effects of aging, mental health disorders, and chronic health problems. It does, however, have the potential to change the quality of life for many individuals." Melinda Suto[76]

Selected Reading Guide Questions

1. When meeting a client for the first time to discuss leisure and social activities, how would you solicit the client's perspective?
2. What are the specific benefits associated with participating in leisure and social activities for all adults, disability or not?
3. What are the concerns of people with disabilities with respect to participating in leisure and social activities?
4. Why is it important for an OTA to consider the timing of when to introduce leisure and social participation during therapy? What could happen that might have a negative impact on a client if activities are introduced too soon, too late, or not at all?

Learning Activities

1. Conduct a mock interview with a classmate or family member using the questions from Table 18-1 as a guide. Audiotape or videotape yourself during the interview and evaluate your skills in eliciting the person's meaning of and experience with leisure and social activities.
2. Keep track of your leisure and social activities for a week. Identify which activities you consider leisure or social, how often you engage in them, their relative value to you according to preference, and the qualities you experience during each activity that make it more leisurely or social. If you could no longer engage in these activities because of a physical disability, which might you give up if you could not do them to your performance standards? Which would you consider continuing even if you had to use an adapted manner?

CASE STUDY

Winnie, Part 4: A Postscript

Winnie was discharged 17 days before the "May Babies" celebration. Although she was grateful to be home at last with her husband, she looked forward to the weekend getaway and to reclaiming some semblance of her life before her stroke. Three days before the celebration, Winnie suffered a second stroke and died. After the funeral, Winnie's family sent a letter to the SNF staff expressing their gratitude and sharing that although Winnie never realized her dream to attend the "May Babies" celebration, hope and joy were a part of her life until the end because of the attention paid to who she was and to what was important in her life.

References

1. Almborg AH, Ulander K, Thulin A, Berg S: Discharged after stroke—important factors for health-related quality of life, *J Clin Nurs* 19(15-16):2196–2206, 2010.
2. American Occupational Therapy Association: Occupational therapy practice framework: domain & process, ed 2, *Am J Occup Ther* 62(6):625–683, 2008.
3. American Occupational Therapy Association: Guidelines for supervision, roles, and responsibilities during the delivery of occupational therapy services, *Am J Occup Ther* 63(6):797–803, 2009.
4. Anke AGW, Fugl-Meyer AR: Life satisfaction several years after severe multiple trauma-A retrospective investigation, *Clin Rehabil* 17(4):431–442, 2003.
5. Awaad T: Culture, cultural competency and occupational therapy: A review of the literature, *Br J Occup Ther* 66(8):356–362, 2003.
6. Ball V, Corr S, Knight J, Lowis MJ: An investigation into the leisure occupations of older adults, *Br J Occup Ther* 70(9):393–400, 2007.
7. Baum CM, Edwards D: *Activity card sort*, ed 2, Bethesda, MD, 2008, AOTA Press.
8. Bier N, Dutil E, Couture M: Factors affecting leisure participation after a traumatic brain injury: An exploratory study, *J Head Trauma Rehabil* 24(3):187–194, 2009.
9. Bonder BR, Martin L, Miracle AW: Culture emergent in occupation, *Am J Occup Ther* 58(2):159–168, 2004.
10. Brown M, Gordon WA, Spielman L, Haddad L: Participation by individuals with spinal cord injury in social and recreational activity outside the home, *Top Spinal Cord Inj Rehabil* 7(3): 83–100, 2002.
11. Bundy AC: Assessment of play and leisure: Delineation of the problem, *Am J Occup Ther* 47(3):217–222, 1993.
12. Bundy AC, Clemson L: Leisure. In Bonder B, Dal Bello-Haas V, editors: *Functional performance in older adults*, ed 3, Philadelphia, 2009, F. A. Davis, pp 290–306.
13. Caldwell LL: Leisure and health: Why is leisure therapeutic? *Br J Guid Counc* 33(1):7–26, 2005.

14. Centers for Medicare & Medicaid Services: Medicare Benefit Policy Manual: Chapter 15-Covered Medical and Other Health Services. 2010, Retrieved from www.cms.gov/manuals/Downloads/bp102c15.pdf.
15. Cipriani J: Altruistic activities of older adults living in long term care facilities: A literature review, *Phys Occup Ther Geriatr* 26(1):19–28, 2007.
16. Cipriani J, Haley R, Moravec E, Young H: Experience and meaning of group altruistic activities among long-term care residents, *Br J Occup Ther* 73(6):269–276, 2010.
17. Clark F, Azen SP, Zemke R, Jackson J, Carlson M, Mandel D, et al: Occupational therapy for independent-living older adults: A randomized controlled trial, *J Am Med Assoc* 278(16):1321–1326, 1997.
18. Clark F, Carlson M, Zemke R, Frank G, Patterson K, Ennevor BL, et al: Life domains and adaptive strategies of a group of low-income, well older adults, *Am J Occup Ther* 50(2):99–108, 1996.
19. Cowdell F, Garrett D: Recreation in stroke rehabilitation part two: Exploring patients' views, *Int J Ther Rehabil* 10(10):456–462, 2003.
20. Crenshaw W, Gillian ML, Kidd N, Olivo J, Schell BAB: Assisted living residents' perspectives of their occupational performance concerns, *Act Adapt Aging* 26(1):41–55, 2001.
21. Dahan-Oliel N, Gelinas I, Mazer B: Social participation in the elderly: What does the literature tell us? *Crit Rev Phys Rehabil Med* 20(2):159–176, 2008.
22. Dedding C, Cardol M, Eyssen IC, Dekker J, Beelen A: Validity of the Canadian Occupational Performance Measure: A client-centred outcome measurement, *Clin Rehabil* 18(6):660–667, 2004.
23. Desrosiers J, Noreau L, Rochette A, Carbonneau H, Fontaine L, Viscogliosi C, et al: Effect of a home leisure education program after stroke: A randomized controlled trial, *Arch Phys Med Rehabil* 88(9):1095–1100, 2007.
24. Fitts HA, Howe MC: Use of leisure time by cardiac patients, *Am J Occup Ther* 41(9):583–589, 1987.
25. Gabriel Z, Bowling A: Quality of life from the perspectives of older people, *Ageing Soc* 24(5):675–691, 2004.
26. Garcia LE, Banegas JR, Pérez-Regadera AG, Herruzo Cabrera R, Rodríguez-Artalejo F: Social network and health-related quality of life in older adults: A population-based study in Spain, *Qual Life Res* 14(2):511–520, 2005.
27. Glass TA, de Leon CM, Marottoli RA, Berkman LF: Population-based study of social and productive activities as predictors of survival among elderly Americans, *Br Med J* 319(7208):478–483, 1999.
28. Griffin J, McKenna K: Influences on leisure and life satisfaction of elderly people, *Phys Occup Ther Geriatr* 15(4):1–16, 1998.
29. Hartman-Maeir A, Soroker N, Ring H, Avni N, Katz N: Activities, participation and satisfaction one-year post stroke, *Disabil Rehabil* 29(7):559–566, 2007.
30. Hatter JK, Nelson DL: Altruism and task participation in the elderly, *Am J Occup Ther* 41(6):379–381, 1987.
31. Herzog AR, Ofstedal MB, Wheeler LM: Social engagement and its relationship to health, *Clin Geriatr Med* 18(3):593–609, 2002.
32. Holt-Lunstad J, Smith TB, Layton JB: Social relationships and mortality risk: A meta-analytic review. [electronic], *PLoS Medicine* 7(7), 2010:e1000316. doi:1000310.1001371/journal.pmed.1000316.
33. Horowitz BP, Vanner E: Relationships among active engagement in life activities and quality of life for assisted-living residents, *J Hous Elderly* 24(2):130–150, 2010.
34. Interest Checklist (UK). (n.d.). Available from www.moho.uic.edu/mohorelatedrsrcs.html.
35. Jackson J, Carlson M, Mandel D, Zemke R, Clark F: Occupation in lifestyle redesign: The well elderly study occupational therapy program, *Am J Occup Ther* 52(5):326–336, 1998.
36. Jongbloed L, Morgan D: An investigation of involvement in leisure activities after a stroke, *Am J Occup Ther* 45(5):420–427, 1991.
37. Kielhofner G: *Model of human occupation: Theory and application*, ed 4, Baltimore, 2008, Lippincott Williams & Wilkins.
38. Korner-Bitensky N, Desrosiers J, Rochette A: A national survey of occupational therapists' practices related to participation post-stroke, *J Rehabil Med* 40(4):291–297, 2008.
39. Larson R, Mannell R, Zuzanek J: Daily well-being of older adults with friends and family, *Psychol Aging* 1(2):117–126, 1986.
40. Law M: Participation in the occupations of everyday life, *Am J Occup Ther* 56(6):640–649, 2002.
41. Law M, Baptiste S, Carswell A, McColl MA, Polatajko H, Pollock N: *Canadian occupational performance measure*, ed 4, Toronto, 2005, Canadian Association of Occupational Therapists.
42. Law M, Steinwender S, Leclair L: Occupation, health and well-being, *Can J Occup Ther* 65(2):81–91, 1998.
43. Litwin H: Social network type and morale in old age, *Gerontologist* 41(4):516–524, 2001.
44. Lloyd KM, Auld CJ: The role of leisure in determining quality of life: Issues of content and measurement, *Social Indic Res* 57(1):43–71, 2002.
45. Madden M: *Older adults and social media [report]*, Washington, D. C, 2010, Pew Research Center.
46. Mars GMJ, Kempen GIJM, Post MWM, Proot IM, Mesters I, Van Eijk JTM: The Maastricht social participation profile: Development and clinimetric properties in older adults with a chronic physical illness, *Qual Life Res* 18(9):1207–1218, 2009.
47. Matsutsuyu JS: The interest check list, *Am J Occup Ther* 23(4):323–328, 1969.
48. McColl MA, Paterson M, Davies D, Doubt L, Law M: Validity and community utility of the Canadian Occupational Performance Measure, *Can J Occup Ther* 67(1):22–30, 2000.
49. Meyer A: The philosophy of occupation therapy. [reprint], *Am J Occup Ther* 31(10):639–642, 1922/1977.
50. Modified Interest Checklist. (n.d.). Available from www.moho.uic.edu/mohorelatedrsrcs.html.
51. Morgan D, Jongbloed L: Factors influencing leisure activities following a stroke: An exploratory study, *Can J Occup Ther* 57(4):223–229, 1990.
52. Mosey AC: *Applied scientific inquiry in the health professions: An epistemological orientation*, ed 2, Bethesda, MD, 1996, American Occupational Therapy Association.
53. Nour K, Desrosiers J, Gauthier P, Carbonneau H: Impact of a home leisure educational program for older adults who have had a stroke (Home Leisure Educational Program), *Ther Recreation J* 36(1):48–64, 2002.
54. O'Sullivan C, Chard G: An exploration of participation in leisure activities post-stroke, *Austral Occup Ther J* 57(3):159–166, 2010.
55. Odawara E: Cultural competency in occupational therapy: Beyond a cross-cultural view of practice, *Am J Occup Ther* 59(3):325–334, 2005.
56. Parham LD, Fazio LS: *Play in occupational therapy for children*, St. Louis, MO, 1997, Mosby.
57. Parker C, Gladman J, Drummond A: The role of leisure in stroke rehabilitation, *Disabil Rehabil* 19(1):1–5, 1997.
58. Pereira RB, Stagnitti K: The meaning of leisure for well-elderly Italians in an Australian community: Implications for occupational therapy, *Austral Occup Ther J* 55(1):39–46, 2008.

59. Primeau LA: Work and leisure: Transcending the dichotomy, *Am J Occup Ther* 50(7):569–577, 1996.
60. Primeau LA: Play and leisure. In Crepeau EB, Cohn ES, Schell BAB, editors: *Willard & Spackman's occupational therapy*, ed 10, Philadelphia, 2003, Lippincott, pp 354–363.
61. Radomski MV: There is more to life than putting on your pants, *Am J Occup Ther* 49(6):487–490, 1995.
62. Ragheb MG, Beard JG: *Idyll Arbor Leisure Battery*, Enumclaw, WA, 1993, Idyll Arbor.
63. Reinseth L, Espnes GA: Women with rheumatoid arthritis: Non-vocational activities and quality of life, *Scand J Occup Ther* 14(2):108–115, 2007.
64. Rochette A, Desrosiers J, Bravo G, St-Cyr/Tribble D, Bourget A: Changes in participation after a mild stroke: Quantitative and qualitative perspectives, *Top Stroke Rehabil* 14(3):59–68, 2007.
65. Roelofs LH: The meaning of leisure, *J Gerontol Nursing* 25(10): 32–39, 1999.
66. Rogers N: Family obligation, caregiving, and loss of leisure: The experiences of three caregivers, *Act Adapt Aging* 24(2):35–49, 1999.
67. Rudman D, Cook J, Polatajko H: Understanding the potential of occupation: A qualitative exploration of seniors' perspectives on activity, *Am J Occup Ther* 51(8):640–650, 1997.
68. Schweitzer JA, Mann WC, Nochajski S, Tomita M: Patterns of engagement in leisure activity by older adults using assistive devices, *Technol Disabil* 11(1/2):103–117, 1999.
69. Sellar B, Boshoff K: Subjective leisure experiences of older Australians, *Austral Occup Ther J* 53(3):211–219, 2006.
70. Shaw S: The measurement of leisure: A quality of life issue, *Soc Leisure* 7:91–107, 1984.
71. Shaw S: Leisure, recreation or free time? Measuring time usage, *J Leisure Res* 18(3):177–189, 1986.
72. Smith NR, Kielhofner G, Watts JH: The relationships between volition, activity pattern, and life satisfaction in the elderly, *Am J Occup Ther* 40(4):278–283, 1986.
73. Specht J, King G, Brown E, Foris C: The importance of leisure in the lives of persons with congenital physical disabilities, *Am J Occup Ther* 56(4):436–445, 2002.
74. Stephens M, Yoshida KK: Independence and autonomy among people with rheumatoid arthritis, *Can J Rehabil* 12(4):229–243, 1999.
75. Stevens AB, Coon D, Wisniewski S, Vance D, Arguelles S, Belle S, et al: Measurement of leisure time satisfaction in family caregivers, *Aging Ment Health* 8(5):450–459, 2004.
76. Suto M: Leisure in occupational therapy, *Can J Occup Ther* 65(5):271–278, 1998.
77. Suto M: Exploring leisure meanings that inform client-centred practice. In Carpenter C, editor: *Qualitative research in evidence-based rehabilitation*, Edinburgh, 2004, Churchill Livingstone, pp 27–39.
78. Sveen U, Thommessen B, Bautz-Holter E, Wyller TB, Laake K: Well-being and instrumental activities of daily living after stroke, *Clin Rehabil* 18(3):267–274, 2004.
79. The Next Big Thing. (January 21, 2005 episode). Heard on the phone: Public Radio International.
80. Turner H, Chapman S, McSherry A, Krishnagiri S, Watts J: Leisure assessment in occupational therapy: An exploratory study, *Occup Ther Health Care* 12(2/3):73–85, 2000.
81. Ward GE, Jagger C, Harper WM: The Canadian Occupational Performance Measure: What do users consider important? *Br J Ther Rehabil* 3(8):448–452, 1996.
82. Whiteford GE, Wilcock AA: Cultural relativism: Occupation and independence reconsidered, *Can J Occup Ther* 67(5):324–336, 2000.
83. Widen-Holmqvist L, de Pedro-Cuesta J, Holm M, Sandsrom B, Hellblom A, Stawiarz L, et al: Stroke rehabilitation in Stockholm: Basis for late intervention in patients living at home, *Scand J Rehabil Med* 25(4):173–181, 1993.
84. Wikstrom E, Isacsson A, Jacobsson L: Leisure activities in rheumatoid arthritis: Change after disease onset and associated factors, *Br J Occup Ther* 64(2):87–92, 2001.
85. Williams AL, Haber D, Weaver GD, Freeman JL: Altruistic activity: Does it make a difference in the senior center? *Act Adapt Aging* 22(4):31–39, 1997.
86. Wise EK, Mathews-Dalton C, Dikmen S, Temkin N, MacHamer J, Bell K, et al: Impact of traumatic brain injury on participation in leisure activities, *Arch Phys Med Rehabil* 91(9):1357–1362, 2010.
87. Yamada T, Kawamata H, Kobayashi N, Kielhofner G, Taylor RR: A randomised clinical trial of a wellness programme for healthy older people, *Br J Occup Ther* 73(11):540–548, 2010.
88. Zoerink DA: Exploring the relationship between leisure and health of senior adults with orthopedic disabilities living in rural areas, *Act Adapt Aging* 26(2):61–73, 2001.

Resources

Activity Card Sort (ACS)
www.aota.org

Canadian Occupational Performance Measure (COPM)
www.caot.ca
www.aota.org

Leisure Attitude Measure (LAM), Leisure Interest Measure (LIM), Leisure Satisfaction Scale (LSS), and Leisure Motivation Scale (LMS)
www.idyllarbor.com

Occupational Questionnaire (OQ), Modified Interest Checklist, Interest Checklist (UK)
www.moho.uic.edu

PART VI

Interventions for Performance Skills and Client Factors

CHAPTER 19

The Older Adult

MICHELE D. MILLS AND KERBY COULANGES

Key Terms

Aging
Age-related changes
Polypharmacy
Long-term care
Pharmacokinetics
Adult daycare
Home and community care
Assisted living
Subacute care
Resident Assessment Instrument (RAI)
Minimum data set (MDS)
Physical restraints
Chemical restraints
Restorative programs
Maintenance program
Enhanced environments

Chapter Objectives

After studying this chapter, the student or practitioner will be able to do the following:

1. Recognize the varied functional abilities of the older adult.
2. Discuss the developmental psychology theories regarding the older adult.
3. Describe various stages of aging.
4. Recognize the common age-related changes in the older adult.
5. Discuss the common pathological conditions that influence health and function in the older adult.
6. Understand the potential effect of medication on the functioning of the older adult.
7. Describe occupational therapy interventions for the older adult.
8. Discuss the variety of settings that provide services to the older adult.
9. Describe the methods used in a fall prevention program.
10. Explain the federal regulation concerning restraint-free environments.
11. Describe various interventions for the reduction of restraint use.
12. Use communication strategies with family, client, supervisor, and other staff members in long-term care.
13. Discuss the purpose and makeup of the minimum data set.

The term *elderly* is a commonly used label for the population of adults 65 years of age and older, yet this is a heterogeneous population. It is important to understand that members of this population have different experiences in aging. Some have significant financial and health problems, while others spend winters skiing and summers mountain climbing. Some stay in the paid work force until death, while most others have much leisure time filled with volunteer work, care of children or the frail elderly, puttering about, or other activities that are personally satisfying. Others are bored or depressed. In short, "the elderly," like other age groups, are mixed in needs, abilities, and resources.[15] Occupational therapy (OT) practitioners provide services to promote participation in occupation to this heterogeneous group of older adults across the continuum of function from frail to well.[7]

According to Data Sources on Older Americans, as of 2008, 39 million people were aged 65 and older.[2] The population of older adults is expanding. By 2050, the number of older Americans is expected to reach 90 million.[7] The aging American population presents a special challenge for the OT practitioner. Despite the myth that most older adults live in nursing homes, in actuality "only 4% to 5% of those persons 65 and older are in a nursing home at any one time."[1,7] The majority remain in the community, receiving assistance from family members and significant others.[20] These individuals will seek medical care and rehabilitation services on an as-needed basis. This growing number of persons 65 and older will place significant demands on all aspects of the continuum of health care services.[37] According to Data Sources on Older Americans in 2009, the percentage of adults 65 and older who were limited in activity was 42%.[19] However, the majority of older adults continue to live in their homes.[20,21]

Health factors greatly influence how a person will experience older age. "Some gerontologists distinguish between the *young-old* (persons 65 to 74) and the *old-old* (persons 75 years of age and older). The young-old tend to be more vigorous and have fewer health concerns than the old-old."[21] The old-old tend to be the largest consumers of health care services.[20]

*Angela M. Peralta contributed to the first edition of this book.

However, aging is an inevitable and complex process that begins as soon as an individual is conceived. Health and disease determine the quality of life individuals will have as they reach maturity.[2] Aging by itself does not necessarily precipitate an increase in disease.[48] Rather, age-associated changes in various organs and age-associated diseases contribute to the belief that old age means illness, dependency, and dementia.

It is important to view illness separately from reduced abilities. Disease should not be confused with normal aging. Generally, changes from normal aging cause a slowdown in normal functioning, whereas changes from illness and disease may cause temporary or permanent functional limitation.

Many of us know people who are extremely healthy and productive through their 80s and 90s and others who are totally dependent at age 65 or younger. Despite this range in ability to participate in life roles, normal aging continues to be associated with physiological and functional change. Rowe and Kahn challenge that "many usual aging characteristics are due to lifestyle … "[45] Understanding that older age is not synonymous with illness is important because it clarifies the importance of a healthy lifestyle. Nutrition, exercise, rest, good relationships with others, and participation in life through engagement in occupation are the foundation of healthy aging.[41]

Lewis[34] described four stages of older age. Stage I, from 50 to 65 years, is the preretirement age, when a person begins to plan for the use of leisure time and may begin to assume new roles such as grandparent or caretaker of elderly parents. In stage II, from 65 to 74 years, the individual may begin to encounter increased health problems and may experience grief as his or her spouse, friends, and/or siblings die. Stage III, from 75 to 84 years, may be when independent living is jeopardized. The person may begin to require assistance in life tasks. In stage IV, 85 years and older, the individual may become increasingly dependent on others. Institutional living arrangements may need to be made, or the individual may need to live with a family member.

Developmental Factors

For OT practitioners, understanding developmental psychology theories can help in anticipating some of the needs of the older adult.

Human development is widely described in the literature and is often presented in a model that goes from birth to childhood to adolescence to early adulthood to adulthood and to old age. Traditional theories postulate that a person must first master the tasks required of each stage before progressing to the next. Contemporary theories recognize that tasks may be mastered in isolation and/or may be carried over to another developmental stage.

Havighurst[47] defines a developmental task as one "which arises at or about a certain period in the life of the individual, successful achievement of which leads to his happiness and to success with later tasks, while failure leads to unhappiness in the individual, disapproval by the society, and difficulty with later tasks." Havighurst identified the following six tasks related to "later maturity": (1) adjustment to decreased physical strength and health; (2) adjustment to retirement and reduced income; (3) adjustment to the death of a spouse; (4) establishment of affiliation with own age group; (5) flexible adaptation to social role in a flexible way; and (6) establishment of satisfactory physical living arrangements.[47]

Havighurst argues that development is a cognitive learning process. Tasks develop out of a combination of pressures arising from physical development, cultural expectations, and individual values and goals. He postulates that "teachable moments" of a special sensitivity or readiness to learn arise from the unique combination of physical, social, and psychic readiness.[47]

Erik Erikson's theory of human development includes a model of eight stages of psychosocial development a healthy individual will traverse while experiencing life from infancy to mature adulthood. Within each stage, the individual is challenged to confront and master new skills. The last two stages of the model represent middle to mature adulthood. Generativity versus stagnation, the stage of middle adulthood (ages 35 to 65), focuses on individual understanding about one's own value in society. Ego integrity versus despair, the stage of later adulthood (65 years and beyond), involves a retrospective review of life, evaluating accomplishments and considering unachieved goals.[47]

Biological and sociological theories also seek to explain the aging process. Biological theories are generally concerned with how the cells age and how the aging process affects the various organs. Sociological theories are concerned with the types of activities in which the elderly engage and how the elderly disengage from familiar roles.

Expected biological changes are well documented in the literature. As age increases, various body functions decrease. The type and rate of change, however, vary with the individual. Many of these changes do not necessarily affect an individual's ability to function except when illness or disease occurs.

OT practitioners must be aware of how normal aging and pathological conditions affect the individual client in order to develop an OT intervention that (1) does not aggravate the condition; (2) promotes remediation of functional limitation; (3) provides compensatory strategies for participation in occupation; and (4) respects individual and familial goals, roles, and values.[4]

Common Age-Related Changes

The common age-related changes are not pathological and should not be seen as inevitable. When they occur, these changes are the bases on which specific pathological conditions are superimposed. Physiological aging may modify significantly the signs and symptoms and clinical course of disease processes. Pneumonia can be used to illustrate how the aging person's body reacts to disease in comparison with a younger person's body. In a younger person, pneumonia may resolve in a few weeks, whereas it may be fatal in an older person.

The common age-related changes in various systems include decreased functioning of the heart in times of stress and exercise. The strength of the heart muscle is reduced; the heart needs a longer time to relax between contractions. Normal aging also reduces the elasticity of the cardiovascular system.[35]

Decalcification causes the bones to become more porous, thus reducing the normal quantity and quality of bone structure.[23] As the demineralization of bone proceeds, bones become brittle; fractures may be common.[23]

Decreased hormone levels, decreased basal metabolic rate, decreased overall use of glucose, and decreased adrenal activity under stress are some of the endocrine changes seen in the older adult.

With advancing age, changes occur at all levels of the nervous system. A gradual decrease in bulk of individual muscles occurs, although the changes in muscle seen with aging do not produce clinically symptomatic muscle weakness. Nerve conduction velocity and oxygen consumption slow as well.

In the older adult, the body becomes less efficient in receiving, processing, and responding to stimuli. The older person experiences neurologic changes related to temperature regulation and ability to perceive pain. The older adult may feel cold more easily; it is common to see an older person wrapped in blankets and keeping the room temperature quite warm. Pain perception and reaction to painful stimuli are decreased with age. The number and sensitivity of sensory receptors are reduced in the aging process. The sense of balance and the ability to use fine movements are affected by the aging process. The aged person may reach for doorways, chairs, and hand railings to maintain balance and ensure stability.[23]

Older persons may experience a decrease in function of various senses. Visual acuity usually decreases with age. The incidence of cataracts increases with age. The lenses of the eye also become somewhat rigid; therefore the eye accommodates less efficiently. Table 19-1 suggests environmental adaptations for vision impairment.

Sexuality or sexual function should not be ignored when establishing interventions with the older adult. Sexual activity, engaging in activities that result in sexual satisfaction, is a basic ADL. It is important to be mindful that many older adults maintain desire (libido), sexual capacity, and satisfaction as long as they have their health and a capable partner.[31] The older adult continues to experience the same four stages of human sexual response during sexual stimulation: excitement phase, plateau phase, orgasmic phase, and resolution phase.[8] Common physiological changes in the sexual function of the older adult usually manifest as a gradual slowing. For instance, men may experience a longer time needed for arousal (erection) and women may require more time to develop lubrication. Unlike women, healthy men remain fertile until the end of life. The most common barriers to sexual activity in later life are declining medical status, physiological concerns, and social obstacles.[8]

Rest and sleep are influential when exploring an individual's physiological functioning and psychosocial well-being. According to the *Occupational Therapy Practice Framework II: Domain and Process,* edition 2, "rest and sleep include activities related to obtaining restorative rest and sleep that supports healthy active engagement in other areas of occupation."[4] Both older and younger adults spend an average of 6.5 to 7.5 hours sleeping during a 24-hour period, but older adults spend an additional 3 to 4 hours resting in order to achieve the same amount of sleep attained by younger adults.[16] Poor quality of sleep puts the older adult at risk for depression, adverse effects to medication, and pathological conditions.[13,35] OT practitioners assisting older adults dissatisfied with their sleep should identify the risk factors that can be addressed to

Table 19-1 Environment Adaptations for Visual Impairments

Condition	Problem	Intervention
Glare	May distract older people, especially those who have difficulty concentrating	Reducing glare will make it easier to recognize faces, which may improve communication.
Dark/light adaptation	Delayed for the older person when moving from a light to a darker area or vice versa	Freeing the entrance of furniture or other objects will make it easier to move from light to dark areas.
Color perception	Decreased for the aged	If colors are being used to enhance orientation, contrasting colors should highlight only those areas that are important to the person. For example, the utility room door may be painted the same color as the wall and the bathroom door may be painted in a contrasting color. Color contrast is helpful not only in public areas but also in activities of daily living such as dressing. Other tasks can also be made easier by creating a contrast between objects such as a toothbrush and a sink, a handrail and a wall, and a plate and a tablecloth.
Depth perception	Decreases with age and is more dependent on brightness and contrast	With age, more attention must be given to floor surfaces and steps. Figure-ground illusions are created when patterns are used. For example, when a floor surface is patterned, it may appear to be an object or several objects. Older people who have a cognitive impairment may perceive patterns as objects but not be able to ask questions or otherwise determine which objects are truly present in an environment.

Modified from Christenson MA: Adaptations for vision changes in older persons, *OT Pract* 1:1, 1996.

improve sleep quantity and quality, rather than viewing this as a consequence of aging.

Overlaid on these normal changes are a number of pathological conditions that can affect the older person's health status.

Common Pathological Conditions That Influence Health and Function

Cardiovascular Conditions

The cardiovascular system undergoes several physiological alterations with advancing age. Gerontologists and exercise physiologists suggest that physiological deconditioning is the major causative factor for heart disease in the older adult. Cardiovascular disease accounts for a large number of adult deaths in the United States, with the greatest percentage attributed to atherosclerosis.[35]

Common cardiovascular conditions in the older adult include hypertension, congestive heart failure (CHF), arteriosclerotic heart disease (ASHD), valvular problems that can necessitate a pacemaker, peripheral vascular disease (PVD), and cardiac arrest.

Pulmonary Conditions

The most common pulmonary condition associated with aging is chronic obstructive pulmonary disease (COPD). COPD results in airflow obstruction and often in hyperreactive airways, usually with bronchitis or emphysema. COPD is a functional diagnosis that includes a variety of disease processes that affect the upper and lower respiratory tracts and are characterized by cough, expectoration, wheezing, and dyspnea, first on exercise and later at rest.[35,51] These conditions may severely limit the person's stamina and endurance, thus impairing the ability to participate in self-care, work, and leisure activities.

Musculoskeletal Conditions

Pathological changes that develop with aging include osteoarthritis and osteoporosis. These conditions affect the bones and joints. Decreased mobility, joint stiffness, and deformities contribute to difficulty with participation in occupation.

Endocrine System Conditions

The most prevalent disorder of the endocrine system in the aged is diabetes mellitus (DM). Diabetic neuropathy commonly results in segmental injury to nerves and may cause decreased sensation, most commonly in the hands and feet of the individual.

Nervous System Conditions

Nervous system disorders include cerebrovascular accidents (CVAs), multiple sclerosis, and Parkinson's disease. These conditions significantly affect the person's ability to engage in occupation and participate in society.

Sensory Changes

Sensory changes may include decreased visual acuity, hearing loss, changes in taste and smell, decreased proprioception, decreased sensory awareness, decreased sensory processing, difficulties with perception, and deficits in the vestibular system. A pathological condition can lead to sensory change.

Vision

Changes in vision can result from glaucoma, cataract, or DM. The older person may have difficulty adjusting to changes in light and may experience impaired depth perception. These conditions can severely limit the person's engagement in occupation.[40,44] Table 19-1 offers suggestions on how to modify the environment.

Hearing

Changes in hearing often affect a person socially and physically. Even a slight hearing loss can be emotionally upsetting, particularly if it interferes with understanding family, friends, or television. Hearing loss can lead to isolation, depression, and anxiety.[44] People with impaired hearing may withdraw from group situations because listening is a chore.

Taste and Smell

Decreasing ability to taste and smell food is compounded by disease or use of medications, both of which can adversely affect these senses. Changes in the taste mechanism include difficulty in perceiving and identifying odor. Smelling food is a large part of enjoying it. Because of these decrements, many older people do not eat enough food to meet their nutritional needs. In addition, changes in the sense of taste and smell may lead the person to unknowingly eat spoiled food. These problems, of course, can result in poor health.

Sensorimotor

Sensorimotor changes may include decreased sensory awareness, sensory processing, and perceptual skills.

Cognitive Changes

Some pathological conditions that occur more commonly in the older adult are dementias such as Alzheimer's disease, memory disorders, and delirium.[15,40]

Dementia

Dementia is a permanent or progressive structural decline in several dimensions of intellectual function that interferes substantially with the individual's normal social or economic activity. Conditions such as drug intoxication, hyperthyroidism, and insulin shock also result in symptoms of dementia. When these conditions are treated, the symptoms of dementia are usually resolved. Several types of dementia are often seen in the elderly, the most common being Alzheimer's-type dementia. Memory loss is the most prominent early symptom. Multi-infarct dementia is more common in men than women and begins most often in the seventh decade. It tends to progress in a steplike manner, each step accompanied by intellectual worsening and perhaps the development or aggravation of neurologic signs. In the early stages of the illness, personality and insight tend to be better preserved than in Alzheimer's dementia. Depressive symptoms are common, and suicide is possible. As the condition advances, neurologic features, especially hemiplegia, pseudobulbar palsy, lability (pathological laughing and crying), or other signs of extrapyramidal dysfunction, may develop.[51]

Delirium

Delirium is characterized by extreme disturbances of arousal, attention, orientation, perception, intellectual function, and affect; delirium is commonly accompanied by fear and agitation. It is occasionally seen with large right hemispheric parietal occipital infarcts in the older person.[51]

Memory

Memory disorders involve partial or total inability to encode (process), store, or retrieve information. Encoding determines which stimuli are noticed or addressed and which are stored. Retrieval concerns the recall of information from a memory store. Memory can be divided into the following three major psychological components: immediate—the past few seconds; intermediate—the period from a few seconds past to a few days before; and remote or long-term—extending further back in time.[15,51]

Potential Effects of Medication on Functioning

When a pathological condition is irreversible, the individual is left with a chronic illness. The limiting factors of one chronic illness predispose the individual to other illnesses. The OT practitioner often treats an older adult with multiple chronic medical conditions. Management of these medical conditions can lead to concerns about the effect of medication on the individual's function.[28]

Older adults in the United States use a disproportionate amount of prescription and nonprescription medications: They represent 13% of the total population but account for more than 30% of the total drug expenditures.[21,27,29] Many take more than one drug. Use of prescription drugs tends to increase with age.[21] Older adults are at a higher risk for adverse drug reactions than other groups because of age-related changes in physiology, decrements due to chronic diseases, and use of multiple drugs.[21]

The practice of using multiple medications at the same time is termed **polypharmacy**. Polypharmacy is common among both institutionalized and community-dwelling older adults.[27] Multiple medications may be taken to treat multiple medical conditions. This intake can cause a number of side effects and/or secondary impairments, the result of excessive drug concentrations in the body and drug-to-drug interactions.[27]

Pharmacokinetics studies what happens to a drug after it enters the body: its absorption into the bloodstream, its distribution to the body tissues, its metabolism by the liver, and its excretion by the liver or kidney. The physiological changes of the body associated with aging are hypothesized to influence drug absorption, distribution, metabolism, and excretion.[34] It is imperative that older adults and their caregivers pay close attention to medication dosage and frequency to avoid toxic effects.[12,21,27]

The OT practitioner providing services to the older adult must remain informed about the effects of medication on the functioning of the older adult client. Medication used to treat medical conditions can significantly influence occupation and the older adult's safe participation in society."[12] The client's actual functional capacity may be altered by adverse medication effects. Knowledge (gained by the practitioner) will allow for an increased understanding of medication usage (and anticipation of effects), assessment of the client's functional status, devising prevention strategies, and potentially facilitating aging in place.

Communicating with Older Adults and Their Caregivers

Because of the number and severity of conditions that can affect the older adult, communication is especially important. The older adult and his or her caregiver may be of a different culture than the practitioner and have strongly held values and beliefs derived from a lifetime of experiences.[19] OT practitioners constantly communicate verbally and nonverbally with their clients and clients' significant others. Verbal communication provides directions, explains a treatment method, or expresses an idea. Nonverbal communication such as smiles, frowns, and posture reinforces or discourages a behavior or provides information regarding pleasure or displeasure.

The OT practitioner's mode of communication can enhance the intervention process by providing the client, the family, and other caregivers with information regarding the expected outcome of the intervention and by discussing questions or fears in a nonthreatening environment.[49] By explaining methods, suggesting alternatives, and promoting client/practitioner collaboration, we empower the older adult client, the family, and the caregiver to participate in the treatment process (Box 19-1).

Recently, associations between religious and spiritual factors and health and wellness outcomes have been reported by both the popular and scientific community. Most Americans continue to hold positive attitudes and beliefs about the efficacy of spiritual-related intervention (i.e., prayer).[16,17,42] *The Occupational Therapy Practice Framework: Domain & Process,* edition 2, defines spirituality as "a personal quest for understanding answers to ultimate questions about life, about meaning and about relationship with the sacred or transcendent, which may lead to or arise from the development of religious rituals and the formation of community."[4] James suggests prayer provides meaning, which may lessen depression/anxiety, paving a way to better long-term adjustments to a newly acquired pathology.[13] Furthermore, prayer can be used as a coping strategy to provide comfort or motivation to overcome a task that would appear to be achievable. It is important for practitioners to consider an individual's spirituality when designing and establishing interventions.

Communicating with Family and Significant Others

For many older adults, family members and significant others are the most trusted people in their lives. This trust is based on a common history. OT practitioners can use these trusted individuals to encourage a client to participate in the treatment process and to monitor follow-through.[49] The literature also shows support for collaborating with both the client and the caregiver when making environmental modification and assistive device recommendations[11] (Boxes 19-1 and 19-2).

Health care regulations require that both the client and specified family members or significant others be informed about the type of intervention the client receives.[36] The occupational therapy assistant (OTA) must develop skill in conveying information to the family and the client's significant others.

When communicating with families and significant others, the practitioner should explain in simple terms. Jargon and medical terminology should be minimized and clearly explained. Respectful explanations are crucial. The therapist must remember that the purpose of communicating with the family is to enhance the intervention process.[49]

OT practitioners must also understand the potential impact of a client's functional limitation on the family unit (i.e., familial role changes).[30] According to the *Occupational Therapy Practice Framework: Domain & Process*, edition 2, "caregiving is a co-occupation that involves active participation on the part of the caregiver and the recipient of care."[4] Caregiver burden has been recognized as a major concern for the families and significant others of older adults with significant functional limitations (i.e., community-dwelling older adults). Through effective communication and inclusion of the family and significant other in intervention and goal development, the practitioner can significantly reduce caregiver burden.[18,22,30]

Box 19-1

Techniques for Communicating

The following is a selection of techniques that can be used to enhance the communication process between therapist and patients authored by Cheryl Joiner and Mary Hansel.

Use active listening techniques. Let people know you are interested in what they have to say and that you want to fully understand them. Free the area of distractions. Positioning yourself at their level and making eye contact tells them that you are attentive. Once patients know that you are interested in them as people and care about their needs, they are often more willing to engage in therapy.

Give choices. No matter how trivial they may seem, choices are important. If possible, offer selections among predetermined modalities. This practice helps patients have more control over what happens to them.

Problem solve to encourage involvement in the therapy process. Encourage **clients** to brainstorm to reinforce their worth and primary importance in the treatment effort.

Be consistent whenever possible. Having the same practitioners and schedules helps patients feel secure. If a decision must be made to change therapists or treatment times, the patients must be informed before the change occurs.

Educate. Education helps patients feel more comfortable in the long-term care setting. Providing them with as much information as possible helps them to understand their illness and know what to expect from treatment. Some clients are not familiar with nursing homes and need instruction in routine policies and in their own rights.

Modified from Joiner C, Hansel M: Empowering the geriatric client, *OT Pract* 1:2, 1996.

Developing Appropriate Occupational Therapy Goals

Goal development, although broad in nature, must reflect the client's goals and values. The OT practitioner must be well versed in a variety of intervention approaches (including health promotion, remediation, maintenance, compensation, and disability prevention) that are theoretically based and grounded in sound research and evidence.[4] Interventions are best conducted when the occupational therapist, OTA, client, and their caregivers collaborate on the plan.[10] In accordance with the *Occupational Therapy Practice Framework II: Domain & Process*, edition 2, this process is dynamic and interactive.[4] The framework's process of service delivery includes (1) evaluation (gathering an occupational profile and analysis of client occupational performance); (2) intervention (intervention plan, intervention implementation, and intervention interview); and (3) outcomes (determining success in reaching targeted client outcomes and assessing client program for future planning). The framework encourages client-practitioner interaction throughout the evaluation, intervention, and outcomes assessment to promote client engagement in occupation. The successful intervention engages the client in occupation to support participation.[4]

Box 19-2

A Person-Centered Approach to Adaptive Equipment

Introducing Adaptive Equipment and Devices: A Person-Centered Approach

- Provide education
- Identify the person in need
- Identify potential risk factors/behaviors
- Listen
- Provide education
- Promote person-environment fit
- Listen
- Provide choices
- Implement realistic solutions
- Provide education
- Follow up

Tips for Promoting Person-Environment Fit

Major points to consider when making recommendations for the modification of the home of an older adult are the following:

- Is the suggested adaptation acceptable to the person?
- Does the person understand why the adaptation is suggested?
- Is the adaptation aesthetically pleasing?
- Is the adaptation affordable, easy to obtain, and easy to apply?
- Is the person physically, emotionally, and cognitively capable of accepting the adaptation?

In OT, the occupational therapist is responsible for determining when an evaluation is indicated. The occupational therapist is also responsible for verifying the competency of the OTA in performing specific procedures. The occupational therapist can assign the OTA specific areas of occupation, performance skill, performance patterns, and client factors to assess following a structured format. Although the occupational therapist maintains the responsibility for the intervention plan, it should be a collaborative effort between both practitioners. OT practitioners ensure that the intervention plan is clear and that the OTA has the knowledge and expertise to carry out the intervention program.

One of the challenges of working with the older adult is developing an intervention plan that addresses normal aging when it is accompanied by several pathological and/or chronic medical conditions.

As noted earlier in this chapter, the practitioner who is developing intervention plans for persons with multiple diagnoses must be aware of how one diagnosis will affect another and of how one medication may affect or cause symptoms that interfere with functional abilities. For example, someone who is recovering from a CVA may also have a diagnosis of ASHD, CHF, and DM. If the person is to perform light cooking or meal preparation, the intervention plan may require diabetes education for meal planning and compensatory strategies for sensory loss. Rest periods and energy conservation techniques are necessary to minimize CHF-related shortness of breath. The individual must be taught to recognize additional adverse symptoms such as swelling of the feet. Moreover, safety precautions with the use of kitchen knives are essential; a simple cut may take a longer period to heal because of the DM, thereby increasing the risk of infection.

The following case studies may help the reader integrate the information on theoretical frameworks/practice models.

Intervention Settings

Role of Occupational Therapy Assistant in Long-Term Care

The overwhelming majority of OTAs work in long-term care settings (Table 19-2). In response to a growing population of older adults, the OT practice community has developed programs to address their varied occupations, roles, and interests. The older adult may be seen in multiple environments including the home, rehabilitation centers, extended care facilities, daycare centers, senior centers, nursing homes, assisted living facilities, and varied wellness and health promotion programs. These programs are considered part of the continuum of care.

Table 19-2 Number of Occupational Therapy Practitioners Working in Long-Term Care Settings*

Year	Occupational Therapist	Occupational Therapy Assistant
1986	5.8%	20.1%
1996	18.2%	42.2%
2007	18%	42%

*Skilled nursing facility/intermediate care facility.

Modified from American Occupational Therapy Association: *Member survey*, Bethesda, Md, 1996, The Association. Results from *NBCOT Practice Metrics Survey*, Fall 2004 Newsletter. Metrics updated with permission from Bent MA: The value of certification: a retrospective of certification renewal findings. AOTA Conference Presentation, Long Beach, Calif., 2008.

CASE STUDY

A Lesson Learned about Client-Practitioner Collaboration: Ms. O.

Ms. O. was an 82-year-old woman who lived alone in a small, one-bedroom, walk-up apartment. As part of a falls prevention study, Marsha, an occupational therapist, was assigned to visit Ms. O. to perform a home safety assessment and assessment of select ADL (basic activities of daily living [BADL] and instrumental activities of daily living [IADL]). The goal of assessment was to determine environmental modification recommendations, assistive devices, and equipment that would promote Ms. O.'s occupational performance and personal safety within her home.

The study enabled Marsha to recommend, order, and train individuals with varied devices and equipment to promote fall prevention. Knowing that she could recommend and order equipment for a study participant without cost to the individual was a perk for Marsha during her participation as an OT consultant within the study. Within previous practice experiences, Marsha had come across clients for whom affordability of adaptive equipment and devices had been a concern.

After the assessment, Marsha informed Ms. O. of all of the devices and equipment from which she would benefit to support her independence and safety. Unexpectedly, Ms. O. proceeded to cry upon completion of Marsha's report. Marsha was not prepared for the expression of emotion that poured from Ms. O. Amidst the tears, Ms. O. cried out "all of these things ... I can't believe that I need all of these things ... I feel so old."

This experience helped Marsha realize the significance and importance of client-practitioner collaboration. It became apparent to Marsha that she had informed Ms. O. about her device and equipment needs. However, she had not included Ms. O. in the decision-making process.

Marsha's experience with Ms. O. was invaluable, influencing all aspects of her clinical practice and service delivery. Marsha learned the value of providing client education, listening to the client, providing choices, listening again, providing education, and recommending respectful and realistic solutions.

The significance of client-practitioner collaboration can be easily missed, even in the case of an experienced practitioner, when the practitioner does not initiate the interaction using a client-centered approach. This revelation led Marsha to formulate a systemized method for introducing environmental modifications, adaptive equipment and devices, and tips for promoting person-environment fit (Box 19-2).

CASE STUDY

Biomechanical Model: Mrs. I.

Mrs. I. is an 81-year-old woman with a diagnosis of DM, ASHD, and hypertension. She was recently hospitalized for CHF and has been discharged to a nursing home for rehabilitation. She now requires assistance with self-care activities because of generalized weakness. Mrs. I. is expected to return to the community. She reports interest in returning to an independent self-care status.

After the occupational therapist and OTA gathered an occupational profile, analyzed Mrs. I.'s occupational performance, and collaborated effectively with the client, the following OT goals were determined:

1. Mrs. I. will be independent in dressing, grooming, and bathing.
2. Mrs. I. will be able to select, don, and doff her dress independently.
3. Mrs. I. will be able to brush her hair independently.
4. Mrs. I. will be able to reach for her clothing in the closet and grooming supplies in the cabinet independently.

The intervention plan includes the following:

1. Practice sessions in dressing, grooming, and bathing
2. Therapeutic activities to address client factors interfering with occupational performance (i.e., range of motion, muscular endurance, respiratory capacity)
3. Problem solving and active client participation in forming strategies during occupational performance
4. Incorporating energy conservation and work simplification techniques during occupational performance

Outcomes of Intervention

1. Participation in meaningful occupations to support participation in society
2. Client participation in assessment of intervention outcomes

Long-term care refers to services provided over a long period of time to persons with chronic illnesses or conditions requiring extended medical and rehabilitation management. These individuals often require assistance with BADL such as eating, bathing, dressing, and mobility-related ADL (MRADL). Long-term care can be provided in the home (e.g., by a visiting nurse), in the community (e.g., as adult day care), or in an institution (e.g., nursing home).

Long-term services and support encompass a wide spectrum including assistance with BADL and IADL and facilitating full functioning in family, work, school, and leisure. Long-term services may also include skilled and therapeutic care for the treatment and management of chronic conditions.[5]

The OTA or occupational therapist might also coordinate services or provide case management to assist clients with long-term services and supports. OT practitioners are qualified to provide specialized services such as training and consultation on assistive technology and modification of homes and other environments.[5]

After an occupational therapist has conducted a client-centered evaluation and established a collaborative intervention plan, the OTA, supervised by the occupational therapist, can provide services to the clients in any of the settings described in the following discussion. The OTA may treat individuals onsite without the occupational therapist's physical presence (assuming state or other local jurisdictions permit this). The OTA provides intervention activities to improve abilities in identified areas of occupation, performance skills, and body functions—with the final goal of returning the individual to optimal functioning within the most appropriate environment. The OTA may administer standardized tests in a noninterpretive manner with the occupational therapist's supervision once service competency has been established. Other aspects of the OTA's role may include assisting in ADL evaluation, ordering equipment, providing adaptations to equipment and the environment, and training caregivers.

Daycare Centers

Adult daycare is a program of care during the day for the adult with declining function in a group setting away from home. These older adults are often affected by physical, mental, or social problems and sometimes require medical and rehabilitation services that are not offered in senior centers available to the general population.[50]

Home Health Care

Home and community care for functionally disabled older adults is generally defined as care provided to financially eligible people 65 years of age or older who require substantial human assistance in performing two of three specified ADL. Individuals with Alzheimer's disease may qualify for the program under somewhat more liberal eligibility criteria: requiring assistance in two of five specified ADL or being sufficiently cognitively impaired as to require substantial supervision because of inappropriate behaviors that pose serious health or safety hazards to themselves or others. Home care and community care include homemaker, home health aide, household chore, and personal care services; nursing care services provided by or under the supervision of a registered nurse; rehabilitation services; respite care; training for family members in managing the individual; adult daycare; and for the chronically mentally ill, day treatment partial hospitalization, psychosocial rehabilitation services, and clinic services.[50]

Assisted Living

Assisted living is an innovative approach to meeting the housing and care needs of frail older persons and individuals with disabilities in a residential rather than an institutional environment, while maximizing independence, choice, and privacy.

CASE STUDY

Rehabilitation Model: Mrs. C.

Mrs. C. is a 73-year-old widow with diagnoses of COPD, arthritis, hypertension, and depression. She lives in a two-story home with her daughter, two grandchildren, and her mother who lives in the second-floor apartment. Her mother is homebound and receives full-time home care. Mrs. C's daughter Alicia works full time, cares for her children, and assists with her mother and grandmother's care. Mrs. C. stopped working as a bookkeeper 8 years ago and retired this year from her part-time job at the library. Mrs. C. presents with +2 edema in both ankles, ROM within functional limits for all joints, and 3/3+ muscle strength in both upper extremities. At this time, she exhibits a significant decrease in ADL participation. Mrs. C. rarely goes outside the house and makes infrequent visits to her mother due to shortness of breath and joint pain when climbing the stairs. She no longer participates in housekeeping activities. Mrs. C. has become fearful about her declining independence. She would like to regain active participation within her immediate environment (including modified independence in self-care and ability to perform light home maintenance tasks).

After gathering an occupational profile, analyzing her occupational performance, and collaborating on goals with Mrs. C. and her family, the occupational therapist, the OTA, and Mrs. C arrived at the following OT goals:

1. Mrs. C. will engage in grooming, dressing, and bathing activities with modified independence on a daily basis.
   - She will retrieve clothing from the closet and drawers.
   - She will don/doff clothing with adaptive devices.
   - She will enter the bathtub and shower with adaptive equipment.
2. Mrs. C. will engage in light home maintenance while using energy conservation techniques on a daily basis.
   - She will be out of bed for at least 3 hours in the morning and 3 hours in the afternoon.
   - She will make the bed in the morning on a daily basis.
   - She will engage in light meal preparation.
   - She will wash and put away dishes at least one time per day.
3. Mrs. C. will engage in an exercise routine at least four times per week.
   - She will walk to the front stoop and pick up the mail daily.
   - She will visit with her mother, going up one flight of stairs, at least once per day.
   - She will walk to the neighborhood senior center at least three times per week with another person.
   - She will engage in modified yoga exercises using paced breathing techniques three times per week.

The intervention plan includes the following:

Practice Sessions in Self-Care Skills

1. Problem solving and active client participation in strategy formation during occupational performance
2. Client participation in adaptive equipment, device, and home modification choices (see Box 19-2)
3. Client education and provision of adaptive equipment to assist with housekeeping, bathing, and dressing
4. Client education and training in energy conservation and work simplification activities
5. Client education and instruction in health maintenance and safety

Outcomes of Intervention

1. Participation in meaningful occupations to support participation in society
2. Client participation in assessment of intervention outcomes
3. Familial support to decrease caregiver burden and preserve familial roles and values

Assisted living is defined as a group residential program that is not licensed as a nursing home but provides personal care to individuals with needs for assistance in ADL (bathing, dressing, feeding, transferring, toileting, continence) and that can respond to unscheduled needs for assistance. For many individuals with modest to substantial care needs, assisted living offers an alternative to nursing homes and board-and-care homes.[50]

Subacute Care

Subacute care is defined as a comprehensive inpatient program designed for the individual who has had an acute event as a result of an illness, injury, or exacerbation of a disease process; has a determined course of treatment; and does not require intensive diagnostic and invasive procedures. The severity of the individual's condition requires an outcome-focused interdisciplinary approach that employs a professional team to deliver complex clinical medical interventions and rehabilitation.

The majority of individuals in subacute care settings have conditions with diagnoses associated with rehabilitation such as stroke, cardiac conditions, orthopedic conditions (including joint replacements and fractures), general and degenerative neurologic disorders (including multiple sclerosis, muscular dystrophy, Parkinson's disease), amputations, severe arthritis, neuromuscular disorders, and general debilitation. The goal of rehabilitation is to return the individual to his or her previous level of function and natural setting.[50]

Skilled Nursing Facility

Skilled nursing facilities (SNFs), formerly known as *nursing homes*, are residential facilities that provide skilled nursing care, rehabilitative services, or health-related care on a daily basis to individuals who are injured, disabled, or sick. Services include daily basic nursing care or other rehabilitative services that reasonably can be provided only in a nursing facility on an inpatient basis. These include nursing and related services; specialized rehabilitative services; medically related social services; and activities to attain or maintain to the fullest extent possible the physical, mental, and psycho-social well-being of each individual.[50] An individual may return to her natural living environment or remain as a resident based on safety concerns or limited functional ability.

Senior Centers and Wellness Promotion Centers

With an increasingly aging America, a number of young and not so young older adults attend senior centers and wellness promotion centers to promote health, wellness, and socialization.[8,18] This is an emerging practice area for the health care practitioner, despite the fact that health maintenance organizations seldom directly reimburse practitioners for services rendered in these settings. Many well older adults seek these services to support participation in occupation.[32,39] OT practitioners are among the growing number of health care professionals who provide individualized programs, education, leisure management, and consulting services to this growing consumer population.

Medicare, Medicaid, and the Resident Assessment Instrument

Medicare

The Medicare program helps pay medical costs for people 65 years and older and a vast number of disabled individuals who are younger. Medicare Part A covers inpatient hospital services, home health services, and other institution-based services. Part B covers physician, outpatient hospital, and various other health services such as diagnostic tests. Practitioners should check with individual state Medicare providers because guidelines often change.[6,50]

Medicaid

Medicaid is a federally aided, state-administered medical assistance program intended, among other things, to provide low-income individuals with access to health care. The services provided by the Medicaid program include inpatient and outpatient hospital, home health, physician, and skilled nursing facility services.[50]

Medicare and Medicaid are the largest third-party reimbursers of medical and ancillary care for those persons 65 and older in the United States. These federal, state, and local funding sources provide reimbursement for services used by older Americans throughout the continuum of care. Knowledge of the Medicare and Medicaid reimbursement systems, methods of patient assessment, and service inclusions is crucial for the OT practitioner providing services to the older adult.[24,36,50]

Resident Assessment Instrument

Medicare has developed a joint assessment form and reimbursement strategy with Medicaid. With this program, long-term care reimbursement rates are based on patient grouping called Case Mix. The Case-Mix classification system is called the Resource-Utilization Groups (RUGs IV). Both Medicaid and Medicare patients are grouped based on the level of care needed when a patient enters a long-term care program.[36,50]

Patients entering long-term care are assessed using the Resident Assessment Instrument (RAI) (Box 19-3), which is a Congressionally mandated resident assessment tool used to conduct a comprehensive assessment of all residents in federally certified nursing homes. It includes the minimum data set (MDS) and the care area assessment (CAA). The MDS provides data for classifying residents into RUG IV groups. The CAA provides guidelines for the clinician to assess the patient, concentrating on conditions that affect physical, cognitive, and psychosocial functioning.[36,43,50]

Communicating with Supervisors

Nursing home practice in the United States has seen a rapid change in the way OT services are provided. Before 1990, when the Omnibus Budget Reconciliation Act of 1987 (OBRA 87) became law, many OT programs in nursing homes were staffed by OTAs with OT consultants. This model required that the OTA coordinate the OT service with the occupational therapist providing overall supervision. The requirement that restorative OT services be provided with the occupational therapist on the premises has changed this model because the OTA now has more regular access to OT supervision. The OTA must have a clear job description and develop a mutually effective communication strategy with the occupational therapist. Regular supervision sessions are recommended. These sessions should not be limited to establishing client-centered intervention programs, but they should also include

Box 19-3

How the Resident Assessment Instrument Is Used in Clinical Practice

A. Perform initial assessment with RAI.
   1. Perform a comprehensive assessment encompassing completion of the MDS 3.0 and problem identification CAA.
   2. Develop a care plan.
B. Begin to deliver care.
   1. Implement a care plan.
   2. Evaluate care provided; reassess based on time frames for each goal/approach to care established in the care plan.
   3. Modify plan of care as necessary.
C. Review resident status at least every 3 months (quarterly review) to ensure that assessment remains accurate, revising plan of care as necessary.
D. Reassessments (including MDS 3.0 and CAA) are conducted according to the utilization guidelines.
   1. Identify problems using CAA.
   2. Evaluate whether care plan addresses current needs of resident.
   3. Review and revise the care plan as needed.

From Lee S, Dichter B: *The multistate nursing home case mix and quality demonstration,* Natick, Mass, 1996, Eliot Press.

discussion regarding professional growth and development to promote effective OT and OTA collaboration.

Communicating with Other Professionals

OTAs are expected to communicate with other professionals within the facility including doctors, nurses, social workers, physical therapists, and speech pathologists.

The OTA often demonstrates or teaches nursing assistants specific methods for working with the patient. Communication also may entail teaching passive ROM, splint application, or the use of an assistive device. Communication with others may also include gathering information about how a client manages a specific activity, learning the funding source for the individual, or participating in intervention planning meetings.

Environmental Safety/Fall Prevention and the Restraint-Free Environment

Fall Prevention

According to the National Safety Council, falls are a leading cause of injury-related death in the older adult.[38]

Each year approximately 30% of community-dwelling persons older than the age of 65 and 50% of those older than the age of 80 will fall. Among older adults living in institutional settings, more than 50% percent will fall each year. An estimated 5% of falls result in a fracture. Of the older adults admitted to a hospital after a fall, only 50% will be alive 1 year later. Often, older adults who have fallen develop a fear of falling and avoid activity performance in order to avoid falling. Compared with older adults who have not experienced a fall, those who have fallen tend to experience more functional decline in ADL and social activity. Falls have been shown to be a strong predictor of nursing home placement.[46]

Older persons are highly susceptible to falls because of health problems such as arthritis, poor eyesight and hearing, frailty, poor balance and coordination, senility, dementia, and weakness or dizziness caused by medications.[33,46] Recent literature questions whether the high-risk behaviors of the vigorous older adult who participates in sporting activities, heavy household chores, and so on may increase their risk of falling[21] or decrease risk of falling.[14] The high-risk behaviors of the vigorous older adult often coincide with a reluctance to use home safety equipment and an unwillingness to consider activity modification strategies. However, participation in sporting activities, exercise, and household activities has also been found to enhance bone density, muscle strength, balance, and endurance.[14,21,38,46]

Brungardt and other researchers[9, 20,38,47] have described the following as increasing the risk factor for falls in the elderly: mental status factors including disorientation, depression, and dementia; medical factors including more than one disease, acute illness, or orthostatic hypotension; medication; sensory factors including changes in vision or vestibular or proprioceptive dysfunction; musculoskeletal factors including increased activity, decreased mobility, foot disorders, and cervical disk disease; neurologic factors including changes in gait and peripheral neuropathy; environmental factors including stairs, undifferentiated steps, slippery surfaces, poor lighting, and unexpected obstacles; and other factors including confinement, history of falls, and ill-fitting shoes.

OT practitioners participate in the fall prevention program by assessing and developing a plan of care for individuals who are at high risk for falls.

The OT assessment includes information on the sensorimotor, cognitive, and psychological functions.

The OTA, in conjunction with the occupational therapist, assists in developing a plan of care geared toward the remediation of deficits or compensation for any loss of function.

OT practitioners provide intervention in environmental safety and fall prevention by assessing individuals in their environments. Intervention includes the remediation of deficits; instruction in compensatory techniques; the provision of adaptive equipment such as reachers, stocking aids, or carts for carrying heavy loads; and collaboration with the team regarding appropriate mobility devices.

OT practitioners also assess and plan intervention in home design and modification. Because of the importance of facilitating client education and collaboration, home modification may include the removal of obstacles such as throw rugs; the rearrangement of cabinets to place heavier things on the bottom rather than on top shelves; and bathroom aids such as a call bell, bathtub seat, grab bars, and raised toilet seats (Figure 19-1, Box 19-2).

Restraint Use

OBRA 87 made restraint use the exception rather than the rule. The law requires nursing homes to provide quality care and quality of life for each individual. This includes maintaining the well-being of each individual and ensuring to the greatest practical extent a good quality of life by providing services and activities.

Physical restraints are any manual method or any physical or mechanical device, material, or equipment attached or adjacent to the individual's body that the individual cannot remove independently; they restrict freedom of movement or normal access to the body. Physical restraints include vests, belts, wheelchair seat belts, wheelchairs, hand mitts, wheelchair safety bars, bed rails, and other devices used to position an individual.

Chemical restraint is also a method for restricting an individual's movement.[21] **Chemical restraints** are medications that restrict an individual's interaction with the environment. For the older adult certain medications can produce the effect of chemical restraint.

Since the 1990s there have been widespread efforts to reduce the use of physical and chemical restraints and to find alternatives to prevent falls in nursing homes.[33]

Risks of Restraint Use

In 1994 Haddad[26] described several risks of restraint use. The individual may become agitated and more disoriented. The individual might be embarrassed, which would diminish

CASE STUDY

Fall Prevention: Mr. G.

Mr. G. is an 86-year-old man who sustained a hip fracture 2 weeks ago while changing a light bulb and was admitted to the nursing home for rehabilitative care. Mr. G.'s family hopes to be able to take him home as soon as he is able to walk again. Mr. G. and his family hope that he will be able to continue to participate in social activities such as going to the senior center and independently performing ADL such as dressing, grooming, bathing, and light meal preparation. Mr. G. lives alone in a barrier-free (i.e., no steps) senior citizen building. Before the fall he was independent in all self-care activities, attended tai chi classes, and regularly traveled by bus.

He also met with friends weekly at the senior center and attended community events with his girlfriend. During his hospitalization, Mr. G. underwent a right total hip replacement. Because of his diabetes, healing was slow. During his hospitalization, Mr. G. spent the days alone and was visited by family and friends in the late afternoon and evening.

On admission to the nursing home, Mr. G. was assessed as being disoriented (a reaction to anesthesia and pain medication), unable to participate in any self-care activity except eating, and unable to transfer from the bed independently. He had decreased ROM on the right hip and exhibited poor endurance and impaired postural control. He was incontinent and nonambulatory. Because of his disorientation, Mr. G. made several attempts to climb out of bed and staff feared that he might fall and reinjure himself. Mr. G.'s behavior triggered a CAA, and a fall risk assessment was performed by the interdisciplinary team.

Each discipline assessed Mr. G., and a plan of care was instituted. The recreational staff formulated and implemented an activity plan that included a variety of social activities. The OT staff was able to suggest mentally and physically stimulating activities that were identified in his occupational profile. The nursing and social service staff provided reality orientation and encouragement for continued participation in therapy and activities.

The OT evaluation included the gathering of an occupational profile and assessment of Mr. G.'s basic ADL skills including dressing, grooming, bathing, and transfer skills. The evaluation of client factors and performance skills included assessment of ROM, muscle strength, endurance, mobility, orientation, ability to follow directions, and ability to conceptualize safety issues. The interview included familial and client discussions about Mr. G.'s goals, interests, and expectations.

The OT intervention plan included increasing ROM, muscle strength and endurance, topographical orientation, and mobility while providing practice sessions in self-care activities such as dressing, bathing, grooming, and transfer training. The anticipated outcome of Mr. G.'s intervention plan was to promote participation in meaningful occupation with reentry into the community.

As Mr. G.'s mental and physical status improved, he increasingly could make his own decisions and could collaborate with the OT staff to develop an activity schedule for home. Mr. G. expressed concern about his ability to return to his prior level of functioning without becoming a burden on his family. He could describe his apartment and where his furniture was located and was able to make decisions about what could and could not be moved. He participated in the rearrangement of the home to eliminate obstacles and increase safety. Mr. G. was discharged from the nursing home and was referred to a home health service that provided OT. The home-care occupational therapist assisted Mr. G. in readjusting to community life by assessing his ability to perform self-care activities and use public transportation and by offering suggestions for modifying the home.

self-esteem. Restrained individuals may experience increased injuries while attempting to break free from the restraints. The individual may suffer the effects of immobility including skin breakdown, decreased circulation, and incontinence. The nursing staff may end up with more work, not less, if the individual becomes injured while trying to remove the restraints or develops skin and other problems from restraints.

Most practitioners who work in long-term care settings would agree that these risks continued to be associated with restraint use.

Occupational Therapy Role

Today long-term care facilities are required to provide a restraint-free environment. Restraints are used in only the most extreme cases. These patients require constant monitoring and reassessment of the individual, family notification, and multidisciplinary case management to limit or eliminate the use of a restraint. Long-term care facilities are required to use a multidisciplinary team approach to limit and/or eliminate the use of restraints.

Among the varied multidisciplinary assessments that are performed to reduce or eliminate use of a restraint, most facilities require that an OT evaluation be completed to determine alternatives to physical restraint. The evaluation will determine the individual's positioning needs and transfer skills, as well as other needs associated with the individual's ability to negotiate the environment safely. In many instances individuals are restrained because they slide out of their wheelchairs. The clinician will need to assess whether this problem is caused by an inappropriate seating and positioning system, an inappropriate type of wheelchair, or other physiological, neurologic, or orthopedic factors.

In evaluating and determining alternatives to physical restraint, the practitioner must consider the needs of the individual, as well as any problems, conditions, and risk factors. If a restraint must be used, the clinician must explain why the

Patient ______________________ **Age** __________ **Room** __________

Triggered problems ______________________

Assessment goals are (1) to ensure that a treatment plan is in place for patients with history of falls, and (2) to identify patients who are at risk for falls and are not currently enrolled in a fall prevention program.

1. Is there a previous history of falls? Yes_____ No_____
2. Was the fall an isolated event? Yes_____ No_____

Internal risk factors

Does patient have?	Yes	No
Cardiovascular abnormalities		
Cardiac dysrhythmia		
Hypotension		
Syncope		
Neuromuscular impairments		
Cerebrovascular accident		
Hemiplegia		
Unsteady gait		
Incontinence		
Seizure disorder		
Parkinson's diesase		
Chronic/acute condition causing instability		
Loss of leg or arm movement		
Decline in functional status		
Orthopedic impairments		
Arthritis		
Osteoporosis		
Joint pain		
Hip fracture		
Perceptual abnormalities		
Impaired hearing		
Dizziness or vertigo		
Psychiatric or cognitive impairments		
Alzheimer's/dementia		
Decline in cognitive skills		
Delirium		
Manic depression or other affective disorder		
Other dementia		

Figure 19-1 Sample of a falls protocol worksheet.

restraint is being used; the type of restraint being used; and when, where, for how long, and under what circumstances the restraint is used. Once the underlying problem is identified and resolved, it is the obligation of the multidisciplinary team to eliminate the restraint. If the restraint is used to control a behavior, the clinician must bear in mind that many behaviors are caused by unmet needs and can often be eliminated by meeting those needs. The OT practitioner will be expected to participate as a team contributor to aid in managing the individual's behavior without restraints. The MDS restraint

External factors

	Yes	No
Medications		
Psychotropic medications		
Cardiovascular medications		
Diuretics		
Was medication administered before fall		
Was medication administered after the fall		

If medications were administered before the fall, how much time before the fall were they first administered? ____________

List all medications and note possible side effects ____________

____

____

____

Appliances and devices

	Yes	No
Pacemaker		
Walker or cane		
Physical restraints		
Other		
Restraints before fall		

Observe patient's use of the device for possible problems and describe performance ____________

____

____

Environmental and situational hazards

	Yes	No
Glare		
Poor illumination		
Slippery floors		
Uneven floors		
Patterned carpets		
Objects in walkway		
Recent move		
New arrangement of objects		
Proximity of aggressive residents		
Type of activity		
Standing still/walking		
In a crowded area		
Responding to bladder/bowel urgency		
Reaching/not reaching		

Figure 19-1, cont'd

Is there a pattern of falls in any of the above circumstances (environmental and situational hazards? ______

______

______

______

If you know what the resident was doing immediately leading to the fall, have resident repeat the activity and observe ______

______

______

______

Vital signs

Measure patient's blood pressure and heart rate:

Supine ______

1 minute after standing ______

3 minutes after standing ______

Resident interaction with the environment

Observe resident and check "able" or "not able" and "safe" or "unsafe."

Activity	Able	Not able	Safe	Unsafe
Moving in and out of bed				
Walking				
Turning				
Transferring				
Toileting				

Identified problems ______

______

______

______

______

______

______

______

Suggested multidisciplinary treatment interventions

Nursing ______

______

______

OT/PT ______

______

______

______

______

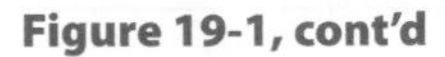
Figure 19-1, cont'd

protocol guidelines include a review of the individual's record and the conditions that seem to precipitate restraint use including problem behaviors, risk of falls, and treatment regimens.[36] The MDS protocol also includes conditions under which a restraint may be used. These include enhancement of independent ADL performance. For example, although a full-length rail on an individual's bed is intended to reduce the risk of injury by preventing him from getting out of bed, it would nonetheless be considered a restraint. Although still a restraint, a half bed rail that assists an individual with performance of independent transfers would be considered an ADL enhancement.

Activities

Medical

Social services

Figure 19-1, cont'd

Alternatives to Restraints

Alternatives to restraints include restorative and maintenance programs, supportive devices, enhanced environment, and a variety of staff approaches.

Restorative Programs

Restorative programs are individualized programs that address and remediate underlying impairments such as proprioceptive deficits and problems with balance, mobility, positioning, and ADL.

Maintenance Programs

Maintenance programs are designed to maintain the individual at the highest possible level by providing exercise and cognitive programs, as well as activity programs.

Enhanced Environments

Enhanced environments may include changes in the individual's room and immediate environment such as color-coding walls, arranging furniture to reduce obstacles, decreasing glare in corridors, labeling doors, reducing noise, providing conversational seating, and allowing furnishings to be brought from the home.

Adaptive Equipment and Devices

Adaptive equipment and devices provide alternatives to restraint use. The following is a sampling of adaptive equipment and devices commonly used in skilled nursing facilities as alternatives to restraint: bed and chair alarms, low beds, mats placed on the floor next to an individual's bed, and hip protectors.

Staff Approaches

Each member of the interdisciplinary team should be trained to support the individual. Team members should learn about the individual's interests and desires. Some staff will be better at interacting with certain individuals than others will be.[33] Family and significant others who are close to the individual can be questioned (within the allowable boundaries of client confidentiality) to assist with gaining an understanding of the individual's values, interests, and desires.

Summary

Aging is a complex process that begins as soon as the individual is conceived. Health, lifestyle, and disease, however, determine quality of life as individuals reach maturity. Illness must be viewed separately from reduced abilities. Although some diseases are more common in the older adult, the disease process should not be confused with normal aging.

OT practitioners must understand the developmental needs of the older person. In addition, practitioners must be aware of what constitutes normal aging and how superimposed pathological conditions and adverse medication reactions affect the older person. The practitioner must appreciate cultural and value differences and take care to communicate information clearly to the older adult, their families, and other persons involved in their care. OT practitioners must be prepared to initiate their interactions and interventions from a client-centered approach that incorporates client-practitioner collaboration throughout all aspects of the service delivery process.

OTAs collaborate with the occupational therapist in developing intervention plans for the older adult. When developing intervention plans for older clients with multiple diagnoses, the practitioner must be aware of how one diagnosis will affect another and of how one medication may affect or cause symptoms that interfere with functional abilities.

OT practitioners may work in a variety of settings within the long-term care continuum. These settings may include daycare centers, the home, assisted living centers, subacute care units, nursing homes, and community wellness centers.

OT services may be funded under a variety of programs including Medicare and Medicaid. Older adult clients residing at federally or state-funded nursing facilities receive a comprehensive, multidisciplinary assessment—the RAI. This assessment process includes the completion of the MDS form and the development of a multidisciplinary treatment plan. OT practitioners are involved in facility-wide, federally mandated programs such as fall prevention and the promotion and assessment of environmental adaptations that promote a restraint-free environment.

Selected Reading Guide Questions

1. List three theories that address the developmental needs of the older adult.
2. Describe four common age-related changes.
3. List four pathological conditions that are commonly seen in the older adult.
4. List four sensory changes common in the older adult.
5. Discuss potential effects of medication on the function of the older adult.
6. Describe three practice models used when working with multidiagnosis patients.
7. Describe four intervention settings in which the OTA may provide services to the older adult.
8. Describe one method that may be used to prevent falls in the older adult.
9. Define restraints.
10. List the risks of restraint use.
11. Describe three interventions that may be used to prevent restraint use.
12. Describe the importance of communicating with the family.
13. Describe one method of communicating with a supervisor.
14. Name and discuss techniques that can be used to communicate with patients.
15. What is the Resident Assessment Instrument? What are its inclusions?
16. What is the minimum data set?
17. Define CAA.
18. Who is responsible for completing the MDS 3.0?
19. Name the components of the comprehensive care plan.

References

1. *Administration on Aging: A Profile of Older Americans*, 2009, http://www.aoa.gov/AOARoot/Aging/. Accessed 2/4/11.
2. *Administration on Aging: Promoting healthy lifestyles*, 2004, http://www.aoa.gov/prof/healthy_lifestyles/phl.asp. Accessed 2/8/05.
3. Ai AL, Ladd KL, Peterson C, et al: Long-term adjustment after surviving open heart surgery: the effect of using coping replicated in a prospective design, *Gerontologist* 50(6):798–809, 2010.
4. American Occupational Therapy Association: *Occupational therapy practice framework: Domain and process, ed 2*, Bethesda, MD, 2008, Author.
5. American Occupational Therapy Association: Position paper: occupational therapy and long-term services and supports, *Am J Occup Ther* 48:1035, 1994.
6. Brooks S, Anderson M, Esslinger L: The Health Care System. In Ham R, Sloane PD, Warshaw G, et al: *Primary care geriatrics: a case-based approach*, ed 5, Philadelphia, 2007, Mosby.
7. Brummel SK, Gunderson A: Caring for older patients and an aging population. In Ham R, Sloane PD, Warshaw G, et al: *Primary care geriatrics: a case-based approach*, ed 5, Philadelphia, 2007, Mosby.
8. Butler RN, Lewis M: Sexuality in old age. In Saunders E, editor: *Geriatric medicine and gerontology*, ed 7, Philadelphia, 2010, Brocklehursts.
9. Brungardt GS: Patient restraints: new guidelines for a less restrictive approach, *Geriatrics* 49:44, 1994.
10. Byers-Connon S, Park S: Opportunities for best practice in various settings. In Byers-Connon S, Lohman H, Padilla R, editors: *Occupational therapy with elders: strategies for the COTA*, ed 2, St. Louis, 2004, Mosby.
11. Chen A, Mann WC, Tomita M, et al: Caregiver involvement in the use of assistive devices by frail older persons, *Occup Ther J Res* 20(3):179–199, 2000.
12. Classen S, Mann W, Wu SS, et al: Relationship of number of medications to functional status, health, and quality of life for the frail home-based older adult, *OTJR: Occup Particip Health* 24(4):151–160, 2004.
13. Cohen ZM, Ancoli IS: Sleep disorder. In Halter JB, Ouslander JG, Tinetti ME, et al: *Hazzards geriatric medicine and gerontology*, ed 6, San Francisco, 2009, McGraw Hill Medical.
14. Cook C, Shroyer J: Vigorous physical activity and fall occurrence, *Phys Occup Ther Geriatr* 21(1):1–19, 2002.
15. Craft S, Cholerton B, Reger M: Cognitive changes associated with normal and pathological aging. In Halter JB, Ouslander JG, Tinetti ME, et al: *Hazzards geriatric medicine and gerontology*, ed 6, San Francisco, 2009, McGraw Hill Medical.
16. Crowther MR, Parker MW, Achenbaum WA, et al: Rowe and Kahn's Model of Successful Aging Revisited: Positive Spirituality - The Forgotten Factor, *Gerontologist* 42(5), 2002.
17. Daaleman TP: Spirituality. In Halter JB, Ouslander JG, Tinetti ME, et al: *Hazzard's geriatric medicine and gerontology*, ed 6, San Francisco, 2009, McGraw Hill Medical.
18. Dooley RH, Hinojosa J: Improving quality of life for persons with Alzheimer's disease and their family caregivers: brief occupational therapy intervention, *Am J Occup Ther* 58(5):561–569, 2004.
19. Federal Interagency Forum on Aging Related Statistics: Data Sources on Older Americans 2009: National Center for Health Statistics, http://www.agingstats.gov/. Accessed 2/4/11.
20. *Federal Interagency Forum on Aging Related Statistics: Older Americans 2004: key indicators of well being, Health Care*, 2004, http://www.agingstats.gov/. Accessed 2/8/05.
21. Ferrini AF, Ferrini RL: *Health in the later years*, ed 3, Boston, 2000, McGraw-Hill.
22. Fitzgerald MH: A dialogue on occupational therapy, culture, and families, *Am J Occup Ther* 58(5):489–498, 2004.
23. Flynn JE, Mabry ER: Biophysical development of later adulthood. In Schuster CS, Asbum SS, editors: *The process of human development*, ed 2, Canada, 1986, Little, Brown.
24. Glantz CH, Richman NR: The regulation of public policy for elders. In Byers-Connon S, Lohman H, Padilla R, editors: *Occupational therapy with elders: strategies for the COTA*, ed 2, St. Louis, 2004, Mosby.
25. Goldstein A, Damon B, Taeuber TM: *We the American. Elderly, U.S Department of Commerce Economics and Statistical Administration*, September 1993.
26. Haddad A: Acute care decisions: ethics in action, *RN* 57:19, 1994.
27. Ham RJ: Illness and aging. In Ham R, Sloane PD, Warshaw G, et al: *Primary care geriatrics: a case-based approach*, ed 5, Philadelphia, 2007, Mosby.
28. Hanlon JT, Fillenbaum GG, Kuchibhatla M, et al: Impact of inappropriate drug use on mortality and functional status in representative community dwelling elders, *Med Care* 40(2): 166–176, 2002.

29. Hilmer SN, Ford GA: General principles of pharmacology. In Halter JB, Ouslander JG, Tinetti ME, et al: *Hazzard's geriatric medicine and gerontology*, ed 6, San Francisco, 2009, McGraw Hill Medical.
30. Humphrey R, Corcoran M: Exploring the role of family in occupation and family occupations, *Am J Occup Ther* 58(5):487–488, 2004.
31. Johnson LE, Alline KM: Sexual Health. In Ham R, Sloane PD, Warshaw G, et al: *Primary care geriatrics: a case-based approach*, ed 5, Philadelphia, 2007, Mosby.
32. Kaminsky T: The role of occupational therapy in successful aging, *OT Practice*, April, 2010.
33. King MB: Falls. In Halter JB, Ouslander JG, Tinetti ME, et al: *Hazzard's geriatric medicine and gerontology*, ed 6, San Francisco, 2009, McGraw Hill Medical.
34. Lewis SC: *Elder care in occupational therapy*, Thorofare, NJ, 1989, Slack.
35. Miller CA: *Nursing for wellness in the older adult*, ed 5, Philadelphia, 2009, Walters Kluwen Health & Lippincott Williams and Wilkins.
36. *Minimum Data Set (MDS) - Version 3.0 Resident Assessment and Care Screening Nursing Home Comprehensive (NC) Item Set*, 2010, Myers & Stauffer.
37. *National Center for Chronic Disease Prevention and Health Promotion: Healthy aging for older adults, Health Information for older adults*, 2004, http://www.cdc.gov/aging/. Accessed 2/8/05.
38. National Safety Council, 2010, *http://www.nsc.org/safety_home/Resources/Pages/Falls.aspx.*
39. Oswald F, Jopp D, Rott C, et al: Is aging in place a resource for or risk to life satisfaction? *Gerontologist* 51:238–250, 2011.
40. Perlmutter M, Bhorade A, Gordon M, et al: Cognitive, visual, auditory, and emotional factors that affect participation in older adults, *Am J Occup Ther* 64(4), July/August 2010.
41. Phelan EA, Paniagan MA, Hazzard WR: Preventive gerontology: strategize for optimizing health across the life span. In Halter JB, Ouslander JG, Tinetti ME, et al: *Hazzard's geriatric medicine and gerontology*, ed 6, San Francisco, 2009, McGraw Hill Medical.
42. Phillips I: Infusing spirituality into geriatric healthcare, *Top Geriatr Rehabil* 19(4):249–256, 2003.
43. *Preparing for MDS 3.0*, 2011, *http://www.keanecare.com*. Accessed 2/5/2011.
44. Reuben D, Rosen S: Principles of geriatric assessment. In Halter JB, Ouslander JG, Tinetti ME, et al: *Hazzard's geriatric medicine and gerontology*, ed 6, San Francisco, 2009, McGraw Hill Medical.
45. Rowe JW, Kahn RL: Successful aging, *Gerontologist* 37(No 4):433–440, 1997.
46. Schneider DC, Scott M: Falls. In Ham R, Sloane PD, Warshaw G, et al: *Primary care geriatrics: a case-based approach*, ed 5, Philadelphia, 2007, Mosby.
47. Schuster CS, Ashburn SS: *The process of human development: a holistic life-span approach*, ed 2, Boston, 1986, Little Brown.
48. Stalworth M, Sloane PD: Clinical implications of normal aging. In Ham R, Sloane PD, Warshaw G, et al: *Primary care geriatrics: a case-based approach*, ed 5, Philadelphia, 2007, Mosby.
49. Strauss SE, Tinetti ME: Evaluation, management, and decision making with the older patient. In Halter JB, Ouslander JG, Tinetti ME, et al: *Hazzard's geriatric medicine and gerontology*, ed 6, San Francisco, 2009, McGraw Hill Medical.
50. The Center for Medicare and Medicaid Services: 2010. *http://www.cms.gov/*. accessed 2/5/11.
51. The Merck Manual Online Medical Library for Healthcare Professionals: 2010. *http://www.merckmanuals.com/professional/index.html*. Accessed 2/5/11.

CHAPTER 20 Hand Splinting

SERENA BERGER

Key Terms

Splints
Arches
Radial
Ulnar
Creases
Distal
Proximal
Dorsal
Volar
Extrinsic muscles
Intrinsic muscles
Thenar
Hypothenar
Phalanx
Tenodesis action
Low-temperature thermoplastics

Chapter Objectives

After studying this chapter, the student or practitioner will be able to do the following:

1. Locate important landmarks in the anatomy of the hand including arches and other structural elements that contribute to hand function.
2. Identify normal prehension and grasp patterns and describe the three basic positions of the hand.
3. Understand the primary purposes for splinting an extremity.
4. Understand the biomechanical, physiological, and patient compliance considerations involved in splint selection and fabrication.
5. Determine what low-temperature thermoplastic handling and performance characteristics are useful for fabricating different splints.
6. Recognize indications for soft splinting.
7. Explain basic pattern-making, fabrication, and strapping principles and techniques.
8. Draw patterns for and fabricate three basic upper extremity splints.

The hand serves to obtain information, execute motor activities, and express emotions. The hand requires sensation, mobility, and stability to interact effectively with the environment. Any defect in sensory, neuromuscular, skeletal, articular, vascular, or soft tissue structures affects the functioning of the hand and its appearance.[2,4] The function of the proximal joints (shoulder, elbow, forearm) is to place and stabilize the hand for functional activities. Thus the hand must be assessed in relation to function of the entire arm.

Because of its primary role in daily activities and interaction, the appearance of the hand is important. Use of skin moisturizers, manicures, and jewelry testifies to the importance of its attractiveness in interpersonal contact. The exquisite sensibility of the hand permits an amazing level of coordinated activity, and it transmits enormous amounts of information about the environment to the brain. People use their hands to prepare for and perform all activities of daily living (ADL) and to express themselves. The hand may caress or slap. The hearing-impaired person uses the hand to speak, and the blind person uses it to see.

Psychosocial problems may be associated with dysfunction or injury that disrupts the hand's primary role in daily interactions with both the physical world and other people.[13] Splinting is one of several treatment modalities used to restore normal function and appearance of the hand. The occupational therapy assistant (OTA) is often called on to fabricate splints (i.e., orthopedic devices used to immobilize, mobilize, or protect a body part) and to assist with the assessment of patient positioning. This chapter briefly reviews the structures and function of the hand, introduces basic principles and goals of hand splinting, and provides basic instruction on fabrication of three common hand splints.

Structures of the Hand

Bones

The wrist and hand are composed of 27 bones: 8 carpals (wrist), 5 metacarpals (palm), and 14 phalanges (fingers). The proximal row of carpals articulates with the radius and ulna of the forearm. Combined movements of hand, wrist, and forearm permit an amazing variety of positions during activity.

Alignment

The precise relationship of length, mobility, and position of each finger and between the thumb and fingers is the key to functional use. The fingertips converge toward the pad of the thumb during palmar prehension. When individually flexed, they converge toward the center of the wrist (capitate bone), but when simultaneously flexed, they contact the palm parallel to each other. Alignment of the digits must be respected during splint design and fabrication.

Arches

Three arches (curves) are present in the hand: the longitudinal, the proximal transverse, and the distal transverse. The longitudinal arch follows the lines of the carpal and metacarpal bones down along the third finger. The ability to flex and extend the digits occurs along this arch. The proximal transverse arch is a bony, fixed arch formed by the proximal row of carpal bones and annular ligaments. This arch is deep; through it pass all the nerves, blood supply, and tendons of the extrinsic hand muscles. This arch also acts as a fulcrum for the finger flexors, preventing them from bowing during flexion. The distal transverse arch (also called the *metacarpal arch*) lies across the metacarpal heads (knuckles). The dexterity and functional use of the hand rely on the mobility of this arch.

Place your left thumb on the palm side of the fourth and fifth metacarpal heads of your right hand and push them back to where they are flat across with the second and third metacarpal heads. When you attempt to make a fist with your right hand, you will see that it is not possible. Flattening of the distal transverse arch is not a functional position. Flattening may be caused by many conditions including intrinsic muscle paralysis, edema, scarring, contractures, or poor positioning in a splint. A splint must be formed to preserve the distal transverse arch to ensure maximal functional use of the hand while the splint is on or off.

Dual Obliquity

The dual obliquity (or two nonparallel lines) (Figure 20-1) in the hand occurs because the length of the second to fifth metacarpals gradually decreases from the radial (thumb) side of the hand to the ulnar side of the hand. A line drawn through the metacarpal heads forms an oblique angle with a line drawn through the wrist. A second oblique angle occurs at the distal transverse arch. The second and third metacarpals are relatively fixed, stable bones, whereas the fourth and fifth move more freely. Functionally, this means that an object, when grasped cylindrically, is higher on the radial side of the hand and not parallel to the floor when the hand is in full pronation. An easy way to remember this is simply that the radial (thumb) side of the hand is longer and higher than the ulnar (small finger) side. Any hand or forearm-based splint must respect this anatomy.

Creases

The skin creases (folds) (Figure 20-2) can act as guides when the occupational therapy (OT) practitioner is designing and fitting splints. The creases indicate where the axis of motion for the joint occurs. The wrist, palmar, thenar, and proximal, middle, and distal finger creases deepen when the associated joint is moved. For the palmar creases the distal crease is associated with metacarpophalangeal (MP) flexion of digits III, IV, and V, and the proximal crease with digits II and III. Dorsal (on the back of the hand) splints should be constructed so that the splint extends to the midpoint of the next proximal joint. The volar (on the palm side) splint extends up to but does not include the next distal crease.

> **CLINICAL PEARL 20-1**
>
> The splint pattern is drawn to the crease and then shortened approximately ⅛ inch (0.3 cm) to accommodate skin folds.

Skin

The dorsal skin of the hand on the extensor surface is fine, supple, and mobile to allow it to move freely during flexion and extension of the fingers. Scarring and edema limit hand function by destroying skin mobility. The palmar skin

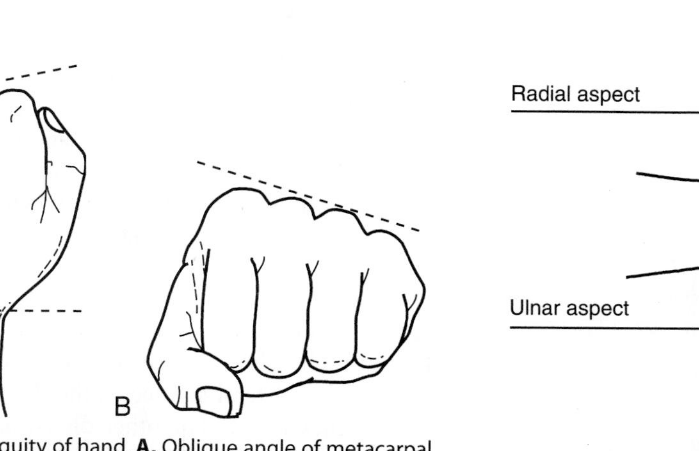

Figure 20-1 Dual obliquity of hand. **A,** Oblique angle of metacarpal heads in relation to axis of wrist joint. **B,** Oblique angle of metacarpal heads from radial to ulnar side of hand. (From Fess EE, Gettle KS, Philips CA, et al: *Hand and upper extremity splinting: principles and methods,* ed 3, St Louis, 2005, Mosby.)

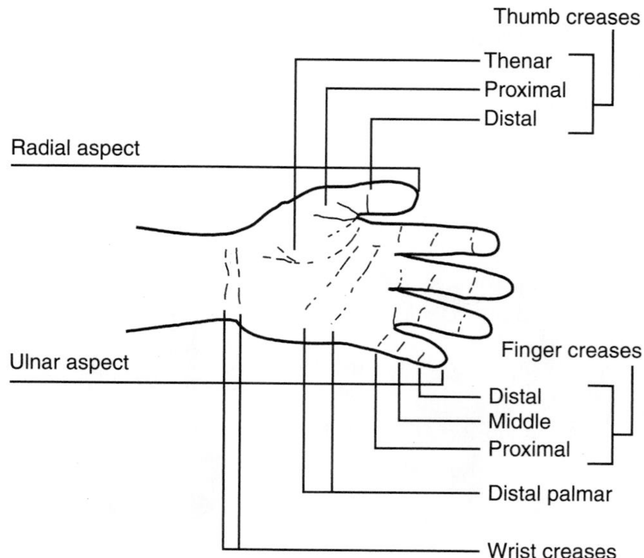

Figure 20-2 Palmar creases of hand. (From Malick MH: *Manual on static hand splinting,* Pittsburgh, 1972, Harmarville Rehabilitation Center.)

(on the flexor surface) by comparison is tough, thick, and inelastic. It protects and supports the underlying structures and prevents slippage between the skeleton and an object grasped.[13] The integrity of the skin is affected by many factors including medical and neurologic conditions, hydration, and job tasks.

Muscles

The movements of the hand and wrist involve 39 muscles: 20 extrinsic (outside the hand) muscles and 19 intrinsic (inside the hand) muscles.[13] The 20 extrinsic muscles include the long flexors and extensors of the wrist and fingers, the pronators, and the supinator and are located in the forearm. The 19 intrinsic muscles include those of the thenar (thumb side) and hypothenar (little finger side) eminences, the lumbricals, and the interossei.[2] An elaborate ligamentous system in the hand and wrist helps bony alignment by providing stability and mobility. A pulley system improves the mechanical advantage of the long finger muscles by keeping the tendons close to the bones as they glide.

Nerve Supply

Three peripheral nerves supply the hand: the radial, median, and ulnar. In general the radial nerve supplies the extensor/supinator muscle group and sensation to the dorsal surface of the radial side of the hand. The median nerve supplies the flexor/pronator muscles, the thenar group, and the first and second lumbricals. This nerve provides sensation to the radial side of the palm and thumb. The median nerve therefore is crucial in grasp, prehension, and tactile discrimination functions. The ulnar nerve innervates most of the intrinsic muscles and supplies sensory fibers to the ulnar side of the hand and digits. Figure 20-3 shows the sensory distribution.

Normal Hand Function

Understanding the normal functions of the hand is fundamental to designing and fabricating effective splints. The hand is the terminal point of the arm. Adequate range of motion (ROM) and sufficient muscle strength in the upper extremity joints are necessary for full use of the hand. Shoulder motions are critical for reaching and for such hand-to-body activities as eating and performing personal hygiene and grooming tasks. Elbow motion and supination/pronation of the forearm permit hand-to-face activities. The wrist, which is used chiefly to stabilize the hand during activity, contributes significantly to functional grip strength (see later section on tenodesis).

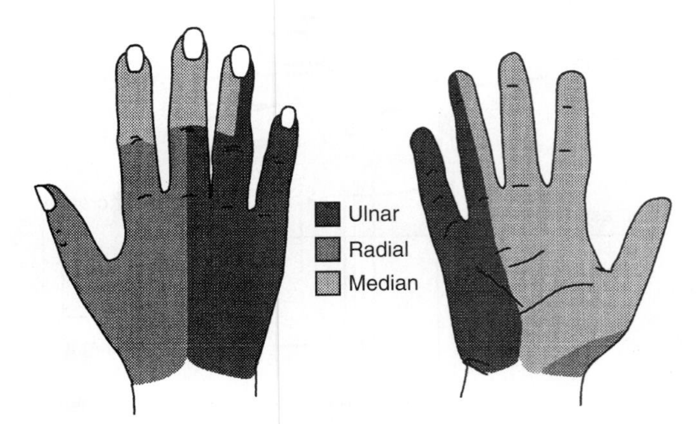

Figure 20-3 Sensory distribution in hand. Median nerve distribution includes most of the prehensile surface of the palm.

MP and interphalangeal (IP) joint flexion and stabilization are critical to grasp and prehension, and joint extension is necessary for release. The distal palmar arch formed by the metacarpals ensures the motion and opposition of the thumb and little finger, the ability to grasp round or large objects, convergence of the fingers during flexion, and the ability to press with the palm against resistance.

Opposition of the thumb is the basis of all prehension patterns. Thumb rotation at the carpometacarpal (CMC) joint is necessary to perform pad-to-pad prehension. Hand splints are typically fabricated to stabilize and position the thumb so that grasp and prehension can occur.

The normal hand is capable of mobility and stability at all joints. A splint can provide one or the other but rarely both.[7,10] A splint ultimately may aid in the recovery of dexterity, but hand function is hindered while it is worn due to decreased sensory input and limited mobility.

The normal hand can perform a variety of prehension and grasp patterns. Splinting can assist these patterns when muscle function is impaired or deformity is present.[10]

Prehension and Grasp Patterns

Hand movements are complex and occur in smooth sequence and combinations; however, they can be reduced to six basic patterns.[7,8,10]

Fingertip Prehension

Fingertip prehension (Figure 20-4, *A*), or tip-to-tip pinch, is the contact of the thumb pad with the pad of the index or middle finger. Fine, coordinated movement allows the fingertips to pick up small objects, fasten snaps and buttons, or hold a needle for sewing.

Palmar Prehension

Palmar prehension (Figure 20-4, *B*), also known as three jaw chuck, is contact of the thumb, middle, and index fingers. It is the most common prehension pattern and requires a high degree of coordination. It is the prehension pattern used for holding a pen, utensil, or small object of any shape (e.g., paper clip).

Lateral Prehension

Lateral prehension (Figure 20-4, *C*) is contact of the thumb pad with the lateral surface of the distal or middle phalanx of the index finger. The other digits may support the index finger, but the stability provided by the contraction of the first dorsal interosseus is essential. This pattern requires less coordination than the others but is stronger. Examples include turning a key or carrying a mug by its handle.

Cylindrical Grasp

Cylindrical grasp (Figure 20-4, *D*) occurs when an object is stabilized against the palm by finger flexion. Intrinsic and thenar muscles are essential to the power of this grasp. Examples include holding a drinking glass, hammer, or pot handle.

Spherical Grasp

Spherical grasp (Figure 20-4, *E*), or ball grasp, is used to hold round objects against an arched palm. Wrist stability and intrinsic and extrinsic hand muscle strength contribute to the ability to hold an apple, a ball, or a round doorknob.

Hook Grasp

Hook grasp (Figure 20-4, *F*) can be accomplished using the fingers only. It requires flexor strength and stability of the IP joints, MP joints, and wrist remaining in neutral. Examples include carrying a briefcase or shopping bag or pulling open a drawer.

Tenodesis

The tendons of the intrinsic hand muscles are held close to the bones of the wrist and hand by connective tissue. This close association between tendon and bone results in tenodesis action. In the normal hand when the wrist is flexed, the fingers are passively pulled into extension (Figure 20-5). The tendons of finger extensors are too short to permit simultaneous flexion of all the joints that the finger extensors cross: wrist, MP, proximal IP, and distal IP. The opposite is also true. With wrist extension the fingers are slightly pulled into flexion (Figure 20-5, *A*). This tenodesis action (wrist flexion with finger extension, wrist extension with finger flexion) is easily seen if you relax your fingers and move your wrist into flexion and extension rapidly. Tenodesis action results in a passive prehension pattern.

For a patient with quadriparesis, a tenodesis splint may cause passive finger flexion through active wrist extension. Release is accomplished by relaxation of wrist extension. See case study of Mr. R on the following page. For a patient with radial nerve palsy, a dynamic splint may take advantage of tenodesis to increase wrist extension passively during active finger flexion.

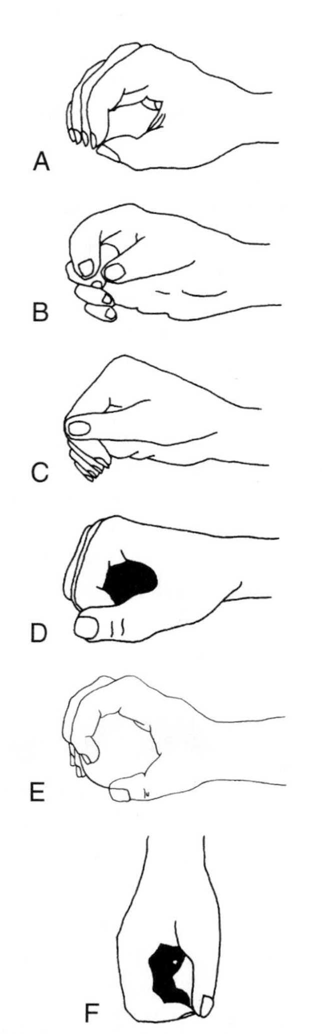

Figure 20-4 Basic types of prehension and grasp. **A,** Fingertip prehension. **B,** Palmar prehension. **C,** Lateral prehension. **D,** Cylindric grasp. **E,** Spherical grasp. **F,** Hook grasp.

Basic Positions of Hand

Functional

The functional position (Figure 20-6) is the hand position most often used during activity. It is similar to holding a soda can or ball. The wrist is in 20 to 30 degrees of extension; the thumb is abducted and opposed to the pad of the middle finger; metacarpals are flexed to approximately 30 degrees; and IP joints are flexed to approximately 45 degrees. In this position tension is equal in all muscles; the hand is in its mechanically most efficient posture.

Resting

Resting position (Figure 20-7) is the position a normal hand assumes when resting passively. In this position the wrist is in 10 to 20 degrees of extension. All finger joints are slightly flexed, and the thumb is midway between opposition and abduction, with the thumb's pad facing the side of the index

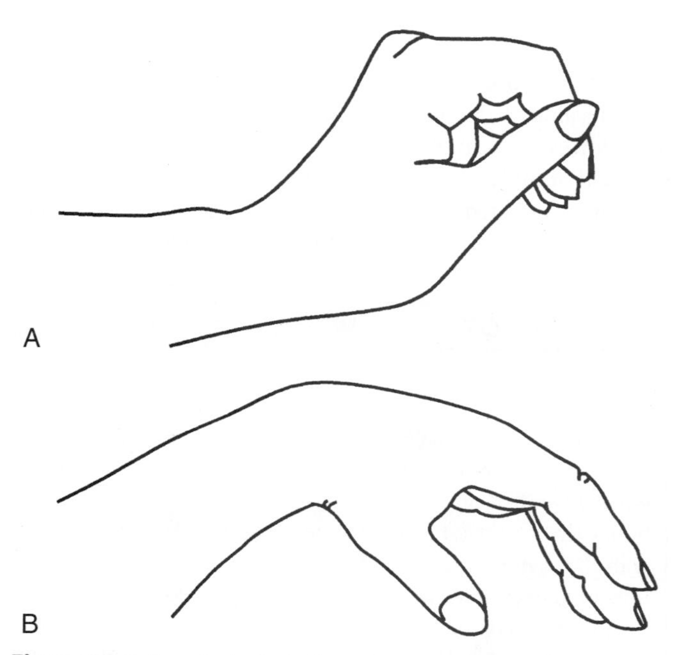

Figure 20-5 Tenodesis. **A,** Active wrist extension results in passive finger flexion. **B,** Active wrist flexion results in passive finger extension.

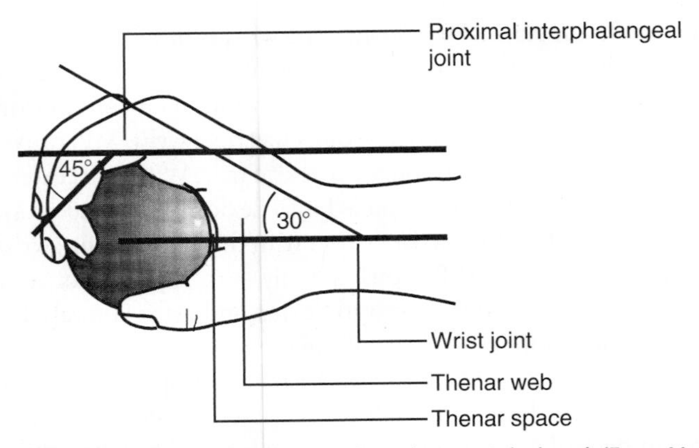

Figure 20-6 Functional position, lateral view, right hand. (From Malick MH: *Manual on static hand splinting,* Pittsburgh, 1972, Harmarville Rehabilitation Center.)

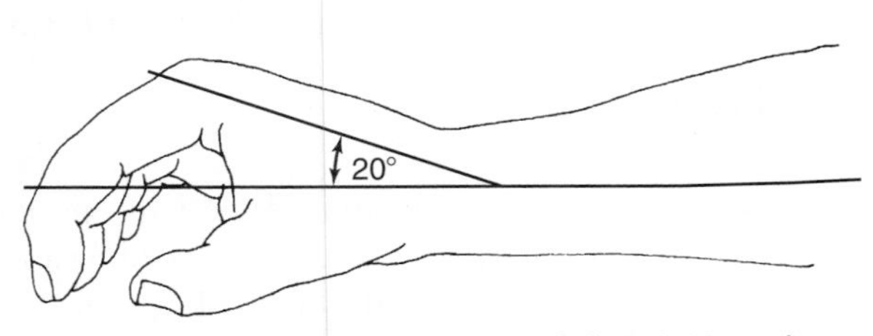

Figure 20-7 Resting position. (From Malick MH: *Manual on static hand splinting,* Pittsburgh, 1972, Harmarville Rehabilitation Center.)

finger. The proximal, distal, and longitudinal arches are maintained in this position. Splints are often fabricated in this position to rest joints or to prevent deformity.

CLINICAL PEARL 20-2

The occupational therapist often uses the resting position when splinting the hand of an older person who has arthritic changes of the CMC joint that may cause pain on full opposition.

Safe

The safe position maintains optimal stress on metacarpal, phalangeal, and IP collateral ligaments,[2] thereby "saving" the hand for eventual motion. In this position the MP joints are flexed; IP joints are in full extension; and the wrist is in 10 to 30 degrees of extension. This position is common after thermal injuries (burns), trauma, and invasive surgery.

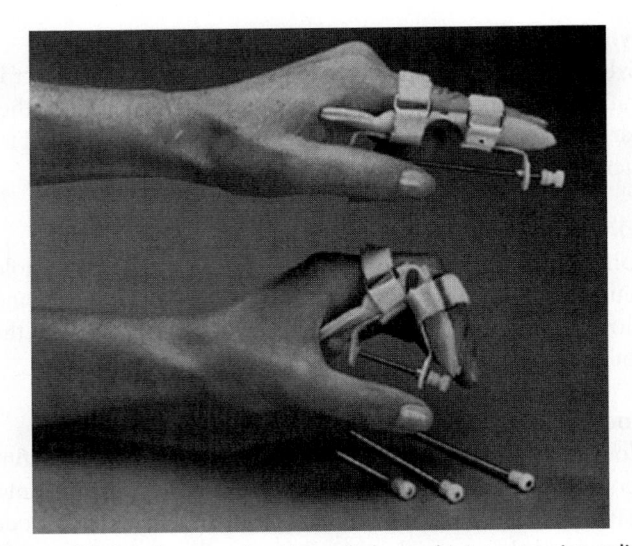

Figure 20-8 Rolyan proximal interphalangeal joint extension splint for static progressive splinting. (Courtesy Smith and Nephew Rolyan.)

Principles of Hand Splinting

Types of Splints

In the past, splints were often classified according to form rather than function. These classifications were called *static, dynamic,* and *static progressive.* The Splint Classification System (SCS), which was created by the American Society of Hand Therapists (ASHT) in 1992, "describes splints through a series of six predefined divisions that guide and progressively refine splints' technical names, working from broad concepts to individual splint specifications"[3] (Figure 20-8). In 2004 Fess and colleagues[3] further expanded and refined the SCS to create the Expanded Splint Classification System (ESCS). Some settings, particularly chronic care and general physical disability settings, continue to use the older system of terms.

The four ESCS purpose classifications for splints are immobilization, mobilization, restriction, and torque transmission. The main objective of immobilization splints is to immobilize the primary joints being splinted; mobilization splints move the primary joints. Restriction splints restrict motion of the primary joints, whereas torque transmission splints transmit torque to the primary joint(s).

CASE STUDY

Mr. R.

Mr. R., a 32-year-old male, has a history of substance abuse. After a night out, he awakes the next evening, unable to move his right wrist or hand, having slept with his head on his arm for nearly 24 hours. The next day, he goes to a medical clinic and is diagnosed with radial nerve palsy, confirmed by electromyography. He is unable to extend his wrist or fingers actively. He is immediately referred to occupational therapy. Over the months of his recovery, three splints will be fabricated for him to preserve the orthopedic integrity of his hand, as well as to improve his function.

A safe position splint will be fabricated for Mr. R. at his first appointment. The goal of using this splint is to preserve the structural integrity of his wrist and hand due to the unopposed active flexion of his wrist and fingers. The patient will be instructed in ROM; however, his reliability about positioning and performing his home exercise program is questionable at this time. The patient has agreed to wear the splint at night to prevent overstretching of his extensor muscles, which, in the long term, will limit his hand function on nerve recovery. The anatomy of the wrist and hand must be maintained during the many months it will take for nerve regeneration to achieve active ROM.

These ESCS classifications eliminate the ambiguity of the old system, in which the classifications referred to the structure of the splint components. Under the new ESCS, a single splint can have more than one purpose, thus allowing accurate and precise naming of splints according to the specific functions they perform. An example of a splint with a dual purpose is a flexion restriction splint, which can be used for trigger finger.

Purposes of Splinting

The goal of all splinting is to enable the patient to perform daily life tasks as easily as possible. Static, dynamic, and static progressive splints may be used to achieve any combination of the following[2,12]:

1. To protect, support, or immobilize joints to permit healing after inflammation or injury to the tendons, joint, soft tissue, or vascular/nerve supply. An arthritis resting mitt, which immobilizes the MP and wrist joints (of an inflamed arthritic hand), permits IP movement to allow for function (Figure 20-9).
2. To position and maintain alignment to keep the integrity of the arches, the ligamentous structures, and joint relationships. This goal can be accomplished with resting, functional, and safe positions and footdrop splints. An adjustable outrigger on a splint ensures alignment of the MP joints after surgical replacement.
3. To correct deformity or to prevent further deformity. An ulnar drift positioning splint (see Figure 30-16) is used to align the fingers of a patient with rheumatoid arthritis in a neutral position. In the early stages of the disease the splint acts to prevent the rapid progression of the deformity. Later on, it positions the digits for more effective functional use.
4. To substitute for weak or absent muscle function caused by neuromuscular disease and spinal cord or peripheral nerve injury. A radial nerve splint (Figure 20-10) amplifies the strength of the tenodesis action for the patient who cannot actively extend the wrist or fingers. With active finger flexion the wrist is passively extended, thus functionally increasing prehensile strength.
5. To maximize ROM by preventing contractures caused by adhesion formation. A dorsal blocking splint assists flexion yet blocks extension to decrease stress and stretch on the surgical repair side while permitting tendon excursion (see Chapter 30).
6. To increase ADL independence by acting as a base for the attachment of devices or compensating for decreased hand function. It is easier for the patient, for example, to have a splint attached to a razor to allow him or her to hold it or use a walker splint (Figure 20-11) to compensate for weakness or sensory loss.
7. To exercise, which can be accomplished with mobilization or torque transmission splints that either assist or strengthen the patient's own active motion, depending on the direction of pull of the splint.
8. To enhance positioning and functional performance in patients with abnormal tone (Figure 20-12). This may serve two different purposes, generally not at the same time—either to prevent malalignment or to improve function through low load stress or positioning. There is significant controversy over the fabrication and use of splints for patients after stroke, with regard to timing and effectiveness of use. The supervising therapist is obliged to keep well informed on current intervention strategies before deciding on a splinting intervention.[4]

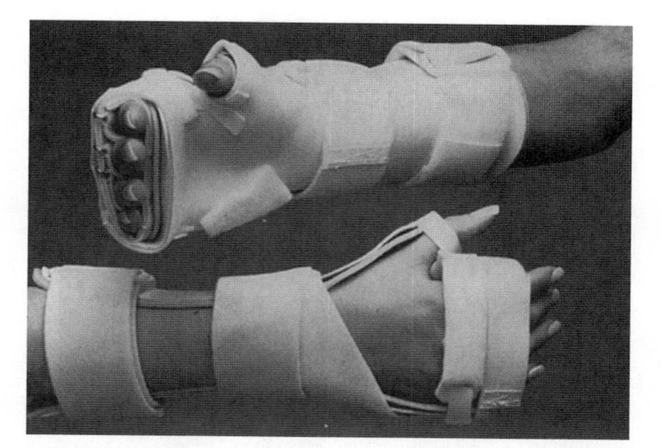

Figure 20-9 Arthritis resting mitt splint. (Courtesy Smith and Nephew Rolyan.)

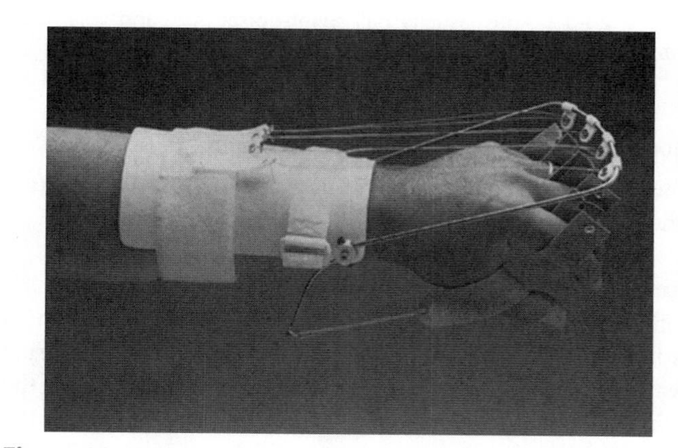

Figure 20-10 Rolyan static radial nerve splint. (Courtesy Smith and Nephew Rolyan.)

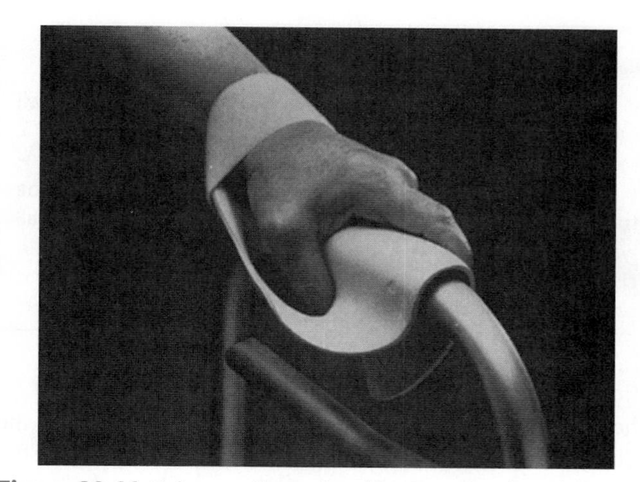

Figure 20-11 Rolyan walker splint. (Courtesy Smith and Nephew Rolyan.)

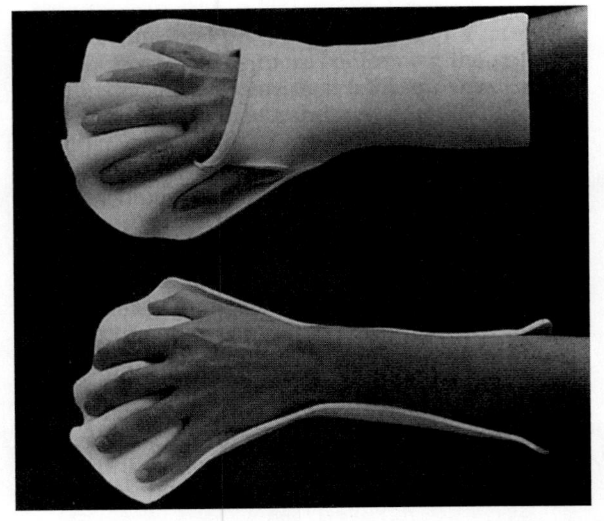

Figure 20-12 Antispasticity ball splint-dorsal *(top)* and volar *(bottom)* versions. (Courtesy Smith and Nephew Rolyan.)

Biomechanical Considerations

The OT practitioner must bear in mind the following factors when constructing a splint.

Bony Prominences

Soft tissue is particularly thin over bony prominences such as the radial and ulnar styloids, the pisiform, the metacarpal heads, and the base of the thumb's metacarpal. Because of the lack of natural padding over these areas, significant potential for skin breakdown due to pressure exists.[9] If possible, the practitioner should avoid splint contact with bony prominences by trimming and flaring the thermoplastic.

CLINICAL PEARL 20-3

If the OTA chooses to pad an area, a self-stick circle of closed-cell padding is placed on the bone before molding the thermoplastic so that the OTA can either put the padding back onto the thermoplastic, to ensure consistent pressure, or leave a "bubble" where the thermoplastic will be flared out, to avoid the prominence. A small wad of exercise putty may be used for the "bubble" technique. A circle of sticky-back foam may be used when padded consistent contact is indicated (Figure 20-13).

Alignment

The normal alignment of the digits should be maintained in the splint. The digits, when flexed, are parallel across the palm. At the wrist, 10 degrees of ulnar deviation is the normal resting posture.

Dual Obliquity

The radial side of the splint is longer and higher than the ulnar side to match the hand's anatomy (Figure 20-14).

Joints

Exact positioning of the joints varies and depends on the patient's diagnosis and the purpose for which the splint is used. For example, the wrist is usually placed at −7 to 9 degrees of extension for carpal tunnel syndrome,[3] at 30 degrees of extension for functional position, or at 20 degrees of extension for resting. For the patient with increased flexor tone, wrist extension is sometimes compromised to permit adequate finger extension. The angle of the wrist also affects tone.[5] Diagnosis, common sense, and physician preference all enter into the decision. The OTA should consult the supervising occupational therapist to ensure that positioning is as desired.

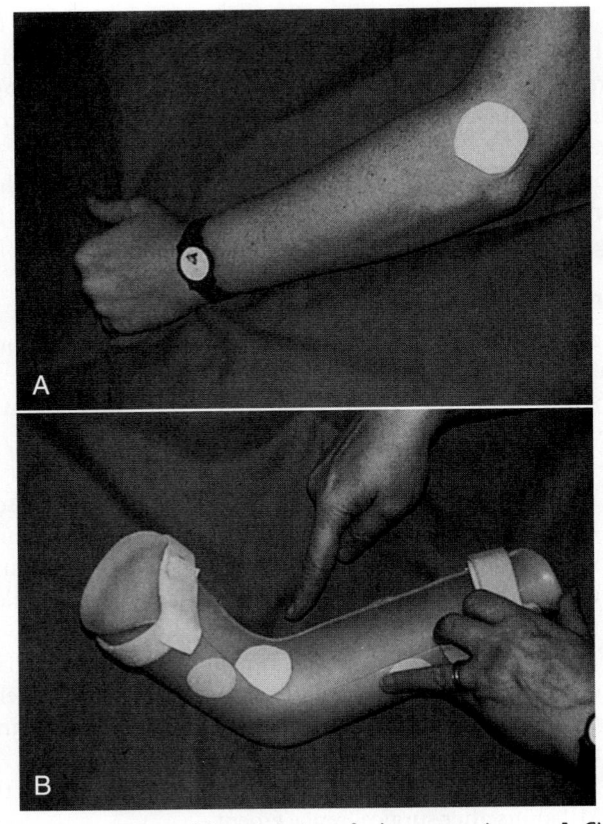

Figure 20-13 Prepadding technique for bony prominence. **A,** Circle of self-adhesive foam applied to patient before application of thermoplastic. **B,** Self-adhesive foam pad in splint ensures consistent pressure.

Preformed and soft splints are commonly set at 30 degrees of wrist extension, making them an inappropriate choice for a patient with carpal tunnel syndrome. You must modify these should a patient purchase one or be provided one by his or her physician/insurance carrier.

Preventing the adverse effects of immobilization is extremely important. To a joint, motion is lotion. Static splinting can cause joint stiffness with a resulting decrease in ROM. Thus two important points: (1) static splints must be removed periodically for active or passive exercise unless contraindicated by surgery, infection, or trauma; and (2) unless absolutely unavoidable, joints that do not require immobilization should not be included in or restricted by the splint.

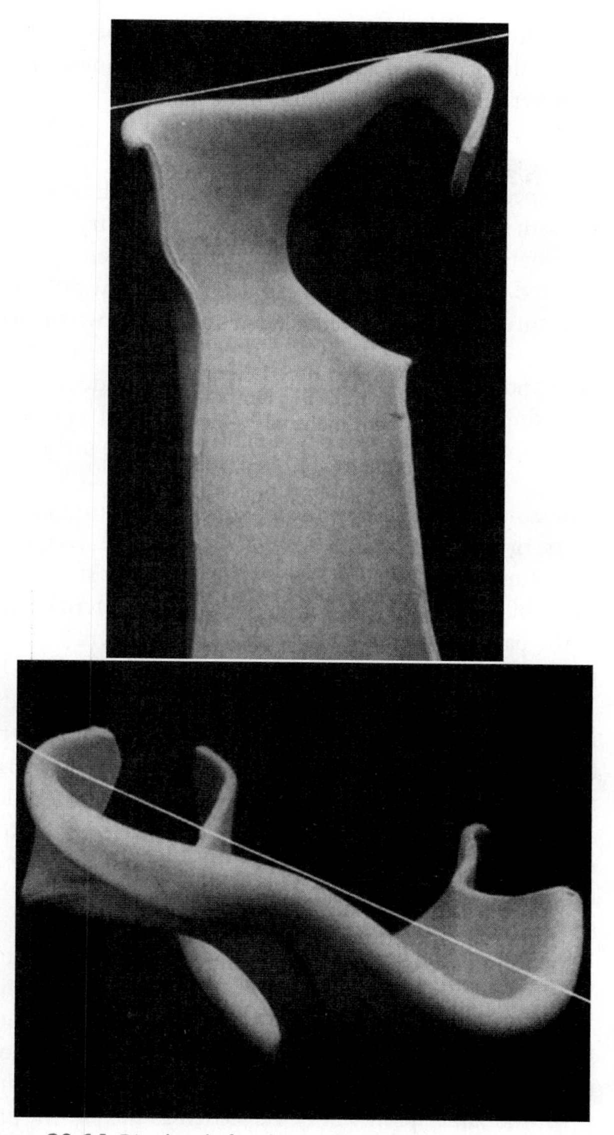

Figure 20-14 Distal end of cock-up splint demonstrates dual obliquity.

Creases

The skin creases must be acknowledged as described earlier. Exceptions to this rule are (1) when including a joint because a muscle or tendon passes over it (e.g., immobilization of the wrist after flexor tendon repair in the digit); and (2) when the splint physically needs to be made longer to counterbalance the distal force.

In the normal hand, joints have an amazing capacity for stability or mobility. A splint cannot provide both; therefore the supervising occupational therapist must choose between stability and mobility based on the patient's dysfunction, purpose of splinting, potential deformity, and functional use of the hand. The patient may be given both dynamic and static splints for the same diagnosis.

Collateral Ligaments

Maintaining the maximal length of collateral ligaments whenever possible is important. IP extension and MP flexion preserve this length. If the ligaments are allowed to shorten, restrictions in ROM may result.

Skin

As discussed earlier, more padding exists on the volar surface of the hand and forearm than on the dorsal surface; therefore it is the preferred splinting surface if skin condition and functional needs can be met. The sensory input received through cutaneous receptors is the key to functional use of the hand. A secretary might prefer a dorsal cock-up splint for carpal tunnel syndrome so that writing is not inhibited by decreased sensory input from the wrist and the ulnar border of the hand.

Open wounds and incision sites should be avoided whenever possible. Pressure or friction results in microtrauma to underlying structures. This trauma increases circulation to the area, and a red spot is seen after the patient has worn the splint for approximately 20 minutes. All splints should be checked for fit after 20 minutes of wear in the clinic to assess potential pressure areas.

Generally, the patient's arm is warm from wearing the splint or may look pinker in appearance. This is normal after several minutes; it is warm under the plastic. The OTA or occupational therapist typically provides the patient with some stockinette to wear under the splint to absorb perspiration. Thermoplastic materials do not breathe; however, perforated material does permit some air exchange. Antimicrobial-coated materials may also have applications for specific populations.

Pressure is probably the greatest overall problem with fabricating a splint. In addition to potential spots over bony prominences, pressure may also be caused by poor fit and design. Wider, longer splints fit better than short, narrow ones.

General rules for avoiding pressure areas during splint fabrication are the following:

1. The splint should be two-thirds the length of the forearm.
2. The splint should cover approximately half the circumference of the extremity (midbone trim marks work well).
3. Splint up to but do not include the next skin crease in the wrist/hand area, in order to leave room for skin folds during ROM.
4. Fold or flare proximal and distal edges so that they are rounded.
5. Round all internal and external corners. Sharp corners wear poorly and will dig into the patient's skin.
6. Reduce unequal pressure by means of a more conforming fit. The more conforming the splint, the better the pressure is distributed. What is more comfortable: a brand new pair of stiff, leather dress shoes or a pair of soft, conforming running shoes?

CLINICAL PEARL 20-4

For patients with darker pigmentation, the OTA runs a finger over the bony prominences to check for "hot spots" and then makes modifications as needed. Should a pressure spot be evident, place a dab of dark lipstick on the area and reapply the splint. This will mark the spot for adjustment (flaring).

Sensorimotor Function

Sensory information and feedback are essential components of normal movement. Splinting reduces sensory input from the area covered with thermoplastic and therefore may contribute to the patient's discomfort. Many patients requiring a splint have decreased sensation because of central or peripheral nerve deficits, and their risk of developing pressure areas with resulting skin breakdown is greater. Because their sensation is diminished, they may not complain that the splint is uncomfortable. These patients must be taught to compensate visually or to use their other hand to check for hot spots. Not uncommonly, a caregiver must be instructed to assess ongoing fit because the patient is unable to do so.

Precautions

Significant precautionary measures have already been covered in this chapter, especially the risks involved with a poorly fitting splint. In addition, the skin's integrity is influenced by general medical conditions such as diabetes (sensory loss and atrophy), dehydration, and congestive heart failure (vascular compromise and edema).

Edema occurs, to a slight degree, whenever an extremity is immobilized, because the splint prohibits active ROM. Active motion is the muscle pump that keeps fluids moving. Therapists often must splint an edematous extremity. Significant edema can occur after trauma and may also be seen in patients with compromised cardiac status. The splint must be large enough to accommodate the edema. The patient is instructed to keep the arm elevated whenever possible by placing it up on a pillow when resting or by using a sling when standing for extended periods.

Patient compliance is essential, but many reasons for noncompliance exist. The OTA should address these from the start. First, the splint must fit well; no one wants to wear something uncomfortable. Second, it must be cosmetically acceptable. Splints should be clean and neat, not marred by ragged edges and fingerprints. The patient pays a significant sum of money for the splint, and the splint is a reflection of the practitioner and the clinic. Third, splints are generally an inconvenience to the patient. They limit motion and sensation, are warm, and often seem "in the way." The OTA must explain that the temporary inconvenience is necessary for long-term gain in function. A carpal tunnel splint that sits atop a computer does no one any good.

CLINICAL PEARL 20-5

If the patient swells during the course of the day, the OT practitioner should fabricate the splint later in the day. If this is not possible, the practitioner can allow for the anticipated swelling by using multiple layers of stockinette on the arm during fabrication.

Material Selection

A tremendous variety of splinting material is available in the market today. Low-temperature thermoplastics are generally used for rigid splints. Flexible materials such as heavy fabric, neoprene, knitted elastics, and foam laminates may be used alone or in combination with rigid metal or thermoplastic stays. A quick overview of these "soft splints" follows later in this chapter.

Low-Temperature Thermoplastics

Low-temperature thermoplastics are generally heated in a water bath (splint pan, hydrocollator, electric fry pan) to approximately 160° F (71.1° C), their molding temperature. The heated thermoplastic is applied to the patient dry. Low-temperature thermoplastic selection is based on two primary criteria: (1) how it handles during the forming (fabrication) process; and (2) how it performs as a finished product.

Handling characteristics when the material has been heated to the recommended molding temperature include the following:

1. Moldability refers to how the material shapes around contours, or how easy it is to form. Moldability allows the OT practitioner to have the material take a specific shape.
2. Drapability refers to how easily the warm material forms to the patient with only gravity to mold it down. The drapier the material, the gentler the clinician's touch must be. These materials must be stroked—not poked or pushed—into place. By keeping his or her hands moving during the forming process, the clinician will not leave fingerprint marks behind. The more drapey the material, the less appropriate it is for large splints. Generally the less experienced splinter prefers a low to moderate drape material. *Rebound* is the term used for a nondrapey material that springs back slightly during molding.
3. Elasticity refers to how much the material resists stretch. When pulled or tugged, does it follow easily or does it resist?
4. Memory materials, when reheated, return to their original size and shape. They are usually more elastic than nonmemory materials. These are often used for serial splinting, when the same splint will be remolded as the patient progresses, for example, to increase wrist or digit extension.
5. Heating is how much time is required in the water bath to reach molding temperature. Usually, 1 to 3 minutes will heat material ⅛ inch (0.3 cm) thick.
6. Edge finishing is the ease of finishing the edges in a smooth manner. Generally, synthetic (all-plastic) materials edge more easily than rubber-based thermoplastics.
7. Self-bonding materials bond to each other when they are warm and dry. Coated materials tack together at the edges, but once the material hardens, they can be popped apart. For a more permanent bond, the coating must be scraped off or removed with a solvent before bonding. A coated material, once stretched, is tackier and more likely to self-bond.
8. Shrinkage may occur in some materials during the cooling process. The final adjustments must compensate for shrinkage.
9. Working time averages 3 to 5 minutes for solid ⅛-inch thick material. The thinner or more perforated the material, the faster it cools. In some materials, the conformability during cooling may slowly ease off; in others it cuts off quickly. This is also influenced by the temperature of the room you are working in.

CLINICAL PEARL 20-6

Very drapey materials should only be used on cooperative patients—those who can hold their extremity in the appropriate position so that gravity can assist the practitioner during forming.

Performance characteristics relate to the end results or how the splint works once it has hardened. Performance characteristics include the following:

1. Conformability is how intimately the splint fits into contoured areas. The OTA may see the imprint of the patient's fingerprints and hand creases with a very drapey material. More conforming splints are usually more comfortable and less likely to migrate during use.
2. Rigidity is the strength of the splint. Will it bend under stress (from the patient's weight, muscle tone, or strength)? Rigidity of the splint also increases with the number of arches and contours built into the splint. Note that rigidity and drape are not related, although some OT practitioners use these terms interchangeably. A very drapey material may produce a very rigid end product, and vice versa.
3. Flexibility relates to how much repeated stress a splint can take. This quality is important in a circumferential (going around the arm) splint design, in which the splint is pulled open for application or removal. A thumb spica, seen in Figure 20-31, is an example of this.
4. Durability is how long the splint will last. Natural rubber-based materials are more likely to become brittle with age and use than are all-plastic materials. Low-temperature thermoplastic splints are most often used for a temporary condition.
5. Finish on the material may be smooth or slightly textured. Coated materials are slightly easier to keep clean.
6. Moisture permeability (air exchange) is affected solely by the amount of perforation (if any). Memory materials are available in superperforated versions for maximum air exchange.
7. Colors have an effect on patient compliance. The darker thermoplastic colors and patterned materials are less likely to become lost in institutional bedsheets and show less dirt.
8. Thickness. The thinner the material, the more responsive it is to handling during the forming process, and the lighter it is in weight. Ultra-thin materials are not recommended for a novice splinter. Thicker materials are usually stronger than thinner ones. Material ⅛-inch thick is generally used for most splints.

Manufacturers' catalogs assist the clinician in selecting appropriate materials for specific splint types and for the fabricator's level of skill. Materials change, new ones appear, former ones are retired, features change, and a clinician must keep up to date. The practitioner should mold a sample of material before using it to fabricate a splint so that he or she can acquire some experience with its handling characteristics.

Soft Splints

Soft splints, because they are fabricated from more flexible materials, may permit partial motion at a joint. These semi-flexible splints are used to limit motion or protect an area. They may be used for patients who "just won't tolerate" rigid immobilization. Other uses are for joint protection to ease chronic pain syndromes and for patients with arthritis in whom total immobilization would cause painful joint stiffness.

Soft splints are often fabricated for geriatric patients, who have an increased potential for skin breakdown because of fragile skin or poor carryover of the wearing regimen. Figure 20-15 provides examples of soft splints.

Strapping and Padding Principles

Straps hold the splint in place and are fastened down with hook and loop material, adhesive, or rivets. Most splints are fastened with a hook and loop at three points to ensure that they do not migrate or rotate on the extremity. Hook fasteners and loop strapping (Velcro) are available with and without self-adhesive backing. The loop strapping is always applied

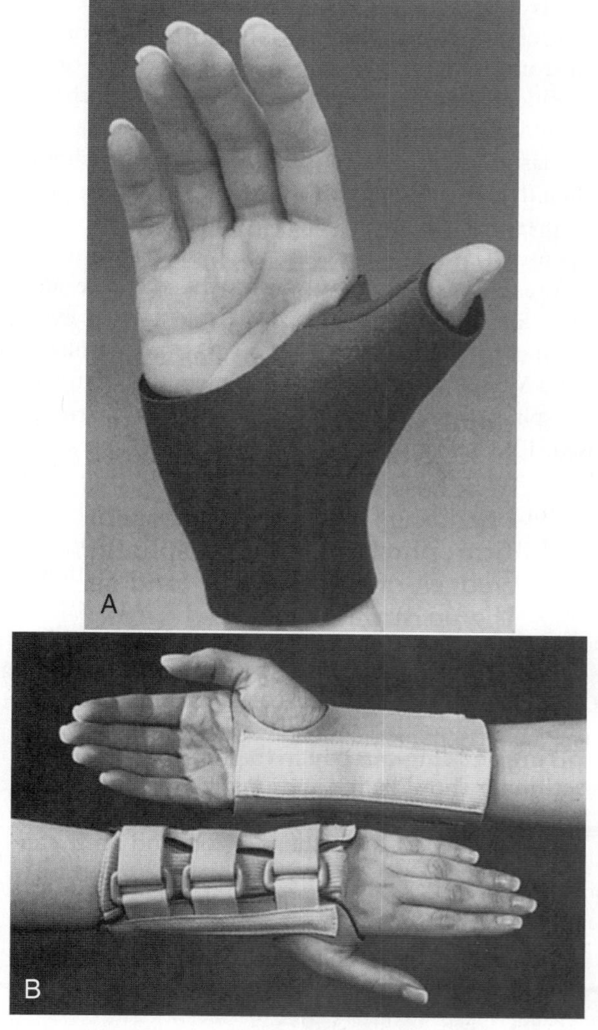

Figure 20-15 **A,** Rolyan neoprene pull-on-thumb support. Warmth and compression of neoprene help reduce pain due to overuse of thumb and wrist. **B,** Rolyan D-ring wrist brace with metal support bar in a sleeve on flexor surface. (Courtesy Smith and Nephew Rolyan.)

facing the skin to prevent abrasion. Soft straps with foam laminate are used when increased softness is necessary and are compatible with hook fasteners. They can collapse somewhat to accommodate edema. Stretchy strapping may be used to reduce constriction.

D-ring straps may be used for a more secure fit or for a patient with decreased coordination. A variety of colors and widths of strapping materials is available. Wider straps may help distribute pressure more evenly. When acute edema is present, a splint may be bandaged on to ensure even pressure distribution.

CLINICAL PEARL 20-7

Straps in which a self-adhesive hook is sewn onto the loop strap decrease the risk of losing the strap, which is beneficial in institutional settings.

Padding is available in two basic types: closed-cell or open-cell. Closed-cell paddings are nonabsorbent and can be wiped clean and dry. They do not absorb moisture or bacteria. Closed-cell foams may be applied directly to the thermoplastic before heating (the material floats in the heat pan, foam side up). This technique is desirable when additional insulation from heat is necessary, as for burn patients or babies. Polycushion padding, for example, is soft and stretchable and easily molded around contours, whereas self-adhesive padding (Plastazote) is less stretchable. The clinician should use padding that resists bottoming out (completely compressing) under pressure.

Open-cell cushioning is absorbent, similar to a sponge. Therefore it needs to be changed regularly to ensure adequate hygiene. Slow-recovery foams that "mold" to the extremity are often used to compensate for lack of splint contour. Moleskin and Molestick are thin paddings often used to reduce the risk of splint migration when a noncontouring thermoplastic is used. PPT™ foam padding is a durable, shock-absorbing padding. Although it is open-cell, it has a nylon top skin that allows for easy washing.[11]

Most padding materials are available in ¹⁄₁₆-, ⅛-, ¼-, and ½-inch (0.15- to 1.25-cm) thicknesses, with or without self-adhesive backing. The ¹⁄₁₆- and ⅛-inch sticky-back paddings are the most commonly used. To ensure a firm purchase on the splinting material around the edges of the padding (and self-adhesive Velcro), the glue surface is heated with a heat gun before applying to the splint.

CLINICAL PEARL 20-8

When applying sticky-back foam directly to a bony prominence, one should use a circular shape; it is easier to replace the foam in the indentation left in the thermoplastic.

Before applying padding directly to the patient's skin, the OT should stick and unstick the glued side on a towel to decrease its adhesive power; thus it will not stick too firmly to the patient's skin and can be removed easily.

Patient Instruction

The patient instruction handout should always include wearing schedules, care instructions, and a precaution statement. When possible, wearing time should be built up over a few days so that the patient can become accustomed to the splint. The clinician must perform frequent skin checks and ensure that the patient knows how to clean the splint with mild soap and warm—not hot—water and knows to dry the splint thoroughly before reapplying. The patient should be cautioned not to put splints in the washing machine or dishwasher or leave them in a hot car in the summer or on a radiator. The splint will begin to melt at 135° F (57.2° C).[6]

Correct positioning is crucial and should be reviewed with the patient. Straps should be snug, not tight. The patient should be able to insert a finger under the strap once it is fastened.

CLINICAL PEARL 20-9

Instruct the patient to secure the strap "watchband tight."

After instruction, the patient (or the caregiver) should be able to do the following: (1) tell the clinician the purpose of the splint and when it should be worn; (2) demonstrate the home exercise program (see Chapter 30); (3) don and doff the splint independently; (4) perform skin checks; and (5) explain how to care for the splint.[6]

Other Considerations

Clinical reasoning takes into account each patient's individual care need. Treatment goals and lifestyle considerations (age, dominance, medical/social history, home and work environments) help the clinician determine the best splint option. Examples are using black material for a construction worker or perforated material for someone in a warm climate. Ease of donning and doffing and caregiver instructions are essential for those who rely on others for their care. Weakness, diminished dexterity, and visual acuity issues in the geriatric client will influence the weight of material selected, as well as the type of strapping and closures. Vitality of the skin must also be considered.[1]

Splint Fabrication

Specific pattern-making techniques, material suggestions, fabrication instructions, and strapping patterns are provided for each of the three splints discussed in this chapter. To start, the following supplies are necessary: (1) a heat pan; (2) a plastic spatula; (3) a towel; (4) sharp, clean scissors; (5) paper towels; (6) a grease pen or awl; and (7) a heat gun. The heat pan needs a minimum of 2 to 3 inches of water heated to 160° F (71.1° C) (just beyond the simmer setting). It should have an unscratched, nonstick coating.

CLINICAL PEARL 20-10

If the bottom of the splinting pan does not have a nonstick coating, or if the coating is scratched, line the bottom of the pan with a pillowcase or paper toweling to prevent the material from sticking.

The following general technical tips will aid the reader in cutting, molding, and finishing various types of splints.

Pattern Making

Patterns are usually made on a paper towel. The OTA or occupational therapist cuts out and checks the fit on the patient, then traces the pattern onto the thermoplastic. Precut splint blanks are popular because they significantly decrease fabrication time and cost.

CLINICAL PEARL 20-11

When drawing a pattern, if it is difficult to position the extremity because of the patient's muscle weakness, abnormal muscle tone, or pain, the pattern may be made on the opposite extremity and then inverted.

Cutting

1. Place the pattern on the thermoplastic. Trace it with an awl or marker slightly wider than the pattern itself. You want to be able to cut inside your pattern lines so that the markings are not on the actual splint.
2. Using a utility knife, score a rectangular shape around the pattern and snap off the piece.
3. Heat the thermoplastic to the correct temperature by leaving it in the heat pan until it is uniformly flexible.
4. Remove the thermoplastic from the heat pan using the spatula. A plastic spatula will help prevent marring the nonstick coating of the pan.
5. Place the material promptly on the towel and gently swipe it dry. Repeatedly flip the stickier materials over during drying so that they do not adhere to the towel.
6. Support the excess material with one hand and the working surface to prevent stretching. Cut out the marked splint. Use the scissors as if you were cutting paper, leaving the blades slightly open between cuts and perpendicular to the material. Round all the corners (Figure 20-16).

Never cut splinting material when it is cool because the splint edges will be jagged and the force needed may strain the clinician's thumb.

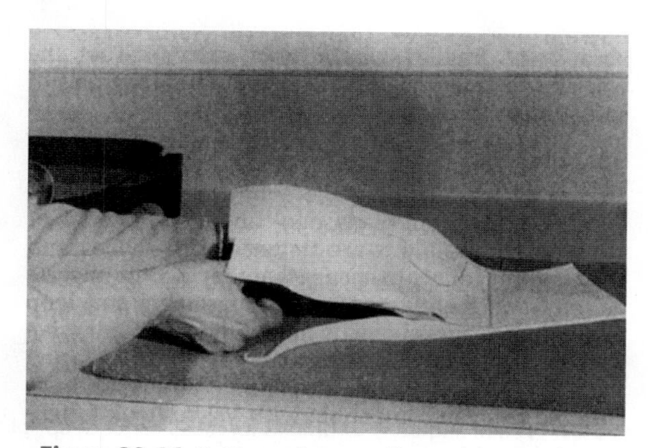

Figure 20-16 Cutting splint out of heated thermoplastic.

When removing material from the splinting pan, do not hold the material vertically in an effort to allow the excess water to drip off because some materials may stretch in this position.

CLINICAL PEARL 20-12

To avoid having the towel texture become imprinted on warm splinting material, cover the towel with a pillow case.

Molding

1. Heat a thermoplastic precut splint blank (or reheat the custom-cut splint) to the appropriate temperature. Remove the material from the heat pan, dry it, and let it cool for several seconds until it is comfortable to touch.
2. Position the patient, preferably so that gravity will assist the thermoplastic draping.
3. Place the thermoplastic material on the arm/hand. Be sure to align the pattern properly. Stroke it into place. Use firm yet gentle strokes with the pads of the fingers or the side of the hand to mold the plastic. Do not poke at the material or grasp it because this may leave behind fingerprints and affect the contour of the splint as well. Keep your hands moving when they are on the thermoplastic to prevent imprinting. Make sure to acknowledge the arches and to contour them into the splint carefully.
4. Flare the proximal edges of the splint and any other edges where pressure might occur. Flared or folded edges are more comfortable and increase the splint's strength.
5. Allow the splint to set until it is fairly rigid. Total working time is usually 3 to 5 minutes. Make sure to maintain the patient's position while the material sets.
6. If the splint was molded in supination, pronate the patient's forearm and check the fit.
7. Mark any trim lines that are indicated (e.g., midbone on the forearm, crease clearance, two-thirds length of the forearm).

Thermoplastics with memory need to be consistently molded until the material is firm because of their tendency to return to their original flat shape.

CLINICAL PEARL 20-13

If the forearm trough is not centered, grasp the dorsal end and twist it to center the trough. ("Off-centering" occurs because the contour of the forearm changes as gravity pulls on the flexor muscles.)

CLINICAL PEARL 20-14

Make your pattern marks a tad wide and cut them off when trimming so that no ink stains remain on the splint.

Finishing

1. Hold the splint up vertically and dip the area to be trimmed repeatedly in and out of the heat pan. When slightly softened, trim to the marked length and gently flare the proximal end toward the outside of the splint with a sweeping stroke using the palm of the hand. This flare prevents the proximal end from digging into the forearm musculature.
2. To trim the sides or top, heat the side or top edge either by dipping the material in and out of the heat pan, pouring warm water over the spot to be trimmed, or using a heat gun. Once the material is slightly warm, cut along the trim lines. Do not heat the material to full molding temperature to do this step; it may disfigure the edge.
3. If necessary, smooth rough or jagged edges, again by dipping in and out of the water to slightly heat the material. Polish carefully with the fingertip or palm while the material is still wet.
4. If major fit changes are required, reheat the entire splint and remold it. Do not attempt to spot-heat large areas such as the wrist or thumb.

> Beware of the heat gun. It is difficult to control the flow of hot air with a heat gun, and it is easy to accidentally heat a portion of the splint that does not need adjustment.

Strapping

Straps are applied last. Refer to strapping methods and technical information discussed earlier in this chapter. Remember that three points of control are usually necessary to hold a splint in place, so at least three straps are customarily used on a forearm-based splint (see Figure 20-26).

Evaluation

On completion, the splint must be analyzed for function, fit, and appearance.

Function

1. Are the arches of the hand maintained? Looking at the splint directly on, is the metacarpal area properly arched? Is the radial side of the palm higher than the ulnar side? Looking at the splint from the side, is the longitudinal arch obvious?
2. Is the hand splinted in the proper position? Use a goniometer to check joint angles.

Fit

1. Are the straps correctly placed to promote stability and to avoid pressure points?
2. Do the sides of the splint extend at least to midbone?
3. Is the splint long enough to effectively support the body parts involved? Are the appropriate joint creases visible to permit full joint ROM?
4. Could any edges or corners press into the patient's skin? Do any potential pressure sites over bony prominences, such as the ulnar styloid, exist? Check for reddened or warmer areas on the skin after 20 minutes of wearing time.

Appearance

1. Is the splint surface smooth and free of marks, dents, and rough edges?
2. Are all the corners rounded, edges smooth, and proximal and distal ends flared where appropriate?
3. Are the straps neat and aligned correctly? Is the self-adhesive hook fully covered by the strap?
4. Is it cosmetically acceptable to the clinician and the patient?

Directions

Radial Bar Wrist Cock-Up Splint

A cock-up splint is used to support and/or position the wrist. For functional positioning the wrist is aligned at 20 to 30 degrees of extension. In patients with carpal tunnel syndrome the wrist is positioned at −7 to 9 degrees. Use a drapey splinting material with moderate resistance to stretch.

Pattern

1. Mark the following landmarks: the MP heads on the radial and ulnar sides of the hand, the base of the web space, the wrist joint on the radial side, and two-thirds the length of the forearm.
2. Draw the pattern as shown in Figure 20-17, allowing sufficient excess for the width of the splint to wrap halfway around the forearm.
3. Remove the patient's arm and connect, with a circular arc, the web space and wrist markings as seen in Figure 20-18.
4. Cut out the pattern and check the fit on the patient. Make adjustments as needed.

Fabrication

1. Trace the pattern onto the thermoplastic and heat it. Cut out the splint blank and reheat to molding temperature if necessary.
2. With the patient's forearm supinated, position the wrist at the appropriate angle of extension and ulnar deviation. Drape the material over the hand/forearm, taking care to line up the distal end with the palmar crease. Wrap the radial bar through the web space around to the dorsum of the hand.

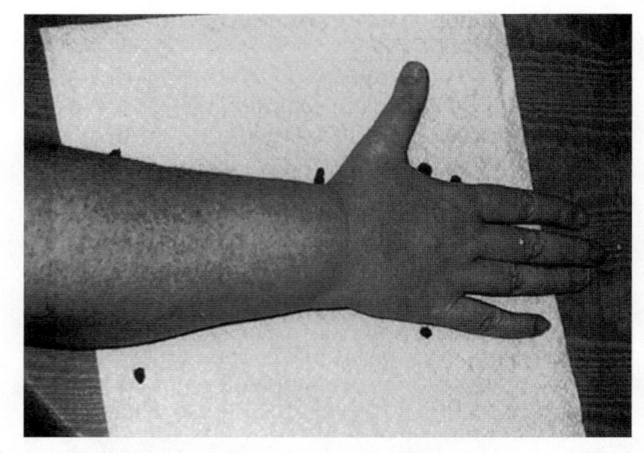

Figure 20-17 Marking bony landmarks for radial bar cock-up splint on paper towel.

3. Smooth the wrist area of the material by stroking it into place laterally and continue proximally up the forearm, taking care not to twist the trough to either side (Figure 20-19).
4. Place the thumb gently in the palmar arch area to ensure contour and stroke into place. Flare or fold the distal edge so that the palmar crease (proximal crease at the second MP, distal crease for third to fifth MP) is visible and continues through the web space. Have the patient oppose the thumb to the tip of the index or middle finger. This position will cause a fold at the thenar eminence. Flatten this fold down and continue along the radial bar into the web space area as seen in Figure 20-20.

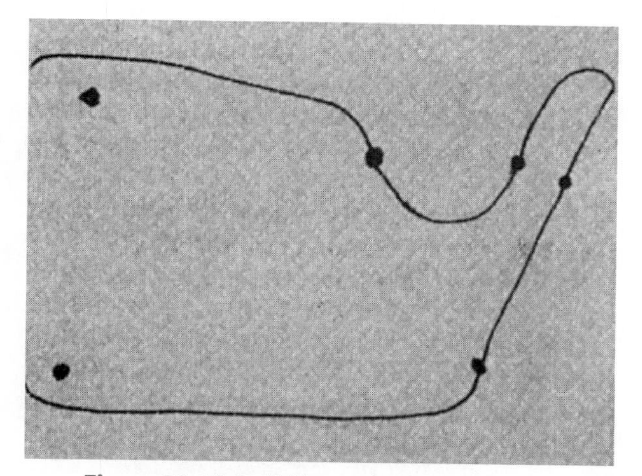

Figure 20-18 Radial bar cock-up splint pattern.

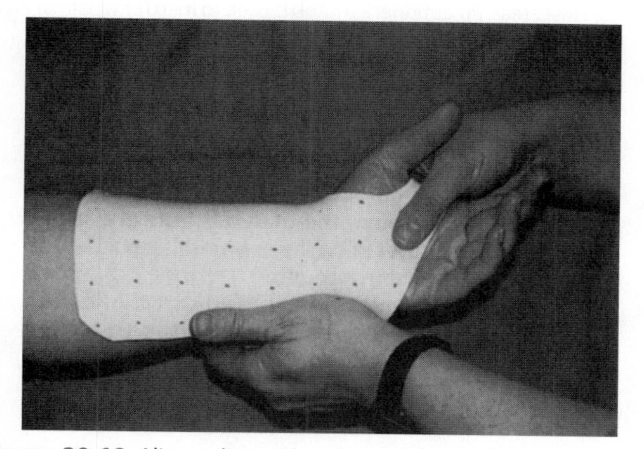

Figure 20-19 Align splint with palmar arch and begin to mold in contours.

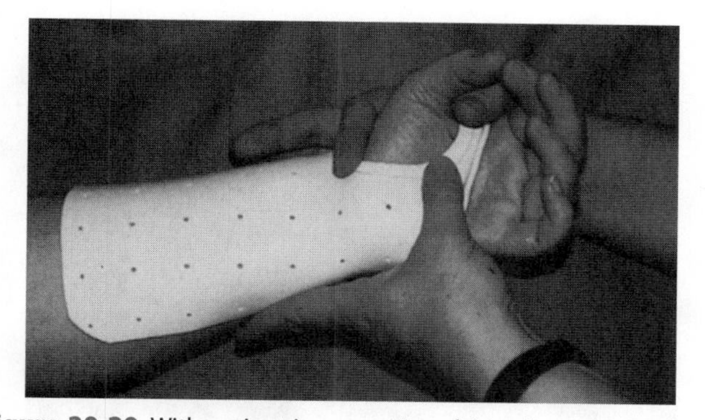

Figure 20-20 With patient in opposition, fold splint at palmar and thenar creases.

5. Allow the splint to set.
6. Apply straps (Figure 20-21) to the splint proximally, across the wrist and across the dorsum of the hand to the radial bar tab.

CASE STUDY

Mr R.; Part 2

A radial bar wrist cock-up splint will be fabricated for Mr. R. early in his treatment. It will support his wrist, and it is easier to wear "all day," as when putting your hand in a shirt of coat sleeve. It is both cosmetically and socially more acceptable to Mr. R. as he goes through his day. At work, he is also using a dynamic outrigger that has been fabricated on a similar base splint. The dynamic portion of the splint is used for finger extension, so he is better able to use his keyboard at work. The patient has stated that he "would not be seen wearing this thing in public." Nonetheless, he is willing to use it for keyboarding so that he can function better at work. He is managing his other ADL using his nondominant hand. As the nerve regenerates over several months, he will no longer need the dynamic splint but will continue to use the radial bar cock-up as he waits for his wrist extensor muscles to regain innervation and strength sufficient to support the weight of his hand.

Resting Hand Splint

Resting hand splints are used for positioning the wrist and fingers. Common goals for using resting splints are to decrease joint inflammation or prevent joint contractures. Use a material with moderate drape and rigid performance. Ezeform splinting material is a popular choice for this type of splint.

Pattern

1. Trace the hand, leaving approximately ½-inch excess width around the hand area and 1½ inches in the forearm area. Mark two thirds the length of the forearm. Your pattern should resemble a mitten (Figure 20-22).
2. Cut it out of the paper towel and check the fit on the patient before transferring the pattern to the thermoplastic. Once the splint blank is cut out of the thermoplastic, reheat to molding temperature if necessary.

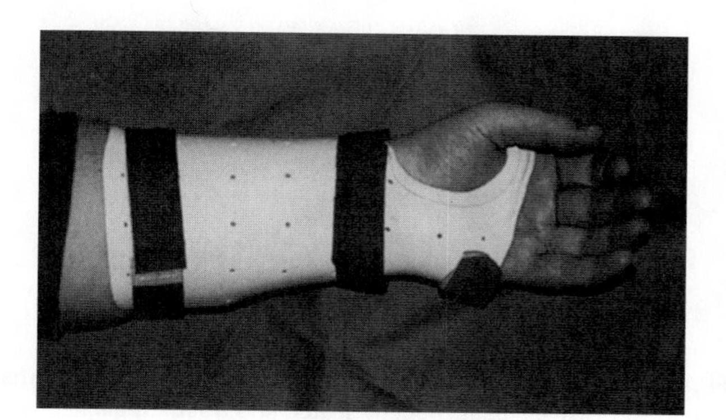

Figure 20-21 Completed radial bar cock-up splint.

Fabrication

1. Place the warm splinting material on the patient as seen in Figure 20-23, preferably with the patient's forearm in a supinated position so that gravity assists in holding the material in place. Make sure the thumb/web space area is seated properly, and flare the thermoplastic to create the flange on the splint in the thumb/web area.
2. Stroke the material into position at the wrist. This technique creates a waist in the material and helps keep it from sliding. Continue molding up the forearm.
3. Using two hands, one to ensure correct anatomic position of the wrist/hand and the other to mold, gently form the material. Create a flange along the sides of the fingers to increase material strength in the hand area as seen in Figure 20-24. Use alternate hands: one to position, the other to mold. Use your thumb to ensure proper forming in the palmar arch area.
4. Once the material is semirigid, pronate the forearm (Figure 20-25) and proceed as previously described to trim and finish.
5. Apply straps proximally, at the wrist, across the dorsum of the hand or proximal phalanges, and at the thumb (Figure 20-26).

Short Opponens Splint

A short opponens splint is used to support the CMC (knuckle) joint of the thumb when it is inflamed from overuse or arthritic changes. A forearm-based version of this splint is used for de Quervain syndrome, a commonly seen tendonitis of the long extensor and abductor tendons of the thumb, which cross the wrist. Use a moderately drapey material with a high degree of contour. In some cases, because of an enlarged IP joint or a bulbous distal phalanx, opening the thumb spica area may be necessary to allow donning and removal of the splint. For such patients, a resilient, memory splinting material would be a good choice. Such materials are slightly flexible and hold up well under the repeated stress of being pulled open.

Pattern

1. Mark the following landmarks on the paper toweling: the MP heads on the radial and ulnar sides of the hand, the radial and ulnar sides of the wrist, and the IP crease of the thumb (Figure 20-27).

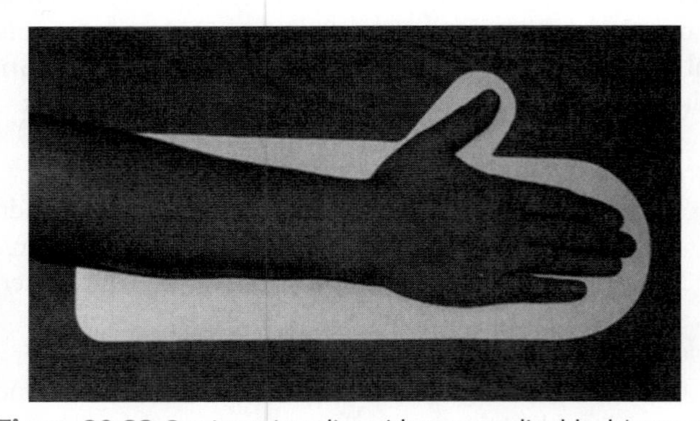

Figure 20-22 Resting mitt splint with precut splint blank/pattern.

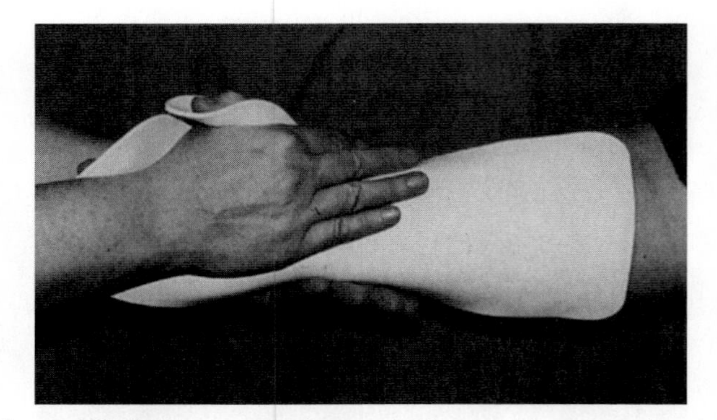

Figure 20-23 Place warm thermoplastic on patient, ensuring that thumb/web space area is properly seated and trough is aligned with forearm.

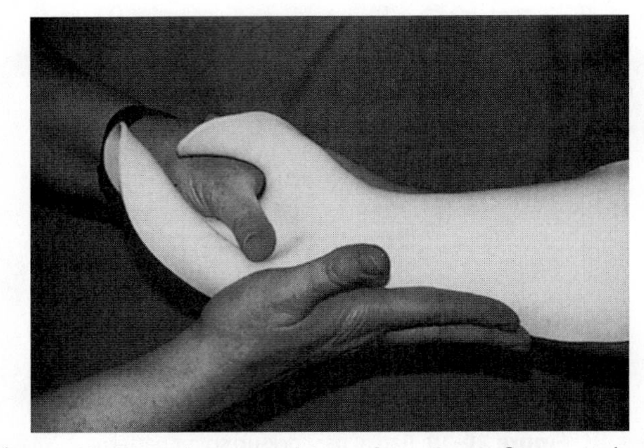

Figure 20-24 Stroke material into place. Create flanges in hand/thumb/wrist areas. Practitioner's thumb is used to help form palmar arch.

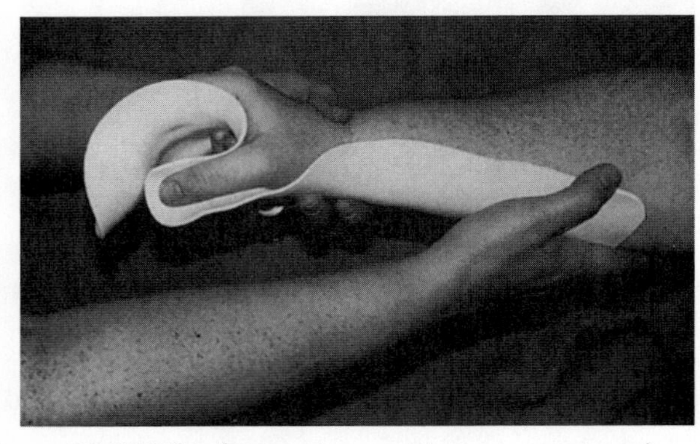

Figure 20-25 With forearm in pronation, grasp proximal end of splint and twist it to center the trough.

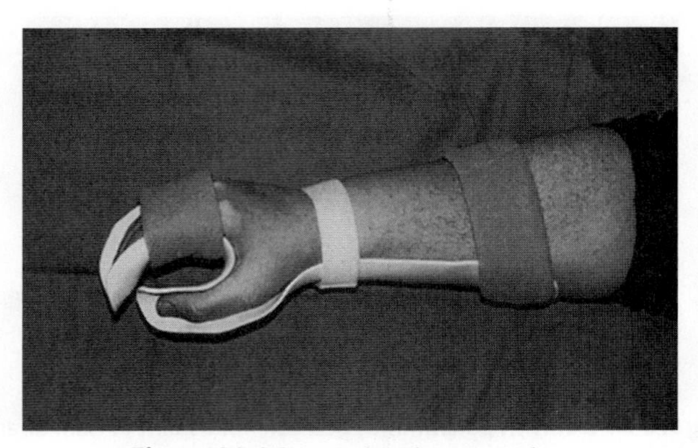

Figure 20-26 Completed resting splint.

2. Draw the pattern as shown in Figure 20-28 and cut out the pattern. Check the fit on the patient. The bulbous end of the pattern wraps circumferentially around the thumb. Trace the pattern onto the splinting material and proceed as described earlier.

Fabrication

1. Reheat the splint to molding temperature. Position the patient's elbow on the table with the forearm straight up. Align the edge of the splinting material with the IP crease and wrap the splinting material snugly around the thumb, as seen in Figure 20-29.
2. Wrap the narrow end of the splint around the ulnar border of the hand (Figure 20-30). Keep this part centered. Ask the patient to oppose the thumb to the second digit while you smooth the material into place. Make sure the splint contours well into the web space.

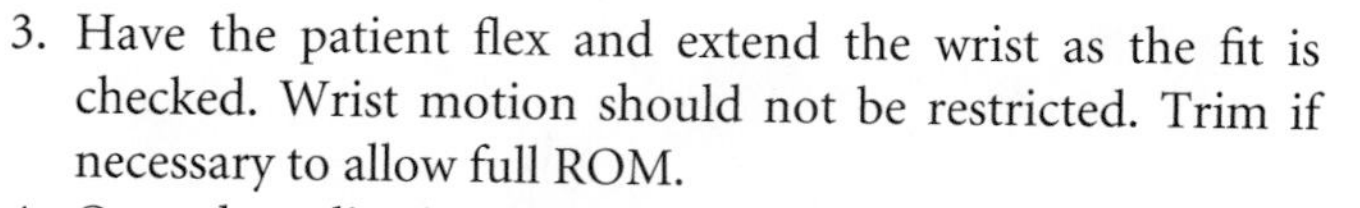

3. Have the patient flex and extend the wrist as the fit is checked. Wrist motion should not be restricted. Trim if necessary to allow full ROM.
4. Once the splint is set, trim if necessary around the thenar crease.
5. Apply a strap to secure the ulnar border to the thenar area (Figure 20-31).

CLINICAL PEARL 20-15

To ensure that the splint contours well into the web space, give the patient a quarter to pinch. This technique prevents the thumb from moving out of alignment while the splint hardens.

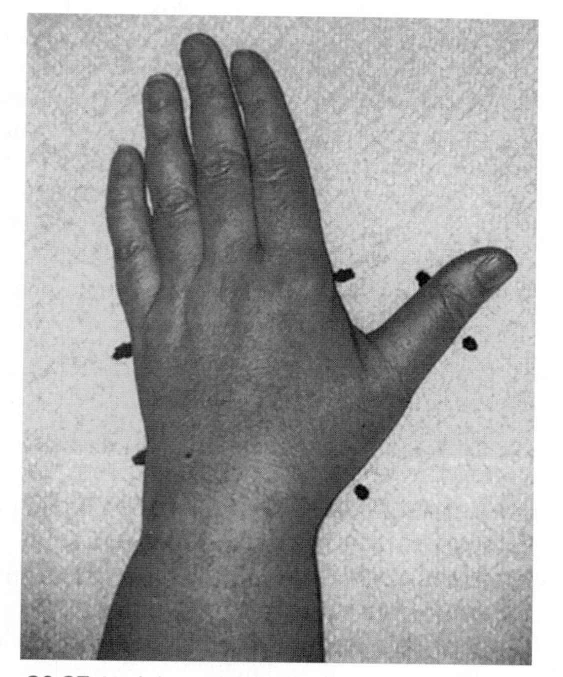

Figure 20-27 Mark bony landmarks for short opponens splint on paper towel.

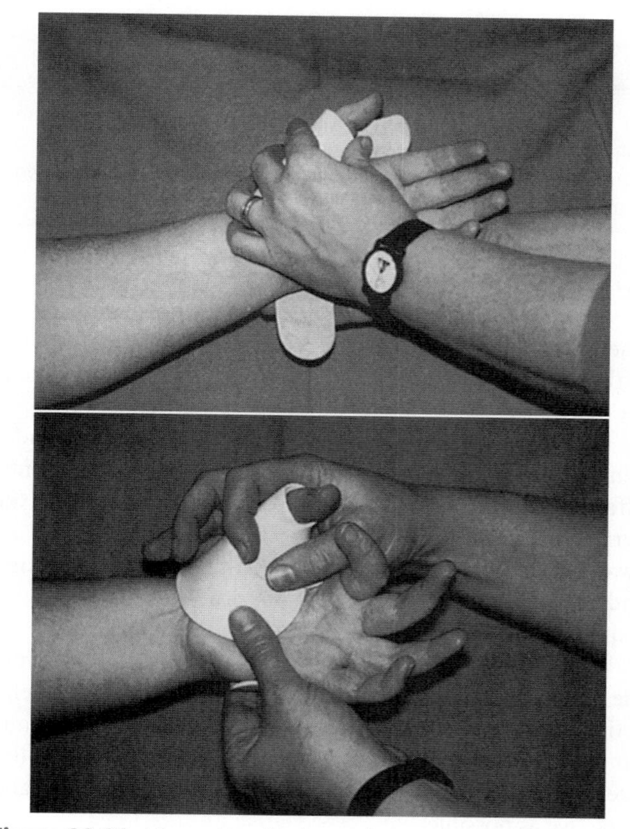

Figure 20-29 Align edge of splint with interphalangeal crease and wrap snugly around thumb.

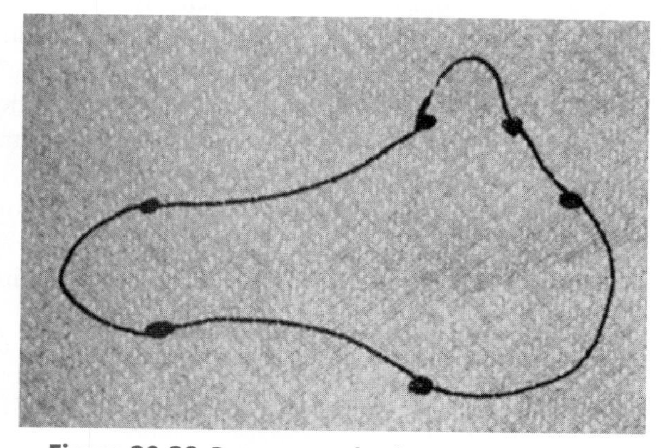

Figure 20-28 Draw pattern for short opponens splint.

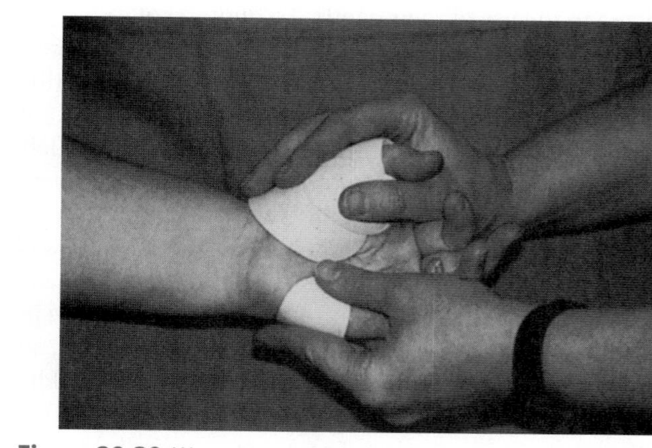

Figure 20-30 Wrap narrow end of splint dorsally around hand, over ulnar border.

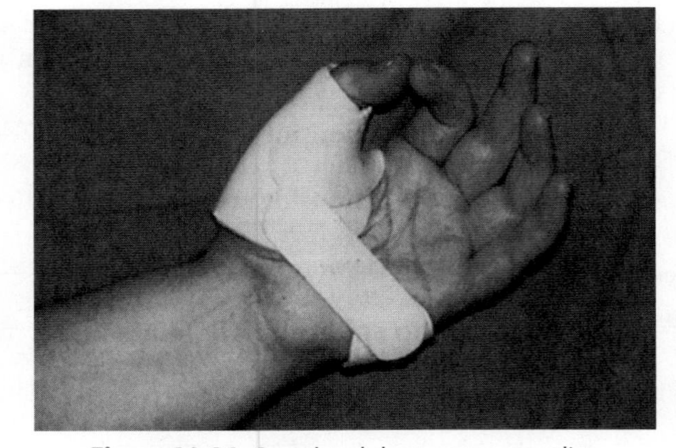

Figure 20-31 Completed short opponens splint.

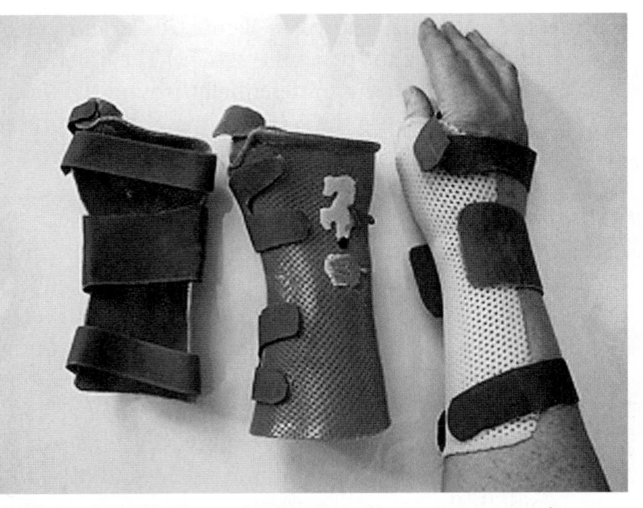

Figure 20-32 The author's cache of long opponens splints.

CLINICAL PEARL 20-16

If the patient has difficulty inserting and removing the thumb through the splint, pop the overlapped area open by twisting it once the material is completely cool. Secure with hook-and-loop strapping material.

Summary

The purpose of splinting is to preserve or enhance the use of the hand. Thus the construction of every splint must respect the hand's natural arches, contours, and mechanics.

The OTA who has achieved service competency may independently construct resting splints and other static splints. Effective splint construction requires an understanding of the performance and handling characteristics of the materials, an awareness of precautions, and expertise in pattern making and use of materials. The actual physical skill of splinting is acquired with patience and practice.

When possible, the splint should be designed to best ensure the client's maximal participation in his or her purposeful activities and occupations. The clinician should address any functional issues that wearing the splint will create. The splint affects the appearance of the hand and should be as neat and attractive as possible.

The author of this chapter is keenly aware of how difficult it may be for patients with repetitive stress injuries to be restricted in the use of their hands. To quote a colleague, "It is a temporary inconvenience for a long-term gain." Please refer to Figure 20-32 to view the variety of splints that this chapter author wore during a course of de Quervain disease (extensor tendonitis of the thumb). The splint on the left is a typical long opponens splint—a forearm-based version of the short thumb opponens splint described in this chapter. Given the strength of the writer's hands, she was unintentionally aggravating the repetitive stress of her tendons by fighting against the splint during her work hours in a hand therapy office. She kept popping the straps open, so a colleague made her a circumferential splint (the middle splint), which was more restrictive and decreased her "fighting" the limitation in motion. The decoration on the splints was done to decrease her patients' concerns about having a therapist with a problem hand, as well as to add some humor to the situation. The splint on the right was a gutter-style long opponens splint, which she wore while at leisure and when she needed to write legible chart notes! This personal experience of needing splints and having them adjusted to accommodate occupational and personal concerns was highly illuminating. The outcome of the splinting process and the additional clinical interventions was completely satisfactory, demonstrating to me that indeed splinting is an effective tool in occupational therapy practice when used appropriately.

Selected Reading Guide Questions

1. What is the role of the OTA in hand splinting?
2. List five functions of the normal hand.
3. Describe the relationship of shoulder, elbow, and wrist function to hand use.
4. Which type of prehension is used to pick up a straight pin?
5. Which type of prehension is used to turn a key in a lock?
6. Which type of grasp is used to hold a soda can?
7. What happens to the hand if the metacarpal transverse arch is flattened?
8. In which position are the muscles of the hand at the best mechanical advantage to function efficiently?
9. Describe and demonstrate the dual obliquity of the hand. Why is it an important consideration in hand splinting?
10. Name the three nerves that supply sensation and motion to the hand. Which one is most critical to tactile discriminative function?
11. Name the three major classifications of splints. Give one example of each.
12. How are the adverse effects of immobilization by splinting best prevented?
13. What is the optimal position for splinting the wrist for function?
14. What is the optimal position for splinting the wrist for carpal tunnel syndrome?

15. What effect does wrist flexion have on hand function?
16. Why is it important to splint the MP joints in some flexion if these joints are to be splinted?
17. State six purposes of splinting.
18. List and discuss three limitations of splints.
19. What are the two main characteristics that influence selection of thermoplastic material? Give several examples of each.
20. List six general guidelines for achieving optimal fit and function of the splint.

References

1. Amini D: Splinting the geriatric hand, *OT Pract* 9(3):CE1, 2004.
2. Fess EE, Gettle KS, Strickland JW: *Hand splinting: principles and methods*, St. Louis, 1987, Mosby.
3. Fess EE, Gettle KS, Philips CA, et al: *Hand and upper extremity splinting: principles and methods*, ed 3, St. Louis, 2005, Mosby.
4. Gillen G: *Stroke rehabilitation, a function-based approach*, ed 3, St. Louis, 2011, Elsevier Mosby.
5. Gillen G, Goldberg R, Muller S, Straus J: The effect of wrist position on upper extremity function while wearing a wrist immobilizing splint, *J Prosthet Orthot* 20(1):19–23, 2008.
6. Jacobs ML, Austin N: *Splinting the hand and upper extremity: principles and process*, Baltimore, 2003, Lippincott Williams & Wilkins.
7. Kiel JH: *Basic hand splinting: a pattern designing approach*, Boston, 1983, Little, Brown.
8. Malick M: *Manual on dynamic hand splinting with thermoplastic materials*, Pittsburgh, 1982, Harmarville Rehabilitation Center.
9. Malick M: *Manual on static hand splinting*, Pittsburgh, 1972, Harmarville Rehabilitation Center.
10. *Principles of hand splinting*, Downey, CA, 1962, Occupational Therapy Department, Ranchos Los Amigos Hospital, (unpublished).
11. Sammons Preston: *Hand rehabilitation catalog*, Bolingbrook, IL, 2010, Patterson Medical.
12. *Static splinting workshop*, Germantown, WI, 1995, Smith and Nephew Rolyan, (unpublished).
13. Tubiana R: Architecture and functions of the hand. In Tubiana R, Thomine J, Mackin E, editors: *Examination of the hand and upper limb*, Philadelphia, 1984, WB Saunders.

Recommended Reading

Brand P: The forces of dynamic splinting: ten questions before applying a dynamic splint to the hand. In Hunter JM, Mackin EJ, Callahan AD, editors: *Rehabilitation of the hand*, ed 4, St. Louis, 1995, Mosby.

Coppard BM, Lohman HL: *Introduction to splinting: a clinical-reasoning and problem-solving approach*, ed 2, St. Louis, 2001, Mosby.

Hardy MA: Preserving function in the inflamed and acutely injured hand. In Moran CA, editor: *Hand rehabilitation*, New York, 1986, Churchill Livingstone.

Jacobs M, Austin N: *Splinting the hand and upper extremity: principles and process*, Philadelphia, 2003, Lippincott Williams & Wilkins.

McKee P, Morgan L: *Orthotics in rehabilitation*, Philadelphia, 1998, FA Davis.

Melvin JL: *Rheumatic disease: occupational therapy and rehabilitation*, Philadelphia, 1977, FA Davis.

VanLede P, Veldhoven G: *Therapeutic hand splints: a rational approach*, Volume 1, Antwerp, Belgium, 1998, Provan.

CHAPTER 21 Neurotherapeutic Approaches to Treatment

PATRICIA ANN GENTILE AND ELZA GUZMAN

Key Terms

Muscle tone
Spasticity
Flaccidity
Proprioceptive stimulation
Cutaneous stimulation
Cerebrovascular accident (CVA)
Neurodevelopmental treatment approach (NDT/Bobath)
Proprioceptive neuromuscular facilitation (PNF)
Rood approach
Movement therapy
Brunnstrom approach
Limb synergies
Manual contact
Stretch
Traction
Approximation
Repeated contraction
Rhythmic initiation
Relaxation techniques
Facilitation techniques
Inhibition techniques

Chapter Objectives

After studying this chapter, the student or practitioner will be able to do the following:

1. Describe in general terms what is meant by a neurotherapeutic treatment approach.
2. Name the four traditional neurotherapeutic treatment approaches.
3. Describe the basic goals and focus of each of the four neurotherapeutic treatment approaches.
4. Discuss common sensorimotor deficits seen in patients with neurologic dysfunction, and provide examples of how these problems can interfere with function.
5. Provide an example of how each of the neurotherapeutic treatment approaches can be incorporated into activities of daily living training.

Occupational therapy (OT) practitioners often work with adults who have sustained damage to the central nervous system (CNS). For these patients the outcome of treatment is directed toward promoting and maximizing functional movement to allow engagement in their desired occupations. Neurotherapeutic treatment approaches are adjunctive techniques directed toward motor performance skills that can assist in achieving this outcome. This chapter provides the occupational therapy assistant (OTA) with an introduction to and practical information about the neurotherapeutic approaches used in OT treatment.

Neurotherapeutic treatment approaches are used with patients who have CNS dysfunction. The CNS consists of the brain and spinal cord. When damage to these structures occurs, an individual's motor performance skills are affected and difficulties in movement will occur. The patient's ability to produce controlled, coordinated movement is often lost because of abnormal changes in muscle tone, balance, posture, and reflexive movement. Muscle tone, which refers to the natural tension within a muscle, can become either too high (spasticity) or too low (flaccidity).

Changes in muscle tone can affect the ability to move. In normal movement, muscle tone adjusts to the demands of the task on hand. When CNS damage occurs, the ability of muscle tone to accommodate to the demands of a task is often lost and muscle tone may stay at a constant state of spasticity or flaccidity. When this happens, functional movement is impaired. Patients with spasticity may decrease their movement or be unable to initiate movement. Joint contractures may result from lack of movement. On the other hand, if muscle tone is too low (flaccid), a patient may have difficulty maintaining an upright position or lifting an arm or leg against gravity.

Balance and posture are typically affected in patients with CNS dysfunction. A patient's posture may appear asymmetrical or uneven because of low tone of the trunk muscles, giving the person the appearance of leaning toward one side. Balance, which depends on the ability to shift weight and react to changes in positioning, may also be affected. Because of the inability to maintain balance while sitting or standing, patients may experience difficulty performing self-care activities. Poor balance may also put patients at risk for falling.

The reappearance of reflexes after CNS dysfunction is common. Reflexes are stereotypical, automatic movements present in all individuals. During normal motor development, reflexes become integrated, allowing an individual to perform controlled movements. When damage to the CNS occurs, reflexes may lose their integration and become more powerful, limiting the available types of movement. For example, placing an object in the palm of the hand may result in automatic closing of the fingers and the inability to open the hand. This reflex action can affect task-oriented movement.

Finally, CNS damage can adversely affect a patient's sensation. Some patients may report "not feeling" the affected limbs or may describe the arm or leg as feeling heavy and clumsy. Others may not be able to distinguish where the arm is in relationship to objects or other body parts, resulting in decreased coordination.

Neurotherapeutic treatment approaches are geared toward reducing the abnormal changes just described. These approaches are based on the idea that abnormal motor responses can be reduced and that the CNS can relearn more normal motor responses. This outcome is the ultimate goal of all the neurotherapeutic approaches. Neurotherapeutic treatment approaches use sensory stimuli to influence motor responses. Proprioceptive and cutaneous stimuli are commonly used.

Proprioceptive stimulation affects joint and muscle receptors and employs techniques such as stretching, weight bearing, and resistance.[9] **Cutaneous stimulation** acts on the exteroceptors of the skin.[1,4,37] *Exteroceptors,* located immediately under the skin, respond to stimuli such as touch, temperature, and pain.[30,41] Cutaneous stimuli can be used to facilitate or inhibit muscle responses. Combined with proprioceptive stimulation, cutaneous stimulation may be used to elicit voluntary control of specific muscles.

Reflex mechanisms may also be used in some treatment approaches. As described earlier, reflexes are automatic, stereotypical motor responses. In some approaches, reflexes may be used early in treatment to elicit movement. For instance, when a patient with poor balance is encouraged to lean toward the weak side, the person may demonstrate a reflexive extension of the affected arm to prevent falling. This situation is an example of a specific reflexive response known as a *protective reaction.*

Neurotherapeutic treatment approaches are used with individuals who have sustained injury to the CNS. This injury could be the result of a disease process, a structural or genetic defect, or a traumatic event. Such CNS injuries include **cerebrovascular accident (CVA)**, traumatic brain injury, and cerebral palsy. Neurotherapeutic treatment approaches work to normalize muscle tone, to facilitate symmetrical posture, and to improve balance. Achievement of these objectives can help to restore coordinated and purposeful movements and a return to independence.

When treating patients with CNS dysfunction, the occupational therapist begins by selecting a specific neurotherapeutic approach. Selection depends on several factors including the patient's strengths and weaknesses, the therapist's preference, and the philosophy of a particular treatment setting. Using the evaluation procedures for the approach selected, the occupational therapist performs a comprehensive evaluation that establishes a baseline for the patient. This baseline is the starting point for treatment. In general, any neurotherapeutic evaluation procedure that the occupational therapist uses should examine motor performance skills within the context of a functional activity. For example, when observing a patient reach for a shirt hanging in a closet, the occupational therapist would assess the patient's ability to maintain balance and ability to maintain upright trunk posture while coordinating forward reach to retrieve the shirt.

When working together with the OTA, the occupational therapist directs and oversees the OTA in aspects of the selected approach in treatment. Both occupational therapist and OTA must recognize that many neurotherapeutic techniques can affect the patient adversely; therefore all clinicians using these techniques must demonstrate sufficient knowledge and skills for safe application. Before initiating a neurotherapeutic treatment technique with a patient, the OTA must have demonstrated the sufficient clinical competence to safely use the technique.

To implement treatment plans effectively for persons with neurologic dysfunctions, the OTA should be familiar with the various neurotherapeutic approaches, their basic principles, and the specific techniques used in each. The OTA who treats patients with CNS damage and intends to use any of these techniques can do so only with specific directions from the occupational therapist. The OTA always must be thoroughly trained and properly supervised when he or she is using these techniques. Instruction about the nature of the technique, the specific procedure for application, the expected response, and possible risks and contraindications must be provided to the OTA by the occupational therapist.

This chapter discusses the four neurotherapeutic treatment approaches most commonly used in practice: the Rood approach, the Brunnstrom (movement therapy) approach, the **proprioceptive neuromuscular facilitation approach (PNF)**, and the **neurodevelopmental treatment approach (NDT/Bobath)**.

Rood Approach

Margaret S. Rood was both an occupational therapist and a physical therapist. She began to develop her theory in the 1940s, drawing from the developmental and neurophysiological literature of the previous decade.[41] Rood integrated this literature with her own clinical observations to create an approach based on the use of sensory stimulation to effect motor responses.

Rood did not write extensively, seeming to prefer clinical teaching to disseminate her ideas. Most of the literature that describes the Rood approach is based on interpretations by accomplished physical and occupational therapists such as Ayres,[2,3] Farber,[14,15] Heininger and Randolph,[18] Huss,[20] and Stockmeyer.[36] Despite some controversy about the efficacy of Rood's techniques, current neuroscience research continues to support the importance of sensory stimulation.

The basic assumption of Rood's theory is that appropriate sensory stimulation can elicit specific motor responses. Rood combined controlled sensory stimulation with a sequence of positions and activities that replicate normal ontogenic motor development (i.e., the normal progression of motor skills) to achieve purposeful muscular responses.[20]

Basic Assumptions

The basic assumptions of Rood's theory are the following:

1. Normal muscle tone is a prerequisite to movement.

Patients with CNS dysfunction may exhibit changes in muscle tone, ranging from *hypertonicity* (too much tone) to *hypotonicity* (too little tone). This abnormal tone interferes with movement, and the achievement of normalized muscle tone is essential for controlled movement.

Normal muscle tone flows smoothly and is constantly changing, depending on the demands of a motor act. For example, to turn on the ignition of a car, a person must have good eye-hand coordination, postural control of the trunk muscles, co-innervation of the proximal arm muscles, forearm pronation and supination, and moderately fine prehension and dexterity in the hands.

In addition, the demands placed on the various muscle groups are different. Rood recognized this when she stated, "Muscles have different duties."[32] Some muscles are used predominantly for heavy work and others for light work. *Light-work muscles* are called *mobilizers* and are primarily the flexors and adductors. The primary function of the light-work muscles is directed toward skilled movement patterns. *Heavy-work muscles,* however, act as *stabilizers* and consist of the extensors and abductors.[16] The primary function of heavy-work muscles is to allow maintenance of posture and holding patterns of movement. Heavy-work and light-work muscles act together to allow coordinated movements to occur. For example, when a person is putting on a necklace, the heavy-work muscles are responsible for co-contraction proximally at the trunk, shoulder, and forearm, thereby maintaining the arm up against gravity. The light-work muscles, located more distally, are responsible for the coordination and dexterity needed to manipulate the clasp.

Rood[32] also believed that reflexes are the foundation of any voluntary motor act. These reflexes are modified, controlled, and integrated by the CNS. She began therapy by eliciting motor responses on a reflex level and using developmental patterns to improve the motor response.

2. Treatment begins at the developmental level of functioning.

Rood believed that movement occurs in a developmental sequence. Patients are evaluated developmentally, and treatment follows a developmental sequence. Because one skill builds on the other, patients do not proceed to the next level of sensorimotor development until some degree of voluntary control is achieved. This principle follows the *cephalocaudal rule.* Treatment begins from the head and proceeds downward segment by segment, from proximal to distal, to the sacral area. When adhering to this rule in treatment (e.g., when working with a patient on feeding), the clinician would first direct treatment on controlled reaching for the utensil before focusing on holding the utensil.[1]

3. Motivation enhances purposeful movement.

Rood realized that motivation plays an important role in rehabilitation. Activities that are meaningful for the patient encourage practice of desired movements. This results in greater patient participation in treatment.

4. Repetition is necessary for the reeducation of muscular responses.[4]

Repetition helps develop coordination.[22,23] Repetition assists the brain in developing an internal "memory" of a specific motor activity. Repetition, however, can be monotonous. To avoid boredom, the occupational therapist should provide various activities that incorporate similar motor patterns.

Principles of Treatment

Rood suggested the following four general principles in the treatment of neuromuscular dysfunction[33]:

1. Reflexes can be used to assist or retard the effects of sensory stimulation.

According to Rood, reflexes can be used to influence muscle tone. Two commonly mentioned mechanisms are the *tonic neck reflexes* (TNRs) and *tonic labyrinthine reflexes* (TLRs). The TNRs are triggered by changes in the relationship of the head to the neck; TLRs occur with changes in the relationship of the head to gravity. Consequently, any changes in the position of the head to the neck, or in relationship of the head to gravity, can result in increases or decreases in muscle tone. Clinicians must therefore be aware of the position of the head and neck and the potential effects of gravity on the body. For example, in wheelchair seating, symmetrical alignment of the head and neck will promote normal muscle tone in the arms and legs.

2. Sensory stimulation of receptors can produce predictable responses.

Responses to sensory stimulation to specific receptors are predictable. Clinicians using sensory stimulation can use this predictability to achieve a desired outcome. For example, a slow rocking stimulus produces a calming effect and may be beneficial for patients with high tone or agitation.

3. Muscles have different duties.

As discussed earlier, some muscles predominate as stabilizers (heavy-work muscles), whereas others undertake the duties of mobilization (light-work muscles). According to Rood, each group has distinct functions and characteristics.

4. Heavy-work muscles should be integrated before light-work muscles.

The principle of integrating heavy-work muscles before light-work muscles refers primarily to the use of the upper extremities (UEs). For example, fine fingertip manipulation (which involves light-work muscles) is not functional if the proximal muscles (heavy-work muscles) are not strong enough to lift or stabilize the position of the arms.

Sequence of Motor Development

Rood proposed the following four sequential phases related to the development of motor control[3,33,34]:

1. *Reciprocal inhibition (innervation).* Reciprocal inhibition is an early mobility phase that serves a protective function. The muscle acting on one side of a joint *(agonist)* quickly contracts while its opposite *(antagonist)* relaxes. An example of reciprocal innervation is seen in infants who randomly flex and extend their arms and legs.
2. *Co-contraction.* Co-contraction occurs when opposing muscles (usually those surrounding a joint) contract simultaneously, resulting in stabilization of the joint. The co-contraction phase allows an individual to hold a position or an object for a longer time. Standing upright is a result of co-contraction of the trunk muscles, as well as muscles acting on the hips, knees, and ankles.
3. *Heavy work.* The heavy-work phase has been defined as "mobility on stability."[35] In this phase the proximal muscles move, and the distal segments are fixed. An example of this phase is creeping. During creeping the infant is in a quadruped (all-fours) position. The hands and feet are in a fixed position, but the shoulders and hips move.
4. *Skill.* Skill is the highest level of control and combines the efforts of mobility and stability. In a skilled movement pattern the proximal segment is stabilized while the distal segment moves freely. Reaching overhead to unscrew a light bulb is an example of this pattern.

Ontogenic Movement Patterns

The sequence of motor development described previously occurs as the patient is put through a specific sequence that Rood called *ontogenic motor patterns.*[16] Figure 21-1 illustrates the eight ontogenic motor patterns.

Supine Withdrawal (Supine Flexion)

Supine withdrawal is a total flexion response toward the navel. This position is protective. Supine withdrawal is a mobility posture that requires reciprocal innervation; it also requires heavy work of the proximal muscles and trunk.[33] Rood recommended this pattern for patients who do not have the reciprocal flexion pattern and for those dominated by extensor tone (Figure 21-1, *A*).

Roll Over (Toward Side-Lying)

When the patient rolls over, the arm and leg flex on the same side of the body (Figure 21-1, *B*). Rolling over is a mobility pattern for the UEs and lower extremities (LEs) and activates the lateral trunk musculature.[36] This pattern is encouraged for patients who are dominated by reflexes or who need segmental movements of the extremities.

Pivot Prone (Prone Extension)

The pivot-prone position demands a full range of extension of the neck, shoulders, trunk, and LEs (Figure 21-1, *C*). This pattern has been called both a mobility pattern and a stability pattern. The position is difficult to assume and hold. It plays an important role in preparation for stability in the upright position.

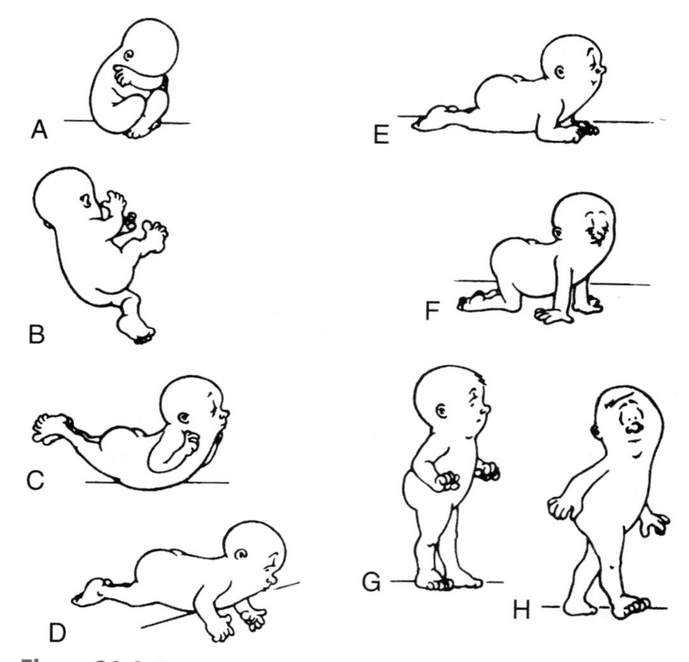

Figure 21-1 Ontogenic motor patterns. **A,** Supine withdrawal. **B,** Roll over toward side-lying. **C,** Pivot prone. **D,** Neck contraction. **E,** Prone on elbows. **F,** Quadruped pattern. **G,** Static standing. **H,** Walking.

Neck Co-Contraction (Co-Innervation)

Neck co-contraction is the first real stability pattern. It is used to develop head control and stability of the neck (Figure 21-1, *D*). This pattern is necessary to raise the head against gravity.

On Elbows (Prone on Elbow)

Following co-contraction of the neck and prone extension, weight bearing on the elbows is the next pattern to achieve. This pattern helps develop stability in the scapular and glenohumeral (shoulder) regions. This position gives the person a better view of the environment and an opportunity to shift weight from side to side (Figure 21-1, *E*).

All Fours (Quadruped Position)

The quadruped position develops stability of the lower trunk and legs. Initially the patient holds the position. Eventually, weight shifting forward, backward, side to side, and diagonally is added. The weight shifting may be preparatory for balance responses (Figure 21-1, *F*).

Static Standing

Static standing is thought to be a skill of the upper trunk because it frees the UEs for prehension and manipulation.[36] At first, weight is equally distributed on both legs; then weight shifting begins. This position requires higher-level integration such as maintaining and achieving balance (Figure 21-1, *G*).

Walking

Walking unites skill, mobility, and stability. Walking is a complicated process that requires coordinated movement patterns of the various parts of the body (Figure 21-1, *H*).

Specific Techniques Used in Treatment

Rood described in detail the use of cutaneous and proprioceptive stimulation in treatment. Stimuli typically used in clinical practice are briefly described next. Before using any of these techniques with patients, the OTA must be properly trained and demonstrate clinical competency. During these techniques, the occupational therapist is responsible for providing proper supervision to the OTA. Emphasis during supervision should be on safe application, precautions, and awareness of the expected outcome of the technique.

When applying any of the cutaneous or proprioceptive techniques, the OTA should always remember that these techniques are adjunctive treatment techniques and are preparatory to functional activity. Whenever possible, the application should be followed immediately by the patient's involvement in an activity performed in a functional context. For example, applying deep pressure to the tendon of the biceps may help relax the elbow so that the patient can place his or her arm in the sleeve of a shirt with less difficulty.

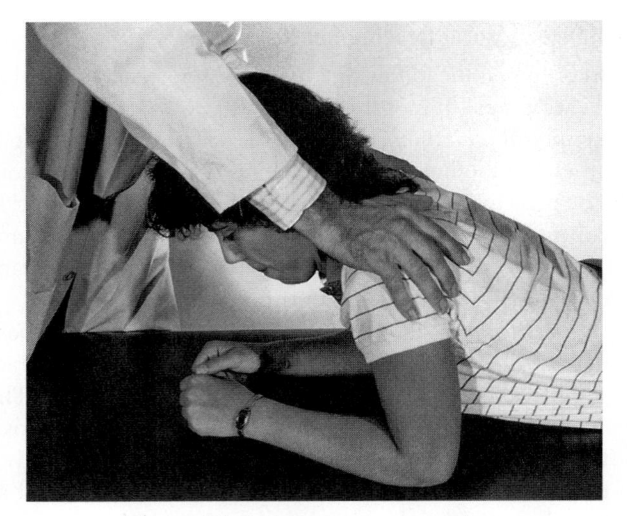

Figure 21-2 Heavy joint compression.

Cutaneous Stimulation

Cutaneous stimulation is applied to the skin. Light-moving touch, fast brushing, and icing are examples of cutaneous stimulation. *Light-moving touch,* or slow stroking of the skin, has been used to activate superficial muscles. The clinical result is a reflexive withdrawal response. *Fast brushing,* applied through a battery-operated brush, can be performed over the muscle belly of these muscles to be facilitated.[16,36] The results of fast brushing are delayed and do not have a maximal effect until 30 minutes after application.

Icing, a thermal stimulus, has also been used for facilitation of muscle activity.[32] Icing is a powerful stimulus, and the results can be unpredictable. Icing can facilitate a flexor withdrawal response in superficial muscles.[36] Icing can also facilitate opening and closing of the mouth and induce swallowing.[20]

Strict precautions must be followed for icing or fast brushing; improper use can adversely affect the patient. All clinicians using these techniques must be familiar with and strictly adhere to these precautions.

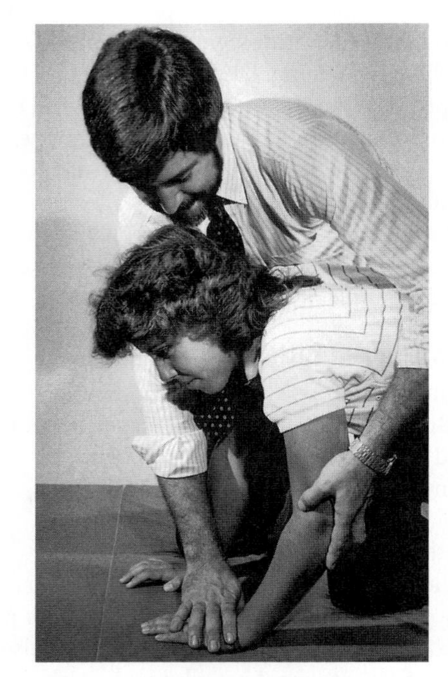

Figure 21-3 Joint compression in quadruped position.

Proprioceptive Stimulation

Proprioceptive stimulation refers to the facilitation of joint and muscle receptors and the vestibular system.[24,27,35] In general, proprioceptive stimulation gives the clinician more control over the motor response. The motor response lasts as long as the stimulus is applied.[13,35] Several proprioceptive stimulation techniques are used.

Heavy joint compression (Figure 21-2) facilitates contraction at the joint undergoing compression. This technique can be combined with developmental patterns such as prone on elbows, quadruped (Figure 21-3), sitting, and standing. Joint compression is clinically most effective when applied through the longitudinal axis of long bones such as the humerus (glenohumeral joint) and the femur (acetabulum).

Quick stretch is applied by holding the proximal bony prominences of the limb to be stretched while moving the distal joint in one direction. For example, the triceps is stretched by securing the elbow while the forearm is pushed into flexion. The response is immediate and short-lived.

The *tapping* technique involves tapping over the belly of a muscle with the fingertips. The occupational therapist or OTA percusses (taps) three to five times over the muscle to be facilitated. This technique may be done before or during the time a patient is voluntarily contracting the muscle. Tapping on spastic muscles, or muscles that are likely to develop spasticity, should be avoided. Prolonged or excessive tapping can also result in spasticity and should be avoided.

Vestibular stimulation is another type of proprioceptive input.[8] Extreme caution should be taken with vestibular stimulation because it can have a profound effect on the body. Any clinician planning to use vestibular stimulation must be adequately trained and must monitor the patient closely during treatment. The OTA who has been instructed in vestibular stimulation by the occupational therapist must receive close supervision to ensure the patient's safety.

Vibration, applied with a hand-held vibrator, has been used to produce tonal changes in muscles.[15,18,20] Vibration over spastic muscles, or muscles prone to developing spasticity, should be avoided. The patient's age may be a factor in using vibration. For example, vibration should not be used with children younger than 3 years of age and must be used with caution in persons older than age 65. OTAs using vibration in treatment must be properly trained and supervised.

Neutral warmth, an inhibitory technique, has been successful for general relaxation and to reduce muscle tone. It may also be helpful for children with attention deficit disorders.[15]

To inhibit spastic or tight muscle groups in which the tendons are accessible, the practitioner can apply *manual pressure* to the tendinous insertion of a muscle or across long tendons.[3,18] Pressure provided by hard surfaces is more effective than that provided by soft surfaces.[11] In the hand a hard cone with the tapered end toward the thumb side to inhibit the flexors can be used.[15] This principle has been used in various orthotic devices to manage muscle imbalance and contracture resulting from spasticity.

To inhibit spastic muscles around a joint, the occupational therapist can use *light joint compression* (approximation) with patients who are hemiplegic to alleviate pain and to offset muscle imbalance temporarily around the shoulder joint.[15]

Rood also recommended positioning hypertonic extremities in the *elongated position* for various periods.[26,34] Maintaining stretch in this position has an inhibitory effect. This principle is the basis for inhibitory casting, which is often used with patients who demonstrate severe spasticity of the extremities.

Finally, Rood suggested the use of olfactory and gustatory stimuli to facilitate cranial nerves and to influence the autonomic nervous system.[34,40] Odors could be used to facilitate a response. Pleasant odors such as vanilla may have a calming effect. Unpleasant and noxious substances such as sulfa and ammonia could trigger protective responses including coughing and sneezing.[16] Rood did not provide specific guidelines for the stimulation of special senses.

Sensory stimulation in patients with neurologic dysfunction can have a powerful effect. OTAs must be properly trained and appropriately supervised when using any of the cutaneous or proprioceptive modalities described in this chapter. Patients to whom these modalities are applied must be closely monitored.

Occupational Therapy Application

The OT treatment process begins with the occupational therapist's evaluation. The evaluation identifies the patient's level of motor development. Treatment starts at this level and is directed toward progressing the individual along the developmental continuum. Initially, if severe neurologic damage is present, the patient may need to begin with reflexive movements. The occupational therapist then progresses the patient along the ontogenic development patterns. Sensory stimulation can reinforce these patterns and can be used to inhibit or facilitate specific muscle activity as needed. The sensory stimulation techniques described are used primarily to prepare the patient for purposeful activities.

In treatment the OTA should consider ontogenic patterns when he or she is positioning patients for activities. For example, the roll-over pattern can be reinforced by having the patient turn in bed to reach bed controls. Prone-on-elbows positioning can be adapted for tabletop use by having the patient sit at a table and lean on his or her elbow and forearm while playing a recreational game. Grooming activities such as shaving or makeup application can also be positioned so that the patient must lean on the affected elbow and forearm while reaching for objects. The standing position often provides the best position for activities of daily living (ADL) and purposeful activities. While standing, the patient can use his or her arms to explore and manipulate the environment. For example, while performing a homemaking activity, the individual can reach up to place objects in a cabinet. As the patient develops stability in standing, activities that require more weight shifting and balance reactions can be provided.

Movement Therapy: Brunnstrom Approach to Treatment of Hemiplegia

Signe Brunnstrom was a physical therapist from Sweden. Her practice, teaching, and theory development in the United States extended from the World War II years through the 1970s. Her clinical observations and research led to the development of the treatment approach she called **movement therapy**. Her book, *Movement Therapy in Hemiplegia,*[6] was published in 1970 and applied movement therapy, also known as the **Brunnstrom approach**, to the treatment of hemiplegia.

Theoretic Foundations

Brunnstrom evolved her treatment approach after study of the literature in neurophysiology, CNS mechanisms, effects of CNS damage, sensory systems and related topics, and clinical observations and application of training procedures.[6] Brunnstrom based her intervention on the concept that the damaged CNS has undergone an "evolution in reverse" and regressed to former patterns of movement. These patterns include the **limb synergies**, which are gross patterns of limb flexion and extension that originate in primitive spinal cord patterns and primitive reflexes.[6] In the normal individual these primitive movement patterns are thought to be modified through the influence of higher centers of CNS control. After a CVA, because the influence of higher centers is disturbed or destroyed, motor function reverts to this primitive state.[6] Reflexes present in early life reappear, and normal reflexes become exaggerated.

The Brunnstrom approach to the treatment of hemiplegia uses the motor patterns available to the patient at any point in the recovery process. The goal is to allow progress through the stages of recovery toward more normal and complex movement patterns. Brunnstrom saw synergies, reflexes, and other abnormal movement patterns as a normal part of the process through which an individual with CNS dysfunction must go before normal voluntary movement can occur. Brunnstrom noted that able-bodied people use synergistic movements all the time, but with control, and in a variety of patterns that can be modified or stopped at will. Brunnstrom maintained that the synergies appear to constitute a necessary intermediate stage for further recovery. She believed that the gross movement synergies of flexion and extension always precede the restoration of advanced motor functioning after hemiplegia.[6] During the early stage of recovery, Brunnstrom recommended that the patient should be aided to gain control of the limb synergies and that selected sensory stimuli can help the patient initiate and gain control of movement. Once the synergies can be performed voluntarily, they are modified and movement combinations that deviate from the synergy pattern can be performed.[6]

Limb Synergies

A limb synergy of flexion or extension, seen in hemiplegia, is a group of muscles acting as a bound unit in a primitive and stereotypical manner.[6] The muscles acting in synergy are linked and cannot act alone. If one muscle in the synergy is activated, each muscle in the synergy responds partially or completely. As a result, the patient cannot perform isolated movements when bound by these synergies.

The *flexor synergy* of the UE consists of scapular adduction and elevation, shoulder abduction and external rotation, elbow flexion, forearm supination, wrist flexion, and finger flexion. Hypertonicity (spasticity) is usually greatest in the elbow flexion component and least in shoulder abduction and external rotation (Figure 21-4). The *extensor synergy* consists of scapular abduction and depression, shoulder adduction and internal rotation, elbow extension, forearm pronation, and wrist and finger flexion or extension. Shoulder adduction and internal rotation are usually the most hypertonic components of the extensor synergy, with much less tone in the elbow extension component (Figure 21-5).

In the lower extremity (LE) the flexor synergy consists of hip flexion, abduction, and external rotation; knee flexion; ankle dorsiflexion and inversion; and toe extension. Hip flexion is usually the component with the highest tone, and hip abduction and external rotation are the components with the least tone. The extensor synergy is composed of hip abduction, extension, and internal rotation; knee extension; ankle plantar flexion and inversion; and toe flexion. Hip abduction, knee extension, and ankle plantar flexion are usually the most hypertonic components, whereas hip extension and internal rotation are usually less hypertonic.

Characteristics of Synergistic Movement

The flexor synergy is more often seen in the arm, and the extensor synergy is more common in the leg. When the patient performs the synergy, the components with the greatest degree of hypertonicity are often most apparent, rather than the entire classical patterns just described. Moreover, the resting posture of the limb, particularly the arm, is usually characterized by a position that represents the most hypertonic components of both flexor and extensor synergies (i.e., shoulder abduction, elbow flexion, forearm pronation, and wrist and finger flexion). With facilitation or voluntary effort, however, the more classical synergy pattern can usually be evoked.[6]

Motor Recovery Process

After a CVA resulting in hemiplegia, Brunnstrom observed that the patient progresses through a series of *recovery steps* or *stages* in fairly stereotypical fashion (Table 21-1). The progress through these stages may be rapid or slow.

The recovery follows an ontogenic process, usually proximal to distal, so that shoulder movement can be expected before hand movement. Flexion patterns occur before controlled volitional movement, and gross movement patterns can be performed before isolated, selective movement.[6]

Patients' recoveries vary and are influenced by factors such as cognitive deficits, visual-perceptual deficits, family support, motivation, and mood. Few patients make a good recovery of arm function, and the greatest loss is usually in the wrist and hand. Also, no two patients are exactly alike; much individual

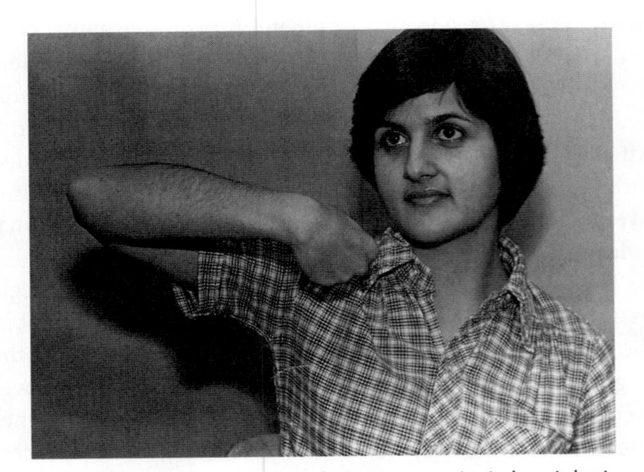

Figure 21-4 Flexor synergy of upper extremity in hemiplegia.

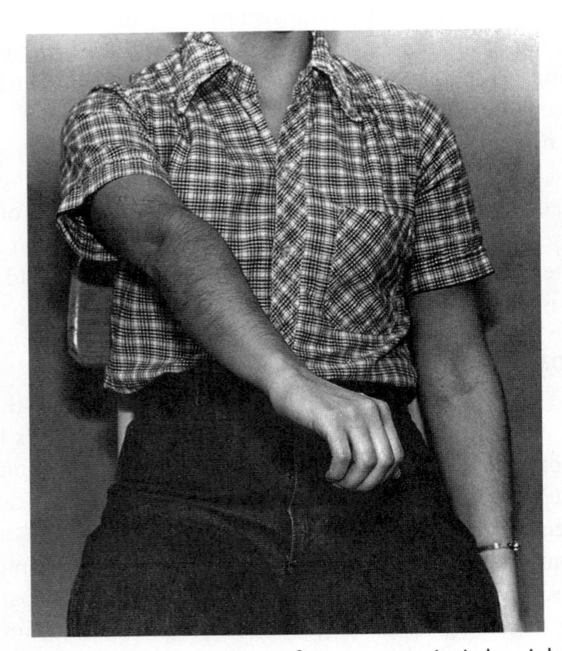

Figure 21-5 Extensor synergy of upper extremity in hemiplegia.

Table 21-1 Motor Recovery after Cerebrovascular Accident (CVA)

	CHARACTERISTICS		
Stage	Leg	Arm	Hand*
1	Flaccidity	Flaccidity; inability to perform any movements	No hand function
2	Spasticity develops; minimal voluntary movements	Beginning development of spasticity; limb synergies or some of their components begin to appear as associated reactions	Gross grasp beginning; minimal finger flexion possible
3	Spasticity peaks; flexion and extension synergy present; hip-knee-ankle flexion in sitting and standing	Spasticity increasing; synergy patterns or some of their components can be performed voluntarily	Gross grasp, hook grasp possible; no release
4	Knee flexion past 90 degrees in sitting, with foot sliding backward on floor; dorsiflexion with heel on floor and knee flexed to 90 degrees	Spasticity declining; movement combinations deviating from synergies are now possible	Gross grasp present; lateral prehension developing; small amount of finger extension and some thumb movement possible
5	Knee flexion with hip extended in standing; ankle dorsiflexion with hip and knee extended	Synergies no longer dominant; more movement combinations deviating from synergies performed with greater ease	Palmar prehension, spherical and cylindric grasp and release possible
6	Hip abduction in sitting or standing; reciprocal internal and external rotation of hip combined with inversion and eversion of ankle in sitting	Spasticity absent except when performing rapid movements; isolated joint movements performed with ease	All types of prehension, individual finger motion, and full range of voluntary extension possible

Data from Brunnstrom S: *Movement therapy in hemiplegia,* New York, 1970, Harper & Row.
*Recovery of hand function is variable and may not parallel six recovery stages of arm.

variation occurs in the recovery process. The motor behavior and recovery process described represent common characteristics that may be observed in most persons after CVA occurs.[6]

Principles of Treatment

The goal of Brunnstrom's movement therapy is to facilitate progress through the recovery stages that occur after the onset of hemiplegia (see Table 21-1). Because reflexes represent normal stages of development, they can be used to assist and/or initiate movement. *Associated reactions,* which are movements seen on the hemiplegic side in response to forceful movements on the normal side, can be used to initiate or elicit synergies by giving resistance to the contralateral (opposite-side) muscle group on the unaffected side. With the asymmetrical tonic neck reflex (ATNR), head rotation to the left causes extension of the left arm and leg and flexion of right arm and leg. With the symmetrical tonic neck reflex (STNR), flexion of the neck results in extension of the arm and flexion of the legs.

Proprioceptive stimuli can also be used to evoke desired motion or tonal changes.[19] To facilitate a synergy pattern, the therapist can rub skin over the muscle belly with his or her fingertips, thus producing a contraction of the muscle and eliciting the synergy pattern to which the muscle belongs. For example, briskly rubbing the triceps muscle while the patient attempts to push the arm through the sleeve of a shirt can promote extensor synergy.

Synergistic movement may be reinforced by the patient's voluntary efforts through visual feedback such as mirrors or videotapes or auditory stimuli such as loud and repetitive commands.

General Treatment Goals and Methods

Before initiating any intervention strategies, the occupational therapist performs a thorough evaluation of the patient's motor, sensory, perceptual, and cognitive functions. The motor evaluation yields information about stage of recovery, muscle tone, passive motion sense, hand function, and sitting and standing balance.[6]

The occupational therapist outlines a treatment plan based on the results of this evaluation. The OTA can easily incorporate many of Brunnstrom's techniques into this plan. The treatment goals and methods summarized in this chapter are directed primarily to the rehabilitation of the UE. The treatment goals and techniques chosen depend on the stage of recovery and muscle tone of the individual patient.

Bed Positioning

The OTA often instructs the patient and caregivers on positioning strategies. Proper bed positioning begins immediately when the patient is in the flaccid stage.[6] Proper positioning promotes normal alignment and can decrease the influence of hypertonic muscles. This is important in the prevention of contractures and deformity. For example, the LE often tends to assume a position of hip external rotation and abduction and knee flexion. This position mimics the LE's flexor synergy. If the extensor synergy is developed in the LE, a different position may be present. In this case the LE's posture is characterized by extension and adduction at the hip, knee extension, and ankle plantar flexion.

If the extensor synergy dominates in the LE, the recommended bed position for patients in the supine position is slight hip and knee flexion maintained by a small pillow under the knee. Lateral support of the leg at the knee with pillows or a rolled blanket or bolster should be provided to prevent abduction and external rotation.

If the flexor synergy dominates in the LE, the knee must be maintained in extension. Hip external rotation can be prevented with supports as described.

To position the affected UE, the practitioner supports the arm on a pillow in a position comfortable for the patient. Abduction of the UE should be avoided because this position can contribute to shoulder subluxation. While moving the patient, the OTA avoids pulling on the affected UE. The patient is instructed to use the unaffected hand to support the affected arm when moving in bed.

Bed Mobility

Turning toward the affected side is easier than turning toward the unaffected side. For turning in bed, the OTA can instruct the patient to raise the affected arm to a position of forward shoulder flexion with the elbow in extension. The affected LE is then positioned in partial flexion at the knee and hip; the clinician may need to stabilize it in this position. The patient turns by swinging the arms and the affected knee across the body toward the unaffected side. As control improves, the patient may perform this technique independently to roll toward both sides of the bed.

Balance and Trunk Control

Early in treatment the patient needs to develop balance, a prerequisite for functional activities. Patients with hemiplegia may have poor postural/trunk control, often demonstrating a "listing" (leaning) toward the affected side. To facilitate upright posture, treatment should focus on improving trunk control through a variety of sitting balance exercises with focus on anterior and posterior pelvic tilts and lateral weight shifting. The clinician should support the affected arm to protect the shoulder during these balance-challenging activities. Supporting the arm also prevents the patient from grasping the supporting surface during the activity. As trunk control improves, the clinician initiates and assists the patient to bend the trunk in various directions. If balance is poor, the clinician can stabilize the patient's knees. In this position the clinician can guide the patient while moving the trunk in various directions. The clinician can also incorporate passive range of motion (ROM) at the shoulder by raising the patient's arms up as the trunk bends forward.

Shoulder Range of Motion

The maintenance of pain-free shoulder ROM is important in patients with hemiplegia. Brunnstrom believed that traditional passive exercises may actually contribute to pain in these patients.[6] Instead, the shoulder joint should be mobilized through guided trunk motion without forceful stretching.

To accomplish this motion, the patient sits erect, cradling the affected arm. The clinician supports the arm under the elbows while the patient leans forward. The more the patient leans, the greater the range of shoulder flexion can be obtained. The clinician guides the arm gently and passively into shoulder flexion while the patient's attention is focused on the trunk motion. In a similar manner the clinician can guide the arms into abduction and adduction while the patient rotates the trunk from side to side. Later, active-assistive movements of the arm in relation to the trunk can begin.

Shoulder Subluxation

Glenohumeral subluxation appears to be a result of dysfunction of the rotator cuff muscles. These muscles maintain the humeral head in the glenoid fossa. Activation of the rotator cuff muscles is necessary if subluxation is to be minimized or prevented. Slings have been used in an effort to hold the humeral head in the glenoid fossa, but they do not activate the muscles needed to protect the integrity of the shoulder joint.[6] Slings have been found to be of little value and may be harmful.[7] Therapeutic taping (kinesiotaping) has also been used to lift the shoulder into alignment.

Methods of Treatment

The training procedures for improving arm function are geared to the patient's recovery stage. These procedures are performed primarily by the occupational therapist. During stages 1 and 2, when the arm is essentially flaccid or when some components of the synergy patterns are beginning to appear, the aim is to elicit muscle tone and the synergy patterns on a reflex basis. This aim is met through a variety of facilitation procedures.

The occupational therapist does not employ treatment methods in any set order but varies them depending on the patient's needs. Because the flexor synergy usually appears first, it may be useful to begin trying to elicit the flexor patterns. This attempt should be followed immediately with facilitation of the extensor synergy components, which tend to be weaker and more difficult to perform in later stages of recovery.[6,31] Overtraining of either synergy should be avoided.

When the patient has recovered to stages 2 and 3, the synergies are present, and components can be performed voluntarily. During this period the goal is for the patient to achieve voluntary control of the synergy patterns.

The treatment aim during stages 4 and 5 is to move away from the synergies by mixing components from both synergies to perform new and complex patterns of movement.

In the final recovery period, stage 6, the goal is to achieve ease in performance of movement combinations, to increase isolated motions, and to increase speed of movement. Activities that encourage varying motions and increasing speed of performance can be introduced during this stage.

For retraining hand function, Brunnstrom described separate techniques. As in treatment of the rest of the UE, the concept of helping the patient progress through the stages of hand recovery is the same. For example, patients are first provided with activities to promote gross grasp, followed by wrist fixation for grasp, then active release.[6]

Occupational Therapy Application

The focus of OT in the Brunnstrom technique is helping the patient use newly learned movement patterns for functional and purposeful activities. Using this principle, the OTA can

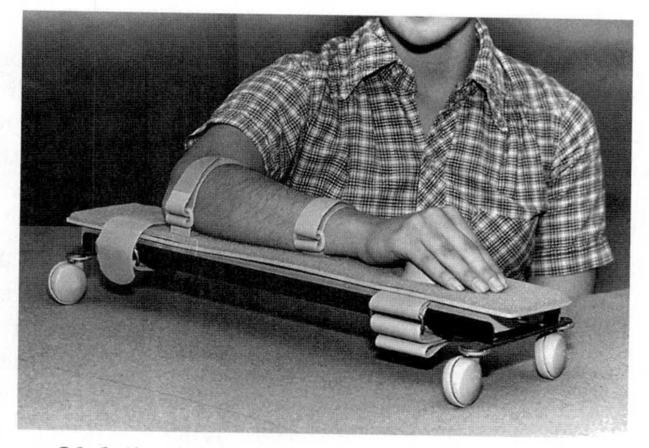

Figure 21-6 Skateboard activities for synergy or combined movement patterns.

consider incorporating whatever movement the patient demonstrates into treatment activities. For instance, during stage 3, when the patient can perform synergy voluntarily, the extensor synergy can be used to stabilize an object on a table while the unaffected arm is performing a task.

During stage 4 the OTA can provide activities that encourage movements deviating from synergy such as skateboard activities (Figure 21-6), sponging off tabletops, or finger painting.

Practice in functional movement patterns for self-care can also be performed. They might include hand-to-mouth motions used in eating finger foods, combing hair, washing the face, washing the unaffected arm, and reaching the opposite axilla for washing or application of deodorant.[6] The clinician's role is to analyze activities for movement patterns the patient can perform and to select meaningful and interesting activities with the patient.

The OTA should always reinforce and encourage any voluntary movement of the affected limb during the performance of self-care activities. Using the arm for dressing and hygiene skills translates the movements to purposeful use. If the patient moves beyond stage 4, the number of activities that can be performed increases and more movement combinations are possible. The involvement of the affected limbs in ADL should be encouraged. Gardening, rolling out dough, sweeping, dusting, and washing dishes are a few of the activities that may enlist the affected arm purposefully if hand recovery is adequate.

Proprioceptive Neuromuscular Facilitation

PNF originated with Dr. Herman Kabat, a physician and neurophysiologist, in the 1940s. Kabat applied neurophysiological principles to the treatment of paralysis resulting from poliomyelitis and multiple sclerosis. In 1948 Kabat and Henry Kaiser founded the Kabat-Kaiser Institute in Vallejo, Calif. At the institute Kabat worked with physical therapist Margaret Knott to develop the PNF method of treatment. By 1951 the diagonal patterns and several PNF techniques were established. In 1952 Dorothy Voss, a physical therapist, joined the staff at the Kabat-Kaiser Institute. She and Knott undertook the teaching and supervision of staff therapists. In 1956 the first edition of Knott and Voss' *Proprioceptive Neuromuscular Facilitation* was published.[38,39]

PNF is based on normal movement and motor development. In normal motor activity the brain registers total movement and not individual muscle action.[21] The PNF approaches use mass movement patterns that resemble normal movement during functional activities. Facilitation techniques are superimposed on these movement patterns and postures through manual contacts, verbal commands, and visual cues.

Principles of Treatment

Voss presented specific principles of treatment at the Northwestern University Special Therapeutic Exercise Project in 1966. These principles were developed from concepts in the fields of neurophysiology, motor learning, and motor behavior. Examples of some core concepts from these principles are the following[34]:

1. *Normal motor development proceeds in a cervicocaudal and proximodistal direction.* During evaluation and treatment, the cervicocaudal (head to "tailbone") and proximodistal (body center to extremities) directions are followed. Attention is given first to the head, followed by the neck, trunk, and finally the extremities. For clinicians, this order is of particular importance in treatment that facilitates fine motor coordination in the UEs. Without adequate control of the head, neck, and trunk region, fine motor skills cannot be developed effectively.
2. *Early motor behavior is dominated by reflex activity.* Mature motor behavior is supported or reinforced by postural reflexes. As a person matures, primitive reflexes are integrated and available for reinforcement to allow for progressive development such as rolling, crawling, and sitting. Reflexes also affect tone and movement in the extremities, and head and neck movements affect arm and leg movements.[18] For example, reaching for an object can be reinforced by having the head turned toward the object.
3. *Motor behavior is expressed in an orderly sequence of total patterns of movements and posture.* Motor skills develop progressively. For example, an infant learns to roll, to crawl, to creep, and finally to stand and walk. Throughout these stages the infant also learns to use the extremities in different patterns and postures. Initially the hands are used for reaching and grasping within the most supported postures such as supine and prone. As control in these postures develops, the infant begins to use the hands in side-lying, sitting, and standing. Coordination develops as a result.
4. *The growth of motor behavior has a rhythmic and cyclical trend, as evidenced by shifts between flexor and extensor dominance.* These shifts help to develop muscle balance and control. One of the main goals of the PNF treatment approach is to establish a balance among opposing (antagonistic) muscle groups. In treatment the clinician must establish a balance between muscles by first observing where imbalance exists and then facilitating the weaker component. For example, if a patient demonstrates a flexor synergy, extension should be facilitated.

5. *Normal motor development has an orderly sequence but lacks a step-by-step quality.* Overlapping occurs; the child does not perfect performance of one activity before beginning another, more advanced activity. Normal motor development follows a predictable pattern, which the practitioner must consider when positioning a patient. If one posture technique is not effective in obtaining a desired result, the OTA may need to attempt the activity in another developmental posture. For example, if a patient with ataxia cannot write while sitting, the person may practice writing in a more supported posture such as prone on elbows. If the patient has not perfected a motor activity such as walking on level surfaces, however, the person may benefit from attempting a higher-level activity such as walking up or down stairs. This activity in turn can improve ambulation on level surfaces. Moving up and down the developmental sequence is a natural occurrence that allows for multiple, varied opportunities for practicing motor activities.
6. *Establishing a balance between antagonists is a main objective of PNF.* As movement and posture change, continuous adjustments in balance are made. When these adjustments are not made, an imbalance in muscles occurs, such as seen in the patient with a head injury who cannot maintain adequate sitting balance during a table-top activity because of a dominance of trunk extensor tone. In treatment, emphasis would be placed on correcting the imbalance. In the presence of spasticity, this correction may have to be done by first inhibiting (reducing) the spasticity, then facilitating the antagonistic muscles, evoking reflexes, and promoting stable posture.
7. *Improvement in motor ability depends on motor learning.* Multisensory input facilitates the patient's motor learning and is an integral part of the PNF approach. For example, when working with a patient on a shoulder flexion activity such as reaching into the cabinet for a cup, the clinician may say "reach for the cup." This verbal input encourages the patient to look in the direction of the movement to allow vision to enhance the motor response. Thus tactile, auditory, and visual inputs are used. Motor learning has occurred when these external cues are no longer necessary for adequate performance. Practice and repetition enhance motor learning. In treatment, opportunities for practice must be afforded to patients. Practice should be varied and occur in different positions and patterns. This repetition builds skill and coordination.
8. Goal-directed activities coupled with techniques of facilitation are used to hasten learning of total patterns of walking and self-care activities. When facilitation techniques are applied to ADL, the objective is improved functional ability. This improvement requires more than instruction and practice alone. Correction of deficiencies is accomplished by directly applying manual contacts and techniques to facilitate the desired response.[39] Examples include applying stretch to finger extensors to release an object and providing joint approximation through the shoulders and pelvis of a patient with ataxia to provide stability while standing to wash dishes.

Motor Learning

Motor learning requires a *multisensory* approach; auditory, visual, and tactile systems are all used to achieve the desired response. The correct combination of sensory input for each patient should be identified and altered as the person progresses.

Verbal commands should be brief and clear. Timing of the command is important. Tone of voice may influence the quality of the patient's response. Strong, sharp commands are used when maximal stimulation of motor response is desired. A soft tone of voice is used to encourage a smooth movement (e.g., in the presence of pain). *Verbal mediation,* whereby patients say aloud the steps of an activity, has also been found to enhance learning.[25]

Visual stimuli help to initiate and coordinate movement. Visual input should be monitored to ensure that the patient is tracking in the direction of movement. The clinician's position and the treatment activity must be considered. For example, if the treatment goal is to increase head, neck, and trunk rotation to the left, the activity should be located in front and to the left of the patient.

The use of *tactile input* is essential to guide and reinforce the desired patterns of movement. Manual contacts by the clinician provide this input.

Finally, to increase speed and accuracy in motor performance, the patient needs the opportunity to *practice.* Practice should include part-task and whole-task practice. In part task, emphasis is placed on the parts of the task that the patient is unable to perform independently. For example, the patient learning to transfer from a wheelchair to a tub bench may have difficulty lifting the leg over the tub rim. This part of the task should be practiced with repetition and facilitation techniques to the hip flexors during performance of the transfer. When the transfer becomes smooth and coordinated, it is no longer necessary to practice parts individually.

Evaluation

PNF evaluation of the patient requires keen observational skills and knowledge of normal movement. The occupational therapist completes an initial evaluation to identify the patient's abilities, deficiencies, and potential. After the treatment plan is established, ongoing assessment is necessary to determine the effectiveness of treatment; modifications are made as the patient changes. The PNF evaluation follows a sequence from proximal to distal. Special attention is given to muscle tone, alignment (midline or a shift to one side), and stability/mobility.[28]

When examining the trunk and extremities, the clinician evaluates each segment individually in specific movement patterns, as well as in developmental activities that use interaction of body segments. For example, shoulder flexion can be observed in an individual UE movement pattern, as well as during a total developmental pattern such as rolling.

During the evaluation the occupational therapist should note the facilitation techniques and sensory inputs (auditory, visual, tactile) to which the patient responds most effectively. Once identified, these techniques and sensory inputs are used to promote controlled movements.

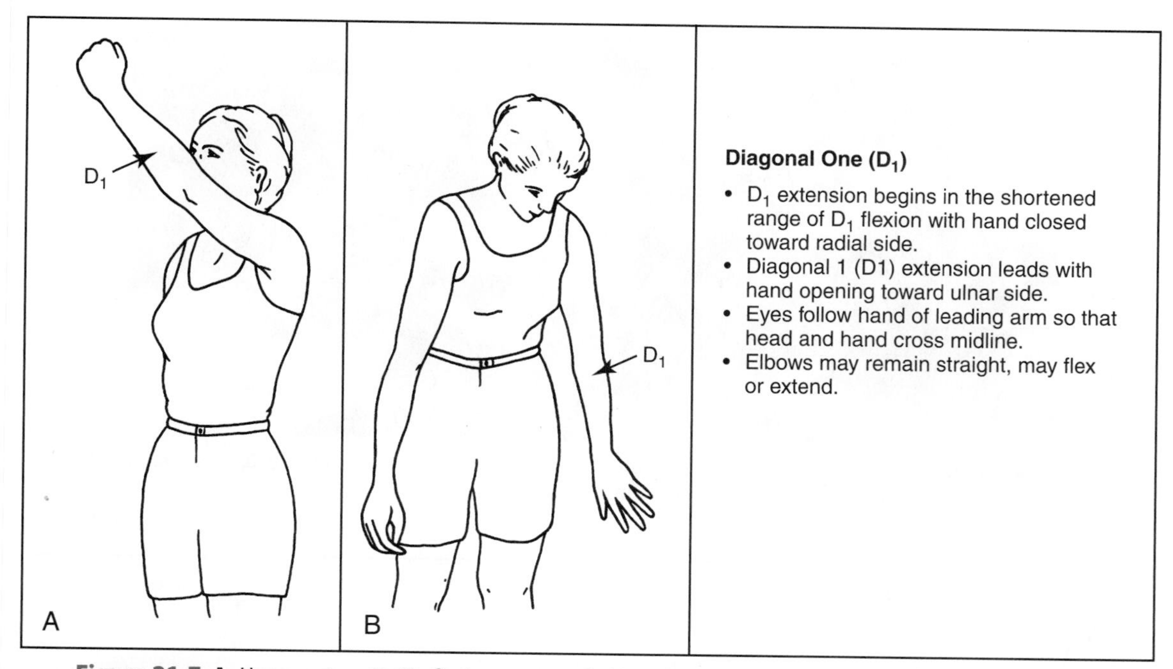

Figure 21-7 **A,** Upper extremity D_1 flexion pattern. **B,** Upper extremity D_1 extension pattern. (From Myers BJ: *PNF: diagonal patterns and their application to functional activities,* Chicago, 1982, Rehabilitation Institute of Chicago [videotape].)

Evaluation should be performed during self-care and other ADL to determine whether performance patterns are adequate within the context of a functional activity. Because performance may vary from one setting to another, the treatment plan must allow for practice of motor skills in a variety of settings and in locations appropriate to the specific activity.

Treatment

Once the evaluation is completed, a treatment plan is developed including goals the patient hopes to accomplish. The clinician uses the techniques and procedures identified in the evaluation as having favorably influenced movement and posture. Similarly, appropriate total patterns and patterns of facilitation are selected to enhance performance.

The treatment techniques used in the PNF approach are diagonal patterns, total patterns, and facilitation techniques.

Diagonal Patterns

The diagonal patterns used in the PNF approach are mass movement patterns observed in most functional activities. Part of the challenge in using this approach is recognizing the diagonal patterns in ADL. Two diagonal motions (D_1, D_2) are present for each major part of the body: head and neck, upper and lower trunk, and extremities. Each diagonal pattern has a flexion and extension component together with rotation and movement away from or toward the midline. Both unilateral and bilateral diagonal patterns are described for the extremities. Only UE patterns are discussed in this chapter.

The movements associated with each diagonal pattern and examples of these patterns seen in ADL are described next. Not all components of the pattern or full ROM are necessarily seen during functional activities. Furthermore, the diagonals interact during functional movement, changing from one pattern or combination to another.[29]

Upper Extremity Unilateral Patterns

1. *UE D_1 flexion (antagonist of D_1 extension).* Scapular elevation, abduction, and rotation; shoulder flexion, adduction, and external rotation; elbow in flexion or extension; forearm supination; wrist flexion to the radial side; finger flexion and adduction; thumb adduction (Figure 21-7, *A*). Examples in functional activity: hand-to-mouth motion in feeding, combing hair on left side of head with right hand (Figure 21-8, *A*).
2. *UE D_1 extension (antagonist of D_1 flexion).* Scapular depression, adduction, and rotation; shoulder extension, abduction, and internal rotation; elbow in flexion or extension; forearm pronation; wrist extension to the ulnar side; finger extension and abduction; thumb in palmar abduction (Figure 21-7, *B*). Examples in functional activity: pushing car door open from inside (Figure 21-8, *B*).
3. *UE D_2 flexion (antagonist of D_2 extension).* Scapular elevation, adduction, and rotation; shoulder flexion, abduction, and external rotation; elbow in flexion or extension; forearm supination; wrist extension to radial side; finger extension and abduction; thumb extension (Figure 21-9, *A*). Examples in functional activity: combing hair on right side of head with right hand (Figure 21-10, *A*), swimming the backstroke.
4. *UE D_2 extension (antagonist of D_2 flexion).* Scapular depression, abduction, and rotation; shoulder extension, adduction, and internal rotation; elbow in flexion or extension; forearm pronation; wrist flexion to the ulnar side; finger flexion and adduction; thumb opposition (Figure 21-9, *B*). Examples in functional activity: pitching baseball; buttoning pants on left side with right hand (Figure 21-10, *B*).

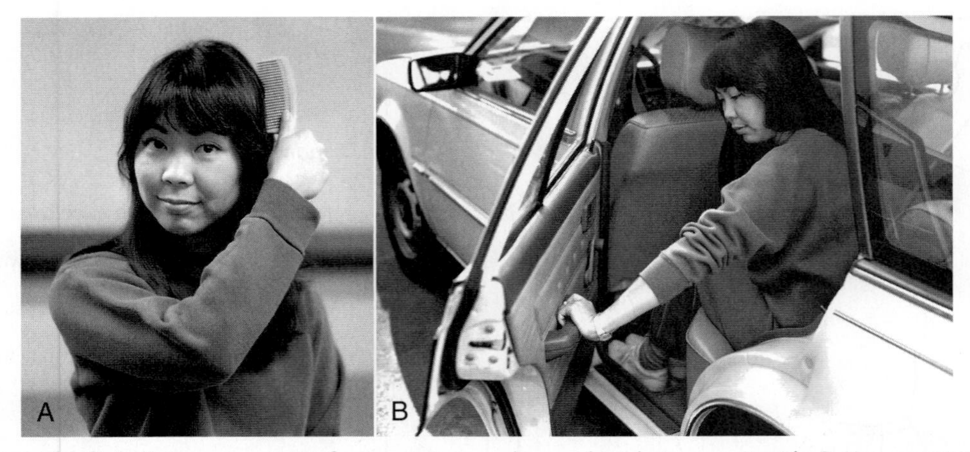

Figure 21-8 **A,** Upper extremity D_1 flexion pattern used in combing hair, opposite side. **B,** Upper extremity D_1 extension pattern used in pushing car door open.

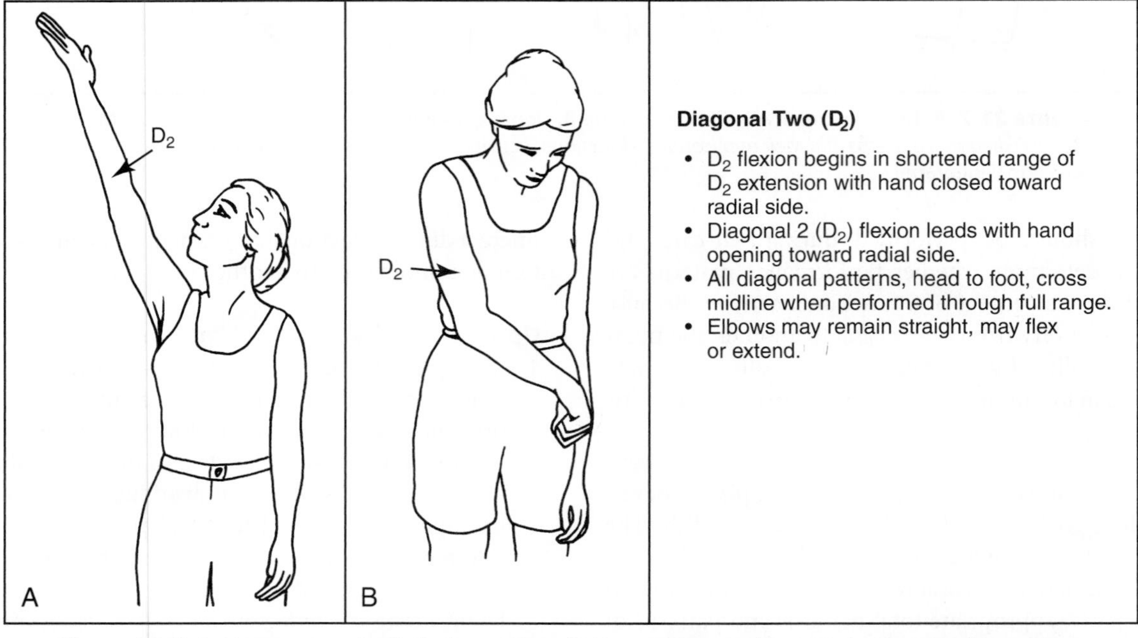

Figure 21-9 **A,** Upper extremity D_2 flexion pattern. **B,** Upper extremity D_2 extension pattern. (From Myers BJ: *PNF: diagonal patterns and their application to functional activities,* Chicago, 1982, Rehabilitation Institute of Chicago [videotape].)

Bilateral Patterns

Movements in the extremities can be reinforced by combining diagonals in the following bilateral patterns:

1. *Symmetrical patterns.* Paired extremities perform like movements at the same time (Figure 21-11). Examples are bilateral symmetrical D_2 extension such as starting to take off pullover sweater (Figure 21-12, *A*); and bilateral symmetric D_2 flexion such as reaching to lift large item off high shelf (Figure 21-12, *B*).
2. *Asymmetrical patterns.* Paired extremities perform movements toward one side of the body at the same time. Asymmetrical patterns facilitate trunk rotation. The asymmetrical patterns can be performed with the arms in contact or not (Figures 21-13 and 21-14). Examples are bilateral asymmetrical flexion to the left, with the left arm in D_2 flexion and right arm in D_1 flexion such as putting on a left earring (Figure 21-15) or bilateral asymmetrical extension to the left, with the right arm in D_2 extension and left arm in D_1 extension such as zipping a left-sided skirt zipper.
3. *Reciprocal patterns.* Paired extremities perform movements in opposite directions at the same time. Reciprocal patterns have a stabilizing effect on the head, neck, and trunk. Examples are pitching in baseball or walking on a balance beam with one extremity in a diagonal flexion pattern and the other in a diagonal extension pattern (Figure 21-16). During activities requiring high-level balance, reciprocal patterns come into play to maintain balance and prevent a fall.

Diagonal patterns offer several advantages in OT treatment. First, crossing of the midline of the body occurs. Most functional activities require crossing the midline, which can also be important in the remediation of visual perceptual deficits such as unilateral neglect, in which integration of both sides of the

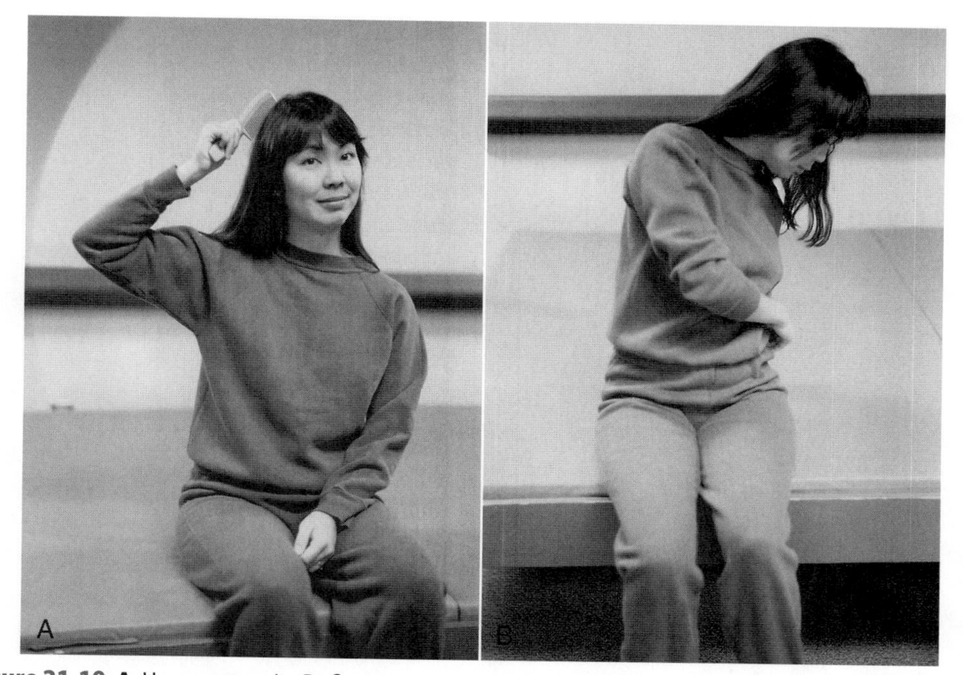

Figure 21-10 **A,** Upper extremity D_2 flexion pattern used in combing hair, same side. **B,** Upper extremity D_2 extension pattern used in buttoning trousers, opposite side.

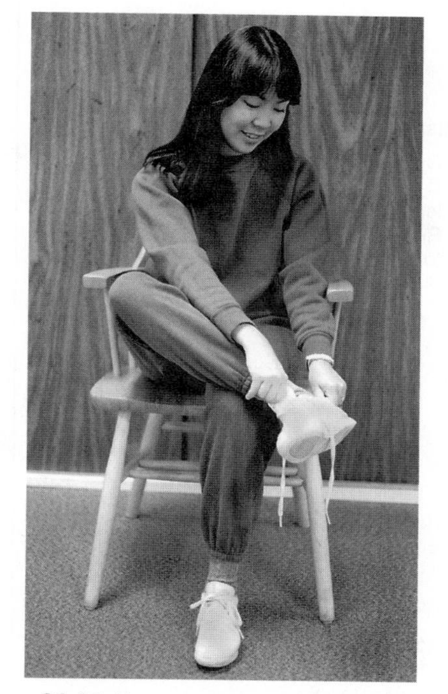

Figure 21-11 Upper extremity symmetrical pattern.

body and awareness of the neglected side are treatment goals. Second, because each muscle has an optimal pattern in which it functions, the total pattern can be used to strengthen weaker ones. Third, the diagonal patterns use groups of muscles; this movement is typical of functional activities. Finally, rotation is always a component in the diagonals. With an injury or the aging process, rotation is often impaired and can be facilitated with movement in the diagonals.

In treatment the occupational therapist or OTA would place activities so that movement occurs in a diagonal. For example, if the patient is working on a simple homemaking task such as preparing a meal, trunk rotation with extension can be facilitated by placing all the ingredients and utensils on a cupboard located above and diagonal from the patient.

Total Patterns

In PNF, developmental postures are called *total patterns of movement* and posture.[28] Total patterns require interaction between proximal (head, neck, trunk) and distal (extremity) components. Maintenance of postures is important. When posture cannot be maintained, emphasis is placed on the assumption of posture.[39] The active assumption of postures can be incorporated into functional activities. For example, a reaching and placing activity could be designed so that the patient must reach for the object while in a supine posture and then move into a side-lying posture to place the object. The use of total patterns also can reinforce individual extremity movements. For example, in an activity such as wiping a tabletop, wrist extension is reinforced while the patient leans forward over the supporting arm.

Procedures

PNF techniques are superimposed on diagonal movements and posture. Two procedures, verbal commands and visual cues, have been discussed previously. Other common procedures include manual contact, stretch, traction, and approximation.

Manual contact refers to the placement of the clinician's hands on the patient. Pressure from the clinician's touch is used as a facilitating mechanism and provides a sensory cue to help the patient understand the direction of the anticipated movement.[39] The amount of pressure applied depends on the specific technique and the desired response. Location

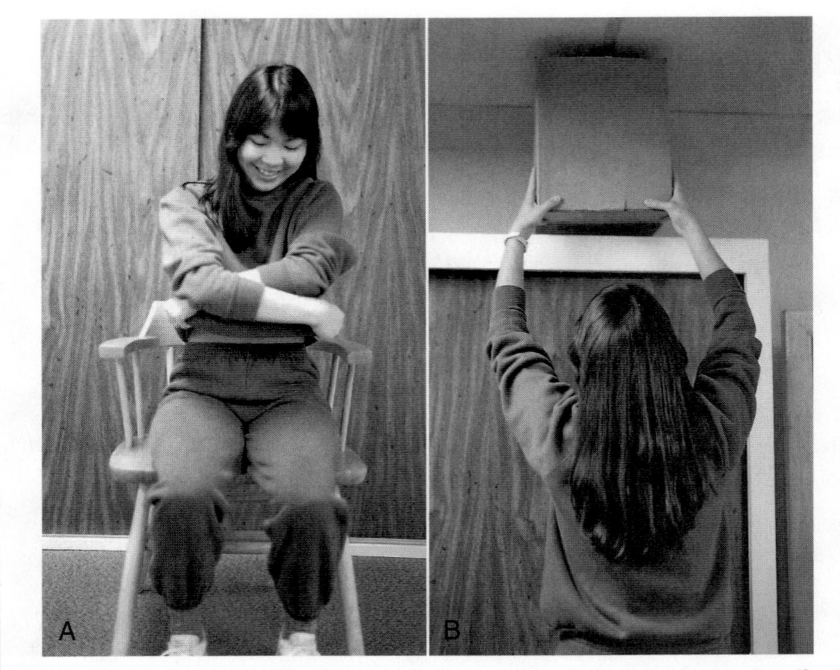

Figure 21-12 **A,** Upper extremity bilateral symmetrical pattern used when starting to take off pullover shirt. **B,** Upper extremity bilateral symmetrical pattern used when reaching to lift box off high shelf.

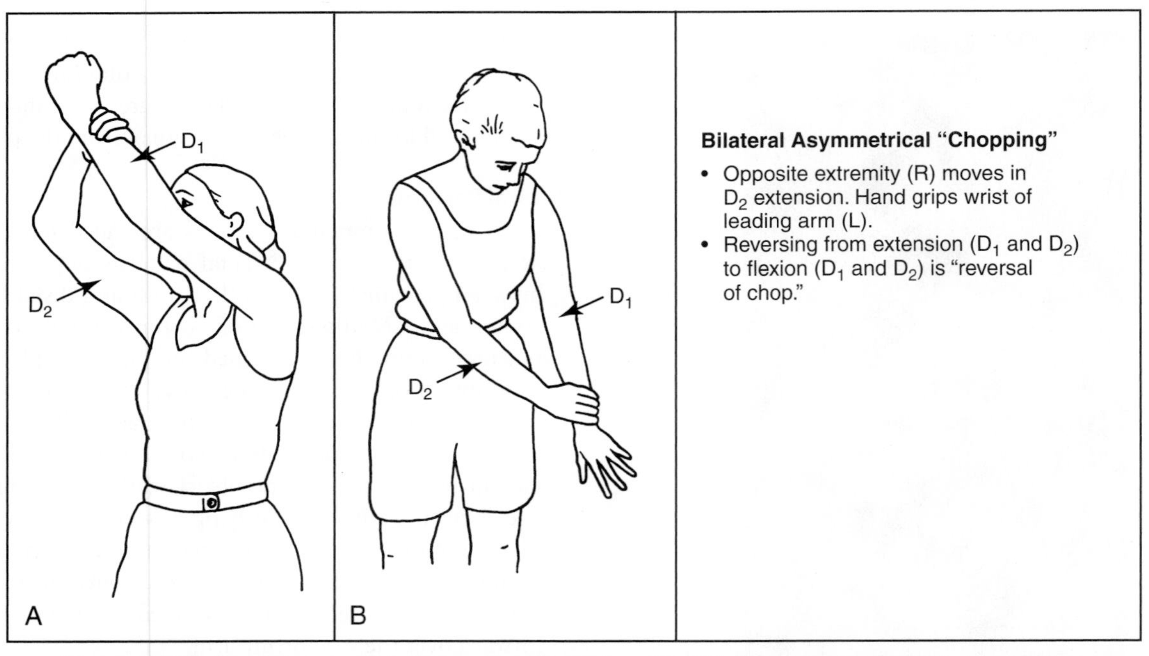

Figure 21-13 Bilateral asymmetrical chopping. (From Myers BJ: *PNF: diagonal patterns and their application to functional activities,* Chicago, 1982, Rehabilitation Institute of Chicago [videotape].)

of manual contacts is chosen according to the groups of muscles, tendons, and joints responsible for the desired movement patterns. For example, if a patient is having difficulty reaching to comb the back of the hair because of scapular weakness, the desired movement pattern would be D_2 flexion. Manual contacts would be on the posterior surface of the scapula to reinforce the muscles that elevate, adduct, and rotate the scapula.

Stretch is used to initiate voluntary movement and enhance speed of response and strength in weak muscles. When stretch is used in this approach, the part to be facilitated is placed in the extreme lengthened range of the desired pattern (or where tension is felt on all muscle components of a given pattern). After the correct position for the stretch stimulus has been achieved, stretch is superimposed on the pattern. The patient should attempt the movement at the exact time that the stretch reflex is elicited. Verbal commands should coincide with the application of stretch to reinforce the movement. Using stretch, the OTA must take care to prevent increasing pain or muscle imbalances. The OTA who plans to use the

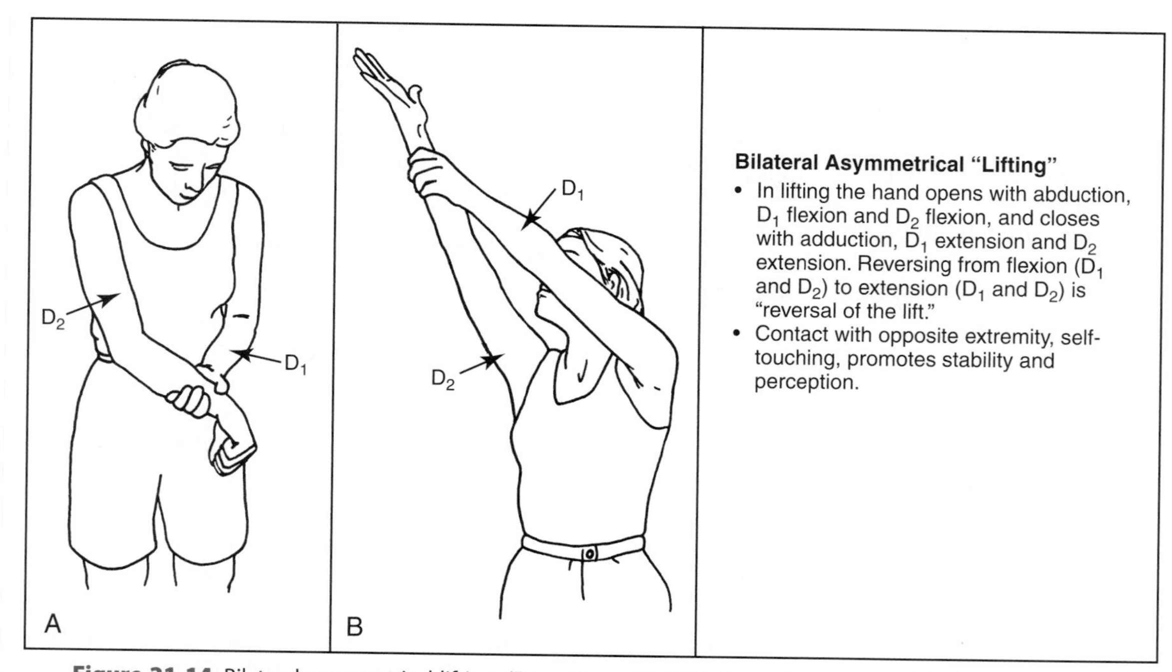

Figure 21-14 Bilateral asymmetrical lifting. (From Myers BJ: *PNF: diagonal patterns and their application to functional activities,* Chicago, 1982, Rehabilitation Institute of Chicago [videotape].)

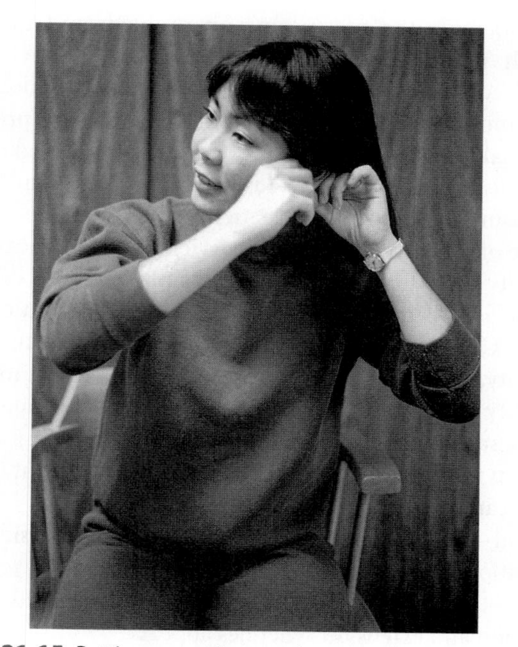

Figure 21-15 Putting on earring requires use of upper extremity bilateral asymmetrical flexion pattern.

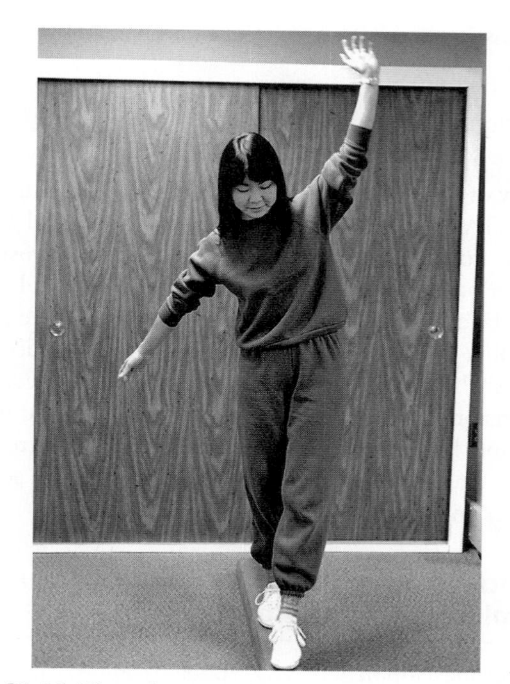

Figure 21-16 Bilateral reciprocal pattern of upper extremities used to walk balance beam.

stretch technique must be thoroughly trained in proper application and precautions.

Traction facilitates the joint receptors by separating the joint surfaces. Traction promotes movement and occurs in pulling motion.[40] In an activity such as carrying a heavy suitcase, traction can be felt on joint surfaces. Traction may be contraindicated in patients after surgery or fractures or in patients with a subluxed shoulder.

Approximation facilitates joint receptors by creating a compression of joint surfaces. It promotes stability and postural control and occurs in pushing motion.[40] Approximation is usually superimposed on a weight-bearing posture. For example, to enhance postural control in the prone on elbow position, approximation may be given through the shoulders in a downward direction.

Techniques

Several specific techniques are used with these basic procedures; a few have been selected for mention here. Before incorporating any of these techniques into treatment, both the occupational therapist and the OTA must be trained in safe applications and precautions and must demonstrate the appropriate level of competence. Improper application can result in spasticity, pain, and abnormal movement patterns.

Repeated contraction is a technique based on the assumption that repetition of an activity is necessary for motor learning and helps develop strength, ROM, and endurance.

Rhythmic initiation is used to improve the ability to initiate movement, a problem that may be seen in patients with Parkinson disease or apraxia.

Relaxation techniques are an effective means of increasing ROM, particularly when pain or spasticity increases with passive stretch. Two examples of PNF relaxation techniques are contract-relax and hold-relax. *Contract-relax techniques* involve a holding contraction of the antagonistic pattern against maximal resistance, followed by relaxation and then passive movement into the agonistic pattern. This procedure is repeated at each point during the ROM in which limitation is felt to occur.[40] Contract-relax is used when no active ROM in the agonistic pattern is present. *Hold-relax techniques* are performed in the same sequence as contract-relax techniques but involve an isometric (holding) contraction of the antagonist, followed by relaxation and then active movement into the agonistic pattern. This technique may benefit patients with pain.

Occupational Therapy Applications

The PNF approach can be incorporated into OT practice in a variety of ways. Whenever feasible, the occupational therapist or OTA should incorporate appropriate diagonal patterns into functional treatment activities. Tasks can be positioned so that a patient can perform a particular diagonal needed for function. During homemaking, for example, the process of reaching into a bag to retrieve items that are placed on a kitchen shelf could be set up to incorporate the D_1 flexion and D_2 extension patterns. Verbal and tactile cues should be used to promote functional movement patterns. Specific treatment techniques and procedures could be used with these activities to further enhance function.

Neurodevelopmental Treatment of Adult Hemiplegia: Bobath Approach

The neurodevelopmental (NDT/Bobath) approach was first developed in the 1940s by Bertha Bobath, a physical therapist, and her husband, Dr. Karel Bobath, a neurologist.[5] The Bobaths coined the term *neurodevelopmental treatment* to describe their work with children with cerebral palsy. Also known as the *Bobath approach,* NDT has been used successfully by occupational and physical therapists to treat adult hemiplegia.

The Bobaths believed strongly in the potential of the hemiplegic side for normal function. On the basis of this belief, they established a treatment program that focused on relearning normal movement. NDT is geared toward encouraging the use of both sides of the body. Development of alignment and symmetry of the trunk and pelvis is emphasized; these conditions are thought to be necessary for normal function of the extremities. When therapists use an NDT approach, patients should be trained to use methods other than compensatory techniques. Relying only on compensatory techniques may lead to overuse of the uninvolved side and underuse of the involved side. This pattern will ultimately interfere with functional recovery of the hemiplegic side.

Typical Problems of Hemiplegia

Motor Problems

The Bobaths suggest that the major motor problem in hemiplegia is the lack of motor control affecting voluntary movement. *Flaccidity* is most common at the onset of a CVA. During this time the patient demonstrates low endurance and low activity tolerance. The period may last a few days or several months. Although no movement in the affected extremities is displayed at this time, a proper treatment program can strongly alter the eventual functional outcome.[5]

After the flaccid stage the patient enters a stage of *mixed tone,* displaying a combination of flaccidity and spasticity. For example, the UE might have an increase in tone proximally at the scapula and shoulder but a decrease in tone distally at the wrist and hand. If treatment does not address the problems of high tone at this stage, the patient progresses to the next stage of spasticity.

Spasticity is the most common problem and the most difficult motor problem to manage after a CVA. If not treated correctly, spasticity can severely compromise functional mobility and ADL performance. Spasticity produces abnormal sensory feedback and contributes to weakness of antagonist muscles. It can cause contractures, pain, and an all-consuming fear in many patients. Fear, pain, and spasticity are often so intertwined that a vicious cycle appears. The spasticity can cause an increase in pain, which can cause an increase in fear, which in turn increases the amount of spasticity.[10] Conversely, a reduction in pain and fear can reduce spasticity. Other factors that may influence the amount of spasticity are emotional stress, physical effort, temperature, and the rate of activity.

The typical posture in the adult hemiplegic patient (Figure 21-17) can be described as follows:

- Head—Lateral flexion is toward the involved side with rotation away from the involved side.
- UE—Combination of the strongest components of the flexion and extension synergies appears.
  1. Scapula—depression, retraction
  2. Shoulder—adduction, internal rotation
  3. Elbow—flexion
  4. Forearm—pronation
  5. Wrist—flexion, ulnar deviation
  6. Fingers—flexion
- Trunk—Lateral flexion is toward the involved side.
- LE—Typical extensor posture
  1. Pelvis—posterior elevation, retraction
  2. Hip—internal rotation, adduction, extension
  4. Knee—extension
  5. Ankle—plantar flexion, supination, inversion
  6. Toes—flexion

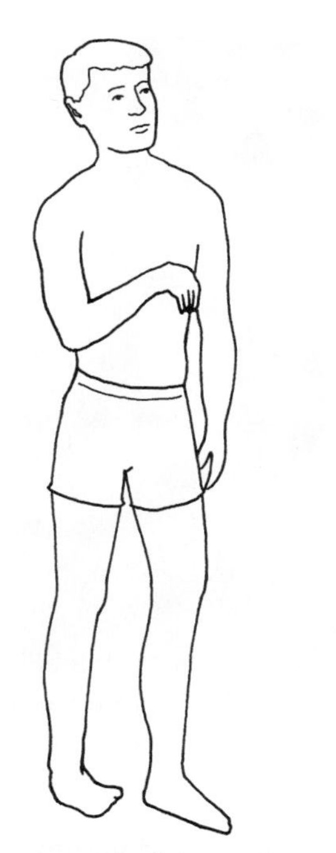

Figure 21-17 Typical posture of adult with hemiplegia in standing position.

Additional Problems

With these motor problems, patients often have other deficits that can affect function including diminished weight bearing on the hemiplegic side, sensory loss, neglect, and fear.

Patients with hemiplegia commonly avoid bearing weight on the affected side. When sitting or standing, the patient shifts weight to the nonhemiplegic side, thus causing an asymmetrical posture that cues patient to lean toward the side. Sensory loss, visual perceptual impairments, and cognitive deficits can contribute to this problem.

Sensory loss varies and may include the loss of stereognosis, kinesthetic awareness, light touch, and light pressure. Abnormal sensation in an extremity, even with good motor control, can render that extremity useless.[5,10] Unilateral body or unilateral spatial neglect can occur after a CVA. It is defined as an inattention to or neglect of visual stimuli presented to body side contralateral to a lesion.[17] It can result from defective sensory processing or attention deficit, which causes neglect or impaired use of extremities.[17] For example, the patient does not dress affected body parts, the patient forgets to shave or wash one side of face, or the patient may run into furniture, doorways, or walls located on affected side.

Fear can also be a major limiting factor for many patients. Fear can be related to loss of sensory awareness; poor balance reactions; lack of protective extension, resulting in a fear of falling; and perceptual or cognitive problems.[10]

Many other problems related to CVA including aphasia, apraxia, and visual-perceptual problems may occur and affect a patient's functional abilities.

Evaluation

When evaluating a patient, the occupational therapist emphasizes the *quality of movement,* or how the patient moves. During evaluation of coordination, changes in overall muscle tone and postural reactions (rather than specific muscles and joints) are the focus of observation.[5] During the evaluation and treatment the clinician must understand normal posture and movement to identify abnormal patterns. Each patient may have a different clinical picture based on age, premorbid physical condition, and normal degenerative changes. Observations should be performed in a functional context because muscle tone may change on the basis of specific task demands.

Observation is a key component in an NDT evaluation. The patient is observed from the front, back, and both sides. Comparison of the body's hemiplegic and nonhemiplegic sides provides information about the patient's symmetry. The clinician should observe the patient at rest; during sitting, standing, and lying; and while the patient is performing various functional activities. During movement any changes in posture and muscle tone of the head, neck, trunk, and extremities should be noted.

When asymmetries are noted, the occupational therapist begins to identify possible underlying causes. The practitioner moves the body part through the normal ROM, noting pain and deviations from movement. If resistance is felt, it is likely the result of abnormally high tone. If no resistance is felt but the arm feels heavy, abnormally low tone is the probable cause.

The clinician also observes any movement initiated by the patient on the weak side. *Associated movements,* which are normal, may occur when the patient attempts to move the weak side and the strong side responds by making the same movement. *Associated reactions,* in which the patient moves using compensatory movements or movements influenced by abnormal synergy patterns, are abnormal and should be avoided. The patient should also avoid excessive effort because the exertion can trigger abnormal reactions and movement patterns.

Comparison of the patient's movement pattern to the normal movement required for the same task reveals problem areas. For example, when a patient reaches for an object, the occupational therapist may note that the hemiplegic arm elevates and retracts at the shoulder, flexes at the elbow, supinates at the forearm, and flexes at the wrist and fingers. The trunk may also flex forward to position the hand nearer the object (Figure 21-18, *A*). In comparison, a normal pattern of movement might include trunk stability with scapular protraction, selective elbow extension with pronation, wrist extension, and finger flexion (Figure 21-18, *B*). When comparing the two sides, the OT practitioner can identify elements of abnormal patterns of movement. Understanding the components of normal movement, both in isolation and within the context of an activity, is essential to identifying abnormal patterns.

In NDT the evaluation and treatment processes are intertwined and integrated. While evaluating the patient's movement patterns, the clinician performs techniques to promote normal tone and facilitate controlled patterns of movement. The occupational therapist continuously assesses the effects of these techniques on the patient's movement pattern and adjusts treatment accordingly. The OTA receives information from the occupational therapist's evaluation so that activities that reinforce normal movement patterns can be provided in treatment. In addition, the OTA's observation skills should be

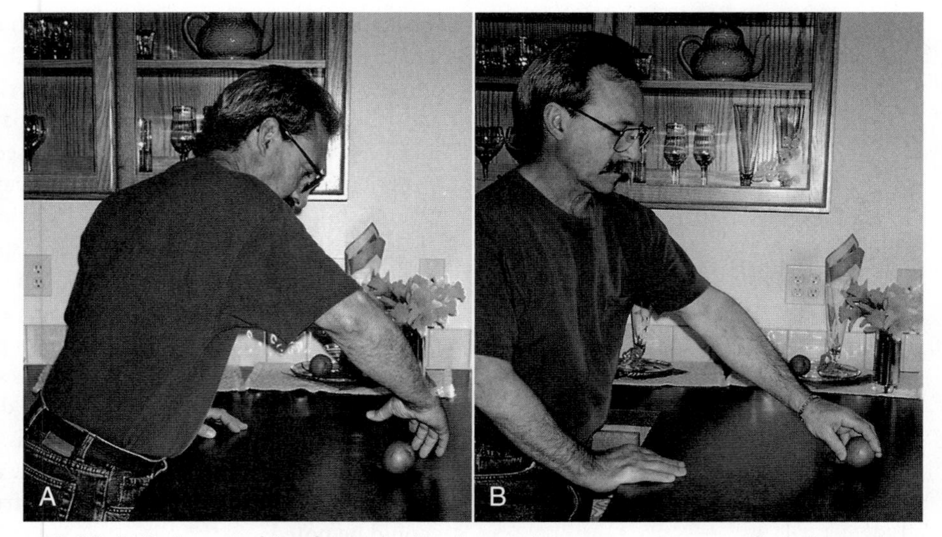

Figure 21-18 **A,** Patient reaching forward with abnormal movement patterns. **B,** Patient using normal movement patterns while reaching forward with uninvolved side.

developed so that adjustments in treatment can be made "in the moment," on the basis of actual patient performance.

Principles of Treatment

The goal of NDT is to normalize tone, inhibit primitive patterns of movement, and facilitate automatic, voluntary reactions and subsequent normal movement patterns. The amount of movement a patient demonstrates is not as important as the *quality* of movement performed. The quality of the movement evoked is more important than the amount of movement. During an examination of the quality of movement, the primary concerns are whether the patient exhibits good trunk control while moving, whether the movement is free from abnormal muscle tone and synergies, and whether the movement is coordinated.

Facilitation techniques and **inhibition techniques** are important tools in NDT. These techniques are used to normalize, or balance, tone. Normal tone fluctuates on the basis of activity demands; however, if tone is abnormally high or abnormally low, tone problems in movement can occur. The clinician must determine where tone is too high or too low and use techniques to normalize the tone. Therefore abnormally high tone is reduced (inhibited), and abnormally low tone is increased (facilitated). Once normalization of tone occurs, patterns of movement are used to allow the patient to experience the sensation of normal movement. These normal movement patterns are guided from proximal points of the body, primarily at the shoulder and pelvis ("key points of control"). The reduction of abnormal patterns of movement must be accomplished before normal, selective isolated movements can occur. Normal movement is impossible in the presence of abnormal tone.[6]

According to the Bobaths, normalization of muscle tone can be accomplished by using one or more of the following techniques[5,10,12]:

- Weight bearing over the affected side
- Trunk rotation
- Scapular protraction
- Anterior pelvic tilt/forward positioning of pelvis
- Facilitation of slow, controlled movements
- Proper positioning
- Incorporating the UE into activities

These techniques provide the foundation for NDT treatment. The techniques are most effective in rehabilitation when initiated in the acute (early) phase but can be used at any time in the treatment regimen.

Weight bearing over the hemiplegic side is an effective way to help regulate or normalize tone and is one of the most common techniques seen in the clinic. Weight bearing can be either facilitory or inhibitory. Weight bearing also provides sensory input to the hemiplegic side, which can increase the patient's awareness of the hemiplegic side.

Weight bearing through the UE while sitting or standing helps to normalize tone throughout the arm. Weight bearing is most effective with patients who display a flexor synergy of the UE. The patient can be brought into a weight-bearing position in preparation for a functional task during a treatment session.

Before weight bearing through the UE, the occupational therapist or OTA must prepare the UE and shoulder girdle. Preparations include scapular mobilization (gliding scapula into abduction, adduction, elevation, depression, and upward rotation). During UE weight-bearing activities, the patient's hand should be placed on a mat or bench several inches away from the hip to prevent wrist hyperextension. The humerus is placed in external rotation, with the elbow in extension. As the patient shifts weight over the hemiplegic side, the clinician should not allow the UE to rotate internally or the elbow to collapse. The patient should not hang on the arm during weight bearing but instead should move the body over the arm. This position will avoid undue stress on the elbow joint (Figure 21-19). Weight bearing should not be painful to the patient and should be avoided when hand pain or edema is present.

Trunk rotation, or the disassociation of upper and lower trunk, is another effective way of normalizing tone and facilitating normal movement. Patients with hemiplegia often have a

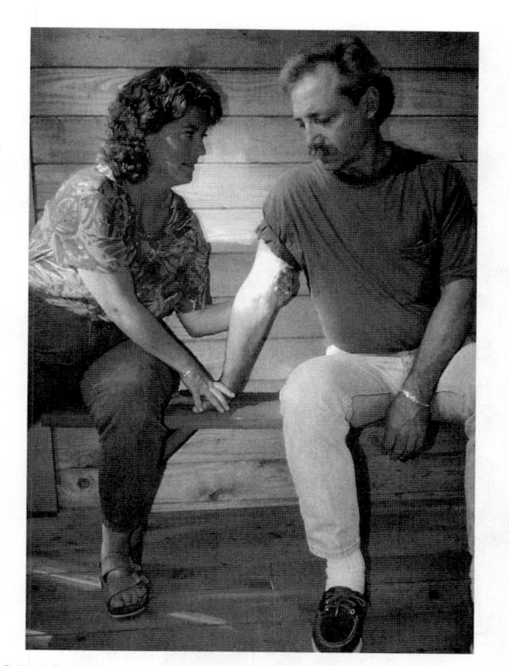

Figure 21-19 Proper position for weight bearing over hemiplegic side during functional activity.

difficult time separating shoulder movements from the pelvic girdle, thus exhibiting a "blocklike" pattern. To promote disassociation, the clinician should introduce activities that incorporate or facilitate trunk rotation. This activates trunk musculature and aids in trunk stability, which will enhance UE movement.

Trunk rotation performed in the sitting or standing position promotes weight shifting to the hemiplegic side. Additional benefits from trunk rotation activities include increased sensory input and improved awareness of the hemiplegic side and trained compensation for visual field deficits (Figure 21-20). Often the easiest and most effective way to facilitate trunk rotation is during functional daily activities.

Scapular protraction (scapular abduction) benefits patients who display a flexor synergy of the UE. Following the rule of working proximal to distal, the scapula should always be guided into forward protraction before the patient attempts to raise the hemiplegic arm or open the hand. The scapula can be protracted if the clinician cradles the arm with one hand while placing the other hand along the scapula's medial border and then brings the arm forward. Once it is forward, this position should be maintained for a few seconds before returning to the starting position. Care should be taken not to glide the scapula back into retraction. *Pelvis in anterior pelvic tilt position* is the optimal sitting position for patients with hemiplegia. This position provides proper alignment of the pelvis, shoulder, and head. Patients often assume a posterior pelvic tilt, which promotes abnormal posture such as thoracic spine flexion, scapular abduction, and cervical flexion. Such a posture has an adverse effect on swallowing, breathing, and visual-perceptual input. It also promotes misalignment of the shoulder girdle and encourages the flexor synergy of the UE. When performing reaching activities in sitting, the clinician may help the patient adjust the pelvis into a greater anterior tilt to promote more effective reaching patterns.

Slow, controlled movements should be facilitated in patients with high tone. Quick movements increase tone and tend to trigger an associated reaction, thus resulting in a flexor synergy of the UE; they should be avoided. Patients with high muscle tone should be instructed to perform activities slowly and in a controlled manner. The OT or OTA should provide feedback to help the patient recognize when an activity is performed well.

Proper positioning of the patient in bed, sitting, or standing facilitates the development of normal movement throughout the recovery process. It also helps to normalize muscle tone and provide normal sensory input to the body. For example, the preferred position for lying in bed is on the hemiplegic side[6,13] (Figure 21-21), with the patient's back positioned parallel to the edge of the bed; head placed on a pillow, avoiding extreme flexion; shoulder fully protracted with at least 90 degrees of shoulder flexion; forearm supinated and elbow flexed; and hand placed under the pillow. An alternate position is with the elbow extended and the wrist either supported on the bed or slightly off the bed. The unaffected leg should be placed on a pillow. The affected leg is slightly flexed at the knee, with hip extended. To prevent the patient from rolling onto the back, a pillow is placed behind the back and buttocks for support.

The proper position for sitting is with the patient placing both feet flat on the floor, the hips near 90 degrees of flexion, the knees and ankles at less than 90 degrees of flexion, and the trunk extended. The head should be in midline and the affected arm fully supported when working at a table. During standing, the weight should be equally distributed on both LEs, the trunk symmetrical, and the head in midline.[6]

Incorporating the UE into activity is important in promoting functional use of the involved UE. The involved UE can be incorporated via weight bearing, bilateral activities, or guided use. For example, during a writing activity, the patient can use the involved arm to bear weight and stabilize the pad. Also, the patient can assume a clasped hand ("prayer") position of both UEs to perform bilateral, assisted self-ROM, or therapists can guide and place the UE onto the arm of the chair when the patient is pushing up to stand. Incorporating the involved UE into the activity will help develop selective use and bring NDT strategies into daily activities.

Occupational Therapy Application

In the NDT approach the OTA should design activities that can incorporate the hemiplegic UE into routine daily activities. This practice helps to reinforce techniques and interventions that the occupational therapist uses in designing the treatment plan. As previously discussed, the OTA can incorporate the hemiplegic UE into activities in three ways: (1) weight bearing through the involved UE during functional activities (Figure 21-22, *A*); (2) bilateral activities (Figure 21-22, *B*); and (3) guided use (Figure 21-22, *C*).

Bilateral activity (see Figure 21-22, *B*) and guiding the affected UE (see Figure 21-22, *C*) help to discourage the flexion synergy and allow the hemiplegic arm to participate in purposeful activities. In addition, when performing bilateral

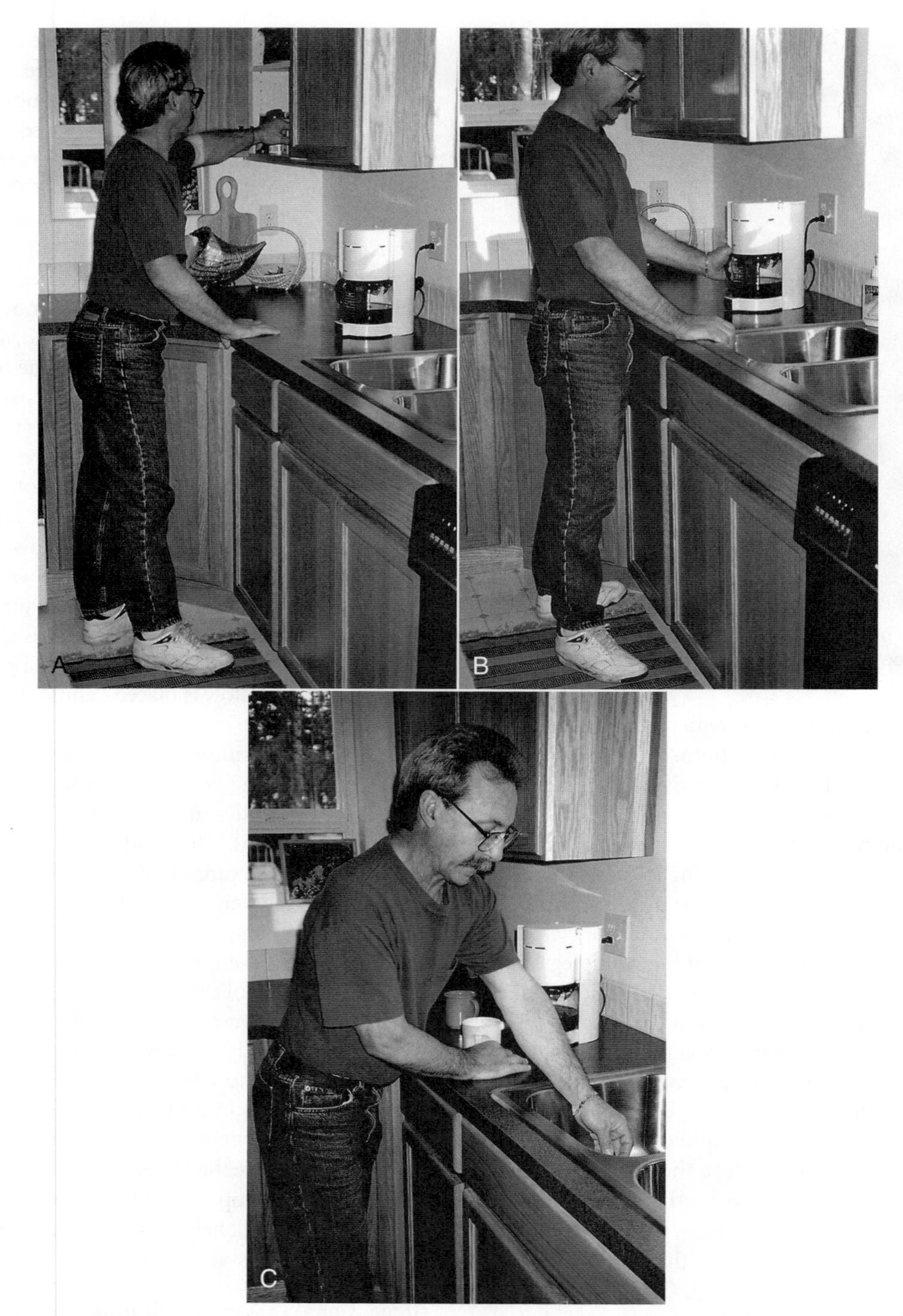

Figure 21-20 **A,** Trunk rotation, side to side, to high surface. **B,** Trunk rotation, side to side, to counter height. **C,** Trunk rotation, side to side, to lower surface.

activities, the patient experiences sensory input to the hemiplegic side and the hemiplegic UE is brought into the visual field. Seeing the UE can be beneficial to patients who have unilateral neglect or visual inattention. Guiding the affected UE is another way to incorporate the hemiplegic UE into activities and can help the patient experience normal movement patterns during purposeful activities.

When engaging patients in treatment activities using the NDT approach, the OTA should offer meaningful and practical tasks to enhance carry-over from selected normal movement patterns to functional performance. Patients can more easily attend to and be motivated by activities that relate to real-life situations.

Dressing Activities

Dressing and grooming activities are a part of almost every OT program. These activities are familiar, purposeful, and necessary for independent functioning. The following methods illustrate how NDT principles can be used in ADL training.

The patient should sit in a chair with a firm back when dressing. The chair provides stability and can improve balance. The same sequence should be followed to enhance learning.

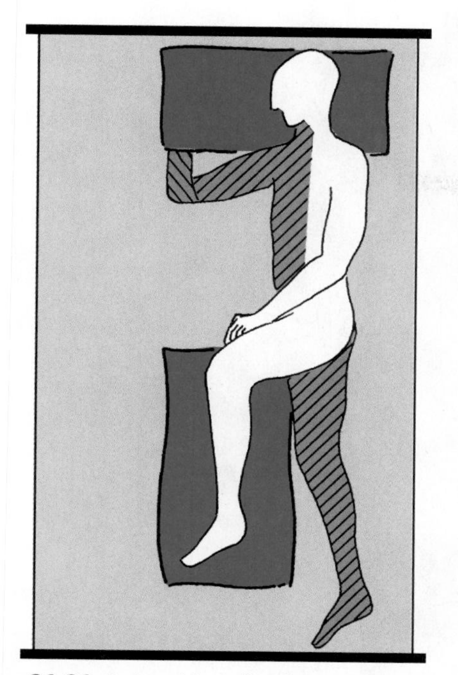

Figure 21-21 Bed position when lying on affected side.

Donning Shirt

1. Position shirt across patient's knees with armhole visible and sleeve between knees (Figure 21-23, *A*).
2. Patient bends forward at hips (inhibiting extensor synergy of LE), placing affected hand in sleeve (Figure 21-23, *B*).
3. Arm drops into sleeve; shoulder protraction and gravity inhibit UE flexor synergy.
4. Bring collar to neck.
5. Sit upright; dress nonhemiplegic side.
6. Button shirt from bottom to top.

Donning Underclothes and Pants

1. Clasp hands, and cross affected leg over nonhemiplegic leg (Figure 21-24). (Clinician helps when needed.)
2. Release hands. Hemiplegic arm can dangle and should not be trapped in lap. When able, patient can use affected hand as needed.
3. Pull pant leg over hemiplegic foot.
4. Clasp hands to uncross leg.
5. Place nonhemiplegic foot in pant leg (no need to cross legs). This step is difficult because patient must bear weight on hemiplegic side.
6. Pull pants to knees.
7. While holding onto waistband, patient stands with clinician's help.
8. Zip and snap pants.
9. Clinician helps patient return to sitting position.

Donning Socks and Shoes

1. Clasp hands and cross legs (as before) (Figure 21-25).
2. Put sock and shoe on hemiplegic foot.
3. Cross nonhemiplegic leg; put on sock and shoe.

Summary

CNS dysfunction, such as from a CVA or traumatic brain injury, can result in muscle imbalance and abnormal muscle tone, poor posture, decreased balance, and loss of controlled movements. Neurotherapeutic treatment approaches are used with patients who exhibit these deficits. These approaches link neurophysiological principles to the rehabilitation of patients with CNS dysfunction by targeting motor performance skills. In today's clinical practice, many of the techniques described in this chapter are used as adjunctive or preliminary techniques or are integrated into occupation-based treatment activities.

The four traditional neurotherapeutic approaches are the Rood, the Brunnstrom (movement therapy), PNF, and Bobath/NDT approach.

The Rood approach emphasizes the use of controlled sensory stimulation to achieve purposeful motor responses.[20] Rood's work laid the foundation for the use of sensory stimulation in clinical practice.

The Brunnstrom (movement therapy) approach describes stages of motor recovery after a CVA and applies treatment methods that help a patient progress through the recovery stages.

PNF uses a multisensory approach in which mass patterns of movement, usually performed in diagonals, help strengthen weak components of movements.

The NDT (Bobath) approach emphasizes relearning normal movement while avoiding abnormal movement patterns. Principles include the normalization of muscle tone, avoidance of synergistic movement, and incorporation of the affected side into purposeful activities.

These neurotherapeutic treatment approaches are valuable tools for the occupational therapist and OTA. Whenever possible, these techniques should be applied within an occupational context. OTAs planning to use these approaches should be trained and supervised until they achieve service competency. The challenge for all clinicians who use these approaches is to apply them in contexts that are meaningful and purposeful for the patient and that will promote independent functioning.

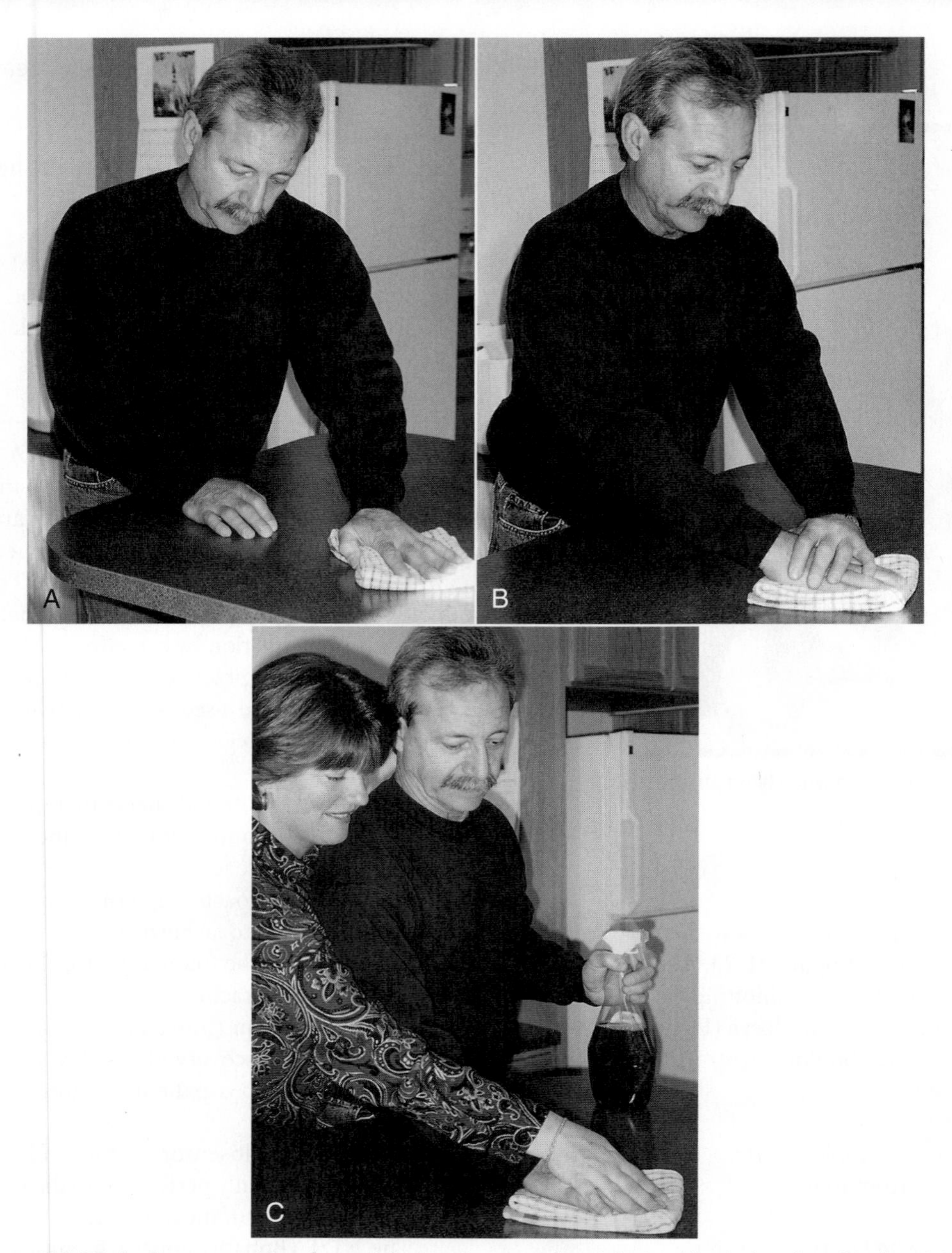

Figure 21-22 **A,** Proper position for weight bearing over hemiplegic side during functional activities. **B,** Bilateral use of upper extremity (UE) during functional activities. **C,** Guiding UE during functional activities.

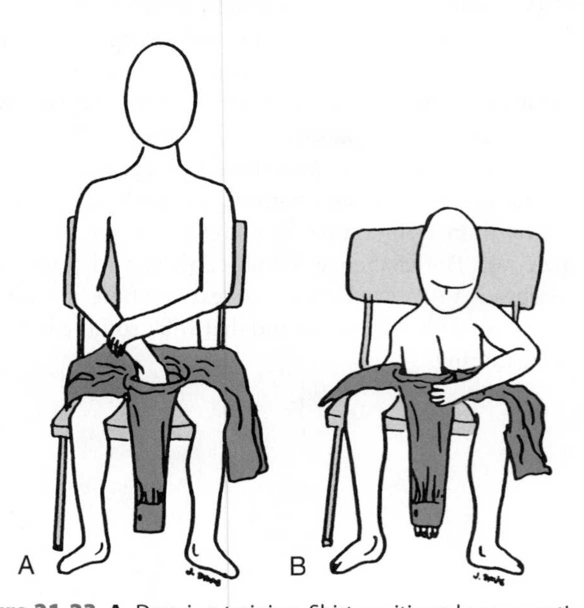

Figure 21-23 **A,** Dressing training. Shirt positioned across patient's knees; armhole visible; sleeve dropped between knees. **B,** Patient bends forward at hips (inhibiting extension synergy of lower extremity) and places affected hand into sleeve.

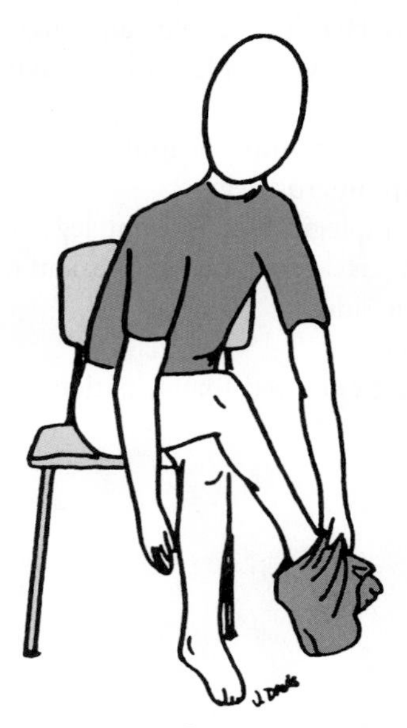

Figure 21-24 Proper position for putting on undergarments and pants.

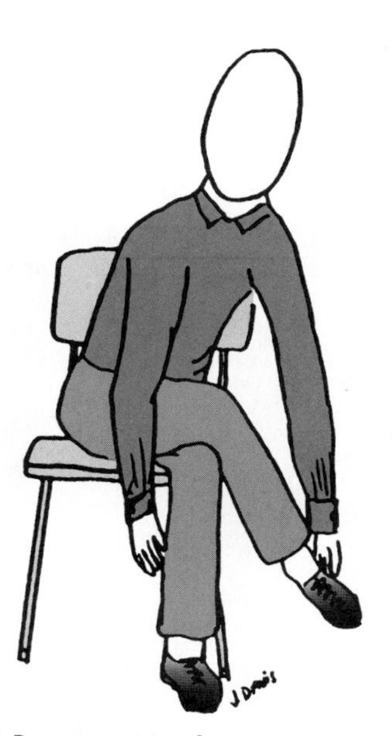

Figure 21-25 Proper position for putting on socks and shoes.

Selected Reading Guide Questions

1. Give two examples of patients for whom neurotherapeutic approaches are used.
2. List two basic goals of the Rood approach.
3. List the stages of recovery of arm function after a CVA, as described by Brunnstrom.
4. Describe the UE flexor and extensor synergy patterns.
5. Describe how tone of voice can be used in PNF treatment.
6. Identify the UE PNF diagonal used to bring the hand to the mouth during feeding.
7. Identify the primary goal of the NDT approach.
8. On the basis of the NDT approach, identify the recommended position in bed for a patient with hemiplegia.
9. Describe how the NDT techniques can be incorporated into a basic daily living task.

References

1. Alpern M, Lawrence N, Wolsk D: *Sensory processes*, Belmont, CA, 1976, Brooks/Cole.
2. Ayres J: *Sensory integration and learning disorders*, Los Angeles, 1972, Western Psychological Services.
3. Ayres J: *The development of sensory integration theory and practice*, Dubuque, IA, 1974, Kendall/Hunt.
4. Barr ML: *The human nervous system*, ed 2, New York, 1974, Harper & Row.
5. Bobath B: *Adult hemiplegia: evaluation and treatment*, London, 1978, Heinemann.
6. Brunnstrom S: *Movement therapy in hemiplegia*, New York, 1970, Harper & Row.
7. Calliet R: *The shoulder in hemiplegia*, Philadelphia, 1980, FA Davis.
8. Clark B: The vestibular system. In Mussen PH, Rosenweig MR, editors: *Annual review of psychology*, New York, 1970, Harper & Row.
9. Crepeau EB, Cohn ES, Boyt Schell BA, editors: *Willard & Spackman's occupational therapy*, ed 10, Philadelphia, 2003, Lippincott Williams & Wilkins.
10. Davis P: *Steps to follow*, Berlin, 1985, Springer-Verlag.
11. Dayhoof N: Re-thinking stroke: soft or hard devices to position hands? *Am J Nurs* 7:1142, 1975.
12. Eggars O: *Occupational therapy in the treatment of adult hemiplegia*, Rockville, MD, 1984, Aspen.
13. Eldred E: Peripheral receptors: their excitation and relation to reflex patterns, *Am J Phys Med* 46:69, 1967.
14. Farber S: *Sensorimotor evaluation and treatment procedures for allied health personnel*, Indianapolis, 1974, Indiana University—Purdue University Medical Center.
15. Farber S: *Neurorehabilitation: a multisensory approach*, Philadelphia, 1982, WB Saunders.
16. Goff B: The Rood approach. In *Cash's Textbook of neurology for physiotherapists*, ed 4, Philadelphia, 1986, Lippincott.
17. Gillen Glen: *Stroke rehabilitation: a function-based approach*, ed 3, New York, 2011, Mosby.
18. Heininger M, Randolph S: *Neurophysiological concepts in human behavior*, St. Louis, 1981, Mosby.
19. Hellebrandt FA, Schacle M, Carns ML: Methods of evoking the tonic neck reflexes in normal human subjects, *Am J Phys Med* 4:139, 1962.
20. Huss J: Sensorimotor treatment approaches. In Hopkins HL, Smith HD, editors: *Willard and Spackman's occupational therapy*, ed 6, Philadelphia, 1983, Lippincott.
21. Jackson JH: *Selected writings*, vol 1, London, 1931, Hodder & Staughton. J Taylor, editor.
22. Kotte F: From reflex to skill: the training of coordination, *Arch Phys Med Rehabil* 61:551, 1980.
23. Kotte F, Lehmann J: *Krusen's handbook of physical medicine and rehabilitation*, ed 4, Philadelphia, 1990, WB Saunders.
24. Loeb GE, Hoffer JA: *Muscle spindle function in muscle receptors in movement control*, London, 1981, Macmillan.
25. Loomis JE, Boersma FJ: Training right brain damaged patients in a wheelchair task: case studies using verbal mediation, *Physiother Can* 34:204, 1982.
26. Matthews PBC: Muscle spindles and their motor control, *Physiol Rev* 58:763, 1978.
27. McCloskey DI: Kinesthetic sensibility, *Physiol Rev* 58:764, 1978.
28. Myers BJ: *Proprioceptive neuromuscular facilitation: concepts and application in occupational therapy as taught by Voss*, Chicago, September 8-12, 1980, Rehabilitation Institute of Chicago (course notes).
29. Myers BJ: *PNF: patterns and application in occupational therapy*, Chicago, 1981, Rehabilitation Institute of Chicago (videotape).
30. Nolte J: *The human brain: an introduction to its functional anatomy*, ed 5, St. Louis, 2002, Mosby.
31. Perry C: Principles and techniques of the Brunnstrom approach to the treatment of hemiplegia, *Am J Phys Med* 46:789, 1967.
32. Rood M: Neurophysiological reactions as a basis for physical therapy, *Phys Ther Rev* 34:444, 1954.
33. Rood M: Neurophysiological mechanisms utilized in the treatment of neuromuscular dysfunction, *Am J Occup Ther* 10:4, 1956.
34. Rood M: The use of sensory receptors to activate, facilitate and inhibit motor response, automatic and somatic, in developmental sequence. In Sattely C, editor: *Approaches to the treatment of patients with neuromuscular dysfunction*, Dubuque, IA, 1962, Brown.

35. Schmidt RA: Motor learning principles for physical therapy. In Lister MJ, editor: *Contemporary management of motor control problems, Proceedings of the 11 Step Conference*, Alexandria, VA, 1991, Foundation for Physical Therapy.
36. Stockmeyer SA: An interpretation of the approach of Rood to the treatment of neuromuscular dysfunction, *Am J Phys Med* 46:900, 1967.
37. Vallbo A, Hagbarth H, Torebjard H: Somatosensory, proprioception sympathetic activity in human peripheral nerves, *Physiol Rev* 59:919, 1979.
38. Voss DE: Application of patterns and techniques in occupational therapy, *Am J Occup Ther* 8:191, 1959.
39. Voss DE: Proprioceptive neuromuscular facilitation: the PNF method. In Pearson PH, Williams LE, editors: *Physical therapy services in the developmental disabilities*, Springfield, IL, 1972, Thomas.
40. Voss DE, Ionta MK, Myers BJ: *Proprioceptive neuromuscular facilitation*, ed 3, Philadelphia, 1985, Harper & Row.
41. Williams P, Warwick R: *Functional neuroanatomy of man*, Philadelphia, 1975, WB Saunders.

CHAPTER 22

Interventions for Visual and Other Sensory Dysfunction

LORI M. SHIFFMAN

Key Terms

Somatosensory
Special sensory systems
Vision
Visual perception
Visual acuity
Oculomotor control
Visual fields
Visual attention
Visual scanning
Pattern recognition
Visual memory
Visual cognition
Cataracts
Macular degeneration
Glaucoma
Diabetic retinopathy
Age-related macular degeneration (ARM or ARMD)
Homonymous hemianopsia

Chapter Objectives

After studying this chapter, the student or practitioner will be able to do the following:

1. Explain how sensory dysfunction or the absence of sensation affects areas of occupation.
2. Understand the process of recovery from peripheral nerve dysfunction.
3. Give examples of compensatory strategies for clients with sensory loss caused by central nervous system or peripheral nervous system lesions.
4. For a client who lacks protective sensation, describe how the OTA would educate the client and his/her significant other(s).
5. Explain the importance of the client's visual history.
6. Understand the functional effects of common visual conditions and diseases.
7. Identify some remedial and compensatory strategies used for treatment of visual dysfunction.
8. Explain the role of the OTA when treating clients with visual-perceptual dysfunction.

Engagement in occupation relies on the ability to see, hear, feel, smell, taste, and balance; to organize sensations into meaningful representations of the world; and to plan and sequence responses.[2] Impairments in client factors (body functions and body structures) can affect functional performance.[2,52] Sensation is unique to each person.[18] The occupational therapist is trained to assess all areas of occupation within each client's context[2] and establish a treatment plan to address all problem areas. The occupational therapy assistant (OTA) should be aware of deficit areas in considering the approach to clients with sensory dysfunction. The extent of the OTA's role depends on the nature of the client's impairment. This chapter presents techniques the OTA might employ at entry level and also introduces interventions that the more experienced OTA practitioner, who has acquired service competency under qualified supervision, would provide.

This chapter has two sections: sensation and vision. Each section examines the treatment of that client factor, and each may be studied separately. However, the OTA will need to integrate considerable information from this chapter and from Chapter 23 to provide effective interventions in complex cases, such as the case study of Mr. J.

Normal Sensory Function

The sensory receptors receive information from the person's internal body structures and the external environment and send it to the brain for interpretation. When sensation is normal, this process works quickly and smoothly and is often not consciously perceived. Sensation is important for learning, motor performance, and protection.[9] Persons are often unaware of the importance of sensation until it is impaired or absent. When sensation is abnormal the process of receiving information can be slowed and disorganized, causing impairment.[52] Sensation is divided into the somatosensory and special sensory systems.[24] The somatosensory components include the primary senses (i.e., tactile, deep pressure, pain, proprioception, kinesthesia) and the cortical senses (i.e., two-point discrimination, stereognosis).[24] The special sensory system includes vision, hearing, smell, taste, and balance.[24]

CASE STUDY

Mr. J.

Mr. J. is a 48-year-old man diagnosed with multiple sclerosis 10 years ago. He was recently discharged from the acute care medical floor of the hospital to a home-based rehabilitation program after a recent exacerbation. At discharge, symptoms included blurred vision, numbness and mild spasticity of all extremities, mild intention tremors of the right dominant side, moderate intention tremors of the left side, overall weakness, balance issues, and limited endurance. Mr. J. is married and has two sons, aged 9 and 11. Mrs. J. works outside the home as a nurse consultant for an insurance company. Mr. J. did not receive any occupational therapy (OT) services before leaving the hospital. The referral for home services was for evaluation and treatment. The occupational therapist completed an evaluation at home and recommended treatment once weekly. The J. family lives in a one-floor ranch-style home especially designed for Mr. J. to accommodate his functional and mobility needs.

The occupational profile showed that before his most recent flare-up, Mr. J. was responsible for his own activities of daily living (ADL) and selected instrumental activities of daily living (IADL). He prepared breakfast and dinner for his family, worked as a website designer 16 to 20 hours a week from his home office, volunteered for his church by updating their website monthly from home, played board games or computer games with his sons, and read computer magazines and websites. Mr. J. attended church services every Sunday morning with his family.

Mrs. J. performs the majority of household tasks. The children help with some of the chores. Other family members provide assistance in tasks such as lawn care, home maintenance, home repair, and transportation. After Mr. J.'s most recent hospitalization, in the analysis of occupational performance the occupational therapist noted that Mr. J. feeds himself but spills his food and drink, washes his face and hands, partially dresses himself, and performs functional mobility independently. He toilets himself but requires assistance with bathing in the shower despite having a walk-in shower with built-in seat, grab bars, and shower hose. Mr. J. requires assistance to put on his socks and shoes. He requires much more time to perform these ADL and can no longer stand while performing any tasks. The only IADL he can now perform are heating up a prepared lunch in the microwave and "watching" his sons when they return home from school. Before his hospitalization he could walk short distances with forearm crutches, but he currently uses an electric scooter for all mobility.

Regarding performance skills, Mr. J. showed reduced attention and concentration, blurred vision with corrective lenses, double vision, decreased light touch and proprioception of both sides (left greater than right), lack of protective sensation of left hand, impaired memory, impaired body scheme, and visual agnosia. The client can stay up out of bed for about 60 minutes and then has to rest in bed about 2 hours afterward. Mr. J. stated that he values all of his life roles and would like to be able to prepare meals, play games with his children, read, volunteer for his church, and return to work. Mrs. J. has already returned to work because she has no more vacation days to use. The client is receiving physical therapy in the home once a week for management of increased tone, strengthening, and functional mobility.

Interventions for Sensory Dysfunction

Sensory dysfunction can result from damage to or diseases of the central nervous system (CNS), peripheral nervous system (PNS), or cranial nerves. Sensory dysfunction of CNS origin can be more generalized and cause sensory changes that affect the entire body, as occurs with multiple sclerosis (MS). CNS lesions may affect the entire contralateral (opposite to brain hemisphere) side of the body as a result of a cerebrovascular accident (CVA, stroke) or traumatic brain injury. Sensory changes that affect the PNS and cranial nerves are specific to the affected nerves. For example, palsy of cranial nerve III, the oculomotor nerve, may cause drooping of the eyelid, thus blocking vision. The spinal nerves innervate specific areas of the skin called dermatomes. Lesions can cause dulled or absent sensation in affected areas.

Some of the terms associated with sensory dysfunction are anesthesia (complete loss of sensation), paresthesia (abnormal sensation such as tingling or "pins and needles"), hypoesthesia (decreased or dulled sensation or hyposensitivity), hyperesthesia (increased tactile sensitivity or hypersensitivity), analgesia (complete loss of pain sensation), and hypalgesia or hypoalgesia (diminished pain sensation). Clients with hyposensitivity are at higher risk for injury because protective sensation is lacking, as in Mr. J.'s case. Clients with hypersensitivity may find touch so painful that they avoid it.

Sensory impairments severe enough to require treatment can make performing everyday occupations difficult.[2,52] Mr. J. has numbness of all four extremities, which causes him to require more time to complete tasks. He spends more time lying down after his flare-ups of MS symptoms. He is at higher risk for injury when performing tasks. He is prone to develop pressure sores, which can result from being in one position too long. The occupational therapy (OT) practitioner will educate him on the importance of protective techniques and weight-shifting every 30 minutes when sitting and changing position every 2 hours while lying in bed.

OT can improve the performance of persons with sensory changes or loss by teaching compensatory strategies and facilitating recovery (in some clients) of absent sensory function. The roles of the occupational therapist and the OTA in this area are complementary. The occupational therapist evaluates, plans treatment, and carries out remedial programs; the OTA teaches compensatory techniques and may assist in remedial treatment.

Because sensory changes or loss may have a significant effect on the patient's ability to function and to achieve fulfillment in everyday activities, the occupational therapist and OTA must promote sensory recovery or reeducation to the extent possible and teach safety precautions and compensatory techniques.

Treatment Guidelines

Before evaluation of sensory dysfunction can begin, the occupational therapist must know and understand the medical diagnosis, the cause of the sensory impairments, the prognosis for return of sensation, and the current progression of recovery. The results of the occupational therapist's sensory evaluation guide all treatment planning. Information from review of the client's chart and the evaluation will suggest whether the treatment approach should be remedial, compensatory, or both.

Remedial treatment employs the plasticity of the human nervous system to change the sensory response itself and to restore more normal sensory function. This objective is more successful with clients with reversible conditions (usually involving the PNS). Candidates for sensory reeducation programming should understand the purpose of the training. They should also be able to learn and practice the techniques and incorporate use of the involved body part in functional tasks.[9]

Compensatory treatment employs strategies for adjusting and adapting to sensory changes or losses. Such strategies include precautions to avoid injury, using other senses to obtain information, and environmental modifications. The OTA would teach Mr. J. (and his family) how to adapt the environment to compensate for blurred vision by increasing contrast (e.g., placing reflective tape on edges of tables, counters); adding proper lighting; and spacing objects in the home to allow for easier mobility and access. The OTA might suggest that Mr. J. use a magnifying mirror to see his face clearly when washing and an electric razor with a strap to help keep the tool on his hand. For his computing needs, if financially feasible, Mr. J. might consider an enlarged keyboard with tremor-dampening keys (and mouse control or alternatives), padded wrist support, and highlighted letters, as well as a larger monitor screen with enlarged font (print) and high contrast. These adjustments are only a few of the possible compensatory strategies.

This section now considers treatment approaches for the two major types of sensory dysfunction: CNS and PNS.

Central Nervous System Dysfunction

Effects of Sensory Changes

CNS damage can occur from trauma to the brain, conditions such as CVA, and diseases such as MS or Parkinson disease (PD). Resulting sensory changes or losses will diminish function. The inclination to move is based on how well sensory information is received and interpreted by the brain. Persons with poor sensation have little urge to move; those with dulled sensation such as Mr. J. have even less urge to move. Attempted movement may be clumsy or uncoordinated, even when muscle recovery is good. An example is trying to walk on a leg that has "fallen asleep." Although the leg muscles are still working, the sensation has changed, and the movements are awkward. Clients with sensory dysfunction are at much higher risk for injury, especially if they have cognitive deficits such as impulsivity, reduced safety awareness, or impaired memory. Such clients will require supervision for all tasks in order to prevent injury.

Sensory dysfunction can create functional difficulties in some or all of the areas of occupation.[2,52] Appetite may diminish because of changes in smell and taste. Loss of visual fields may result in bumping into door frames. Clients may cease attending community events because of hearing loss. Reduced tactile sensation may result in inability to feel the zipper pull when dressing or failure to notice that a brace is too tight, which could cause pressure sores of the lower leg. Hands may become frostbitten because of cold exposure. The client may stop playing piano because of an inability to feel the keys with one hand and the pedals with one foot. Severe chronic pain may prevent the client from working. Sensory dysfunction may worsen the effects of other deficits such as loss of motor control, reduced coordination, or left unilateral neglect.

In the case study, Mr. J. has shown impairments in ADL, IADL, work, play, leisure, and social participation. These impairments ensue from several deficits in body function including sensory function.[2,52] Mr. J. requires assistance in self-care, can perform only minimal caregiver and home management chores, has suspended his work role, has reduced play and leisure roles, and has experienced social isolation as a consequence of being alone at home and resting due to fatigue.

Client Education

Sensory recovery is a slow process that may stop at any time. Many clients may not have awareness of their sensory dysfunction and the effect on function. Because safety is primary, the clinician must teach clients, family members, or significant others about the sensory changes and how to protect the affected body parts while the client is performing all tasks. The first step is to help the client increase self-awareness by recognizing symptoms and then learning how to self-monitor. Therapy aims to increase the client's vigilance about safety issues. The clinician reinforces safety factors throughout all self-care training sessions. For example, Mr. J. can learn to check the water temperature with an unaffected body part such as an elbow before washing his face. The clinician's repeated verbal, visual, and tactile cueing may be necessary. The client should have many opportunities to practice skills and use them in daily tasks. If the client cannot self-monitor because of cognitive dysfunction such as inattention, reduced self-awareness, impaired memory, or poor judgment, the client will require constant supervision. The OT practitioner would teach the caregiver(s) how to modify the environment to help the client function safely despite sensory dysfunction.

> ***Safety Precautions for Clients with Sensory Impairment***
>
> The OTA should be aware of the type of sensory impairment for each individual client such as absent, dulled, hypersensitive, or mixed and understand all precautions and contraindications for treatment planning to promote function and prevent injury (such as compensating with vision).

Remedial Treatment

The purpose of remedial treatment for sensory loss due to CNS lesions is to promote recovery of sensation using at first preparatory methods, then purposeful activity and progressing to occupation-based activity. Traditional sensorimotor approaches have focused on promoting the return of muscle function of involved extremities using various forms of sensory input such as light touch, deep pressure, vibration, proprioception, and weight bearing.[7,8,34,41] Eggers[19] combined sensory reeducation using graded tactile discrimination training of the affected hand with neurodevelopmental treatment (NDT) of the involved upper extremity. Carr and Shepherd[10] used task performance to promote motor relearning, which they believe also assists sensory integration. The effectiveness of these techniques has not been conclusively proven. Other practitioners[54] have used sensory reeducation techniques to treat clients with sensory changes from CNS dysfunction (Box 22-1) with limited success as well. Health care providers untrained in sensory reeducation techniques can unintentionally injure clients. The OTA would not generally be providing these treatments but might participate in some aspects of treatment incorporating sensory retraining into functional activities as instructed, only under close supervision of the OT until service competency is well established. Care should be given to ensure that any sensory input does not increase spasticity.

Box 22-1

Elements of a Sensory Reeducation Program for Impairments of Central Nervous System[14,19,53]

Electrical Stimulation—Activation of sensory nerves to promote feeling and awareness of movement through functional electrical stimulation.

Progressive object discrimination—The practitioner presents a graded series of objects so that the client can see and hear the object while feeling it. The series begins with larger, three-dimensional, heavier, and more texturally distinct familiar objects. Later, vision is occluded, but the client is allowed to hear any sound the object might make when being felt. The client progresses to identifying smaller two-dimensional objects. Finally, the client is asked to identify the object through touch only, without visual or auditory information.

Functional activities—The client learns how to incorporate the involved body part(s) in purposeful activities leading to the ability to participate in areas of occupation.

Compensatory Treatment

Compensatory strategies help the client maximize safe performance in occupation by working around problems associated with sensory deficits.

Callahan[9] proposed guidelines for clients who lack protective sensation of the hand. The following is a modification of those suggestions, applicable to clients with CNS or PNS impairment.

- Avoid or limit exposure of the involved body part(s) to hot, cold, and sharp objects.
- Avoid tasks that require use of one tool for extended periods, especially if the hand cannot adapt by changing the manner of grip.
- Be conscious not to apply more force than necessary when holding a tool or object.
- Distribute forces evenly when using tools or objects, by enlarging the handle or using different tools. Change tools frequently to avoid too much friction, and rest involved areas.
- Use the uninvolved or less involved hand to perform household management tasks such as testing the bath water temperature, eating, and ironing.
- Use vision to observe movement and positioning of body parts such as looking behind the body to visually locate the commode seat.
- Observe the skin for signs of stress (redness, edema, warmth) from excessive force or repetitive pressure, and rest the area if these signs occur.
- Avoid wearing restrictive clothing, jewelry, braces, etc. over involved areas.
- Enlist help from caregivers to check for pressure sores in places that the client cannot see or feel.
- Follow a daily routine of skin care as recommended by the physician to keep skin soft and pliant.

Peripheral Nervous System Dysfunction

Effects of Sensory Changes

Peripheral nerve injury (PNI) may affect the nerve "cell body, the myelin sheath, axons, or neuromuscular junction."[35] Nerve fiber damage usually results from reduced circulation and is the mildest and most temporary form of PNI.[24] Complete recovery occurs within 3 months.[24] When the myelin (the outer coating of the nerve that insulates the axon) is damaged, regeneration occurs at a rate of about 1 mm per day.[35] The most severe injury involves the nerve cell body and results from penetrating wounds, crushing, or stretching.[24] Cell body regrowth is slow—about 8 mm per day[6]—and because several of the branches from the nerve trunks can be over 1 m in length, recovery may take several months to a year. Clinicians should always be aware of the type of peripheral nerve damage and the expected recovery period. During recovery, clients often experience increased sensitivity of the affected parts and may be tactilely defensive. They may guard sensitive areas and avoid using the affected part in bilateral functional tasks.

PNS dysfunction caused by PNI can result from a variety of causes: injury such as carpal tunnel syndrome; entrapment such as spinal stenosis; ischemia such as thoracic outlet syndrome[24]; metabolic diseases such as diabetes; infections such as Lyme disease or HIV; or inflammation such as Guillain-Barré syndrome. Damage can occur in one set of nerves or in several, depending on the cause. Symptoms of PNI include muscle weakness, hyperesthesia, hypoesthesia, lack of sensation, pain, muscle atrophy, loss of the ability to perspire, and changes in the quality of the skin and nails innervated by the affected nerves.[24] The skin can dry out and may be more easily injured. If the client has no open wounds or infection, early treatment of hypersensitivity is best—before sensory reeducation begins.[37] Desensitization is most often performed in hand and burn rehabilitation, which require advanced education and experience. Specific details of desensitization programs are beyond the scope of this chapter and the OTA's usual service competencies. A service-competent occupational therapist would use desensitization, a graded program including massage, vibration, tapping, or rolling over the involved areas with varied textures as tolerated by the client. This method aims to raise and normalize the client's pain threshold.

Client Education

The occupational therapist has the primary role in educating the client, family, or significant others by reinforcing information provided by the physician about recovery from PNI. The occupational therapist and the OTA act as a team, the OTA reinforcing what the occupational therapist has explained. The OTA has a more direct role during treatment involving ADL training; he or she explains the benefits of using the involved body parts as one way to help reduce hypersensitivity.[4] Use of involved parts in functional tasks may help clients reduce pain and increase comfort with movement. Clients usually perform better when they are in control and can move the involved body parts on their own with their uninvolved arm (in contrast to having someone else help them move). The OTA can also teach the client how to instruct others to help him or her move without causing discomfort. If cognitive dysfunction prevents the client from learning how to protect the involved part and perform functional tasks safely, the clinician will recommend that the caregiver(s) provide constant supervision. In this situation, the occupational therapist teaches the caregiver(s) how to modify the environment to help the client function safely. For example, the clinician might recommend Mr. J. install an antiscald valve on his water heater to prevent accidental burns when showering or using the bathroom or kitchen sinks.

Remedial Treatment

Remedial treatment or sensory reeducation is introduced after desensitization treatment is completed.[46] The purpose of remedial treatment or sensory reeducation is to promote recovery of dulled or absent sensation via appropriate sensory input. Sensory reeducation may also reduce sensory hypersensitivity and allow sensory desensitization through graded sensory input. Individuals with hypersensitivity overreact to "normal" sensations such as touch, light, and sounds, finding them unpleasant or noxious. The program begins with teaching the client how to use sensation.[46] When nerves in the hand are repaired or recover after injury, the messages to the brain are altered. The new pattern of neural impulses may be so different that the brain fails to identify the sensory stimulus, and the client may incorrectly interpret the sensory information. Sensory reeducation instructs the client how to reinterpret the sensory impulses reaching the consciousness and enhances the client's potential for functional recovery after nerve injury.[16,53] Although the occupational therapist generally provides sensory reeducation, the OTA with proven advanced proficiency could provide it under the occupational therapist's direct supervision. Box 22-2 shows some of the elements of a sensory reeducation program for deficits originating in PNI.[16] The OTA may assist, under close supervision, by incorporating specific techniques into activities that simulate those of the client's occupational roles.

Box 22-2

Elements of a Sensory Reeducation Program for Impairments of the Peripheral Nervous System[9,15,53]

Graded stimulation—First with client's eyes open, then with eyes closed, stimuli are graded to match recovery of different kinds of sensation during nerve regeneration. For example, the clinician moves an object such as a pencil eraser up and down the affected area to enhance sensation of moving touch. As this sense recovers, the clinician introduces constant touch, then gentle pressure.

Localization of stimuli—The client is asked to identify where the involved body part is being touched by the eraser.

Tactile discrimination, visual and tactile integration—The practitioner presents a grade series of objects so that the client can see and hear the object while feeling it beginning with larger, three-dimensional, heavier, and more texturally distinct familiar objects. The client works with vision occluded but can open the eyes if he or she cannot identify the item through touch. The client is asked to compare the sensation with how the object feels in the uninvolved hand. The task can also be graded by asking the client to locate items buried in rice, beans, or sand, while using touch only. This description helps the client to integrate visual and tactile information using both sides of the body.

Frequency of training—Training occurs two to four times daily for 10-minute sessions.

Compensatory Treatment

In addition to increasing the client's awareness of the specific sensory deficits associated with PNS dysfunction, safety is the first and major focus of compensatory training for clients with reduced or absent sensation, especially protective sensation. The OT would determine recommendations for each client. In some cases, it may be a better choice for the client to avoid using the involved limb during functional activities that are potentially unsafe, especially if the person is impulsive, inattentive, or lacks safety awareness. The client would then learn how to function safely with the lifelong impairment, which may or may not cause permanent disability.[52]

Summary of Interventions for Sensory Dysfunction

The skin receptors and sensory organs send information from the environment to the brain through the peripheral and spinal nerves and the spinal cord. Sensation provides information to the brain about the external environment necessary to guide purposeful and effective motor action. Sensory dysfunction disrupts the link between sensation and movement. The clinician should be aware of the type and extent of sensory dysfunction and expected recovery for each client. Lack of protective sensation can increase the client's risk for injury of the involved body part. OT practitioners can help improve the daily lives of persons with sensory impairments by maximizing safe, functional use of the involved extremity by providing remedial and compensatory treatments. There may be lifelong changes in sensation to which the client with sensory loss will need to adapt. Sensory reeducation and remediation require advanced training and should not be performed by the entry-level OTA.

Treatment of Vision Deficits and Visual-Perceptual Dysfunction

Understanding and using visual information require vision and visual perception. Vision is a sensory function,[2,52] referring to the reception of sensory information through the visual receptors. Visual perception is the process by which information from vision receptors is integrated with information from the other senses and interpreted by the brain. This process requires the brain to combine information from all of the senses: visual, proprioceptive (pressure), kinesthetic (sense of movement), tactile (touch), vestibular (balance and equilibrium), olfactory (smell), and auditory (hearing). In adapting to the environment, the brain puts together the separate pieces of sensory information it receives, integrating them to form a visual image of the environment. Because sensory information coming into the CNS is constantly changing, the picture, likewise, is dynamic and constantly changing as well. A person's decision on how to respond to a situation changes moment by moment with alterations in the person's sensory context (experience). Clients with altered vision or perception may require more time to make decisions or may make decisions on the basis of erroneous information.

Mr. J. has problems with blurred and double vision and the perceptual problems of impaired body scheme and visual agnosia (inability to recognize objects by sight). Visual, physical, and cognitive problems increase Mr. J.'s performance time for ADL. To address visual problems, the OTA could incorporate compensatory strategies into ADL training. For example, when working on upper body bathing, the clinician could spread out the supplies, increasing contrast by placing a white washcloth on a dark countertop or towel and using a colored liquid soap container. The client is encouraged to perform the task in the same sequence each time while identifying each body part in front of a mirror to improve body scheme awareness. The OTA could limit the number of items used, arrange to keep items in the same place at all times, and apply large-print waterproof labels to address visual agnosia.

Visual acuity—how clearly the human eye can discriminate detail and contrast—can be affected by nearsightedness, farsightedness, presbyopia, astigmatism, eye diseases, trauma to the eye, or CNS dysfunction. These eye conditions can cause damage to the eye structure or function.[52] In the United States, more than 30 million adults older than 40 are nearsighted and more than 11 and a half million are farsighted.[13] About 1 in 28 Americans aged 40 and older have low vision or blindness, a proportion that has increased due to the aging of the U.S. population.[13] Corrective lenses are usually required for nearsightedness and farsightedness. The OT practitioner should be aware of the client's preexisting visual acuity and whether the client wears corrective lenses. If so, the occupational therapist should know the type of lenses.

Nearsightedness, farsightedness, and astigmatism are often easily corrected with prescription corrective lenses (i.e., eyeglasses or contact lenses). As adults age, they typically require corrective lenses to read because of presbyopia or farsightedness associated with age-related changes of the lens. Clients who require correction for both nearsightedness and farsightedness wear bifocal lenses that correct both problems within the same lens. Occasionally some clients choose to wear contact lenses for distance viewing and reading glasses for near viewing or may wear two different contact lenses, one for distance and one for near. Other clients may need to wear only one contact lens for distance and can read without correction with the other eye. Some clients require trifocal lenses, which include a midrange distance. The lens of the eyeglasses may show a distinct demarcation of the different corrections within the glass lenses or may be unnoticeable, as with progressive lenses. Many modifications such as ultraviolet protection tinting, lightweight lenses and frames, lenses that stay light indoors and darken in the sunlight, and glareproofing are available. Laser eye surgery is an option some clients may have chosen to free themselves from need for any corrective lenses. However, everyone should wear sunglasses when outside to protect the retinas from the damaging ultraviolet rays of the sun.

The evaluation performed by the occupational therapist includes exploring the client's visual history, investigating the presence of visual symptoms, whether corrective lenses are used and for what purpose, the age the client began wearing glasses and for what purpose, age of current glasses and their condition, date of the last professional vision examination by a vision specialist, name of the vision specialist, the presence of eye diseases, and any history of eye injury or eye surgery. The OT then assesses visual functions including visual acuity, oculomotor control, and visual field testing. All clients who wear or need corrective lenses should have current eyeglasses or contact lenses that provide optimal corrected vision. It is not unusual for clients to have lost their glasses, attend therapy wearing outdated glasses, or have ill-fitting glasses or ones that require repairs. The occupational therapist shares his or her findings with the client and may consult with the client's physician to request a referral for a complete vision examination. The client may require a current vision examination to update a prescription or for other visual problems. The OT practitioner should consider vision problems including recommendations and devices recommended by the optometrist in treatment planning for every client.

Because Mr. J. has blurred and double vision with his glasses, he might benefit from a vision assessment to determine the most appropriate options to improve vision. The OT practitioner would assist the client in using his or her eyeglasses appropriately (e.g., wearing them to all therapy sessions as indicated). Reminders such as signs in a client's room or notes in the client's daily planner or memory notebook would remind the client and inform others that the client should always have his or her glasses. The clinician also includes eyewear use and care in therapy. Clients may need to practice putting on and taking off their glasses, cleaning them, putting them in and out of their case, etc. For clients who tend to misplace or lose their eyeglasses, a headband can secure the glasses and prevent loss. Damage to the brain can impair visual-perceptual functioning. Clients like Mr. J. gain more from visual-perceptual training when their vision has been corrected.

Visual Perception Organization and Processing

Visual-perceptual skills are organized in a hierarchy of levels that work together (Figure 22-1).[42] The ability to use visual-perceptual skills to adapt to the environment depends on the interaction of all of these skills at all levels.

One should read Figure 22-1 from the bottom. First, at the foundation level, the brain must receive clear, concise visual information from the environment. The three primary visual functions at this basic level are visual acuity, oculomotor control, and the visual fields.

Visual acuity ensures that the visual information sent to the brain is sharp, clear, and accurate. Oculomotor control occurs with effective coordination of eye movements by the eye muscles. The visual fields represent reception of complete information in the environment in all areas of vision. These primary visual functions act together so that humans can focus on and follow moving targets in the environment. These functions also provide the basis for all higher-level skills. In the case study, Mr. J. has blurred vision, thus indicating reduced visual acuity. Mr. J. also has double vision that may indicate eye misalignment or eye coordination deficits. Both these issues occur commonly in individuals with MS.

Visual attention, the next level in the hierarchy, involves fixating gaze on an image for as long as required and shifting to other objects as needed. When processing speed is reduced, the client must attend visually long enough to process all of the information. Mr. J. has reduced attention and concentration, suggesting that he has reduced visual attention as well.

Visual scanning consists of shifting attention from one vision target to another in smooth succession so that the person continues to see the image clearly no matter how much the eyes move. Scanning allows a person to focus vision gaze on a chosen object on the area of the retina with the greatest ability to process detail, even when the eyes, the head, or the object is moving. Mr. J.'s blurred and double vision may slow scanning speed.

Pattern recognition is the ability to identify the important features of objects and the environment and to use these features to distinguish an object from its surroundings[26] and objects from each other.

Visual memory is the next skill level in the hierarchy. The brain must be able to create and retain a mental image of the observed object in the mind's eye and store the visual image temporarily in short-term memory. The brain processes visual information in working short-term memory to produce a response. The brain also must be able to store the image in long-term memory and then remember the information from a selection of choices (recognition) or retrieve it from memory (recall), when needed. The difficulties with attention, concentration, and visual problems that Mr. J. has demonstrated would interfere with memory, which is also impaired.

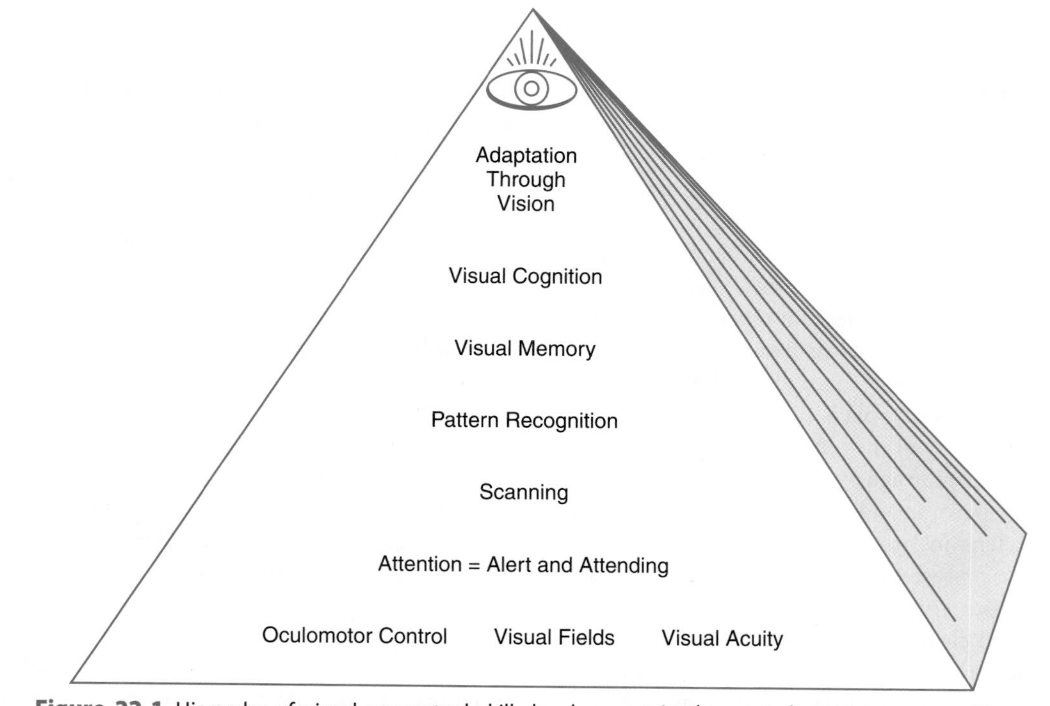

Figure 22-1 Hierarchy of visual perceptual skill development in the central nervous system. (Courtesy Josephine C Moore. From Warren M: A hierarchical model for evaluation and treatment of visual perceptual dysfunction in adult-acquired brain injury. Part I, *Am J Occup Ther* 47:42, 1993.)

The highest skill in the hierarchy is visual cognition, the ability to manipulate visual information mentally, understand the mental image, and integrate it with other sensory information, using all the other skills described in the hierarchy. Visual cognition serves as a foundation for all learning (i.e., reading, writing, mathematics, work, academic, leisure pursuits, etc.).

The brain works most efficiently only when all systems work together and allow clients to adapt to all environments. A disruption of any of the skills at any level in the hierarchy will reduce performance at that level and all the levels above as seen with Mr. J.

The evaluation of visual function requires an understanding of the role of vision at each skill level, which is the responsibility of the occupational therapist. Treatment for visual dysfunction focuses first at the level that has been disrupted. The following information is provided to prepare the OTA to provide treatment under supervision of the OT.

Deficits in Primary Visual Functions

Visual Acuity

Visual acuity is more than just the ability to read a line on the letter chart. It represents a complex interaction between the optical system, which focuses light at the back of the eye on the retina, and the CNS processing, which transforms that light into the visual images seen. The first stage of CNS visual processing begins at the retina, where the sensory receptors of the eye or photoreceptors respond to specific visual information in the environment and activate only when that stimulus occurs. The retinal field contains an estimated almost 1 million discretely coded photoreceptors that send detailed information on the spatial components of objects to the CNS for visual processing. This neural specificity enables the CNS to detect minute differences between patterns.

For the retina to resolve spatial information, visual images must be focused precisely. A defect in the external eye structures such as the cornea, lens, and optic media can result in poor focusing of images on the retina.

The four most common optical defects reducing acuity are myopia (nearsightedness), hyperopia (farsightedness), presbyopia (farsightedness associated with aging), and astigmatism (variations in curvature of the cornea). In myopia the image of an object is focused at a point in front of the retina and is blurred when it reaches the retina. Myopia is corrected by placing a concave lens in front of the eye. In hyperopia the image comes into focus behind the retina, causing blurred vision.[50] Presbyopia is caused by age-related changes or reduced elasticity of the lens of the eye. It occurs for many adults older than the age of 40 years and eventually affects most adults. Hyperopia and presbyopia are corrected by placing a convex lens in front of the eye. Persons with myopia, hyperopia, or presbyopia require a bifocal lens, which contains correction for each problem. In astigmatism, light cannot be focused clearly because the cornea is spoon shaped rather than spherical. This results in a blurring of the image and can be corrected with a prescription lens.

The clinician may see clients with conditions or diseases that affect vision such as cataracts, macular degeneration, glaucoma, and diabetic retinopathy. Preexisting vision conditions, which previously may have affected visual function minimally, may be a bigger factor in cases of neurologic dysfunction such as with CVA or traumatic brain injury.

Conditions affecting the lens such as cataracts can reduce the quality of the image projected onto the retina. More than 20 million adults older than 40 have cataracts[13] caused by aging, trauma, smoking, alcohol use, exposure to x-rays, systemic diseases such as diabetes, genetic factors, and exposure to UV light.[11] Cataracts affect one or both eyes and first develop in middle age or later. The incidence is expected to increase significantly in the next 20 years. Cataracts result in a gradual, painless loss of vision,[5] as if the person is seeing through plastic wrap. Early symptoms include loss of contrast, issues with glare, difficulty differentiating blue from black, and needing more light to see.[11] Treatment involves wearing thick lenses (because of severely reduced visual acuity) or surgical removal of the affected lenses, which are then replaced with an intraocular lens implant,[11] which restores significant if not all lost vision.

The health and integrity of the retina also influence the image quality sent on to the CNS. The macular area of the retina is particularly critical for identification of visual detail. Unfortunately, this structure is also vulnerable to several diseases that destroy its function including age-related macular degeneration (ARM or ARMD) and systemic diseases (e.g., diabetic retinopathy, hypertension).

ARMD is the leading cause of loss of central vision for older adults[21] and affects more than 1.75 million adults in the United States.[21] This number is expected to increase to 3 million by 2020.[20] There are two types: 90% of cases have dry and 10% have wet ARMD. Macular degeneration accounts for 90% of individuals who experience blindness.[21] Central visual loss is gradual and painless,[5,21] but peripheral vision stays intact. Central visual acuity is often 20/200 and is considered legally blind.[5] Macular damage also significantly reduces the ability to distinguish visual details and color[38] because the CNS does not receive sufficient information to identify main features. For example, human faces have little contrast between the features—that is, the nose is the same color as the forehead, cheeks, and chin, and eye and hair color blend with skin tones. For this reason, clients with macular loss almost universally have difficulty identifying faces, even of close friends and family members. They must rely on other characteristics of the person such as height, weight, hair color, clothing preferences, and voice to identify him or her. Individuals with ARMD can ambulate using their residual vision[38] but do not have sufficient vision to drive. There is no effective medical treatment to cure ARMD, but drug and laser treatment may slow its progression.[21] Clients with ARMD who require occupational therapy would be provided by the OT with advanced training in low-vision rehabilitation.[38]

Glaucoma, the second leading cause of blindness in the United States, affects more than 3 million adults and is caused by damage to the optic nerve, usually from increased pressure in the eye.[33] Peripheral or side vision loss occurs first, and central vision remains intact until the advanced stages of the disease.[33] Two types of glaucoma exist: open angle and closed angle. Open-angle glaucoma is the most common, painless type, occurring slowly as the result of clogged drainage canals of the eye.[33] Closed-angle glaucoma has a sudden painful onset. Risk factors include a family history of glaucoma, diabetes, African-American descent, and age 40 and older.[33] Medical treatment includes the lifelong use of eyedrops, surgery,[33] and oral medications. Although glaucoma is treatable, any visual loss is permanent and clients with glaucoma may require low-vision rehabilitation, provided by the OT with advanced training.

Diabetic retinopathy affects both eyes and is caused by dilation and leakage of blood from retinal vessels[13] or the growth of abnormal blood vessels on the retina.[30] The first symptom of retinal damage is often floaters or small spots of missing vision, progressing to blurred vision and then visual loss.[30] About 40% to 45% of Americans with diabetes are estimated to have diabetic neuropathy.[30] Control of blood sugar slows the progression of symptoms.[30] Laser surgery can be effective in treating the condition.[13,30] Clients with diabetic retinopathy usually have advanced diabetes and may have accompanying complications such as distal sensory loss, stroke, amputations, and heart disease. The OT practitioner should be aware of any low-vision needs in treatment programming. Again, low-vision rehabilitation might be provided by the OT.

The conditions discussed earlier affecting visual acuity are progressive to varying degrees and generally can be corrected by lenses, medications, or surgery. These interventions are provided by a vision specialist such as an ophthalmologist or an optometrist. The OT's role is to help clients compensate for reduced vision and maximize safety and functioning in all relevant areas of occupation. The OTA who wants to develop service competency can complete all the necessary requirements to achieve Low Vision Specialty Certification through the American OT Association.

Treatment Strategies for Visual Acuity

Reduced ability to see contrast or color and the loss of central or peripheral vision cannot be resolved by prescribing a pair of lenses. Instead, the OT practitioner teaches the client active compensatory strategies and helps him or her adapt the environment. Factors can be manipulated to make the environment more user-friendly to the individual with reduced acuity: background contrast, illumination, background pattern, size, and spacing.

The key to using contrast effectively is first to identify the critical items needed for orientation or identification in the environment and then to increase their contrast with surrounding features (e.g., by placing a light-colored object on a dark background). Individuals with low vision have difficulty distinguishing groups of colors that fall in the same value range such as the dark colors navy blue, brown, and black. Similarly, they will have difficulty differentiating light or pastel colors when used with each other.[40] Mixing colors of different values (light to dark) is more effective. Using a light plate with a dark edging might help Mr. J. see his plate more easily because of the increased contrast.

CLINICAL PEARL

To experience the dark-light value range, place a variety of objects that are similar in shape or kind but different in color next to each other on a table. Step back and squint. You will see that darker colors are hard to tell apart. And pastel colors tend to blend together. To achieve high contrast for a person with vision impairment, choose colors that look different when you squint (e.g., cream with navy blue, or yellow with black).

Increasing the intensity of available light for better illumination enables objects and environmental features to be seen more clearly and reduces the need for high contrast between objects. For example, facial features can be identified more easily if the person's face is fully illuminated. The challenge in providing light is to increase illumination without increasing glare. Natural and white lighting provide the best sources of high illumination with minimal glare and are recommended over standard fluorescent lighting for both room and reading illumination.

In addition to reducing glare, minimizing shadows is also important. The use of single bulb or recessed "can" lighting in hallways and rooms should be avoided; instead, long panels of fluorescent lights should be used. For reading, direct "white" (pure) lighting in the form of desk lamps or natural lighting provides the best illumination.

Patterned backgrounds have the effect of camouflaging objects lying on them. Even people with excellent vision have trouble locating an earring back or a small screw on a patterned carpet. Solid colors should be used for background surfaces such as bedspreads, bed sheets, placemats, dishes, countertops, rugs, towels, carpets, and furniture coverings.

Individuals with reduced visual acuity can more easily see information such as maps, photos, and print if the size is increased. Standard font size of print for the sighted population varies from 8 to 13.[27,51] Print size ranging from 16 to 20 is considered "large" and at 28 or greater is considered super large.[51] Specific changes in print proportions, character thickness, edging, or style can improve readability.[27] Given that most people have computer access, it can be quite easy to find and select the most appropriate font characteristics for each client with reduced visual acuity, which can be used to customize large-print reading materials, therapy instructions, client education materials, etc. Mr. J. might benefit from using large-print recipe instructions with color coding.

Spacing objects farther apart can further improve visibility. Clutter in an environment causes the same problems as pattern. A person who has difficulty identifying objects will perform better when asked to scan a kitchen shelf with a few orderly items rather than one with dozens of items. The same is true of closets, drawers, sewing baskets, desks, bookshelves, countertops, and clinic areas.

Oculomotor Control

The process by which the eye muscles control eye movements is oculomotor control. Oculomotor skills include alignment, range of motion, speed, and coordination. Deficits in oculomotor control can cause severe problems. To maintain a single visual image, the eyes must always line up evenly and move together. If the muscles of one eye are paretic (weakened), the eye may drift toward one side of the eye socket (i.e., drift either in or out). When the movement of one eye does not match that of the other, the person often sees a double image. This condition is known as *diplopia,* or double vision.[31] To eliminate the double image, the patient often holds the head in a position that reduces the need to use the paretic muscle (usually in the same direction as the weak muscle) or closes one eye. If the range of motion is affected, the person may not be able to move his or her eyes in all planes as quickly, causing difficulty with using the eyes together in a coordinated manner. Dysmetric eye movement, in which the eye undershoots or overshoots a target, may also be observed.[3,29]

These disturbances in the control of the eye muscles affect functional performance. Visual images may appear blurred or doubled, and the client may have difficulty focusing at different distances from the body, which would reduce depth perception. Compensating for double vision by closing one eye can further reduce depth perception. Deficits in oculomotor control create significant visual stress for the client, reducing attention and concentration and endurance for activities. In response to this increased visual stress, the person may complain of headaches, eye pain, eye strain, or neck strain. The client may be slower in scanning the environment, taking in visual information, and responding to the environment. In response, the client may become frustrated, agitated, and less cooperative in therapy. Treatment for oculomotor dysfunction should be coordinated by the occupational therapist with the guidance of vision specialists.[22,31]

Visual Fields

Numerous visual field deficits, some of which can limit the client's independence and functional mobility within the environment, exist. Homonymous hemianopsia, the loss of visual field in the corresponding right or left half in each eye, is the most common visual impairment observed after a CVA,[45] and one example of a "field cut." The OTA should observe the client with CVA for signs of a visual field deficit including (1) changing head position when asked to view objects placed in a certain plane; (2) consistently bumping into objects; (3) placing objects in one field; (4) problems finding easily seen items in the environment; and (4) making consistent errors in reading. Such observations should be reported to the occupational therapist. Clients with visual field deficits experience changes in several areas of performance that affect their ability to complete daily activities safely and effectively.

The most significant change occurs in visual scanning. Instead of spontaneously adopting a wider scanning strategy, turning the head farther to see around the blind field, clients tend to narrow their scope of scanning.[48] They adopt a more protective strategy, turning the head less; limiting their scanning to areas immediately adjacent to the body; and relying more on sensory input from the tactile, proprioceptive, and vestibular senses. This strategy for field loss occurs because the brain fills in (perceptually completes) any portion of the visual field that is missing, thus providing the viewer with the illusion of seeing a complete visual scene.[47] The person experiencing visual field loss is often unaware of any absence of vision[29] and may not be aware of the boundary between the seeing and nonseeing field. Instead, they (incorrectly) perceive a complete visual scene in which objects always seem to be appearing, disappearing, and reappearing without warning. Clients are less aware of objects and the environment because they have reduced the space in their world only to what they see, often directly in front of them. Therefore they have difficulty in tasks requiring awareness and scanning, especially in wider environments such as shopping malls.

If the central and particularly the macular portion of the visual field are affected, the client tends to miss or misidentify detail when viewing objects. Reading can present a challenge and cause frustration for the client. Words may often be guessed from context. Inaccurate reading of numbers is the more functionally limiting problem because numbers appear without context. Because Mr. J.'s visual problems would interfere with his ability to perform one of his favorite pastimes, reading, as stated previously in this chapter, the OT clinician might suggest alternatives such as large-print materials, an e-book reader with enlarged larger font and higher contrast, and perhaps audio books.

Depending on the size of the visual field loss and the side on which the loss occurs, the client may experience difficulty guiding the hand in writing and other near-vision tasks such as cutting. The top envelope in Figure 22-2 illustrates the handwriting of a client with right visual field loss. In attempting to address the envelope, the client would lose sight of the hand in the hemianopsic field on the right side and subsequently begin to drift downward on that side. The bottom envelope in Figure 22-2 illustrates the client's performance after training.

As part of the evaluation process, the occupational therapist would identify the presence of visual field deficits and recommend complete testing by a vision specialist such as an optometrist or ophthalmologist, who has the expertise to diagnose visual field cuts.

Intervention Strategies

In providing interventions for clients with visual field deficits, education and a combination of strategies are used. First the clinician works with the client to increase awareness of the dysfunction and effect on functional performance. Remedial strategies focus on increasing the speed, scope, and effectiveness of the scanning and saccadic patterns. The client must first learn the recommended head movements to compensate for any limitations in the visual field. Some clients will require special lenses prescribed by a vision specialist to help them compensate for field cuts.

Visual field deficits can affect all functional areas but have a primary effect on near tasks such as reading and writing, as well as on far tasks such as driving. Under the direction of the OT, the OTA would use activities relevant to the client that incorporate the recommended techniques to improve scanning and saccades in all visual fields including the involved ones. OT would work in conjunction with speech-language pathologists to address reading and writing issues.

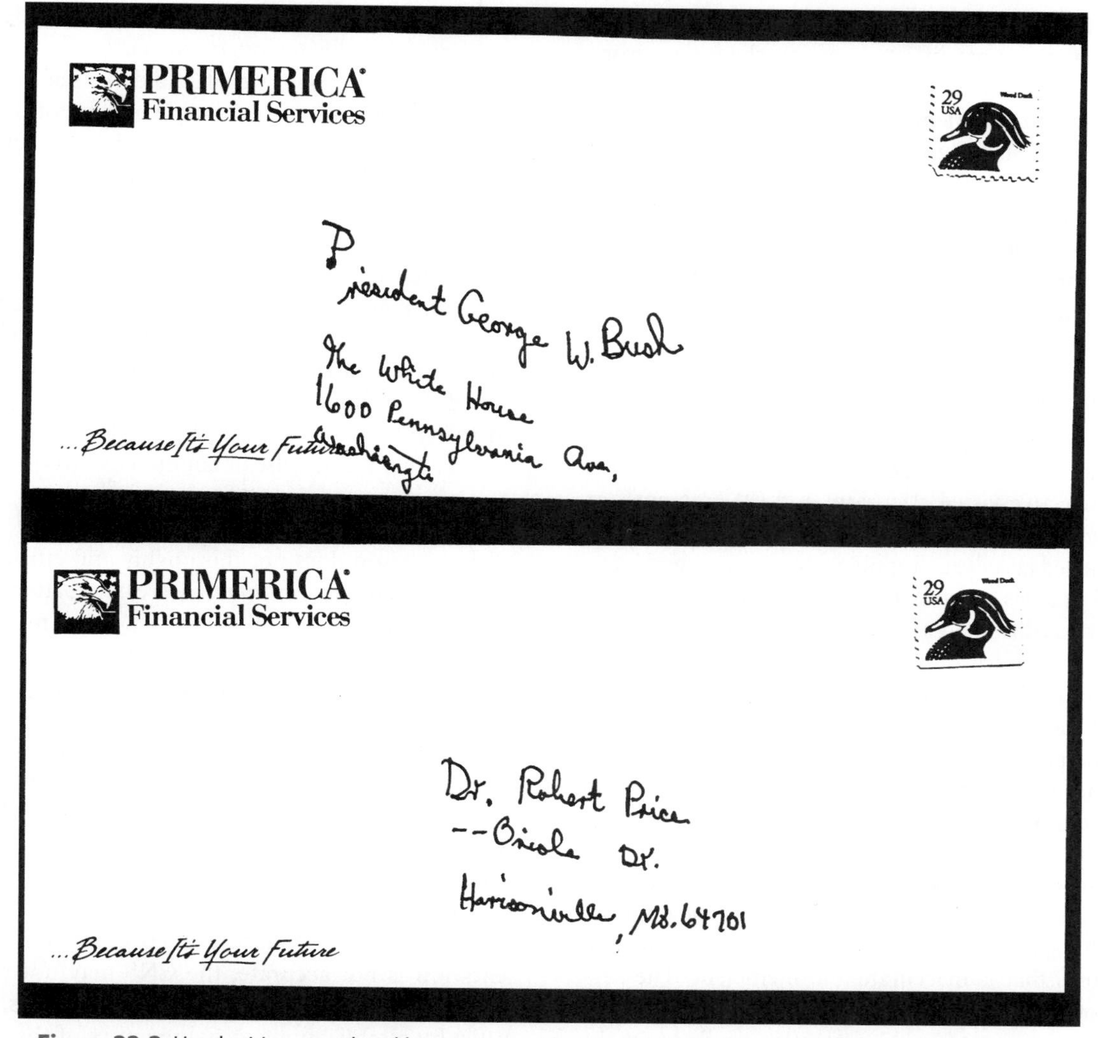

Figure 22-2 Handwriting completed by a patient with right-sided hemianopsia (hemianopia). Upper drawing depicts typical slant as pen moves into hemianopic field. Lower drawing shows improvement after training. (From Warren M: Visuospatial skills: assessment and intervention strategies. In Royeen CB, editor: *AOTA self-study series: cognitive rehabilitation,* Rockville, Md, 1994, American Occupational Therapy Association.)

When reading, clients with visual field deficits have difficulty locating the correct line of print, staying on the line, seeing all of the words, etc. For clients with hemianopsia, the OTA would address visual-perceptual and motor skills first because these are necessary for normal visual reading skills.[28] Clients with left visual field deficit typically do not move their eyes to the far left-hand margin of the reading material to begin a new line of text. Using boundary markers (e.g., lines, cards with red edges) and techniques such as teaching clients to look for the last letter of a word (rather than the first) are effective for hemianopsia.[51] The clinician teaches the client to move his or her eyes until he or she finds the red line to avoid missing any of the written material. If the client has difficulty staying on the line or moving down to the correct line, a ruler or card can be held under the line of print. These techniques can be employed when the patient is required to read a bill, financial statement, recipe, or cooking instructions. The client can also check off each line to help keep his or her place.

To learn how to stay on the line when writing, the OT practitioner teaches the client to watch the pen tip and maintain visual fixation as the hand moves across the page and into the area of visual field loss. Activities that require the client to trace lines toward the side of the field loss are effective in reestablishing the eye and hand connection. Contrast in writing can be heightened by using black felt-tip pens and boldly lined paper. Devices that offer feedback, such as a talking pen, also work well to train the client to monitor the pen tip while writing.

Driving "is a complex task requiring the integration of visual-perceptual stimuli, information processing, good judgment and decision making, and the performance of appropriate motor responses."[12] It is highly valued because it enables individuals to participate in a variety of areas of occupation.[12] Physicians usually recommend that clients with visual field cuts cease driving. In some states, such individuals are denied driving privileges. A client's ability to resume driving safely requires a specialized evaluation completed by qualified personnel (see Chapter 15). The extent of the difficulties depends on the size of the field deficit, the client's awareness of the problem, and the client's demonstrated ability to compensate for the deficit.

Additional compensatory strategies can enhance functional performance by modification of the client's environment. Adding color and contrast to the key structures in the environment needed for orientation (e.g., door frames, furniture, stair edges) assists the client in locating these structures. Reduction of pattern in the environment by decluttering it and using solid-colored objects can enhance the client's ability to locate items. For functional mobility in the community, the clinician instructs the client to walk in noncongested well-defined areas (e.g., grocery stores with shelving in high contrast with the floor).

Deficits in Central Nervous System Visual Skills

Visual Attention and Scanning

Visual attention can be divided into two categories: (1) focused[32] or selective visual attention; and (2) ambient[32] or peripheral visual attention. Focused or selective attention is used for structured tasks[32] such as object recognition and identification and enables persons to discriminate visual details accurately, such as differences between letters and numbers. It contributes greatly to learning. Ambient or peripheral attention is more useful in unstructured tasks[32] and allows people to detect and locate items in the environment. It relies on input from the peripheral visual field and mostly attends to moving objects. To have a fully functional and efficient visual system, the two modes of visual attention must work together.

Injury to the brain can disrupt normal scanning strategy. Visual scanning deficits associated with brain injury are characterized by avoidance in shifting the eye toward the opposite half of the visual space. The avoidance creates an asymmetrical scanning pattern that is inaccurate and inefficient. The person misses both detail and configuration in viewing objects and may fail to note some visual information needed to make accurate identification and decisions. When reading, clients with right hemianopsia experience the field cut as a blind spot moving down the line that can block the end of the line or long words.[51] Those with left hemianopsia may show difficulty starting at the beginning of each line.[51]

Visual inattention associated with right-sided brain injuries is often labeled visual neglect, left unilateral spatial neglect, hemi-inattention,[23] or hemispatial neglect.[51] Although neglect is often used to describe inattention to visual space occurring after left or right hemisphere lesions, research indicates that the condition primarily occurs with right-sided brain injuries.[51] Neglect is often confused with visual field deficits. Although both conditions may cause the client to miss visual information, they are distinctly different and do not have the same effect on the client's performance. When a visual field deficit occurs, the client may direct eye movements toward the side of the vision loss in an attempt to gather visual information from that side. Because of the field deficit, however, the client may not move the eyes far enough to see the needed visual information and thus miss visual information on that side. This performance may create a false impression of hemi-inattention or neglect. In contrast, the client with true hemi-inattention or neglect has lost the attentional CNS mechanisms that drive the search for visual information. The inattentive client makes no attempt to search for information on the left side of the visual space (as if that side no longer exists).[49]

The client with both visual field deficits and neglect misses visual information on the left side because of the field deficit and has no means to compensate for it by directing attention toward the left side. The presence of a visual field deficit exaggerates the inattentive behavior observed in the patient with neglect.[25]

Research has shown that normal adults scan in an organized, systematic, and efficient pattern.[22,44] The type of scanning pattern used depends on the demands of the task. In reading, a left-to-right and top-to-bottom rectilinear strategy is used. In scanning an open array (e.g., a room), a circular, left-to-right strategy is generally employed, with the eye following either a clockwise or counterclockwise pattern.

Pattern Recognition

When a person does not thoroughly and efficiently scan for objects in the environment, decreased pattern recognition results. Clients with right-sided brain injury may fail to recognize an object or pattern because they do not perceive or "see" all of it. Clients with left-sided brain injuries may be aware of objects but have difficulty identifying them.[17,36] Mr. J. has visual agnosia (inability to recognize and name objects), suggesting that he has left-sided brain involvement.

Visual Memory

Visual memory depends on accurate pattern recognition. When an important aspect of an object is overlooked, the brain generates an inaccurate representation. If the representation is not accurate, the CNS may not recognize the object or may misidentify it. When this occurs, the CNS has difficulty establishing a visual memory of the object. Mr. J. has demonstrated memory problems in conjunction with deficits in attention, concentration, and visual function. Therefore he probably would have difficulty remembering ADL sequences or recipes and would benefit from large-print signs (visual cues) posted in places in which he can easily see.

Because humans do not store information through vision alone, information stored in memory can be retrieved through other sensory channels. If a person does not recognize an object by looking at it, the person can pick it up and feel it or can ask someone to explain what it is. Thus a client with a visual deficit that results in inaccurate pattern recognition may still function reasonably well in ADL provided a variety of sensory information is available. However, as discussed earlier, function is likely to be impaired in the three daily living skills that rely almost exclusively on vision for performance (reading, writing, and driving). Given Mr. J.'s problems, the OT practitioner would address reading, functional mobility (instead of driving, which is contraindicated), and likely writing. Incoordination and sensory dysfunction would affect handwriting. Mr. J may benefit from using a weighted marker pen, which is easier to hold and requires less pressure, to practice writing, perhaps beginning with his signature, needed for daily functioning.

Visual Cognition

Visual cognition is the final product of the integration of all the foundation skills—visual attention, visual scanning, pattern recognition, and memory. Any deficit in these lower-level skills reduces the person's ability to apply these skills cognitively to function and adapt to environmental demands.

Deficits in visual cognition result in problems identifying the spatial properties of objects and mentally manipulating these properties in thought. Many terms are used to describe the deficits that occur in visual cognition. They include spatial agnosia, alexia, impaired visual closure, spatial relations, and figure-ground discrimination. Assessment of visual cognition is done by the occupational therapist[43]; the OTA provides treatment under supervision with guidelines directed by the OT.

Treatment Strategies

Treatment of visual-perceptual deficits is aimed at teaching the client to take in visual information in a consistent, systematic, and organized manner. Clients with inattention caused by right-sided brain injuries learn to reorganize their scanning pattern by beginning scanning in the impaired space (or left side) first.[48] Two scanning strategies are taught: a left-to-right rectilinear pattern for reading and a left-to-right circular pattern for scanning an unstructured array. Any therapeutic activity chosen to reestablish an organized scanning pattern is more effective if the patient is required to physically manipulate the objects scanned. Research has shown that a stronger mental representation of a visual image is formed if what is seen is verified by tactile exploration.[13] The OTA can incorporate the training of systematic scanning into ADL and other interactive tasks such as games (e.g., solitaire card games, dominoes, ball games, jigsaw puzzles, checkers).

Clients with left-sided brain injuries benefit from engaging in activities that emphasize conscious attention to detail and careful review and comparison of objects. These include any type of matching or sorting activity such as laundry, form boards, puzzles, or dominoes.

To improve the client's ability to scan, every activity should require the person to scan as broad a visual space as possible. The working field should be large enough to require the client to either turn the head or change body positions to accomplish the task. Some smaller spaces such as a closet in which the client looks for clothing do not require adaptation. Activities and games can be enlarged to require head turning for scanning; one example is playing tic-tac-toe on a chalkboard, with the letters at least 5″ tall.

To improve selective attention, the OTA teaches clients to study objects consciously, emphasizing items placed in the impaired space. Matching activities that require discrimination of subtle details are especially effective. Treatment may begin by using pairs of common objects such as toothbrushes, combs, etc., which may be easier to match because they are familiar. Also effective are games such as Concentration, Connect Four, checkers, Scrabble, dominoes, and 300- to 500-piece puzzles, word or number search workbooks, crossword puzzles, and crafts such as mosaic tiles. The OT practitioner encourages the client to double check his or her work to ensure that critical details are not missed. Success in regaining selective attention is related to the client's ability to learn and employ a conscious strategy to compensate for the deficits created by inattention.

According to Toglia,[39] clients with brain injury may overestimate their abilities, believing them unaffected by injury. Without a real understanding of their limitations, clients may not be able to understand fully the purpose of compensatory strategies. Overestimation of ability may contribute to reduced safety awareness, necessitating constant supervision for safety. To increase insight, Abreu and Toglia[1] advocate teaching clients how to monitor and control performance by learning to recognize and correct for errors. The clinician gives the client immediate feedback about performance and points out problems. The client is taught self-monitoring techniques such as activity prediction, in which the client predicts how successfully an activity will be performed and identifies aspects of the activity in which errors are likely to occur. The client then compares actual performance with predicted performance. Employing this technique helps the client become aware and anticipate how the deficit will affect functional performance.

A final treatment guideline is to practice the skill within context to ensure carryover to functional activities. Research has shown that brain-injured clients generally do not transfer skills spontaneously from one learning situation to the next. The OT practitioner therefore must have the client apply the learned strategy to different ADL contexts. Mr. J. could use the strategy of initiating organized search when selecting and gathering his supplies for upper body bathing or searching for items in a refrigerator or on a shelf. Repetition and practice in a variety of circumstances help the client generalize the skill and transfer it to new situations. Independent-living apartments, simulated work areas, and kitchens within the clinic may be used regularly in treatment. However, real-life situations, preferably in the community environment, are most likely to help the client develop insight into abilities and learn compensation for limitations. Cafeterias, gift shops, and office areas within the health care facility, and streets, fast-food restaurants, and shops near the facility can be used to expose the client to more realistic and demanding visual environments.

Mr. J. has several deficits within the visual-perceptual hierarchy. These changes can cause him to make errors in viewing and manipulating simple and complex visual information. In dressing training, Mr. J. could participate in a graded dressing program, beginning with the aspects he can perform without assistance and progressing to aspects in which he requires minimal assistance. Because of visual impairments, incoordination, and sensory deficits, he would not be a candidate for using a buttonhook to fasten buttons and would more likely benefit from wearing loose-fitting pullover shirts, adapting the shirt closure with a Velcro strip with buttons sewn on the outside to look like a buttoned shirt. He could benefit from learning how to arrange his clothing so that he can see the items to identify them more easily, which will also help him remember the dressing sequence. Initially, the OT practitioner would limit ADL training time to just over Mr. J.'s attention span to reduce frustration and fatigue and gradually increase training time with progress.

Vision Loss: Compensatory Techniques for Activities of Daily Living

Performing ADL may be overwhelming for the person with a new vision loss. Clients should be encouraged to use the remaining senses (hearing, taste, touch, smell) to gather and filter information. The occupational therapist or OTA teaches safety techniques first, breaking each activity into small parts and organizing all materials before beginning each activity. Starred items (*) could be incorporated into Mr. J.'s OT treatment program.

Eating

The newly vision-impaired individual may be concerned about whether his or her eating behaviors will be socially acceptable. Lack of confidence may lead the person to avoid social situations that involve eating foods that require the use of utensils. Initially, self-feeding with finger foods is recommended but should progress to eating food with utensils.*

General Suggestions

The client should learn the following:

1. Establish a point of reference with an object at the table such as a dinner plate. From this object, the placement of other objects can be determined. The place setting should be the same at every meal. Using the plate as a "clock" can help clients learn a frame of reference to recall the location of items.
2. Place the plate on a contrasting colored placemat.*
3. If meat is on the plate, it should be placed at the 6-o'clock position, where cutting will be easier.
4. Always maintain tactile contact with the table.*
5. Bend forward while eating (if there are no feeding problems) so that any food falling from the fork will land on the plate.
6. Estimate the weight, temperature, and texture of the food from the way it feels on the fork or spoon before placing it in the mouth.
7. Use a "pusher" (e.g., piece of bread or roll) to stabilize food so that the fork will pick it up.

Exploring Contents of a Plate

1. Depending on other factors, use of a spoon is recommended for all self-feeding.*
2. Check the location of contents on the plate using a fork or spoon periodically while eating. Ask others to cut meat and pour liquids as needed* until proficiency is achieved.
3. Hold fork with the tines turned downward.
4. Insert fork into food starting with the 12-o'clock position and working around the plate clockwise.
5. Identify food by texture and smell before placing it in the mouth.*

Cutting Food with a Knife and Fork

1. Locate knife and turn cutting edge downward toward the table. Hold knife in the right hand.
2. Hold knife in the right hand with index finger firmly along the handle and thumb by the side of the handle.
3. Hold fork in the left hand with the tines turned downward to the table and the index finger along the top surface of the handle.
4. Use knife to locate food (preferably placed at the 6-o'clock position) to be cut.
5. Place fork about 1 inch (2.5 cm) from the outer edge of the food to be cut, and cut bite-sized pieces by placing knife against the back of fork's tines and sawing back and forth firmly and slowly.

Simple Food Preparation

A large tray should be used to prepare foods; it should be a different color than the dishes, cups, and utensils. This strategy keeps all items together, minimizes the area to be cleaned, and makes carrying items to the sink easier.*

Pouring Cold Liquids

1. Use a thermal cup with a lid with spout or cut-out and straw for all liquids.*
2. Use a tall glass and center the container of liquid over the glass.
3. Before pouring, place the glass in the sink or a bowl to catch spills.
4. To estimate the level of the liquid as the glass fills, place the index finger (up to the first joint) over the lip of the glass. Electronic liquid level indicators are also available.
5. Note changes in weight, temperature, and sound as glass is being filled.

Opening a Container of Milk

1. Locate the seam of the milk carton. The side that should be opened is directly opposite this seam. Milk cartons are easier to open when taken directly from the refrigerator when the wax is stiffer.
2. Alternatively, locate the two indented lines on the top of the milk carton. These lines indicate that this is the side to be opened.

Buttering a Piece of Bread

1. Use softened tub butter or butter substitute that is easier to spread.
2. Use fingers or the feel of the knife's weight to determine the amount of butter on the knife.
3. Place bread either in the palm of the hand or on a plate. Spread the butter from the top right-hand corner to the lower right-hand corner. Then turn the bread 90 degrees counterclockwise and repeat the procedure.

Making a Sandwich

1. Apply sandwich spreads in same manner as for butter.
2. Use presliced cold cuts.
3. Cut a sandwich safely by first placing the thumb and index finger on either side of the bread so that an arch is formed. Then place the knife under the fingers in the center of the arch and cut the bread.

Mobility and Safe Travel

Most significantly vision-impaired persons receive training in techniques of orientation and mobility. This is a specialized program, with separate training, available to interested OTAs.

However, all OT practitioners should understand the basics of trailing and sighted guiding, techniques that can be used with the client inside and outside the home.

Trailing

This technique involves the use of the hands to trail along a smooth, stationery object in a straight line such as a wall or table edge.

1. Use the arm closest to the smooth trailing surface.
2. Person should hold the arm straight but not rigid, extending down in a diagonal.
3. The hand should lightly touch the trailing surface.

Sighted Guiding

The following is the recommended technique for a sighted person to guide a vision-impaired person when they are traveling together.

1. Guides should always ask the vision-impaired client to take their arm.
2. The client grasps the guide's arm lightly but firmly above the elbow, with thumb outside and fingers wrapped to inside of arm.
3. The guide holds arm relaxed, with elbow bent.
4. The client stands at the side of the guide, who walks in front with the client following a half step behind to ensure safety.
5. The guide should try to set a comfortable pace. If the client's grip tightens or if the client pulls back, slow down.

Protective Techniques for Safe Functional Mobility

These protective techniques are used to warn the vision-impaired person of unexpected and potentially harmful objects. These techniques are used most often in unfamiliar areas or in areas that may have been changed by others (e.g., repositioning of furniture). The two techniques given may be used separately or together.

Upper Body Protection (Upper Chest, Head)

For upper body protection the clinician teaches the client to do the following:

1. Bend forearm across the chest and touch the opposite shoulder.
2. Move hand forward so that it is about 12 inches (30 cm) from the shoulder, with the palm facing outward and the fingers held loosely.

Lower Body Protection

For lower body protection the clinician teaches the client to do the following:

1. Extend one arm forward and downward, placing it about 12 inches (30 cm) in front of the opposite thigh.
2. Turn palm to face the body, with fingers pointing toward the feet.

Telling Time

Low-vision aids such as magnifying glasses and telescopes may be used to view watches or clocks. Special timepieces with Braille, talking features, and large numbers with contrasting background colors can be obtained from the American Foundation for the Blind. However, the client will require training with any new device; therefore the OT practitioner should be familiar with low-vision aids. The occupational therapist may recommend the devices, and the OTA with service competency could perform the training.

Money Identification

The ability to manage money independently is an important functional skill.

Bills

U.S. currency of different denominations is the same size and color. The numbers have recently been enlarged but individuals who do not have sufficient vision to differentiate numbers can learn to use a system of folding. After someone tells them the domination, the system is as follows:

1. Singles should remain flat in the wallet.
2. Fives can be folded in half horizontally.
3. Tens can be folded in half vertically.
4. Twenties can be folded in half twice.

Coins

Coins can be identified through stereognosis, as follows:

1. Quarters are large and have rough edges.
2. Dimes are small and thin and have rough edges.
3. Nickels are thicker and wider than dimes and have smooth edges.
4. Pennies are smaller and thinner than nickels and have smooth edges.

Clothing Identification

Various methods may be used to mark clothing to assist in color matching such as the following:

1. Safety pins (e.g., one for red, two for green) may be attached to the label. Alternatively, French knots or iron-on patches may be used. Braille labels from the American Foundation for the Blind are also available.
2. Texture or identifying marks (e.g., fasteners, trimmings) may be used to identify certain garments.
3. Small dots of clear nail polish simulating Braille letters can be applied on the inside of the heel of shoes to identify color.

Summary

A variety of structures in the eye and brain are responsible for the processing of visual information. Whether a deficit in visual processing requires therapeutic intervention depends on the patient's lifestyle (i.e., their individual contexts) and whether the visual deficit prevents successful participation or causes permanent disability.[2,52]

OT evaluation and treatment of visual perception are based on a hierarchy of skill levels that are so interrelated that a skill function cannot be disrupted at one level without negatively affecting all perceptual processing. Intervention focuses on increasing the accuracy and organization of the sensory input into the system by remediating skills, adapting the environment, and teaching clients compensatory strategies to minimize the effect of deficits on functional performance. In addition, the experienced OTA might teach compensatory techniques to persons with vision loss to maximize functional performance and mobility.

Treatment of clients with visual and visual-perceptual dysfunction requires experience, expertise, and clinical reasoning skills. Although clients with visual and visual-perceptual deficits can recover, they may have residual lifelong losses to which they will need to adapt.[52] Some clients, such as Mr. J, may have accompanying deficits which may further reduce their ability to participate in areas of occupation.[2] The OT practitioner plays an important role in helping clients set and meet achievable short-term goals and long-term goals (Quote Box 22-1) in order to maximize health and participation through engagement in meaningful occupations.[2,52]

Long-Term Occupational Therapy Goal Identified by Case-Study Client Mr. J.

"Most important to me is taking care of my boys, helping out my wife some around the house, then maybe the church website. I think I could work in a few months when I'm not so tired all the time."

Selected Reading Guide Questions

1. Describe how sensory changes can cause problems in performance skills and body functions.
2. Compare and contrast the roles of the OT and the OTA in the treatment of clients with CNS and PNS dysfunction.
3. List some safety precautions used for clients with total sensory loss of one hand.
4. Explain how the OTA would treat a client who has sensory changes on the left side of the body and poor self-awareness of deficit areas. How would the OTA instruct the client's significant other(s)?
5. List three environmental modifications that would help a client with a severe deficit in visual acuity brush his teeth.
6. Explain what techniques a client with ARMD might use to play cards. How would her performance differ from a client who has advanced glaucoma?
7. A client tells the OTA that his glasses "don't work anymore." How might the OTA best handle the situation?
8. Describe how the OT practitioner would coordinate treatment with the client's vision specialist.
9. What happens to the eye that lacks oculomotor control? What happens to vision as a consequence?
10. Contrast the effects of a visual field loss with the effects of true hemi-inattention.
11. Describe the scanning pattern used to train clients with right-sided brain injuries to compensate for inattention.
12. Identify some strategies the client with a new and severe visual loss of both eyes would use on a trip to the grocery store.

References

1. Abreu BC, Toglia JP: Cognitive rehabilitation: a model for occupational therapy, *Am J Occup Ther* 41(7):439–448, 1987.
2. American Occupational Therapy Association: Occupational therapy practice framework: domain and process (ed 2), *Am J Occup Ther* 62:625–683, 2008.
3. Baker RS, Epstein AD: Ocular motor abnormalities from head trauma, *Surv Ophthalmol* 35(4):245–267, 1991.
4. Barber LM: Desensitization of the traumatized hand. In Hunter JM, Mackin EJ, Callahan AD, editors: *Rehabilitation of the hand*, ed 4, St. Louis, 1995, Mosby.
5. Beers MH, Berkow R, editors: *Merck manual of diagnosis and therapy*, Cataract, Hoboken NJ, 2004, John Wiley & Sons.
6. Beers MH, Berkow R, editors: *Merck manual of diagnosis and therapy, Disorders of the Peripheral Nervous System*, Hoboken NJ, 2004, John Wiley & Sons.
7. Bobath B: *Adult hemiplegia: evaluation and treatment*, ed 3, Oxford, 1990, Buttersworth-Heinemann, Ltd.
8. Brunnstrom S: *Movement therapy in hemiplegia*, New York, 1970, Harper & Row.
9. Callahan AD: Methods of compensation and re-education for sensory dysfunction. In Hunter JM, Mackin EJ, Callahan AD, editors: *Rehabilitation of the hand*, ed 4, St. Louis, 1995, Mosby.
10. Carr JH, Shepherd RB: *A motor relearning programme for stroke*, ed 2, London, 1987, Heinemann Medical Books.
11. Colby K: *Cataract, The Merck manuals online medical libraries*, July, 2008. http://www.merck.com/mmpe/sec09/ch104/ch104a.html. Accessed October 30, 2010.
12. Classen S, Levy C, McCarthy D, Mann WC, Lanford D, Waid-Ebbs JK: Traumatic brain injury and driving assessment: an evidence-based literature review, *Am J Occup Ther* 64:580–591, 2009.
13. Congdon N, O'Colmain B, Klaver CC, et al: Causes and prevalence of visual impairment among adults in the United States, *Arch Ophthalmol* 122(4):477–485, 2004.
14. Dannenbaum RM, Dykes RW: Sensory loss in the hand after sensory stroke: therapeutic rationale, *Arch Phys Med Rehabil* 69:833–839, 1988.
15. Dellon AL: *Evaluation of sensibility and reeducation of sensation in the hand*, Baltimore, 1981, Williams & Wilkins.
16. Dellon AL, Curtis RM, Edgerton MT: Reeducation of sensation in the hand after nerve injury and repair, *Plast Reconstr Surg* 53:297–305, 1974.
17. DeRenzi E: *Disorders of space exploration and cognition*, New York, 1982, Wiley & Sons.
18. Dunn W: The sensations of everyday life: empirical, theoretical, and pragmatic considerations (Eleanor Clarke Slagle Lecture), *Am J Occup Ther* 55:608–620, 2001.
19. Eggers O: *Occupational therapy in the treatment of adult hemiplegia*, Rockville, MD, 1984, Aspen.
20. Friedman DS, O'Colmain BJ, Muñoz B, et al: Prevalence of age-related macular degeneration in the United States, *Arch Ophthalmol* 122:564–572, 2004.
21. Garg SJ: *Age-related macular degeneration, The Merck manuals online medical libraries*, December, 2008. http://www.merck.com/mmpe/sec09/ch106/ch106b.html?qt=age related macular degeneration&alt=sh. Accessed October 30, 2010.
22. Gianutsos R, Matheson P: The rehabilitation of visual perceptual disorders attributable to brain injury. In Meier MJ, Benton AL, Diller L, editors: *Neuropsychological rehabilitation*, New York, 1987, Guilford.

23. Gianutsos R, Ramsey G, Perlin RR: Rehabilitative optometric services for survivors of acquired brain injury, *Arch Phys Med Rehabil* 69(8):573–578, 1988.
24. Gutman SA, Schonfeld AB: *Screening adult neurologic populations*, Bethesda, MD, 2003, AOTA.
25. Halligan PW, Marshall JC, Wade DT: Do visual field deficits exacerbate visuo-spatial neglect? *J Neurol Neurosurg Psychiatry* 53(6):487–491, 1990.
26. Jules B: Preconscious and conscious processing in vision. In Chagas C, Gattass R, editors: *Pattern recognition mechanisms*, 1985, Exp Brain Res III (suppl).
27. Kitchel JE: *Large Print: Guidelines for Optimal Readability and APHontTM, a font for low vision*, 2004. http://www.aph.org/edresearch/lpguide.htm. Accessed October 31, 2010.
28. Leff AP, Scott SK, Crewes H, Hodgson TL, Cowey A, Howard D, Wise RJS: Impaired reading in patients with right hemianopia, *Ann Neur* 47:171–178, 2000.
29. Leigh RJ, Zee DS: *Neurology of eye movements*, Philadelphia, 1983, FA Davis.
30. National Eye Institute—National Institutes of Health: *Facts about diabetic retinopathy*, October, 2009. http://www.nei.nih.gov/health/diabetic/retinopathy.asp. Accessed October 31, 2010.
31. Neger RE: The evaluation of diplopia in head trauma, *J Head Trauma Rehabil* 4(2):27–34, 1989.
32. Rensink RA: Seeing seeing, *Psyche* 16(1):68–78, 2010.
33. Rhee DJ: *Glaucoma, The Merck manuals online medical libraries*, August, 2008. http://www.merck.com/mmhe/sec20/ch233/ch233a.html. Accessed October 31, 2010.
34. Rood M: Neurophysiological mechanisms utilized in the treatment of neuromuscular dysfunction, *Am J Occup Ther* 10(4), 1956.
35. Rubin M: *Peripheral nervous system and motor unit disorders—Introduction*, February, 2008. http://www.merckandcoinc.net/mmpe/sec16/ch223/ch223a.html. Accessed October 25, 2010.
36. Scheiman M: *Understanding and managing vision deficits: a guide for occupational therapists*, Thorofare, NJ, 1997, Slack.
37. Schutt AH, Opritz JL: Hand rehabilitation. In Goodgold J, editor: *Rehabilitation medicine*, St. Louis, 1988, Mosby.
38. Sokol-McKay DA, Michels: Facing the challenge of macular degeneration: therapeutic interventions for low vision, *OT Practice* 10(9):10–15, 2005. http://www.aota.org/Pubs/OTP/1997-2007/Features/2005/f-052305. Accessed October 30, 2010.
39. Toglia JP: Generalization of treatment: a multicontext approach to cognitive perceptual impairment in adults with brain injury, *Am J Occup Ther* 45(6):505–516, 1991.
40. Vision Aware: *Home modifications for people who are blind or have low vision*, 2010. Accessed on October 31, 2010.
41. Voss DE: Proprioceptive neuromuscular facilitation: the PNF method, *Am J Occup Ther* 8:191, 1956.
42. Warren M: A hierarchical model for evaluation and treatment of visual perceptual dysfunction in adult acquired brain injury, parts 1 and 2, *Am J Occup Ther* 47(1):42–66, 1993.
43. Warren M: Evaluation and treatment of visual deficits. In Pedretti LW, editor: *Occupational therapy: practice skills for physical dysfunction*, ed 5, St. Louis, 2001, Mosby.
44. Warren M: Identification of visual scanning deficits in adults after cerebrovascular accident, *Am J Occup Ther* 44(5):391–399, 1990.
45. Warren M: Pilot study on activities of daily living limitations in adults with hemianopsia, *Am J Occup Ther* 63:626–633, 2009.
46. Waylett-Rendell: Sensory reeducation. In Crepeau E, Cohn E, Boyt Schell B, editors: *Willard & Spackman's occupational therapy*, ed 10, Baltimore, 2003, Lippincott Williams & Wilkins.
47. Weil RS, Watkins S, Rees G: Neural correlates of perceptual completion of an artificial scotoma in human visual cortex measured using functional, *MRI NeuroImage* 42(4):1519–1528, 2008.
48. Weinberg J, Diller L, Gordon WA, et al: Visual scanning training effect on reading-related tasks in acquired right brain damage, *Arch Phys Med Rehabil* 58(1):479–486, 1977.
49. Wikipedia: *Hemispatial neglect*, August 28, 2010. http://en.wikipedia.org/wiki/Hemispatial_neglect. Accessed November 6, 2010.
50. Wikipedia: *Hyperopia*, October 28, 2010. http://en.wikipedia.org/wiki/Hyperopia. Accessed on November 6, 2010.
51. Wikipedia: *Large-Print*, July 2010. http://en.wikipedia.org/wiki/Large-print. Accessed on October 31, 2010.
52. World Health Organization: *International classification of functioning, disability and health (ICF)*, Geneva, Switzerland, 2001, World Health Organization.
53. Wynn Parry CB: *Rehabilitation of the hand*, London, 1981, Butterworth.
54. Yekutiel M, Guttman E: A controlled trial of the retraining of the sensory function of the hand in stroke patients, *J Neurol Neurosur Psychiatry* 56:241–244, 1993.

CHAPTER 23

Intervention for Disturbances in Cognition and Perception*

REGI ROBNETT

Key Terms

Orientation
Attention
Memory
Thought functions
Higher-level cognitive functions
Remedial approach
Adaptive approach
Transfer-of-training approach
Generalization
Functional approach
Categorization
Domain-specific training
Executive functions
Neurodevelopmental treatment
Astereognosis
Apraxia
Ideational apraxia
Ideomotor apraxia
Compensatory approach

Chapter Objectives

After studying this chapter, the student or practitioner will be able to do the following:

1. Describe basic cognitive deficits and how they may affect functional performance.
2. Compare and contrast remedial and adaptive approaches for the cognitive impairments that affect occupational performance.
3. Describe strategies for the treatment of specific cognitive deficits.
4. Identify intervention strategies used to assist the client with deficits in executive function such as reasoning, judgment, awareness, and behavioral control.
5. Identify the effects of perceptual deficits on functional skills.
6. Compare and contrast remedial and adaptive approaches for perceptual impairments affecting occupational performance.
7. Articulate the challenges of working with clients who have cognitive and perceptual impairments.

"The human brain is the most magnificent system in the universe."[45]

Our brains control everything we do, from breathing, to complex movement sequences, to solving complicated problems. Cognition (i.e., thinking, learning, and memory skills) and perception (i.e., interpretation of in-coming sensory information) are challenging client factors to address in occupational therapy (OT) practice. Whereas physical client factors such as decreased range of motion or strength can be observed directly, impaired cognitive or perceptual skills can only be *inferred* through the client's behavior. Performance skills are "observable, concrete, goal-directed actions"[21] that form the building blocks of tasks within various areas of occupation. The occupational therapist focuses on evaluating and treating cognitive and perceptual performance skills (bottom-up approach) or engagement in occupations (top-down approach).

The occupational therapy assistant (OTA) has a distinct role working with clients who have cognitive and perceptual impairments. The range of services provided in this role depends on various factors: the OTA's experience level and service competencies, familiarity and skill level in this practice area, the intervention setting, and the geographic location including the influence of state practice laws. Where a shortage of medical personnel exists (e.g., in rural communities and general medical settings), the OTA may work with people who have cognitive and perceptual disorders more frequently. Clients present with cognitive and/or perceptual deficits in all intervention settings; therefore all OTAs should be familiar with these problems and know appropriate cognitive and perceptual intervention techniques to enhance performance skills.

Recognizing the OTA's important and variable role in intervention for deficits in client factors related to cognition and perception, as well as their effect on performance

*Doreen Olson, Lorraine Williams Pedretti, Barbara Zoltan, and Carol J. Wheatley contributed large portions of this chapter to the first and second editions of this book.

skills in relation to activity demands, this chapter presents a number of important concepts OTAs should understand and techniques OTAs might use. It is understood that the OTA will take responsibility to acquire the necessary service competency under qualified supervision and/or gain the required knowledge through educational opportunities before implementing these techniques. Settings and jurisdictions differ in guidelines for OTA services; the OTA is responsible for learning relevant guidelines and for following them to ensure compliance with state and national regulatory agencies.[1,2,67]

This chapter is divided into two sections: cognition and perception. Although these are not isolated from one another (and often are intertwined), the chapter separates them for ease of understanding. Each section examines foundational concepts and intervention techniques related to client factors, performance skills, and areas of activity in varied contexts. The section on perception includes a discussion of the interaction between perception of sensory input and subsequent motor actions because these are intricately linked in producing occupational performance outcomes.

Occupational Therapy Intervention for Those with Cognitive Impairments

This section outlines basic intervention for clients with deficits in cognitive functioning. The goal is positive functional change.[55] The OTA would not be expected to design an individualized cognitive retraining program but certainly may assist in its implementation. An understanding of basic intervention techniques is essential.

According to the *OT Practice Framework 2nd Ed* (OTPF-2e),[1] client factors related to cognitive performance skills include the following:

- *Global mental functions* such as level of alertness and orientation, energy, motivation, and emotional stability;
- Attention including sustained, selective, alternating, and divided;
- Memory (short to long term) including working memory and various types of memory such as procedural, prospective, semantic, and episodic;
- Thought functions including recognition, categorization, and being able to generalize ideas;
- Higher-level cognitive functions such as insight/judgment, awareness, concept formation, metacognition, and mental flexibility.[1]

The OTA might consider cognition in relation to the underlying skills necessary for planning and carrying out performance in activities of relevance to the client, be these in the occupational areas of activities of daily living (ADL), instrumental ADL (IADL), rest and sleep, education, work, play, leisure, and/or social participation.[1] These underlying skills include, but are not limited to, the following:

- *Judging* such as deciding on appropriate clothing for the weather or deciding on a life partner;
- *Selecting* such as choosing ingredients for a recipe or the correct amount of change for a cup of coffee;
- *Sequencing* such as determining the correct order of dressing (e.g., socks before shoes) or repairing a broken faucet;
- *Organizing* such as planning a party or making sure all school assignments are done by the deadline;
- *Prioritizing* such as deciding how much time is necessary to complete a task and how important it is to get the task done in relation to other commitments (e.g., work or volunteer duties);
- *Identifying* such as coming up with solutions to a life problem (e.g., finding transportation to an event); and
- *Creating* such as engagement in artistic endeavors for pleasure.[1]

The *Framework*[1] also includes *multitasking,* which would be doing a combination of skills simultaneously. However, because people with no impairment often have difficulty doing more than one task at a time effectively, the OTA should consider what might be a reasonable expectation for a client with neurologic impairments. In general, completing one skill at a time is probably as much as can or should be expected.

Two primary intervention approaches are used: the remedial approach, which focuses on restoring cognition to its former level (or as close as is feasible), and the adaptive approach, which focuses on adapting the task and/or the environment to enhance occupational performance. The occupational therapist who is designing the intervention for the specific client may decide to use one or the other or both approaches simultaneously. With regard to the realms of cognition and perception, OT practitioners may also use health promotion, maintenance, and prevention approaches.[1] (See pp 657-659 in the OTPF-2e for details on the different types of OT approaches.)[1]

Remedial Approaches for Cognitive Deficits

"Cognitive rehabilitation is goal oriented, and while problem focused, builds on strengths."[55]

Remedial approaches seek to improve or restore cognitive skills. Remediation involves engagement in tasks that will enhance recovery from an acquired brain injury. Alternately, brain "exercises" may be used to promote cognitive performance in tasks requiring certain cognitive skills. The underlying assumption is that the brain can reorganize itself and new learning can take place. Sometimes this approach is also referred to as the transfer-of-training approach.[23] Pencil-and-paper and tabletop activities may include various cognition-based worksheets such as word problems, crossword puzzles, word/letter finds, mazes, math computations/problems, copying designs, sequencing tasks, and image replications. These activities are intended to be introduced at a level just above the client's present cognitive level. Given encouragement and support from the practitioner as needed, the clients are encouraged to challenge their current level of thinking and responding and aspire to a higher level (e.g., more accurate or quicker). The activity is scored for accuracy; deficits or improvements in the areas of motivation, attention, and concept formation are noted. Additional distractions may be added during the activities, as improvement occurs, to test the extent to which the client can continue to perform in a more complex context. The key to success with remedial cognitive approaches is the ability of the client to "transfer" this improving ability with paper and pencil exercises to real-life situations. For example, doing math computations on paper would be expected to also help in calculating the amount of money needed to purchase items at a store.

The remedial approach is also used while the client is engaged in real-life tasks of interest (not contrived cognitive exercises). For example, intervention to improve money management may actually involve purchasing items and counting change. In this case the assumption is that repeated practice in a task at a level that is challenging, but not overwhelming, can also lead to improvements in the cognitive performance of that task. Neistadt[42] long ago promoted the use of functional tasks such as meal preparation as superior to contrived exercises. The occupational therapist would be expected to design interventions to include the "just-right" cognitive challenge. The OTA would be involved in carrying through these interventions and noting details of the client's successes or difficulties.

Computer-based activities provide a means to practice cognitive skills and may be a valuable tool for rehabilitation. However, evidence indicates that cognitive retraining software used in isolation, rather than under the direction of a skilled professional, is not necessarily an effective means to enhance life skills.[11,12] Similarly, Dickenson and colleagues,[17] in a randomized controlled trial of computer-based training for people with schizophrenia, found that although the computer-based skills of their participants improved, these skills were not carried over to improved performance in everyday tasks. Computer-based cognitive games and exercises such as Brain Train or Captain's Log are available (Figure 23-1). Commercial educational programs and specialized software can provide graded treatment modules focusing on specific areas of cognition such as remediation of arithmetic skills, attention, concentration, concept formation, memory, reasoning, association, categorization, cause-and-effect reasoning, problem solving, organization, generalization, level of abstraction, judgment, safety awareness, spatial orientation, sequencing, and verbal memory. Software programs can be used in the clinic as an adjunct to therapy or as a home program but should be used in the context of skilled intervention.

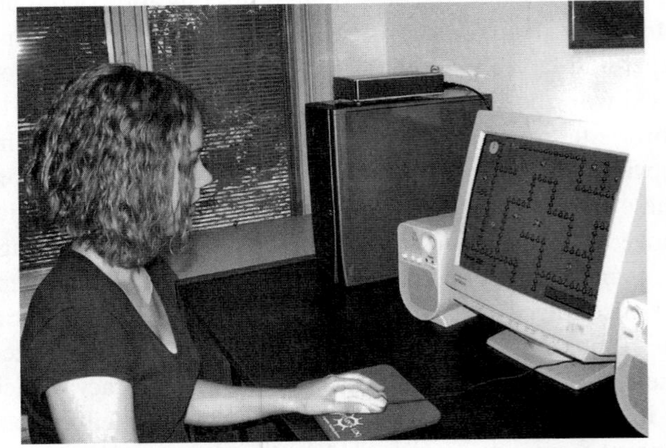

Figure 23-1 Various computer games or activities target cognitive skills such as problem solving, generalization, categorization, and attention. (Courtesy BrainTrain, Inc., Richmond, Va.)

"To improve cognitive functioning, 'the ideal time to intervene is throughout the entire lifespan before functional problems emerge' (Vance, Roberson, McGuinness, Fazeli, 2010, p. 24)."

Adaptive Approach

The adaptive approach (also called the functional approach) uses intact cognitive skills to compensate for deficits. Variations of the adaptive approach focus on context, activity demands, and performance patterns such as habits and routines. Engaging in occupations that are meaningful to the client is fundamental to the adaptive approach.[23] The assumption is that impairments are likely to be long term, so the goal is to maximize performance by adapting to or working around the deficits. Using the adaptive approach in the realm of cognitive intervention can involve many aspects, individualized for the client by the treating occupational therapist. Global examples include written reminders for decreased memory, sequence lists for enhancing ADL performance, and referring to "what-if" scenarios to handle emergencies. In providing intervention, the occupational therapist or OTA considers the context in which the individual will ultimately perform tasks and assists in adapting the situation for successful performance. See Table 23-1 for additional examples.

Optimal intervention may involve shifting roles for clients, altering or reducing demands placed on them, or giving them less challenging responsibilities in relation to other members of the family, while maintaining their participation to the fullest extent possible. For example, a client who can no longer safely

Table 23-1 Examples of Treatment Approaches

Approach	Activity Example: Buttoning
Adaptive approach (also known as *functional* and *compensatory*)	Change physical context such as simplify object (use colored buttons) Change performance pattern such as habit or routine (grade the task down into a simple perceptual sequence by starting to button at the bottom of the shirt) Change activity demands or modify the intervention (sewing up part of a button shirt to eliminate buttoning)
Remedial approach	
Sensory-integrative	Repetitive movement sequence with added tactile input, weight, and soft music playing during dressing
Neurodevelopmental	Manual tactile cueing with facilitation and approximation toward midline during buttoning/dressing intervention
Transfer-of-learning	Use a button board or buttoning game before learning buttoning on self

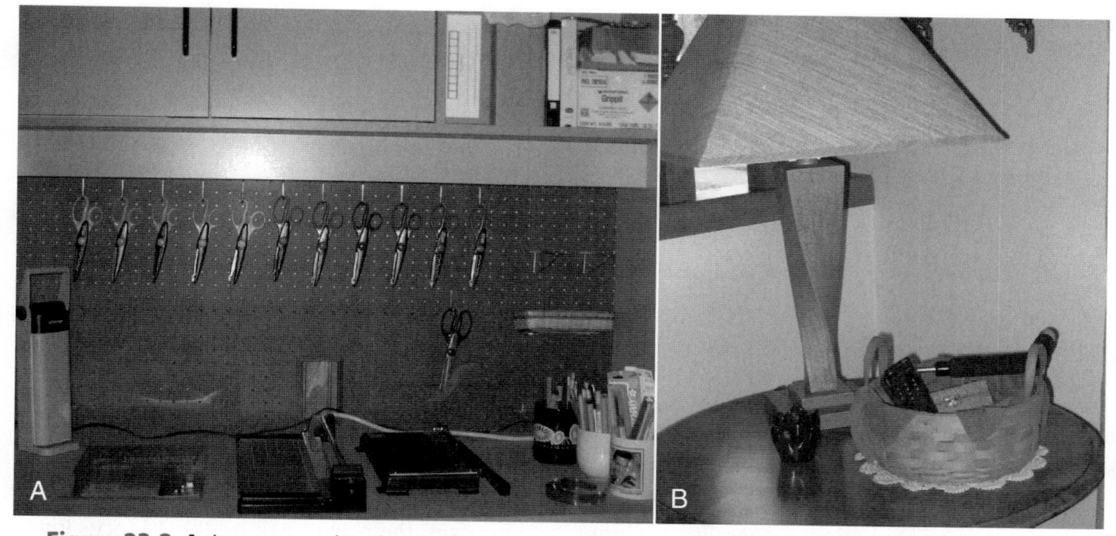

Figure 23-2 **A,** Items on and in the desk are arranged by use, labeled, and clutter free. This environment assists the patient to maintain or recall the use of various tools for the leisure task of scrapbooking. **B,** Exercise tools and remote controls are stored in the basket near the couch to remind the patient to complete his or her exercises when watching television.

sequence the steps for laundry completion may benefit from shifting responsibility to another family member. Perhaps the client could fold the clothes or do other individual steps of completing laundry instead of the entire chore. If cooking is no longer safe, then engagement in portions of meal preparation such as peeling potatoes or setting the table may be more appropriate. Programs such as "Meals on Wheels" may provide a nutritious alternative. Remediation involving returning to cooking in a graded or adapted format might be possible if cognitive skills are likely to improve. Again, using the adaptive approach does not preclude using remediation for some skills at the same time or at some point in the intervention process.

"Habits hold together the patterns of ordinary action that give life its familiar character."[30]

Intervention may focus on establishing routines to enable successful participation in daily tasks. Habits and routines that provide order and consistency in the flow of activities will reduce demands for decision making by the client.[30] To assist in establishing routines, the OTA may use daily checklists, introduce a systematic filing system, set up a regular and perhaps simplified ADL schedule, and/or set up the environment for the client to easily complete specific tasks in a predetermined sequence (Figures 23-2 and 23-3). Routines are "patterns of behavior that are observable, regular, repetitive, and that provide structure for daily life."[1] Repetition and consistency over time are necessary for a routine to become fully established into an automatic behavior. Habits, which are internal repetitive behaviors with little or no conscious awareness, may be produced as a result of the establishment of routines. As the routine and habits are established, the client should be able to complete the task with greater ease, accuracy, speed, and better overall performance.[30]

Internal strategies may be used if the client has sufficient awareness and is motivated to improve performance.[49,50] The OTA can assist by reinforcing these strategies. For example,

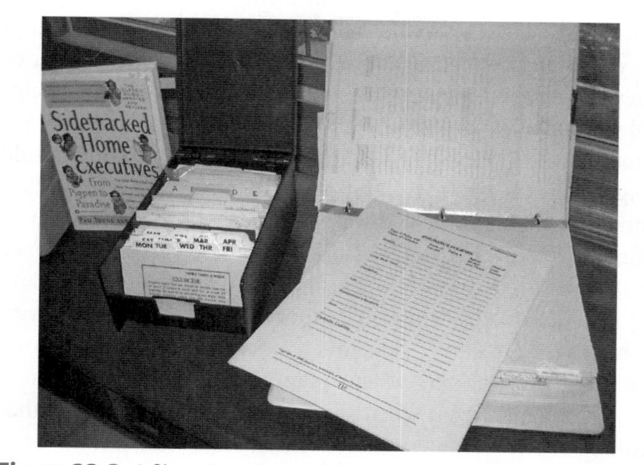

Figure 23-3 A file system listing daily activities and logs of important documents and their location maintains the patient's participation in higher-level cognitive function.

to enhance memory performance the client may use visual imagery, mental rehearsal, chunking, association, and repetition.[35,55,65] To improve attention to task, the client may use sensory strategies such as wearing earplugs or headphones, taking sensory breaks, or reading the material aloud. Many people who are cognitively impaired find these strategies difficult to initiate on their own; consequently, external strategies initiated by others such as the practitioner or family members are more common.

Intervention for Specific Cognitive Deficit Areas

Orientation Functions

Basically, orientation is classified as (1) alert and oriented to self (A & O × 1), (2) oriented to self and place (A & O × 2), or oriented to self, place, and time (A & O × 3). Time is the most abstract and difficult construct and therefore most easily lost.

Staff and family members who come into contact with a person who is not oriented can assist in orienting the person

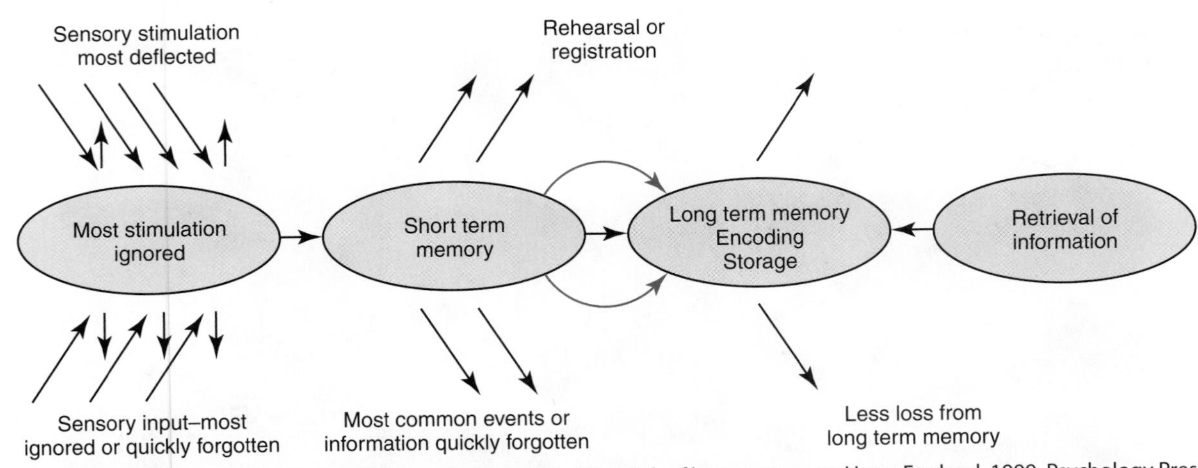

Figure 23-4 Path of memory. (Modified from Baddeley AD: *Essentials of human memory,* Hove, England, 1999, Psychology Press.)

to self, others, place, time, and situation. Generally, it is not helpful to quiz the person about orientation information because this can easily lead to frustration. External aids such as calendars, bulletin boards, and "orientation boards" with pertinent information such as the facility's name, the date, the season, and current events are often used in long-term settings or rehabilitation centers. These must be kept up-to-date, or they can easily contribute to further disorientation. One helpful strategy is to use photographs, especially with captions for those who can read.[7] For example, a photo of a young child might have the caption, "Ted, my son, at age 3, in 1948." This can assist those who are disoriented because they can refer to photos whenever they feel confused. There is some evidence that structured orientation groups can be helpful in delaying institutionalization and cognitive decline in people with dementia.[36] However, definitive guidelines for providing orientation information, either on an individual or group basis, are lacking, and even when gains are made in cognitive functioning test scores, these improvements may not carry over to daily functional performance.[52]

CLINICAL PEARL

Never argue or debate with someone who is confused or disoriented. You cannot win the argument, and frustration will surely ensue. Instead, redirect attention to another topic that is less distressing.

Attention Functions

Attention functions include sustained attention to task (focusing), alternating attention between two or more tasks, divided attention (attending to more than one task simultaneously), and selective attention (focusing under distracting circumstances). Attention difficulties occur more frequently in distracting environments. Most people find it easier to focus their attention when the environment is not overloaded with various types of auditory, visual, or other sensory stimuli. The initial goal of treating attention impairments is to identify the optimal environment that enables the client to attend to task for the longest possible time. As attention and level of concentration improves, the person will be able to focus longer under more distracting conditions. However, not all people can improve (or remediate) their level of attention. Those who cannot improve are likely to function more effectively in a low-stimulus environment or an environment individualized for level of stimulus and conducive to their specific needs with regard to stimulation. Music of particular interest may be used to promote attention skills.[54] Also, if clients are having difficulty focusing, keeping chatter to a minimum during therapeutic sessions can help. For example, if the client needs to concentrate on walking with a cane following a stroke, carrying on even normal everyday conversations while walking may distract the client enough to cause a fall. Formalized attention training models are available both electronically and through specific learning systems.[55] These require additional training for use.

Memory Functions

Memory is not one simple construct. Often when people talk about poor memory, they are referring to short-term memory, or the ability to remember facts for a brief period of time (e.g., names, grocery lists, telephone numbers). One consideration with short-term memory is that it relies heavily on adequate attention. One cannot remember what one did not attend to initially[35] (Figure 23-4). Asking someone if he or she has good memory skills yields little reliable information, precisely because people with memory difficulties have difficulty remembering.[15,31] In general, people can remember seven digits for a short period of time (with a standard deviation of ± 2). This is based on Miller's research in the 1950s and still holds true today.[23,39] Most people can remember a phone number long enough to dial it. This kind of remembering activates the "working memory" system, which involves simultaneously activating other skills in the realms of cognition and perception (e.g., interpretation of the stimulus, attention, problem solving, goal setting).[35] One actively uses, interacts with, or manipulates the information with the intention of retaining it. Other activities that require intact working memory include cooking (especially using recipes), playing games with rules (especially calculating scores midplay), and recalling and implementing multiple-step driving directions just obtained from a helpful person on the street.

Procedural memory concerns recall of procedures or motor skills such as driving (the motoric aspects), riding a bicycle, or dressing. Procedural memory is often retained in persons who have acquired brain injury or even Alzheimer's disease and may be able to be used as a strength, for example, when reestablishing habits.[35,55]

Prospective memory is concerned with memory for tasks to be completed at some point in the future. A common example is remembering to take medications at the prescribed times. Many people have developed techniques to help them remember these essential tasks (e.g., linking taking medications with another established routine such as brushing teeth or eating breakfast).

Episodic memory is simply memory for episodes or events in one's life (e.g., first day of school, birthday parties, weddings). Semantic memory concerns our deep-seated memory of language and basic facts that most of us know (e.g., multiplication tables, grammar, geographic facts).

These differing types of memory are related to one another, but a client may have more difficulties with one type than another. It is helpful for the OTA to consider the pathways involved in developing and using memories because clients may have difficulty at any point in the process. See Figure 23-4 for a schematic of the process. The person must first pay attention to the incoming stimulus, then store the information, and ultimately retrieve it. People generally have more success recognizing information than recalling it outright. Retention of information improves when the person repeats and manipulates it.[35] For example, if a client needs to remember hip precautions following hip surgery, involving the person in practicing these precautions during daily tasks, writing them down, and talking about them (versus just hearing or reading about them once) will certainly promote improved recall.

Thought Functions

Recognition is the skill by which a person identifies something seen or encountered in the past. Recognition is involved in the many types of memory described earlier. Categorization allows us to chunk information (place it in groups), thereby promoting understanding. Without this, sensory information can be overwhelming. Categorization of things we are familiar with is relatively easy, whereas categorization of novel situations or new items is more challenging as we seek to impart meaning by associating it with something we have come in contact with in the past.[69] Some common examples of categorization include grouping items of clothing by type or season, sorting playing cards into suits or colors, and differentiating foods in groups according to protein or fat content.

One way to use categorization in treatment would be to practice dividing objects into different groups (by features such as color, shape, size, etc.). Another way is to generalize information through the reasoning process. An example of this is comprehending, after having experienced a fall on the ice, that one should walk carefully on slippery surfaces. We learn in this way using our past experience to better understand the world around us and to enhance our safety and comfort.

Principles of Cognitive Retraining to Enhance Learning and Memory

"The process of synapse development and growth is 'not only sensitive to experience, it is driven by experience' (National Research Council, p. 117, in Metz & Robnett, 2011). In other words: engagement in meaningful occupations promotes brain health."

An intervention task can be analyzed and modified in several ways to improve performance.[56] One way is to provide increased structure or less ambiguity. A simple example would be to offer a client two or three choices rather than the whole array of possibilities (e.g., perhaps in choosing clothing for the day). In this way the client still maintains a level of control but is not overwhelmed with the decision-making process.

Intervention activities can be graded by changing some aspect of the activity demands. Many possibilities are presented in the *Framework*.[1] One example would be to alter the social demands of the task, either to ease the social expectations placed on the client to engage with others or to challenge the client socially by encouraging increased group participation. Other aspects of the activity demands that might be altered include task space demands, familiarity/novelty of the task, types of directions needed for successful completion of the task, number and types of objects used, spatial arrangement of the items, and the required response skills including rate of response. The OTA and the occupational therapist can collaborate to optimize learning and cognition by considering how aspects of the activity support or hinder occupational performance.

During intervention, the OT practitioner systematically provides verbal and physical cues through interpersonal interaction and modifies cueing according to the client's response. Cues can be used to direct attention to a particular aspect of a task, to guide problem solving, and to facilitate recall. Some examples of cueing techniques are imitation (e.g., "do what I do"); repetition ("try again"); problem solving ("what do these objects have in common?"); general ("what do you think you do next?"); specific ("you have food on your chin, you need to wipe it"); checking and verification ("are you sure of your answers on this?"); and direction of attention ("look here on your left").[56,57] The occupational therapist or OTA should bear in mind the ultimate goal of intervention. If remediation is possible for the client, the potential would be to move toward internalizing these cues, thus reducing the need for extrinsic cueing to ensure successful performance.[18,70] Progressing from using external cues designed by the clinician, to using internal and/or external cues established either jointly or independently and maintained by clients on their own, is optimal, though not always possible. A group approach that empowers clients to guide the intervention process has also been shown to be effective.[4,51]

To promote learning and memory of important information, a person's preferred learning style should be considered. To understand more about learning styles in general, the following Vark Questionnaire website is helpful.[22] It offers a questionnaire that will help readers determine their own learning style or learning style combination (visual, aural, reading/

writing, or kinesthetic). Although the VARK questionnaire is considered an instructional tool rather than a test, preliminary psychometric analysis shows limited but positive results.[34] The clinical team (psychologist, occupational therapist, speech-language pathologist, and others) can attempt to identify the patient's optimal learning style. Visual learners prefer visual stimulation to promote learning (e.g., pictures, photos, videos), whereas aural learners prefer to listen to instructions or hear other needed information. Aural learners enjoy stories and examples to enhance their retention, and they often want to talk about what they have learned in therapy. Those who prefer reading and writing may also choose to take notes and write down what they want to remember from the therapy session. For these avid readers, suggesting websites for further information can be beneficial, and they value written handouts.[25]

Consideration of the readability of any written information is crucial for all clients. Handouts need to be written in plain, direct, and concise language, using bullets when appropriate to convey information. Kinesthetic learners use a "hands-on approach to learning."[25] They benefit from demonstrations, the use of models, and interacting with the material to be learned through their various senses. As the characteristics of the optimal teaching methods are uncovered, this information can be communicated to the client, to others who work with the client (the client is unaware), and the client's family. All can then provide pertinent information in the preferred way, which is most likely to promote learning and retention.

Memory performance can sometimes be remediated for those with only mild impairments, although remediation has not been shown to be effective for those with moderate or severe memory losses.[12] Remediation involves practicing memory tasks such as word lists or remembering names. These exercises seem to work most effectively if the person is motivated to improve his or her performance and if the items to be remembered are meaningful to the person (versus meaningless word lists).[35] Memory training may have potential for increasing memory functioning and other cognitive skill. Training may be in the form of "mental aerobics" in a group.[26] If the person is not able to improve memory performance, various external strategies such as cue cards or signs can be employed (Table 23-2).

Domain-specific training, or task-specific training, may be used for the client who has global memory deficits. This client may be able to learn new skills in a particular situation (usually after much repetition) but cannot transfer or generalize the learning process and skills to a new environment.[24] An example is the client who is taught one-handed cooking skills in the OT department's kitchen but cannot implement those skills in the home environment. Home instruction, in this case, would be preferable. If home OT is not an option, then the problem of transfer must be addressed during intervention. Gillen[23] suggests the following techniques: practicing techniques in various settings, especially in the client's natural environments; practicing strategies (e.g., for remembering) during multiple meaningful tasks; and making the client aware of the intention of the intervention (e.g., using self-awareness or metacognition). Transfer of learning will occur more easily if the new setting or altered task is just slightly different (known as a "near transfer of learning").[43,57] Job coaching, a type of supported employment in which OTAs may provide services, is based on promoting new learning through these techniques. For best results, the skills needed for the job are taught to the client at the job site.[62]

Table 23-2 Examples of Adaptive and Compensatory Strategies

Task	Impairment	Strategy
Dressing	Sequencing deficit	Consistently place garments in the sequence to be donned, provide laminated check list, develop routine
Bathing	Sequencing deficit	Provide a pictorial of the sequence of washing—starting distally and progressing proximally (laminated if necessary in shower)
Feeding	Sequencing deficit or lack of judgment	Provide smaller utensils that assist the intake of smaller portions with each bite; encourage putting down utensil between bites
Safety and emergency maintenance	Judgment deficit	Provide step-by-step instructions for handling emergency by phone or wherever needed; obtain and encourage use of automatic button for summoning assistance (e.g., on wall, worn on wrist or around neck)
Job performance	Impaired short-term memory	Employ calendars or day-to-day planners; Morse[40] suggests using small daily planners with insert 3″ x 5″ cards for daily to-do lists
Grooming	Impaired short-term memory	Purchase devices that shut off automatically
Meal preparation	Impaired alternating attention	Set timers on the oven; check off what has been completed (can use laminated sheets with dry erase markers)
Social participation	Disorientation	Have people wear name tags; start conversation with statement of who the visitor is; display schedule boards that include who will visit
Reading	Visual field loss	Use a red marker or ribbon to mark the edge of the page[14]
Bathing	Unilateral neglect	Make sure water heater is turned down to 120° F or lower, for safety, because the hot water faucet is generally on the left[14]
Home maintenance	Figure-ground impairment	Use high contrast between foreground and background, simplify and organize

Higher-Level Cognitive Functions

Higher-level cognitive functions include insight and judgment, awareness, concept formation, time management, organization, problem solving, and decision making.[3] Sometimes these skills are called executive functions because they manage and control other cognitive processes. The client's level of awareness of higher-level cognitive function deficits will determine the type of intervention to be used. At one extreme is the client who is aware of the problem and realizes the impact of the deficit. This client may learn to respond to internal strategies for self-monitoring or to environmental compensatory cues. For example, the client may develop a mnemonic or jingle to assist in organizing and remembering information or keep a notebook, calendar, to-do-lists, and other reminders to stimulate initiation of activity.

Those with less self-awareness do not understand or cannot admit that any deficits exist. These clients may need cueing from trusted others. A peer group approach can also be useful in obtaining feedback from others to build awareness.[57] Videotaping can provide a visual record of behavior that can be discussed with the client so that he or she may be able to learn to use internal techniques to control behavior.

"[Any] problem may at first seem confusing—that the way to work the problem may not at first be obvious—but that through carefully breaking the problem down, by pinpointing first one piece of information and then another, a difficult problem can be gradually analyzed."[63]

The focus of intervention for higher-level cognitive dysfunction is generally to promote effective reasoning and problem solving. The process for proficient problem solving is still useful today, although it is not an easy fix for those with higher-level cognitive dysfunction. The OTA should model the step-by-step process and help the client to use the sequence of problem solving when challenges occur during daily tasks.

The steps are:

1. Defining the main points of the problem in relevant terms
2. Organizing or structuring the information into easy and difficult portions of the problem (e.g., breaking down the problem)
3. Developing possible solutions
3. Choosing one best solution
4. Executing the solution
5. Evaluating the outcome[6,59,60,68]

The client may be able to learn this sequence along with instructions to follow the steps when a problem is encountered in therapy or during day-to-day tasks. Along a similar vein, Parente and Herrmann[50] offer steps in decision making, which also may be impaired in those with cognitive deficits.

They use the mnemonic of DECIDE in the following way:

D = Deciding to get going and to not procrastinate

E = Evaluating options (looking for options that offer win-win solutions)

C = Creating new options if none are found to be suitable

I = Investigating the best options

D = Discussing potential choices with others (initially avoiding sharing one's own opinion) and listening to their advice

E = Evaluating your feelings (thinking twice before taking action)

The OTA can use these sequences in assisting clients to transfer and apply decision making and problem solving to a variety of situations within the context of OT intervention and beyond into their personal everyday lives.

"Getting all the necessary information is essential in making the right decision." (Michaud & Wild, 1991, p. 120)

CLINICAL PEARL

The occupational therapy practitioner can help the client with decision making by ensuring that several or many options are considered. Rarely is either "yes" or "no" the only way to go.

Awareness impairments are addressed in OT intervention using various approaches. Remediation of awareness deficits may be appropriate for those who do not have severe problems in this realm and who have the cognitive capacity to learn new information. Awareness level may be increased through the use of self-estimation by asking the client to predict the outcome of a question or task performance and then together processing the discrepancies that may exist between what actually occurred and what was expected.[28] The practitioner and client can also reverse roles within the context of intervention to promote increased awareness of safety issues. Toglia[57] suggests using the technique of self-evaluation both before a task and following the completion of the task to problem solve errors in performance and to build self-awareness. This not only gives the practitioner a sense of the client's self-awareness level but also imparts information about the person's level of self-confidence. Intervention may focus on the client's ability to question and evaluate his or her own or others' performance.

Behavioral Problems

A deficit in higher-level cognitive functioning (including decreased self-awareness) may result in behavioral or social problems due to the client's lack of insight or judgment and deficient problem-solving skills. These deficits may occur during recovery in persons who have experienced head trauma. Behavioral management strategies may be helpful to control or restrict behavioral outbursts. Staff members may need to give consistent, client-specific, direct feedback regarding the inappropriateness of the behavior. If the client's level of insight and self-control warrant, internal strategies (such as personal time-out or actively removing oneself from the situation) can be incorporated into the client's plan. External controls may be used as needed. For example, a staff member may escort the patient to a quiet area until behavioral control once again is established. The staff member must remain calm and provide consistent verbal cues related to the situation. A strong emotional response including arguing with the client on the part of the staff can exacerbate the situation. Training programs such as the Mandt system[8] may be helpful in facilities and at worksites in which behavioral issues are more common.

Summary of Intervention for Those with Cognitive Impairments

Cognition is always a factor in OT intervention. For those who are functioning at a high cognitive level, learning new tasks and problem solving comes easily. For those who have deficits, the challenge is to make the most of their cognitive strengths while managing their deficits. Due to the complexity of factors and the compounding effect of multiple impairments in cognition, interventions involving cognitive training or retraining can be convoluted and time consuming. Those with impaired cognition may require more time to learn new skills or to consistently use compensatory measures. Clients with significant cognitive impairments specifically require team intervention to promote optimal functioning.

CLINICAL PEARL

Always think biopsychosocially—do what you can to make sure that the client's environment, physical condition, and emotional state are optimally primed for learning.

Intervention for Perceptual and Perceptual Motor Deficits

"Perception is not simply the registration and evaluation of sense data, but rather an active taking hold of the world"[30]

Perceptual skills allow people to interpret and impart meaning to the input arriving through their sensory systems. Adept performance of daily tasks in all areas of occupation requires intact perceptual and cognitive skills. Accurate perceptual processing (based on incoming sensory data) provides a foundation for appropriate motor actions. Due to the direct impact on motor actions, remediation or compensation for perceptual deficits (specifically visual) may result in improved functional performance.[42] OT practitioners can focus on retraining specific perceptual skills and/or incorporating perceptual retraining into functional tasks such as ADL, IADL, education, and work.

As with intervention for cognitive deficits, the two most common approaches are remedial and adaptive. The remedial approach uses the transfer-of-training approach or perceptual retraining, through practice, exercises, and engagement in activities related to the deficient areas.[66] Typically these practice drills have involved tabletop, pencil-and-paper, and computer activities. The adaptive approach uses client skills that are relatively intact to compensate for skills that are deficient. Intervention activities should be client centered and related to functional, real-life, and meaningful tasks.[42,43]

Intervention Approaches

Remedial or restorative intervention approaches focus on repairing the underlying perceptual impairment(s) through a potential reorganization of the central nervous system. The goal is to improve the accuracy of interpretation of incoming visual information.[69] This approach is based on the assumption that the brain remains plastic and capable of making positive changes (with regard to neuronal regeneration, growth, and development) even after sustaining an injury or illness. The occupational therapist identifies and selects techniques that might improve the client's ability to function. The remedial approaches touched on in this chapter include the following:

- Neurodevelopmental treatment
- Perceptual skills remediation (practicing skills during meaningful tasks)
- Transfer of training approach (practicing skills in skill-based tasks)

In neurodevelopmental treatment (NDT) the practitioner works on the restoration of normal movement patterns, through handling techniques and repetitive movement patterns.[69] Originally developed by the Bobaths, this approach is still used throughout the world. NDT attempts to retrain perceptual functions by promoting the experience and sensation of normal movement and the resulting sensory feedback by controlling motor performance. For example, bilateral activities used in the motor retraining program stimulate total body awareness and may be able to help remediate problems of unilateral neglect and homonymous hemianopsia (a visual deficit of the right or left visual field). Weight bearing, manual facilitation or handling, and tactile cueing to enhance proprioception are important elements of the motor retraining program.[16] Although advanced certification is not necessary for an OT practitioner to use NDT techniques, advanced training is available for those with years of experience (see http://www.ndta.org/ for more information).

After an acquired brain injury (ABI), visual perception is often affected. Zoltan[69] outlines restorative techniques for improving visual search, scanning, and attention strategies. One technique that has demonstrated success in retraining those with ABI to attend to the full spectrum of visual space is "the lighthouse strategy" in which the client emulates being a lighthouse to fully scan the environment.[44] When body scheme perception is impaired, constraint-induced therapy (CIT) may be used to help the client learn to use a hemiplegic limb if it has the capacity or potential for improved function.[47,54] This is accomplished through engagement in everyday tasks that focus on affected limb use (often for several hours per day), while constraining the use of the preferred or stronger limb. Evidence for the success of CIT is mounting, although it does require intensive therapy and may be detrimental if undertaken too early in the rehabilitation process (e.g., during the acute rehabilitation phase).[27]

The transfer-of-training approach assumes that practice and subsequent improvement in specific perceptual skill drills will generalize to better performance in everyday perceptual activities that require the same perceptual skills. For example, practice in reproducing pegboard designs or parquetry puzzles for spatial relations training might carry over to dressing skills that require spatial judgment (e.g., matching shirt components to the corresponding body parts, front and back of pants and shirt, discriminating right from left shoe). Formerly this approach was in widespread use for treating perceptual problems in OT clinics. However, transfer of learning or generalization may be more reliable when functional activities are used throughout.[43] Practitioners have begun using an occupation-based approach in the clinic to facilitate transfer of training from the clinic to the client's home or work environment. The use of practice tasks (paper and pencil worksheets, puzzles) for specific perceptual skill development is still common.

This chapter offers just a few examples of possible intervention strategies. OTAs typically carry out these intervention techniques under the supervision of the occupational therapist except when the OTA has additional training in these skills and/or has proven service competency as determined by the facility or state regulatory board.

The adaptive approach uses environmental change or adaptation to enhance performance of daily tasks. Interventions involve engagement in the client's occupations of interest. The adaptive approach includes two types of intervention: compensation and adaptation.[69] Compensation entails making the client aware of the perceptual problem and teaching the client to take compensatory measures to improve performance. In the case of visual field loss (homonymous hemianopsia), for example, a male client can be taught to compensate for loss of vision by making sure he turns his heads both ways before crossing the street. If he has difficulty distinguishing colors or subtle features of clothing, items of clothing that go together could be stored together for ease of recognition. The client can then learn to pick out piles of clothing rather than individual pieces of clothing to wear.

Adaptation involves changing the environment with the goal of improved performance (Figure 23-5). In the case of visual neglect, all ADL items would be presented in the field of vision that is currently available (e.g., to the right of midline for those with left neglect). Another example would be arranging for intervention sessions to occur in a quiet, uncluttered room to minimize distractions. If the client tends to become distracted with excess auditory or visual stimulation, providing a calm environment will promote thinking and learning. If the client has *dressing apraxia* (inability to dress due to body scheme and spatial relations deficits, not problems with motor performance per se), colored tabs could be sewn into clothing to provide cues for top, bottom, inside, and/or outside of the clothing item.[69] If the client has difficulty dressing due to a body scheme deficit, the occupational therapist or OTA may work with the client to establish a regular dressing sequence and routine, ideally providing fewer cues over time as practice improves performance. The OTA can work with the occupational therapist and other team members to determine which environmental adaptations are most likely to optimize functional performance in ADL, IADL, and other activities of interest.

Selected Perceptual Deficits—Descriptions and Interventions

Perception and cognition are intricately related. Perceptual deficits may be misinterpreted as cognitive deficits by the casual observer who observes flawed motor responses brought on by impaired perception and assumes this means that the person cannot understand what is being asked of him or her. Fascinating reading that explores the sometimes devastating impact of perceptual difficulties is presented in the book by Oliver Sacks, *The Man Who Mistook His Wife for a Hat and Other Clinical Tales*.[53] Even highly experienced OT practitioners can find perceptual deficits extremely challenging to address.

Visual Processing

Zoltan[69] includes basic visual skills such as acuity, contract sensitivity, visual fixation and attention, oculomotor control, and eye movements including scanning (pursuing objects) and saccades (moving eyes to new objects, e.g., from word to word in reading) under visual processing. These are primarily basic vision skills (under Warren's visual hierarchy),[61] so only visual fields are addressed in this chapter. (See Chapter 22 for related information.)

Visual field loss can occur in any portion of all four quadrants of space (inferior, superior, left, and right). If the damage has occurred only in the eye or the nerves around the eye itself before reaching the processing centers in the brain, then the field loss is generally easier to manage. However, when damage has occurred deeper in the brain where interpretation

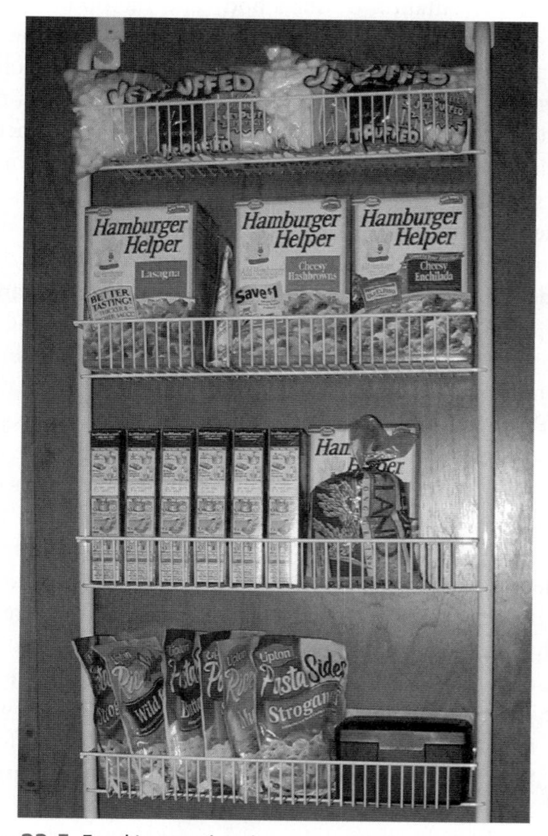

Figure 23-5 Food is stored and organized in the same direction and location to accommodate for perceptual deficits.

of visual stimuli takes place, the affected person may not be able to comprehend that a loss has occurred. Once the health care team has determined the type of visual loss, then remediation and/or compensation can commence. For example, the person could practice being a lighthouse as described earlier, to work on restoring vision in all directions. Engagement in meaningful tasks that "stretch" vision just beyond where the person usually gazes might also be restorative. Having the person point and follow his or her finger may also be helpful in that the pointing finger can provide an "anchor" to show the person where to look.[14] If comprehension of the deficit is absent, the practitioner will need to make sure all needed objects (for ADL or eating or other tasks) are available in the usable visual space. Using "anchors" to draw attention to the edge of the visual field can also be helpful (e.g., using a marker to mark the edge of a page, safety tape around the home).[69]

CLINICAL PEARL

If the practitioner can "stretch" the client's vision to the neglected side, great! But if not, the practitioner must ensure that stimulation takes place on the sighted side. Otherwise, the client is at risk for sensory deprivation and social isolation.

Visuospatial Impairments

Visuospatial functions involve understanding space and spatial relations using information from vision. *Body scheme,* a mental representation of one's body and the bodies of others, is one example. Body scheme disorders are common after sustaining a stroke in either hemisphere, although Paolucci, McKennam, and Cooke[48] found body scheme deficits more common after a left hemisphere stroke. Body scheme functions include being able to identify body parts of self and others, understanding right and left sides of the body, understanding the relationships of body parts to one another (e.g., distal, proximal, above, below), and position in space. Body scheme disorders show up frequently during ADL tasks. For example, body parts may be neglected during bathing or dressing. The client may demonstrate anger at his or her hemiplegic limb or seem not to understand how to move a limb for ease of dressing. "Postural body geometry," which is necessary to keep our bodies in alignment gravitationally, seems to be more often impaired after right brain damage.[32] This impairment is often associated with spatial neglect (generally left) and can result in poor postural control, loss of balance, and a "pushing syndrome" in which the person pushes contralateral to the side with the lesion. These body scheme deficits, if severe, can greatly affect the person's potential for rehabilitation. Zoltan[69] and Corbin and Unsworth[14] offer a number of intervention strategies for body scheme disorders including the following:

- Providing tactile stimulation to the body parts affected. Stimulation may be given by the practitioner, or preferably by the client herself
- Facilitating normal bilateral movements using NDT handling techniques
- Using a mirror to augment the visual awareness of the neglected parts
- Educating clients (and their families) about the disorder to the level they can understand, with an emphasis on safety

Kempler[28] suggests avoiding the use of the words "right" and "left" in giving directions if these are confusing to the client, but rather providing a visual cue (e.g., colored tape) on one side or the other to remind the client the difference between the two sides (e.g., shoes).

Visual Agnosia

Agnosia is a condition in which a person does not recognize common everyday objects. *Visual agnosia* is a failure to recognize items that can be seen. The person can see the objects, but this is a "perception without meaning."[69] The problem may be specific to one type of item (e.g., faces, utensils) or more global. Dense agnosia results in a general and extremely debilitating inability to interact appropriately with visually perceived items. Clients may carry out unusual or even bizarre acts such as donning underwear on their heads or using a comb as a toothbrush. Visual perceptual functions sometimes improve spontaneously. Not much is known about intervention because only a few single-case studies exist. Zoltan[69] shares some helpful hints in management of this deficit including promoting the use of other sensory modalities such as touch to add "texture or edge orientation cues," providing labels, and giving verbal cues as needed.

Visual Discrimination Deficits

Visual discrimination includes several subskills such as discrimination by form, depth perception, figure-ground perception, and spatial relations. *Form discrimination* is the ability to group and to differentiate various forms of the same type of item (e.g., various makes of cars are still identified as vehicles) and to identify an item when viewed from various vantage points such as from the side or the back. Helpful techniques may include practice in identifying objects not only by sight but also through tactile manipulation. The therapist must make sure that the item is presented in the most common position (upright, forward facing). Labeling and organizing items are adaptations that may make it easier for the person to recognize items of interest.

Depth perception is the ability to recognize and understand differences in distances between objects. This skill requires vision in both eyes to get the true binocular effect of perceiving three-dimensional space. However, people can and do use other cues besides binocular vision to determine depth or spatial relations between objects. One cue is the relation of size to distance, in that same-sized items that are farther away appear smaller. Learning about the typical relationships between different-sized objects over time is also helpful. In addition, light, shadows, and movement in relation to the observer can play into the understanding of distance and depth.

Figure ground perception is the ability to distinguish an object from its background such as a fork in a bunch of silverware or a certain type of leaf in a pile of leaves. Practicing finding objects at the level the client is able to, starting

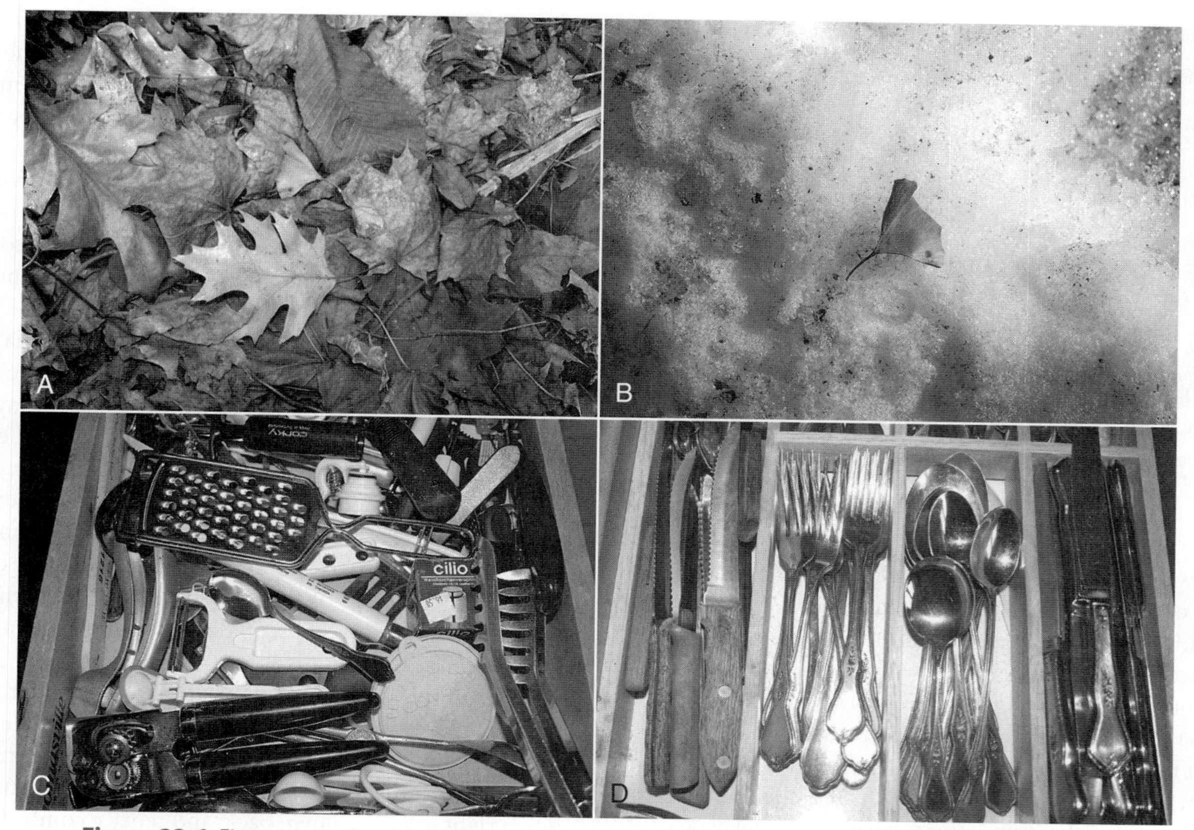

Figure 23-6 Figure-ground examples. **A,** It is difficult to identify the figure of a ginkgo leaf among many different leaves. **B,** Increasing contrast and simplicity makes the task easier. **C,** It is difficult to find a soup spoon in a cluttered drawer. **D,** Organizing utensils can help the client find needed items.

with few objects and obvious contrast if necessary and gradually introducing more complexity to challenge the person to improve, may enhance these perceptual skills. If the client is unable to understand how these perceptual factors affect daily performance and how to compensate for their absence, educating the family and trusted others is certainly necessary (Figure 23-6).

Astereognosis

Stereognosis is the perceptual skill of identifying familiar objects and geometric shapes through touch, proprioception, and cognition without the aid of vision. Astereognosis, or *tactile agnosia,* is a deficit of this skill. The person is unable to perceive identity of objects due to the loss of capacity to sense or organize shape, texture, temperature, or weight.[9] Vision is often used to compensate. Astereognosis may occur after a lesion on either side of the brain in the somatosensory perception areas, which is a common lesion site in cerebrovascular accident (CVA) and in neurologic conditions such as cerebral palsy.[13] Stereognosis or "seeing with the hands" is integral to the typical performance of everyday activities such as finding a key in a pocket or a specific coin in a purse. Evidence-based intervention for astereognosis is lacking in the scientific literature, but it follows common sense that a client could work on practicing identifying objects first using vision and then with vision occluded, describing the object and carefully exploring its tactile features (Figure 23-7). A tub of sand, uncooked rice, or beans can be used to hide objects, which clients can then try to locate and retrieve with their affected hand.[33] Practicing stereognosis during tasks that are meaningful for the client should take precedence. A sample task for a homemaker might be finding specific utensils while doing the dishes in soapy water (with sharp knives removed for safety). Similar games or object-finding activities can be devised for whatever task in which the client has complained of having difficulty.

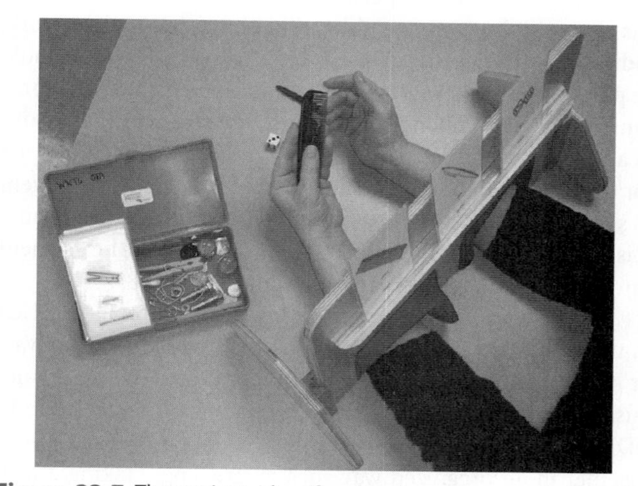

Figure 23-7 The patient identifies familiar objects verbally or by pointing to the card during intervention for astereognosis.

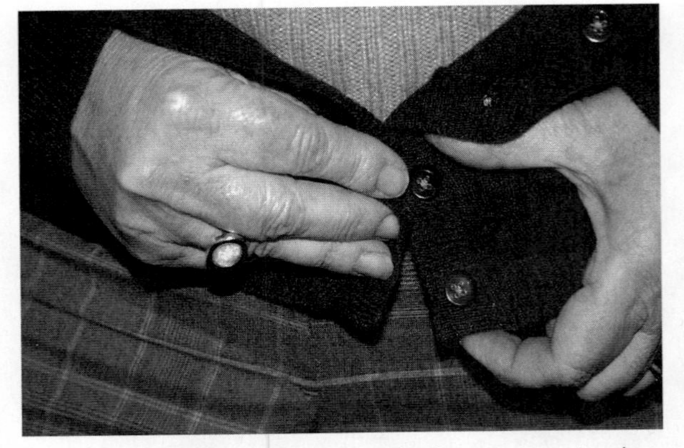

Figure 23-8 Buttoning starting from the bottom is easiest because one can see and line up the bottom edges of the sweater.

Apraxia

Apraxia is the inability to plan and perform the motor acts necessary to complete an ordinary task such as dressing or brushing teeth, even though there are no obvious motoric deficits or significant muscular weaknesses. Intervention involves the occupational therapist or OTA teaching a set routine for dressing, in the case of dressing apraxia, and providing cues to assist the client in distinguishing clothing item features such as right arm from left arm or front from back.[69] The client is encouraged to look for distinctive features such as the collar or label to orient the clothing item correctly. One method is to have the client position the garment the same way each time, as in laying out a shirt with the buttons face down and top away from the client to promote a specific routine. To assist a client who has difficulty buttoning a shirt, different tactics might work; individualized trial and error is often necessary. The shirt could be partially buttoned and the client could finish the task of buttoning. Or, to compensate, the buttoned shirt could be worn as a pullover shirt.[46] A pullover or zipper shirt might be easier for the client, or another technique could be to cue the patient to start buttoning at the bottom of the shirt or sweater because it is easier to match the right and left halves when the garment can be seen and the edges are distinct (Figure 23-8).

A related type of apraxia is *constructional apraxia,* a deficit in the ability to copy, draw, or construct a design, either two- or three-dimensional, whether on command or spontaneously. Constructional apraxia causes significant dysfunction in ADL tasks that require constructional ability or putting things together in an organized way such as dressing, making a bed, folding clothes, organizing food on a shelf, or food preparation.[46]

Apraxia is evident when perceptual impairments affect functional performance. Ideomotor and ideational apraxia are two types of apraxia that may occur after stroke. *Ideomotor* or *ideokinetic apraxia* is an inability to plan or perform a motor skill. The patient may understand the concept, may even be able to describe the intended motion and attempt to carry out the task, but cannot execute the motor act at will. Some skills such as waving goodbye or brushing teeth may be performed spontaneously but cannot be executed on demand.[19] *Ideational or conceptual apraxia* is an inability to comprehend the concept of the required movement or to execute the act in response to a command or automatically. In ideational apraxia it is as if the "mental representation about the concept required for performance"[23] has been lost. Clients may seem confused and display hesitant motor actions, or they may not be able to initiate the task at all. It is difficult to distinguish between ideational and ideomotor apraxia in individual clients, especially those who also have aphasia or comprehension difficulties. However, those who have not lost the concept of the task (i.e., those with ideomotor apraxia) may be able to complete tasks, especially those that are automatic.

Treatment of ideational and ideomotor apraxia is challenging. The therapy practitioner should use short, clear, concise, concrete, and repetitive instructions. It may help to break down tasks into component steps and teach each step separately. Verbal and demonstrated instructions may be ineffective. Guiding the patient through the correct movements, while giving intermittent tactile and proprioceptive input with short instructions, may be more successful. After the client has performed each step of the task separately, the clinician can begin to combine the steps, grading the complexity and number of steps as the client is able.[46]

An example of a complete task is combing hair. The OT practitioner can break the task into a motor sequence with or without hand-over-hand guidance: pick up comb; bring comb to hair; move comb across top of head, down left side, down right side, and down back; and replace comb on table. It may help for the client to verbalize (or think about) each step as he or she completes it. The clinician instructs the client to watch as each step is completed[10] (in the case of hair combing by looking in the mirror). Repetition is necessary for effective results. Ideomotor apraxia is less severe than ideational because comprehension of the task has not been entirely lost. Those who have ideomotor apraxia may do better attempting the entire task rather than the individual components, especially if this is an automatic task that is completed in a typical context (e.g., environment, time of day, familiar items). To complete the hair combing task, the practitioner may try handing the comb to the client while he or she is in the bathroom standing in front of the sink. A client with ideomotor apraxia may be able to complete the task spontaneously.

Overview of Intervention for Cognitive and Perceptual Deficits

Effective restoration or management of cognitive and perceptual skill impairments requires understanding the underlying mechanisms and identifying the point of breakdown in a particular action or task. A competent OT practitioner has the ability to conduct activity analyses as needed to determine the usual demands of any pertinent task, as well as the specific client factors including the requisite levels of those factors needed to successfully complete the task. Through this analysis process, the practitioner can determine what skills are lacking and when performance breaks down during the steps of the task. A strong OT evidence base for intervention in cognition and perception has not yet been firmly established. Despite this, OT practitioners throughout the world regularly provide successful interventions in the areas of cognition and perception, both restorative and adaptive or via the compensatory approach. It is expected that these talented practitioners will eventually collaborate with one another and with OT researchers to publish and disseminate optimal interventions so that clients with deficits in cognition and perception will receive treatment that is based on strong research.

"Personal perceptions and responses to stressful life events are crucial elements to survival, recovery, and rehabilitation, often transcending the reality of the situation or the interventions of others. The inner life (affective and cognitive processes and content) holds the potential for transforming traumas into varying degrees of triumph."[20]

Summary

Cognitive and perceptual dysfunction is complex and can seem overwhelming to the novice practitioner. Working in this realm requires the OTA to develop astute observational skills, an awareness of providing optimal cueing, therapeutic use of self, and the ability to understand the impact of context on functioning. Breaking down the functional performance deficits by the impact of specific client factors can make this complex realm of OT more manageable. Many theories have been developed to assist practitioners in providing thoughtful and cohesive intervention using restoration techniques and/or compensation and adaptation. The occupational therapist is responsible for evaluation, planning, and designing interventions for clients with cognitive and perceptual deficits. The OTA can contribute by carefully observing patient behavior and by applying general intervention principles and techniques, in consultation with the occupational therapist. Detailed intervention methodology in cognition and perception is beyond the scope of this textbook, but the interested OTA should educate himself to the possibilities. OTAs are encouraged to obtain continuing education and sufficient clinical experience to refine their skills so that they can competently and confidently work with clients who have cognitive and/or perceptual dysfunction.

CLINICAL PEARL

Have hope. Convey hope. People are resilient and can work to make positive changes. As a client-centered occupational therapy practitioner, you can be a catalyst for this transformation.

Selecting Reading Guide Questions

1. Compare and contrast the roles of the occupational therapist and the OTA in the intervention of clients with deficits in cognition and/or perception.
2. Come up with examples of how several different cognitive and perceptual impairments affect daily performance by relating them to areas of occupation in the *Occupational Therapy Practice Framework,* edition 2.
3. Compare remedial and compensatory/adaptive intervention techniques.
4. List three strategies used for patients with problems in orientation.
5. Give at least three examples (beyond those mentioned in the chapter) of each of the different types of memory described using everyday activities (short-term, working, long-term, prospective, episodic, and semantic). Explain how these types differ.
6. Describe how context (as many aspects as are pertinent, see the *Occupational Therapy Practice Framework,* edition 2, p. 645) would affect the intervention approach for patients with memory deficits, and give two or three examples of intervention that might be helpful.
7. Explain what is meant by *categorization,* and describe ways you use this skill when you learn something new.
8. Give examples of strategies and activities used for the patient with unilateral neglect.
9. Describe how you might work with a client with ideational or ideomotor apraxia in relearning to brush his or her teeth.
10. Explain how astereognosis might affect the completion of a skill you do everyday, and suggest intervention techniques.
11. Discuss the Clinical Pearl by Kielhofner on page 458 about thinking biopsychosocially. Considering a client or person with whom you are familiar, give examples using the *Occupational Therapy Practice Framework,* edition 2 (AOTA, 2008) of how you would ensure optimal learning.

References

1. American Occupational Therapy Association: Occupational Therapy Practice Framework: domain and process, 2nd ed, *Am J Occup Ther* 62:625–683, 2008.
2. American Occupational Therapy Association: Guidelines for supervision, roles, and responsibilities during the delivery of occupational therapy services, *Am J Occup Ther* 58:663–667, 2004.
3. American Occupational Therapy Association: Occupational therapy practice framework: domain and process, *Am J Occup Ther* 56:609–639, 2002.
4. Averbuch S, Katz N: Cognitive rehabilitation: a retraining model for clients with neurological disabilities. In Katz N, editor: *Cognition & occupation across the life span*, Bethesda, MD, 2005, AOTA Press, pp 113–138.
5. Baddeley AD: *Essentials of human memory*, Hove, England, 1999, Psychology Press.
6. Beyer BK: *Practical strategies for the teaching of thinking*, Boston, 1987, Allyn & Bacon.
7. Bourgeois M: *Memory books and other graphic cuing systems*, Baltimore, 2009, Health Professions Press.
8. Bowen B: Moving away from coercion and enhancing patient dignity and respect. In Privitera M, editor: *Workplace violence in the mental and general health care setting*, Sudbury, MA, 2011, Jones and Bartlett, pp 135–150.
9. Bradshaw JL, Mattingly JB: *Clinical neuropsychology: behavioral and brain science*, San Diego, 1995, Academic Press.
10. Butler JA: Evaluation and intervention with apraxia. In Unsworth C, editor: *Cognitive and perceptual dysfunction*, 1999, pp 257–298.

11. Cicerone KD, Dahlberg C, Kalmer K, Langenbahn DM, Malec JF, Bergquist TF, et al: Evidence-based cognitive rehabilitation: recommendations for clinical practice, *Arch Phys Med Rehabil* 81:1596–1615, 2000.
12. Cicerone KD, Dahlberg C, Malec JF, Langenbahn DM, Felicetti T, Kneipp S, Ellmo W, et al: Evidence-based cognitive rehabilitation: updated review of the literature from 1998 through 2002, *Arch Phys Med Rehabil* 86(8):1681–1692, 2005.
13. Connell LA, Lincoln NB, Radford KA: Somatosensory impairment after stroke: frequency of deficits and their recovery, *Clin Rehabil* 22:758–767, 2008.
14. Corbin L, Unsworth C: Evaluation and intervention with unilateral neglect. In Unsworth C, editor: *Cognitive and perceptual dysfunction*, Philadelphia, 1999, F.A. Davis, pp 357–392.
15. Craik FIM, Anderson ND, Kerr SA, Li KZH: In Baddeley AD, Wilson BA, Watts FN, editors: *Handbook of memory disorders*, Chichester, UK, 1995, John Wiley & Sons.
16. Davies P: *Steps to follow*, ed 2, Berlin, Germany, 2000, Springer Verlag.
17. Dickinson D, Tenhula W, Morris S, Brown C, Peer J, Spencer K, et al: A randomized, controlled trial of computer-assisted cognitive remediation for schizophrenia, *Am J Psychiatry* 167(2): 170–180, 2010.
18. Doughtery PM, Radomski MV: *The cognitive rehabilitation workbook*, ed 2, Gaithersburg, MD, 1993, Aspen.
19. Duchenne PM: Rehabilitation involving the senses, sensation, perception, and pain. In Hoeman SP, editor: *Rehabilitation nursing: process and application*, ed 3, St. Louis, 2002, Mosby.
20. Fine SB: 1990 Eleanor Clarke Slagle Lecture. Resilience and human adaptability: who rises above adversity? *Am J Occup Ther* 45:493–503, 1991.
21. Fisher A: Overview of performance skills and client factors, *Cited in AOTA (2008)* , 2006.
22. Fleming N: The Vark Questionnaire V7.1, http://www.vark-learn.com/english/page.asp?p=questionnaire, Accessed February 3, 2012.
23. Gillen G: *Cognitive and perceptual rehabilitation: optimizing function*, St. Louis, 2009, Mosby Elsevier.
24. Glisky EL, Schacter DL: Remediation of organic memory disorders: current status and future prospects, *J Head Trauma Rehabil* 1:1–96, 1986.
25. Hamilton S: How do we assess the learning style of out patients? *Rehabil Nurs* 30(4):129–131, 2005.
26. Hayslip B, Paggi K, Poole M, Pinson MW: The impact of mental aerobics on memory impaired older adults, *Clin Gerontol* 32:389–394, 2009.
27. Humm JL: Use-dependent exaggeration of brain injury: is glutamate involved?, *Exp Neurol* 157(2):349–358, 1999.
28. Katz N, Hartman-Maeir A: Higher-level cognitive functions. In Katz N, editor: *Cognition & occupation across the life span*, Bethesda, MD, 2005, AOTA Press, pp 3–25.
29. Kempler D: *Neurocognitive disorders of aging*, Thousand Oaks, CA, 2005, Sage Publications, Inc.
30. Kielhofner: *Model of human occupation theory and application*, ed 4, Baltimore, 2008, Lippincott, Williams & Wilkins.
31. Knight RG, Godfrey HPD: Behavioral and self-report methods. In Baddeley AD, Wilson BA, Watts FN, editors: *The handbook of memory disorders*, Chichester, UK, 1995, John Wiley & Sons Ltd.
32. Lafosse C, Kerckhofs E, Vereeck L, Troch M, Van Hoydonck G, Moeremans M, et al: Postural abnormalities and contraversive pushing following right hemisphere brain damage, *Neuropsychol Rehabil* 17(3):374–396, 2007.
33. Laver A, Unsworth C: Evaluation and intervention with simple perceptual impairment (agnosias). In Unsworth C, editor: *Cognitive and perceptual dysfunction*, Philadelphia, 1999, F.A. Davis, pp 299–356.
34. Leite WL, Svinicki M, Shi Y: Attempted validation of the scores of the VARK: learning styles inventory with multitrait-multimethod confirmatory factor analysis models, *Educ Psychol Meas* 70:323–339, 2010.
35. Levy L: Cognitive aging in perspective. In Katz N, editor: *Cognition & occupation across the life span*, Bethesda, MD, 2005, AOTA Press, pp 305–325.
36. Metitieri T, Zanetti O, Geroldi C, Frisoni GB, De Leo D, Buono MD, et al: Reality Orientation Therapy to delay outcomes of progression in patients with dementia. A retrospective study, *Clin Rehabil* 15:471–478, 2001.
37. Metz A, Robnett R: Engaging in mentally challenging occupations promotes cognitive health throughout life, *Gerontol Spec Interest Sect News AOTA* , 2011, June, in press.
38. Michaud E, Wild R: *Boost your brain power*, Emmaus, PA, 1991, Rodale Press.
39. Miller G: The magical number seven, plus or minus two, *Psychol Rev* 63:81–97, 1956.
40. Morse P: Memory Notebook, *Building bridges in occupational therapy: clients across the lifespan with neurological impairments*, 2010, September 13:Portland, ME.
41. National Research Council: *How people learn: brain, mind, experience, and school*, Washington, D.C, 2000, National Academy Press.
42. Neistadt ME: A critical analysis of occupational therapy approaches for perceptual deficits in adults with brain injury, *Am J Occup Ther* 44:299, 1990.
43. Neistadt ME: Perceptual training for adults with diffuse brain injury, *Am J Occup Ther* 48:225–233, 1994.
44. Niemeier JP, Cifu DX, Kishore R: The lighthouse strategy: improving the functional status of patients with unilateral neglect after stroke and brain injury using a visual imagery intervention, *Top Stroke Rehabil* 8(2):10–18, 2001.
45. Nussbaum P: *Brain health and wellness*, Tarentum, Pa, 2003, Word Association Publishers.
46. Okkema K: *Cognition and perception in the stroke patient: a guide to functional outcomes in occupational therapy, Rehabilitation Institute of Chicago*, Gaithersburg, Md, 1993, Aspen.
47. Page SJ, Sisto S, Levine P, Johnston MV, Hughes M: Modified constraint induced therapy: a randomized feasibility and efficacy study, *J Rehabil Res Dev* 38(5):583–590, 2001.
48. Paolucci A, McKenna K, Cooke DM: Factors affecting the number and type of impairments of visual perception and praxis following stroke, *Austral Occup Ther J* 56:350–360, 2009:doi: 10.1111/j.1440-1630.2008.00743.x.
49. Parente R, Anderson-Parente J: *Retraining memory: techniques and applications*, Houston, 1991, CSY.
50. Parente R, Herrmann D: *Retraining cognition: techniques and applications*, Gaithersburg, 1996, Md: An Aspen Publication.
51. Parente R, Stapleton M: An empowerment model of memory training, *Appl Cogn Psychol* 7:585, 1993.
52. Patton D: Reality orientation: its use and effectiveness with older person mental health care, *J Clin Nurs* 15:1440–1449, 2006:doi: 10.1111/j.1365-2702.2005.01450.x.
53. Sacks O: *The man who mistook his wife for a hat and other clinical tales*, New York, 1985, Harper & Row.
54. Shih Y, Huang R, Chiang H: Correlation between work concentration level and background music: a pilot study. Work 33: 329–333, 2009:DOI 10.3233/WOR-2009-0880.

55. Sohlberg MM, Mateer CA: *Cognitive rehabilitation: an integrative neuropsychological approach*, New York, 2001, The Guilford Press.
56. Toglia JP: Visual perception of objects: an approach to assessment and treatment, *Am J Occup Ther* 43:587, 1989.
57. Toglia JP: A dynamic interactional approach to cognitive rehabilitation. In Katz N, editor: *Cognition & occupation across the life span*, Bethesda, Md, 2005, AOTA Press, pp 29–72.
58. Vance DE, Roberson AJ, McGuinness TM, Fazeli PL: How neuroplasticity and cognitive reserve protect cognitive functioning, *J Psychosocial Nurs* 48(4):23–30, 2010.
59. von Cramon D, Matthes-von Cramon G: Recovery of higher-order cognitive deficits after brain hypoxia or frontomedial vascular lesions, *Appl Neuropsychol* 1:2–7, 1994.
60. von Cramon D, Matthes-von Cramon G, Mai N: Problem solving deficits in brain injured adults: a therapeutic approach, *Neuropsychol Rehabil* 1:45–64, 1991.
61. Warren M: A hierarchical model for evaluation and treatment of visual perceptual dysfunction in adult acquired brain injury, *Am J Occup Ther* 47(1):55, 1993.
62. Wehman PH: Cognitive rehabilitation in the workplace. In Kreutzer JS, Wehman PH, editors: *Cognitive rehabilitation for persons with traumatic brain injury: a functional approach*, Baltimore, 1991, Brookes.
63. Whimbey A, Lochhead J: *Problem solving and comprehension*, ed 5, Hillsdale, NJ, 1991, Lawrence Erlbaum Associates.
64. Wolf SL, Thompson PA, Winstein CJ, Miller JP, Blanton SR, Nichols-Larsen DS, et al: The EXCITE stroke trial: comparing early and delayed constraint-induced movement therapy, *Stroke* 41(10):2309–2315, 2010.
65. Wilson BA: *Rehabilitation of memory*, New York, 1987, Guilford.
66. Wilson BA: Cognitive rehabilitation: how it is and how it might be, *J Int Neuropsychol Soc* 3:487–496, 1997.
67. Youngstrom MJ: Evolving competence in the practitioner role, *Am J Occup Ther* 52:716–720, 1998.
68. Ylvisaker M, et al: Topics in cognitive rehabilitation therapy. In Ylvisaker M, Gobble EM, editors: *Community re-entry for head injured adults*, Boston, 1987, Little Brown.
69. Zoltan B: *Vision, perception, and cognition*, ed 4, Thorofare, NJ, 2007, Slack Inc.
70. Zoltan B, Siev E, and Frieshtat B: The adult stroke patient: a manual for evaluation and treatment of perceptual and cognitive dysfunction, rev ed 2, Thorofare, NJ, 1986, Slack.

PART VII

Clinical Applications

CHAPTER 24 Cerebrovascular Accident

PATRICIA ANN GENTILE

Key Terms

Cerebrovascular accident (CVA, stroke)
Hemiplegia/hemiparesis
Flaccid paralysis/hypotonicity
Deep venous thrombosis (DVT)
Subluxation
Hypotonic
Synergies
Spasticity/hypertonicity
Constraint-induced movement therapy (CIMT)
Robotic-assisted therapy
Hemianopsia
Apraxia (dyspraxia)
Perseveration
Emotional lability
Dysphagia
Aphasia

Chapter Objectives

After studying this chapter, the student or practitioner will be able to do the following:

1. Define cerebrovascular accident and list potential causes of cerebrovascular accident.
2. Discuss modifiable and nonmodifiable risk factors for cerebrovascular accident.
3. Explain the role of the occupational therapy practitioner in preventing common complications after cerebrovascular accident.
4. Understand how stroke may affect performance skills including motor, sensory-perceptual, cognitive, communication, and social (behavioral) and performance patterns; identify occupational therapy treatment strategies to address this.
5. Describe the effects of deficits commonly experienced after left-sided cerebrovascular accident and right-sided cerebrovascular accident in performance of familiar and new tasks.
6. Identify occupational therapy treatment strategies for clients with stroke in the following areas of occupation: activities of daily living, instrumental activities of daily living, work, leisure and social participation.
7. Explain the role of the occupational therapy practitioner in providing client-centered services to stroke survivors across the rehabilitation continuum of care (e.g., from acute management to inpatient rehabilitation, to home care, to outpatient).
8. Understand the need to involve and include caregivers in occupational therapy interventions.
9. Identify the role of the occupational therapy practitioner in health management and health maintenance as it pertains to stroke prevention.

Cerebrovascular accident (CVA, stroke) is the leading cause of serious long-term adult disability[2]; more than 4 million stroke survivors live in the United States alone.[2,15] Each year approximately 795,000 people experience a new or recurrent stroke; an average of 30% of these strokes result in death within 30 days.[2] At least half of stroke survivors report permanent disability, resulting in complete or partial dependence in activities of daily living (ADL).[11] The economic impact of stroke on society is enormous. Estimates place the direct and indirect economic cost of stroke in the United States at well over $73 billion.[2] Adult stroke survivors are the single largest diagnostic group seen by occupational therapy (OT) practitioners in physical dysfunction.[75] OT plays an important role in the rehabilitation of stroke survivors across the continuum of care, beginning in the acute care phase of stroke and continuing through community reintegration. Occupational therapy assistants (OTAs) play an important role in helping stroke survivors gain maximal functional independence and return to desired role participation.

Definition

CVA, or stroke, is a sudden loss of blood supply to the brain that damages and kills brain cells, thus resulting in neurological deficits related to the involved areas of the brain.

Stroke commonly results in **hemiplegia** (one-sided paralysis) or **hemiparesis** (partial motor loss on one side of the body); stroke may also affect the trunk, face, and oral muscles. Stroke effects are experienced in the side of the body opposite to the hemisphere of the brain that suffered the lack of blood supply. A lesion on the left side of the brain produces right-sided hemiplegia, and a right-sided CVA produces left-sided hemiplegia. Incomplete strokes or transient ischemic attacks (TIAs) are temporary. The symptoms of TIA are usually mild, develop suddenly, and last from a few minutes up to 24 hours. There are no remaining symptoms. Approximately a third of persons with TIAs will go on to have a stroke. Because of this risk, recognizing the symptoms of a TIA and seeking immediate treatment is important in reducing the incidence of future strokes.[2]

Etiology

A stroke generally occurs in either of two ways: from sudden blockage of a blood vessel in the neck or brain, causing brain tissue to be deprived of oxygen, or from a blood vessel bursting in the brain. These two types of stroke are known as ischemic and hemorrhagic. Ischemic strokes, which cause 87% of total strokes,[2] may be caused by a thrombus (blood clot that causes blockage) or an embolus (traveling blood clot). Hemorrhagic strokes occur when a rupture of a blood vessel results in bleeding into the brain. Hemorrhagic strokes account for approximately 10% of strokes but result in a significantly higher death rate.[2] The temporary or transient strokelike condition of TIA occurs when the blood supply to the brain is temporarily reduced.

Risk Factors

Several risk factors for stroke have been identified.[2,35] Stroke risk factors are classified as modifiable (controllable) and nonmodifiable (uncontrollable) and are listed in Table 24-1. The risk of stroke increases with age, especially into late adulthood, when most strokes occur.[2,35] Men have a slightly higher risk of stroke than women do.[2,35] African Americans tend to have a much higher frequency of stroke than other racial groups because of the increased incidence of predisposing diseases such as hypertension and diabetes.[15,56,58]

Prevention of stroke focuses on measures that reduce the risk and help to prevent CVA including control of blood pressure and diabetes, elimination of smoking and obesity, regular exercise, proper diet, and reduction of high cholesterol levels. Stroke prevention education should be provided to all individuals who have risk factors for stroke.

Table 24-1 Risk Factors for Stroke

Modifiable/Nonmodifiable	Risk Factors
Nonmodifiable Risk Factors	Age Gender (male) Race (African American and Hispanic) Genetic predisposition
Modifiable Risk Factors	Hypertension Cardiac disease Diabetes mellitus Obesity Diet High cholesterol Use of oral contraceptives with high dose of estrogen Cigarette smoking Alcohol abuse

Effects

Stroke can cause severe loss of function of many body systems and can affect most body function categories including mental functions, sensory functions, neuromuscular and movement-related functions, and voice and speech functions.

Warning Signs

Before stroke, many adults experience warning symptoms that are often ignored.[2,4] This situation is unfortunate because early identification of acute stroke allows health care providers to initiate early administration of effective and appropriate stroke therapies that can reduce stroke progression and residual deficits.[4] Early warning signs of stroke are listed in Box 24-1.

Dysfunction

Immediately after stroke, there is flaccid paralysis (absence of muscle tone), or hypotonicity (low muscle tone) of the affected side with reduced or absent reflexes.[44] Other losses may include impaired postural control, sensory deficits, visual impairments, perceptual dysfunction, cognitive dysfunction, behavioral and personality changes, and impaired speech and language skills.[11,44]

The outcome and severity of CVA depend on the type, size, location, and density of the brain damage; the timing and success of medical care; other medical or neurological problems; and the client's state of health before the stroke.[55,69] Associated diseases of aging such as arthritis, diabetes, and osteoporosis often make recovery from stroke more difficult and affect outcome.[11,31]

The area of the brain affected by stroke is determined by the cerebral blood supply involved.[55] Spontaneous recovery of motor function occurs mostly in the first 3 months after CVA[55] but can continue for up to 1 year. Improvement in functional abilities may continue years after stroke. Factors associated with a poor prognosis are advanced age, coma, seizures, poor perceptual or cognitive functions, lack of motor return, absent sensation, prior history of CVA, and chronic diseases and depression.[11,44,49]

Medical Management

The development of dedicated stroke centers has improved survival rates and reduced secondary complications from stroke in the period immediately after the CVA.[4] Emergency

Box 24-1

Warning Signs of Stroke

- Sudden numbness or weakness of the face, arm, or leg, especially on one side of the body
- Sudden confusion
- Sudden difficulty speaking or understanding, slurred speech
- Sudden blurred vision or loss of vision
- Sudden difficulty walking, dizziness, loss of balance or coordination
- Sudden severe headache with no known cause

medical treatment of CVA includes maintaining an open airway, establishing fluid balance, and treating medical problems. Medications are often used to prevent or reduce damage to cerebral tissues.[4] These medications work by helping reestablish blood flow to the brain. Timing of when these medications are given is critical, so it is important that individuals seek medical care immediately. Surgery may be indicated to repair damaged blood vessels to reduce bleeding and to prevent additional damage to intact cerebral tissues.

Medical Complications

Stroke survivors are prone to developing a wide range of multiple complications.[11,69] Many complications can be prevented by early mobilization. Interventions to prevent complications should begin on the day of admission. The most common complication after CVA is deep venous thrombosis (DVT), which usually develops in the veins of the legs.[12,24] DVT is most likely to occur in the paretic leg. Blood clots called pulmonary emboli, released from deep veins and lodged in the lungs, are the most common cause of death within the first month after CVA.[12,24,55] Some clients with DVT may present with fever, pain, tenderness and swelling, and tenderness in the lower extremity (LE). Other clients may demonstrate no clinical symptoms. Diagnosis of DVT can be done through medical imaging. After a DVT is diagnosed, the affected limb must be elevated and non weight-bearing until the clot is resolved. DVT may be prevented by early exercise, medication, or use of elastic stockings.[62] Low-dose anticoagulation medications, which prevent blood from clotting, may be prescribed to prevent DVT.

Damage to brain tissue after stroke can result in seizures in about 10% to 18% of stroke survivors.[49] The risk for seizure is highest in the first year after the stroke. Medical care stresses prevention or control of seizure activity with anticonvulsant drugs. Side effects from seizure medication may result in drowsiness and may impair thinking skills.[6]

Subluxation commonly occurs in the glenohumeral (GH) joint of the affected upper extremity (UE). The GH joint is between the glenoid fossa of the scapula and the head of the humerus. Subluxation is a separation of the joint as a result of paralysis or weakness of the rotator cuff muscles and spasticity of the scapular muscles. Shoulder subluxation may cause pain in the joint, and, if not treated, can lead to deformity and adhesive capsulitis. The OT practitioner can palpate shoulder subluxation; the presence of a subluxation can be confirmed with an xray. Shoulder subluxation can be prevented through supportive positioning and by avoiding traction when handling the affected UE.

For clients with cardiac problems and stroke, treatment should be individualized, with precautions taken to avoid straining the heart (see Chapter 34). After CVA, the client is at increased risk for lung infections such as pneumonia because of impaired mobility, poor inhalation because of weakness of respiratory muscles from hemiparesis, and impaired swallowing.[8,11]

After stroke, bowel and bladder incontinence is common. Retention of urine can lead to urinary tract infection. Maintenance of continence and prevention of urinary tract infection are common goals early in the medical management of stroke. Medical care is directed toward regular toileting, bowel and bladder retraining, diet, and fluid control. Medication may aid in regulating digestion and elimination and in reducing fluid retention.

Several risk factors for the development of skin breakdown and decubitus ulcers (pressure areas that tend to develop over bony prominences) are present after stroke. Specific contributing factors that affect stroke survivors include prolonged immobility, contracture, sensory loss, malnutrition, and perceptual-cognitive impairments.[6] Regular weight shifting, turning, early exercise, daily skin checks, proper nutrition, and the monitoring of all positioning and pressure relief mattresses and cushioning devices can significantly reduce the risk of pressure damage.[6]

Aspiration can occur in clients with stroke who present with difficulty swallowing (dysphagia).[8,11,46] Aspiration occurs when food or liquid goes into the lungs rather than the stomach. Most, but not all, clients who aspirate will present with clinical signs and symptoms such as coughing, throat clearing, and gurgly speech. Fever may also occur in these clients. Modified diets and close monitoring during meals may prevent aspiration from occurring.

Once the client is medically stable, rehabilitation is the primary treatment for clients recovering from stroke.[4] Effective rehabilitation for the stroke survivor is multidisciplinary, with client and caregivers actively involved in treatment planning and goal setting at each stage.

Occupational Therapy Intervention

Role of Occupational Therapy

OT in the treatment of CVA focuses on the following:

- Improving motor function of the affected side
- Integrating sensory-perceptual and cognitive functions
- Facilitating maximum level of functional independence
- Encouraging resumption of life roles and return to participation as soon as possible
- Promoting health management and maintenance behaviors to prevent recurrent stroke

OT treatment occurs throughout the continuum of care for the stroke survivor. In the acute care management of stroke, a referral for OT can be requested to begin at the bedside. Clients in this early stage may be medically fragile, and it is important that treatment be individualized and precautions be followed. At this early stage, OT stresses early mobility, graded exercise to the client's activity tolerance, prevention of complications, basic self-care training, and gathering of information in order to make appropriate recommendations for the next level of rehabilitation care. Inpatient and subacute rehabilitation OT focuses on ADL and instrumental ADL (IADL), work, and leisure skills. Outpatient services and home health care continue rehabilitation goals until maximum functional performance is achieved, which may involve special programming such as job reentry or driver's training. Home evaluation and modification are also important to successful return to community independence.

Box 24-2

General Occupational Therapy Goals for Clients with Stroke

1. Prevention of secondary complications and injury
2. Encouragement of normal postural and movement patterns
3. Achievement of maximum active and passive range of motion (AROM, PROM) strength and coordination
4. Achievement of maximum functional use of the affected side
5. Remediation and/or compensation of visual perceptual and cognitive dysfunction
6. Achievement of maximum level of independence in all areas of occupation
7. Achievement of maximal mobility skills
8. Achievement of functional communication skills and social interactive skills
9. Facilitation of realistic adaptation to residual problems
10. Facilitation of reentry into meaningful social participation

Goals of Occupational Therapy

OT services for the client with stroke focus on preventive and rehabilitative goals in occupational performance. Overall OT goals are listed in Box 24-2.

Occupational Therapy Programming Considerations

Consistent with the *Occupational Therapy Framework,* edition 2,[3] the OT intervention program is based on a client-centered evaluation of performance skills (i.e., motor and praxis skills; sensory-process skills; and emotional regulation, cognitive, and communication social skills) and areas of occupation (ADL, IADL, education, work, leisure, and social participation). Client factors including values and beliefs must be identified in the evaluation because they will help direct treatment priorities and planning.[3] The occupational therapist uses assessment tools that focus on task performance during ADL to identify client strengths and weaknesses. OT assessment of contextual factors including environmental, social support, and cultural considerations should be considered in the programming process to develop interventions that will support successful engagement in occupation. An understanding of the client's needs, goals, priorities, and concerns further enhances the OT process.

Clients with stroke typically receive OT treatment earlier than similar clients did in the past. OTAs working in the acute stages of stroke must demonstrate the necessary clinical competence for the acute care practice setting. This competence should be assessed regularly because protocols for acute care practice frequently change.

Confounding Factors

More clients with stroke are surviving, and many have a higher level of medical acuity or illness. In the early phase of stroke, medical status can change daily. Frequent reassessment by the occupational therapist may be necessary to provide direction to the OTA. The Black Box on this page provides considerations for this initial phase of rehabilitation. All OT practitioners treating clients with stroke must know signs and symptoms of all diagnoses, as well as current emergency procedures. Careful attention must be given in treatment planning to avoid activities that may worsen symptoms. OTAs should monitor clients with stroke carefully during treatment and be ready to adjust interventions if the client demonstrates fatigue or increased difficulty with movement. Consultation and communication with the medical team are essential at this stage to ensure safe treatment.

Black Box Warning: Safety Considerations in the Early Phase of Stroke Rehabilitation After Stroke

- Review chart prior to each treatment session and consult with supervising OT whenever there are changes in client status or new medical orders are written.
- Be aware of the presence of all feeding tubes, catheters and IV line placements and adhere to precautions regarding same.
- Check and adhere to all precautions related to vital signs (e.g. blood pressure, heart rate and oxygen saturation rates).
- Begin each session with an assessment of vital signs, mental status and activity tolerance.
- Monitor vital signs closely throughout treatment session and proceed based on client's tolerance.

The majority of clients with stroke are older persons with high rates of concurrent disabilities because of chronic medical problems.[15,64] Although older clients do benefit from rehabilitation, increasing age has been associated with more severe symptoms, more recovery time, and overall greater disability in ADL.[43,69]

Gradation of Treatment

Treatment is graded by increasing the length and complexity of the activity. The starting level of difficulty is based on the evaluation results. Time for completion, extent of setup, number of steps, amount of physical assistance, number and frequency of verbal cues, and use of adaptive equipment are adjusted as needed. Age, medical status, and symptoms of disease or other complications may change the gradation of treatment. Stroke survivors may experience setbacks and require readjustment of the treatment program, restarting at a lower level of skill demand. As improvements in endurance and skills increase, task complexity increases until maximum benefit has been achieved.

Occupational Performance Domain of Concern for Treatment

OT treatment for the client with stroke is based on occupational performance (see Chapter 1 and the *Occupational Therapy Practice Framework: Domain and Process,* edition 2).[3] Treatment begins with tasks to prepare the client for occupation and activities and leads to practicing desired previous roles and community reintegration in context.

Dysfunction Characteristics and Occupational Therapy Interventions

Abnormal Reflexes and Postural Mechanisms

CVA often alters postural mechanisms. Normal righting, equilibrium, and protective responses can be delayed or absent on the hemiplegic side. Without the ability to maintain and recover balance, stability, body alignment, and mobility skills can be significantly impaired. These impairments also put clients with stroke at an increased risk for falls.

Positioning Techniques

Proper positioning after CVA is important to minimize the effects of abnormal muscle tone.[26] Individualized positioning interventions should be implemented based on specific client need. General objectives of positioning should be to promote normal alignment of the trunk and extremities and prevent contracture and skin breakdown.

Positioning of the spastic extremities can reduce the risks of developing contractures or skin ulcers. Positioning of the hypotonic (low muscle tone) extremities can reduce the risk of overstretching muscles. In bed, alternating between supine, side-lying on the affected side, and side-lying on the unaffected side at 2- to 4-hour intervals is recommended. Symmetry of trunk alignment is desirable in all positions. The affected arm should be supported in supine and in side-lying while on the unaffected side to reduce edema and prevent injury. The affected leg should be positioned to encourage hip and knee flexion in all positions. During positioning changes, excessive effort should be avoided to prevent the influence of abnormal muscle tone on the affected side. Clients may require adaptive devices such as wedges, bolsters, extra pillows, towel rolls, or splints to maintain proper alignment and positioning. Frequent change of position should be incorporated to encourage awareness of both sides of the body and promote good skin care.

In upright sitting, the trunk should be symmetrical and erect. The affected arm should be supported with pillows, a bedside table, or a lap tray. The affected leg should be positioned in flexion at the hip and knee joints. A properly fitting wheelchair significantly improves a client's sitting posture (see Chapter 15). A lumbar support, a solid seat and back, or a custom cushion can maximize comfortable and symmetrical sitting. The feet should be supported at all times while the client is sitting. Wheelchair lapboards or an arm trough may be required (Figure 24-1).

The resting hand splint is the splint used most commonly to protect the affected forearm, wrist, and hand and for prevention of contractures or deformities (Figure 24-2). Resting hand splints are commonly employed to maintain and support the hand in clients with hypotonia. In cases in which spasticity is present, a resting hand splint may be used to maintain tissue length and provide a gentle stretch. Whether prefabricated or custom-made, the resting hand splint supports the distal arm in a functional position (see Chapters 20 and 25). If provided to the client with stroke, the wearing schedule for the resting hand splint should be individualized. The splint must be removed periodically during the day to prevent learned nonuse, to promote sensory awareness of the hand, and to encourage functional use.[54] Client and caregivers must be instructed in proper technique for application and care of splint including accurate return demonstration.

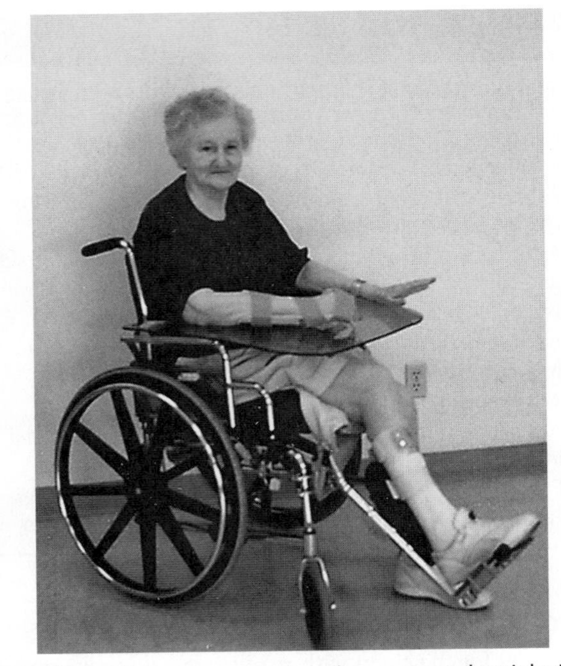

Figure 24-1 Client using a lapboard to support hemiplegic arm while sitting in a wheelchair. A lapboard promotes proper wheelchair positioning and symmetrical trunk alignment.

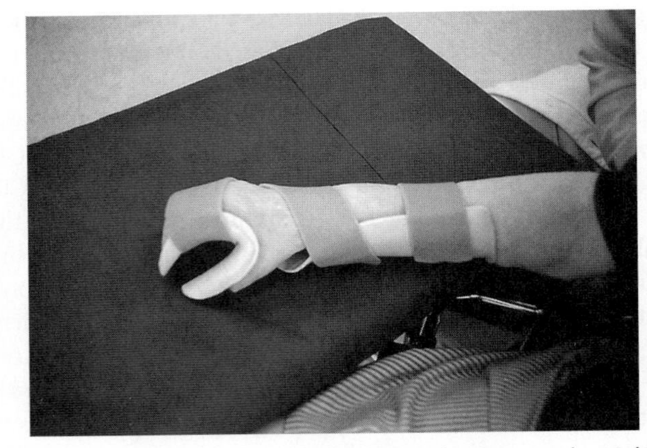

Figure 24-2 A resting hand splint properly supports hemiplegic forearm, wrist, and hand in a functional position.

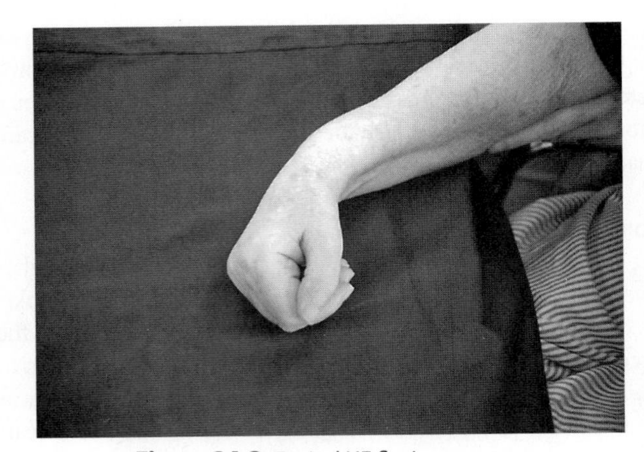

Figure 24-3 Typical UE flexion synergy.

Abnormal Muscle Tone

After CVA, flaccid paralysis is often replaced by spastic paralysis or paresis, resulting in a nonfunctional extremity. Clients move the affected extremities in flexion or extension patterns called synergies. Flexor spasticity of the arm musculature is more dominant and can result in a strong involuntary adducted and flexed positioning of the UE (Figure 24-3). Prolonged posturing in these positions can shorten muscle length and should be avoided.

Functionally, synergy influence or overlay is more obvious in movements against gravity, especially those requiring more effort and reach. Extension synergy is more dominant in the LE. In walking, as the client attempts to flex the hip, knee, and ankle to step, the unintended responses are hip extension and adduction, knee extension, and plantar flexion of the ankle. Without intervention, synergy patterning may progress to contractures and deformities in the affected extremities, as well as asymmetries in the trunk.

Spasticity can be described as minimal, moderate, or severe and may fluctuate daily. Hypertonicity (high muscle tone) tends to increase with stressful bodily changes such as pain, fatigue, infections, injury, ulcers, and bowel dysfunction and in response to some medications. A significant increase in tone may indicate a urinary tract infection, a developing decubitus pressure sore, or bowel impaction. In these cases, spasticity usually reduces to previous levels after successful medical treatment of the underlying problem. The presence of spasticity may interfere with the client's and caregiver's ability to perform hygiene activities and can lead to secondary complications. For example, finger flexor spasticity may result in posturing in a clenched fist, which can cause skin breakdown. Tone may decrease during rest or sleep. In cases in which severe spasticity persists, medical interventions including the use of nerve blocks and oral antispasticity medication may be used in conjunction with therapy interventions.[23,26]

Motor Skills Deficits

Immediately after stroke, voluntary control of the affected UE is usually absent. Motor function returns in stages and may stop at any stage. As motor function returns, it typically develops from the trunk, into the shoulder and hip, and down into the extremities (proximally to distally). Motor recovery often begins with partial active movements and may progress to stronger, more coordinated movements against gravity. Many clients experience some return in scapular retraction, shoulder horizontal adduction, and shoulder elevation. Although complete recovery is rare, some clients regain full functional UE use, especially when sensation is intact and awareness of the hemiplegic side is normal.[9]

Balance Impairment

After a stroke, the client may have problems sitting or standing erect. Because of poor automatic and postural adjustments against gravity, clients tend to compensate by reluctance or decreased ability to bear weight on the hemiplegic side, often leaning away from that side.[10] Balance is poorer if sensation is impaired. Clients unaware of their poor vertical sense may assume they are upright and may need to correct positioning visually. Balance training that incorporates the affected UE will encourage more automatic use of motor and cognitive perceptual skills.[1] While sitting, clients may benefit from supportive devices such as lateral trunk supports, seat belts, or lapboards; these devices can increase stability and may be required for safety until balance improves. Balance impairments significantly increase the risk for falls, especially for clients with multiple problems. Decreased balance can affect UE movement by limiting the ability to reach. The client's ability to participate actively in self-care may be affected by balance impairment.

Common Motor Problems

The person with hemiplegia cannot perform a wide variety of normal movement combinations.[10] The available movements become less selective because of the dominance of synergy patterns. As motor function returns, gross and fine motor coordination problems or incoordination such as ataxia may occur. Chapters 6 and 21 discuss the coordination problems that can occur in a person with hemiplegia. The quality of movement is also affected by muscle weakness, fatigue, infection, and certain drugs. Quicker, fine, skilled movements are usually the last to recover.

Occupational Therapy Treatment Techniques

Treatment of the motor dysfunction focuses on improving balance and voluntary control of the hemiplegic side to support task performance and maximum function.

Passive and Active Range of Motion

Maintenance of full joint range of motion (ROM) and prevention of deformity are important early goals in OT. Passive ROM (PROM) exercises should be performed at least twice daily and continued indefinitely if sufficient active movement does not return. ROM can be limited by fluctuating tone, subluxation, pain, edema, fractures, joint diseases, and reduced scapular and clavicular mobility. Full mobility of the scapula, clavicle, and humerus is required for pain-free shoulder motion. If the scapula does not protract (abduct) and rotate upward and outward with shoulder movements, ROM exercises past 90 degrees of shoulder flexion are contraindicated because of the risk for injury.

PROM exercises of the affected UE are performed by the client (using the unaffected arm) or by another person. PROM or self-ROM (SROM) exercises are required when active movement is weak or absent. During SROM exercises the unaffected UE fully supports the affected UE through all exercises. Care must be taken when performing SROM to the spastic UE to avoid further increasing abnormal muscle tone (Box 24-3). When there is minimal active movement, active assisted ROM (AAROM) exercises are performed. These exercises involve partial assist from the unaffected UE, another person, or an assistive/robotic device. Active ROM (AROM) is performed only by the client and requires voluntary movement of the hemiplegic UE. Incorporation of individually designed home ROM exercise programs has been found to increase motor recovery.[76]

Box 24-3

Self-ROM (SROM) of the Spastic UE

Should be pain free
Should be performed in a slow, controlled manner; avoid quick movements.
Should take each joint through its full ROM; if possible hold for a few seconds at end of range to maintain stretch.

Treatment of Shoulder Subluxation and Pain

As discussed previously, when the hemiplegic shoulder moves and normal scapular motion does not occur, the GH joint can become subluxed. Factors that contribute to increased risk for subluxation include severe sensory loss, poor UE support, poor alignment of GH joint during ROM exercises, arthritic shoulder joint, and incorrect handling of the involved UE by staff or untrained family members.[23,30] Overhead pulley exercises past 90 degrees should be avoided for clients with subluxation.

Pain in a subluxed GH joint may or may not be present. When it occurs, shoulder pain can be present during movement and/or at rest and may range from minimal to severe. Shoulder pain can be prevented through proper positioning; PROM exercises; and education of client, staff, and family on proper handling techniques. The affected UE should be fully supported at all times. In bed, pillows can be used to maintain proper alignment; while in a wheelchair, the client can use a lapboard. When upright during functional ambulation, the client may benefit from kinesiotaping the arm at the shoulder. Kinesotaping involves a hypoallergenic tape applied so as to lift the head of the humerus back into the glenoid fossa.

The use of arm slings to support the shoulder is controversial because most tend to increase the flexed adducted posture while reducing sensory feedback, without reducing the risk for subluxation.[30] Clients who have severe edema, have a heavy flaccid UE, or are at high risk for injury may require a sling temporarily during transfers or gait training.[30,44] If a sling is provided, the client and caregiver must be given clear instructions as to the purpose of the sling, when it should be worn, and proper technique for sling application. Continued assessment of whether the sling is meeting its intended purpose is essential.

Motor Retraining

Motor retraining programs encourage normal postural mechanisms, normal movement, and use of the affected side in functional activities. Retraining is accomplished with sensorimotor (see Chapter 21) or with task-oriented, functionally based approaches.[16,21,23,31] Some basic considerations for motor retraining activities are listed in Box 24-4.[16,20,23,30,57,61]

Box 24-4

General Considerations for Motor Retraining Activities After Stroke

- Select and engage client in activities that are goal-directed, task-oriented, and meaningful.
- Match activities with client's skill level and grade activity up as client improves.
- Teach client to think about movement before and while performing an activity (mental practice).
- Provide opportunities for client to perform activities in different positions (e.g., sitting, standing), at varying speeds and in different contexts.
- Allow client ample opportunities for both mental and motor practice.

Constraint-induced movement therapy (CIMT) techniques have been found to be beneficial in improving arm function and use in clients with stroke with learned nonuse.[25,33,47,60,74] CIMT combines forced use of the affected arm via intensive training through active participation in specific functional activities. CIMT helps to overcome learned nonuse of the affected upper extremity. Robotic-assisted therapy has also been used for retraining upper arm movements after stroke and has been found to improve effectiveness of rehabilitation in selected populations. The use of robotic-assisted devices in therapy provides the opportunity for high-intensity, repetitive, task-specific, and interactive treatment of the impaired upper limb, as well as an objective, reliable means of monitoring patient progress.[48,51,77] Virtual reality systems such as the Wii or Kinect also provide opportunities for motor retraining after stroke by directing automated, real-time feedback to the client.[70]

Influencing Muscle Tone

OT treatment techniques may influence muscle tone. Active movement of hypotonic muscles can be facilitated through stimulation of various sensations. Inhibition (reduction of tone) of hypertonic muscles can be accomplished through positioning and handling. Tactile and proprioceptive input can help to decrease high tone. In the presence of increased muscle tone, slow and controlled movements should be encouraged; clients should be discouraged from excessive effort, which may only further increase muscle tone. Whenever possible, clients should be taught appropriate techniques to normalize muscle tone on their own. OTAs looking to address muscle tone in treatment should collaborate closely with the occupational therapist. Specialized training in this area is required.

Bilateral Integration

Bilateral integration of the UEs is an early and important goal in stroke rehabilitation, even if the affected arm is nonfunctional. Increased tactile and visual input will encourage development of movement sense. The affected UE should be properly positioned and kept within the client's view at all times including during one-handed activities.[10] UE activities with hands clasped such as pushing a ball on a tabletop,[10] or "towel on table activities,[30] can incorporate the affected arm into activity. As motor functions return, the affected arm initially serves as a stabilizer and progresses to being a gross assist, then a partial assist, and may eventually become functional in all tasks.

Strengthening and Endurance

Clients may exhibit muscle weakness after stroke, even in the presence of abnormally high muscle tone.[30,31] Stroke survivors often demonstrate an overall loss of strength and a significant reduction of endurance. Therapeutic goals directed toward strength and endurance for clients after stroke should be a carefully planned element of OT treatment. Assessing strength in the presence of abnormal muscle tone can be difficult. If spasticity is present in the affected UE, resistive activities may increase tone and should be prescribed with caution.

Strengthening of the unaffected side is appropriate if increased resistance does not increase spasticity of the hemiplegic side. If prescribed, resistive exercises should focus on both agonist (targeted) and antagonist (opposing) muscle groups. Clients should be monitored closely so that exercises can be graded down and modified if increased spasticity is observed.

Nearly one half of all stroke survivors report fatigue as a factor that interferes with participation in daily activities and exercise programs.[41] Endurance training should be included in every stroke program and should be graded according to each client's abilities and lifestyle needs. Inclusion of rest periods is essential. Monitoring of vital signs (e.g., blood pressure, pulse, respiration) during exercise may be required for clients with cardiovascular precautions (see Chapter 34). For these clients, the OTA should demonstrate clinical competence for monitoring vital signs and be sure to adhere to specific vital sign parameters prescribed by the referring physician.

Elevation and Retrograde Massage

Edema or fluid accumulation is a common preventable complication after a stroke. Edema can be caused by various factors including immobility, poor circulation, dependent positioning and poor posture, sensory loss, and overexercise. Swelling increases the diameter of the skin, which becomes soft and puffy. Prolonged edema results in shiny hard skin, stiff joints, pain, and loss of ROM. The presence of severe edema may be an early sign of complex regional pain syndrome (CRPS), formally known as *reflex sympathetic dystrophy* (RSD). If CRPS is suspected, early diagnosis of and treatment for CRPS should be addressed immediately.

Edema can be prevented by elevating extremities. AROM tasks, especially those involving upward reach, are most effective in preventing or reducing edema. Retrograde manual massage of the elevated hand, beginning at the fingertips and moving toward the elbow, can be performed by the client, the caregiver, or a clinician. Elastic stockings or sleeves, self-adherent wraps (Coban), and pneumatic compression devices such as air splints reduce edema through constant pressure. Splints and positioning devices should be closely monitored to prevent edema.

Compensatory Techniques

For some stroke survivors, the dominant side is also the hemiplegic side. Such clients may require training in one-handed performance and possibly dominance retraining because they may have to rely permanently on one hand.[10] Strategies for one-handedness include learning methods of stabilizing objects and compensating with adapted equipment. During the performance of these one-handed activities, the affected UE should be incorporated into the activity as much as possible (e.g., as a stabilizer).

Sensory System Dysfunction

Stroke can cause absent or impaired sensation. If sensation returns, it usually does so in a proximal to distal pattern.

Visual Deficits

OT practitioners should be aware of many factors that affect visual performance. Because stroke usually occurs in the elderly, many clients with stroke may exhibit age-related visual deficits such as cataracts, macular degeneration, and glaucoma[43] (see Chapter 22). Obtaining information about any preexisting visual deficits can aid in realistic treatment planning.

Stroke can affect many aspects of vision, and visual losses after stroke usually reduce safety. A stroke often reduces visual functions related to distance vision, peripheral awareness, and accommodation (the ability to use eyes together to focus on images at any distance). Diplopia (double vision) may also occur. Clients are not always aware of their visual deficits, and when they are unaware, their functioning and safety may be compromised.

The occupational therapist may perform a visual screening after stroke. If visual problems are identified during screening, the client should be referred to an ophthalmologist or optometrist.

The ability to see objects in the center of vision is usually not affected by CVA, but peripheral vision losses are common. **Hemianopsia** is a permanent visual defect after stroke that results in loss of vision on the contralateral half of the visual field. Homonymous hemianopsia is a loss of the visual field of the lateral (temporal) aspect of the hemiplegic side and the medial (nasal) aspect of the unaffected side, resulting in a loss of one half (R or L) of the visual field. Clients with visual field loss may not see objects in the affected area of vision. Visual deficits related to perception are discussed later in this chapter.

Auditory Deficits

Stroke generally does not seem to affect hearing, even in clients with aphasia (language disorders); if hearing deficits exist in clients after stroke, they are usually a result of normal aging.[50] To avoid erroneously labeling clients with hearing loss "confused," documentation of hearing loss by the audiologist is important.

Tactile Deficits

Changes in the senses of touch, pain, pressure, temperature, vibration, and proprioception (position sense) are common after CVA.[44] Without sensory feedback, clients experience difficulty using affected extremities, even when motor recovery is good. Risk for injury increases with increased sensory loss.

Olfactory and Gustatory Deficits

After stroke, brain damage may dull the senses of smell and taste.[28] OT practitioners can instruct clients about changes in taste or smell that could contribute to poor appetite, hygiene problems, safety problems (e.g., inability to smell dangerous odors), or a reduced enjoyment of pleasurable odors and tastes. These deficits may affect nutrition and quality of life for some clients.

Occupational Therapy Treatment Considerations

Sensory Retraining and Compensatory Techniques

The OT program for the client with stroke may include sensory reeducation and compensatory techniques, as described in Chapter 21.

Perceptual Dysfunction

Perception is the complex process of interpreting sensory information from the environment. Stroke may affect a variety of visual-perceptual and perceptual motor skills. Changes in visual perception seen after CVA result from the stroke rather than from normal aging.[73,74]

Visual Perceptual Impairments

Normal human visual behavior involves visual attention and search. Visual attention is a purposeful visual response to the environment and in normal adults can be sustained as desired. Visual search, or tracking, is the process of selecting objects on which to focus attention by scanning the environment. A common visual-perceptual problem after CVA is hemi-inattention. Clients with a visual attention deficit have difficulty shifting their gaze or attending to objects.[71] Their eye movements tend to be slower. When clients cannot attend, search, and scan, the ability to identify objects or people is diminished. Hemi-inattention can affect function and safety significantly.

Spatial Relations Deficits

The ability to identify shapes and recognize the relationship between objects and between object and self is affected by CVA. Clients may have trouble judging the distance between objects or following a familiar route.[81] Deficits in understanding concepts such as over, under, through, and behind can cause dressing problems.[67]

Visual figure-ground perception is the ability to distinguish forms hidden within a complicated background.[81] Clients with figure-ground problems appear distractible but could be responding to irrelevant visual information.[8,79]

Difficulty with vertical or horizontal orientation (directionality) may be present, especially in clients with left-sided hemiplegia, who tend to see vertical objects as tilted left of center.[9] Because visual orientation is important to the righting reactions for upright posture, directional disturbances interfere with balance and ambulation.[9,21] Because clients with these deficits have a distorted perception of the vertical plane, tactile cues may be more effective than verbal when prompting them to assume an upright position in sitting or standing.

Color Discrimination Deficits

Problems discriminating color after CVA are less common. However, because the majority of stroke survivors are elderly, age-related changes in color vision may be present.[19]

Perceptual Motor Impairments

Perceptual motor skills rely on the processing of sensation to develop adaptive motor responses. A person who has suffered a CVA may have perceptual motor deficits that interfere with functional independence.

Unilateral Neglect

Unilateral neglect is the inability to interpret perceptual messages from the hemiplegic side of the body or space. Unilateral neglect is more common in persons with left-sided hemiplegia and can occur with or without visual inattention and hemianopsia. Clients show a gaze preference, keeping the head turned away from the affected side and ignoring the affected half of the body and of space. Clients with unilateral neglect often demonstrate difficulties in ADL, and safety can be compromised. Unilateral neglect that persists past the acute phase of stroke has been associated with a poorer functional outcome in therapy.[18]

Apraxia (Dyspraxia)

Apraxia (dyspraxia) is an impaired ability to plan motor acts. Clients can have difficulty performing purposeful movement on command, understanding the concept of a task, or drawing or constructing two- or three-dimensional designs. Apraxia occurring with body scheme problems can cause dressing apraxia and problems with ADL.[79]

Body Awareness Deficits

Body scheme disorders affect knowledge of body construction, spatial relationships, awareness of bodily parts in relation to one another, and right and left discrimination.[5,52] Because bodily awareness is basic to all motor function, poor body scheme causes many functional deficits, which are particularly evident in basic self-care.[45,52]

Agnosia

Agnosia refers to the inability to recognize objects by vision, hearing, touch, or proprioception (position sense) despite intact senses. Symptoms are worsened when the client has an impaired body scheme and unilateral neglect.[34] One of the more common problems is tactile agnosia or astereognosis, the inability to recognize familiar objects by touch without vision. Additional information on these and other sensory and perceptual problems can be found in Chapters 9, 22, and 23.

Occupational Therapy Treatment Considerations

Remediation of Visual-Perceptual Deficits

Perceptual difficulties are often not well understood by clients and their families or caregivers. Remediation of deficits focuses on the goal of restoration of skills (see Chapters 22 and 23). Clients and significant others need to be educated about visual perception and perceptual motor impairments to understand the treatment process.

Compensatory Strategies for Visual-Perceptual and Perceptual Motor Impairments

Compensatory strategies are important for clients with perceptual impairments. Compensatory strategies use intact skills to substitute for deficits. When using compensatory strategies, some elements of a task may be enhanced to provide cues and other elements masked to reduce distractibility.[3] Selection of treatment activities should be based on the client's interests, previous lifestyle, remaining strengths and deficits, living situation, and goals. Caregivers should be trained in the use of compensatory strategies to allow for carryover when the client is not in therapy.

Some clients can compensate automatically and may require minimal or no intervention, whereas others may need repetitive practice to learn a compensatory strategy. Clients with gaze preference can learn to turn their heads toward the affected side and use auditory and tactile cues and remaining vision. Clients with apraxia can learn a task using environmental cues or tactile cues from others to assist them through familiar basic functional tasks until performance becomes more automatic. Persons with mild neglect can learn strategies such as verbally cueing themselves to attend to the affected side or wearing a watch on that side. Persons with persistent neglect require continual supervision for safety. For clients with unilateral neglect, use of functional activities and feedback from videotaping such activities can improve awareness.[65,67]

In some cases the use of a mirror and clothing labels to identify parts (e.g., right sleeve) can compensate for body awareness deficits. Clients with spatial relations problems may learn routes in their environments by using the same route each time and taking notice of signs to mark the way. Clients with agnosia can learn to use other senses to compensate for problems. For example, clients who do not recognize their family members by sight may identify them by their voices. Labeling family pictures can be useful.

Garments can be labeled to avoid mismatching clothing for individuals with impaired color discrimination. Customizing treatment materials and the environment to address color-contrast needs of the older adult is recommended.[19] Color or texture contrasts in self-care tasks may also help clients with figure-ground impairments.

Cognitive Dysfunction

Cognition requires the integration of numerous abilities, many of which may be impaired by CVA.

Initiation and Motivation Deficits

Impaired initiation is characterized by difficulty starting and finishing tasks. Clients require physical assistance or verbal cues to begin and often cannot restart after stopping. These behaviors may be mistaken for noncompliance or poor motivation and this can be quite frustrating for client's caregivers. Step-by-step assistance to complete even familiar basic self-care tasks may improve skills. Many clients show a decrease in intrinsic motivation, or the inner drive to act spontaneously. Such clients should not be labeled "unmotivated" or "resistant" because the lack of drive is a result of brain damage.

Attention and Concentration Deficits

Deficits in the abilities to attend to information and to maintain that focus affect every aspect of performance. Distractibility is common, especially in a stimulating environment. Attention problems are worsened by fatigue, depression, illness, disinterest, and certain medications.

Disorientation and Confusion

Orientation involves awareness of person, place, time, and situation. Awareness of person includes being aware of information such as full name, birth date, age, marital status, telephone number, number of children, and education. Place concepts involve knowing current location (e.g., hospital), address, city, state, and country. Time orientation includes day, date, time, month, year, season, and next holiday. Situational information includes identifying the reason for hospitalization or verifying employment or general knowledge such as naming the President. Orientation is often documented as the abbreviation "O" times the number of oriented areas (e.g., O × 2). Clients tend to retain personal information longest and forget situational information first.

Memory Deficits

CVA can affect reception, integration, and retrieval of information for short- or long-term memory skills. Memory deficits after stroke are more commonly seen in older clients, and deficits can range from minimal to severe.[27] Clients may have difficulty recalling persons, objects, and procedures.

Sequencing and Organization Deficits

Sequencing involves planning, organizing, and completing the steps of a task in correct order. It includes temporal concepts such as first, second, and third and spatial ordering such as top, bottom, left to right, and around.[5] Sequencing errors can occur in any task, even familiar ones. The more complex the activity, the greater the number of errors.

Effective organization requires higher levels of attention, concentration, orientation, memory, and correct sequencing. Clients who are disorganized have severe difficulty in activities such as maintaining schedules, fulfilling responsibilities, and completing projects. Categorization involves the organizational ability to group similar objects or concepts. Deficits in this area can affect IADL such as shopping or budgeting.

Abstract Reasoning and Problem-Solving Deficits

When abstract thinking is impaired, clients show concrete literal thinking. Clients with deficits may have difficulty planning ahead, recognizing problems, or generating solutions. They may propose extremely ineffective, unrealistic, or unsafe answers to questions or solutions to problems.

Thought Inflexibility

Thinking involves the flow of thoughts or ideas and may be affected by stroke. Thought inflexibility or rigidity is the inability to adapt thinking patterns or behavior in response to change. The client may be labeled as "difficult" as a result of problems accepting new concepts. Changing from one activity to another, changing environments, or following more complex conversation is also impaired.

Insight Deficits

After stroke, insight into lifestyle changes and limitations may be reduced. Dysfunction may be denied despite obvious disability. Continued denial can prolong or prevent the client's progress toward adjustment to disability. Problems with insight may also reduce a client's safety awareness and increase risk for injury.

Judgment and Safety Awareness Deficits

Poor judgment and decreased safety awareness impair the ability to understand consequences of behavior. Clients may be unreceptive to feedback and become argumentative or noncompliant. Family and caregiver education is important for client safety.

Generalization and Learning Deficits

One of the main focuses of stroke rehabilitation is generalization for use after discharge of all skills learned during the rehabilitation program. If learning ability is impaired, carryover of new techniques may be reduced. To effectively plan treatment to maximize learning, the clinician must understand previous and current learning styles. Challenging the client to apply skills from one task to another promotes generalization. Treatment sessions should be structured so that the client performs tasks in various contexts to allow training for generalization.

Cognitive Fatigue

Performance errors due to cognitive fatigue are common after CVA. OT practitioners should be familiar with signs of fatigue and make adjustments in programming accordingly. Signs may include decreased attention and concentration, increased lethargy, increased distractibility, increased performance errors, decreased quality control, decreased performance speed, decreased frustration tolerance, and complaints of fatigue. Clients and caregivers should also be taught to recognize early signs of fatigue. In those clients with cognitive fatigue, frequent rest periods should be built into treatment sessions.

Occupational Therapy Treatment Considerations

OT intervention for cognitive deficits focuses on maximizing long-term generalization of learned skills and safety procedures. Providing opportunities for clients to actively work on generalizing skills from one task to another is key for true learning to occur.

Cognitive Retraining

Neuropsychologists, speech-language pathologists, and OT practitioners provide different aspects of cognitive rehabilitation. Treatment methods for cognitive dysfunction are described in Chapter 23.

Compensatory Strategies for Cognitive Deficits

Verbal and tactile cues may stimulate clients with decreased initiation to begin an activity. The need for cues diminishes as skills improve. Establishing realistic, meaningful, achievable treatment goals and giving frequent positive feedback improve motivation. The client and therapist should plan and modify treatment goals together.

Clients with impaired attention can benefit from brief, frequent sessions in activities of high interest in a nondistracting environment. Time and difficulty are increased as the client's capacity increases. These activities can be provided in a group format or individually. Orientation methods include reality orientation, reminiscence therapy, use of family pictures, labeling client's belongings, using calendars and watches, or using props for holidays. Family members and friends can help to individualize the treatment program.

Memory strategies often involve devices. Some of the many commercially available products include notebooks, daily calendars, watches, posted schedules, labels, smart phones, and personal digital assistants. Clients may also be taught "memory tricks" such as mnemonics for retaining information.

OT intervention for organizational deficits focuses on gradual increase of task complexity. Treatment for sequencing and categorization errors involves building skill level from one step to multiple step tasks. Problem solving also involves a graded approach with the use of simulations. Clients who are concrete problem solvers benefit more from a functional approach. A step-by-step training should include recognizing a problem, generating solutions for the problem, selecting and implementing a solution, and then assessing the effectiveness of the solution selected.

Easing transitions from one activity to another and increasing client control can reduce anxiety for clients with rigid thinking. Clients with thought inflexibility perform better when breaks between activities are longer to allow time for adaptation. Intervention for insight deficits involves gradual introduction to performance problems, beginning with nonthreatening information and progressing as the client tolerates. A matter-of-fact approach addressing safety issues is useful. Training should take place in the real-life situations relevant and meaningful to the client.

Increasing instruction time, repeating instructions, and using written instructions are helpful in addressing learning problems. Understanding the cause of functional problems will prompt treatment strategies. For example, clients may experience difficulty in UE dressing primarily as a result of perceptual and cognitive problems, and deficits in LE dressing may be more related to motor recovery deficits.[79]

Behavioral Manifestations

After CVA, cognitive deficits may lead to behavioral problems that impair interaction skills. Clients have a limited understanding of the motives and consequences of their behavior. Inappropriate behavior reduces the ability to participate in rehabilitation, impairs safety, and may damage the quality of social interactions.

Impulsivity and Perseveration

Decreased insight can lead to impulsive behavior. The client makes quick decisions without fully considering the consequences.

Motor perseveration is the meaningless, nonpurposeful repetition of an action.[36] Clients with perseveration have difficulty terminating a task and will usually continue until someone or something intervenes. Perseveration is more obvious during activities that are repetitive in nature such as writing, combing hair, or shaving.

Mood and Emotional Impairments

Mood and emotional problems including lability, depression, and anxiety are common in the first year after a stroke but can occur at any time.[14,22,41] Estimates of the frequency of these problems vary and appear to depend on the type of stroke, the timing of assessments, presence of a social support system, and severity of physical disability from stroke.[22,39]

Shortly after stroke occurs, many clients show emotional lability, which is the inability to control the expression of emotions.[14] Inappropriate, uncontrolled outbursts of laughing (euphoria) or weeping are common. Emotionally charged situations, whether pleasant or unpleasant, can cause such responses. Some clients may become combative and agitated, often as a result of confusion. Medications and behavior modification programs can reduce these behaviors. In the most severe cases of agitation, some clients may need to be restrained for safety.

Depression after stroke is common, affecting approximately 20% to 70% of clients annually.[14,39] Depression can be reactive, an appropriate grieving response to losses, but it is more often the result of cerebral damage.[14] Strokes of the left hemisphere are much more likely to result in major depression.[40] Poststroke depression can adversely affect long-term functional outcomes.[17,63] Early identification and medication management can be effective. Symptoms of depression include lethargy, apathy, extreme fatigue, excessive sadness, forgetfulness, disorganization, loss of appetite, and sleep disturbance. Anxiety often accompanies depression and may also need to be addressed.[14] Anxiety may result in overdependence on staff and reduced frustration tolerance.

Behavioral Implications

Behavioral problems that result from CVA may reduce a client's ability or willingness to participate in therapy. A history of previous behavior and usual coping methods during crisis helps the OT practitioner understand the current behavior of the client with cognitive deficits. Shifts in behavior may be viewed as losses by client and family. Significant others and caregivers need to understand why behavioral problems occur and need to learn how to implement effective strategies to respond to behavioral problems. Providing education to significant others and caregivers early and often about this can help with their understanding of these problems.

Psychosocial Adjustment and Adaptation

An important role of the OT practitioner is to aid in the client's and family's adaptation to disability. A lack of independence may affect the client's performance patterns and disrupt daily habits and routines. It is essential that the occupational therapist and the OTA understand how each client's participation and satisfaction with activities and occupations have been affected by stroke. Client-centered treatment approaches are crucial to this process. OT practitioners need to understand and incorporate client and caregiver goals and expectations into the treatment. Discharge planning should be directed toward helping clients prepare for the impact of their limitations on previous habits and routines.[66,78]

Dealing with the effects of stroke can be difficult, and clients and families make take many months to learn how to cope with the many personal and social changes. Repetition may be necessary to clarify questions and reduce concerns. Coping with extreme reversals in functional abilities after the CVA is challenging for all involved. Allowing families and future caregivers to actively participate in the therapy process is critical, especially in preparation for discharge from a rehabilitation program. Predischarge home visits and self-care days, where families come and spend the day as an active caregiver for client, can help with this preparation. Providing client and family education information and teaching them how to access information on their own is vital.

Caregivers are at risk for stress-related conditions and burnout. OT intervention should include support and recognition of the caregiver's contribution, addressing caregiver needs, and offering strategies to avoid burnout.[59] Options such as taking turns in the family, hiring professional help in the home, or using respite care can reduce stress. Some stroke survivors and families choose to participate in community or online stroke support groups, often after discharge (online support resources for caregivers can be found at the end of this chapter). Engaging family and friends throughout the rehabilitative process can reduce stress levels and help to improve generalization of skills to the home environment.

Occupational Therapy Treatment Considerations

OT programming for behavioral problems of adult clients with stroke focuses on the development of appropriate behaviors and generalization to daily life.

Behavioral Intervention Strategies

Strategies for impulsivity include giving directions slowly, verbally, or in written form one step at a time and using a calm approach in a nondistracting environment. Verbal and tactile cues and avoidance of repetitive tasks can reduce perseveration. Some clients with reduced frustration tolerance perform better with new activities in which they have no preconceived ideas about expected performance. The OT practitioner should provide activities that involve choice, using a matter-of-fact approach and immediate positive reinforcement. To improve attention to detail, a graded approach would initially focus on recognizing errors and then progress to correcting errors and finally to checking quality of performance. Prior to performance of a task, asking clients to predict performance and then engaging them in comparing predictions to actual performance can also help improve insight into abilities.

When treating agitated or combative clients, OT practitioners should obtain information regarding their current behavioral state before every session and decide whether treatment is possible at that time. If agitation increases, treatment should be discontinued immediately and reattempted only when the client is calmer. Consulting and collaborating with the psychologist can also be helpful.

Many clients and families are unfamiliar with OT services. They may question the value of therapy or express reluctance to participate in activities that seem simple or tedious. OT practitioners can avoid much resistance by clients and families by providing treatment activities that are meaningful and relevant to the client's goals. Many clients focus on the possibility of full recovery despite the fact that it is likely problems may remain. The therapist may approach this matter by discussing it openly and honestly in objective terms but without eliminating hope. Repeated discussions may be necessary before the client begins to apply the information to personal recovery.

Social Skills Training

The multiple deficits resulting from stroke can have a major impact on social skills. Common behaviors include acting out, emotional outbursts, interrupting others, seeking constant immediate reinforcement, flirting, or other attention-seeking behaviors. These behaviors can be minimized with consistent limit setting. Social skills training individually or in a group setting can be effective in improving appropriate behavior.

Oral-Motor Dysfunction

Oral-motor control is the coordination of movement for speech, facial expression, sucking, chewing, and swallowing. It involves the muscles and other structures of the face, throat, and tongue.

Dysarthria

Normally, the coordination of facial muscles, lips, tongue, and jaw produces articulated speech that can be understood by listeners. After stroke, oral-motor weakness on the affected side causes facial palsy or drooping, especially of the corner of the mouth. Reduced sensation often accompanies muscle weakness. Clients with dysarthria have difficulty pronouncing many sounds or combinations of sounds, causing slurred speech. These clients may be difficult to understand.

Dysphagia

Dysphagia (difficulty in swallowing or the inability to swallow) is caused by sensory loss and muscle weakness in the structures of the mouth and throat that control swallowing.[13] Clients often exhibit dysphagia immediately after stroke, especially when the stroke occurs in the area of the brainstem.[29,36] Assessment of dysphagia may be done by the occupational therapist or speech-language pathologist. The assessment process includes clinical observation of the client during meals or the use of videofluoroscopy or fiberoptic endoscopic studies.[42] Clinicians who evaluate and treat clients with dysphagia require specialized training. It is not an entry-level practice area for the OTA; OTAs who carry out dysphagia programs must demonstrate clinical competence in this area and be supervised closely by the occupational therapist.

Common observable clinical signs of dysphagia include drooling, pocketing of food in the mouth, coughing, or a gurgly voice. Clients with dysphagia are at high risk for aspiration of saliva or food,[46] which can lead to aspiration pneumonia. To protect the airway, some clients receive a temporary or permanent tracheostomy ("trach") tube—a tube surgically placed through the skin of the neck and into the trachea. The primary physician and the dysphagia therapist together determine whether a client can eat orally or must be fed by tube. Many clients with stroke with dysphagia are given nutrient liquids and medications by a nasogastric (NG) tube, which passes through the nose into the stomach. NG tubes can cause increased gagging and irritation of the nasal passages and upper gastrointestinal tract.[24] Confused clients often tug at and remove their NG tubes unless they are restrained. Gastrostomy tubes (G tubes) placed surgically through the abdominal wall into the lower stomach are used by clients with dysphagia who cannot eat anything by mouth (NPO). Maintaining adequate hydration can be a challenge to the medical team treating the client with dysphagia.

Occupational Therapy Treatment Considerations

Dysphagia often occurs in association with dysarthria and cognitive impairments.[53] These problems contribute to poorer oral control, increased communication difficulties, and decreased safety while eating. Clients, staff, and families need to be educated early and often about a client's specific swallowing problems and any dietary restrictions that might be imposed—especially for those clients who may not show any visible signs of problems swallowing.

Oral-Motor Control

Clients who have difficulty keeping their lips closed tend to drool saliva and leak food from the affected corner of the mouth. This problem can be minimal to severe and is worsened by impaired sensation. Many clients, especially those with unilateral neglect, may be unaware of the problem. Treatment for dysphagia involves a feeding program; modified diet; and ongoing instruction of client, family, and staff to promote carryover of feeding techniques. Frequent consultation with nursing, nutrition and speech-language pathology is essential when working with this population. General eating/feeding considerations are listed in the Black Box below.

Black Box Warning: Safe Eating/Feeding for Clients with Dysphagia

- Determine proper positioning for eating, including the use of necessary equipment to promote the best position for eating.
- Understand and comply with prescribed food and liquid consistencies of diet.
- Be knowledgeable about specific eating/feeding precautions.
- Observe and monitor client closely while he or she is eating.
- Educate and involve client, family, and caregivers in client feeding program.
- Demonstrate competence for emergency procedures for choking and aspiration.

Safe eating is also related to diet and food choices. Items such as dry foods (bread, crackers, chips), chewy foods (meat, candy), thin liquids (water, soda), and foods with mixed consistencies (casseroles, soups) are problematic. Softer foods such as cream of wheat, gelatin, mashed potatoes, applesauce, custards, puddings, popsicles, and ice cream are easier to chew and swallow. Sensory loss may reduce ability to detect hot and cold foods. A variety of diet types and diet modifications can be offered to clients based on individual needs, as determined by the physician, dysphagia therapist, and dietitian.

Safety Issues

All clients with dysphagia should be supervised by staff at all times to prevent complications and maximize safety. Some clients may be self-conscious about their appearance while eating and may prefer a more private dining setting. Clients with visual-perceptual and cognitive problems may show impaired safety, increased spillage (especially with hotter foods or liquids), and noncompliance with dietary changes. OT practitioners should be familiar with all client precautions, dietary restrictions, symptoms of dysphagia, and emergency procedures in case of choking. Facilities that treat clients with dysphagia should have the proper emergency equipment such as a suction machine readily available. Both client and caregiver must understand and be trained in dysphagia precautions and safe eating/swallowing techniques so that they can effectively carry this over at discharge.

Speech and Language Dysfunction

CVA causes several language disorders, varying from mild to severe, often in combination with speech problems. Language dysfunction occurs most commonly in left-sided CVA but can occur with damage to the right hemisphere. The speech-language pathologist recommends the best communication techniques. The OT practitioner's role is to promote communication by reinforcing these techniques and adapting augmentative communication devices.

Aphasia

Aphasia is an acquired language disorder that may result in a wide variety of deficits in verbal comprehension, reading comprehension (alexia), oral expression, written expression (agraphia), ability to interpret gestures, or mathematical skills (acalculia).[38] Several different types of aphasia exist. Anomia, or word-finding difficulty, occurs in all types. Clients with expressive aphasia (Broca's aphasia) have difficulty speaking, and those with receptive aphasia (Wernicke's aphasia) have problems understanding language. Global aphasia is characterized by a loss of both language skills. The ability to speak is often absent. Clients with global aphasia often may appear to respond to gestures, voice tone changes, and facial expression. Careful consideration of what clients actually understand is important because clients with global aphasia may appear to understand more than they actually do.[80]

Occupational Therapy Treatment Considerations

Recovery from aphasia varies. Education designed to improve understanding of aphasia by caregivers and others may help the client manage with adjustment.[72]

Box 24-5

Suggestions for Improving Communication with Clients Who Have Aphasia

- Be patient.
- Reduce environmental distractions.
- Use face to face communication; establish and maintain eye contact during communications.
- Stress the important words in sentences.
- Speak clearly in simple direct sentences; do not shout.
- Ask "yes/no" or forced choice questions.
- Allow adequate time for a response to questions; do not interrupt.
- Observe and respond to non-verbal communications from client (body language, gestures).
- Let the client know you do not understand; if necessary take a short break to avoid client from getting too frustrated.

Communication Guidelines for Clients with Aphasia

Most clients with aphasia use a variety of communication methods including alphabet boards, notebook computers, picture boards, gestures, and writing. Some can speak single words or phrases. Client responses may be less than totally accurate and become less so with fatigue. Box 24-5 provides for suggestions for communicating with clients with aphasia.[32,75]

Hemispheric Lateralization

Left-Sided Cerebrovascular Accident

The left cerebral hemisphere of most right-handed persons is primarily responsible for language, time concepts, and analytical thinking.[17,36] Clients with right-sided hemiplegia (left brain damage) often demonstrate aphasia and apraxia. They commonly achieve self-care independence earlier than clients with left-sided hemiplegia (right brain damage) but are more likely to experience depression.

Right-Sided Cerebrovascular Accident

The right cerebral hemisphere primarily controls visual-perceptual skills and perception of the whole.[36] It plays an important part in interpreting information from the environment and one's own body.[36] Damage to this hemisphere results in difficulties in tasks that require spatial analysis and orientation and dressing praxis.[65,68] Clients with left-sided hemiplegia (right brain damage) may retain good verbal skills, which may tend to hide perceptual dysfunction, and may show poorer functional performance. Because of the many deficits often seen in clients with right brain damage, implementation of environmental safety precautions is essential.

Comparison of Left- and Right-Sided Cerebrovascular Accident

Although the left and right cerebral hemispheres show specialization, both control several of the same abilities, which

Table 24-2 Differences and Similarities between Left- and Right-Sided Cerebrovascular Accident

Left-Sided Cerebrovascular Accident and Right-Sided Hemiplegia	Skills	Right-Sided Cerebrovascular Accident and Left-Sided Hemiplegia
Right-sided paralysis/paresis, decreased motor control of repetitive movements (dysphagia*)	Motor	Left-sided paralysis/paresis, more severe motor problems, decreased motor response time (dysphagia)
Right-sided sensory loss	Sensory	Left-sided sensory loss
Right visual field cuts (visual neglect)	Visual	Left field cuts, visual neglect
Impaired right/left discrimination, verbal apraxia (hemi-inattention, motor apraxia)	Perceptual	Unilateral neglect, hemi-inattention, motor apraxia, constructional apraxia, dressing apraxia, agnosia, disorientation for directionality, difficulty crossing midline
Decreased analytic thinking, impaired logic, impaired time concepts, impaired memory associated with language	Cognitive	Impaired attention span, impaired understanding of the whole, decreased creativity, impaired memory for performance, poor insight, poor safety awareness, poor judgment
Slow performance, cautious behavior, depression	Behavioral	Impulsivity, emotional lability
Aphasia, agraphia, dyscalculia, decreased understanding of gestures, impaired reading, decreased ability to learn new information	Speech and language	Decreased ability to differentiate between gestures, decreased learning for familiar (old) information

*Conditions in parentheses play a lesser role.

may explain how clients who apparently have permanently lost brain function for certain skills can regain function. Left-hand-dominant adults tend to exhibit less specialization than right-handed adults.[44] Similarities and differences between left and right CVA are shown in Table 24-2.[34,36,68,71]

Bilateral Cerebrovascular Accident

Some clients experience multiple strokes that affect both hemispheres. Clients with significant left- and right-sided hemiplegia and numerous deficits may have functional losses that are more like those of clients with traumatic brain injuries than of clients who have had left- or right-sided CVAs. Treatment interventions for clients with head injury may be used after bilateral CVA (see Chapter 25).

Cerebellum and Brainstem Stroke

A stroke that takes place in the cerebellum can cause a wide variety of deficits. Common problems include abnormal reflexes of the head and torso, coordination and balance problems, dizziness, problems with swallowing and articulation, and cranial nerve deficits.[36]

Strokes in the brainstem are often life threatening because the brainstem is the control center for essential life functions such as breathing, heart rate, blood pressure, and arousal. As with a cerebellum stroke, survivors of brainstem stroke may also present with dizziness, problems with swallowing and articulation, cranial nerve deficits, and paralysis.[36]

Recurrent Cerebrovascular Accident

Rates of stroke recurrence are high, and approximately one third of stroke survivors will have a second stroke.[2] Risk of recurrence increases with more strokes and with advanced age.[2] OT treatment programs should include education related to health management of modifiable risk factors for stroke. Box 24-6 offers suggestions for incorporating this information into OT interventions.

Box 24-6

Examples of Ways to Incorporate Stroke Health Management and Maintenance into OT Interventions

Diet / Weight Management

- Provide client/caregivers information on how to make heart healthy food choices.
- Teach client/caregivers how to read food labels to identify low sodium and low fat choices.
- Work with client/caregiver on how to locate heart healthy recipes on line or in magazines.
- Provide home exercise and conditioning programs based on client's activity tolerance.

Medication Compliance

- Work with medical team on simplifying medication regimen for clients with cognitive impairments.
- Teach client/caregivers reasons for medication, side effects, importance of timely refilling of medication.
- Train client in use of adaptive devices (e.g. pill splitter, medication organizers, one-handed syringe) when indicated.
- Recommend telemonitoring of medication compliance in the home, if necessary.

Areas of Occupation and Occupational Therapy Treatment Techniques

Treatment of the client with stroke focuses primarily on areas of occupation including ADL, IADL, work, and leisure and social participation.[3] Functional skills in these areas are often severely impaired. Suggestions for functional treatment interventions for these areas are provided in Table 24-3.

Activities of Daily Living

The performance of self-care activities after a stroke often requires extra time. Besides mastering new self-care skills, clients need time to reflect on how changes in their bodies from the stroke may affect their performance.[37] It is essential that

Table 24-3 Areas of Occupation and Suggested Treatment Strategies

Selected Area of Occupation[3]	Treatment Considerations and Activities	Adaptive/Compensatory Strategies and Techniques
Activities of Daily Living		
Bathing and Showering		
Obtaining and using supplies; soaping, rinsing, and drying body parts; maintaining safe position and balance while bathing; transferring to and from bathing positions	Maintaining balance while reaching to wash body parts, practice turning water on and off and adjusting temperature; transfer training into tub and shower; sequencing activities.	Wash mitt, soap-on-a-rope, pump-style soap dispenser, long-handled sponge, bath bench, handheld shower, grab bars; establish routine for bathing regimen
Bowel and Bladder Management		
Complete, intentional control of bowel movements and urinary bladder and, if necessary, use of equipment for bladder control	Manage and empty leg bag, self-catherization training, bladder/bowel retraining program	Leg bag straps, catheter clamps, suppository inserter, digital stimulator, panty liners/incontinence pads
Toilet Hygiene		
Obtaining and using supplies, managing clothing, maintaining toileting position, toilet transfer, cleaning body, caring for menstrual and continence needs	Mobility activities such as rolling side to side, bridging and lifting hips to use bedpan, transfer training onto/off toilet, reaching body parts to clean self, raise/lower and adjust clothing	Use of grab bars, raised toilet seat, bedside commode, bidet to assist with hygiene, toilet tissue aid, loose fitting clothing with elastic fastenings
Dressing		
Selecting appropriate clothing and accessories; obtaining clothing; dressing/undressing including fastening and adjusting, applying, and removing personal devices, prosthesis, or orthosis	Practice undressing first in loose fitting garments, use full-length mirror while sitting supported in chair and then progress to unsupported sitting (e.g., at edge of bed); use clothing in contrasting colors, select clothing and lay out in advance	Teach adaptive/one-handed dressing techniques, Velcro fastenings, elastic waistbands and shoelaces, shoe horn, provide adaptive straps on splints to improve to don and doff.
Eating, Feeding		
Setting up food, using utensils, cups (follow direction of dysphagia therapist)	Monitor client for swallowing problems, follow dietary and dysphagia guidelines and restrictions when indicated, oral motor intervention	Use of plate guards or scoop dish, adapted cups with lids or easy grip handles; cup and straw holders, adapted utensils, rocker knife, antiskid placemat, proper positioning at table, teach strategies for one-handed technique to open food containers and packages. For clients with hemianoposa, place food tray in intact visual field.
Functional Mobility		
Bed mobility, wheelchair mobility, transfers, functional ambulation	Provide progressive mobility training on a variety of surfaces; teach bed mobility, including rolling, bridging, moving from supine to sit; teach indoor wheelchair mobility over even, uneven, and inclined surfaces. Transfer training to a variety of surfaces, including the bed, chair, toilet, tub, floor. Train on safe indoor functional ambulation, including reinforcing the use of ambulatory device, instruction on how to transport objects during ambulation activities.	Use of bedrails, overhead trapeze bars, pull straps to assist with bed mobility, patient lift for dependent clients. Specialized wheelchair assessment and training, including hemi-wheelchair that is lower to ground for eaiser propulsion; wheelchair modifications (e.g., removable armrests, brake extension, swing-away leg rests), recliner; lightweight, one-arm drive; power mobility. Use portable ramps/chair lifts for patients unable to manage stairs; use walker basket, backpack, lidded cups while transporting objects during functional ambulation; adaptive wheelchair propulsion (e.g., use of the unaffected UE and LE to propel and steer).
Personal Care Device		
Using, cleaning, and maintaining personal care items such as hearing aids, glasses, orthotics, adaptive equipment	Practice cleaning, caring for, and learning sources for repair or replacement of eyeglasses, splints, braces, slings, edema gloves, communication devices, and durable medical equipment, such as wheelchairs or bath seats	Wash mitt; magnifying lens; notebook with written directions, address book with phone numbers and contact persons for service and repair

Continued

Table 24-3 Areas of Occupation and Suggested Treatment Strategies—cont'd

Selected Area of Occupation[3]	Treatment Considerations and Activities	Adaptive/Compensatory Strategies and Techniques
Personal Hygiene and Grooming		
Shaving, cosmetic application; hair, nail and skin care; deodorant application; cleaning mouth; brushing and flossing teeth; removing, cleaning, and reinserting dental orthotics and prosthetics	Use mirror during grooming activities Organizing and sequencing activities Promote the proper positioning during hygiene and grooming activities Comb or brush hair, and practice putting on and taking off hair clips, bobby pins, headbands Scrub nails with stationary brush, file nails with stationary nail file, cut nails with stationary nail clipper, and paint nails with stationary nail polish brush Open and close deodorant, adjust deodorant level, and apply deodorant Open and close mouthwash containers and rinse mouth; open and close toothpaste and brush teeth; remove, reinsert, and clean dentures.	Small, adjustable double-sided mirror with magnifying and regular sides; angled wall mirror, electric safety razor, razor holder with strap (for higher-level clients using a manual razor); aerosol can dispenser, handles for can such as shaving cream; electric hair trimmers, air dry hair to avoid having to manipulate blow dryer, large or extended-handle comb/brush, comb/brush with Velcro strap, suction nail brush, suction nail file, pump-style toothpaste dispenser, denture brush, denture tablets (reduced need for brushing), suction denture brush, glycerin swabs to clean mouth, use stick or cream deodorant
Toilet Hygiene	Mobility activities such as rolling side to side, bridging and lifting hips to use bedpan, transfer training onto/off toilet, reaching body parts to clean self, raise/lower and adjust clothing	Use of bidet to assist with hygiene, loose fitting garments with elastic fastenings, toilet tissue aid. Use of grab bars, raised toilet seat, bedside commode.
Instrumental Activities of Daily Living		
Care of others, care of pets, child rearing	Direct care of adults may not be possible depending on level of impairment. Improve safe ability to care for children and pets. Train in assertive techniques in order to direct and supervise home health aides, attendants, and housekeepers who might assist in care for others	Modified baby doll with added weight cuffs, adapted games and stories to use with children, one-hand release crib and high chair Adapted pet care products (e.g., single packet foods, larger-handle bushes and leashes with solid grips)
Communication management		
Use of writing equipment, telephones, computers, communication boards, call lights, emergency systems, Braille writers, telecommunication devices, and augmentative communication devices	Dominancy retraining, if indicated, establish effective pen/marker grip patterns; graded writing exercises; look up and dial phone numbers, one-handed typing Practice emergency training/call light use.	Built-up writing utensils, writing aids. Clipboards, phone holders, speaker phone and head sets, programmable cell phone, modifications to keyboards and computer adaptations (e.g., touch pads, expanded keyboard, "sticky keys"), smart phones.
Community Mobility		
Moving in the community; using public and private transportation	Outdoor wheelchair/functional ambulation training, including practice going in/out all types of doors; using the elevator; performing car transfers. Sequencing and planning activities for taxi rides or gettingg information regarding the bus/train/paratransit schedules, using public transportation, if appropriate. Obtain a wheelchair sticker for car or license plate for disabled from state Department of Motor Vehicles if approved by doctor	Treated wheelchair tires, appropriate footwear for outdoor terrains, transfer board, reachers, notebook/smart phone or tape recorder for information, Wheelchair carrier for car, ramp for van. Refer for driving evaluation, including assessment for adaptive controls for driving car or van. Assist with completion of paratransit application process, if appropriate
Financial Management		
Using fiscal resources; making financial transactions, including budgeting, paying bills	Perform commercially available budgeting exercise, practice writing checks, paying bills online and balancing accounts	Calculator with large number keyboard, flow chart of monthly bills, computer software for financial management, direct deposit with online and automatic bill-paying systems, smart phones with budgeting applications.

Table 24-3 Areas of Occupation and Suggested Treatment Strategies—cont'd

Selected Area of Occupation[3]	Treatment Considerations and Activities	Adaptive/Compensatory Strategies and Techniques
Health Management and Maintenance		
Developing, managing, and maintaining routines for health and wellness promotion, including medication routines	Identify client's risk factors for stroke and strategies to reduce modifiable ones (e.g., smoking cessation, stress reduction groups, walking for weight reduction); improve and apply knowledge of nutrition and of prescribed diet; and develop home-exercise programs for self range of motion, and general conditioning s indicated; use of Wii video games for fitness and mobility training Understand medication use and precautions; understand how to adhere to schedule; practice opening and closing medication containers, practice simulated administration; use consumer skills to learn to ask questions about medications, report side effects, and obtain refills. Introduce activities to maintain cognitive fitness and flexibility (e.g., word puzzles, word searches).	Cookbooks/online resources for low-salt, low-fat, and low-sugar recipes; provide individualized home exercise program, which may include Theraband, light weights, relaxation tapes, referral to wellness and exercise groups. Smart phones with medication schedule applications. Tele-monitoring for medication management, glucometer use. Pill sorters, adaptive insulin synergies, speak with physician regarding single dose medication regimes, easy-open medication containers.
Home Establishment and Management		
Developing, managing, and maintaining personal and household possessions and environments, including maintaining and repairing personal possessions (clothing and household items) and knowing how to seek help or whom to contact	Home management activities such as folding clothing, towels, sheets, practicing sorting and measuring laundry detergent, using washer and dryer, putting clothing in closet, vacuuming, making bed, mopping, emptying trashcans and sorting recyclables Practice simple household responsibilities such as changing a lightbulb, replacing batteries, watering plants, and cleaning refrigerator—progress as possible; determine capabilities for certain jobs and assistance options for the remaining jobs	Rolling cart to transport heavy items; premeasured laundry detergents, front-loading washer and dryer for wheelchair users, labeling closets to organize storage Reachers, pull-down ironing board, lightweight iron; work station for laundry; sweep, dust, mop from wheelchair or while ambulating; straighten up room; remove linens from beds; handheld vacuum, lightweight upright vacuum cleaner, long-handled dust pan, wonder-mop (for use with one hand), long-handled cleaning sponge, fitted bed sheet, trash bags with built-in tie, recyclable sorters
Meal Preparation and Cleanup	Graded cooking program beginning with planning and preparing a table-top, cold snack, moving to hot meals in oven and cleanup. Full training should incorporate the use of the appliances the client will use at home, as well as kitchen organization and mobility activities.	Adaptive one-handed cutting boards, jar openers, pot handle holders, use of rolling cart, one-handed electric can openers, angled wall mirror over stove, built-up utensils, long arm oven mitt. Label drawers and refrigerator; rearrangement of items with those the most used more accessible, One-pot meals, timers, preplanning and organizing meals in advance.
Safety and Emergency Management	Practice responding to emergencies, including how to recognize hazards and taking action to reduce threat to safety. Brainstorm emergency management plans, prepare a "go" bag for emergencies, recommend clients carry valuables on body rather than in backpack on back of wheelchair to prevent theft, assist clients in identifying "back-up" for equipment (e.g., power w/c users) and assistance in event of emergency.	Programmable cell phone and emergency call systems; obtain stickers from local firehouse to put on windows indicating that a person with a disability resides in household.

Continued

Table 24-3 Areas of Occupation and Suggested Treatment Strategies—cont'd

Selected Area of Occupation[3]	Treatment Considerations and Activities	Adaptive/Compensatory Strategies and Techniques
Shopping		
Preparing shopping lists, selecting and purchasing items, selecting method of payment, competing transaction	Perform simulated shopping activities, including online and telephone ordering; money management skills, including counting money, making change.	Store money in accessible purse or wallet, use debit card, adaptive shopping cart; automated online grocery ordering (i.e., Fresh Direct®).
Work		
Employment interests and pursuits, seeking and acquisition of employment, job performance, retirement preparation and adjustment, volunteerism	Perform simulated work tasks and work samples; work hardening program as appropriate; explore retirement options and plan for retirement activities, assist with identifying potential community volunteer experiences that might be appropriate.	Adapt work environment for wheelchair and ambulatory device user; make recommendations for reasonable accomodations based on specific client needs and job responsibilities (e.g., adaptive keyboard, phone head set.
Leisure		
Leisure exploration and participation	Identify and practice previous leisure tasks adapt technique or equipment of these tasks. Assist client In developing and exploring alternative leisure tasks.	Adaptive book holders, audio books, automatic card shufflers, adaptive games and equipment such as bowling ramps, one-handed needlepoint hoops, large print books and playing cards, Wii games.
Social Participation		
*Engaging in characteristic and expected activities with community, family, peers and friends.	Social skill training, role playing, videotaping; identify and make appropriate community referrals. Participation in online social networking, blogging, etc. to maintain social interactions.	Assist client in exploring and identifying community resources. Make referrals to community support groups. Identify and offer strategies to address environmental barriers to community groups.

OT treatment sessions allow extra time for client reflection and practice. OT intervention for improving self-care often begins with basic activities and progresses to higher-level skills. Treatment strategies for clients with stroke should be adapted for use of the unaffected dominant UE (one-handedness), use of the unaffected nondominant UE (dominance retraining), and use of both UEs (bilateral integration). The affected limbs should be incorporated into treatment as much as possible, and active problem solving should be encouraged. Opportunities for practice in self-care are critical for clients to refine skills and achieve maximal independence. OTAs should educate nursing staff and caregivers to understand the need for practice so that they can build time for this into daily routines.

Instrumental Activities of Daily Living and Work Activities

IADL and work activities are unique, complex tasks; OT intervention in these areas requires an understanding of the stroke survivor's previous performance pattern in these areas. Obtaining information about the client's home environment and daily routines in these areas is critical to this understanding. Because lengths of stay at rehabilitation units have been decreased, a home evaluation early in the rehabilitation process can assist with treatment planning. A home evaluation allows the OT practitioner to gain a clearer understanding of the discharge setting. Home care is an important part of the rehabilitation process for the client with stroke because it allows training in his or her real-life environment.

Leisure Activities

After stroke, disability may prevent participation in previously enjoyed leisure activities. The therapist can provide the client with information, skills training, and adapted equipment. Emphasis on reintegrating the client into community activities should be included in the treatment plan whenever possible. Continued participation in enjoyable activities can reduce stress, improve coping skills, and maximize quality of life after CVA.

Social Participation

Numerous barriers to social participation may occur as a result of stroke. Lack of mobility and environmental barriers may limit access in the community. Communication and behavioral problems may affect opportunities for social interaction. Changes in body image as a result of physical impairments, such as a facial droop or a limp, may decrease self-esteem. Depression may reduce desire to maintain and develop social contacts. Clients' perceived low expectation of what they can perform may affect their social participation as well.[7]

OT practitioners play an important role in addressing these barriers, with the goal of facilitating a client's reentry into social activities and resumption of social roles after a stroke.

CASE STUDY 24-1

Mr. L

Mr. L. is a right-handed 57-year-old male who recently retired from the police force. Mr. L. is divorced and lives in a single family home that he owns with his daughter, Maria. Since his retirement 6 months ago, Mr. L. has been enjoying his newfound free time by completing a variety of small home improvement projects that he had been putting off because of his former work schedule.

Three days ago, Mr. L. woke up with a headache; at breakfast that same morning Maria noticed that Mr. L.'s speech was slurred and that he was dragging his left foot when he walked. She immediately took him to the hospital emergency room. Medical work-up revealed Mr. L. had suffered a right CVA with left hemiplegia and he was admitted to the stroke unit. His medical history is significant for high blood pressure and cigarette smoking. Mr. L's daughter Maria reported to the medical team that her father has not been compliant with taking his blood pressure medicine and still smokes a pack of cigarettes a day.

The stroke team evaluated Mr. L., and a referral to rehabilitation was made. The occupational therapist completed an initial evaluation and determined that Mr. L. had significant problems in all areas of occupation, including eating, personal hygiene, showering, dressing, and functional mobility. Mr. L. was not ambulatory and was using a wheelchair for mobility on the stroke unit.

The occupational therapist's assessment of performance skills revealed that Mr. L. had deficits in both motor and process skills. Specifically, he demonstrated decreased balance, which contributed to an asymmetrical posture while he was sitting and standing. Mr. L.'s left UE had flaccid muscle tone and no active range of motion. Tactile sensation was, however, intact throughout his entire left side.

Cognitively, Mr. L. was alert and oriented X 3 and followed directions. When fatigued, however, he became easily distracted. During functional activities, Mr. L. exhibited a decreased awareness of his left side; as a result, his left arm was often dangling at his side.

The occupational therapist noted that Mr. L. was motivated for therapy and expressed interest in improving his ability to perform personal self-care. When discussing his problems, Mr. L. became tearful and expressed sadness about the amount of assistance he needed to perform simple tasks like shaving.

When Mr. L. is ready for discharge from the hospital, the current plan is for him to return home with home care services. Mr. L. agrees with this plan but is concerned about how he would manage at home while his daughter was at work.

1. How might Mr. L.'s balance problems be affecting his ability to perform self-care activities, especially dressing and bathing? What compensatory techniques could he learn to increase independence in these areas?
2. What are some potential complications of Mr. L.'s having a flaccid arm? What preventive strategies could address these complications? Should he be provided with a sling? Why or why not?
3. How might Mr. L.'s decreased awareness of his left arm affect his safety during performance of functional mobility?
4. What information would you need about Mr. L.'s home environment to assist with planning for discharge?
5. How would you involve Mr. L's daughter in his OT program at this time?
6. How might you incorporate health management and stroke prevention education into MR. L's OT program?

CASE STUDY 24-2

Mrs. M

Mrs. M is a right- handed, 70 year old female who sustained a left CVA, resulting in right hemiparesis, 6 weeks ago. She is currently receiving home care occupational therapy services and has a home health aide 7 days a week 4 hours a day. The home health aide will not be covered by her insurance once skilled OT services are completed in 2 weeks.

Mrs. M lives with her husband in a first floor walk-up apartment. Prior to her CVA, she was independent in all BADL and IADL and was the primary homemaker for the family. Mrs. M misses this role and is looking forward to resuming her home management tasks as soon as possible.

At this time, Mrs. M presents with mild right UE weakness and deceased sensory awareness in her right hand. She ambulates independently indoors with a cane, but needs contact guarding to negotiate steps. She is easily fatigued.

Cognitively, Mrs. M is alert, oriented X3, can follow directions, but can become distracted when performing multi-step tasks.

At this time, Mrs. M has achieved independence in all BADL. She would like to resume involvement in simple home management tasks and has identified participation in meal preparation and clean-up as a short term goal.

1. What safety concerns are raised by Mrs. M's sensorimotor and attention deficits as they relate to her participation in meal preparation activities?
2. Describe two treatment considerations and/or adaptive strategies for meal preparation and clean-up that can be incorporated into Mrs. M's treatment session.
3. Describe a graded sequence of tasks that might be used during treatment with Mrs. M to work towards increasing her independence in meal preparation.
4. How would you involve Mrs. M's husband and home health aide in her OT program at this time?

Summary

CVA results in a complex disability that can significantly affect all areas of occupational performance. Reaching client goals depends on multiple factors including extent of damage to the brain, rate of client recovery, client motivation and adjustment, client support systems, and the timely application of appropriate treatment by health professionals. Inpatient rehabilitation stays for clients with stroke continue to shorten, and there is increased emphasis on providing rehabilitation services to clients in the community. Community settings may include the home, adult day programs, and outpatient settings. In addition to providing direct treatment to clients with stroke, occupational therapists and OTAs can also play an important role in designing health maintenance programs directed toward prevention and education in this area.

Selected Reading Guide Questions

1. Explain the difference between a CVA and a TIA.
2. Name three common warning signs of CVA.
3. Explain why stroke survivors are at higher risk for developing medical complications.
4. Describe how OT treatment would change for a client who develops a DVT of the unaffected LE.
5. Describe the effects of long-standing edema of the hemiplegic forearm and hand.
6. How are the OT goals of prevention of deformity and injury important to the achievement of rehabilitation goals for the client with a stroke?
7. Discuss the differences in roles of the OT practitioner treating the stroke survivor in acute care and home health settings.
8. What are the effects of abnormal reflexes and impaired postural mechanisms on the sitting balance of the client who has experienced a CVA?
9. State and discuss the important considerations for positioning a client with a stroke in bed and in the wheelchair.
10. What factors would prevent a client from using adaptive equipment for dressing?
11. Why is it important in self-care training to allow opportunities for practice?
12. What are the purposes of the lapboard and resting hand splint for the client with hemiplegia?
13. Explain why PROM is recommended for the client with a flaccid UE.
14. Why is scapular mobility required for pain-free ROM activities for the shoulder?
15. What strategies can be implemented to prevent subluxation of the shoulder?
16. What causes a reduction in strength and endurance after CVA?
17. Describe some methods of positioning the affected arm and leg to reduce edema.
18. How does stroke affect vision?
19. Explain how to increase the attention of a client who is easily agitated.
20. Explain why early and frequent inclusion of the family and caregivers is important to OT treatment planning and implementation.
21. Describe how the OTA could incorporate health maintenance and management into treatment interventions.

References

1. Abreu B: The effect of environmental regulations on postural control after stroke, *Am J Occup Ther* 49(6):517–525, 1995.
2. American Heart Association: *Heart disease and stroke statistics: 2010 Update*, Dallas, 2010, the Association.
3. American Occupational Therapy Association: Occupational therapy practice framework: domain and process, ed 2, *Am J Occup Ther* 56:609–639, 2008.
4. American Stroke Association: Recommendations for the establishment of stroke systems of care, *Stroke* 36:690–703, 2005.
5. Ayres A: Perceptual motor training for children. In *Approaches to the treatment of clients with neuromuscular dysfunction.* Proceedings of study course IV, Third International Congress, World Federation of Occupational Therapists, Dubuque, Iowa, 1962, William C Brown.
6. Bartels MN, Duffy CA, Belhand HE: Pathophysiology and medical management of stroke and acute rehabilitation of stroke survivors. In Gillen G, editor: *Stroke rehabilitation: a function-based approach*, ed 3, St. Louis, 2011, Mosby.
7. Baseman S, Fisher K, Ward L, Bhattacharya A: The relationship of physical function to social integration after stroke, *J Nurs Neurol* 42:237–244, 2010.
8. Jamison PW, Orchanian DP: Cerebrovascular accident. In Atchison B, Direte DK, editors: *Conditions in occupational therapy: effect on occupational performance*, ed 3, Baltimore, 2007, Williams & Wilkins.
9. Birch GH, et al: Perception in hemiplegia: judgment of the vertical and horizontal by hemiplegic clients, *Arch Phys Med Rehabil* 41:19, 1960.
10. Bobath B: *Adult hemiplegia: evaluation and treatment*, ed 3, Oxford, 1990, Butterworth-Heinemann Ltd.
11. Brandsater ME: Stroke rehabilitation. In Delisa JA, Gans BM, Walsh NE, et al, editors: *Physical medicine and rehabilitation: principles and practice*, ed 4, Philadelphia, 2005, Lippincott Williams & Wilkins.
12. Brandsater ME, Roth EJ, Siebens HC: Venous thromboembolism in stroke: literature review and implications for clinical practice, *Archs Phys Med Rehabil* 73(Suppl 5):S379–S391, 1992.
13. Buchholz DW: Dysphagia associated with neurological disorders, *Acta Otorhinolaryngol Belg* 48(2):143–155, 1994.
14. Carota A, Bogousslavsky J: Mood changes after stroke. In Bogousslavsky J, editor: *Long-term effects of stroke*, New York, 2002, Dekker.
15. CDC: *Stroke facts. America's stroke burden*, Atlanta, GA, 2010, US Department of Health and Human Services, CDC. Available at http://www.cdc.gov/stroke/facts.htm.
16. Charness A: *Stroke/head injury*, Rehabilitation Institute of Chicago Procedure Manual, Rockville Md, 2004, Aspen.
17. Chemerinski E, Robinson RG, Kosier JT: Improved recovery in activities of daily living associated with remission of post stroke depression, *Stroke* 32(1):113–117, 2001.
18. Clark S: Right hemisphere syndrome. In Bogousslavsky J, Caplan L, editors: *Stroke syndromes*, ed 2, New York, 2001, Cambridge Press.
19. Cooper BA: A model for implementing color contrast in the environment of the elderly, *Am J Occup Ther* 39(4):253–258, 1985.

20. Davis J: Improving UE function in adult hemiplegia. *OT Practice Online.* Retrieved April 5, 2005 from http://www.aota.org//featured/area2/links/link16DE.asp.
21. Davies PM: *Steps to follow: the comprehensive treatment of clients with hemiplegia*, ed 2, New York, 2000, Springer-Verlag.
22. Dennis M, O'Rourke S, Lewis S, et al: Emotional outcomes after stroke: factors associated with poor outcome, *Neurol Neurosurg Psychiatry* 68:47–52, 2000.
23. Dobkin BH: Rehabilitation and recovery of the client with stroke. In Mohr JP, Choi DW, Grotta JC, et al, editors: *Stroke: pathophysiology, diagnosis, and management*, ed 4, Philadelphia, 2004, Churchill Livingstone.
24. Dorsher PT, McMichan JC: Pulmonary considerations in rehabilitation. In Sinaki M, editor: *Basic clinical rehabilitation medicine*, ed 2, St. Louis, 1993, Mosby.
25. Dromerick AW, Edwards DF, Hahn M: Does the application of constraint-induced movement therapy during acute rehabilitation reduce arm impairment after ischemic stroke? *Stroke* 31(12):2984–2988, 2000.
26. Elovic E, Bogey R: Spasticity and movement disorders. In Delisa JA, Gans BM, Walsh NE, et al, editors: *Physical medicine and rehabilitation: principles and practice*, ed 4, Philadelphia, 2005, Lippincott Williams & Wilkins.
27. Ferro JM, Martins JM: Memory loss after stroke. In Bogousslavsky J, Caplan L, editors: *Stroke syndromes*, ed 2, New York, 2001, Cambridge Press.
28. Foulkes MA: Design issues in chemosensory trials, *Arch Otolaryngol Head Neck Surg* 116(1):65–68, 1990.
29. Fuller KS: Stroke. In Goodman CC, Fuller KS, editors: *Pathology: implications for the physical therapist*, ed 3, Philadelphia, 2008, WB Saunders.
30. Gillen G: Upper extremity function and management. In Gillen G, editor: *Stroke rehabilitation: a function-based approach*, ed 3, St. Louis, 2011, Mosby.
31. Gillen G, editor: *Stroke rehabilitation: a function-based approach*, ed 3, St. Louis, 2011, Mosby.
32. Gillen G, Rubio KB: Treatment of cognitive and perceptual deficits: a function-based approach. In Gillen G, editor: *Stroke rehabilitation: a function-based approach*, ed 3, St. Louis, 2011, Mosby.
33. Gillot AJ, Holder-Walls A, Kurtz JR, et al: Perceptions and experiences of two survivors of stroke who participated in constraint-induced movement therapy home programs, *Am J Occup Ther* 57(2):168–176, 2003.
34. Goldberg E: Associative agnosias and the functions of the left hemisphere, *J Clin Exp Neuropsychol* 12(4):467–484, 1990.
35. Goldstein LB, editor: *A primer on stroke prevention and treatment: an overview of AHA/ASA*, Hoboken, NJ, 2009, Wiley-Blackwell.
36. Gutman S: *Quick reference neuroscience for rehabilitation professionals: the essential neurological principles underlying rehabilitation practice*, ed 2, Thorofare, NJ, 2007, Slack.
37. Guidetti S, Asaba E, Tham K: The meaning of context in recapturing self-care after stroke and spinal cord injury, *Am J Occup Ther* 63, 2009:323-322.
38. Halpern H: *Language and motor speech disorders in adults*, ed 2, Austin, TX, 2000, Pro-Ed.
39. Herrmann M, Black SE, Lawrence J, et al: The Sunnybrook stroke study: a prospective study of depressive symptoms and functional outcome, *Stroke* 29(3):618–624, 1998.
40. Herrmann M, et al: Poststroke depression: is there a pathoanatomic correlate for depression in the post acute stage of stroke? *Stroke* 26(5):850–856, 1995.
41. Ivey FM, Macko RE, et al: Prevalence of deconditioning after stroke. In Stein J, editor: *Stroke recovery and rehabilitation*, New York, 2009, Demos Medical.
42. Logemann JA: Management of dysphagia after stroke. In Barnes M, Dobkin B, Bogousslawsky J, editors: *Recovery after stroke*, New York, 2005, Cambridge University Press.
43. Kalra L: Does age affect benefits of stroke unit rehabilitation? *Stroke* 25(2):347–351, 1994.
44. Kaplan PR, Caillet R, Kaplan CP: *Rehabilitation of stroke*, Philadelphia, 2003, Butterworth-Heinemann.
45. Khader MS, Tomlin GS: Change in wheelchair transfer performance during rehabilitation of men with cerebrovascular accident, *Am J Occup Ther* 48(10):899–905, 1994.
46. Kidd D, Lawson J, Nesbitt R, MacMahon J: Aspiration in acute stroke: a clinical study with videofluoroscopy, *Q J Med* 86(12):825–829, 1993.
47. Kunkel A, Kopp B, Muller G, et al: Constraint-induced movement therapy for motor recovery in chronic stroke clients, *Arch Phys Med Rehabil* 80(6):624–628, 1999.
48. Kwakkel G, Knollen Bj, Kregs HI: Effects of robot-assisted therapy on upper limb recovery after stroke: a systematic review, *Neurorehabil Neural Repair* 22(2):111–121, 2008.
49. Labott A, Bladin CF, Donnan GA: Seizures and stroke. In Bogousslavsky J, Caplan L, editors: *Stroke syndromes*, ed 2, New York, 2001, Cambridge Press.
50. Lavine R, Hausler R: Auditory disorders after stroke. In Bogousslavsky J, Caplan L, editors: *Stroke syndromes*, ed 2, New York, 2001, Cambridge Press.
51. Lo AC, Guarino PD, Richards LG, et al: Robot-assisted therapy for long-term upper-limb impairment after stroke, *N Engl J Med* 362:1772–1783, 2010.
52. MacDonald JC: An investigation of body scheme in adults with cerebral vascular accidents, *Am J Occup Ther* 14:75–79, 1960.
53. Martin BJ, Corlew MM: The incidence of communication disorders in dysphagic clients, *J Speech Hear Disord* 55(1):28–32, 1990.
54. Milazzo S, Gillen G: Splinting applications. In Gillen G, editor: *Stroke rehabilitation: a function-based approach*, ed 3, St. Louis, 2011, Mosby.
55. Mohr JP, Choi DW, Grotta JC, et al: *Stroke: pathophysiology, diagnosis, and management*, ed 4, Philadelphia, 2004, Churchill Livingstone.
56. Morbidity and Mortality Weekly Report Supplements: *CDC health disparities and inequities report*, Jan 14, 2011. Available at http://www.cdc.gov/mmwr/preview/mmwrhtml/su6001a13.htm
57. Nilsen DM, Gillen G, Gordon AM: Use of mental practice to improve upper-limb recovery after stroke: a systematic review, *Am J Occup Ther* 64:695–708, 2010.
58. Office of Minority Health: *Closing the health gap: reducing health disparities affecting African-Americans.* [DHHS Fact Sheet.] Washington DC, 2001, Department of Health and Human Services. Available at http://www.hhs.gov/news/press/2001pres/20011119a.html
59. O'Sullivan A: AOTA's statement on family caregivers, *AJOT* 61(6):710, 2007.
60. Page SJ, Sisto S, Johnston MV, et al: Modified constraint-induced therapy after subacute stroke: a preliminary study, *Neurorehabilitation Neural Repair* 16(3):223–228, 2002.
61. Page SJ, Levine P: Effects of mental practice on affected limb use and function in chronic stroke, *Arch Phys Med Rehabil* 86(4):399–402, 2005.

62. Piambianco G, Orchard T, Landau P: Deep vein thrombosis: prevention in stroke clients during rehabilitation, *Arch Phys Med Rehabil* 76(4):324–330, 1995.
63. Pohjasvaara T, Vataja R, Leppavuouri A, et al: Depression is an independent predictor of poor long-term functional outcome post stroke, *Eur J Neurol* 8(4):315–319, 2001.
64. Roth ER, Harvey RL: Rehabilitation of stroke syndromes. In Braddom RL, Buschbacher RM, editors: *Physical medicine and rehabilitation*, ed 3, Philadelphia, 2011, WB Saunders.
65. Rubio KB, Van Deuson J: Relation of perceptual and body image dysfunction to activities of daily living of persons after stroke, *Am J Occup Ther* 49(6):551–559, 1995.
66. Schlesinger B: *Higher cerebral functions and their clinical disorders*, New York, 1962, Grune & Stratton.
67. Söderback I, Bengtsson I, Ginsburg E, Ekholm J: Video feedback in occupational therapy: its effects in clients with neglect syndrome, *Arch Phys Med Rehabil* 73(12):1140–1146, 1992.
68. Sterzi R, et al: Hemianopsia, hemianesthesia, and hemiplegia after right and left hemisphere damage: a hemispheric difference, *J Neurol Neurosurg Psychiatry* 56(3):308–310, 1993.
69. Stein J, Harvey R, Macko R, et al, editors: *Stroke recovery and rehabilitation*, New York, NY, 2009, Demos Medical.
70. Stein J, Krebs HI, Hogan N: Technological aids for motor recovery. In Stein J, Harvey R, Macko R, et al, editors: *Stroke recovery and rehabilitation*, New York, NY, 2009, Demos Medical.
71. Stone SP, Halligan PW, Green RJ: The incidence of neglect phenomena and related disorders in clients with acute right or left hemisphere stroke, *Age Aging* 22(1):46–52, 1993.
72. Sundin K, Jansson L: 'Understanding and being understood' as a creative caring phenomenon in care of clients with stroke and aphasia, *J Clin Nurs* 12(1):107–116, 2003.
73. Su CY, et al: Performance of older adults with and without cerebrovascular accident on the test of visual-perceptual skills, *Am J Occup Ther* 49(6):491–499, 1995.
74. Taub E, Uswatte G, Pidikiti R: Constraint-induced movement therapy: a new family of techniques with broad application to physical rehabilitation—a clinical review, *J Rehabil Res Dev* 36(3):237–251, 1999.
75. Trombly CA, Radomski MV: *Occupational therapy for physical dysfunction*, ed 6, Baltimore, 2007, Lippincott Williams & Wilkins.
76. Turton A, Fraser C: The use of home therapy programmes for improving recovery of the upper limb following stroke, *Br J Occup Ther* 53:457–462, 1990.
77. Volpe BT, Krebs HI, Hogan N: Robot-aided sensorimotor training in stroke rehabilitation, *Adv Neurol* 92:429–433, 2003.
78. Wallenbert I, Jonsson H: Waiting to get better: a dilemma regarding habits in daily occupation after stroke, *Am J Occup Ther* 59:218–229, 2005.
79. Walker MF, Lincoln NB: Factors influencing dressing performance after stroke, *J Neurol Neurosurg Psychiatry* 54(8):699–701, 1991.
80. Whitworth A, Webster J, Howard D: *A cognitive neuropsychological approach to assessment and intervention in aphasias: a clinician's guide*, New York, 2005, Psychology Press.
81. Zoltan B: *Vision, perception, and cognition: a manual for the evaluation and treatment of the adult with acquired brain injury*, ed 4, Thorofare, NJ, 2007, Slack.

Recommended Reading

Bolte J: *My stroke of insight: a brain scientist's personal journey*, New York, 2008, Penguin Group.

Carr JH, Shepherd RB: *Stroke rehabilitation: guidelines for exercise and training to optimize motor skill*, ed 2, Oxford, 2003, Butterworth-Heinemann.

Duncun PW, Zorowitz B, Bates B, et al: Management of adult stroke rehabilitation care: a clinical practice guideline, *Stroke* 36(9):e100–e143, 2005 Sep. PPMID: 16120836 [PubMed - indexed for MEDLINE].

Gillen G, editor: *Stroke rehabilitation: a function-based approach*, ed 3, St. Louis, 2011, Mosby.

Gutman S: *Quick reference neuroscience for rehabilitation professionals: the essential neurological principles underlying rehabilitation practice*, ed 2, Thorofare, NJ, 2007, Slack.

Kime SK: *Compensating for memory deficits: using a systematic approach*, Bethesda, Md, 2001, American Occupational Therapy Association.

Sabari J: *Occupational therapy practice guidelines for adults with stroke*, Bethesda, Md, 2008, American Occupational Therapy Association.

Siebert C: *Occupational therapy practice guidelines for home modifications*, Bethesda, Md, 2001, American Occupational Therapy Association.

Stein J, Harvey R, Macko R, et al: *Stroke recovery and rehabilitation*, New York, NY, 2009, Demos Medical.

Online Resources for Stroke Survivors and Caregivers

American Heart Association *www.americanheart.org*
Caring.com *www.caring.com*
Family Caregiver Alliance *www.caregiver.org*
Medix Health Information, Medical Questions and Patient Community *www.imedix.com*
National Alliance for Caregiving *www.caregiving.org*
National Association of Area Agencies on Aging *www.n4a.org*
National Family Caregivers Association *www.nfcacares.org*
National Stroke Association *www.stroke.org*
The Stroke Network *http://www.strokenetwork.org/*

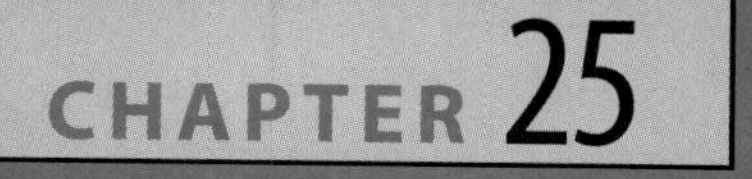

Traumatic Brain Injury

LORI M. SHIFFMAN

Key Terms

Traumatic brain injury (TBI)
Open brain injury
Closed brain injury
Primary injury
Diffuse axonal injury (DAI)
Secondary injury
Posttraumatic amnesia (PTA)
Decorticate posturing
Decerebrate posturing
Dysphagia
Post-traumatic vision syndrome (PTVS)
Impaired initiation
Disinhibition
Emotional lability
Sensory regulation treatment

Chapter Objectives

After studying this chapter, the student or practitioner will be able to do the following:

1. Define traumatic brain injury and identify its common causes.
2. Discuss the impact of posttraumatic amnesia on function.
3. Explain the purpose of sensory regulation and how it is used in treatment of a client with traumatic brain injury who is functioning at a lower level.
4. Identify treatment activities for clients with traumatic brain injury at each level of the revised Rancho Los Amigos Level of Cognitive Functioning.
5. Identify how engagement in occupation, participation, and health are affected by traumatic brain injury.
6. Explain the role of OT in behavior management programming.
7. Identify and describe appropriate remedial, functional, and compensatory treatments for specific client factors caused by traumatic brain injury.
8. Describe the role of the family and significant others in the recovery process of the client with traumatic brain injury.

Traumatic brain injury (TBI) results from a penetrating (open) or nonpenetrating (closed) injury to the brain. TBI is a life-altering experience that causes physical, cognitive, behavioral, and emotional changes affecting the person's ability to engage in occupations, participation, and health. Survivors of TBI may show a variety of problems because the range of disability after a TBI is more varied than in other central nervous system dysfunction. No two clients present with exactly the same symptoms, even if they have common diagnoses. Some brain injuries cause immediate death, whereas others result in mild damage. One TBI client may emerge from coma, respond inconsistently and nonreactively to painful stimuli (as presented when tested by a physician), and eventually require assistance the remainder of his or her life. Another may be able to complete all activities of daily living (ADL) but have difficulty with instrumental activities of daily living (IADL), rest and sleep, education, work, play/leisure, or social participation without external structure, cues, or assistance from others. All clients with TBI will have to make the necessary adjustments.

This chapter begins with a brief overview of the incidence, pathophysiology, and medical management related to changes in body structures[53] as the result of TBI and its evaluation. The occupational therapy (OT) evaluation, as performed by the occupational therapist, is discussed briefly. The main focus of this chapter is on interventions in which the occupational therapy assistant (OTA) might be expected to participate. Changes in client factors and performance skills and their effect on performance patterns are presented in more detail to help the reader to understand the differences between clients functioning at a lower level from those functioning at an intermediate to advanced level (Table 25-1).

Changes in Body Structures and Functions

Incidence of Traumatic Brain Injury

In the United States, there are more than 5.3 million survivors of traumatic brain injury.[35] More than 1.7 million persons sustain a new TBI every year. Three percent are fatal, 16.3% require hospitalization, and 80.7% are treated and released from the emergency room.[26] Seventy-five percent of these injuries result in concussion and other forms of mild TBI.[34] An estimated 3.2 million Americans are living with impairments[53] after being hospitalized following a TBI.[10] In the United States the leading cause of TBIs is falls, followed by motor vehicle accidents (MVAs).[26] TBI is increasing in third world countries because of the increased use of motor vehicles but has steadily decreased in the United States since the 1970s due to improved safety laws and standards in automobiles.[31] The number of fatal and severe TBIs has been declining, a trend that is attributed to a decreased incidence of drunk driving; increased use of seatbelts, airbags, and motorcycle helmets; and increased public education on prevention of TBI.[47] The increased use of airbags and the extreme velocity at which they are deployed have increased the incidence of mild TBI. Consider the case of Mr. B. His injuries might have been much less serious if he had been wearing his seatbelt at the time of impact.

Table 25-1 Levels of Cognitive Functioning

Level of Cognitive Function	Characteristics
I. No Response: Total Assistance	Appears to be in a deep sleep Completely unresponsive to any stimuli presented
II. Generalized Response: Total Assistance	Reacts inconsistently and nonpurposefully to stimuli in a nonspecific manner Responses are limited in nature and are often the same regardless of stimulus presented Responses may be physiologic changes, gross body movements, and/or vocalization Earliest response may be to deep pain Responses are likely to be delayed
III. Localized Response: Total Assistance	Reacts specifically but inconsistently to stimuli Responses are directly related to the type of stimulus presented in the environment such as head turning toward a sound Withdrawal of extremity and/or vocalization when presented with a painful stimulus May follow simple commands in a delayed and inconsistent manner such as closing eyes or squeezing or extending an extremity Responds to auditory and visual stimuli (in the visual fields at near distances) After external stimulus is removed, client may lie quietly and may also show a vague awareness of self and body by responding to discomfort by pulling at nasogastric tube or catheter May show bias by responding to some persons (especially family, friends) but not to others
IV. Confused-Agitated: Maximal Assistance	Heightened state of activity with severely decreased ability to process information Detached from the present and responds primarily to own internal confusion Behavior is often bizarre and nonpurposeful relative to immediate environment May cry out or scream out of proportion to stimuli even after removal, show aggressive behavior, attempt to remove restraints or tubes, or crawl out of bed in a purposeful manner Lack of discrimination between persons or objects Unable to cooperate directly with treatment effort Verbalization is often incoherent and/or inappropriate to the environment Confabulation may be present; patient may be euphoric or hostile Attention is very short; selective attention is often minimal at best Lack of awareness of present events Lacks short-term recall but may react to past events Needs maximum assistance to perform basic self-care (feeding, dressing) If not disabled physically, the client may be able to perform motor activities as in sitting, reaching, and ambulating as part of agitated state, but not purposefully on request May show mood shifts from euphoric to agitated without any relationship to environmental events
V. Confused-Inappropriate, Nonagitated: Maximal Assistance	Appears alert Able to respond to simple commands fairly consistently Responses are nonpurposeful and random in more complex situations and with less structure May be agitated, but not on an internal basis (as in Level IV) but rather as a result of external stimuli—and usually out of proportion to the stimulus Gross attention to the environment but is highly distractible Lacks ability to focus attention on a specific task without frequent redirection back to it With structure, the client may be able to converse on a social, automatic level for short periods of time Verbalization is often inappropriate; confabulation may be triggered by present events Memory is severely impaired, with confusion of past and present in reaction to ongoing activity Lacks initiation of functional tasks and often shows inappropriate use of objects without external direction May be able to perform previously learned tasks when structured but cannot learn new information Responds best to self, body, comfort—and often family members Usually can perform self-care activities with assistance and may accomplish feeding with maximum supervision May wander off either randomly or with vague intention of "going home"

Continued

Table 25-1 Levels of Cognitive Functioning—cont'd

Level of Cognitive Function	Characteristics
VI. Confused-Appropriate: Moderate Assistance	Goal-directed behavior but depends on external input for direction Response to discomfort is appropriate and the client tolerates unpleasant stimuli (e.g., nasogastric tube) when need is explained Follows simple directions consistently and shows carryover for relearned tasks (such as self-care) Needs less supervision with familiar tasks (old learning) Shows little or no carryover for new learning Responses may be incorrect because of memory problems, but they are appropriate to the situation Responses may be delayed Decreased ability to process information with little or no anticipation or prediction of events More depth and detail in past memories than recent memory Beginning awareness of situation by realizing an answer is unknown No longer wanders and is inconsistently oriented to time and place Selective attention to tasks may be impaired, especially with difficult tasks and in unstructured settings, but is now functional for common daily activities (30 minutes with structure) Shows at least vague recognition of some staff and has increased awareness of self, family, and basic needs (such as food), again in an appropriate manner as in contrast to Level V
VII. Automatic-Appropriate: Minimal Assistance for Daily Living Skills	Appears appropriate and oriented within hospital and home settings Completes daily routine automatically but often does so in an almost robotic way Minimal to absent confusion but has shallow recall of what has been done Shows increased awareness of self, body, family, foods, people, and interaction in the environment Superficial awareness of but lacks insight into his condition, demonstrates decreased judgment and problem solving, lacks realistic planning for the future Shows carryover for new learning but at a decreased rate Requires at least minimal supervision for learning and for safety purposes Independent in self-care activities and supervised in home and community skills for safety With structure, can initiate tasks in social and recreational activities of interest Unaware of needs and feelings of others Oppositional/uncooperative Judgment remains impaired, such that client cannot drive a car Unable to recognize inappropriate behavior in social interactions
VIII. Purposeful and Appropriate: Standby Assistance	Completes familiar tasks in a distracting environment for 1 hour Aware of and responsive to culture Shows carryover for new learning if acceptable to life role and needs no supervision after activities are learned Within physical capabilities, client is independent in home and community activities including driving Vocational rehabilitation to determine ability to return as a contributor to society (perhaps in a new capacity) is indicated Shows continued impairments in comparison to previous level of function in abilities, reasoning, tolerance for stress, judgment in emergencies, or unusual circumstances Irritable Argumentative Self-centered Depressed Social, emotional, and intellectual capacities may continue to be decreased but are functional for society Recognizes and corrects inappropriate behavior in social interactions but needs standby assistance to make corrections Alert and oriented Recalls and integrates past and recent events
IX. Purposeful and Appropriate: Standby Assistance on Request	Can shift back and forth between tasks, complete them accurately for about 2 hours Uses assistive memory devices such as planners, "to do" lists Performs familiar personal, household, work, and leisure activities, independently Performs new personal, household, work, and leisure activities, with assistance as needed Aware of problems that interfere with performance after they occur and can take corrective action but may need standby assistance to anticipate problems Thinks of consequences of actions with standby assistance May become easily irritated and have a low frustration tolerance Depression may continue Monitors self for appropriateness of social interaction with standby assistance

Table 25-1 Levels of Cognitive Functioning—cont'd

Level of Cognitive Function	Characteristics
X. Purposeful and Appropriate: Modified Independence	Multitasks in all environments and may require periodic rest breaks Initiates use of assistive memory devices independently Performs new personal, household, work, and leisure activities but may need more time and use of compensatory strategies Anticipates problems but may need more time and use of compensatory strategies Estimates abilities accurately and can make changes as indicated Recognizes the needs of others and socially interacts appropriately all of the time Periodic episodes of depression Irritability and lowered frustration tolerance when stressed, fatigued, or ill

Modified from Rancho Los Amigos Medical Center: *Original scale: levels of cognitive functioning,* Downey, Calif, 1995, Ranchos Los Amigos Medical Center, Adult Brain Injury Service.

CASE STUDY

Mr. B.: A Client Functioning at Low Level

Mr. B. is a 19-year-old, right-handed male who was involved in a motor vehicle accident (MVA) in which he was sitting without a seatbelt in the front passenger seat. The car was hit on the passenger side by a delivery truck that ran a stop sign. All airbags deployed. Mr. B. had a positive loss of consciousness and began to experience seizures at the scene of the accident. The emergency medical technician noted decerebrate posturing. Mr. B. had no previous medical problems and was not on any medications. He was immediately transported to the intensive care unit (ICU) of a level I trauma medical center. A computed tomography scan of the head showed bilateral intraventricular hemorrhage with multiple shear lesions. The Glasgow Coma Scale score was 6. Within 24 hours, Mr. B. underwent emergency surgery or ventriculostomy (insertion of tube through skull into brain) to reduce brain swelling. A Foley catheter was placed, and a bowel management program (using medications) was initiated. Two days after the accident, Mr. B. underwent a craniotomy for evacuation of a right frontal lobe subdural hematoma. A tracheostomy tube and parenteral nutrition tube were placed within a few days after the injury. Mr. B. stayed in the ICU for the next 3 weeks. He was unconscious for 14 days and awoke from the coma 1 week before being transferred to the rehabilitation unit.

Initial Occupational Therapy Evaluation

The occupational therapist obtained the following information from Mr. B's mother:

Mr. B. lives in a two-story home with his parents and his 16-year-old sister. At the time of the injury, he was enrolled in the spring semester at a local community college, where he was majoring in criminal justice, but had to withdraw for the semester because of his injury. In the fall, he had achieved a B+ average, completing 12 credits. He has no history of learning disabilities or academic difficulties. He worked 12 hours most weekends at a local restaurant as a short-order cook and played soccer once a week in an adult league. Before his injury, Mr. B. was completely independent in all activities of daily living, managed his own money, kept his room clean, did his own laundry, and cooked breakfast for the family on Sundays after church. On awaking from coma, Mr. B. responded to pain and showed purposeful movement of his nondominant left upper extremity (UE) but could not follow commands or verbalize at all. His eyes were open during his wake cycle, but he did not visually attend or track. His sleep patterns were abnormal (i.e., sleeping most of the day and night). Increased tone was noted in both UEs (right greater than the left). There was some movement of his right extremities, but the UE showed flexor patterning. Right hemiparesis was present. Medications were prescribed to prevent seizures, reduce spasticity, regulate the wake/sleep cycle, reduce gastric discomfort, and increase alertness. In the third week in the ICU, Mr. B. began sitting up in a bedside chair with a reclined high back, leg rests, tilted seat, and lapboard for 30 minutes twice a day. Mr. B. required maximal assist of two persons to transfer from the bed to the chair and back. Postural control and static sitting balance were fair to poor, and dynamic sitting balance was very poor. Mr. B. began verbalizing (answering simple questions) and moving his left upper and lower extremities (LEs) purposefully. Mr. B. was given a helmet to wear at all times when out of bed. Dysphagia prevented him from eating or drinking anything by mouth. He had difficulty swallowing his saliva at times and was partially aware that he drools. All feeding supplements, fluids, and medications were being given through the feeding tube. When medically stable, Mr. B. was transferred to the inpatient rehabilitation program.

Inpatient

In the rehabilitation unit, Mr. B. required maximal assistance with all activities of daily living and functional mobility. He could not complete any other areas of occupation. The speech-language pathologist and the respiratory therapist worked with Mr. B. to

Continued

CASE STUDY—cont'd

improve his ability to breathe normally without using the tracheostomy tube. Through oral-motor and swallowing training by the speech-language pathologist, Mr. B. progressed to eating pureed foods but still cannot drink fluids by mouth. All nutritional needs are met through tube feedings. The only self-care task the client could perform was to wash his face using his left hand with moderate assistance from the clinician. He continues to use the Foley catheter for bladder management and is on a bowel management program.

Mr. B. has been wearing corrective lenses for distance since he was 10 years old. His glasses were broken in the MVA, but the family brought to the hospital a second pair with an up-to-date prescription. Every time staff or family has tried to put his glasses on him, he has become agitated and removed them. Mr. B. can visually attend about 10 to 15 seconds and track objects for 10 to 15 seconds.

Mr. B. has reduced active and passive range of motion (ROM) of the right UE and LE due to paresis and spasticity. He has full functional use of the left extremities, has some movement of the right lower extremity, and lacks functional use of the right UE. Sensory and perceptual testing could not be performed fully because of his limited cognition and inability to communicate and participate in objective testing. From observation, Mr. B. seems to have reduced tactile sensation of the right side and pain with passive ROM of the right UE. Cognitively, Mr. B. is at a Level IV on the Ranchos Los Amigos Scale. Posttraumatic amnesia (PTA) is resolving slowly. The client requires 24-hour supervision for safety. Mr. B.'s mother has taken a leave of absence from her full-time job and has been at the hospital 7 to 9 hours daily since his accident. She participates in most of his therapy sessions.

Outpatient Therapy

After several weeks of therapy as an inpatient, Mr. B. made such significant progress that he was referred for outpatient OT 5 days a week through the same hospital rehabilitation program. His seizures are now controlled, and the tracheostomy, gastric tube, and catheter have been removed. Mr. B. eats primarily fluids and softer foods, completes basic hygiene and uses a shower chair and hose for bathing, grooms himself, feeds himself with occasional spills, and dresses with minimal assistance to put on his right AFO and right shoe. He walks with a hemi-cane and requires minimal to standby assistance. He needs moderate verbal and visual reminders to wear his helmet at all times when he is out of bed, especially when ambulating. Both parents provide assistance as needed. Mr.B.'s mother has stopped working so that she can take care of her son.

Mr. B. is bowel and bladder continent. He wears his glasses at all times. He is currently participating in a serial casting program to increase passive ROM of his right elbow, which is limited due to moderate spasticity. He still has no functional use of his right (dominant) extremity. Visual tracking and visual processing speed is slowed. Perceptual deficits include visual agnosia (reduced ability to recognize objects visually), reduced ability to recognize faces, right-left discrimination deficits, impaired figure-ground, topographical disorientation, and depth perception deficits. Language problems include auditory processing deficits, reading problems, and impaired word finding. He has improved to a Level VII on the Ranchos Los Amigos scale and still requires supervision at home. At times, his frustration tolerance is reduced. Mr. B. wants to be able "take care of [himself] without help, go back to school, and drive a car again."

Clients with mild TBI may have other diagnoses such as bruising, fractures, or other complications attributable to injuries at the time of the TBI. Because mild TBI can be underreported, the OTA who is familiar with the signs and symptoms should report any questionable observations to the occupational therapist for further review by the physician. Improved education of health care professionals concerning the signs and symptoms has also led to increased recognition, diagnosis, and treatment of mild TBI.[34] Since the onset of Operation Enduring Freedom/Operation Iraqi Freedom (U.S. military efforts in Afghanistan and Iraq) there has been an increase in TBI in the military. It is estimated that among military personnel serving in combat who experience battle-related injuries, about 30% sustain some form of TBI, most commonly caused by blast injuries.[49] Statistics show that TBI occurs twice as often in males as in females.[26] The risk is higher among children 0 to 4 years old, adolescents aged 15 to 19 years old, adults aged 75 and older,[26] and people who have had previous brain injuries. Adolescents are most likely to sustain traumatic brain injuries in motor vehicle accidents, while adults older than age 75 have the highest rate of hospitalization and fatalities due to TBI.[26] About one third to one half of persons admitted with TBI are found to be legally intoxicated, and it is estimated that nearly two thirds of persons admitted for TBI have a history of drug and alcohol abuse.[9] The OT practitioner should be aware that some clients with TBI may have coexisting conditions that will affect treatment. Some research indicates that women with TBI tend to recover better than men do,[43] but other studies do not support the finding that gender differences exist.[12] The prognosis for younger persons is better than for older persons with similar injuries.[32]

Pathophysiology

Two mechanisms of injury disrupt body structures,[53] causing both primary and secondary damage to the brain. An **open brain injury** typically results from direct trauma to the head by an object that penetrates the skull and brain. Examples are bullets and fragments, pieces from exploding objects, and other flying projectiles. A **closed brain injury** occurs when acceleration, deceleration, and rotational forces are applied to the head and cause brain tissue to shear (tear apart). Closed brain injuries often result from falls (including sports related) and MVAs. In both types of injuries, damage can be caused by coup (the direct hit on the head) and contrecoup (the result of the brain moving inside the skull from the coup impact). Contrecoup injuries often occur on the side of the brain opposite the impact but can occur in other areas as well, depending on the severity of the forces acting on the brain inside the skull.

Primary injury occurs at the time of the trauma and is caused by localized contusions (bruises) that result in diffuse axonal injury (DAI). Contusions often occur in the frontal and temporal regions when the brain slides and strikes the rough skull. The damage is often asymmetrical. Most damage occurs at the site of the first hit, where localized contusions may also be present. DAI results from stretching and shearing forces occurring in the tissues of the brain. The white matter of the cerebral hemispheres, the corpus callosum, and the brainstem are the most commonly affected areas.[1] DAI causes widespread brain damage. Damage may be severe enough to induce a coma or so mild that only a concussion or brief loss of consciousness results. Both Mr. B. and Mrs. R. in the case studies sustained closed brain injuries caused by being thrown around the inside of their cars on impact. Both had coup and contrecoup injuries. Mr. B.'s coup injury caused a subdural hematoma, which required surgery to remove a large blood clot to save his life, and Mrs. R. had a laceration that required stitches to close. Because the impact of the crash was on Mr. B.'s side of the car and he was not wearing a seatbelt, he experienced a much more significant injury and more impairments[53] than Mrs. R.

Secondary Injury

Secondary injury results from a series of chemical reactions in the brain that can occur immediately after the injury, hours or days later, and can significantly worsen the damage caused by primary injury.[39] These secondary effects include intracranial hematomas, cerebral edema, raised intracranial pressure, hydrocephalus, intracranial infection, and posttraumatic seizures. They account for the greatest number of deaths associated with TBI in hospitals.[14]

Early diagnosis and medical management of secondary changes during the acute phase of the injury help minimize impairments of bodily structures, reducing the risk of further brain damage. After a significant rise in intracranial pressure, Mr. B. had to undergo a ventriculostomy to reduce pressure on the brain and to limit the risk of further brain damage. Again, Mr. B's injuries were more severe than Mrs. R's; his head moved around much more in the car because he was not restrained by a seatbelt. The airbag blocked him from going forward but did not limit movement in other directions.

Medical Management

The priorities in the medical and surgical management of the person with a TBI are to minimize effects of the immediate injury, reestablish normal bodily functions, and prevent secondary complications.[29] The paramedics initiate life-saving medical procedures with the person with brain injury at the scene of the injury. When the person arrives at the hospital emergency room, the medical team continues to address life-threatening injuries and works to stabilize the patient medically. For severely injured individuals, this process may take hours to days. The person with a severe TBI may experience medical complications and require emergency treatment for shock or respiratory arrest. Advances in critical care of persons with TBI have led to better outcomes.[29]

The medical team evaluates the client to assess for other injuries such as spinal and soft tissue injuries, fractures, wounds, and/or internal injuries. Suctioning, intubation, or a tracheostomy may be required for a blocked or damaged airway. The person may require stitches or immobilization such as splints, a cervical collar, a halo vest, casts, or traction. A craniotomy, performed by a neurosurgeon, may be necessary to decrease rising intracranial pressure and bleeding.[33] Medical intervention also involves the use of medications for pain, seizures, etc.[29]

Mrs. R.'s injury was mild; she was medically stable when she arrived at the emergency room. Her most immediate medical problem was her forehead wound, which required stitches. Mr. B.'s severe injuries required several medical interventions. Despite the introduction of a tube to drain fluid off his brain, Mr. B. required a craniotomy, in which a portion of his skull bone was removed and saved for future replacement. With an open area of the brain, Mr. B. needed to wear a protective helmet at all times when out of bed to prevent damage to the brain in case of a fall. Because of memory deficits, Mr. B. needed verbal and visual reminders provided by others in order to use the helmet as prescribed.

Initial nutritional needs are usually met with intravenous fluids. For unconscious clients or persons who cannot take in food orally in sufficient quantity, a nasogastric tube is inserted through the nose into the stomach. If the problem continues, a gastrostomy tube may be placed surgically through the abdomen into the stomach. The client receives nutrients through these tubes until he or she can consume sufficient calories or fluids orally. Mr. B. initially could not take in any food or fluids by mouth because of his light coma, or later after awakening, because of dysphagia. As he recovered and received treatment by the speech-language pathologist (SLP) in conjunction with the OT practitioner, Mr. B. progressed to eating foods with softer textures.

After the initial medical evaluation and treatment (management in the emergency room and operating room), the client is typically transferred to the intensive care unit (ICU). In the ICU the client is monitored for response to treatment and for possible complications. The medical status including neurological functioning is frequently reassessed. When medically stable, the client is usually transferred to the acute care neurological service or to a rehabilitation unit.

Occupational Therapy in the Intensive Care Unit

Clients in the ICU who receive OT early in the rehabilitation process have better functional outcomes.[45] In the ICU setting the OT practitioner completes the evaluation, which is often modified to accommodate the needs of the client with reduced cognition, medical, and neurological issues. The OT practitioner would establish a baseline cognitive status and may gather information from the client's family or significant

CASE STUDY

Mrs. R.: A Client Functioning at a High Level

Mrs. R., a 36-year-old schoolteacher, was the driver of a car involved in a motor vehicle accident (MVA). She was wearing a seatbelt at the time of the crash. A truck ran a stop sign and struck the car on the passenger side, injuring her 19-year-old nephew, who was riding in the front passenger seat. Mrs. R. sustained a deep laceration over her left eye and briefly lost consciousness. She was transported to the emergency room at a local hospital, where she received 10 stitches for the laceration and complained of a severe headache, dizziness, and neck pain. Her head and neck xrays and the computer tomography scan of her head were negative. Mrs. R. has a history of allergies and uses prescribed medication as needed. At the emergency room, she was diagnosed with a concussion and whiplash and discharged to home, with recommendations to rest. However, she chose to visit the hospital where her nephew was hospitalized. Initially, she was not allowed in the ICU to visit him but spent several hours sitting with her sister, brother-in-law, niece, and other family members. When her headache, neck pain, and dizziness became severe, she went home. She woke up the next day with a severe headache, light sensitivity, fatigue, severe neck and upper back pain, numerous body aches, dizziness, and difficulty attending and concentrating. She stayed home for the next 10 days, leaving her house only to visit her injured nephew and see her doctor, who diagnosed concussion, sleep disturbance, and cervical muscular strain. She was prescribed medication for pain and sleep and physical therapy.

She "felt better" after taking medications and attending six physical therapy sessions and decided to return to work as a fourth-grade teacher. She noticed immediately that the fluorescent lights and noises in the school were difficult to tolerate. By the end of the first day, she was so exhausted that she had to call her husband for a ride home. She ate a quick meal and slept for 14 hours. Her experience for the remainder of the week was similar, and she chose to find a quiet area in the school to rest in the dark as often as she could to get through the day. She also noticed she had difficulties with focusing, remembering, organizing her schedule, thinking of words to say, sleeping at night, and sitting or standing comfortably for more than 30 minutes. At times, she would forget the lesson she was teaching and started using notes to help when teaching. She prefers to type them instead of writing them as she used to because her handwriting quality has decreased significantly. Without provocation, she is likely to burst into tears. When she stopped performing most household management tasks, daily walks, and leisure reading at home, she could perform slightly better at work temporarily. Mrs. R. continued to teach for the next 4 weeks but was always exhausted, had difficulty performing home management chores, made several errors in bill paying, and began falling farther and farther behind in keeping up with her schoolwork. At work and at home, she isolated herself socially, except to visit her nephew in the hospital three times a week. She expressed to her sister repeatedly how she felt responsible for her nephew's serious injuries. Mr. R. noticed that his wife was more irritable, less focused, unable to converse for more than a few minutes, and emotional at times. She got up often during the night because she could not sleep, kept all the lights off, stopped watching television, bumped into objects in the home, and dropped things. Mrs. R. was referred to a neuropsychiatrist, who diagnosed a mild TBI with executive dysfunction, posttraumatic headache, posttraumatic concussive syndrome, posttraumatic stress syndrome, posttraumatic vision syndrome, depression, disorder of initiating and maintaining sleep, fatigue, and sensory hypersensitivity. The doctor confirmed the previous diagnosis of whiplash. He prescribed medications for headache pain, fatigue, depression, alertness, and sleep and recommended that Mrs. R. take a 3-month leave of absence from work, effective immediately. He also referred Mrs. R. to a licensed professional counselor, occupational therapy, physical therapy, and speech-language pathology for evaluation and treatment.

Occupational Therapy Evaluation

Mrs. R. is independent in self-care but requires more time to complete all tasks. She became dizzy when she closed her eyes in the shower. The therapist recommended a shower chair for safety. Mrs. R. is no longer totally independent in instrumental activities of daily living; she relies on her husband and other help. Her husband, Mr. R., works long hours as a mechanical engineer and has always been responsible for home repairs and yard work. He has taken over all the cooking, grocery shopping, laundry, light cleaning, and bill paying. The family hired a cleaning service for the deep cleaning every 2 weeks. Despite using more prepared foods, Mrs. R. still has difficulty with meal preparation and makes errors in timing of different foods, overcooking foods, and leaving the oven on after using it. She becomes distracted easily and often does not complete tasks such as laundry without reminders from her husband. She forgets when to take medications and no longer follows her daily planner, instead requiring reminders from her husband. Mrs. R. is easily fatigued and takes a 2- to 3-hour nap each afternoon when she can. Mrs. R. has eye misalignment, reduced visual tracking, reduced convergence, impaired depth perception, double vision, and impaired saccades, causing reading problems. She does not wear corrective lenses. She avoids driving at night, in heavy traffic or inclement weather, and she tries to drive only on local familiar roads, but she gets lost about twice a week. Her husband has been supportive about the problems associated with her injury and the accident in which her nephew was seriously injured but feels considerable stress. Mrs. R. has been rated Level VIII on the Ranchos Los Amigos Scale. Her goals are to regain all of her previous life roles.

others to initiate the occupational profile. Family members or significant others will be able to provide details about the client's home environment, performance patterns, and areas of occupation that will help in planning interventions. The occupational therapist may be involved in recommending positioning equipment to be ordered or fabricated, especially for the individual client. In addition, a client with an open brain injury or craniotomy defect requires a helmet when he or she is out of bed to protect the open skull from further brain injury. The OT practitioner might be asked to adapt a helmet to optimize its fit. Use of the helmet is not required for individuals who receive a hinged titanium plate because it covers the skull and protects the brain.[45]

Interventions for the client in this phase of recovery would address areas of occupation such basic ADL, performance skills such as posture or coordination, body functions such as mental functions, and neuromusculoskeletal and movement-related functions. The focus would be on preparatory methods, purposeful activity, and the education process. The OTA may be asked to carry out interventions to optimize proper bed and sitting positioning, maintain range of motion (ROM), facilitate responses to stimuli, ensure practice of basic hygiene skills, increase endurance for activity, etc. Mr. B. might best practice washing his face while he is sitting up in the bedside chair because this is a more familiar context than performing the task in bed. The OTA could instruct Mr. B.'s mother in how to perform daily orientation programming. The OTA might also perform ROM for the upper extremities (UEs), assist with basic personal self-care training, and help Mr. B. follow one-step commands.

A person with urinary incontinence may require catheterization. To assist the individual in eliminating the bowels, the physician usually prescribes stool softeners to prevent impaction. Later in the rehabilitation phase, when elimination functions start to return, a bowel and bladder program is initiated. The OT practitioner may be involved in this training. After the initial evaluation and treatment (management in the emergency room and operating room), the client is usually transferred to the ICU. In the ICU the client is monitored for response to treatment and for possible complications. The clinical neurological status is frequently reassessed.[42] When medically stable, the client is usually transferred to the acute care neurologic service or to a rehabilitation unit.

Severity of Injury

Posttraumatic Amnesia

The spectrum of deficits from TBI varies and can be characterized as severe, moderate, or mild. Although no absolute measure of severity of TBI exists, some measures are indexed by duration and depth of unconsciousness (coma) and length of posttraumatic amnesia (PTA). There are two types of PTA. Retrograde amnesia is a decreased ability to recall information occurring before the brain injury,[7] and anterograde amnesia is a decreased ability to recall new information.[6] One of the more accurate predictors in determining the severity of the diffuse brain damage is the duration of PTA. When a person with a severe TBI comes out of coma, PTA can last from a few days to months.[50] More than 45% of persons with acquired brain injury will experience PTA of 28 days or greater,[50] as was true for Mr. B. Longer periods of PTA are associated with lower levels of cognitive and motor ability. Retrograde memory improves over time, but individuals with PTA may be confused, agitated,[54] and inattentive.

In contrast, the injured person with anterograde amnesia cannot store or retrieve new information,[54] cannot remember daily occurrences such as what he had for breakfast, who came to visit that day, the day of the week, and so on. Safety is also a concern because of poor awareness and impulsivity. Medical centers may have their own systems to rate the level of severity (such as the Grade III head trauma rating for Mr. B.). Regardless of the level of injury, the most significant recovery usually occurs during the first 2 years, especially the first 6 months; however, neurological recovery can continue for years.

Functional Assessment

A number of assessment scales are used with persons with TBI for clinical evaluation, program evaluation, prediction of outcome, and to produce data for clinical research. On admission to the hospital for TBI, most people are rated with the standardized Glasgow Coma Scale (GCS)[48] to measure their level of consciousness. The GCS is divided into categories of eye opening, best motor response, and verbal response; 15 items, in total, are scored. A score of 13 to 15 indicates mild impairment, 9 to 12 moderate impairment, and under 8 severe impairment.[8] Mr. B. had a GCS score of 6, indicating a severe injury. The person with a TBI can show a variety of symptoms manifested in many different ways, depending on the type, severity, and location of the injury. The client may have severe limitations in most of the areas described later or may have subtle deficits, evident only in high-level, complex activities.

Other scales and objective measures such as the Disability Rating Scale,[19,42] the Functional Independence Measure,[16] the Functional Status Examination,[11] the Glasgow Outcome Scale-Extended,[52] the Community Integration Questionnaire,[51] and observational assessments such as the Rancho Los Amigos Scale of Cognitive Functioning[41] (see Table 25-1) are used to evaluate the effects of TBI. The occupational therapist might participate with the team in using these assessments, and the OTA should be familiar with the scale(s) used at the facility.

After a TBI, recovery occurs along a continuum from comatose (at one end of the spectrum) to fully functional in all situations. The revised version of the Rancho Los Amigos Scale of Cognitive Functioning[41] divides recovery into 10 stages. In addition to identifying cognitive deficits and skills, the Rancho Los Amigos Scale also includes behavioral and functional deficits and skills occurring at the various stages of recovery. Becoming familiar with these stages will prove useful to the clinician as he or she seeks to recognize and understand the various characteristics of recovery from TBI. The information is also useful for educating caregivers and families.

In addition to the assessments discussed earlier, the occupational therapist assesses performance in areas of occupation, performance skills, performance patterns, contexts, activity demands, and client factors.[2,53] Despite the considerable difference between Mr. B. and Mrs. R. in the severity of their TBIs, both have experienced changes in their ability to perform customary and valued occupations. Mr. B. demonstrates deficits in all areas of performance skills; Mrs. R., despite her higher level of function, also shows diminished performance skills. Both clients have deficits in performance patterns (habits, routines, and roles).[2] Mr. B. requires much more assistance to participate in his occupations, whereas Mrs. R. has changed her habits to accommodate her brain injury (e.g., staying at home and performing fewer chores). She has given up her work role temporarily and has reduced most other roles because her symptoms such as headache, sensory sensitivity, low endurance, and executive dysfunction interfere with her ability to participate.

The occupational therapist also assesses performance in the contexts of each client's life, which includes: cultural (beliefs, activity patterns), physical (environment), social, personal (age, gender, socioeconomic status, educational status), spiritual, temporal (stage of life, time of year, duration of problems), and virtual (computers, radio).[2] At the time of the accident, Mr. B. was a young adult who was just starting his college education, living at home and still financially dependent on his parents. He had not established himself as an independently functioning mature adult. Therefore some of the skills he needs to learn will be new and challenging. He will require lengthy rehabilitation, with emphasis on basic self-care training and performance skills first. The occupational therapist identifies the activity demands (tools and materials used in tasks, space demands and physical environment, social demands, sequencing and timing, motor skills required, and body parts used in the task)[2] and adapts them to promote success for the client. For example, the occupational therapist might observe Mr. B. eating to determine why he spills his food. Perhaps he is using his nondominant left hand and could benefit from further practice in improving coordination.

Mrs. R. has established herself in many roles that she highly values, particularly at her work. Since her injury, she has not been able to maintain any habits, roles, or routines consistently. She will require intervention to reestablish roles, preferably beginning with those in the home, a familiar environment, which should help her feel more comfortable and less fatigued. Finally, the occupational therapist assesses client factors including body functions and body structures.[2,53] Body functions that would be addressed in OT include mental functions (affective, cognitive, perceptual); sensory functions and pain; neuromusculoskeletal and movement-related functions; cardiovascular, hematologic (vascular), immunologic, and respiratory function; and skin and related structures.[2,53] OT practitioners should be aware of body structures including the structures of the nervous system, ears, and eyes, and those structures related to movement, etc.[2,53] Mr. B. has deficits in all body functions as listed. Mrs. R.'s problems are mostly related to cognitive, global mental, and mental functions. The remainder of this chapter explores OT interventions in areas relevant for Mr. B. and Mrs. R. and other clients who have sustained TBI.

Clinical Picture of Persons with Traumatic Brain Injury

The neuromusculoskeletal and movement-related disorders experienced by clients after TBI can vary from severe motor involvement (of the trunk or of one to all four extremities) to minimally impaired coordination and muscle strength and full isolated voluntary control. Most clients who require OT will exhibit deficits in one or more of the following areas: primitive reflexes, muscle tone, postural stability, motor control, ROM, strength, sensation, and endurance. The OTA should be aware of all contraindications when treating any client with TBI.

> ***Safety Precautions for Clients with Brain Injury***
>
> The OTA should be aware of all precautions and contraindications for each client with TBI. This will include level of supervision needed, oral intake restrictions, risk for seizures, precautions/restrictions for weight bearing, impulsivity, or combative behavior.

Abnormal Reflexes

Common reflexes exhibited in severely brain-injured adults are the asymmetrical tonic neck reflex and the symmetrical tonic neck reflex. Treatment focuses on inhibiting these brainstem reflexes and facilitating normal movement patterns. Mr. B. demonstrated patterning of the right side (flexion of the upper extremity [UE] and extension of the lower extremity [LE]) and did not recover functional movement of his right UE. The occupational therapist would facilitate normal movement patterns involving the entire body (head, neck, trunk, and extremities). The OTA would facilitate Mr. B. achieving normalized movement patterns to maximize function and would instruct his family in ways to support normal movement for Mr. B.

Abnormal Muscle Tone

When muscle tone is affected by the TBI, it varies from hypotonicity (flaccidity) to hypertonicity (spasticity) and can affect all skeletal muscles of the head, neck, trunk, and extremities. When muscles are flaccid, the resistance to passive movement is diminished and the stretch reflex is dampened. The affected body part may appear floppy and will require support to prevent subluxation.

The client in a coma may develop decorticate posturing (sustained contraction and posturing of both UEs in flexion and the trunk and both LEs in extension) or decerebrate posturing (sustained contraction and posturing of the trunk and extremities in extension) in the first days or weeks after injury. These postures may diminish over time as the client recovers neurologically. Mr. B. demonstrated decerebrate posturing at the scene of the accident, which resolved over the next several weeks.

Spasticity will fluctuate with changes in the client's position, volitional movement, or medication. Infections, illness, pain, an overfilled bladder, impaction of the bowels, or resistance to the affected or unaffected muscles on the opposite side can increase spasticity. OT intervention for abnormal muscle tone begins with proper positioning and maintenance of full active and passive ROM to prevent contractures. Long-term consequences of severe spasticity include reduced ability to perform ADL, difficulty in maintaining proper bed or sitting positioning, reduced functional mobility (difficulty with transfers, gait deviations), painful spasms, disruption of sleep, increased risk for skin breakdown, contractures, reduced breath control, reduced speech, and pneumonia.[24] Spasticity may range from minimal to severe and increases the risk for joint contractures. Medical treatment options may include oral medications such as Baclofen, intramuscular injections, nerve blocks, or neurosurgery (cutting nerves or nerve roots).[24] Injections of neurotoxin when combined with passive ROM, casting, and the use of modalities can be effective in treating severe spasticity.[55] Mr. B. has increased tone or spasticity of his right side. Although his LE motor function improved enough to allow him to ambulate with an ankle foot orthosis (AFO) and hemi-cane, his right UE remained nonfunctional, requiring him to change his hand dominance.

Muscle Weakness

After a TBI, muscle weakness or below-average muscle strength can be mild to severe. When muscle weakness is present in the head, neck, and trunk, the client may have difficulty with head control or posture while sitting. If weakness is present in both UEs, deficits in gross and fine motor control or coordination will be present. Mr. B. has weakness of his right side (hemiparesis), suggesting that he will demonstrate problems with motor control.

Postural Dysfunction

Postural deficits result from imbalanced muscle tone; delayed or absent righting reactions; impaired motor control; and deficits in vision, cognition, and perception. Abnormal postures frequently exhibited in adults with moderate to severe TBI are listed in Box 25-1.

Box 25-1

Abnormal Postures Associated with Severe to Moderate Brain Injury

1. Head/neck: forward flexion or hyperextension
2. Scapula: humeral depression with protraction, retraction, or downward rotation
3. UEs: possible bilateral or unilateral involvement; typically have elbow flexion, humeral adduction and internal rotation, forearm pronation, and flexion of wrist and fingers
4. Trunk: kyphosis, scoliosis, loss of lordosis
5. Pelvis: posterior pelvic tilt and pelvic obliquity
6. LEs: hip adduction, knee flexion, plantar flexion, and inversion; if in a persistent vegetative state, may have severe extensor spasms

Mr. B. initially demonstrated postural deficits, which were addressed through adaptations when he first began to sit upright. With recovery he gained more postural control, as well as control of his left extremities and right LE, sufficient enough to allow him to ambulate with devices and assistance.

Impaired Motor Control and Motor Speed

Motor control allows for smooth, purposeful movements of body parts during functional tasks. Impairment in voluntary motor control in all of the extremities (quadriparesis) results from an imbalance in muscle tone and muscle weakness. It is not uncommon for only one side of the body to be involved, thus causing hemiparesis, such as occurred with Mr. B. Loss of motor control leads to deficits in head and trunk control, sitting and standing balance, reaching, bending, stooping, and functional ambulation; these functions are necessary for performing both basic and advanced ADL. Many persons with TBI experience reduced gross and fine motor speed. Both Mr. B. and Mrs. R. show slowed motor speed while performing functional tasks.

Ataxia

Ataxia is abnormal movement and disordered muscle tone seen in clients with TBI due to damage to the cerebellum and/or to the sensory pathways. Ataxia can affect movements of the head, neck, and trunk but usually affects the extremities. The client with ataxia has lost the ability to make small, minute adjustments that allow for smooth coordination of movements. Shakiness and incoordination cause problems in fine motor tasks such as writing, fastening, typing on a keyboard, using the keys on a cell phone, and eating.

Limitations of Joint Motion

Loss of active and passive ROM is a common problem. Interventions for loss of ROM vary depending on the cause; the occupational therapist should determine the cause of the loss of ROM before the OTA begins treatment.

Mr. B. has lost active and passive ROM of his nonfunctional right UE, which did not respond either to daily ROM exercises or to medication to reduce spasticity. The spasticity was severe enough to cause a contracture of his right elbow, requiring an injection of botulinum toxin in conjunction with serial casting of the elbow until maximum passive ROM can be achieved (Figure 25-1). Mr. B. may require additional static splinting to be worn as much as possible to maintain gains; once gains are established, he can reduce hours of wear to only when sleeping.

Sensory Changes

Persons with TBI may experience dulling or a loss of the following: light touch sensation, sharp or dull discrimination, proprioception, kinesthesia, or stereognosis of the extremities. Cranial nerve involvement may cause loss of pain and light touch sensation in the face and impaired senses of taste and smell. Mr. B. demonstrated reduced tactile sensation, or hyposensitivity, of the right side. Treatment focuses on increasing his awareness of the lack of protective sensation.

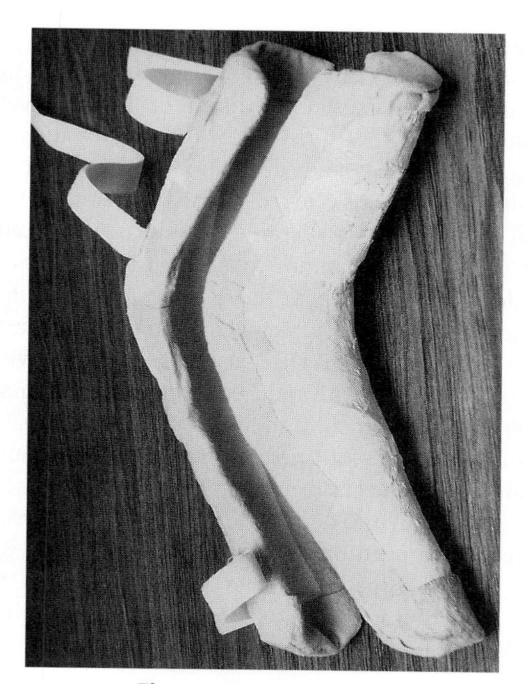

Figure 25-1 Bivalve cast.

For example, Mr. B. should learn to check water temperature with his left hand and check the skin under the AFO for any problems. Mrs. R. has a different sensory problem; she is hypersensitive to noise and visual input. She compensates by isolating herself, keeping all overhead lights off at home, and wearing earplugs when she is with other people in the community.

Decreased Functional Endurance

Decreased endurance usually results from the TBI but may also arise from deconditioning from prolonged bed rest or medical complications such as infections. OT intervention includes a graded program to gradually increase the client's ability to sit up and actively participate. Despite significant differences in the severity of their injuries, Mr. B. and Mrs. R. both have problems with low endurance and fatigue. Although she is participating less in home management, social, and community roles, and no longer working, Mrs. R. still takes a 2- to 3-hour nap every day. Both Mr. B. and Mrs. R. have sleep issues that contribute to fatigue.

Dysphagia

The majority of clients with severe TBI will have dysphagia[46] (problems swallowing). Many may have difficulty controlling oral secretions, handling thin liquids, chewing, or managing food with mixed textures. They may aspirate food or liquid into their lungs and choke easily. Consequently, they are at higher risk for aspiration pneumonia. Clients with dysphagia who are NPO (nothing by mouth) may also drool or experience dry mouth. Such clients will usually have oral hygiene problems. The presence of cognitive, behavioral, and linguistic problems as the result of brain injury further complicates the ability to eat and drink normally.[20] Clients may not understand fully their difficulties with feeding and dietary restrictions. For example, they may attempt to take food off others' trays in the dining room or they may try to take a drink from the water fountain in the hospital, even though both are contraindicated. This behavior is not unusual in clients with impulsivity and lack of insight. The OTA often works in conjunction with the SLP to treat the client with dysphagia. It is important for families and significant others to understand the eating and drinking restrictions specific to the client in each stage of recovery and to guide the client in following a dietary program safely and effectively. The OTA can assist in carrying out the guidelines determined by the OT.

Mr. B. has progressed significantly in eating (i.e., moving from NPO and tube feedings to eating soft foods). He may find it difficult to adhere to his dietary restrictions when discharged to home, especially because his medically restricted diet differs from his peers (i.e., he cannot eat potato chips, chicken wings, tacos, etc. and cannot drink thin liquids such as soft drinks, water, or coffee).

Visual Function

Individuals with TBI may sustain trauma to the vision system that can significantly affect a previously intact visual system. The eye and eyelid can sustain injury. Visual problems that may result from a TBI include eye misalignment, double vision, blurring of vision, inability to smoothly adjust from near to far vision, jerky eye movements, poor tracking (inability to follow objects), field defects (seeing only part of an image), reduced blink rate with dry eye, and ptosis or incomplete eyelid closure, which can also contribute to dry eye.

Many persons with TBI have posttraumatic vision syndrome (PTVS), which affects visual acuity, oculomotor control (eye coordination), binocular vision (eye teaming), and the coordination between the focal (detail oriented) and ambient (peripheral) aspects of the visual and balance systems. Symptoms of PTVS include double vision, reduced gaze stability (perceiving stationary objects as moving), poor attention and concentration, poor visual memory, glare sensitivity, impaired balance, visual-spatial misperceptions, and loss of coordination and postural control.[38] PTVS causes problems with reading, functional mobility, balance, and visual efficiency. Both Mr. B. and Mrs. R. show symptoms of PTVS that reduce their ability to read. Mr. B. is a college student who needs to have good reading skills to be successful. Mrs. R. is a teacher who requires reading for her career to be successful. She no longer enjoys reading, a leisure activity she highly valued. Visual impairments will impair functional performance, depending on the type, severity, and interrelation with deficits in other areas. The occupational therapist evaluates for visual problems occurring as the result of TBI and recommends referral to a vision specialist for a complete evaluation (see Chapter 22). PTVS and other visual deficits caused by TBI respond to vision rehabilitation, which comprises remedial exercises and instruction in and use of compensatory strategies, devices, and modification of the environment.[15] A behavioral optometrist in the College of Vision Development (COVD) most often provides visual therapy in the form of remedial exercises; some occupational therapists are specially trained in this area of functioning (see Chapter 22). The OT practitioner more generally provides interventions for compensation and environmental adaptation.

Perceptual Function

The ability to accurately perceive sensory information and respond to people and objects within the environment is necessary for successful, independent function.[4] Depending on the nature and extent of damage in TBI, impairment may involve visual, tactile, body scheme, language, and motor functions (see Chapter 23). Clients may experience impairments in the following areas: visual agnosia (inability or slowness in recognizing objects by sight), impaired left/right discrimination, impaired figure-ground, reduced topographical orientation (spatial orientation), impaired depth perception, tactile agnosia (astereognosis or inability or slowness in recognizing objects by touch), impaired body scheme (reduced ability to identify body parts), left unilateral neglect (reduced perception of left space), apraxia (impaired motor planning), and others. These deficits may affect the client's ability to interpret sensory information accurately and interact with objects, tools, or people in the environment successfully. Mr. B. has several perceptual problems, which, when combined with his cognitive and neurolinguistic problems, negatively affect his function in his college student role. Mrs. R. shows impaired depth perception and topographical orientation, which create problems with driving and route finding.

Cognitive Function

Varying degrees of cognitive deficits may result from TBI and include disorientation, decreased levels of attention, reduced concentration, impaired memory, **impaired initiation,** diminished safety awareness, decreased ability to process information accurately, and difficulty with executive functions and abstract reasoning.

Disorientation

For clients at a lower level of function, disorientation to varying degrees often occurs in relation to person, place, time, and situation (circumstance). The person appears confused and may need frequent basic reorientation or reassurance through verbal and visual cues while in OT until basic orientation improves consistently. Initially the information should be presented in a matter of fact tone, reminding the client with TBI of the basic orientation information. The clinician should avoid repeatedly asking the person to answer questions because doing so may lead to frustration, reduced cooperation, or agitation. The OTA can teach families and significant others how to provide reorientation cues and help determine relevant environmental cues specific to the client. For example, Mr. B. might be more likely to notice and attend to a large printed sign in his room with the day of the week if this information is written on a large picture of a soccer ball. The reorientation process can take from weeks to months. Although disorientation resolves with recovery for most persons with TBI, for some disorientation may be permanent.

Reduced Attention and Concentration

The client with a TBI often has deficits in the ability to attend to relevant tasks and sustain attention for the time needed to complete the task. TBI often leads to difficulty attending in the presence of any type of distraction, internal or external. Lower-level clients are often distracted by somatic (bodily) internal concerns such as discomfort associated with catheterization or intravenous tubing, pain, or urinary urges. These distractions may cause them to try to remove the tubes any time they can reach the appliances. Such clients require soft physical restraints to limit UE use and 24-hour supervision to avoid injury. Clients with reduced attention and concentration will also have difficulty attending to tasks in a distracting environment because of a reduced ability to mask out irrelevant sounds or visual information. The OT practitioner must select relevant activities to practice with the client to maximize attention and concentration. Both Mr. B. and Mrs. R. have reduced attention spans but have different reactions. Mr. B. is more easily distracted; Mrs. R. is more easily overwhelmed, fatigued, and likely to develop a severe headache.

Impaired Initiation

Impaired initiation—or difficulty in determining and beginning the first actions, steps, or stages of a task—can significantly affect the ability to function. Reduced initiation is not synonymous with impaired motivation. Persons with initiation problems may often stop because they are unsure of the first step in tasks and generally benefit from external written or verbal cues to get going. When they come to a stopping point they may get stuck again and require more cues to continue with the task. Both Mr. B. and Mrs. R. show reduced initiation. Mrs. R. also has depression, which may reduce initiation. Mr. B. requires more structure and moderate verbal cues to initiate most tasks, whereas Mrs. B. needs to have a set schedule with long rest breaks between each brief activity.

Impaired Memory

Several types of memory impairment exist and range from the inability to recall a few words just heard (immediate memory), to forgetting what happened in the last treatment session (short-term memory), to forgetting events that occurred 24 hours ago or years before the injury (long-term memory). Memory loss contributes to confusion and is manifested in the inability to learn and carry over new tasks. If the client does not remember personal information accurately or completely, the OT practitioner must seek other sources of information such as family members.

Establishing a routine using a meaningful cueing system can help the client become more functional. For example, clients who can no longer read words would be better served by an ADL cue sheet with pictures of their own supplies or even of themselves performing tasks such as combing their hair. Mr. B. has more difficulty with new learning and carryover and benefits from lowered expectations, which can be graded up as he succeeds. He could use a one-page daily checklist of his schedule and chores to check off as he finishes each task. He should always wear a large-face watch, which is easier to use.

Mrs. R. could benefit from a few assistive devices such as a main schedule board at home posted in an obvious place, a checklist for chores, and an electronic daily planner that is easier for her than the one she had been using before her injury. A sign could be posted with the day the housecleaning service comes and with all the dates for the next 3 months to help remind her when they will return. Color coding, streamlining information, and using checklists and a visual format with spaces designed so as not to overwhelm might be useful for Mrs. R. The OT practitioner would recommend that both Mr. B. and Mrs. R. set up well-marked areas in their home for belongings to be stored specifically in those locations (e.g., a tray for keys, another for the daily planner).

Decreased Safety Awareness

Unsafe behaviors exhibited by some persons with TBI may result from impulsiveness, decreased insight into deficits, impaired judgment, or a combination of all of these. Disorientation and impaired memory can contribute to the client's inability to recognize limitations for specific situations or analyze consequences of actions. Such clients will require 24-hour supervision for safety. Mr. B. has decreased safety awareness, requiring supervision to prevent injury. The OT practitioner could work with the client and the family to help them learn how to monitor the client (starting in the hospital environment to maintain safety) and how to modify the home situation and environment to maximize safety. For example, the family would need to determine how different members might take turns providing the necessary supervision. In addition, they would need to identify and choose modifications required such as railings on all stairs, unplugging kitchen appliances, or removing controls from the stovetop. Safety compensations for Mrs. R. might include showering on a tub seat to avoid falls and avoiding performing potentially dangerous tasks (such as using kitchen appliances) when she is fatigued.

Delayed Processing of Information

Difficulty with processing visual, auditory, and other sensory information within a normal time frame results in slowed or delayed processing speed. The delay may be a few seconds or minutes. Clients who need more time to respond may seem as if they have additional deficits. Therefore the clinician should allow the client sufficient time to respond during treatment. Both Mr. B. and Mrs. R. have delayed processing. Mr. B. would benefit more from visual and tactile rather than auditory cues. Mrs. R. has difficulty integrating information, especially when it is presented quickly or in groups such as in an automated telephone menu. She would benefit from information presented sequentially but one item a time.

Impaired Executive Functions and Abstract Reasoning

Executive functioning is a prerequisite to functioning in adult roles and is key to setting goals, planning, and effectively completing tasks. This requires high-level problem solving, reasoning, and judgment. Clients with brain injuries tend to view situations in concrete terms, interpreting all information at the most literal level. Functional independence including appropriate social skills and successful return to work demands mastery and control of executive functions.[22] Clients with executive dysfunction usually require assistance or supervision to function.

Mr. B. shows concrete thinking, reduced thought flexibility, and reduced abstract reasoning. Therapy would focus on maximizing his ability to perform functional tasks first and then progressing perhaps to school-related tasks such as introductory college-level mathematics. Mrs. R. has been unsuccessful to varying degrees in home management, work and leisure, and IADL such as money management and medication management, largely because of executive dysfunction. She has compensated by discontinuing or significantly reducing her participation in her daily roles. The OT practitioner would first determine Mrs. R.'s priorities regarding the tasks to which she wishes to return first. Treatment sessions would be graded to increase her ability to participate without becoming overwhelmed by sensation or frustrated or developing a headache. One example might be reinitiating reading, one of her valued leisure pursuits, using large-print books.

Behavioral Function

Behavioral impairments often occur during recovery from a TBI and can challenge both the treatment staff and the families. Behavioral management is a key element of rehabilitation after a TBI. Teamwork is essential because inexperienced individuals who lack prior knowledge of the behavioral problems and the planned strategies may unintentionally reinforce the client's undesirable behavior.

Common behaviors seen in persons after a TBI include lowered frustration tolerance, agitation, combativeness, disinhibition, emotional lability, and refusal to cooperate. After a TBI, some individuals have a reduced ability to tolerate frustration and may act out when challenged. Graded programming that presents the person with tasks that can be accomplished with assistance or cues with success based on the person's specific needs will help reduce frustration levels and acting out. The client who cannot filter distractions, is sensitive to sensory information, or is asked to perform beyond his or her present capability may become agitated in a noisy, visually active environment. An agitated client may become verbally abusive or combative and kick, bite, grab, or spit. These behaviors may be directed at the person the client perceives as the source of agitation or toward others in the environment. Clinicians should be aware of which clients are more easily prone to agitation and should select a treatment environment that will help reduce this problem. Although combative behavior may occur in isolation, some clients go through a period of combativeness that lasts for weeks or months. In such cases, a consistent behavior management program must be immediately established and operationalized by those who interact with the client. The program would include procedures to limit undesirable behaviors and increase desirable behaviors while ensuring the client's safety. This phase can be especially difficult for family members and significant others, who will require encouragement and support.

A client with **disinhibition** lacks proper social awareness of the environmental requirements and consequently acts inappropriately. Disinhibited behaviors can include urinating in public, removing clothing, taking food off others' trays, using obscenities, making inappropriate comments, or making indiscriminate sexual advances to staff members or clients.

Emotional lability is the display of exaggerated and sometimes inappropriate emotional responses to situations. The client reacts by weeping, giggling, or laughing uncontrollably. Lack of cooperation by clients with TBI is often misinterpreted as deliberate, and then the client is mislabeled as noncompliant. Cognitive and behavioral deficits often impair the person's ability to understand the purpose of therapeutic tasks, which may lead to refusal to participate. The cognitive and behavioral aspects of a TBI are complex and interrelated, and the behavior exhibited by the client after a TBI correlates significantly with the level of cognitive function. The lower-functioning client is much more likely to lack self-awareness regarding behavior.

Both case study clients demonstrate behavioral problems related to cognitive deficits that can interfere with social interactions. Mr. B. has reduced insight and pragmatics (social communication skills) and could benefit from participating in small group activities that stress the necessary skills and that provide for positive feedback and constructive criticism. Mrs. R. can be irritable and frustrated when she is overwhelmed, so the OT practitioner must be careful in planning short, successful treatment activities that Mrs. R. finds relevant and that help her feel productive.

Affective Mental Functions

Professional counseling can be invaluable in helping persons with TBI and their family members cope with the numerous changes caused by the injury. Many persons with TBI initially deny their symptoms, which can be considered a coping mechanism, given the serious nature of the losses sustained. Denial becomes dysfunctional when it lasts for more than 2 years.[18] Anger can occur with denial or following that phase. The client's anger may be directed at the health care workers or family[19] and can be stressful for family members. As emotional recovery progresses, the client uses bargaining as a strategy and becomes more cooperative and motivated in therapy.[18] Next, the client may show depression, believing that hope is lost.[18] He or she may experience genuine grieving for the losses resulting from the TBI. The final stage is acceptance, in which the client accepts the residual skills and limitations and is willing to work toward a life with all of these changes.[18]

Clients may move back and forth through these stages and may seem to be involved with several at once. The grieving and depression stage can be especially profound. Mrs. R., with her depression and lowered self-confidence, has withdrawn from the community and her family and is not ready to participate in a group activity with other clients. In addition, she feels responsible for her nephew's injuries. Such feelings of guilt can aggravate her symptoms of depression and posttraumatic stress disorder (PTSD). She may do better with one-on-one treatment with the OT practitioner to create and pursue an individualized plan to improve her functional performance.

One of the strongest predictors of success in rehabilitation after a TBI is social support. Family, friends, and significant others are integral to the rehabilitation process, especially in the beginning stages, because they may be better able to elicit a response from the client than are the health care team members. In addition, they often serve as sources of information regarding the injured person's preinjury roles, habits, routines, and rituals, as well as the person's habitual coping style.

Some clients may have a history of psychiatric or emotional problems, which may be worsened by the injury. Other clients may experience new psychiatric or emotional problems as a result of the injury. Some of these problems such as reactive depression are associated with normal reactions to the losses associated with the TBI, whereas other conditions are organic or caused by the injury (e.g., lability, reduced frustration tolerance, increased anxiety). Understanding the client's previous methods of coping can assist in the selection of treatment activities. For example, a client may have listened to certain types of music to relax and may benefit from continuing to use favorite songs to relax in treatment. Psychiatric or emotional problems worsened or caused by the TBI are generally responsive to medical and psychiatric treatment. Mrs. R. could benefit from assistance in determining what sensory experiences she can tolerate and which ones would be relaxing for her.

It is often difficult for family members and friends to experience changes in the loved one's performance and behavior. No matter how cognizant of the disability the family and the client may be, it does disrupt the family structure. Family members may serve as primary caregivers for the client with a TBI, which can be stressful. Often, clients and their caregivers seek counseling to help them cope with the enormity of the situation. The OT practitioner instructs the client and the caregivers how to assist the client, while minimizing burnout by locating resources to provide transportation, respite care, psychological support, or professional services. Moreover, clients and caregivers choose to participate in groups offered through the local rehabilitation hospital or the state Brain Injury Association. Both Mr. B.'s and Mrs. R.'s families have been stressed and challenged by the severity of Mr. B.'s injury and the changes caused by Mrs. R.'s injury. The OT practitioner would work with the specialists on the team (such as the psychologist or the social worker) in providing a therapeutic, successful, and productive environment for progressing toward their long-term goals.

Occupational Therapy Evaluation

The occupational therapist performs OT evaluations for a TBI adult. The therapist's findings establish a baseline for treatment. The OTA is responsible for reading and familiarizing himself or herself with the OT findings (as stated in the evaluation) and discussing the results with the OT.

Treatment of Clients with Severe Traumatic Brain Injury

OT treatment for the person with a severe TBI or for a client with an injury at a low-level of function[41] (levels I to IV; see Case Study: Mr. B.) aims to increase the person's level of overall responsiveness and awareness through structured graded programming, divided into simple steps. Adequate time must be allowed for a response because low arousal causes delays in processing information. The guidelines that follow can be applied to some individuals with moderate brain injury as well.

Treatment can be broken down into six areas: sensory regulation, bed positioning, wheelchair positioning, use of positioning devices and casting and splinting, dysphagia management, and family and caregiver training. Although the treatments occur simultaneously to optimize the person's progress, the OT practitioner must coordinate treatment with the rest of the team so as not to overwhelm the client. This type of OT program was provided to Mr. B. when he was an inpatient in acute care and in acute rehabilitation.

General Principles

Heinemann and colleagues[21] describe three stages of recovery with the Rancho Los Amigos Level of Cognitive Functioning Scale; these stages are useful for guiding OT treatment planning (see Table 25-1)[2,40,53] and are applicable to persons with severe, moderate, and mild TBI.

1. Stage 1—Coma corresponds to Rancho Los Amigos levels I to III. The OT practitioner focuses on body functions using sensory stimulation and orientation training.[2,21,40,53]
2. Stage 2—Confusion/increasingly goal-directed involves levels IV to VI. The OT practitioner minimizes environmental overstimulation and repeatedly instructs the client in simple goal-directed functional tasks.[2,21,40,53]
3. Stage 3—Cognitive-behavioral rehabilitation addresses levels VII to VIII,[2,17,40,54] and is applicable to levels IX and X. Therapy focuses on higher-level performance in areas of occupation and compensatory strategies and techniques to work around the remaining deficits.[2,8,28,53]

OT treatment begins with preparatory methods. Purposeful activities may simulate performance in occupations. The goal is participation in life occupations. Criteria for discharge from OT for clients with TBI may include the following:

- Goals have been met
- The client has reached a plateau in therapy
- The client cannot participate in treatment because of other complications
- Skilled OT services are no longer required or the client no longer wishes to participate[2,40,53]

Sensory Regulation

For the client who does not respond to pain, touch, sound, or sight or who shows only a generalized response to pain, the goal of OT treatment is to increase his or her level of awareness via controlled sensory input, which activates the limbic system, the part of the brain that controls arousal levels.[13,24]

Sensory regulation treatment is multisensory, incorporating visual, auditory, tactile, and other stimuli into specific functional and familiar tasks such as rolling over in bed. These interventions can be provided by the OTA under direct supervision of the OT. The most effective sensory combinations (termed *multimodal*) are tactile and auditory and visual and proprioceptive.[27,28] The client is engaged actively to maximize the benefit. Treatments are usually brief (initially about 10 minutes) and incorporate both sides of the body. The modalities are common everyday tasks such as hygiene, bed mobility, or using the nurse call system. The clinician continually observes the client during the activity and documents any changes in behavior such as head turning in response to sounds, visual attention and tracking, vocalizations, and following commands. The OT clinician should select tasks that are the most meaningful to the client. For example, the client may prefer using a hairbrush for her hair, rather than a comb.

Bed Positioning

The person with a TBI may not be able to reposition the body spontaneously to relieve pressure as other people do regularly while sleeping. Bed positioning is important because the person with a TBI initially spends most of the time in bed. Although the person may have specialized beds, mattresses, or bed positioning devices designed to distribute weight and maximize positioning for comfort, the goal of OT is to establish a turning and sitting program to reduce risk for development of pressure sores. If possible, the client should rotate through a sequence of different positions: supine, on the right side, on the left side, prone (if possible). Bolsters, pillows, or splints are used as needed, whether the person is awake or asleep. The OT practitioner must be aware of the presence of medical devices and appliances, which may interfere with the client's ability to achieve certain positions. For example, a person with a tracheostomy cannot lie prone.

The person should change positions every 2 hours to avoid constant prolonged pressure on any area. For safety the bedrails should always be up while the person is lying in bed. When positioning the client, the clinician should avoid pressure on bony prominences and other vulnerable areas that are more prone to skin breakdown. These include earlobes, shoulder blades (scapulas), elbows, hips, ankles, and heels. Thinner persons are at higher risk for developing pressure areas over bony prominences, but individuals of all sizes are at risk for decubitus ulcers if they are not turned regularly, especially when there is a loss of sensation. Persons with severe TBI may require maximal assistance of at least two people to turn. When the person is awake, sitting up supported in bed can be added as another position. If the client does not regain the ability to change position during sleep spontaneously, he or she will require a permanent turning program.

Wheelchair Positioning Program

Proper seated positioning of the client with TBI reduces the incidence of skin breakdown and contractures, facilitates normal tone, encourages use of cognitive skills, provides opportunities for social interaction, improves behavior, and enhances safety. Many medical benefits ensue from sitting upright including improved respiratory function and circulation, reduced risk for blood clots in the lower extremities, and reduced isolation. The occupational therapist assesses the client for factors (such as paralysis, weakness, spasticity, or loss of sensation) that would influence the choice of special positioning devices or customized seating. Special attention should be paid to the presence of medical appliances that might interfere with equipment (e.g., certain designs of seatbelts cannot be used with a gastrostomy tube).

Persons who have been on bed rest for an extended time will require a graded program to move from lying supine to sitting erect. If the person gets up too quickly, blood pressure may drop too much and cause the individual to become dizzy, lose consciousness (faint), and fall. The client with a TBI who can sit in a wheelchair is more mobile and can explore and interact with the environment and receive services in other areas of the health care facility.

The occupational therapist establishes the initial seating and positioning program, often in conjunction with other health care team members such as the nurse and physical therapist. The OTA carries out the daily implementation of the program. Effective seating and positioning requires trunk stability, a stable base of support at the pelvis, maintaining the trunk in midline, and holding the head erect in order for the person to use the UEs in functional activities (Figure 25-2).

Graded Seating Program

The person with the TBI begins with sitting upright in bed with the head at the end of the bed and all rails up. As the client becomes comfortable sitting upright, the amount of time the client spends in this position is increased as tolerated.

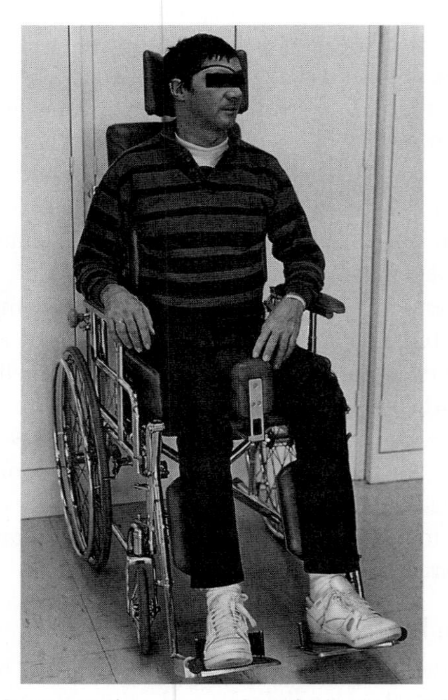

Figure 25-2 Improved posture and trunk alignment achieved with positioning devices.

After each sitting session the skin should be checked for reddened pressure areas, and positioning equipment should be adapted if needed.

Some lower-level individuals who do not have trunk stability and head control to sit upright may be unable to sit in bed and will require transfer to a wheelchair with a high reclining back with head support. For a client who can progress to sitting in a wheelchair, proper positioning should target postural deficits and facilitate postural alignment through choice of the wheelchair design and positioning devices. Often, the client can be positioned using commercially made equipment, but the occupational therapist or OTA may need to fabricate or adapt seating devices. The following are guidelines to consider.

Pelvis

Wheelchair positioning begins with pelvic alignment because poor hip positioning causes poor head and trunk alignment and influences tone throughout the body, especially the extremities. A solid seat insert can be placed on the seat of the wheelchair underneath the client to facilitate a neutral to slight anterior tilt of the pelvis. An insert that is slightly wedged (with the downward slope pointing toward the back of the wheelchair) can be used to flex the hips to help inhibit extensor tone in the hips and LEs. This position can help prevent the client from sliding forward out of the wheelchair. A lumbar support may maintain a natural curve in the spine. A variety of wheelchair cushion choices distribute weight to reduce pressure areas and position the client. A seatbelt angled across the pelvis will help to maintain the hips back up against the back of the wheelchair, the desired position.

Trunk

Positioning the trunk occurs next after the pelvis is properly positioned. The goal is to support the client while sitting to allow the person to sit at midline, while being able to use the UEs without losing balance. A solid back insert or solid contoured back is placed behind the client's back to facilitate a more erect posture of the back. Lateral trunk supports can be used to eliminate leaning to either side; a chest strap or crossed chest straps will decrease leaning forward, pull back the shoulders, and allow for chest expansion. Custom-made trunk support systems may be ordered by the physician and fabricated by an orthotist for clients with severe positioning problems.

Head

For clients with minimal or no active head control, achieving an upright midline head position can be difficult. Most head control devices employ static positioning. The head is kept from falling forward by a forehead strap. Caution must always be taken to avoid overstressing the cervical area or giving excessive resistance to spastic neck muscles. Reclining the patient back will eliminate this problem but also will reduce weight bearing through the trunk and pelvis and limit visual interaction with the environment.

An alternative to static head positioning is dynamic head positioning. The advantages of a dynamic device are that it places the head in good alignment on the trunk and distributes pressure equally. It also allows the client to begin initiating head movements actively (Figure 25-3).

Lower Extremities

Calf supports attached to elevating leg rests can provide additional support for the LEs. Thigh pads placed along the lateral aspect of the thigh may be used to decrease LE adduction. An abductor wedge may be placed between the LEs to eliminate abduction. Proper footwear (e.g., high top athletic shoes) can serve to help position the feet correctly. Use of a foot wedge placed on top of the foot plate under the feet can prevent plantar flexion contractures for one or both feet. Some clients may require calf or toe straps to help them maintain the LEs on the footrests.

Upper Extremities

A lap tray is often used to help support the UEs on a level surface. The UEs should be positioned with the shoulders in slight flexion and external rotation, the elbows in slight flexion, and the wrists and fingers in a functional position. Some clients may benefit from use of a support such as an arm trough or hemi-board for only one UE. Wedges can be used to elevate the affected UE, if needed, to manage edema.

Wheelchair positioning involves constant reevaluation and adaptation of equipment to meet the changing needs of the client. The OTA may be involved in this aspect of treatment as long as he or she is under the close supervision of the occupational therapist.

Splinting and Casting

Splinting is used to properly position a body part or support a part for the client to use it functionally. Casting is used to increase passive ROM when high muscle tone and contractures (or possible contractures) are present. The goals of splinting and casting are to reduce abnormal tone or soft tissue tightness, increase or maintain passive ROM, increase the functional potential of the UE, prevent skin breakdown, and prevent contractures and possible complications.

The most commonly used splint is the resting hand splint. This splint places the wrist and fingers in extension and abducts the thumb (Figure 25-4), which provides passive stretch to the wrist and hand.

A typical splint schedule begins with 2 hours on and 2 hours off, but the wearing schedule depends on the individual client's needs.

A casting program is implemented when other methods for managing spasticity are ineffective. The most common UE cast is designed to increase elbow extension. Casts can be fabricated out of fiberglass or plaster. Fiberglass is preferred because it is lighter in weight, sets (hardens) more quickly, and is easier to apply than plaster. As with splinting, specialized training and practice in casting are required to attain proficiency.

Serial casting uses a series of casts that gradually stretch out the contracture, increasing passive ROM with each new cast getting slightly closer to the desired end position. Serial casting usually requires at least two clinicians, one to position and hold the extremity and one to apply the cast. With training, the OTA may assist the OT practitioner in this process. Serial casts are generally left on the client for several days and then removed. The patient's skin is examined for signs of skin breakdown such as redness. If skin integrity is normal, a new cast (closer to the desired ROM) is applied. Once the desired ROM has been achieved, the last cast is removed and the edges of both halves of the cast are finished (see Figure 25-1). The client wears the bivalved cast to maintain the ROM.

Dysphagia

The patient emerging from coma may have swallowing difficulty and require a feeding evaluation and intervention for specifics. The occupational therapist and SLP would

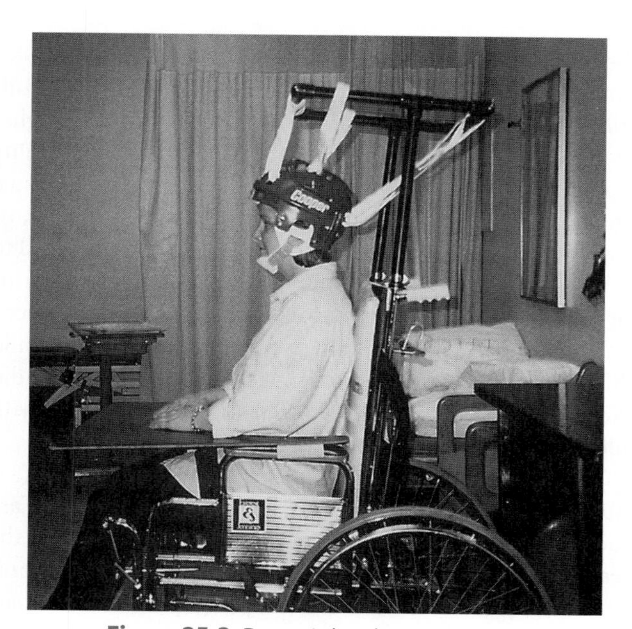

Figure 25-3 Dynamic head control device.

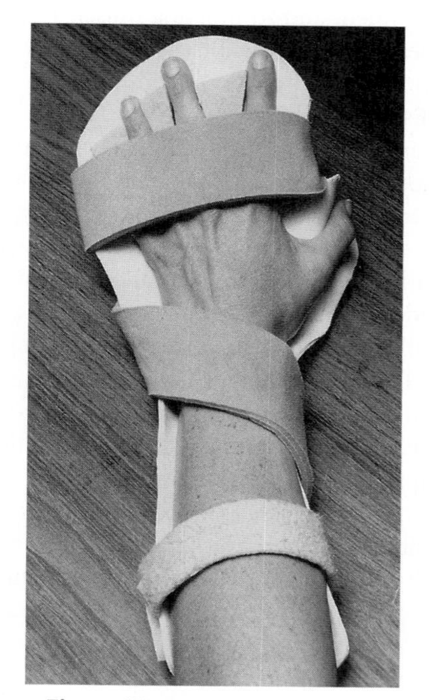

Figure 25-4 Resting hand splint.

work together in developing and implementing a dysphagia program. The experienced OTA practitioner who has demonstrated service competency may work with clients with dysphagia.

Neuromuscular Impairments

Persons with severe and moderate injury can experience a variety of motor impairments. Weakness, spasticity, rigidity, soft tissue contractures, primitive reflexes, reduced or lost postural reactions, impaired sensation, and reduced fine motor coordination will affect speed and accuracy of occupational performance. All treatment should be activity and function based. Any adjunctive technique such as neurodevelopmental treatment (NDT) should be followed by a meaningful and functional activity that requires the same movements.

The prerequisites for normal movement include normal postural tone, normal integration of flexor and extensor control (reciprocal innervation), normal proximal stability, and selective (voluntary) movement patterns.[23] The common principles of treatment are (1) to progress proximal to distal; (2) to establish symmetrical posture; (3) to integrate both sides of the body into activities; (4) to encourage bilateral weight bearing; and (5) to introduce a normal sensory experience. A variety of treatment approaches including NDT, proprioceptive neuromuscular facilitation (PNF), myofascial release, and Rood techniques are used effectively with persons with TBI. Many therapists combine techniques; the occupational therapist should determine the selection and timing of these approaches. These and other such techniques require specialized training including hands-on practice and clinical experience. When the OTA has achieved service competency using these techniques, the OTA may incorporate them into functional training under an occupational therapist's guidance.

Trunk stability is necessary for effective limb movements. Treatment of postural instability of the trunk should focus on achieving alignment and stimulating muscle responses in the trunk muscles. Alignment will facilitate stability. Once trunk control improves, treatment should progress to activities using the UEs while stabilizing the trunk.

The person with severe TBI may have a reduced sense or feeling of movement, which can impair coordination, restrict functional mobility, and increase risk for injury. Changes in taste and smell may affect the appetite. Issues with pain can interfere with attention, concentration, sleep, functional mobility, and cooperation. Ataxia is a common problem that interferes with motor control and can affect one or all four extremities. The degree to which ataxic movements interfere with function is related to which limb is affected and the severity of the ataxia. In ADL training, the OT practitioner should focus on improving function while maintaining safety. Compensatory techniques such as performing tasks as close the body as possible, performing tasks while seated, leaning on the tabletop with either one or both arms to gain stability, moving the UE while still in contact with a surface, and wearing weights can be useful in reducing the severity of the tremors occurring with movement. Using wrist weights may help improve control during performance of functional tasks but may not have carryover when the weights are removed. Weighted eating utensils and cups may help the person with ataxia in self-feeding, as long as they can use the equipment safely.

Caregiver Training

Education of the caregivers (which may or may not include family members or significant others) begins at the first meeting. Initially, the OT practitioner would explain the role of OT and provide information according to each person's ability to handle and process it. Caregivers play an essential part in eliciting the client's responses and can help the client make progress by carrying through with therapy tasks, especially on weekends or holidays. The OT practitioner grades the caregiver education and training so that basic skills are taught first, with more complex skills introduced after the simpler skills are mastered.

The significant changes in the life of the person with a TBI and the impact on the family are important considerations. Because the caregiver provides assistance as well as emotional support, it is easy for caregivers to overlook their own needs such as in the case of Mr. B's mother, who quit her job in order to care for her son. The OT practitioner should encourage the caregiver from the beginning to take time away from the caregiver role to rest and regroup and should reassure the caregiver that he or she need not feel guilty for doing so. Taking personal time will reduce the incidence of caregiver stress and burnout. To help the caregiver establish a larger group of persons to assist with the caregiver role, the clinician can direct the caregiver to additional resources in the community such as other family members, church members, specialty services such as transportation for persons with TBI, or support groups.

Some persons with TBI may return to therapy during a major life transition such as having a child, starting a new job, or losing a loved one because they need additional structure and assistance to work through the transition.[2,40,53]

Treatment of Clients with Mild Brain Injury

The recognition of symptoms and diagnosis of mild (and for some moderate) brain injury is sometimes overlooked initially. Because clients appear to be functioning at a higher level, many health care practitioners assume no loss of ability to perform their daily routines has occurred. It is not unusual for clients with mild TBI to be diagnosed weeks, months, or even years after their injury. As a result, most have adapted to their lives after injury. For example, Mrs. R. stopped performing most instrumental activities and leisure tasks and reduced community participation. However, many clients with mild TBI are dissatisfied that they cannot perform tasks as they did before the injury. No matter when diagnosed, clients with mild brain injury can improve with rehabilitation.

OT treatment for the client with a higher-level injury (see Table 25-1, Rancho Los Amigos levels VIII to IX and Case Study: Mrs. R.) aims to increase the person's abilities in the areas of occupation, addressing issues with body functions, improving performance skills, adapting performance patterns, and activity.

Clients with mild TBI may experience a variety of sensory changes including issues with pain. There is often a hypersensitivity to noise and light and a hyposensitivity to taste, smell, touch, and proprioception. Such is the case with Mrs. R. The OTA would work with the client to compensate for sensory issues (e.g., by adding spices to improve the taste of food).

Most clients with mild TBI have fairly intact motor control. These individuals can ambulate independently (sometimes with assistive devices) and can use both UEs in functional tasks. Closer observation may reveal subtle trunk and UE deficits related to coordination, including ataxia and reduced speed of movement. Mrs. R. no longer writes out her classroom notes due to changes in the quality of her handwriting. OT in such cases would focus on improving the client's accuracy and speed.

Vision

Vision deficits commonly result from TBI. The occupational therapist starts the vision evaluation by getting a complete vision history, which includes whether the client currently uses or needs corrective lenses. In some cases, the glasses may have been broken in the incident that caused the injury. The glasses may be lost, or the prescription may not be current. Clients who usually use contact lenses, depending on the extent of the injury, may not be able to wear them again (due to problems such as dry eye) and therefore may need to revert to the use of glasses. For all persons needing updated corrective lenses, the occupational therapist should recommend a referral to a vision specialist (see Chapter 22). The occupational therapist designs the treatment plan for vision deficits. Most vision problems are addressed in functional activities. The OT practitioner aims to increase the client's awareness of impairments, maximize the client's use of residual vision, and instruct the client in compensatory strategies and how to incorporate these into daily functioning. Providing enlarged print such as with Mrs. R.; spacing objects far apart so that they are easily seen; increasing the illumination on the task; using contrasting colors (e.g., placing a green toothbrush on a white towel); and marking steps, corners of walls, and table edges with reflective tape are some of the adaptations used for vision impairments. If PTVS is present, the occupational therapist would recommend evaluation and treatment by a vision specialist. Care should be given to avoid the use of bifocal or trifocal lenses with clients with visual deficits from TBI because these lenses may increase dizziness due to the multiprocessing requirements.

Perceptual Training

Approaches to treating perceptual dysfunction are remedial, functional, and compensatory. The remedial approach asserts that the adult brain is sufficiently plastic to repair and reorganize itself after injury.[37] For example, to improve figure-ground discrimination, Mr. B. could seek and find objects in photos. The functional approach is based on the theory that recovery results from the use of intact brain areas to perform adapted functional activities, compensating for lost function.[36] The functional approach works better with clients who respond to their environment and situations at a concrete level,[37] such as Mr. B. early in his recovery. Through repeated practice in ADL, Mr. B. would try to locate grooming items on varied backgrounds, to retrain figure-ground perceptual skills. This functional approach encompasses increasing the client's awareness of the perceptual problems, teaching the person how to function with the deficits, and adapting the environment to compensate for deficits. For Mr. B., who has decreased insight into problems, the OT practitioner could instruct the family how to carry over treatment. Compensation involves developing strategies to work around problems.

Cognitive Training

Cognitive retraining is best accomplished in graded programming through a variety of functional tasks. Persons with TBI perform better in tasks that are familiar and meaningful to them. Sequencing, for example, can be practiced in a variety of tasks (dressing, assembling a sandwich); clients may participate more willingly because they understand and value the task. Repetition of skills is important for individuals with cognitive deficits.

The OT practitioner determines with the client which functional activities to address first. Activities should be age appropriate, challenging, and interesting. A computer software and training program is one way to accomplish cognitive training and should be chosen when appropriate for the client. With the increased use of the Internet to search for information, as well as instantaneous communication through e-mail, instant messaging, texting, and so on, using the computer would be considered a functional task for some clients and therefore should be incorporated into the treatment program.

Behavioral Management Strategies

The use of intervention strategies to decrease and eliminate problem behaviors is preferable to the use of medications (chemical restraints) or physical restraints. Consistent behavioral programming among all individuals working with persons with TBI is the most effective. These strategies are divided into two categories: environmental and interactive.

Environmental strategies involve modifying the environment to facilitate appropriate behaviors, inhibit unwanted behaviors, and help to maintain the safety of the client with a TBI. The first step in altering the environment may be to place the client in a quiet, isolated room without a roommate. The television and radio are turned off, and the door is closed, if possible. The walls should be plain, and all extra furniture should be removed from the room.

Clients who are agitated and unsafe alone may require one-on-one nursing care and extra padding on their hospital bed. The reduction of environmental sensory stimulation helps calm the individual. Some clients require the use of an alarm system to help the health care professional team and family monitor their location at all times and prevent unsafe behaviors such as entering prohibited areas of the hospital or wandering outside the hospital unit. The transmitter may be attached out of reach to the underside of the wheelchair or worn in bracelet form.

To interact with the agitated client, the clinician should speak in a calm voice with a soothing matter-of-fact tone. All communication should be brief to prevent overwhelming the person with details, which might cause frustration and increase confusion. Another behavior management technique is diversion. For agitated clients who cannot redirect themselves, the OT clinician can create a diversion such as changing the subject or creating a harmless distraction.

Self-Care

ADL retraining improves the client's functional independence in a familiar and meaningful context. Persons with TBI perform better when tasks are broken down into smaller segments to facilitate learning. Tasks are graded depending on the client's needs. Approaches such as backward chaining, in which the therapist assists the client with the majority of the activity and the client completes the final step, are one way to grade and modify the activity for the individual client. Another is to organize the steps of the activity sequence into visual and written cues. A self-care program should be structured and consistent, with the client following the same daily routine in the same environment, using the same sequence of steps to accomplish the task. As the client makes improvements, the clinician reduces structure and cues and focuses on improving the client's ability to complete the task when the routine is disrupted or altered in some way.

The clinician should employ techniques that increase functional independence and reinforce normal motor patterns. The occupational therapist might recommend the experienced OTA to use a specific neurophysiological approach that helps to normalize tone and integrate both sides of the body into self-care activities. The clinician (OT or OTA) would teach the client how to refine the quality of movement while improving functional performance and maintaining safety at all times.

Self-Feeding

Persons with TBI often have feeding problems, some of which may be too severe for them to take in any fluids or foods orally (NPO). The client who is restricted to NPO initially would have a nasogastric tube; this might later be changed to a gastric tube for all fluid and medication intake. Clients who are NPO are at high risk for choking and aspiration and subsequent aspiration pneumonia if they drink or eat. Individuals with TBI that causes deficits in self-control, insight, safety awareness, and judgment may attempt to drink and eat despite precautions and thus require constant supervision—especially if the client is a silent aspirator and does not show outward signs that he or she has inhaled liquids or foods into the lungs (i.e., choking or holding the throat). Other possible drinking or eating restrictions for persons with TBI include no drinking from a straw, no thin liquids, or only pureed foods. Liquids in the form of ice chips, ice pops, or flavored gelatin may be the only way these clients can safely take in liquids orally. Clinicians educate clients and caregivers on how to help their injured family member adhere to the restrictions.

In some health care settings the SLP may treat the client with dysphagia and work in conjunction with the occupational therapist. The role of the occupational therapist might be to work with oral motor control, swallowing, safe eating, and the feeding process. The OTA may assist with the eating process if service competency is established. In addition to eating issues, the client with a TBI may have other deficits that interfere with self-feeding such as reduced attention, visual changes, left unilateral neglect, impaired memory, reduced sequencing, impulsivity, one-handedness, sensory deficits, incoordination, etc. The OT practitioner would select the most appropriate nondistracting environment for self-feeding training such as the client's room or a quiet area in the dining room. As use of recommended feeding techniques and strategies improves, the client might be able to eat in a more social setting such as in the dining room with other clients or in the kitchen at home with the family. Because persons with swallowing and other eating problems are at risk for choking, the clinician would make sure that additional assistance is readily available nearby if needed.

Persons with TBI require a structured consistent feeding routine to reestablish proper and safe eating. Strategies such as introducing one food item at a time and reminding the client to set the utensil down after each bite and chew thoroughly and then resume eating help persons with TBI reestablish safe self-feeding. Assistive devices such as a plate guard or a cup with a lid may be useful to increase safe independence in self-feeding, depending on the combination of deficits. Some clients may be on eating restrictions initially and then progress, whereas others may need to follow restrictions permanently. The OT practitioner should try to incorporate variety in menu planning and suggest how the food can be presented to make it more visually appealing. Impaired taste and smell can reduce appetite, causing some persons to become disinterested in eating. Individuals who continue to receive tube feedings should participate in self-feeding training prior to tube feeding so as to avoid feeling full and thus reducing the appetite. Some clients will be able to take in some liquids or some foods, but their intake is insufficient to provide adequate nutrition; thus they require supplemental tube feedings until they can drink and eat enough to sustain themselves. Individuals with permanent changes in their ability to drink or eat the foods to which they are accustomed must learn to cope and accept the alterations in their lifestyle.

Functional Mobility

Mobility training for clients such as Mr. B. can be subdivided into bed mobility, transfer training, wheelchair mobility, and functional ambulation. The NDT principles of bilateral involvement, weight bearing, rotation, and tone normalization are used with these activities. The OT practitioner coordinates all programming with the appropriate individuals, the physical therapist, the nurse, and the caregiver (see Chapter 21 for NDT principles.)

Bed Mobility, Wheelchair Management, and Functional Ambulation

When the person with TBI begins mobility training, the OT practitioner starts with bed mobility skills of rolling, moving up and down in bed, bridging, moving from a supine to a sitting position, and the reverse. Safety is always stressed throughout all mobility training. Logrolling is more difficult toward the stronger side because the weaker side may not be able to initiate the roll; thus the client may require more assistance to one side than to the other side. Rolling and moving up and down in bed should be practiced when the bed is in the flattened position, which is easiest for the client. Bed mobility skills are easily adapted according to NDT principles (i.e., the person rolls side to side by putting the stronger leg under the weaker leg, clasps hands, brings the arms up to shoulder height, and initiates the roll). The person may require use of the half bed rails to help in rolling, pushing up, or bridging in bed. Bridging is an important skill because it helps the person manage lower body hygiene and dressing.

When able to sit without complete back support, the person progresses to sitting from supine on the edge of the bed. Because hospital beds may be unusually high, the feet may not touch the floor. In this case the clinician may need to adapt the task by using a sturdy short step stool for the person to place the feet to assist with maintaining balance. Transfer training usually begins with transferring from the bed to and from the wheelchair safely. The amount of assistance and the type of transfer vary with the person. Neuromuscular, visual, visual-perceptual, and cognitive skills dictate the selection of the type of transfer to be used in training. Persons with memory deficits and limited carryover of information would benefit from the same technique and sequence with all persons working with them. If possible, it is preferable for transfers to be practiced by moving to both sides so that the client can transfer to either side in other places (e.g., public restrooms). Some individuals may require the use of a lift, physical assistance of one or more people, use of a sliding board, etc. The NDT approach includes guidelines for transfer training that facilitate the person playing an active role, which helps solidify learning.

All caregivers should be trained to assist the person with TBI in all types of transfer required of that person to fulfill home and community roles. With extensive training, practice, and demonstration in proficiency and safety, the goal is for the caregiver(s) to transfer the client alone. Training alleviates many fears and increases the chances of success in home visits and when the client is permanently discharged.

Many persons with TBI who require the use of a wheelchair for functional mobility will use a manual wheelchair. Use of a power wheelchair involves more extensive training. Wheelchair management includes the ability to manage wheelchair parts (e.g., removing footrests, managing wheel locks, placing a lapboard on and off) and propelling the wheelchair both indoors and outdoors on different types and levels of surfaces safely. The person learns and practices each skill until it is mastered. Initially, endurance for pushing the wheelchair may be quite limited and with practice increases. Some clients may require gloves to protect the hands from blisters caused by using a manual wheelchair.

Functional ambulation refers to the patient's ability to walk to complete all activities. The physical therapist assesses the individual's ability to ambulate and provides graded treatment to improve readiness for ambulation using assistive devices as indicated. The OT clinician facilitates carryover of ambulation into ADL such as dressing, preparing a meal, or mopping a floor while using proper technique, devices, and precautions. Some functionally mobile clients can only walk, but others can carry, hold, move, and use items or tools during an activity. The OT clinician might suggest ways for the client to avoid carrying objects in the hands such as transporting them in an apron, backpack, or rolling cart. The OT practitioner may also teach methods to ambulate safely while performing other daily tasks.

Group Treatment

Initially, the person with a TBI will participate in individualized therapy on a one-to-one basis with the OT clinician. Most therapy programs use group treatment as a supplement to individual treatment; it provides learning experiences not available in individual therapy. Group treatment provides structured socialization in which clients can develop more appropriate communication/interaction and psychosocial skills. The OT practitioner would determine when a client would be able to benefit from group treatment.

Groups allow persons with brain injuries to get feedback from their peers, which can lead to increased self-awareness and problem solving[44] in the "real world," facilitating positive changes in their behavior.[25,30] Group programming for persons with TBI is more successful if it is functionally based. Goals include improving pragmatics, learning appropriate social interaction and behavior, increasing attention and concentration, and working on skills such as counting money and remembering turns. Groups may be facilitated by one discipline but are commonly multidisciplinary. In group treatment, the clinician must understand each client's individual goals so that the person can achieve optimum value from the experience. For example, Mr. B. could tolerate a group activity for about 30 to 60 minutes, but Mrs. R. would not be able to participate until her sensory sensitivity and endurance improves.

Areas of Occupation

As the client regains functional skills and independence in ADL, treatment expands to include instrumental activities of daily living, education, work, play, leisure, and social interaction as indicated.

The OTA will determine the client's previous level of function and goals before initiating treatment interventions. Training is graded to suit the client's functional level. At the end of the session, the next day's activities can be discussed. A session such as this requires simple sequencing, organizing, and memory for the task. As the person progresses, the practitioner increases the task demands until the established long-term goal is met. Prior to his injury, Mr. B. did his own laundry. Initial OT sessions might include sorting and folding a few items of clothing and then subsequently increase in level of difficulty with progress. Prior to her injury, Mrs. R. completed all the household cleaning, but since the injury cleaning is no longer a priority for her; she has hired a cleaning service. Education would be addressed in treatment with Mr. B. but not for Mrs. R. Regarding play and leisure, although Mr. B.

can no longer play soccer, the OT practitioner could help him explore other related options (e.g., helping coach or manage his adult soccer team, playing soccer videogames). OT might work with Mrs. R. to explore options to reinitiate exercise she enjoyed before her injury. Both clients have reduced ability to participate socially. For Mr. B., OT treatment would focus on reestablishing his family roles first before progressing to friends and the community. Mrs. R. has isolated herself from others socially, including her husband. OT could assist her in exploring options to reestablish balance in their lives.

Community Reintegration

Community reintegration must be included in the OT program on admission and throughout the entire program until discharge. In the inpatient phase of the rehabilitation process, the client with a TBI will reach a maximum level of independence or plateau in the protected and structured atmosphere of the hospital environment. A central focus of OT is to assist the client to regain as many home and community roles as possible. Initially, the client gains skills in familiar settings. Clients' independence may not necessarily carry over into the community when the person encounters unfamiliar people, situations, and problems. Focusing on familiar settings in the therapy process increases the likelihood of successful transfer of training from the rehabilitation setting to the home and community. Establishing client-focused goals with the client and family is important. It helps if the family shares the client's goals. The OT practitioner can assist the client with TBI and family members in exploring relevant community resources. The Brain Injury Association of America (BIA) has extensive information and links to resources online at www.biausa.org. Each state has a BIA chapter that provides information, sponsors support groups and other services, and serves as a resource for the brain-injured person and his or her family.

Outcome after TBI

Studies have shown that clients with brain injury tend to have a better prognosis if they have a higher Glasgow Coma Score,[48] shorter duration of PTA, are younger, and have more years of education.[5] The greater the injury to the brain, the more likely there will be residual problems. Both Mr. B. and Mrs. R. showed benefit from OT, but both will have residual problems as the result of their injuries. After completing inpatient and outpatient rehabilitation for possibly 9 to 12 months, Mr. B. can expect recovery to Rancho Los Amigos Level of Cognitive Functioning VIII and is likely to achieve his long-term OT goal, being able to "take care of myself without help, go back to school, and drive a car again." Despite being one-handed, he will be able to complete ADL, learn new skills, return to school, drive, etc., but will require standby assistance from family members with tasks requiring higher-level skills including executive functioning, some IADL, and socialization. It is to his advantage to identify himself as a student with a disability through the Americans with Disabilities Act[3] because this will allow him to receive accommodations to complete his college degree. After participating in 6 months of rehabilitation including outpatient OT, Mrs. R. can expect to recover to Rancho Los Amigos Level of Cognitive Functioning IX, which would fall short of her OT long-term goal (Quote Box).

She will be able to complete all ADL independently with time but may require standby assistance from her spouse for IADL and accommodations for return to work, play, leisure, and social roles. In addition, Mrs. R. may require long-term counseling to help with coping and adjustment to the permanent changes in her life caused by the TBI. Overall, both clients are likely to make significant progress through OT treatment.

Quote Box

Long-Term Occupational Therapy Goal Identified by Case Study Client Mrs. R.

"I want to go back to my old life, when everything was easy to do."

Summary

Treatment of the traumatically brain-injured adult requires experience, expertise, and clinical reasoning skills. Most clients have numerous deficits to varying degrees in areas of occupation, as well as issues with mental functions and behavior that may interfere with treatment at times. Because the central goal of OT treatment is to engage the client in occupation, the process is dynamic and interactive.[2]

All goals should be interdisciplinary and established to meet the specific needs of each client. Treatment of persons with TBI should be meaningful, functionally based, and incorporate meaningful contexts and environments for each client. Also central to treatment is the role of the caregiver and family, who should be involved in the therapeutic process from the beginning of therapy through discharge.

Selected Reading Guide Questions

1. Define TBI and how it affects occupation.
2. List some of the most common causes of TBI.
3. Describe the role of the OTA with a low-level client with a TBI in the ICU.
4. How would abnormal postures of the right UE and LE affect a client's ability to roll in bed?
5. Why might a client with TBI hit, kick, or bite? What are effective strategies to reduce these behaviors?
6. Name an activity that would be a good choice for the first caregiver training session for a client with a severe TBI. Why would transfer training not be a good choice for this situation?
7. Explain how the OTA could help a client with anterograde PTA remember the day of the week.
8. Family members of a client with TBI inconsistently adhere to her eating precautions. Explain how the OTA might handle the situation.

9. How much assistance might a client at a Rancho Los Amigos Scale of Cognitive Functioning level VII require to set the long-term OT goal?
10. What would cause a client with a TBI to refuse to work on a cooking activity?
11. Identify three issues a client with a mild TBI and ataxia of both UEs might encounter when texting on his new touch screen cell phone.
12. Within the first month of treatment, a family member of a client with a moderate TBI is having difficulty accepting the client's limitations and insists he will have complete recovery. What can the OTA do to help that family member?
13. For a client with a TBI who functions at a concrete level, should the OTA pursue a functional or remedial approach to perceptual training? Explain.
14. The mother of a 20-year-old client with TBI is at the hospital every day. Staff has noticed she has started sleeping in a chair in his room while he is at therapy. Her behavior indicates what?
15. A client with TBI who always wears glasses arrives for his outpatient appointment having forgotten them. What could the OTA do so that the client can still participate in therapy that day?

References

1. Adams JH, Doyle D, Ford I, Gennarelli TA, Graham DI, McLellan DR: Diffuse axonal injury in head injury: definition, diagnosis and grading, *Histopathology* 15:49–59, 1989.
2. American Occupational Therapy Association: *Occupational therapy practice framework: domain and process,* ed 2, 2008. Bethesda, Md.
3. Americans with Disabilities Act of 1990(ADA): 42 U.S.C. §§ 12101-12213, 1990.
4. Ayres AJ: *Sensory integration and learning disorders*, Los Angeles, 1972, Western Psychological Services.
5. Bontke CF: Medical advances in the treatment of brain injury. In Kreutzer JS, Wehman P, editors: *Community integration following traumatic brain injury*, Baltimore, 1990, Brookes.
6. Cantu RC: Posttraumatic retrograde and anterograde amnesia: pathophysiology and implications in grading and safe return to play, *J Athl Train* 36(3):244–248, 2001.
7. Cartlidge NEF, Shaw DA: *Head injury*, London, 1981, WB Saunders.
8. Conti GE: Traumatic brain injury. In Hansen AR, Atchison B, editors: *Conditions in occupational therapy-effect on occupational performance*, ed 3, Baltimore, 2000, Lippincott Williams & Wilkins.
9. Corrigan. JD: Substance abuse as the mediating factor in the outcome of traumatic brain injury, *Arch Phys Med Rehabil* 76(4):302–309, 1995.
10. Corrigan JD, Selassie AW, Orman J: The epidemiology of traumatic brain injury, *AJ Head Trauma Rehabil* 25(2):72–80, 2010.
11. Dikmen S, Machamer J, Miller B, Doctor J, Temkin N: Functional status examination: a new instrument for assessing outcome in traumatic brain injury, *J Neurotrauma* 18(2):127–140, 2001.
12. Farace E, Alves WM: Do women fare worse? A meta-analysis of gender differences in outcome after traumatic brain injury, *J Neurosurg* 93(4):539–545, 2000.
13. Freeman W: The neurobiology of multi-modal sensory integration, *Integ Physiol Beh Sci* 33:124–129, 1998.
14. Ghajar J: Traumatic brain injury, *Lancet* 356(9233):923–929, 2000.
15. Gianutsos R: Visual rehabilitation following acquired brain injury. In Gentile M, editor: *Functional vision behavior: a therapist's guide to evaluation and treatment options*, Rockville, Md, 1997, AOTA Press.
16. Goble L, Hier-Wellner S, Lee D: The role of community reintegration activities in a day treatment service, *Phys Disabil Special Interest Section Newsletter* 12(3):7–8, 1989.
17. Gutman SA: The psychosocial sequelae of traumatic brain injury, part I: identification, AOTA Continuing Education Article, *OT Practice* 6(4):CE-1–CE-8, February 5, 2001. American Occupational Therapy Association.
18. Gutman SA: The psychosocial sequelae of traumatic brain injury, part II: Treatment, AOTA Continuing Education Article, *OT Practice* 6(5):CE-1–CE-8, March 5, 2001. American Occupational Therapy Association.
19. Hall K, Cope DN, Rappaport M: Glasgow Outcome Scale, Disability Rating: Scale: comparative usefulness in following recovery in traumatic head injury, *Arch Phys Med Rehabil* 66(1):35–37, 1985.
20. Halper AS, Cherney LR, Cichowski K, Zhang M: Dysphagia after head trauma: the effect of cognitive-communicative impairments on functional outcomes, *J Head Trauma Rehabil* 14: 486–496, 1999.
21. Heinemann AW, Sahgal V, Cichowski K, et al: Functional outcomes following traumatic brain injury rehabilitation, *J Neuro Rehab* 4:27–37, 1990.
22. Huebner RA, Johnson K, Bennett C, et al: Community participation and quality of life outcomes after adult traumatic brain injury, *Am J Occup Ther* 57(2):177–185, 2003.
23. Hulme JB: *Advanced problem solving: the interrelationship of trunk and limb function in abnormal movement patterns. Paper presented at the Seventh Annual Interdisciplinary Bobath Symposium*, April 1994, San Francisco.
24. Ito M: Consciousness from the viewpoint of the structural-functional relationships of the brain, *Int J Psychol* 33:191–107, 1998.
25. Klupt R, Baker E, Patsy D: The importance of functional activities on an inpatient brain injury unit, *Phys Disabil Special Interest Section Newsletter* 12(3):6–7, 1989.
26. Langlois JA, Rutland-Brown W, Thomas KE: *Traumatic brain injury in the United States: emergency department visits, hospitalizations, and deaths. Centers for Disease Control and Prevention*, Atlanta, 2006, National Center for Injury Prevention and Control.
27. Lippert-Gruner M: Terhaag: Multimodal early onset stimulation (MEOS) in rehabilitation after brain injury, *Brain Inj* 14: 585–594, 2000.
28. Lippert-Gruner M, Wedekind C: Klug: Outcome of prolonged coma following severe traumatic brain injury, *Brain Inj* 17: 49–54, 2003.
29. Losiniecki A, Shutter L: Management of traumatic brain injury, *Curr Treat Options Neurol* 12(2):142–154, 2010.
30. Lundgren CC, Persechino EL: Cognitive group: a treatment program for head injured adults, *Am J Occup Ther* 40(6):397–401, 1986.
31. Maas AI, Stocchetti N, Bullock R: Moderate and severe traumatic brain injury in adults, *Lancet Neurol* 7(8):728–741, 2008.
32. Marquez de la Plata CD, Hart T, Hammond FM, Frol AB, Hudak A, Harper CR, O'Neil-Pirozzi TM, Whyte J, Carlile M, Diaz-Arrastia R: Impact of age on long-term recovery from traumatic brain injury, *Arch Phys Med Rehabil* 89(5):896–903, 2008.

33. Miller JD: Early intervention and management. In Rosenthal M, editor: *Rehabilitation of the head-injured adult*, Philadelphia, 1984, FA Davis.
34. National Center for Injury Prevention and Control: *A Report to Congress: Mild Traumatic Brain Injury in the United States: Steps to Prevent a Serious Public Health Problem*, Atlanta, 2003, Centers for Disease Control and Prevention.
35. National Center for Injury Prevention and Control: *A Report to Congress: Traumatic Brain Injury in the United States*, Atlanta, 1999, Centers for Disease Control and Prevention.
36. Neistadt ME: A critical analysis of occupational therapy approaches for perceptual deficits in adults with brain injury, *Am J Occup Ther* 44(4):299–304, 1990.
37. Neistadt ME: Perceptual retraining for adults with diffuse brain injury, *Am J Occup Ther* 48(3):225–233, 1994.
38. Padula WV, Shapiro J: Post-trauma vision syndrome following TBI. In Padula WV, editor: *Neuro-optometric rehabilitation*, ed 3, Santa Ana, Calif, 1988, Optometric Extension Program Foundation.
39. Park E, Bell JD, Baker AJ: Traumatic brain injury: can the consequences be stopped? *Can Med Assoc J* 178(9):1163–1170, 2008.
40. Radomski MV: *Occupational therapy for practice guidelines for adults with traumatic brain injury*, ed 3, Rockville, Md, 2001, American Occupational Therapy Association.
41. Rancho Los Amigos Medical Center: Levels of cognitive functioning, Downey, Calif, Rancho Los Amigos Medical Center, *Adult Brain Injury Service*, 1980. Revised by D. Malkmus and K Stenderup, 1974. Revised by C. Hagen, 1995.
42. Rappaport M, Hall KM, Hopkins K, et al: Disability rating scale for severe head trauma: coma to community, *Arch Phys Med Rehabil* 63(3):118–123, 1982.
43. Ratcliff JJ, Greenspan AI, Goldstein FC, Stringer AY, Bushnik T, Hammond FM, Novack TA, Whyte J, Wright DW: Gender and traumatic brain injury: do the sexes fare differently? *Brain Inj* 21:1023–1030, 2007.
44. Rath JF, Simon D, Langenbahn DM, Sherr RL, Diller L: Group treatment of problem-solving deficits in outpatients with traumatic brain injury: a randomised outcome study, *Neuropsych Rehabil* 13(4):461–488, 2003.
45. Schmidt JH, Reyes BJ, Roopan F, Flaherty BS: Use of hinge craniotomy for cerebral decompression: Technical note, *J Neurosurg* 107(3):678–682, 2007.
46. Schurr MJ, Ebner KA, Maser AL, Sperling KB, Helgerson RB, Harms B: Formal swallowing evaluation and therapy after traumatic brain injury improves dysphagia outcomes, *J Trauma* 46:817–821, 1999.
47. Shilling M: A formula to estimate incidence, *Community Integration* 2(3):8–9, 1992.
48. Teasdale G, Jennett B: Assessment of coma and impaired consciousness. A practical scale, *Lancet* 2:81–84, 1974.
49. VA Health Care—Mild Traumatic Brain Injury Screening and Evaluation Implemented for OEF/OIF Veterans, but Challenges Remain—Government Accountability Office (GAO), GAO-08-276, 2008
50. UAB Traumatic Brain Injury Model System: *Injury Control Recovery System Database. National Institute of Disability and Rehabilitation Research, Office of Special Education and Rehabilitative Services*, Washington, DC, 1999, Dept of Education.
51. Willer B, Rosenthal M, Kreutzer JS, et al: Assessment of community integration following rehabilitation for traumatic brain injury, *J Head Trauma Rehabil* 8(2):75–87, 1993.
52. Wilson JT, Pettigrew LE, Teasdale GM: Structured interviews for the Glasgow Outcome Scale and the extended Glasgow Outcome Scale: guidelines for their use, *J Neurotrauma* 15(8):573–585, 1998.
53. World Health Organization: *International classification of functioning, disability and health (ICF)*, Geneva, Switzerland, 2001, World Health Organization.
54. Xiong Y, Lee CP, Peterson PL: Mitochondrial dysfunction following traumatic brain injury. In Miller LP, Hayes RL, Newcomb JK, editors: *Head trauma: basic, preclinical, and clinical directions*, New York, 2000, John Wiley and Sons, pp 257–280.
55. Yablon SA, Agana BT, Ivanhoe CB, Boake C: Botulinum toxin in severe upper extremity spasticity among patients with traumatic brain injury, *Neurology* 47:939–944, 1996.

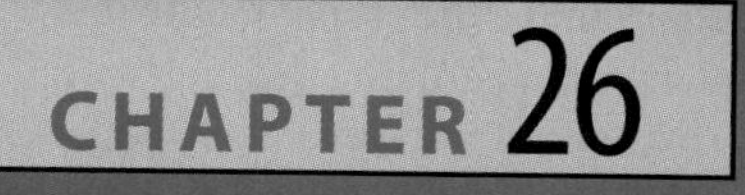

Degenerative Diseases of the Central Nervous System*

GLEN GILLEN

Key Terms

Degenerative neurologic diseases
Multiple sclerosis (MS)
Parkinson's disease (PD)
Amyotrophic lateral sclerosis (ALS)
Alzheimer's disease (AD)
Progressive neurologic diseases
Demyelination
Exacerbations
Remission
Bradykinesia
Rigidity
Dementia
Task segmentation

Chapter Objectives

After studying this chapter, the student or practitioner will be able to do the following:

1. Describe four degenerative diseases.
2. List the signs and symptoms of these diseases.
3. Understand the focus of occupational therapy related to the treatment of degenerative diseases.
4. Describe the precautions that must be observed in the treatment of these diseases.
5. Recognize and describe the occupational therapy interventions used to treat clients with degenerative diseases across the various stages of the disease.

Introduction and General Concerns

Degenerative neurologic diseases cause progressive pathologic changes in the central nervous system (CNS). These changes result in loss of functioning in one or more of the following areas: sensation, motor control, and cognition. The diseases addressed in this chapter are multiple sclerosis (MS), Parkinson's disease (PD), amyotrophic lateral sclerosis (ALS), and Alzheimer's disease (AD). Although no cures exist for these diseases, their debilitating effects can be partially ameliorated with effective medical and rehabilitative management. The role of occupational therapy (OT) in the treatment of degenerative neurologic diseases is to assist in managing symptoms, maintaining function, and optimizing quality of life. Because of the nature of the diseases included in this chapter, compensation/adaptation is a common method used to maximize function.

Because of the progressive and sometimes unpredictable course of the diseases that are discussed later, the occupational therapy assistant (OTA) in conjunction with the occupational therapist must consider the following factors that influence management of this population:

- A probable decline in performance in areas of occupation requires planning ahead. In terms of assessment, periodic reevaluations are necessary to monitor performance. Interventions such as prescription of adaptive devices and/or durable medical equipment should take into account the length of time the equipment will be usable.
- Inconsistent performance in areas of occupation throughout the day due to fatigue issues or cognitive changes, as in delirium in the evening or night ("sundowning").
- Impact of the diagnosis on the family related to role changes, ability to provide care, or potential loss of a loved one.
- Limited medical interventions for some diseases.
- Psychological issues related to coping with a progressive disease including coping with end-of-life issues, fear related to probable future decline of function, anxiety, depression, etc.

Working with those presenting with progressive neurologic diseases is complex and challenging. The focus of interventions varies based on the stage of the disease, as well as the context in which the OT practitioner is interacting with the client (e.g., acute care vs. long-term care vs. home). A client-centered approach is recommended for these reasons: "Client-centered practice is an approach to providing occupational therapy which embraces a philosophy of respect

*Phyllis Ber contributed large portions of this chapter to the first edition of this book.

for, and partnership with, people receiving services. Client-centered practice recognizes the autonomy of individuals, the need for client choice in making decisions about occupational needs, the strengths clients bring to a therapy encounter, the benefits of client-therapist partnership, and the need to ensure that services are accessible and fit the context in which a client lives."[39]

Law and colleagues[39] and Pollack[60] suggest that the therapy practitioners who implement this approach to evaluation consider the advice listed in Box 26-1.

With these strategies the OT process becomes more focused and defined; patients become immediately empowered; the goals of therapy are understood and agreed upon; and an individually tailored treatment plan may be established. The Canadian Occupational Performance Measure[38] is a standardized tool that uses a client-centered approach to allow the recipient of treatment to identify performance areas of difficulty, rate the importance of each area, and rate his or her satisfaction with current performance. It is a particularly useful tool for this population because of the multiple and extensive problems experienced in performance of areas of occupation. In addition, it can be used with family members and caregivers to help prioritize interventions.

In general, after the evaluation is completed, the occupational therapist should have a thorough understanding of the client's strengths and weaknesses, including social supports and environmental factors. In collaboration with the client, the therapist establishes realistic goals with the overall purpose of increasing or maintaining the patient's present functional status. Long- and short-term goals are addressed. General treatment goals for those living with progressive neurologic diseases include the following:

- Maximize the client's ability to engage in meaningful occupations despite disease progression.
- Prevent secondary complications such as decubitus ulcers, contractures, pain, injury, anxiety, and depression.
- Maximize quality of life.

Box 26-1

Client-Centered Practice Considerations[39,60]

1. Recognize that the recipients of OT are uniquely qualified to make decisions about their occupational functioning.
2. Offer the patient a more active role in defining goals and desired outcomes.
3. Make the patient-therapist relationship interdependent to enable the solution of performance dysfunction.
4. Shift to a model in which occupational therapists work with patients to enable them to meet their own goals.
5. Focus evaluation (and intervention) on the contexts in which patients live, their roles and interests, and their culture.
6. Allow the patient to be the "problem definer" so that in turn the patient will become the "problem solver."
7. Allow the client to evaluate his or her own performance and set personal goals.

- Teach clients strategies to self-manage the effects of the disease process (e.g., medication management, dealing with fatigue, coping strategies).
- Teach caregivers safe and effective ways to provide assistance to the client while not undermining the client's abilities.

The success of the OT program depends somewhat on the patient's perceived sense of accomplishment and a positive attitude. The progressive nature of these diseases requires that treatment goals be established in small enough increments that the patient is assured of some measure of progress. Because of the progressive and chronic nature of the diseases included in this chapter, clients in the latter stages of the disease process may require substantial care beyond what is possible within the client's social support system. Placement in a long-term care facility is indicated when the client and family can no longer cope with advancing symptoms in the home. Nursing homes offer (1) comprehensive rehabilitation programs; (2) contracture prevention programs (via positioning, splinting, and range of motion [ROM]); (3) decubitus ulcer prevention and treatment; (4) adjunctive medical interventions such as tube feedings; (5) bowel/bladder management strategies; (6) suctioning of respiratory secretions; (7) palliative care; (8) counseling programs; and (9) the 24-hour supervision necessary for patient safety. In addition, the nursing home will have specific durable medical equipment that may be required to assist those who require substantial physical assistance such as mechanical lifts, electric hospital beds, and pressure-relieving mattresses. End-of-life care may be provided in a hospice setting including home hospice. Hospice care differs from medical care in that it focuses on comfort rather than cure, emphasizes quality of life, promotes personal choice and dignity, and provides care and support to the bereaved.

All clients with a progressive disease can benefit from periodic home evaluations. The foci of the home evaluation are described in the following discussion.

Any hazardous conditions that could trigger a fall should be eliminated. Special care should be taken to remove all throw or scatter rugs. Bathroom rugs should be removed. Doorway thresholds should be even with the floors. On the outside of the home, gravel or cobblestone walkways represent a safety hazard.

Assist in the evaluation of necessary assistive devices or durable medical equipment. In the bathroom, grab bars, a raised toilet seat with a safety frame, and a shower chair or tub transfer bench are recommended. In the bedroom, a sturdy chair with armrests should be used while dressing. A raised bed with a firm mattress and a trapeze over the bed also help with bed mobility. A bedside commode or urinal should be considered when the patient makes frequent nighttime trips to the bathroom.

Consider simple home modifications. In the living room, the patient should be advised not to sit in deep, low chairs. The preferred chair has firm cushions, a straight back, and padded armrests. The height and depth of the chair should allow the patient to maintain feet on the floor with knees flexed at 90 degrees. For those patients who cannot get out of the chair independently, automatic lift chairs are available. In the kitchen, commonly used items should be placed so that excessive bending and reaching are not required. The patient's walker can be fitted with a bicycle basket to make it easier to carry objects.

More substantial home modifications may be necessary. Examples of substantial modifications include the installation of an elevator, stair-glide, stall shower, or ramp.

Accessibility issues may need to be addressed for those clients using a device for gait or wheeled mobility.

Multiple Sclerosis

MS is thought to be an autoimmune disease that affects the CNS including the brain, spinal cord, and optic nerves. Myelin, the tissue surrounding and protecting the nerve fibers of the CNS, helps nerve fibers conduct electrical impulses. In MS, the body mistakenly attacks the myelin, which is then lost in multiple areas (demyelination), leaving scar tissue known as *sclerosis.* These damaged areas are also known as *plaques* or *lesions.* The two processes of demyelination and plaque formation impede the transmission of nerve impulses to and from the brain. Depending on the area(s) that develop plaques, various signs and symptoms occur.[35] Occupational therapy plays a key role in the rehabilitation of those with MS.[15]

Epidemiology

Facts and figures are maintained related to MS. Key facts to consider include the following[5,22,27,35]:

- The typical age of people diagnosed with MS ranges from 20 to 50. However, MS can appear in teens, children, and older adults.
- The disease is more common in women (2 to 3:1).
- It is not hereditary but has a probable genetic aspect.
- There is a 1/750 risk of developing MS in the general population. The risk rises to 1/40 in anyone who has a close relative with MS.
- MS is more common in Caucasians than Hispanics or African-Americans.
- It is more prevalent in higher latitudes.
- Approximately 400,000 are living with MS in the United States, with 2.1 million patients worldwide.

Disease Course

MS is diagnosed when there is evidence of damage in at least two separate parts of the central nervous system. This damage must occur at two separate points in time, and other diagnoses must be ruled out. MS may follow various courses related to progression. The following four courses have been identified[5,22,27]:

1. Relapsing/Remitting: Characterized by acute attacks with full or partial recovery. Between attacks the disease does not progress. Eighty-five percent of those initially diagnosed with MS present with this course.
2. Secondary Progressive: Initially, clients follow a relapsing/remitting course, which is followed by progression at a variable rate. Of those initially diagnosed with a relapsing/remitting course, 50% develop secondary progressive within 10 years and 90% within 25 years.
3. Primary Progressive: Progressive disability without remission from the onset of the disease. Relates to 10% of those diagnosed with MS.
4. Progressive Relapsing: Progressive from the onset with clear acute relapses. Relates to 5% of those diagnosed.

Impact on Client Factors

The signs and symptoms of MS vary depending on the areas of the CNS that have been affected by demyelination and plaque formation. Each patient will present with a unique set of clinical manifestations depending on the locations of the lesions and the stage of the disease process. Symptoms directly caused by demyelination include fatigue; visual disturbances[17]; cognitive disturbances[64] (slowed processing, memory loss including explicit and episodic memory, decreased attention including alternating and divided attention, impairment of executive functions); affective disturbances; (depression, bipolar disorders, lability, euphoria, antisocial behavior)[3,37,38,63]; sensory changes (numbness, tingling, pain); loss of postural control; dizziness and vertigo; tremor; dysphagia; speech disturbances; heat intolerance; spasticity[36]; weakness; ambulation disturbances; sexual dysfunction; and bowel/bladder dysfunction.[30,31]

Medical Management

The treatment of MS focuses primarily on alleviating the patient's symptoms[5,22,27] through, for example, use of antidepressants or antispasmodics. High-dose corticosteroids are often given for acute exacerbations. Immunomodulators are used to reduce the number of relapses and limit the development of new lesions. Typical drugs include Avonex®, Betaserone®, Copaxone®, Novantrone®, Tysabri®, and Rebif®. The OTA can assist the physician by reporting changes in the patient's behavior and physical status.

During the chronic stages of MS, medical management of the disease may include catheterization for urinary dysfunction, tube feeding for swallowing disorders, and nerve blocks or surgical release of tendons for treatment of severe contractures.

Occupational Therapy Management

The patient with MS offers a challenge to the OT practitioner. The disease follows a variable and unpredictable course that changes the patient's functional ability from morning to night, from day to day, and over the course of the disease. These changes demand regular adjustments to the patient's therapy program.

Precautions

The functional status of an MS patient may be affected by a variety of factors such as stress, heat, pain, fatigue, and exacerbations.[49] Considerations include the following:

- Avoiding overfatigue
- Awareness of room temperature; cooler is generally better

- Using heat modalities with caution because of both sensory loss and possible heat intolerance
- Being aware of fluctuations in level of independence. For example, a client who uses a sliding board to transfer may require only supervision in the morning but may require physical assistance by the afternoon
- Guarding against soft tissue injury secondary to sensory loss (e.g., sharp objects, hot water)
- Monitoring for safety issues secondary to loss of postural control and/or cognitive impairment
- Awareness of combined effects of cognitive and physical impairments

Evaluation

The initial evaluation process for the MS patient sets the tone and prepares both the patient and the OT practitioner for the treatment sessions to follow. Principles of a client-centered assessment[60] are necessary because of the multiple areas of occupation that may be adversely affected. It is important that the client and caregivers determine which occupations should be addressed first. In addition, the evaluation reveals the areas amenable to remediation (such as deconditioning) and those for which compensatory techniques should be taught (such as long-standing memory loss). Because the patient may have cognitive deficits or may be experiencing anxiety or stress, the practitioner must be careful to explain the reason for the evaluation and to describe what will occur during the evaluation. Rest periods may be required if the patient becomes fatigued. If necessary, the evaluation may be broken up into two or more sessions. At the conclusion of the evaluation process, the therapist and patient should agree on the goals for the OT program. The practitioner should emphasize that the OT program will be directed toward the improvement and/or maintenance of meaningful occupations—that is, those occupations that the client wants to do, needs to do, or has to do to return home.

The evaluation includes assessment of client factors, areas of occupation, and quality of life issues. Client factors include strength, muscle tone, sensation, coordination, joint ROM, endurance, balance, vision, and cognitive functions.

Performance in areas of occupation including basic and instrumental activities of daily living (ADL, IADL); work; and play/leisure must be evaluated objectively.[15] The ADL evaluation may be administered by an experienced OTA who has demonstrated competency in these evaluation techniques. The coordination and interpretation of the evaluation results is the role of the occupational therapist.

Interventions

The treatment methods selected for MS clients are determined by individual goals for the client and are guided by the client's clinical presentation.

Improving Participation via Fatigue Management

Fatigue is the most common symptom in MS, experienced by 75% to 95% of those living with the disease.[51] Approximately 50% to 60% of those with MS report fatigue as their most troublesome symptom of the disease.[51] Multiple factors may cause a loss of function secondary to fatigue including comorbid medical conditions, psychological issues such as anxiety and stress, disrupted sleep, poor trunk stability, movement disorders, and the environment (increased ambient temperature). MS-related fatigue has been characterized as primary and secondary fatigue.

It is hypothesized that *primary fatigue* is due to the disease process itself: cortical damage, conduction blocks from demyelinated motor pathways, increased energy demands for muscle activation, and increased energy demands from co-contraction of agonist and antagonists. In MS, *secondary fatigue* may be due to deconditioning, respiratory muscle weakness, and pain.[49]

Treatment is a two-step process.[51] The first step is eliminating any secondary causes of fatigue. This includes treating coexisting conditions such as depression; adjustment of medications; improving sleep patterns; managing symptoms that may cause fatigue such as tremor; and education about energy conservation. The second step is managing primary fatigue. This management is achieved via pharmacology in conjunction with energy conservation techniques.

Interventions that may counteract fatigue and result in improved occupational functioning include cooling via use of a cooling garment,[49,65] energy conservation techniques,[43,49,74] and aerobic conditioning.[59] Schwid and colleagues[65] examined the use of a liquid cooling garment worn 1 hour per day for 1 month. Subjects reported less fatigue during the month of daily cooling, and cooling therapy was associated with objectively measurable but modest improvements in motor and visual function, as well as persistent subjective benefits.

Both Mathiowetz and colleagues[43] and Vanage and colleagues[74] have documented the effectiveness of a group format energy conservation program for people living with MS. A six-session, 2-hour-per-week energy conservation course taught by occupational therapists for groups of 8 to 10 participants resulted in less fatigue impact, increased self-efficacy, and improved quality of life. A variety of energy conservation techniques may be used with the MS population (Box 26-2).

Aerobic training has been demonstrated to improve overall fitness and decrease fatigue in the MS population. Petajan and colleagues[59] tested a program of 30 minutes of combined upper extremity (UE) and lower extremity (LE) ergometry plus 5 minutes of warm-up and cooldown (40 minutes total) three times per week. This program resulted in multiple benefits including decreased fatigue. The OTA must work closely with the occupational therapist to determine the correct intensity and duration of any exercise program with this population.

Improving Participation via Control of Tremors and Movement Disorders

Movement disorders such as tremor and ataxia are common problems for people living with MS. Compensatory strategies appear to be the most successful for controlling movement disorders and improve performance despite their presence (Box 26-3).[19,21,32]

Improving Participation via Cognitive Compensations

Decreased cognitive functioning significantly impedes the rehabilitation process because the patient is less able to store and receive new information. Cognitive changes may be present throughout the disease and fluctuate with time of day, task difficulty, and environmental distractions; cognitive function may worsen with fatigue.[4] Short- and long-term memory deficits contribute to confusion and agitation. New information should be presented to the patient simply and repetitively. Consistency in the therapy program as to day, time, and modalities helps to orient the patient and minimize frustration. Compensatory strategies seem to be the most effective intervention because remediation of cognitive deficits (e.g., memory drills) has little research support[22] (Box 26-4).

According to the National MS Society: "Interventions should be designed to improve the person's ability to function in all meaningful aspects of family and community life. Intervention should involve systematic, functionally oriented, therapeutic activities that are based on understanding of specific deficits."[52] Commonly, a compensatory approach is used. This may include strategies such as cognitive structuring, in which cognitive tasks are learned and practiced as a routine. The client might also be encouraged to substitute intact cognitive abilities to compensate for abilities that are impaired. For example, the client who does not remember the words for certain items might use pictures instead. To reduce fatigue the client might use organizers, employ assistive technology, and schedule activities for times of day when energy is higher. A structured environment and structured routines conserve energy and promote organization. Memory strategies (e.g., lists, mnemonics, clustering, visualization techniques) and recording devices might also be used. To improve attention and reduce distractibility, it is helpful to maintain a quiet environment. The specific strategies and solutions should be individual and client centered, focusing on desired areas of participation and providing increased functioning.[52]

Box 26-2

Energy Conservation Techniques Used by Patients with Multiple Sclerosis[43,49,74]

- Pacing
- Successful work/rest ratio
- Use of electronic aids as needed
- Flexible home and work schedules
- Recognition of fatigue warning signals
- Successful use of compensatory strategies
- Acceptance of a request for assistance
- Home/work modifications
- Appropriate ambulatory aids
- Power mobility aids (power wheelchair or scooter)
- Control of spasticity
- Improved trunk control
- Techniques to control tremor
- ADL assistive devices
- Durable medical equipment
- Heat control
- Pharmacologic interventions

Box 26-3

Interventions Related to Ataxia and Tremor[19,20,32]

- Orthotics/splinting (wrist support, thumb support via opponens splints, cervical collar)
- Using the environment for stability (e.g., leaning on the work surface, high back chairs)
- Adaptive devices (Dycem®, long straw, suction devices, built-up handles)
- Assistive technology (speaker phone, adapted mouse/keyboard)
- Weights (wrist weights, weighted gloves, weighted devices, etc.) may be effective for subtle movement disorders.
- Posture/position of activity focused on trunk support
- Minimize the number of joints moving simultaneously during activities
- Keep upper extremities stabilized against the trunk
- Keep the elbow on the work surface (propping)
- Promote a calm/focused emotional state
- Control fatigue
- Adapt activities to eliminate the need to reach into space
- Decrease effort
- Decrease fine motor coordination demands
- Experiment with both slow and fast movements
- Provide exercise for proximal (trunk/scapula) stability
- Pharmacologic management

Improving Participation via Managing Sensory Deficits

The patient with MS may have a variety of sensory and perceptual disorders. In most cases, therapists aim to make the patient and family aware of the problem and to teach the patient to use compensatory techniques. Loss of tactile

Box 26-4

Cognitive Strategies Used by Patients with Multiple Sclerosis[22]

- Use memory aids: timers, watch alarms, personal data assistants, reminder lists, memory books, Post-it notes, computerized organizers, dictation systems.
- Allow extra time for task completion and processing.
- Decrease environmental distractions.
- Avoid multitasking.
- Schedule difficult cognitive tasks during periods of high energy.
- Avoid fatigue.
- Delegate responsibilities.
- Solve problems aloud.
- Check work for accuracy.
- Keep organized and avoid clutter.
- Determine which (visual or auditory) processing system is most effective.

sensation, especially for stereognosis, interferes with performing fine motor tasks such as buttoning, managing utensils, money manipulation, computer use, and writing. If there is no visual loss, the patient may be able to compensate visually. Adaptations such as built-up handles, use of Velcro, and so on may help the client compensate.

Patients with loss of pain and temperature sensation need to be cautioned to avoid situations that could cause burns or other injuries, particularly kitchen and bathroom activities. On the other hand, patients may present with pain secondary to a variety of causes such as decubiti, muscle imbalance, overuse of a particular movement pattern, and postural malalignment. A variety of conservative techniques may be used to decrease pain and include deep breathing, visualization, biofeedback, correcting muscle imbalance, correcting postural alignment, transcutaneous electrical nerve stimulation (TENS), cryotherapy (cooling), and adapting relevant occupations to decrease the use of compensatory movement patterns.

Visual deficits such as double vision, blurred vision, decreased acuity, and nystagmus may make even simple ADL difficult. Patients can be taught compensatory techniques such as covering one eye (full or partial visual occlusion) to minimize double vision or using devices for those with low vision such as magnifying glasses, large-print books, and audiobooks. Consider the following intervention guidelines when working with clients with visual loss[9,22]:

- Magnification/enlargement via magnifying devices, large print, and so on
- Color contrast—for example, using white dishes on a blue placemat
- Decreasing background clutter to increase clarity
- Increased and task-focused illumination. Consider task-specific lighting based on where clients cook, manage medication, and so on.

Improving Participation via Strengthening and Endurance Training

Patients with MS are taught by the OTA to plan their day and pace themselves accordingly (see Box 26-1). Planning and energy conservation help the patient budget strength and endurance to meet daily needs. Important activities including exercises are done in the morning or after a scheduled nap or rest period. Graded resistive exercises increase the strength of key muscle groups and should be targeted to specific muscle groups that are task specific. To increase endurance, emphasis should be placed on increasing repetitions rather than increasing weights. The benefits of aerobic exercise for this population have been documented in terms of improved fitness and quality of life.[59] The OTA should work closely with the occupational therapist to determine the correct duration, frequency, and intensity of exercise to avoid overfatigue.

Patients with severe loss of muscle strength sometimes can perform functional activities with the help of devices that substitute for weak muscles. For example, the OTA may encourage the patient to use an overhead suspension sling or mobile arm support to increase independence.

Contracture Prevention and Treatment

Patients with severe weakness that prevents full active range of motion (AROM), as well as those with spasticity, have the potential to develop soft tissue contractures. Contracture is prevented by deliberate and regular limb movement; active movement is preferred over passive when possible. Moving the patient through complete ROM—and not just the middle ranges—is essential. Therapists must determine what a full ROM is for each individual patient; therefore age-related factors must be considered. A joint that moves or is moved through its full ROM via engagement in daily activities develops almost no deformities. A program of AROM and passive range of motion (PROM) combined with a terminal stretch at least twice per day is recommended if contracture is beginning to develop. Low-load prolonged stretch via splints or positioning must be used if a contracture has developed. During the terminal stretch the proximal body part should be well stabilized.

Whenever possible, the patient should perform self-ranging techniques. PROM of each joint through the full range must be done daily. The occupational therapist may be responsible for teaching the family or a nursing assistant the techniques of ROM. The occupational therapist may administer inhibition techniques (such as icing or positioning to decrease tone before PROM) to patients with severe spasticity. Splints to maintain range or provide sustained stretch may be indicated to treat or prevent contractures of the elbow, wrist, ankle, or hand.

Activities of Daily Living

Independence in ADL promotes self-esteem and quality of life.[37] OT may provide assistive devices and adaptive techniques to enable MS patients to be safer, more independent, and more efficient in both ADL and IADL. Cups with lids, scoop dishes, and adapted utensils assist eating. Long-handled shoe horns, reachers, sock aids, and elastic shoelaces are just some of the devices that can increase independence and ease of dressing. The OTA needs to work with the patient to evaluate the effectiveness of equipment and provide training on an individual basis. As the disease progresses, modifications in equipment and techniques will be necessary. A severely disabled patient may require an environmental control unit (ECU) to operate lights, television, or radio with a simple switch. The OT practitioner may be asked to determine which body part should activate the switch and what type of switch should be used.

Communication

In MS, both written and verbal communication skills may be affected. The occupational therapist often works closely with the speech therapist to devise a method of improving the patient's communication skills. Patients with severe deficits may be given augmentative communication devices such as communication boards or computers that speak for them. The OTA may provide equipment that enables the patient to use these devices, such as splints for UE stabilization or head or mouth pointers. Adaptive writing devices (built-up and weighted pens, pen holders, and magnetized wrist stabilizers) compensate for decreased coordination and weakness. Special computer keyboards and large-button and speech-activated telephones assist independent communication for patients with motor deficits.

Seating and Wheeled Mobility

Many patients with MS will require the use of a wheelchair (manual or electric) or power scooter for mobility as their disease progresses. The primary considerations in recommending a wheelchair for an MS patient are the following:

- Overall endurance
- Trunk control
- LE strength, coordination, sensation, and endurance
- UE strength, coordination, sensation, and endurance
- Disease prognosis

Patients with sufficient UE strength and overall endurance should have a lightweight, high-strength manual wheelchair if they are to propel their own wheelchairs. Patients with a rapidly progressive type of the disease may require wheelchairs with reclining backs or a tilt-in-space[20] frame to compensate for diminished trunk control. In some cases an electric wheelchair or electric scooter may be indicated. Modifications to the wheelchair that are helpful with the MS population include oblique rim projections, lateral supports, solid back and seat inserts, head positioners, and brake extensions.[20] Training in wheelchair mobility and transfer techniques may be taught as part of the patient's OT program. In a long-term care setting, MS patients with poor alignment and no wheelchair mobility skills may be positioned in geri-chairs for proper alignment and comfort.

Proper positioning of the patient both in and out of the wheelchair is under the scope of the OT department in many facilities. MS patients are at high risk for decubitus ulcers because of their diminished sensation, incontinence, and poor ability to reposition themselves. Pressure-relieving cushions and mattresses should be provided to all MS patients. Patients with sufficient strength should be taught and encouraged to do periodic wheelchair push-ups as part of their OT training.

Leisure Skills

Leisure skills provide mental and social stimulation and substitute avocational interests for vocational skills. The OTA can assist the patient by stressing the importance of activity and by recommending adaptive devices such as card holders and shufflers and adapted board games. The patient should be encouraged to manage time effectively, planning for social events with naps and limited exercise on days when evening activities are scheduled.[41]

Work Skills

MS patients may be able to maintain their ability to work during various stages of the disease or during remission, with changes to their schedule and adaptive devices to increase ease-of-work tasks. Worksite modifications for wheelchair accessibility may be required. The OTA may assist the occupational therapist in conducting the vocational evaluation, which may be used to determine a worker's ability to continue the job, and in making recommendations for adaptive equipment.

Psychosocial Issues

The patient and his or her family typically greet a diagnosis of MS with shock, denial, and anger. However, in some cases, the patient may feel some relief in finally knowing that the symptoms were not psychosomatic. As the disease progresses, the client may become depressed.[34,47,48] Incidence of depression is higher for people living with MS than for the general population or for people with other neurologic diagnoses. Other affective conditions include bipolar disorder, lability, and (less commonly) antisocial behavior. Assets and characteristics of those who cope well with MS (and other diagnoses) include the following[3,48]:

- Support
- Connectedness
- Sense of humor
- Spirituality
- Openness

Clinicians may assist in fostering adaptive coping strategies such as active coping, seeking emotional support, seeking instrumental support, positive reframing, planning, humor, acceptance, and religion.[44]

The OTA can offer emotional support to both the patient and family. The patient should be encouraged to maintain a daily schedule of activity. Referral to MS support groups sponsored by the local MS Society may be helpful in dealing with the daily stress of having a chronic progressive disease. Additional support and information are available online at the reference and health sites and in chat groups.

The members of the rehabilitation team including the OTA have an obligation to help the family and the patient adjust to the disease and to provide encouragement, emotional support, training, and exercise programs. OT can help the MS patient function as productively as possible within the limits of the disease.

Parkinson's Disease

PD is a slow, chronic, progressive disease of the nervous system that was first described by James Parkinson in 1817. PD is characterized by four cardinal signs: resting tremor, rigidity in skeletal muscle, bradykinesia, and postural instability. Pathology is characterized by degeneration in dopaminergic pathways in the basal ganglia, particularly in the substantia nigra. The function of the substantia nigra is to produce dopamine, the neurotransmitter that transports signals to motor control areas such as the caudate and putamen. In PD, dopaminergic neurons deteriorate at a fast rate and the amount of dopamine that is produced decreases, resulting in initial impairments. When signs and symptoms are noticed, 80% of the dopaminergic neurons have already deteriorated. Diagnosis is made by the presence of at least two of the cardinal signs, as well as the client's response to levodopa, a dopamine precursor.[8,53]

The symptom complex of PD is termed parkinsonism. Not all clients with parkinsonism have PD. Besides the formal diagnoses of PD, other pathologies that result in parkinsonism include drug-induced parkinsonism (i.e., parkinsonism has been associated with the use of antipsychotics), progressive supranuclear palsy, corticobasal degeneration, multiple system atrophy, and vascular parkinsonism (multiple small strokes).[53]

Epidemiology

At least 500,000 Americans are living with diagnosed PD. Approximately 50,000 individuals are diagnosed each year, and thousands of people live with the disease undiagnosed. PD is more common in men, with a male-female ratio of 3 to 2. Approximately 15% of those living with PD are diagnosed before age 40, although the average age of diagnosis is 60.[8,53,75]

Cause

The cause of PD is not clear. Researchers hypothesize that causes include a combination of genetic and environmental factors. Approximately 15% to 25% of people living with PD have a relative with the disease. Risk of developing PD is increased twofold to threefold if a first-degree relative is affected. Those who sustain serious and recurrent traumatic brain injuries (e.g., professional boxers) may develop a form of PD, as may those living in rural conditions and those exposed to herbicides, pesticides, or some synthetic narcotic agents. Further research continues to attempt to establish the cause of the disease.[8,53]

Impact on Client Factors

PD normally affects the client's motor systems first and foremost. The four primary symptoms, according to the National Institute of Neurological Disorders and Stroke, are[53]:

- **Tremor.** Typically this is a a "pill-rolling" tremor, involving the thumb and forefinger, which move rhythmically back and forth at a rate of four to six beats per second.[53] Although tremor often begins in a hand, it may in some people first affect another body part such as a foot. Generally, the tremor increases with stress and is visible when the person is awake and the body is at rest (not moving). Intentional movement reduces the tremor, which also disappears during sleep.
- **Rigidity.** Most people with PD experience some rigidity (resistance to movement). This rigidity is caused by an imbalance in the innervation of agonist-antagonist coordination. Instead of relaxing when its opposite muscle contracts, the antagonist muscle remains tense. Gait is affected, resulting in a slow and shuffling gait, or a festinating gait in which the patient takes small fast steps that propel him forward faster and faster. The patient has difficulty stopping forward motion. During standing activities the person may fall backwards involuntarily (retropulsion). Muscular rigidity classically manifests as "cogwheel" rigidity. When another person attempts to move the patient's arm, it moves only in short, jerky movements.
- **Bradykinesia.** Bradykinesia manifests as a slowing of voluntary and automatic movements, resulting in difficulty performing ordinary daily activities with ease. Bathing, dressing, and other daily activities take much longer to perform.
- Postural instability. Balance is impaired and patients are at risk of falling. A stooped posture with forward head position may be present.[53]

In addition, loss of gross and fine motor coordination, loss of coordination for writing (presenting as micrographia—small and crowded writing style), and decreased facial expression (mask face) may be present.

Gait and balance are also affected.[79] The client develops a stooped posture and loose arm swing during gait. Episodes of freezing[57] (sudden difficulty in walking through doorways or making turns) are experienced during gait activities. Postural dysfunction and rigidity result in typical gait patterns that are characterized by a stooped-forward posture; a slow, shuffling gait; or a festinating gait that includes small, fast steps, which propel the patient forward with ever-increasing speed. The patient has difficulty in stopping the forward motion. During standing activities the client may experience retropulsion (falling backwards).

As the disease progresses, the patient experiences problems with oral musculature, resulting in drooling, dysphagia, and monotone speech with low volume. The patient may demonstrate disorders in bowel and bladder control. Depression is common in this population.[40] Dementia and other cognitive problems are common. "Some, but not all, people with PD may develop memory problems and slow thinking. In some of these cases, cognitive problems become more severe, leading to a condition called Parkinson's dementia late in the course of the disease. This dementia may affect memory, social judgment, language, reasoning, or other mental skills."[53] Other impairments include emotional changes, urinary problems or constipation, skin problems, sleep problems, orthostatic hypotension, muscle cramps and dystonia, pain, fatigue and loss of energy, and sexual dysfunction.[53] Signs and symptoms are progressive and may be staged for the purposes of developing OT interventions (Box 26-5).[28] All these impairments result in decreased participation and performance in areas of occupation.

Box 26-5

Staging the Advancement of Parkinson's Disease[28]

Hoehn and Yahr Scale

Stage 1: Unilateral tremor, rigidity, bradykinesia, minimal or no functional impairment.

Stage 2: Bilateral tremor, rigidity, bradykinesia, with or without axial signs such as facial involvement, independent with ADL, no balance impairment.

Stage 3: Worsening of symptoms, impaired righting reactions, disability related to ADL, balance changes, may still maintain independence with interventions.

Stage 4: Requires help with some or all ADL, cannot live alone without assistance, able to walk and stand.

Stage 5: Confined to a bed or wheelchair, maximal assistance required.

Medical Management

Although no cure for PD exists, medical management concentrates on relieving the symptoms of the disease primarily through medication and, less often, through surgical techniques. Levodopa is the most widely prescribed medication to manage the symptoms of PD and is usually prescribed in a combined carbidopa-levodopa formula called Sinemet.[53] The OTA should be aware that clients being managed with drugs such as Sinemet will fluctuate in motor and functional status during "on and off" periods. It is helpful to work with clients during periods of both optimal and nonoptimal drug responses to have a full overview of the client's functioning throughout the day. Level of assistance required can vary greatly depending on the timing of drug administration.[13] Dopamine agonists also commonly used with this population include apomorphine, bromocriptine, pramipexole, and ropinirole.[53] All dopamine drugs may cause nausea and decreased blood pressure; therefore clients should be monitored closely. In older adults, dopamine agonists may result in hallucinations. The OTA should report any adverse reactions to the physician as soon as possible.

It is common in the early stages of the disease for the neurologist to prescribe milder medications such as the dopamine agonists or amantadine and add levodopa only when further symptom control is necessary. Similarly, during the early stages of the disease, the physician may prescribe anticholinergic drugs, which reduce rigidity and tremor. In addition to antiparkinsonian drugs, medication for treatment of depression, nutritional supplements, and pain medication may be prescribed.

If patients do not respond well to medications, surgical options include deep brain stimulation, pallidotomy, thalamotomy, and others.[75] Like medication management, surgical interventions are used to manage symptoms, not to cure the disease. Specific symptoms that may be managed via surgical interventions such as deep brain stimulation include tremor, bradykinesia, and rigidity. Loss of balance, gait-freezing episodes, speech deficits, and postural deficits are not amenable to surgery.

Occupational Therapy Management

Participation restriction and activity limitations are substantial problems for those living with PD. Decreased performance in areas of occupation may result from multiple client factors affected adversely in this population. In addition, self-imposed limitations may be a factor as well. Those living with PD may limit their involvement in life situations because of fear of falling and concerns related to continence, drooling, or the amount of time and energy required to participate in meaningful occupations. OT is usually initiated when those living with PD present with a decreased ability to participate in daily life.[18,50]

Precautions

The parkinsonian patient has diminished postural control and may present with orthostatic hypotension as well; therefore risk for falls is significant. Care must be taken during ambulation and transfers. Doorways, elevators, crowds, and surface changes may trigger freezing behavior.[57] The client may have dysphagia and should not be offered food or drink unless the clinician is sure of the client's ability to swallow. The patient's tendency toward immobility (coupled with incontinence) increases the risk of pressure ulcers. Patients need to be encouraged to stand or reposition themselves frequently and will benefit from pressure-relieving wheelchair cushions and mattresses.

Evaluation

The occupational therapist will perform the OT evaluation, focusing on functional performance level related to work, leisure, ADL, and IADL. In addition, measurement of flexibility, strength, quality of movement, rigidity, standing and sitting balance, cognitive skills, and coordination is necessary. The OTA with training may participate in the evaluation of areas of occupation.

Interventions

Evidence-based reviews of rehabilitation strategies including OT interventions have demonstrated a positive effect on both client factors and areas of occupation.[12,13,50,58,68,71] In addition, they have demonstrated the need for further research to solidify the evidence base for OT intervention. In general, reviews have concluded that people living with PD can effectively learn new tasks and improve their functional performance through focused practice of meaningful tasks.[50]

Improving Participation in Areas of Occupation

Patients with PD benefit from learning strategies designed to increase efficiency, safety, and independence.[11] Strategies may be learned via graded task-specific practice and may include the use of adaptive devices and environmental modifications (Box 26-6).[18,58,76]

The patient should attend physical therapy for gait training as a foundation for functional mobility. The occupational therapist can supplement this training by using verbal cues to remind the patient to stand erect, lift the feet, and follow the prescribed gait pattern. Bed mobility skills, transfer training, and wheelchair mobility skills should be taught by the OTA if indicated. As the patient's ambulation status declines, a power or manual wheelchair may be required. The patient should be advised to purchase a lightweight wheelchair. Oblique rim projections, a pressure-relieving cushion, elevating swing-away leg rests, and reclining backs should be considered.

PD often makes it difficult for patients to pursue their hobbies and interests. Adaptive devices for playing cards and board games, gardening, and doing crafts are available through various vendors. The OTA may have to encourage the patient and family to develop new interests.

Motor Skills/Prevention of Deformities

The increased rigidity and tendency toward immobility put the PD patient at great risk for contracture development and general deconditioning. The PD patient requires a daily home exercise program for AROM and stretching, as well as clinic

Box 26-6

Examples of Modifications in Activities of Daily Living for People Living with Parkinson's Disease[7,18,58,76]

Feeding skills may be improved with weighted utensils (for subtle tremors), scoop dishes, Dycem® products, long straws, rocker knives, and cups with lids. Because of the control required for this task, meals should be timed with peak medication effects. See Box 26-3 for suggestions related to tremor control during feeding. Consider safe swallow strategies such as small bites/sips, alternating solids/liquids, staying upright after a meal, and avoiding taking thin liquids by straw. Food consistencies and the thickness of liquids should be considered.

Dressing skills may be enhanced with easy-to-use front fasteners (Velcro closures, elastic shoe laces, elastic waist bands, zipper pulls). Because of balance deficits, patients should be discouraged from bending down to don shoes and socks. Patients should instead be taught to sit and use long-handled shoe horns, reachers, sock aids, and dressing sticks and always to be seated when dressing. Patients with a shuffling gait should not wear rubber- or crepe-soled shoes because they may cause tripping. Flat leather soles are preferred. Ordering clothing one size larger may also ease donning and doffing procedures. Increased time should be scheduled for dressing.

Grooming tasks are simplified with electric toothbrushes, electric razors, and hands-free hair dryers. Bimanual oral care and shaving may be helpful. Suction brushes and soap holders may increase ease of grooming. Grooming tasks should be performed while seated. See Box 26-3 for suggestions about controlling tremors that interfere with grooming.

Bathing can be performed safely and more independently using long-handled brushes, "soap on a rope," soap pumps, and bath mitts. Durable medical equipment such as a bath bench or seat, grab bars, and a handheld shower will decrease fall risks and increase independence as well. No-slip bath mats (inside and outside the tub) should be considered. Sliding doors should be replaced with curtains.

Toileting ability is enhanced and made safer via raised toilet seats, 3:1 commodes, or toilet frames in conjunction with grab bars. Bedside commodes, male/female urinals, or condom-style catheters for men may be options for nighttime toileting needs.

Written communication may be enhanced by rhythmic writing programs, lined paper, or built-up pens. Printing may be easier than cursive writing. Word processors may be an option for some.

appointments in which the exercise program can be closely supervised by the OTA or occupational therapist. The frequency of the therapy is determined by the physician in consultation with the occupational therapist. AROM exercises may be done individually or in a group setting. Passive and/or active stretching exercises are indicated to maintain flexibility. Typical muscle groups and individual muscles that become limited and are a focus for stretching include the following:

- Hip flexors
- Knee flexors
- Gastrocnemius
- Pectoralis major and minor
- Anterior trunk/neck musculature

In the later stages of the disease, splinting may be indicated to maintain joint ranges and skin integrity. Verbal prompting and use of visual cues (sitting patient in front of mirror) can be used to promote improvement in posture. Encourage the patient to take deep breaths, and offer breathing exercises if indicated.

Clinicians can use visual, tactile, and auditory cues to help patients initiate movement.[42,72] Auditory cues should be short, firmly spoken commands such as "stop" and "step up." Rhythmic music and counting can also help to initiate movement. Auditory commands coupled with counting are especially helpful in teaching the patient transfer techniques.

Graded resistive exercises and gross motor activities, particularly sports activities, are used to develop strength and general mobility. Functional fine motor tasks such as jewelry making, manipulating money, and picking up small objects may assist in developing and maintaining hand function and coordination. These tasks can be graded by changing the size of the objects. The clinician should monitor and record the time it takes for the patient to complete the task assigned. Hand-strengthening modalities include repetitions with hand grippers and therapeutic putty exercises.

Communication

Parkinsonian patients often develop a monotone, low-volume speech. OT practitioners can increase the benefits of speech therapy by providing breathing and postural exercises. Diminished blinking responses and disturbances of the ocular muscles impair the patient's ability to read. Large-print books and audiobooks are useful with these patients. Computers and word processors offer an alternative for patients who have difficulty writing. Felt-tip markers are easier to use than are regular pens. A signature stamp is helpful in the workplace. Cordless and automatic dialing telephones simplify communication.

Psychosocial Issues

The person with PD typically tends to withdraw from society because of embarrassment, difficulty in mobility, and depression.[78] The patient and family need a daily schedule that encourages exercise, outside activity, and social contacts. Information and support groups for patients with PD and their families are available through local chapters of the Parkinson's Disease Foundation. The National Parkinson Foundation and the online computer network for PD also offer advice and education. Group counseling and day treatment programs provide emotional and social outlets.

Advanced Parkinsonism

In the latter stages of the disease, patients have severe deficits in communication, mobility, swallowing, and cognition. Social isolation becomes a serious problem. Secondary complications such as decubitus ulcers, aspiration pneumonia, fractures from falls, and contractures may arise. The OTA may help to prevent some of these problems. Use of a pressure-relieving mattress and cushion for the wheelchair, proper head alignment, and use of a flow control cup at meals, daily PROM, and splinting are interventions that should be explored with this population. Group activities at the patient's cognitive level help minimize the social isolation often experienced by those with advanced parkinsonism.

Amyotrophic Lateral Sclerosis

ALS, or Lou Gehrig's disease, is a progressive disease characterized by the degeneration of the motor neurons in the anterior horn cells of the spinal cord, brainstem, and corticospinal tracts. ALS is classified as a *motor neuron disease,* in which motor neurons gradually degenerate and die.[54] Both upper motor neurons and lower motor neurons are affected, eventually losing any ability to send messages to muscles. Consequently, muscles weaken and atrophy. Fasciculations or small twitch movements occur. Death is inevitable once the brain is affected and voluntary movement ceases.[54] Therapy practitioners working with ALS patients should be aware that:

- Patients lose the ability to breathe without ventilatory support once the muscles in the diaphragm and chest wall lose innervation.[54]
- Some individuals may become depressed and experience problems with memory and executive functions.[54]
- ALS does not affect a person's ability to see, smell, taste, hear, or recognize touch. Patients usually maintain control of eye muscles and bladder and bowel functions, although in the late stages of the disease most patients need help getting to and from the bathroom.[54]

Epidemiology

ALS is the most common form of motor neuron disease. Men are 20% more likely to have the disease than women. The usual age for diagnosis of ALS is between the ages of 40 and 70, with an average age of 55. Some cases occur in persons in their 20s and 30s. People of all races and ethnic backgrounds are affected. Approximately 30,000 Americans live with ALS, and an estimated 5600 are diagnosed each year.[2]

Cause

The cause of ALS is unknown. The majority of cases (90% to 95%) occur randomly (sporadic), whereas 5% to 10% of cases are considered familial. The pattern of inheritance requires only one parent to carry the gene that causes the disease. Approximately 20% of familial cases result from a gene defect. Environmental factors such as exposure to toxins or infectious agents are also being researched.[54]

Impact on Client Factors

ALS affects voluntary muscles. Because ALS involves both the upper and lower motor neurons, motor involvement includes both spasticity and stiffness (upper motor neuron) and weakness, low tone, and atrophy (lower motor neuron). In addition, bulbar signs such as speech deficits, swallowing difficulties, and respiratory involvement occur. Eye muscles, external sphincters controlling bowel and bladder management, the five senses, and the heart, liver, and kidneys are usually spared.[54]

Early symptoms of the disease include difficulty walking and/or picking up objects, and/or performing fine motor tasks. The number and side of the limbs affected vary from person to person. The client complains of weakness and stiffness. There is atrophy of the intrinsic muscles of the hands. The client exhibits hyperactive reflexes and fasciculations (twitching) that can be observed under the skin. Complaints of cramping are common. The weakness spreads to other muscle groups relatively quickly and involves all the limbs and the neck and trunk muscles.[54] Eventually the client's muscles become flaccid, resulting in severe disabilities (i.e., requiring total care) in performance in areas of occupation. Although ALS is primarily a disease of the motor system, emerging evidence suggests the presence of some cognitive involvement similar to that of frontal and temporal lobe dementia processes.[1,26,41] Signs may include decreased judgment and decision making.

Because of the severe pattern of weakness that emerges, ALS clients may consider themselves prisoners of their bodies. As the disease progresses, clients, families, and the team must decide whether or not ventilator support will be administered as respiratory muscles fail. Death generally results from respiratory complications.[54]

Medical Management

There is no cure for ALS. Treatment is primarily palliative. The Food and Drug Administration has approved the drug riluzole (Rilutek®) to slow progression of the disease.[54] Medication is also prescribed to reduce uncomfortable symptoms and improve quality of life through control of muscle spasms and pain, minimization of drooling, and treatment of depression. Respiratory and swallowing problems may require tracheotomy and gastrostomy procedures. Frequent suctioning to clear the airway may be necessary. Because of the patient's compromised respiratory system, care should be taken to avoid exposure to respiratory infections.

Occupational Therapy Management

The role of OT with the ALS patient is to enable the client to adapt and maintain the maximal level of functioning throughout the course of the disease, as well as to assist care providers with the necessary skills to safely and effectively assist with daily care issues.[6,11,73]

The initial OT evaluation establishes a baseline of functional abilities and limitations related to areas of occupation, ROM, muscle strength and tone, pain, and chewing and swallowing abilities. In addition, information regarding the home layout is obtained. Frequent reevaluation of the patient's status is required as the disease progresses. Evaluation procedures include standardized evaluations, interviews, and performance-based observations. The ALS Functional Rating Scale[45] is used throughout the country to monitor disease progression in this population.[16,25] It measures the following areas: speech, salivation, swallowing, handwriting, cutting food and handling utensils, dressing and hygiene, turning in bed and adjusting bed clothes, walking, climbing stairs, and respiratory insufficiency. The OTA may assist in the evaluation of occupational performance areas.

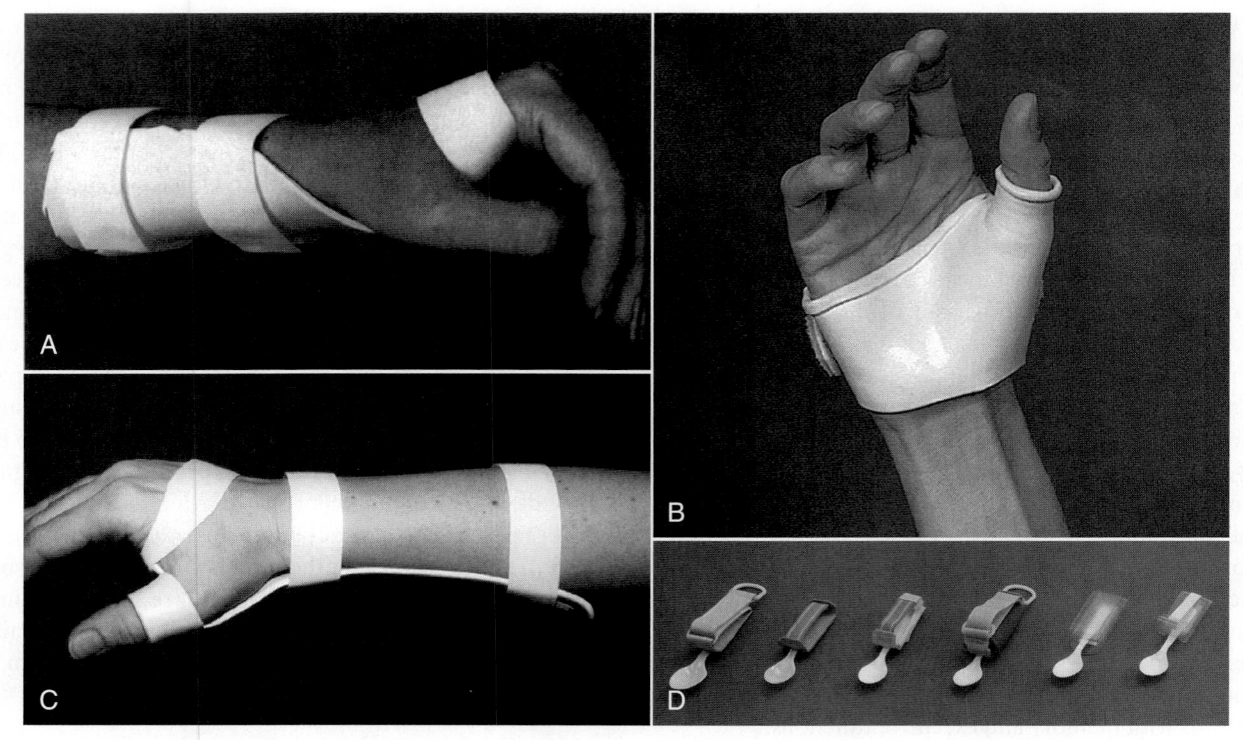

Figure 26-1 Typical splints used to increase or maintain function in those living with amyotrophic lateral sclerosis. The splints provide stability for unstable joints secondary to weakness and place the wrist or hand in a functional position. **A**, Wrist extension splint. **B**, Short opponens splint. **C**, Long opponens splint. **D**, Universal cuff. The universal cuff can be used in conjunction with a wrist support as well. (**A-C** From Fess EE, Gettle KS, Philips CA, et al: *Hand and upper extremity splinting: principles and methods,* ed 3, St. Louis, 2005, Mosby; **D** Courtesy Sammons Preston, Bolingbrook, Ill.)

Interventions

Improving Participation in Areas of Occupation

Intervention will vary depending on the stage of the disease. Early symptoms may include loss of fine motor coordination and hand weakness. Assistive devices such as built-up utensils and writing devices, Dycem®, suction devices, scoop dishes, plate guards, key holders, and devices to open containers may help improve function. Early balance changes due to weakness (i.e., foot drop) may necessitate adaptive ambulation devices or braces (e.g., an ankle foot orthotic) to prevent falls and improve upright function. The OTA should focus on using ambulation devices in functional situations such as kitchen activities and train the patient in relation to daily living problems such as transporting and carrying items.[6] Walker baskets or trays may be useful. Energy conservation techniques (see earlier) should be taught in the early stages of the disease.

As the disease progresses and UE weakness continues to progress, further adaptations are necessary. Functional splints may be necessary to maintain the ability to eat, use a computer, write, use a communication device or ECU, or turn pages. Typical splints that are used to maintain or increase function in this population are wrist extension splints, short or long opponens splints, universal cuff, or dorsal wrist extension splints with a universal pocket (Figure 26-1). In addition, head and neck stability may be compromised, thus requiring a cervical collar. Splints may be used in conjunction with an overhead suspension sling or deltoid aid to compensate for proximal weakness (Figure 26-2).

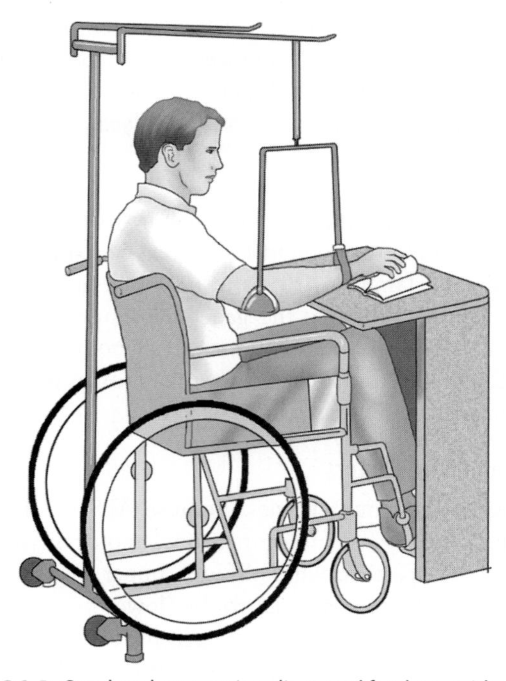

Figure 26-2 Overhead suspension sling used for those with proximal upper extremity weakness to enhance self-feeding, computer use, etc. (From Gillen G: *Stroke rehabilitation: a function-based approach,* ed 3, St. Louis, 2010, Elsevier.)

Trunk and/or LE weakness will affect the client's functional mobility skills. Transfers may be made easier for both clients and caregivers by teaching the use of a sliding board or mechanical lift.

Depending on financial means, home modifications such as ramps, elevators, stair-glides, and ceiling lifts may be necessary. Similarly, bathroom modifications and equipment such as roll-in showers, rolling commodes, pocket doors, offset hinges, removal of glass shower doors, and/or adapted bath seats help maintain independence, increase safety, and facilitate caregiver assistance.

Motor Skills and Prevention of Deformities

When using gentle therapeutic exercises with this population, the OT practitioner should take care to avoid fatiguing the patient. Gentle exercise matched to the patient's current condition will help maintain functional abilities and improve mood. Nonresistive, gradable exercise such as water activities or walking, tai chi, or gentle yoga is appropriate. PROM is provided when the patient cannot move the joint actively to the end of the range; PROM may be used in conjunction with positioning and splints to prevent contracture and control spasticity. Relaxation and deep breathing exercises should be taught. If exercise is an important occupation for the client, it should be done over several short periods throughout the day, rather than in one long session, so as to avoid fatigue. Exercise will not result in increased muscle bulk but may improve aerobic function, decrease fatigue, or help control depression. In the latter stages of the diseases more intensive passive stretching and ranging and splinting (i.e., resting hand splints) are required to prevent contracture development.[46]

Communication

The trauma associated with the loss of verbal communication skills is compounded by the fact that the patient retains significant mental capacity. The OT and speech therapy departments need to work jointly to establish an alternative method to help the patient communicate thoughts and needs. Initially the patient may be able to write. A communication board, an electronic communication aid, and a computer with a voice module offer other alternatives. The OTA may be involved in positioning the patient and fabricating the UE equipment and switches that enable use of these devices. It is important that the patient be able to call for help. Call bells that can be controlled with any part of the body with a minimal amount of pressure are available and will become necessary when the patient can no longer speak.

Assistive Technology

Computers and environmental control units enable the ALS patient to perform a variety of tasks, from speech to turning on lights and appliances. Computers can be activated by a variety of different types of keyboards and switches. The OTA can assist in determining the patient's functional capacity to operate these devices and may be called on to make recommendations as to the type of device to purchase or borrow.[27]

Mobility and Positioning

In the early stages of the disease, the patient will continue to ambulate with the help of a cane or walker but eventually will require a wheelchair. Although initially the patient may have sufficient strength to sit and propel a standard wheelchair, the progressive nature of the disease will inevitably necessitate a reclining or tilt-in-space motorized wheelchair.[70] For financial reasons, it may be wise to plan ahead when consulting on a wheelchair purchase. Proper positioning of the head may require a cervical collar and head support. Lateral supports to the wheelchair may have to be supplied in the latter stages of the disease. Pressure-relieving cushions are indicated. Local ALS care centers may be helpful in terms of procuring equipment via a lending program or suggesting ways to obtain financial assistance.

Psychosocial Issues

Reactive depression and anxiety disorders are common among those living with terminal diseases such as ALS. Medication and counseling may help ameliorate depression. The rehabilitation team needs to provide psychological support to help in coping with the devastating effects of the disease. Independence in meaningful activities may increase the patient's self-esteem in addition to improving functional status. Support groups or individual counseling for clients and their families should be recommended.

Alzheimer's Disease

Dementia is not a disease itself but rather a set of symptoms that accompanies a disease. Dementia refers to the loss of mental function in two or more areas such as language, memory, visual abilities, spatial abilities, or judgment that is severe enough to affect daily life. Many diseases cause dementia including multi-infarct dementia, PD, Huntington's disease, Pick's disease, and Creutzfeldt-Jakob disease. Other conditions such as AIDS, traumatic brain injury, and tertiary syphilis may result in symptoms of dementia. The most common known cause of irreversible dementia in adults is AD. Also known as *senile dementia of the Alzheimer type* (SDAT), this disease was first described by Dr. Alors Alzheimer in 1907. AD is a progressive, slow deterioration of brain tissue that results in decreased cognitive abilities including deficits in language and memory, disturbances in the sense of time and place, personality changes, and emotional instability.[55,67,77]

Epidemiology

AD affects approximately four and one half million Americans. By the year 2050, because of aging of the general population, the number of individuals living with AD could range from 11 to 16 million. Among Americans 1 in 10 has a family member with AD, and 1 in 3 knows somebody with the disease. In addition, 1 in 10 individuals older than 65 years old is affected, as are nearly half of those older than the age of 85. Rarely, inherited forms of the disease can affect individuals in their 30s and 40s.[55,67,77]

A person with AD will live an average of 8 years from the diagnosis but can also live up to 20 years after initial diagnosis. After diagnosis, individuals with AD survive about half as long as those of a similar age without dementia.

Cause

The cause of AD remains unclear. Potential causes and risks for AD include the following[55,67,77]:

- Increasing age. The likelihood of developing AD doubles every 5 years after age 65.
- Family history of the disease. The likelihood of developing AD increases as the number of family members with AD increases.
- Familial AD has been linked to specific genes. Most familial AD occurs before age 60.
- Variations in certain genes are being studied to determine whether they make some individuals more or less susceptible to the disease.

Signs and Symptoms

Early warning signs of AD include memory loss, difficulty performing familiar tasks, problems with language (i.e., as in word finding or word substitutions), disorientation, impaired judgment, decreased abstract thinking, misplacing items, mood or behavior changes, personality changes, and loss of initiative.

Various staging systems have been developed to document the disease progression from early stages to middle stages to late stages (Box 26-7).[61] Understanding the stage of AD will assist in setting goals and planning treatment.

Medical Management

Treatment of the patient with AD is primarily symptomatic. No cure or treatment will slow the progression of the disease. Medications are available to treat some of the behavioral and psychiatric manifestations of the disease but are most effective in conjunction with behavioral interventions and environmental modifications. Examples of medications that may be used include Celexa®, Prozac®, Paxil®, and Zoloft® to ameliorate decreased mood and irritability. For anxiety and restlessness, Ativan® or Serax® may be useful, and for management of hallucinations or delusions Seroquel®, Risperdal®, Clozaril®, and so on may be beneficial.[55,67,77]

Occupational Therapy Management

The role of OT in the treatment of patients with AD varies according to the stage of the disease but aims to maximize independence and to provide guidance and support to the family.[10]

Occupational Therapy Evaluation

The OT evaluation of the patient with AD establishes a baseline related to performance in areas of occupation and in cognitive, motor, and sensory skills. This evaluation is used to establish treatment guidelines and goals and may also help to determine the level of care and supervision necessary for the patient. Additionally, the evaluation will help in determining the timing and type (physical, gestures, verbal) of cues that improve performance. Information from the evaluation may assist the family in making the difficult decision of whether to maintain the patient in the home or to seek placement in an assisted living or long-term care facility.

Evaluation of cognition should be done through formalized assessment tools. Motor functioning should be evaluated by assessing active and passive ROM, coordination, balance, transfer skills, and praxis. The speech-language pathologist and the physical therapist may provide additional information to supplement the OT evaluation. Self-care evaluation includes observation of the patient's ability to feed, dress, groom, and toilet. In the early stages of the disease the OT evaluation may also include the patient's ability to perform housekeeping and work-related tasks.[10]

Leisure skills including the patient's ability to continue to participate in previously enjoyed hobbies should also be assessed. A thorough history should be obtained from the patient's family before evaluation.

The OT evaluation is performed by the occupational therapist. The OTA may be asked to complete the occupational performance part of the evaluation or to assist in determining the patient's perceptual and sensory skills. The occupational therapist coordinates the findings of the evaluation and

Box 26-7

Stages of Alzheimer's Disease[61]

Stage 1: No cognitive impairment

Stage 2: Very mild cognitive decline; subjective complaints of memory loss or word finding, not detected on formal examination.

Mild/Early-Stage Alzheimer's Disease

Stage 3: Mild decline: word-finding deficits, naming objects, misplacing objects, decrease in planning.

Stage 4: Moderate cognitive decline: decreased knowledge of recent events, decreased ability to perform higher-level mental calculations, decreased memory for personal information, inability to participate in complex tasks, socially withdrawn.

Moderate/Midstage Alzheimer's Disease

Stage 5: Moderately severe cognitive decline: major memory gaps, assistance needed for complex daily living tasks, confusion related to orientation, inability to perform simple calculations, still knows own name and names of spouse and children, needs help picking out clothing based on the season and weather.

Stage 6: Severe cognitive decline: memory worsens, personality changes emerge, extensive help required for ADL, occasionally forgets name of spouse, decreased dressing ability, dysfunction of sleep/wake cycle, assistance required for toileting, incontinence, delusions, hallucinations occur, compulsion/repetition of behaviors.

Severe/Late-Stage Alzheimer's Disease

Stage 7: Very severe cognitive decline: does not respond to environment, mutism, inability to control movement, requires feeding assist, loses ability to walk and sit without assistance, dysphagia, skeletal muscle rigidity.

determines the recommendations and treatment goals for the patient.

Interventions

Interventions continue to be developed for this population with positive results. See Box 26-8. The paragraphs that follow summarize essential aspects of OT intervention.

Activities of Daily Living

In the middle stages of AD the patient begins to demonstrate difficulty performing simple ADL. Frequent reminders to initiate a task such as "wash your face" or "put on your shirt" may be required. As the disease progresses, the patient has problems sequencing multistep tasks and benefits from help with breaking the tasks down into one-step segments. This process, known as task segmentation, guides the patient to complete ADL tasks with the verbal prompting of the therapist and also helps to train and refocus on the task at hand. Instead of saying, "Wash your face," the patient is instructed, "Pick up the wash cloth. Put the wash cloth in the water. Now put some soap on the wash cloth. Wash around your mouth." These instructions are offered in a calm, reassuring manner. Positive feedback in the form of praise is provided after each step. Physical prompts (hand-over-hand assistance) may also be given if the patient permits it. The OT should instruct patients' caregivers in these task segmentation methods and may need to remind them of the importance of allowing patients to perform as much of their own daily care as possible.

A patient with AD typically demonstrates poor frustration tolerance. It is important to avoid situations that may trigger catastrophic reactions. Activities should be analyzed and graded to ensure that the patient has sufficient physical and cognitive skill to perform the task requested.

The patient's physical deterioration may contribute to safety problems in the home. Bathroom safety devices should be prescribed if indicated. The family should be advised of hazards in the home or the patient's environment that need to be removed or safeguarded. Scatter rugs, power tools, electric appliances, medications, stairways, windows, balconies, household cleansers, smoking materials, and the kitchen stove are just some of the items that represent a serious potential hazard to the patient.

Mealtimes can be difficult for both the patient and the caregiver. Confused patients are often messy, fussy eaters. Adaptive eating devices such as scoop dishes, spill-proof cups, and built-up utensils may be helpful. If the patient no longer uses utensils, it may be easier to have the caretaker provide finger foods than to try to force use of a fork. The patient may demonstrate swallowing difficulties. The occupational therapist can instruct the caregiver in feeding techniques for the dysphagic patient including changing the food consistency, maintaining the head in neutral position, putting small amounts of food on the spoon, ensuring that the previous mouthful of food has been swallowed before offering the next spoonful, encouraging swallowing with verbal prompting and facilitation techniques, using a thickening agent in liquids, and using a flow control cup.

Environmental Design

The OTA can help the caregiver structure the environment to help maximize the patient's functioning. Eliminating clutter in the environment helps to minimize confusion. Contrasting colors make it easier for the patient to differentiate an object from the background. Simple changes such as eliminating the condiments from the kitchen table and ensuring contrast of color between the plate and table (and the plate and the food) simplify mealtime. Contrasting the color of the toilet seat and bowl with the bathroom floor helps to aid in toileting. Minimizing the amount of furniture and maintaining traffic areas free of obstacles decrease the risk of falls in the home. Gates and locks on stairways and doors may need to be installed for safety. Signs identifying the patient's room and bathroom may be helpful. The OT clinic should also incorporate some of these design features.[33,56,66]

Box 26-8

Evidence Briefs and Alzheimer's Disease/Dementia

- Dooley and Hinojosa[14] (2004): This study examined the extent to which adherence to occupational therapy recommendations would increase the quality of life of persons with Alzheimer's disease living in the community and decrease the burden felt by family members caring for them. Caregivers completed measures of their feelings of burden and the quality of life including level of function of the persons with Alzheimer's disease. The authors concluded that individualized occupational therapy intervention based on the person-environment fit model appears effective for both caregivers and clients.
- Graff, Vernooij-Dassen, Thijssen, et al.[22] (2006): This study set out to determine the effectiveness of community-based occupational therapy on daily functioning of patients with dementia and the sense of competence of their caregivers. The intervention consisted of 10 sessions of occupational therapy over 5 weeks including cognitive and behavioral interventions to train patients in the use of aids to compensate for cognitive decline and caregivers in coping behaviors and supervision. The authors concluded that occupational therapy improved patients' daily functioning and reduced the burden on the caregiver, despite the patients' limited learning ability. Effects were still present at 12 weeks.
- Graff, Vernooij-Dassen, Thijssen, et al.[23] (2007): This study set out to investigate effects of community occupational therapy on dementia patients' and caregivers' quality of life, mood, and health status and caregivers' sense of control over life. The intervention (as described earlier) consisted of 10 sessions of occupational therapy over 5 weeks or no intervention. Cognitive and behavioral interventions were used to train patients in the use of aids to compensate for cognitive decline and caregivers in coping behaviors and supervision. The authors concluded that community occupational therapy should be advocated both for dementia patients and their caregivers because it improves their mood, quality of life, and health status and caregivers' sense of control over life. Effects were still present at follow-up.

Day Care and Group Activities

Programs at adult day care facilities offer the caregiver a respite from the daily pressure and stress of taking care of a loved one with AD. These programs offer a variety of group activities within a structured environment, striving to provide the patient with positive social opportunities. Group activities, whether offered in a day care setting or as part of the activity program in a long-term care facility, may be administered by OT clinicians. The patients often enjoy music-based activities, simple and familiar games, and crafts. Teaching new activities is not recommended. Also enjoyed are sensory stimulation, reminiscing games, and pet therapy visits. Childish activities that may be demeaning to the patient should be avoided. The occupational therapist working in this area should consult the numerous books on activity programs for the dementia patient for further suggestions.

Reality Orientation

Patients with AD become less oriented as the disease progresses. Formal daily orientation programs to review the patient's name, the date, the weather, and the location may be helpful. In addition, the patient should always be addressed by name, and all staff should introduce themselves and tell the patient their function regularly as if they have just met. The practitioner should regularly review the names of the patients' close family members and show them their rooms, the dining room, etc. Clocks and calendars should be clearly displayed. Memory books may also be used.[24]

Exercise Programs

Exercise, whether offered as a group or individual activity, is important to maintain strength, coordination, and ROM. Simple group calisthenics can be done in a standing or sitting position. The addition of rhythmic music helps to keep the patient involved in the activity. Parachute activities and ball, scarf, or balloon tosses are good group exercise activities. Dancing and walking are activities that the caretaker can easily do with the patient. If the patient cannot participate in group exercise programs or if he or she has joint contractures, the patient should be involved in a daily PROM program. It is recommended that exercise programs be offered at the same time each day to help establish a routine.

Psychosocial Issues

Patients with AD may demonstrate a variety of behavior problems including agitation, physical aggression, depression, inappropriate sexual behaviors, "stealing," paranoia, and hallucinations. The patient may receive some form of medication for these problems, but behavioral interventions are frequently preferable to chemical interventions that may have serious side effects.[73] The OT practitioner should always approach the patient while using a calm, reassuring voice. He or she should not become angry or argue with the patient and should redirect and refocus the patient to a different topic. Clear instructions on how to behave or what is acceptable should be offered. Using the name of the patient's spouse in the request often helps to achieve the desired behavior (e.g., "Mary wants you to take a bath now."). Reducing the amount of stimulation, noise, or unstructured time sometimes helps to decrease agitation and antisocial behavior.[62] The patient should be seen in OT when the clinic is relatively quiet and distractions are minimal.

In the final stages of the disease, the patient most often requires long-term and skilled nursing care. The patient may receive OT services in the form of nursing rehabilitation programs for ROM, positioning recommendations, splinting to prevent contractures or maintain ROM and skin integrity, and sensory stimulation.

Throughout the course of the disease, the family will need guidance and support to help cope with the effect of the AD on the patient and the family structure.[29] The nature of the disease demands changes and may necessitate role reversals in the family. The OTA and other team members should be prepared to provide support for these difficult transitions. Families may also seek advice from the Alzheimer's Disease and Related Disorders Association and from online chat groups and informational services.

Summary

This chapter has focused on four degenerative diseases: MS, PD, ALS, and AD. Although other neurologic diseases also result in progressive loss of function, the OT practitioner will find that the treatment goals and interventions for the diseases outlined in this chapter will be helpful in treating all patients with degenerative disorders.

Managing this population is difficult and can take an emotional toll on clients, therapists, and caregivers. Because of the multitude of problems encountered in this population, close collaboration between the occupational therapist and the OTA is necessary. In addition, all people living with these diagnoses can benefit from an interdisciplinary approach for optimal outcomes.

Selected Reading Guide Questions

1. List the precautions that need to be observed when treating a patient with MS.
2. Briefly describe the three clinical signs associated with PD and explain how these signs affect the treatment process.
3. Discuss the psychosocial aspects of treating patients with degenerative diseases.
4. Describe how assistive technology can be used to increase the functional level of the patient with ALS.
5. Describe the treatment goals associated with each of the diseases discussed in this chapter: MS, PD, ALS, and AD.
6. Describe the ways the OTA can help the MS patient cope with fatigue.
7. Explain how the OTA can use adaptive devices to promote independence in feeding skills for patients with degenerative diseases.
8. Describe the techniques used by the OT practitioner to promote proper positioning and the prevention of decubitus ulcers in patients with degenerative diseases.

CASE STUDY

Peter

Peter is a 30-year-old loan officer who enjoys movies, fishing, eating out, and concerts. He was recently engaged to be married. Peter has a 5-year history of multiple sclerosis. One week ago he suffered an exacerbation of symptoms. He is motivated, alert, and oriented × 3. He is able to follow complex directions but lacks concentration on tasks as presented. His speech is understandable. He often loses his train of thought.

Motor function: Peter demonstrates 4/5 strength in both UEs. The greatest limiting factor is fatigue. His LEs are graded as 2/5 on manual muscle testing (MMT).

Sensory: UE sensation is intact, absent light touch, and pinprick is evident from his navel level and below.

Postural control: Peter requires close supervision for static sitting and moderate assistance for all weight shifting and reaching activities beyond his arm span. He falls laterally and posteriorly while seated.

Neurobehavioral deficits: Peter's greatest complaint is loss of short-term memory and feeling "disorganized." He also reports feeling "blue and tired." His greatest fear is that this exacerbation will limit his ability to work. In addition, the occupational therapist notes that he presents with deficits related to sustained attention and short-term memory.

ADL: Peter requires moderate assist for dressing, bathing, and toileting. In addition, all sliding board transfers require minimal assistance. He feels that his dependency in these areas is "humiliating."

Peter has just been transferred to the rehabilitation unit, and you will be the primary OT practitioner working with him. Peter's desire is to return home and to work as soon as possible.

1. Reread the above material. Underline and star the problems of most concern to the patient.
2. Place problems in order of priority and select the first three. State a short-term goal for each. Describe one or more treatment methods the OTA could use to address this goal.
3. Describe the type of wheelchair and the wheelchair features that would be appropriate for Peter at this time.
4. Describe how you would respond to Peter's desire to return to work.

9. Describe the role of the OTA in the treatment and prevention of contractures with patients with MS, PD, ALS, and AD.
10. List some of the environmental changes that the OTA may recommend in the home of a patient with AD.

References

1. Abe K: Cognitive function in amyotrophic lateral sclerosis, *Amyotrophic Lateral Scler Other Motor Neuron Disord* 1(5):343–347, 2000.
2. ALS Association: *About ALS, who gets ALS.* http://www.alsa.org/als/who.cfm. Accessed February 16, 2011.
3. Arnett PA, Higginson CI, Voss WD, et al: Relationship between coping, cognitive dysfunction and depression in multiple sclerosis, *Clin Neuropsychol* 16(3):341–355, 2002.
4. Bobholz JA, Rao SM: Cognitive dysfunction in multiple sclerosis: a review of recent developments, *Curr Opin Neurol* 16(3):283–288, 2003.
5. Calabresi PA: Diagnosis and management of multiple sclerosis, *Am Fam Physician* 70(10):1935–1944, 2004.
6. Casey P: Occupational therapy. In Mitsumoto HM, editor: *Amyotrophic lateral sclerosis: a comprehensive guide to management*, New York, 2001, Denos Medical Publishing.
7. Cianci H, Cloete L, Gardner J, et al: *Activities of daily living: practical pointers for Parkinson's disease*, Miami, 2004, National Parkinson Foundation.
8. Clarke C, Moore AP: Parkinson's disease update, *Clin Evid* 11:1736–1754, 2004.
9. Cohen JR, Dinerstein GR, Katz ER: Living with low vision, *Inside MS* 19(1), 2001.
10. Corcoran MA: Occupational therapy intervention for persons with dementia and their families, *OT Pract* 7(20), 2002.
11. Corr B, Frost E, Traynor BJ, et al: Service provision for patients with ALS/MND: a cost-effective multidisciplinary approach, *J Neurol Sci* 160(Suppl 1), 1998.
12. de Goede CJT, Keus SHJ, Kwakkel G, et al: The effects of physical therapy in Parkinson's disease: a research synthesis, *Arch Phys Med Rehabil* 82(4):509–515, 2001.
13. Dixon L, Duncan DC, Johnson P, Kirkby L, O'Connell H, Taylor HJ, Deane K. Occupational therapy for patients with Parkinson's disease. Cochrane Database of Systematic Reviews 2007, Issue 3. Art. No.: CD002813. DOI: 10.1002/14651858.CD002813.pub2
14. Dooley NR: Hinojosa J: Improving quality of life for persons with Alzheimer's disease and their family caregivers: brief occupational therapy intervention, *Am J Occup Ther* 58(5):561–569, 2004.
15. Finlayson M: *Occupational therapy in multiple sclerosis rehabilitation*, NY, 2008, National Multiple Sclerosis Society.
16. Francis K, Bach JR, DeLisa JA: Evaluation and rehabilitation of patients with adult motor neuron disease, *Arch Phys Med Rehabil* 80(8):951–963, 1999.
17. Frohman EM: *Diagnosis and management of vision problems in MS*, NY, 2008, National Multiple Sclerosis Society.
18. Gillen G: *Cognitive and perceptual rehabilitation: optimizing function*, St. Louis, 2009, Elsevier.
19. Gillen G: Maximizing independence: occupational therapy intervention for patients with Parkinson's disease, *Loss Grief Care J Prof Pract* 8(3-4):65–67, 2000.
20. Gillen G: Improving activities of daily living performance in an adult with ataxia, *Am J Occup Ther* 54(1):89–96, 2000.
21. Gillen G: Improving mobility and community access in an adult with ataxia, *Am J Occup Ther* 56(4):462–466, 2002.
22. Graff MJL, Vernooij-Dassen MJM, Thijssen M, et al: Community-based occupational therapy for patients with dementia and their care givers: randomised controlled trial, *Br Med J* 333(7580):1196, 2006.
23. Graff MJL, Vernooij-Dassen MJM, Thijssen M, et al: Effects of community occupational therapy on quality of life, mood, and health status in dementia patients and their caregivers: a randomized controlled trial, *J Gerontol Series A Biol Sci Med Sci* 62(9):1002–1009, 2007.
24. Hafler DA: Multiple sclerosis, *J Clin Invest* 113(6):788–794, 2004.
25. Han JJ, Carter GT, Hecht TW, et al: The Amyotrophic Lateral Sclerosis Center: a model of multidisciplinary management, *Crit Rev Phys Med Rehabil* 15(1):21–40, 2003.

26. Hanagasi HA, Gurvit IH, Ermutlu N, et al: Cognitive impairment in amyotrophic lateral sclerosis: evidence from neuro-psychological investigation and event-related potentials, *Cog Brain Res* 14(2):234–244, 2002.
27. Hatakeyama T, Okamoto A, Kamata K, et al: Assistive technology for people with amyotrophic lateral sclerosis in Japan: present status, analysis of problem and proposal for the future, *Technol Disabil* 13(1):9–15, 2000.
28. Hoehn M, Yahr M: Parkinsonism: onset, progression, and mortality, *Neurology* 17(5):427–442, 1967.
29. Hogan VM, Lisy ED, Savannah RL, et al: Role change experienced by family caregivers of adults with Alzheimer's disease: implications for occupational therapy, *Phys Occup Ther Geriatr* 22(1):21–43, 2003.
30. Holland NJ: *Bowel management in multiple sclerosis*, NY, 2008, National Multiple Sclerosis Society.
31. Holland NJ, Reitman NC: *Bladder dysfunction in multiple sclerosis*, NY, 2008, National Multiple Sclerosis Society.
32. Jones L, Lewis Y, Harrison J, et al: The effectiveness of occupational therapy and physiotherapy in multiple sclerosis patients with ataxia of the upper limb and trunk, *Clin Rehabil* 10(4): 277–282, 1996.
33. Josephsson S, Backman L, Borell L, et al: Effectiveness of an intervention to improve occupational performance in dementia, *Occup Ther J Res* 15(1):36–49, 1995.
34. Joy JE, Johnston RB: *Multiple sclerosis: current status and strategies for the future. In Committee on Multiple Sclerosis: current status and strategies for the future*, Washington DC, 2001, National Academic Press.
35. Kalb R, Reitman N: *Overview of multiple sclerosis*, NY, 2010, National Multiple Sclerosis Society.
36. Kushner S, Brandfass K: *Spasticity*, NY, 2008, National Multiple Sclerosis Society.
37. Kesselring J: Neurorehabilitation in multiple sclerosis: what is the evidence-base? *J Neurol* 251(Suppl 4):IV25–IV29, 2004.
38. Law M, Baptiste S, Carswell A, et al: *The Canadian Occupational Performance Measure*, ed 4, Ottawa, 2005, CAOT Publications ACE.
39. Law M, Baptiste S, Mills J: Client-centered practice: what does it mean and does it make a difference? *Can J Occup Ther* 62(5): 250–257, 1995.
40. Lemke MR, Fuchs G, Gemende I, et al: Depression and Parkinson's disease, *J Neurol* 251(Suppl 6):VI28–VI32, 2004.
41. Lomen-Hoerth C, Murphy J, Langmore S, et al: Are amyotrophic lateral sclerosis patients cognitively normal? *Neurology* 60(7):1094–1097, 2003.
42. Ma H, Trombly CA, Tickle-Degnen L, et al: Effect of one single auditory cue on movement kinematics in patients with Parkinson's disease, *Am J Phys Med Rehabil* 83(7):530–536, 2004.
43. Mathiowetz V, Matuska KM, Murphy ME: Efficacy of an energy conservation course for persons with multiple sclerosis, *Arch Phys Med Rehabil* 82(4):449–456, 2001.
44. Meyer B: Coping with severe mental illness: relations of the Brief COPE with symptoms, functioning, and well-being, *J Psychopathol Behav Assess* 23:265–277, 2001.
45. Miano B, Stoddard GJ, Davis S, et al: Inter-evaluator reliability of the ALS functional rating scale, *Amyotroph Lateral Scler Other Motor Neuron Disord* 5(4):235–239, 2004.
46. Mitsumoto H, Shockley L: Amyotrophic lateral sclerosis: continuum of care from diagnosis through hospice, *Home HealthCare Consultant* 5(6):20–29, 1998.
47. Mohr DC, Classen C, Barrera M Jr: The relationship between social support, depression and treatment for depression in people with multiple sclerosis, *Psychol Med* 34(3):533–541, 2004.
48. Mohr DC, Dick LP, Russo D, et al: The psychosocial impact of multiple sclerosis: exploring the patient's perspective, *Health Psychol* 18(4):376–382, 1999.
49. Multiple Sclerosis Council for Clinical Practice Guidelines: *Fatigue and multiple sclerosis: evidence-based management strategies for fatigue in multiple sclerosis*, Washington DC, 1998, Paralyzed Veterans of America.
50. Murphy S, Tickle-Degnen L: The effectiveness of occupational therapy-related treatments for persons with Parkinson's disease: a meta-analytic review, *Am J Occup Ther* 55(4):385–392, 2001.
51. National Clinical Advisory Board: *Management of MS-related fatigue*, NY, 2008, National Multiple Sclerosis Society.
52. National Clinical Advisory Board: *Assessment and management of cognitive impairment in multiple sclerosis*, NY, 2008, National Multiple Sclerosis Society.
53. National Institute of Neurological Disorders and Stroke: *Parkinson's disease: hope through research*, Bethesda, Md, 2006, National Institutes of Health.
54. National Institute of Neurological Disorders and Stroke: *Amyotrophic lateral sclerosis fact sheet*, Bethesda, Md, 2003, National Institutes of Health.
55. National Institute of Neurological Disorders and Stroke: *The dementias: hope through research*, Bethesda, Md, 2004, National Institutes of Health.
56. Painter J: Home environment considerations for people with Alzheimer's disease, *Occup Ther Health Care* 10(3):45–63, 1996.
57. Panisset M: Freezing of gait in Parkinson's disease, *Neurol Clin* 22(Suppl 3):53–62, 2004.
58. Patti F, Reggio A, Nicoletti F, et al: Effects of rehabilitation therapy on Parkinson's disability and functional independence, *J Neurologic Rehabil* 10(4):223–231, 1996.
59. Petajan JH, Gappmaier E, White AT, et al: Impact of aerobic training on fitness and quality of life in multiple sclerosis, *Ann Neurol* 39(4):432–441, 1996.
60. Pollock N: Client-centered assessment, *Am J Occup Ther* 47(4):298–301, 1993.
61. Reisberg B, Ferris SH, de Leon MJ, et al: The Global Deterioration Scale for assessment of primary degenerative dementia, *Am J Psychiatry* 139(9):1136–1139, 1982.
62. Rogers JC, Holm MB, Burgio LD, et al: Improving morning care routines of nursing home residents with dementia, *J Am Geriat Soc* 47(9):1049–1057, 1999.
63. Samuel L, Cavallo P: *Emotional issues of the person with MS*, NY, 2008, National Multiple Sclerosis Society.
64. Schiffer RB: *Cognitive loss in multiple sclerosis*, NY, 2008, National Multiple Sclerosis Society.
65. Schwid SR, Petrie MD, Murray R, et al: A randomized controlled study of the acute and chronic effects of cooling therapy for MS, *Neurology* 60(12):1955–1960, 2003.
66. Sheldon MM, Teaford MH: Caregivers of people with Alzheimer's dementia: an analysis of their compliance with recommended home modifications, *Alzheimers Care Q* 3(1):78–81, 2002.
67. Srinivas P: Diagnosis and management of Alzheimer's disease: an update, *Med J Malaysia* 54(4):541–549, 1999.
68. Steultjens EMJ, Dekker J, Bouter LM, et al: Evidence of the efficacy of occupational therapy in different conditions: an overview of systematic reviews, *Clin Rehabil* 19(3):247–254, 2005.

69. Strickland D, Bertoni JM: Parkinson's prevalence estimated by a state registry, *Move Disord* 19(3):318–323, 2004.
70. Trail M, Nelson N, Van JN, et al: Wheelchair use by patients with amyotrophic lateral sclerosis: a survey of user characteristics and selection preferences, *Arch Phys Med Rehabil* 82(1):98–102, 2001.
71. Trend P, Kaye J, Gage H, et al: Short-term effectiveness of intensive multidisciplinary rehabilitation for people with Parkinson's disease and their careers, *Clin Rehabil* 16(7):717–725, 2002.
72. Tse DW, Spaulding SJ: Review of motor control and motor learning: implications for occupational therapy with individuals with Parkinson's disease, *Phys Occup Ther Geriatr* 15(3):19–38, 1998.
73. van den Berg JP, de Groot IJ, Joha BC, et al: Development and implementation of the Dutch protocol for rehabilitative management in amyotrophic lateral sclerosis, *Amyotroph Lateral Scler Other Motor Neuron Disord* 5(4):226–229, 2004.
74. Vanage SM, Gilbertson KK, Mathiowetz V: Effects of an energy conservation course on fatigue impact for persons with progressive multiple sclerosis, *Am J Occup Ther* 57(3):315–323, 2003.
75. Walter BL, Vitek JL: Surgical treatment for Parkinson's disease, *Lancet Neurol* 3(12):719–728, 2004.
76. Ward CD, Robertson D: Rehabilitation in Parkinson's disease, *Rev Clin Gerontol* 13(3):223–239, 2003.
77. Weiner MF: Alzheimer's disease update: using what we now know to help patients, *Consultant* 39(3):675–678, 1999.
78. Welsh M: Parkinson's disease and quality of life: issues and challenges beyond motor symptoms, *Neurol Clin* 22(Suppl 3): 141–148, 2004.
79. Winogrodzka A, Wagenaar RC, Booij J, et al: Rigidity and bradykinesia reduce interlimb coordination in Parkinsonian gait, *Arch Phys Med Rehabil* 86(2):183–189, 2005.

CHAPTER 27 Spinal Cord Injury

CAROLE ADLER

Key Terms

Quadriplegia
Tetraplegia
Paraplegia
ASIA impairment scale
Vital capacity
Hypotension
Autonomic dysreflexia
Spasticity
Heterotopic ossification
Tenodesis
Decubitus ulcers

Chapter Objectives

After studying this chapter, the student or practitioner will be able to do the following:

1. Understand the difference between complete and incomplete spinal cord injury and the classification system used to describe such levels of injury.
2. Recognize and identify the various spinal cord injury syndromes.
3. Briefly describe the medical and surgical management of the individual who has experienced a traumatic spinal cord injury.
4. Identify some of the complications that can limit optimal functional potential.
5. Describe the changes in sexual functioning in males and females after spinal cord injury.
6. Identify the specific assessment tools employed by the occupational therapist before developing treatment objectives.
7. Analyze the critical issues faced by the occupational therapy practitioner in developing treatment objectives during the acute, active, and discharge phases of the rehabilitation process.
8. Identify in detail the functional outcomes including equipment considerations and personal and home care needs that can be reached at each level of complete injury under optimal circumstances.
9. Describe how the normal aging process is accelerated by the effects of spinal cord injury and explain how functional status may change.

CASE STUDY

Mr. S.

Mr. S. is a 44-year-old Caucasian man who sustained a C7-8 complete (ASIA A) spinal cord injury (SCI) as a result of a fall. He also sustained facial lacerations and bilateral radial wrist fractures, which necessitated casting without internal fixation. Mr. S. is divorced with no biological children. He is a firefighter and has a background in auto mechanics. Mr. S. is athletic; he is a triathlete and marathon runner. Just before his accident, Mr. S. had moved into a second-story apartment.

Mr. S. was referred to occupational therapy (OT) on the day of his injury and initially was evaluated in the intensive care unit within 24 hours of injury. He was immobilized in cervical traction and bilateral wrist casts on a kinetic bed. His specific manual muscle test revealed 3+ to 4 strength in deltoids, biceps, and triceps. Wrists could not be tested secondary to bilateral wrist casts, and finger and thumb flexion and extension were noted to be at least 2− bilaterally. Sensory examination was intact to the C7 dermatome. Vital capacity was low secondary to the absence of innervation of intercostal and abdominal musculature, and Mr. S. required respiratory treatments four times daily to mobilize lung secretions. Because of his immobilization, he required assistance for all aspects of his self-care and mobility.

OT treatment objectives included (1) maintaining optimal range of motion (ROM) in all joints for optimal upper extremity (UE) function and seated positioning; (2) achieving optimal strength and endurance in available musculature; (3) achieving optimal independence in all self-care skills including bathing, toileting, and skin care; (4) achieving independent wheelchair mobility on all indoor and outdoor surfaces; (5) receiving appropriate durable medical equipment (DME) to meet both short- and long-term needs (e.g., manual and power wheelchair, cushion, and bathing and toileting equipment); (6) returning to safe and accessible housing; and (7) being educated in all aspects of care and independently instructing caregivers in assistance needed.

CASE STUDY—cont'd

Mr. S. has had a difficult time accepting that he has a complete SCI. He could not imagine how he could function at work and in his community as a quadriplegic. His college and church community offered a tremendous amount of support, yet he continued to be depressed and angry over his loss of mobility and independence. He received regular psychological counseling and attended a weekly peer support group.

On discharge from acute rehabilitation, Mr. S. returned to a newly rented single-story home that required bathroom modifications and ramps at the front and back entrances. Mr. S. initially received 4 hours of attendant care daily. He required assistance only for completion of his daily bath and bowel program, as well as for some homemaking tasks. After Mr. S. received in-home OT for home setup and community transition issues, his need for personal care diminished; he now requires only homemaking assistance. He regularly visits a neighborhood gym to maintain UE strength and endurance, and he will soon be driving a modified van. His vocational plans are on hold until his van and driving training are completed.

Throughout this chapter, consider the muscles that are sufficiently innervated to be clinically functional, the areas of dysfunction, the optimal equipment to enhance mobility, and the long-term consequences of Mr. S.'s injury in relation to his lifestyle.

Rehabilitation of the individual with a spinal cord injury (SCI) is a lifelong process that requires readjustment to nearly every aspect of life. The occupational therapy assistant (OTA) and the occupational therapist play a significant role in physical and psychosocial restoration and in helping the individual achieve maximum independence. Through accurate assessment, retraining, and adaptive techniques and equipment, occupational therapy (OT) practitioners provide their patients with the tools and resources needed to achieve their maximal physical and functional potential.

SCIs occur for many reasons; trauma is the most common. Trauma can result from motor vehicle accidents, violent injuries such as gunshot and stab wounds, falls, sports accidents, and diving accidents.[5,15] Normal spinal cord function may also be disturbed by diseases such as tumors, myelomeningocele, syringomyelia, multiple sclerosis, cancer, and amyotrophic lateral sclerosis. Some of the treatment principles outlined in this chapter may have application to these conditions; however, the emphasis is on rehabilitation of the individual with a traumatic SCI.

Results of Spinal Cord Injury

SCI results in quadriplegia (more recently labeled tetraplegia by the American Spinal Cord Injury Association) or paraplegia. Tetraplegia is any degree of paralysis of the four limbs and trunk musculature. There may be partial upper extremity (UE) function, depending on the level of the cervical lesion. Paraplegia is paralysis of the lower extremities (LEs) with some involvement of the trunk and hips depending on the level of the lesion.[5,15]

SCIs are discussed in terms of the regions (cervical, thoracic, and lumbar) of the spinal cord in which they occur and the numerical order of the neurological segments. The level of SCI designates the last fully functioning neurological segment of the cord. For example, C6 refers to the sixth neurological segment of the cervical region of the spinal cord as the last fully intact neurological segment.[5,13] Complete lesions result in the absence of motor or sensory function of the spinal cord below the level of the injury

Incomplete lesions may involve several neurological segments, and some spinal cord function may be partially or completely intact.[3,13] For example, a C5 injury may have the last intact neurological level at C5 with a zone of partial preservation (ZPP) to C7, with absence of neurological function below C7.

Complete Versus Incomplete Neurological Classifications

The extent of neurological damage depends on the location and severity of the injury (Figure 27-1). In a complete injury, total paralysis and loss of sensation result from a complete interruption of the ascending and descending nerve tracts below the level of the lesion. In an incomplete injury some of the sensory or motor nerve pathways below the level of the lesion are preserved and intact. Pathways must be preserved in the sacral segments to qualify as incomplete. Segments at which normal function is found often differ on the two sides of the body; further, a given segment may have differences between sensory and motor function as revealed by testing.

A very careful neurological examination, performed by trained clinicians, is essential to determine whether an injury is complete or incomplete.

The American Spinal Injury Association (ASIA) impairment scale uses the findings from the neurological examination to categorize injury types into specific categories (Box 27-1).[2]

Clinical Syndromes

Central Cord Syndrome

Central cord syndrome occurs when there is more cellular destruction in the center of the cord than in the periphery. Paralysis and sensory loss are greater in the UEs because these nerve tracts are more centrally located than nerve tracts for the LEs. This syndrome is often seen in older people in whom arthritic changes or developing stenosis have caused a narrowing of the spinal canal; in such cases cervical hyperextension without vertebral fracture may precipitate central cord damage.

Brown-Séquard Syndrome (Lateral Damage)

Brown-Séquard syndrome results when only one side of the cord is damaged, as in a stabbing or gunshot injury. Motor paralysis and loss of proprioception occur below the level of injury, on the ipsilateral side. Loss of pain, temperature, and touch sensation occurs on the contralateral side.

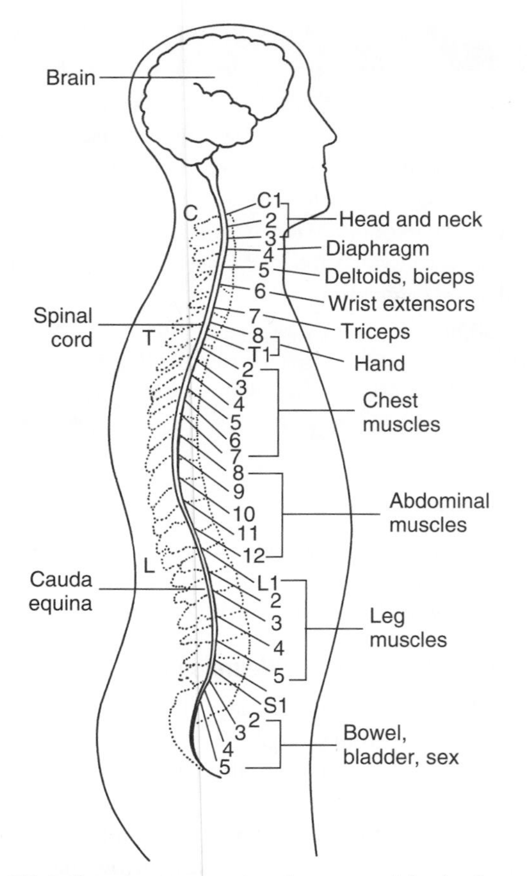

Figure 27-1 Spinal nerves and major areas of body they supply. (From Paulson S, editor: *Santa Clara Valley Medical Center spinal cord injury home care manual,* ed 2, San Jose, Calif, 1994, Santa Clara Valley Medical Center.)

Box 27-1

Standard ASIA Impairment Scale Classification

ASIA classification A indicates a complete lesion; there is no motor or sensory function preserved in the sacral segments S4-S5.

ASIA classification B indicates an incomplete lesion; sensory but not motor function is preserved below the neurological level and includes the sacral segments S4-S5.

ASIA classification C indicates an incomplete lesion; motor function is preserved below the neurological level, and more than half of the key muscles below the neurological level have a muscle grade less than 3.

ASIA classification D indicates an incomplete lesion; motor function is preserved below the neurological level, and at least half of the key muscles below the neurological level have a muscle grade of 3 or more.

ASIA classification E indicates that motor and sensory functions are normal.

Anterior Spinal Cord Syndrome

Anterior spinal cord syndrome results from injury that damages the anterior spinal artery or the anterior aspect of the cord. This syndrome involves paralysis and loss of pain, temperature, and touch sensation. Proprioception is preserved.

Cauda Equina (Peripheral)

Cauda equina injuries involve peripheral nerves rather than directly involving the spinal cord. This usually occurs with fractures below the L2 level and results in a flaccid-type paralysis. Because peripheral nerves possess a regenerating capacity that the cord does not, prognosis for recovery is better with this injury. Patterns of sensory and motor deficits are highly variable and asymmetrical.

Conus Medullaris Syndrome

Injury of the sacral cord (conus) and lumbar nerve roots within the neural canal usually result in an areflexic bladder, bowel, and lower extremities.

Posttraumatic Period

After SCI the victim enters a stage of spinal shock that may last from 24 hours to 6 weeks. This period is one of areflexia, in which reflex activity ceases below the level of the injury.[13] The bladder and bowel are atonic or flaccid. Deep tendon reflexes are decreased, and sympathetic functions are disturbed. This disturbance results in decreased constriction of blood vessels, low blood pressure, a slower heart rate, and no perspiration below the level of injury.[9,15]

The spinal cord is usually not damaged below the level of the lesion. Therefore muscles that are innervated by the neurological segments below the level of injury usually develop spasticity because the monosynaptic reflex arc is intact but separated from higher inhibitory influences. Deep tendon reflexes become hyperactive, and spasticity may be evident. Sensory loss continues, and the bladder and bowel usually become spastic ("upper motor neuron" bladder) in patients whose injuries are above T12. The bladder and bowel usually remain flaccid ("lower motor neuron" bladder) in patients whose lesions are at L1 and below. Sympathetic functions become hyperactive. Spinal reflex activity (mass muscle spasms) usually becomes evident in the areas below the level of the lesion.[3,12,14]

Prognosis for Recovery

The prognosis for substantial recovery of neuromuscular function after SCI depends on whether the lesion is complete or incomplete. If there is no sensation or return of motor function below the level of lesion 24 to 48 hours after the injury in carefully assessed complete lesions, motor function is less likely to return. However, partial to full return of function to one spinal nerve root level below the fracture can be gained and may occur in the first 6 months after injury. In incomplete lesions, progressive return of motor function is possible, yet determining exactly how much and how quickly return will occur is difficult.[14] The longer it takes for recovery to begin, often the less likely it is that it will occur.

The following statements can be used as guidelines to predict the recovery process following a new injury and assist therapists and patients in anticipating what is to come[10]:

- The severity of the original injury determines whether recovery will occur. Unfortunately, no method exists at present to measure this severity, and predictions must be

based on what has happened in past cases with similar neurological findings.
- Incomplete injuries have a better chance of further recovery than complete injuries, but even with incomplete injuries, the extent of the recovery cannot be predicted or guaranteed.
- Most of the recovery that will occur starts within the first few weeks. Therefore as time passes without any return of function, it means that recovery is less likely.
- No amount of hard work will make the nerve function return. If hard work were all it took, very few people would end up with permanent paralysis.
- Rehabilitation will not determine the degree of recovery. The goals of rehabilitation include prevention and minimization of further medical complications through education; maintenance and improvement of strength and skills that are present; maximizing function in self-care activities; facilitating mobility; and optimizing lifestyle options for the patient and his or her family. The overall goal is maintaining the body and general well-being in a "recovery-ready" mode.

Medical and Surgical Management of the Person with Spinal Cord Injury

After a traumatic event in which SCI is likely, the conscious victim should be questioned carefully about cutaneous numbness and skeletal muscle paralysis before being moved. Emergency medical technicians, paramedics, and air transport personnel are trained in SCI precautions and extrication techniques for moving a possible SCI victim from an accident site. Movement of the spine must be prevented during the transfer procedures. A firm stretcher or board to which the victim's head and back can be strapped should be procured before moving the victim. After the victim is transferred to the stretcher or board, he or she should be strapped to the board or stretcher and carefully transferred via air or ground transport to the nearest hospital emergency department. Axial traction on the neck should be maintained, and any movement of the spine and neck should be prevented during this process. Careful examination, stabilization, and transportation of the patient may prevent a temporary or minimal SCI from becoming more severe or permanent. Initial care is directed toward preventing further damage to the spinal cord and reversing neurological damage, if possible, by stabilization or decompression of the injured neurological structures.[5,11,13] Antiinflammatory and steroidal drugs may be administered immediately after injury in an effort to minimize swelling at the site of the lesion and thus minimize neurological damage, although the significance of their effect on neurological recovery is still unclear.

The examining physician performs a careful neurological examination to aid in determining both the bony and neurological type of injury. The patient is in a supine position for this procedure, with the neck and spine immobilized. Typically, a catheter is placed in the patient's bladder for drainage of urine. Anteroposterior and lateral x-ray films may be taken,

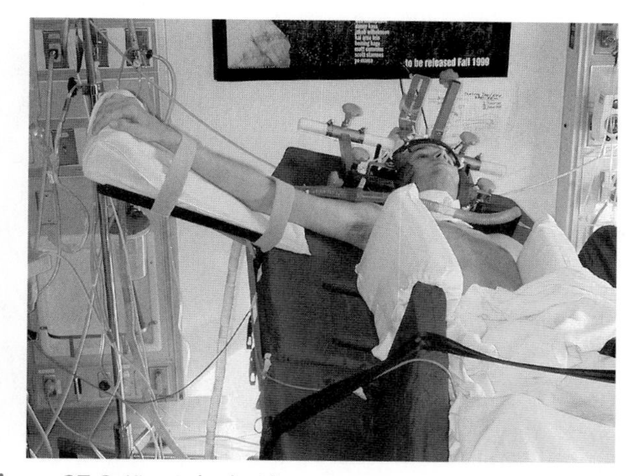

Figure 27-2 Kinetic bed with custom arm positioner. Designed and fabricated by the Occupational Therapy Department, Santa Clara Valley Medical Center of San Jose, Calif. (Courtesy Luis Gonzalez, Media Resource Department, Santa Clara Valley Medical Center.)

with the patient's head, neck, or spine immobilized, to help determine the type of injury. A computed tomography (CT) scan or magnetic resonance imaging (MRI) may be necessary for further evaluation. In early medical treatment the goals are to restore normal alignment of the spine, maintain stabilization of the injured area, and decompress neurological structures that are under pressure.

Bony realignment and stabilization are usually achieved by immobilization and can include placing the patient on a rotating kinetic bed (Figure 27-2) that also allows for skeletal traction. The bed's constant rotation allows continuous pressure relief, mobilization of respiratory secretions, and easy access to the patient's entire body for bowel, bladder, and hygiene care. Patients can also be placed on a standard low air loss mattress and hospital bed.

Open surgical reduction with internal fixation and spinal fusion may be indicated. The goals of surgery are to decompress the spinal cord and to achieve spinal stability and normal bony alignment.[5,13] Surgery is not always necessary, and adequate immobilization may allow the patient to heal. As soon as possible, a means of portable immobilization is provided, usually a halo vest or cervical collar for cervical injuries (Figure 27-3, *A*) and a thoracic, brace, or body jacket for thoracic injuries (Figure 27-3, *B*). Portable immobilization allows the patient to be transferred to a standard hospital bed and subsequently to be up in a wheelchair and involved in an active therapy program in as little as 1 to 2 weeks after injury. Initiating an upright sitting tolerance program shortly after injury can substantially reduce the incidence and severity of further medical complications such as deep vein thrombosis, joint contractures, skin breakdown, and the general deconditioning that can result from prolonged bed rest.

The benefits of early transport to an SCI center have been documented.[6] Patients treated initially in a spinal cord acute-care unit rather than a general hospital had shorter acute-care lengths of stay. Patients treated in general hospitals tended to have a higher incidence of skin problems and spinal instability. It has been found that patients sent to rehabilitation

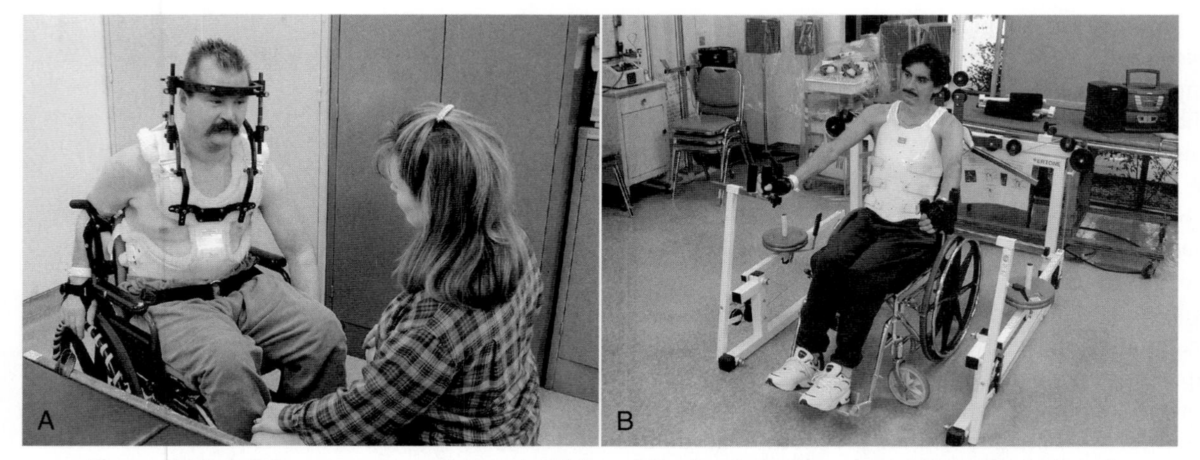

Figure 27-3 **A**, Halo vest, one type of cervical neck immobilization device for patients with quadriplegia and high-level paraplegia (T1 to T4). **B**, Body jacket, one type of immobilization device for paraplegia. (Courtesy Luis Gonzalez, Media Resource Department, Santa Clara Valley Medical Center.)

centers specializing in the treatment of SCI made functional gains with greater efficiency.[15] Spinal cord centers are able to offer a comprehensive, multidisciplinary program executed by an experienced team of professionals who specialize in this unique and demanding disability.

Complications of Spinal Cord Injury

Skin Breakdown, Pressure Sores, or Decubitus Ulcers

Sensory loss increases the risk of skin breakdown. The patient with sensory loss cannot feel the pressure and shearing of prolonged sitting or lying in one position or the presence of pain or heat against the body. Pressure causes the loss of blood supply to the area, which can ultimately result in necrosis (death of tissue) below the surface of the skin. Heat can quickly burn and destroy tissues. Shearing can destroy underlying tissue. Any combination of these issues will hasten skin breakdown. The areas most likely to develop skin breakdown are bony prominences over the sacrum, ischium, trochanters, elbows, and heels; however, other bony prominences such as the iliac crest, scapula, knees, toes, and rib cage are also at risk.

It is important for all rehabilitation personnel to be aware of the signs of developing skin problems. At first the area reddens yet blanches when pressed. Later, the reddened or abraded area does not blanch, which indicates that necrosis has begun. Finally, a blister or ulceration appears in the area. Often the problem is more severe below the level of the skin surface. The visible sore may only be the tip of the iceberg. If allowed to progress, a sore can become severe, destroying underlying tissues even as deep as the bone.

Skin breakdown can be prevented by relieving and eliminating pressure points and protecting vulnerable areas from excessive shearing, moisture, and heat. Turning in bed on a routine basis, using specialized mattresses and pressure-relieving wheelchair seat cushions, protecting bony prominences with various types of padding, and performing weight shifts are some of the methods used to prevent pressure sores.

The use of hand splints, body jackets, and other orthoses can also cause skin breakdowns. The OTA will share in the responsibility for inspecting the patient's skin, and the patient must be taught to examine his or her skin on a consistent, daily basis, using a mirror or caregiver assistance to watch for signs of developing problems. Skin damage can develop within 30 minutes; therefore frequent weight shifting, repositioning, and vigilance are essential for preventing skin breakdown.[13,17]

Decreased Vital Capacity

Decreased vital capacity is a problem in people who have sustained cervical and high thoracic lesions. Such individuals have markedly limited chest expansion and decreased ability to cough because of weakness or paralysis of the diaphragm and the intercostal and latissimus dorsi muscles, which can cause a tendency to develop infections of the respiratory tract. Reduced vital capacity affects the overall endurance level for activity. Endurance can be improved by assisted breathing and by vigorous respiratory and physical therapy. Strengthening of the sternocleidomastoids and the diaphragm, manually assisted coughing, and deep breathing exercises are essential to maintain optimal vital capacity.[12,14]

Osteoporosis

Osteoporosis is likely to develop in patients with SCIs because of disuse of long bones, particularly of the LEs. Osteoporosis may be sufficiently advanced for pathological fractures to occur a year after the injury. Pathological fractures are most common in the supracondylar area of the femur, the proximal tibia, the distal tibia, the intertrochanteric area of the femur, and the neck of the femur. Pathological fractures are usually not seen in UEs. Daily standing with a standing frame may slow the onset of osteoporosis[13,17]; however, this method is controversial and is not embraced in all rehabilitation programs. A standing program must fit into the patient's activities of daily living (ADL) routine after discharge to be effective on an ongoing basis. Not all reimbursement sources will cover the cost of standing equipment.

Orthostatic Hypotension

A lack of muscle tone in the abdomen and LEs leads to pooling of blood in these areas, with a resultant decrease in blood pressure (hypotension). This problem occurs when the patient moves from a supine to upright position or changes body position too quickly. Symptoms are dizziness, nausea, and loss of consciousness.[5] The patient must be reclined quickly and, if sitting in a wheelchair, tipped back with legs elevated until symptoms subside. With time this problem can diminish as sitting tolerance and level of activity increase; however, some people continue to have hypotensive episodes. Abdominal binders, compression garments, antiembolism stockings, and medications can aid in reducing symptoms.

Autonomic Dysreflexia

Autonomic dysreflexia is a phenomenon seen in persons whose injuries are above the T6 level. It is caused by reflex action of the autonomic nervous system in response to some stimulus such as a distended bladder, fecal mass, bladder irritation, rectal manipulation, thermal or pain stimuli, or visceral distention. The symptoms are immediate pounding headache, anxiety, perspiration, flushing, chills, nasal congestion, sudden onset of hypertension, and bradycardia.

Autonomic dysreflexia is a medical emergency and life threatening. The patient should not be left alone.[5,13,17] The condition is treated by placing the patient in an upright position and removing anything restrictive such as abdominal binders or elastic stockings to reduce blood pressure. The bladder should be drained, or the legbag tubing should be checked for obstruction. Blood pressure and other symptoms should be monitored until they return to normal. The OTA must be aware of symptoms and treatment because autonomic dysreflexia can occur at any time after the injury.

Spasticity

Spasticity is a common complication of SCI.[18] It is an involuntary muscle contraction below the level of injury that results from lack of inhibition from the brain. Patterns of spasticity change over the first year, gradually increasing in the first 6 months and reaching a plateau about 1 year after the injury. A moderate amount of spasticity can be helpful in the overall rehabilitation of the patient with an SCI. Spasticity helps to maintain muscle mass, assists in the prevention of pressure sores by facilitating blood circulation, and can assist in range of motion (ROM) and bed mobility. A sudden increase in spasticity can alert the patient to other medical problems such as bladder infections, skin breakdown, or fever.

Severe spasticity can be frustrating to both the patient and the therapist, in that it can interfere with function. It may be treated more aggressively with a variety of medications. In select instances, local injections of nerve blocks or Botox may benefit some patients. In severe cases neurosurgical procedures can be performed.[5,12,14]

Heterotopic Ossification

Heterotopic ossification (HO), also called *ectopic bone*, is bone that develops in abnormal anatomic locations.[18] It most often occurs in the muscles around the hip and knee, but occasionally it can be noted at the elbow and shoulder. The first symptoms are swelling, warmth, and decreased joint ROM. Symptoms are often discovered during physical or occupational therapy treatments despite negative radiologic findings. The onset of HO is usually 1 to 4 months after injury. Early diagnosis and initiation of treatment can minimize complications. Treatment consists of medication and the maintenance of joint ROM during the early stage of active bone formation, to preserve the functional ROM necessary for good wheelchair positioning, symmetrical position of the pelvis, and maximal functional mobility. If HO progresses to the phase of substantially limiting hip flexion, pelvic obliquity while in the sitting position is likely to occur. This problem contributes to trunk deformities such as scoliosis and kyphosis, with subsequent skin breakdown at the ischial tuberosities, trochanters, and sacrum.[5,13]

Sexual Function

The sexual drive and the need for physical and emotional intimacy are not altered by SCI. However, problems of mobility, functional dependency, and altered body image, as well as complicating medical problems and the attitudes of partners and society, affect social and sexual roles, access, and interest and satisfaction. Education is essential for the spinal cord–injured individual and all clinicians and is a critical part of the rehabilitation process.

Lack of sensation over one part of the body is accompanied by increased or altered sensation over other parts of the body. The sexual response of the body after SCI needs to be explored in the same way a person learns what muscles are working and where he or she can feel.

In males, erections and ejaculations are often affected by SCI. However, this problem is variable and needs to be evaluated individually. Often the motility of sperm in men with SCI is decreased even when other function is near normal.[1] Significant advances in treatment are identifying the possible sources of infertility associated with SCI and exploring ways to address the problem.

In women, menstruation usually ceases for an interval of weeks to months after injury. It will usually start again and return to normal in time. Vaginal lubrication during sexual activity may change, but fertility is not affected. Females with SCI can conceive and give birth. Special attention must be given to the interaction of pregnancy and childbirth with SCI, especially in regard to blood clots, respiratory function, bladder infections, dysreflexia, the use of medications during pregnancy, and breastfeeding.

To avoid pregnancy, women with SCI must take precautions and the type of birth control must be considered carefully. Birth control pills are associated with blood clots, especially when combined with smoking, and probably should not be used. The intrauterine device (IUD) is not recommended, even for able-bodied females. Diaphragms may be difficult to position properly when there is loss of sensation in the vagina or decreased hand function. Foams and suppositories are not effective. Use of condoms by the male partner is probably the safest method.

Individuals with disability quickly sense the attitudes of professionals and caregivers toward their sexuality. Awareness and acceptance by professionals are increasing, and sexual counseling and education are a regular part of many rehabilitation programs for all types of physical disabilities. Some patients lack basic sex education. Others feel asexual because of their disability and altered self-esteem and are isolated from peers; thus they may feel uncomfortable with any type of sexual interaction. For these reasons sexual education and counseling must be geared to the needs of the individual patient and his or her significant other. In some instances social interaction skills need improvement before sexual activity can be considered, and occupational therapists play an important role in providing information and a forum to deal with these issues. (See Chapter 16 and the suggested readings and websites at the end of the chapter for more information on sexuality with physical dysfunction.)

Occupational Therapy Intervention

Evaluation

Assessment of the patient is an ongoing process that begins on the day of admission and continues long after discharge on an outpatient follow-up basis. Depending on whether the patient is in an acute inpatient rehabilitation, outpatient, or home setting, the OT staff should continually assess the patient's functional progress and the appropriateness of treatment and equipment. An accurate and comprehensive formal initial evaluation is essential to determine baseline neurological, clinical, and functional status to formulate a treatment program and substantiate progress. Initial data gathered from the medical chart will provide personal information, a medical diagnosis, and a history of other pertinent medical information. Input from the multidisciplinary team will enhance the occupational therapist's ability to predict realistic optimal outcomes accurately.

Discharge planning begins during the initial evaluation. Therefore the patient's social and vocational history, as well as past and expected living situations, is necessary for planning a treatment program that meets the patient's ongoing needs. Treatment should begin as soon as possible. It is possible to gather enough information quickly to begin addressing high-priority areas such as achievable activities, splinting, positioning, and family training without having to wait for the evaluation to be completed.

Physical Status

The occupational therapist performs the evaluation, the results of which will be essential for the OTA in selecting treatment options to meet the patient's needs most appropriately.

Before contact with the patient, the occupational therapist obtains specific medical precautions from the primary and consulting physicians. Skeletal instability and related injuries or medical complications will affect the way in which the patient is moved and the active or resistive movements allowed.

Passive range of motion (PROM) is measured before an ASIA neurological examination or specific manual muscle testing to determine available pain-free movement. This evaluation also identifies the presence of or potential for joint contractures, which could suggest the need for preventive or corrective splinting and positioning.

Shoulder pain, which ultimately causes decreased shoulder and scapular ROM, is extremely common in C4-7 tetraplegic patients. Scapular immobilization resulting from prolonged bed rest and nerve root compression subsequent to the injury is one possible cause. Shoulder pain must be thoroughly assessed and diagnosed so that proper treatment can be provided before the onset of chronic discomfort and functional loss.

Accurate assessment of the patient's muscle strength is critical in determining a precise diagnosis of neurological level and establishing a baseline for physical recovery and functional progress. Using accepted ASIA motor examination and muscle testing protocols ensures accurate technique in this complex evaluation. The motor examination should be repeated as often as needed to provide an ongoing picture of the patient's strength and progress.

Sensation is evaluated for light touch, superficial pain (pinprick), and kinesthesia and to determine areas of absent, impaired, and intact sensation. These findings are useful in establishing the level of injury and determining functional limitations (Figure 27-4).[4]

If the patient is evaluated in the acute stage, spasticity is rarely noted because the patient is still in spinal shock. When spinal shock subsides, increased muscle tone may be present in response to stimuli. The therapist will then determine whether the spasticity interferes with or enhances function.

An evaluation of wrist and hand function will determine the degree to which a patient can manipulate objects. This information is used to suggest the need for equipment such as positioning splints or universal cuffs or, later, for a tenodesis orthosis (wrist-driven flexor hinge splint). Gross grasp and pinch measurements indicate functional abilities and may be used as an adjunct to muscle testing to provide objective measurements of baseline status and progress for patients who have active hand musculature.[7]

Clinical observation is used to assess endurance, oral motor control, head and trunk control, LE functional muscle strength, and total body function. More specific assessment in any of these areas may be required, depending on the individual. The OTA's observation skills in these areas will assist the other team members in their treatment progressions.

An increased number of combined traumatic SCI-head injury diagnoses suggests that a specific cognitive and perceptual evaluation may be necessary.[8] Assessing a patient's ability to initiate tasks, follow directions, carry over learning day to day, and do simple and high-level problem solving contributes to the information base needed for appropriate and realistic goal setting. Understanding the patient's learning style, coping skills, and communication style is also essential.

Functional Status

Observing the patient performing ADL is an important part of the OT evaluation. It is a primary area of treatment intervention and skill of the OTA. The purpose of this observation is to determine present and potential levels of functional ability. If the patient is cleared of bed rest precautions, evaluation and simultaneous treatment should begin as soon as possible after injury. Light activities such as feeding, hygiene at the sink, and

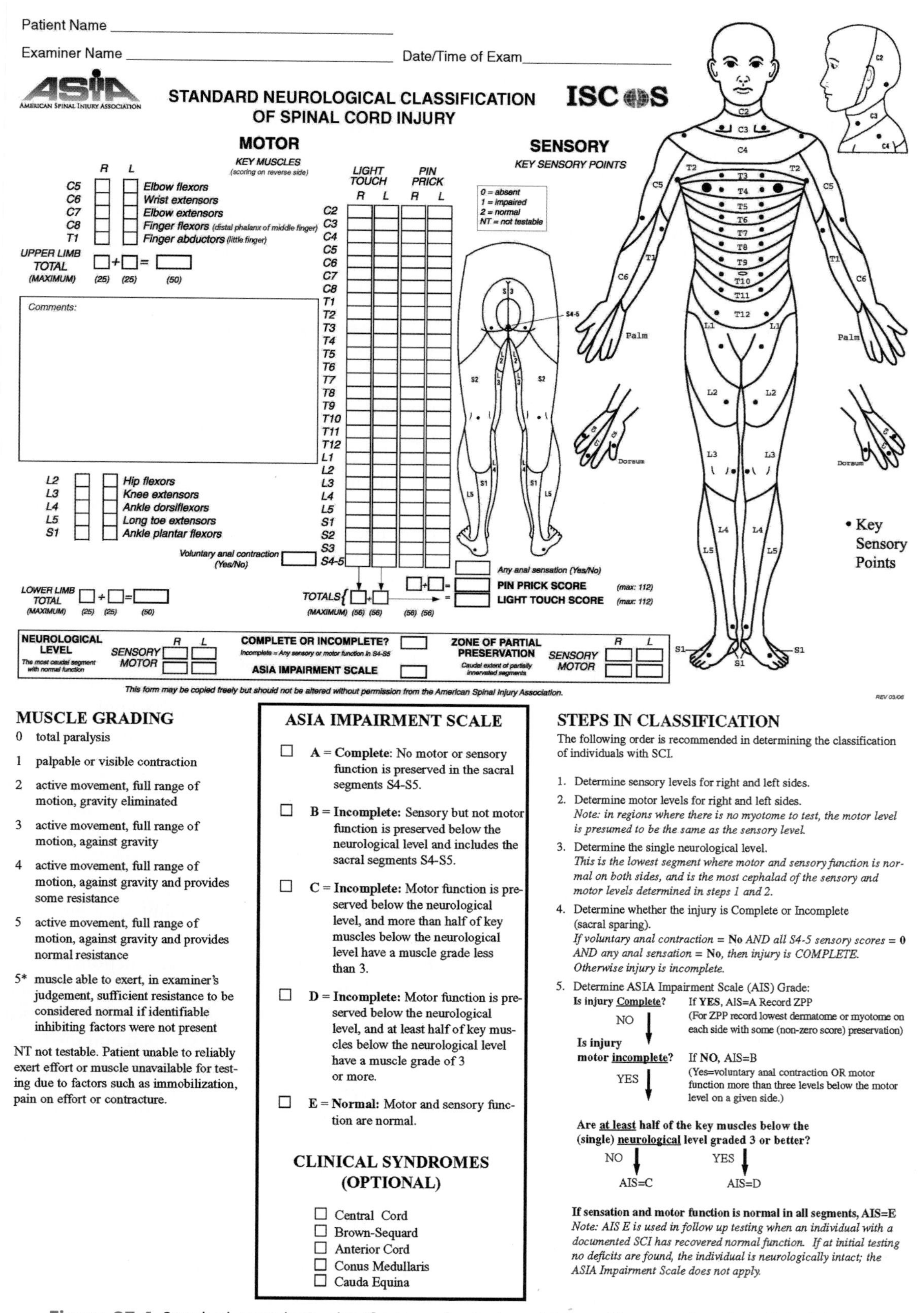

Patient Name ______________________

Examiner Name ______________________ Date/Time of Exam ______________

ASIA — AMERICAN SPINAL INJURY ASSOCIATION

STANDARD NEUROLOGICAL CLASSIFICATION OF SPINAL CORD INJURY

ISCoS

MOTOR

KEY MUSCLES (scoring on reverse side)

	R	L	
C5	☐	☐	Elbow flexors
C6	☐	☐	Wrist extensors
C7	☐	☐	Elbow extensors
C8	☐	☐	Finger flexors (distal phalanx of middle finger)
T1	☐	☐	Finger abductors (little finger)

UPPER LIMB TOTAL ☐ + ☐ = ☐
(MAXIMUM) (25) (25) (50)

Comments:

	R	L	
L2	☐	☐	Hip flexors
L3	☐	☐	Knee extensors
L4	☐	☐	Ankle dorsiflexors
L5	☐	☐	Long toe extensors
S1	☐	☐	Ankle plantar flexors

Voluntary anal contraction (Yes/No) ☐

LOWER LIMB TOTAL ☐ + ☐ = ☐
(MAXIMUM) (25) (25) (50)

SENSORY

KEY SENSORY POINTS

LIGHT TOUCH R L — PIN PRICK R L

C2, C3, C4, C5, C6, C7, C8, T1, T2, T3, T4, T5, T6, T7, T8, T9, T10, T11, T12, L1, L2, L3, L4, L5, S1, S2, S3, S4-5

0 = absent
1 = impaired
2 = normal
NT = not testable

TOTALS ☐ + ☐ ☐ + ☐
(MAXIMUM) (56) (56) (56) (56)

Any anal sensation (Yes/No) ☐

PIN PRICK SCORE (max: 112) ☐

LIGHT TOUCH SCORE (max: 112) ☐

NEUROLOGICAL LEVEL — The most caudal segment with normal function — SENSORY R ☐ L ☐ MOTOR R ☐ L ☐

COMPLETE OR INCOMPLETE? ☐ — Incomplete = Any sensory or motor function in S4-S5

ASIA IMPAIRMENT SCALE ☐

ZONE OF PARTIAL PRESERVATION — Caudal extent of partially innervated segments — SENSORY R ☐ L ☐ MOTOR R ☐ L ☐

This form may be copied freely but should not be altered without permission from the American Spinal Injury Association.

REV 03/06

MUSCLE GRADING

0 total paralysis

1 palpable or visible contraction

2 active movement, full range of motion, gravity eliminated

3 active movement, full range of motion, against gravity

4 active movement, full range of motion, against gravity and provides some resistance

5 active movement, full range of motion, against gravity and provides normal resistance

5* muscle able to exert, in examiner's judgement, sufficient resistance to be considered normal if identifiable inhibiting factors were not present

NT not testable. Patient unable to reliably exert effort or muscle unavailable for testing due to factors such as immobilization, pain on effort or contracture.

ASIA IMPAIRMENT SCALE

☐ A = **Complete:** No motor or sensory function is preserved in the sacral segments S4-S5.

☐ B = **Incomplete:** Sensory but not motor function is preserved below the neurological level and includes the sacral segments S4-S5.

☐ C = **Incomplete:** Motor function is preserved below the neurological level, and more than half of key muscles below the neurological level have a muscle grade less than 3.

☐ D = **Incomplete:** Motor function is preserved below the neurological level, and at least half of key muscles below the neurological level have a muscle grade of 3 or more.

☐ E = **Normal:** Motor and sensory function are normal.

CLINICAL SYNDROMES (OPTIONAL)

☐ Central Cord
☐ Brown-Sequard
☐ Anterior Cord
☐ Conus Medullaris
☐ Cauda Equina

STEPS IN CLASSIFICATION

The following order is recommended in determining the classification of individuals with SCI.

1. Determine sensory levels for right and left sides.
2. Determine motor levels for right and left sides.
   Note: in regions where there is no myotome to test, the motor level is presumed to be the same as the sensory level.
3. Determine the single neurological level.
   This is the lowest segment where motor and sensory function is normal on both sides, and is the most cephalad of the sensory and motor levels determined in steps 1 and 2.
4. Determine whether the injury is Complete or Incomplete (sacral sparing).
   If voluntary anal contraction = **No** *AND all S4-5 sensory scores =* **0** *AND any anal sensation =* **No***, then injury is COMPLETE. Otherwise injury is incomplete.*
5. Determine ASIA Impairment Scale (AIS) Grade:

Is injury Complete? If YES, AIS=A Record ZPP (For ZPP record lowest dermatome or myotome on each side with some (non-zero score) preservation)

NO ↓

Is injury motor incomplete? If NO, AIS=B (Yes=voluntary anal contraction OR motor function more than three levels below the motor level on a given side.)

YES ↓

Are at least half of the key muscles below the (single) neurological level graded 3 or better?

NO ↓ AIS=C — YES ↓ AIS=D

If sensation and motor function is normal in all segments, AIS=E
Note: AIS E is used in follow up testing when an individual with a documented SCI has recovered normal function. If at initial testing no deficits are found, the individual is neurologically intact; the ASIA Impairment Scale does not apply.

Figure 27-4 Standard neurologic classification of spinal cord injury. (Courtesy American Spinal Injury Association, March, 2006.)

object manipulation may be appropriate, depending on the level of injury.

Direct interaction with the patient's family and friends provides valuable information regarding the patient's support systems while in the hospital and, more important, after discharge. This information is relevant to later caregiver training in areas in which the patient may require the assistance of others to accomplish self-care and mobility tasks.

In addition to physical and functional assessments, the OTA has the opportunity to observe the patient's psychosocial adjustment to the disability and life in general through the activities in which the patient participates.[13] Establishing rapport and mutual trust is important to facilitate participation and progress in later and more difficult phases of rehabilitation. An individual's motivation, determination, socioeconomic background, education, family support, acceptance of disability, problem-solving abilities, and financial resources can be invaluable assets or limiting factors in determining the outcome of rehabilitation. The OTA must clearly observe the patient's status and communicate the observations to the primary occupational therapist so that treatment approaches that are effective and consistent for each particular patient are selected.

Establishing Treatment Objectives

Establishing treatment objectives in concert with the patient, family, and rehabilitation team is important. The primary objectives of the rehabilitation team may not be those of the patient. Psychosocial factors, cultural factors, cognitive deficits, environmental limitations, and individual financial considerations must be identified and integrated into a treatment program that will meet the unique needs of each individual. Every patient is different; therefore a variety of treatment approaches and alternatives may be necessary to address each factor that may affect goal achievement.[6] Increased participation can be expected if the patient's priorities are respected to the extent that they are achievable and realistic.

The general objectives for OT treatment of the person with SCI are the following:

1. To maintain or increase joint ROM and prevent deformity via active ROM (AROM) and PROM, splinting, and positioning
2. To increase the strength of all innervated and partially innervated muscles through the use of enabling and purposeful activities
3. To increase physical endurance via enabling and purposeful activities
4. To maximize independence in all aspects of self-care, mobility, and homemaking and parenting skills
5. To explore leisure interests and vocational potential
6. To aid in the psychosocial adjustment to disability
7. To evaluate, recommend, and train the patient in the use and care of necessary durable medical and adaptive equipment
8. To ensure safe and independent home and environmental accessibility through safety and accessibility recommendations
9. To assist the patient in developing the communication skills necessary to train and instruct caregivers to provide safe assistance
10. To educate patients and their families as to the benefits and consequences in relation to long-term function and the aging process of maintaining healthy and responsible lifestyle habits

The patient's length of stay in the inpatient rehabilitation program and ability to participate in outpatient therapy determine the appropriateness and priority of the just-named activities.

Treatment Methods

Acute Phase

During the acute, or immobilized, phase of the rehabilitation program the patient may be in traction or wearing a stabilization device such as a cervical collar or body jacket. Medical precautions must be implemented during this period. Flexion, extension, and rotary movements of the spine and neck are contraindicated.

Optimizing total body positioning and necessary hand splinting should be initiated at this time. In patients with tetraplegia, scapular elevation and elbow flexion (as well as limited shoulder flexion and abduction while on bed rest) cause potentially painful shoulders and ROM limitations. UEs should be intermittently positioned in 80 degrees of shoulder abduction, external rotation with scapular depression, and full elbow extension to assist in alleviating this common problem. The forearm should be positioned in pronation because the patient injured at the C5 level is at risk for supination contractures. At Santa Clara Valley Medical Center a device has been designed and fabricated by the OT department to maintain the arm in an appropriate position while the patient is immobilized on a kinetic bed (see Figure 27-2).

Selection of appropriate splint style by the occupational therapist and accurate fabrication by the OTA will enhance patient acceptance and optimal functional gain. If musculature is inadequate to support the wrist and hands properly for function or cosmesis, splints should be fabricated to support the wrist properly in extension and the thumb in opposition and to maintain the thumb web space while allowing the fingers to flex naturally at the metacarpophalangeal (MP) and proximal interphalangeal (PIP) joints. Splints should be dorsal rather than volar in design to allow maximal sensory feedback while the patient's hand is resting on any surface. If at least F(3) strength of wrist extension is present, a short opponens soft or thermoplastic splint should be considered to maintain the web space and support the thumb in opposition. This splint can be used functionally while the patient is trained to use a tenodesis grasp.

AROM and active-assisted ROM of all joints should be performed within strength, ability, and tolerance levels. Muscle reeducation techniques for wrists and elbows should be employed when indicated. Progressive resistive exercises for wrists and hands may be carried out. The patient should be encouraged to engage in self-care activities such as feeding, hygiene, and keyboard and writing activities, if possible, by using simple devices such as a universal cuff or a custom writing splint. Although the patient may be immobilized in bed, discussion of anticipated durable medical equipment (DME), home modifications, and caregiver training should be initiated to allow sufficient time to prepare for discharge.

Active Phase

During the active, or mobilization, phase of the rehabilitation program, the patient can sit in a wheelchair and should begin developing upright tolerance. A high priority at this time is determining a method of relieving sitting pressure for the purpose of preventing decubitus ulcers on the ischial, trochanteric, and sacral bony prominences. If the patient has quadriplegia yet has at least F(3) shoulder and elbow bilateral strength, leaning forward over the feet will relieve pressure on the buttocks. Simple cotton webbing loops are secured to the back frame of the wheelchair (Figure 27-5). A person with low quadriplegia (C7) or a person with paraplegia with intact UE musculature can perform a full depression weight shift off the arms or wheels of the wheelchair. Weight shifts should be performed every 30 to 60 minutes until skin tolerance is determined.

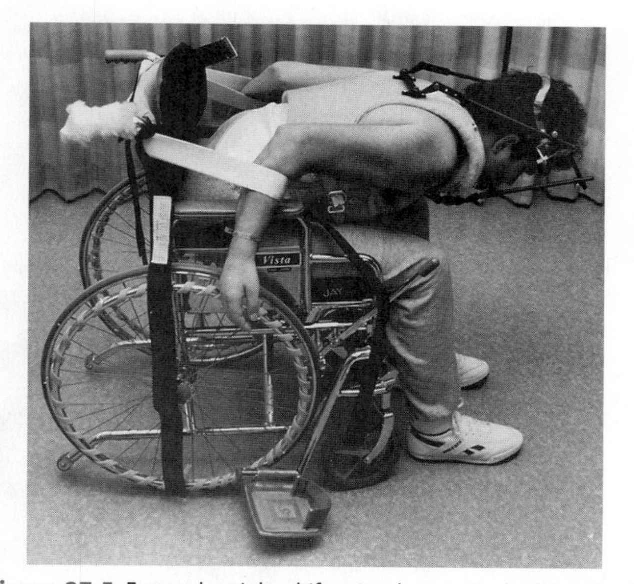

Figure 27-5 Forward weight shift using loops attached to wheelchair frame. This patient has C6 quadriplegia with symmetric grade 4 deltoids and biceps and wrist extensors.

AROM and PROM exercises should be continued regularly to prevent undesirable contractures. Splinting or casting of the elbows may be indicated to correct contractures that are developing. Patients who have wrist extension can learn to substitute for absent grasp through tenodesis action of the long finger flexors. With these patients, some tightness in the wrist extensors is desirable to give some additional tension to the tenodesis grasp. The desirable contracture is developed by ranging finger flexion with the wrist fully extended and finger extension with the wrist flexed, thus never allowing the flexors or extensors to be in full stretch over all of the joints that they cross (Figure 27-6).[17]

Elbow contractures should never be allowed to develop. Full elbow extension is essential for allowing propping to maintain balance during static sitting and for assisting in transfers. With zero triceps strength a person with C6 quadriplegia can maintain forward sitting balance by shoulder depression and protraction, external rotation, full elbow extension, and full wrist extension (Figure 27-7).

Progressive resistive exercise and resistive activities can be applied to innervated and partially innervated muscles. Shoulder musculature should be exercised so as to promote proximal stability, with emphasis on the latissimus dorsi (shoulder depressors), deltoids (shoulder flexors, abductors, and extensors), and the remainder of the shoulder girdle and scapular muscles. The triceps, pectoralis, and latissimus dorsi muscles are necessary for transfers and for shifting weight when in the wheelchair. Wrist extensors should be strengthened to enhance natural tenodesis function, thereby maximizing the necessary prehension pattern in the hand for functional grasp and release.

The treatment program should be graded to increase the amount of resistance that can be tolerated during activity. As muscle power and endurance improve, increasing the amount of time in wheelchair activities will help the patient participate in activities throughout the day.

Many assistive devices and equipment items can be useful to the person with SCI. However, every attempt should be

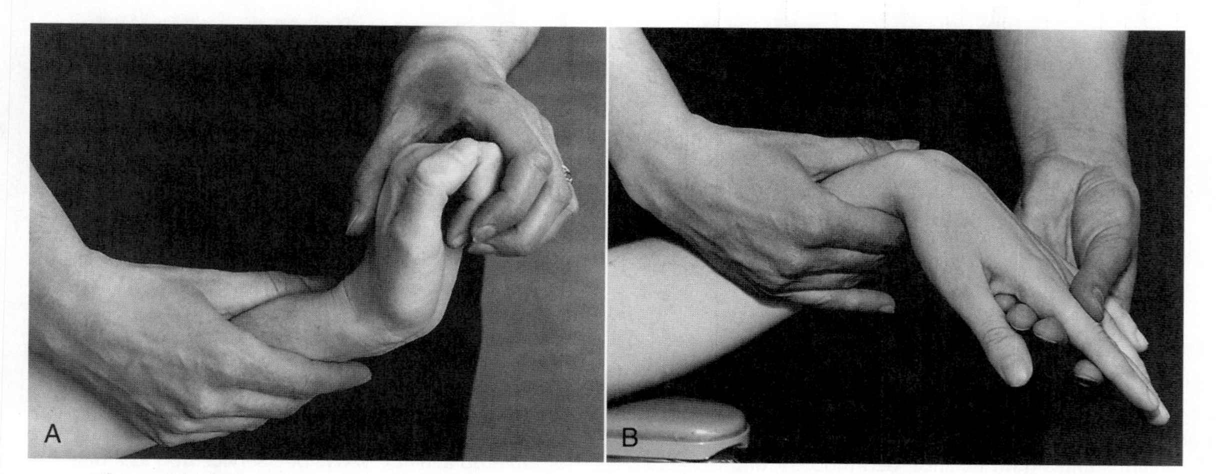

Figure 27-6 Tenodesis action. **A,** Wrist is extended when fingers are passively flexed. **B,** Wrist is flexed when fingers are passively extended.

made to have the patient perform the task with no equipment or with as little as possible. Modified techniques are available that enable an individual to perform efficiently without expensive or bulky equipment.

When appropriate, the universal cuff for holding eating utensils, toothbrushes, pens, and typing sticks offers increased independence. A wrist cock-up splint to stabilize the wrist with attachment of the universal cuff may be useful for persons with little or no wrist extension. A plate guard, cup holder, extended straw with straw clip, and nonskid table mat can facilitate independent feeding. A wash mitt and liquid soap appear to make bathing easier; however, the added difficulty of donning and doffing such equipment must be considered. Many people with quadriplegia can use a button hook to fasten clothing, but pull-over shirts and Velcro closures may be easier to don and doff. A transfer board may facilitate safe transfers. Patients may outgrow the use of initially necessary equipment as they acquire greater strength and coordination.

The ADL program may be expanded to include independent feeding with devices, oral and facial hygiene, and upper-body bathing, bowel and bladder care (such as digital stimulation and intermittent catheterization), UE dressing, and transfers using the sliding board. Developing communication skills in writing and using the telephone, electronic devices, and computer keyboard should be an important part of the treatment program (Figure 27-8). Training in the use of the mobile arm support and overhead slings, wrist-hand orthosis (flexor hinge or tenodesis splint), and assistive devices is also part of the OT program.

The OTA should continue to provide psychological support by allowing and encouraging the patient to express frustration, anger, fears, and concerns.[15] The OT clinic in a spinal cord center can provide an atmosphere where patients can establish support groups with other inpatients and outpatients who can offer their experiences and problem-solving advice to those in earlier phases of their rehabilitation.

The assessment, ordering, and fitting of DME such as wheelchairs, seating and positioning equipment, mechanical lifts, beds, and bathing equipment are extremely important. Such equipment will be specifically evaluated by the occupational therapist, the physical therapist, or occasionally an occupational therapist/physical therapist team and would be ordered only when definite goals and expectations are known. Inappropriate equipment can impair function and cause further medical problems such as skin breakdown or trunk deformity; the therapist must take into account all functional, positioning, environmental, psychological, and financial considerations that

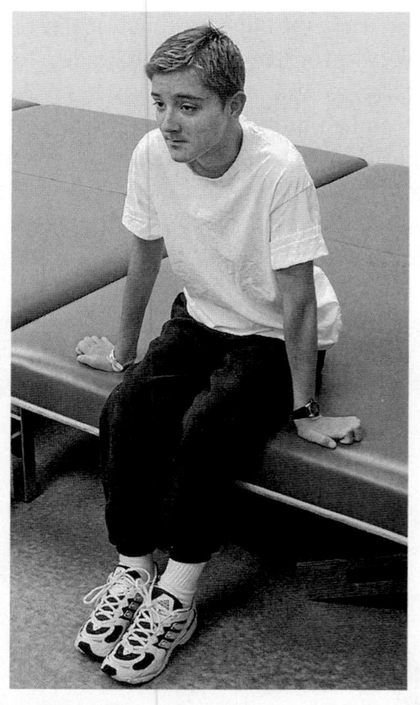

Figure 27-7 A patient with C6 quadriplegia; forward sitting balance is maintained (without triceps) by locking elbows. This technique is valuable for maintaining sitting balance, bed mobility, and transfers. (Courtesy Luis Gonzalez, Media Resource Department, Santa Clara Valley Medical Center.)

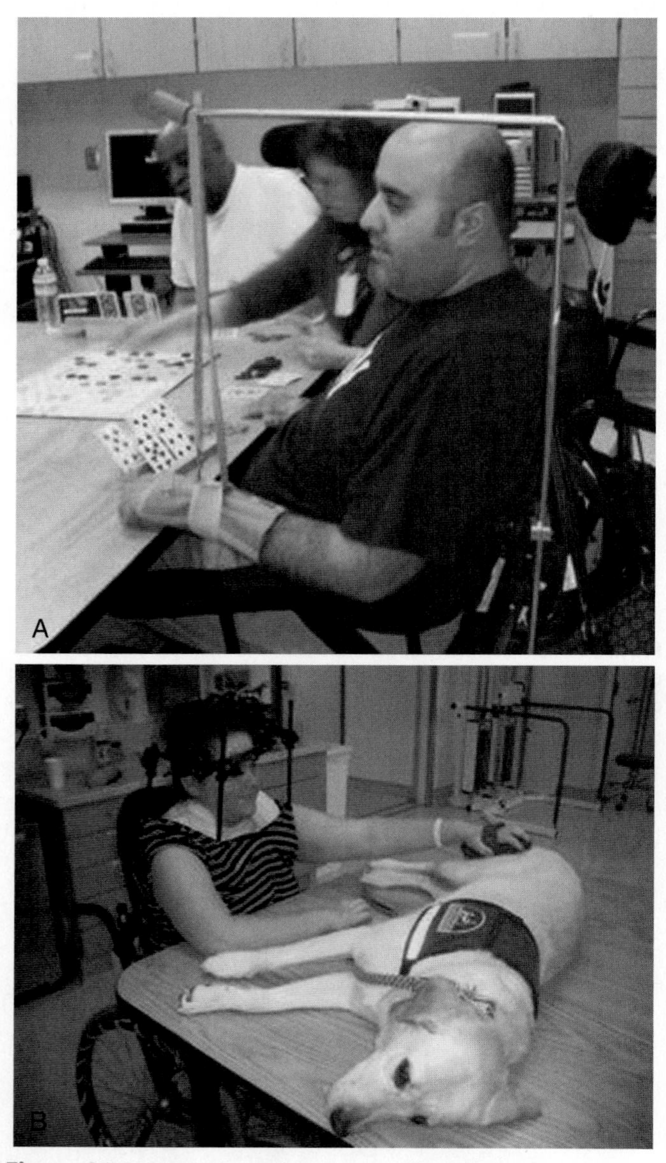

Figure 27-8 A, Patient with injury at C5 utilizing overhead sling for tabletop activity. **B**, Use of a service dog as a treatment option to facilitate bilateral UE use. (Courtesy Luis Gonzalez, Media Resource Department, Santa Clara Valley Medical Center.)

affect the patient's equipment needs. The desired equipment, especially wheelchairs, seat cushions, back supports, positioning devices, and bathing equipment, should be available for demonstration and trial by the patient before final ordering. The OTA involved in the treatment of an individual with an SCI must be familiar with what has been recommended for the patient because he or she will be training with similar equipment to simulate the discharge setting.

In addition to enhancing respiratory function by supporting the patient in an erect, well-aligned position that maximizes sitting tolerance and optimizes UE function, wheelchair seating must assist in the prevention of deformity and pressure sores. An appropriate and adequate wheelchair cushion helps distribute sitting pressure, assists in the prevention of pressure sores, stabilizes the pelvis as needed for proper trunk alignment, and provides comfort. The OTA should work closely with the entire treating team to ensure consistent training and use of the seating system to support each patient.

An increasing number of individuals with high-level SCI-C4 and above are surviving and participating in active

Table 27-1 Expected Functional Outcomes

Expected Functional Outcome		Equipment	FIM/ASSISTANCE DATA		
			Exp	Med	IR
Level C1-3 ***Functionally relevant muscles innervated:*** sternocleidomastoid, cervical paraspinal, neck accessories ***Movement possible:*** neck flexion, extension, rotation ***Patterns of weakness:*** total paralysis of trunk, upper extremities, lower extremities; dependent on ventilator ***NSCISC sample size:*** FIM =15/assist = 12					
Respiratory	Ventilator dependent Inability to clear secretions	Two ventilators (bedside, portable) Suction equipment or other suction management device Generator/battery backup			
Bowel	Total assist	Padded reclining shower/commode chair (if roll-in shower available)	1	1	1
Bladder	Total assist		1	1	1
Bed mobility	Total assist	Full electric hospital bed with Trendelenburg feature and side rails	1	1	1
Bed/wheelchair transfers	Total assist	Transfer board Power or mechanical lift with sling	1	1	1
Pressure relief/ positioning	Total assist	Power recline and/or tilt wheelchair Wheelchair pressure-relief cushion Postural support and head control devices as indicated Hand splints may be indicated Specialty bed or pressure-relief mattress may be indicated			
Eating	Total assist		1	1	1
Dressing	Total assist		1	1	1
Grooming	Total assist		1	1	1
Bathing	Total assist	Handheld shower Shampoo tray Padded reclining shower/commode chair (if roll-in shower available)	1	1	1
Wheelchair propulsion	Manual: total assist Power: independent with equipment	Power recline and/or tilt wheelchair with head, chin, or breath control and manual recliner Vent tray	6	1	1-6
Standing/ ambulation	Standing: total assist Ambulation: not indicated				
Communication	Total assist to independent, depending on work station setup and equipment availability	Mouth stick, high-tech computer access, environmental control unit Adaptive devices everywhere as indicated			
Transportation	Total assist	Attendant-operated van (e.g., lift, tie downs) or accessible public transportation			

Continued

Table 27-1 Expected Functional Outcomes—cont'd

Expected Functional Outcome		Equipment	FIM/ASSISTANCE DATA Exp	Med	IR
Homemaking	Total assist				
Assist required	24-hour attendant to include homemaking Able to instruct in all aspects of care		24*	24*	12-24*

Level C4

Functionally relevant muscles innervated: upper trapezius, diaphragm, cervical paraspinal muscles
Movement possible: neck flexion, extension, rotation; scapular elevation; inspiration
Patterns of weakness: paralysis of trunk, upper extremities, lower extremities; inability to cough, endurance and respiratory reserve low secondary to paralysis of intercostals
NSCISC sample size: FIM = 28/assist = 12

Expected Functional Outcome		Equipment	Exp	Med	IR
Respiratory	May be able to breathe without a ventilator	If not ventilator-free, see C1-3 for equipment requirements			
Bowel	Total assist	Reclining shower/commode chair (if roll-in shower available)	1	1	1
Bladder	Total assist		1	1	1
Bed mobility	Total assist	Full electric hospital bed with Trendelenburg feature and side rails			
Bed/wheelchair transfers	Total assist	Transfer board Power or mechanical lift with sling	1	1	1
Pressure relief/ positioning	Total assist; may be independent with equipment	Power recline and/or tilt wheelchair Wheelchair pressure-relief cushion Postural support and head control devices as indicated Hand splints may be indicated Specialty bed or pressure-relief mattress may be indicated			
Eating	Total assist		1	1	1
Dressing	Total assist		1	1	1
Grooming	Total assist		1	1	1
Bathing	Total assist	Handheld shower Shampoo tray Padded reclining shower/commode chair (if roll-in shower available)	1	1	1
Wheelchair propulsion	Manual: total assist Power: independent	Power recline and/or tilt wheelchair with head, chin, or breath control and manual recliner Vent tray	6	1	1-6
Standing/ ambulation	Standing: total assist Ambulation: not usually indicated	Tilt table Hydraulic standing table			
Communication	Total assist to independent, depending on work station setup and equipment availability	Mouth stick, high-tech computer access, environmental control unit			
Transportation	Total assist	Attendant-operated van (e.g., lift, tie downs) or accessible public transportation			
Homemaking	Total assist				
Assist required	24-hour attendant to include homemaking Able to instruct in all aspects of care		24*	24*	16-24*

Level C5

Functionally relevant muscles innervated: deltoid, biceps, brachialis, brachioradialis, rhomboids, serratus anterior (partially innervated)
Movement possible: shoulder flexion, abduction, and extension; elbow flexion and supination; scapular adduction and abduction
Patterns of weakness: absence of elbow extension, pronation, all wrist and hand movement; total paralysis of trunk and lower extremities
NSCISC sample size: FIM = 41/assist = 35

*Hours per day.

Table 27-1 Expected Functional Outcomes—cont'd

Expected Functional Outcome		Equipment	FIM/ASSISTANCE DATA		
			Exp	Med	IR
Respiratory	Low endurance and vital capacity caused by paralysis of intercostals; may require assist to clear secretions				
Bowel	Total assist	Padded shower/commode chair or padded transfer tub bench with commode cutout	1	1	1
Bladder	Total assist	Adaptive devices may be indicated (electric leg bag emptier)	1	1	1
Bed mobility	Some assist	Full electric hospital bed with Trendelenburg feature with patient controls			
Bed/wheelchair transfers	Total assist	Transfer board Power or mechanical lift	1	1	1
Pressure relief/ positioning	Independent with equipment	Power recline and/or tilt wheelchair Wheelchair pressure-relief cushion Hand splints Specialty bed or pressure-relief mattress may be indicated Postural support devices			
Eating	Total assist for setup, then independent eating with equipment	Long oppenens splint Adaptive devices as indicated	5	5	2.5-5.5
Dressing	Lower extremity: total assist Upper extremity: some assist	Long opponens splint Adaptive devices as indicated	1	1	1-4
Grooming	Some to total assist	Long opponens splint Adaptive devices as indicated	1-3	1	1-5
Bathing	Total assist	Padded tub transfer bench or shower/ commode chair Handheld shower	1	1	1-3
Wheelchair propulsion	Power: independent Manual: independent to some assist indoors on noncarpeted, level surface; some to total assist outdoors	Power recline and/or tilt wheelchair with harm drive control Manual: lightweight rigid or folding frame with handrim modification	6	1	1-6
Standing/ ambulation	Total assist	Hydraulic standing table			
Communication	Independent to some assist after setup with equipment	Long opponens splint Adaptive devices as needed for page turning, writing, button pushing			
Transportation	Independent with highly specialized equipment; some assist with accessible public transportation; total assist for attendant-operated vehicle	Highly specialized modified van with lift			
Homemaking	Total assist				
Assist required	Personal care: 10 hr/day Homecare: 6 hr/day Able to instruct in all aspects of care		16*	23*	10-24*

Level C6

Functionally relevant muscles innervated: clavicular; pectoralis; supinator; extensor carpi radialis longus and brevis; serratus anterior; latissimus dorsi

Movement possible: scapular protraction; some horizontal adduction, forearm supination, radial wrist extension

Patterns of weakness: absence of wrist flexion, elbow extension, hand movement; total paralysis of trunk and lower extremities

NSCISC sample size: FIM = 43/assist = 35

*Hours per day.

Continued

Table 27-1 Expected Functional Outcomes—cont'd

Expected Functional Outcome		Equipment	FIM/ASSISTANCE DATA		
			Exp	Med	IR
Respiratory	Low endurance and vital capacity secondary to paralysis of intercostals; may require assist to clear secretions				
Bowel	Some total assist	Padded tub bench with commode cutout or padded shower/commode chair Other adaptive devices as indicated	1-2	1	1
Bladder	Some total assist with equipment; may be independent with leg bag emptying	Adaptive devices as indicated	1-2	1	1
Bed mobility	Some assist	Full electric hospital bed Side rails Full to king standard bed may be indicated			
Bed/wheelchair transfers	Level: some assist to independent Uneven: some to total assist	Transfer board Mechanical lift	3	1	1-3
Pressure relief/ positioning	Independent with equipment and/ or adaptive techniques	Power recline and/or tilt wheelchair Wheelchair pressure-relief cushion Pressure-relief mattress or overlay may be indicated Postural support devices			
Eating	Independent with or without equipment; except cutting, which is total assist	Adaptive devices as indicated (e.g., U-cuff, tendinosis splint, adapted utensils, plate guard)	5-6	5	4-6
Dressing	Independent upper extremity; some assist to total assist for lower extremities	Adaptive devices as indicated (e.g., buttonhook; loops on zippers, pants; socks, Velcro on shoes)	1-3	2	1-5
Grooming	Some assist to independent with equipment	Adaptive devices as indicated (e.g., U-cuff, adapted handles)	3-6	4	2-6
Bathing	Upper body: independent Lower body: some to total assist	Padded tub transfer bench or shower/ commode chair Adaptive devices as needed Handheld shower	1-3	1	1-3
Wheelchair propulsion	Power: independent with standard arm drive on all surfaces Manual: independent indoors; some total assist outdoors	Manual: lightweight rigid or folding frame with modified rims Power: may require power recline or standard upright power wheelchair	6	6	4-6
Standing/ ambulation	Standing: total assist Ambulation: not indicated	Hydraulic standing frame			
Communication	Independent with or without equipment	Adaptive devices as indicated (e.g., tendinosis splint; writing splint for keyboard use, button pushing, page turning, object manipulation)			
Transportation	Independent driving from wheelchair	Modified van with lift Sensitized hand controls Tie-downs			
Homemaking	Some assist with light meal preparation; total assist for all other homemaking	Adaptive devices as indicated			
Assist required	Personal care: 6 hr/day Homecare: 4 hr/day		10*	17*	8-24*

*Hours per day.

Table 27-1 Expected Functional Outcomes—cont'd

Expected Functional Outcome		Equipment	FIM/ASSISTANCE DATA		
			Exp	Med	IR
Level C7-8					
Functionally relevant muscles innervated: latissimus dorsi; sternal pectoralis; triceps; pronator quadratus; extensor carpi ulnaris; flexor carpi radialis; flexor digitorum profundus and superficialis; extensor communis; pronator/flexor/extensor/abductor pollicis; lumbricals (partially innervated)					
Movement possible: elbow extension; ulnar/wrist extension; wrist flexion; finger flexions and extensions; thumb					
Patterns of weakness: paralysis of trunk and lower extremities; limited grasp and dexterity secondary to partial intrinsic muscles of the hand					
NSCISC sample size: FIM = 43/assist = 35					
Respiratory	Low endurance and vital capacity secondary to paralysis of intercostals; may require assist to clear secretions				
Bowel	Some total assist	Padded tub bench with commode cutout or shower/commode chair Adaptive devices as indicated	1-4	1	1-4
Bladder	Independent to some assist	Adaptive devices as indicated	2-6	3	1-6
Bed mobility	Independent to some assist	Full electric hospital bed or full to king standard bed			
Bed/wheelchair transfers	Level: independent Uneven: independent to some assist	With or without transfer board	3-7	4	2-6
Pressure relief/ positioning	Independent	Wheelchair pressure-relief cushion Postural support devices Pressure-relief mattress or overlay may be indicated			
Eating	Independent	Adaptive devices as indicated	6-7	6	5-7
Dressing	Independent upper extremity; independent to some assist in lower extremities	Adaptive devices as indicated	4-7	6	4-7
Grooming	Independent	Adaptive devices as indicated	6-7	6	4-7
Bathing	Upper body: independent Lower body: some assist to independent	Padded tub transfer bench or shower/ commode chair Adaptive devices as needed Handheld shower	3-6	4	2-6
Wheelchair propulsion	Manual: independent on all indoor surfaces and level outdoor terrain; some assist with uneven terrain	Manual: rigid or folding lightweight or folding wheelchair with modified rims	6	6	6
Standing/ ambulation	Standing: independent to some assist Ambulation: not indicated	Hydraulic or standard standing frame			
Communication	Independent	Adaptive devices as indicated			
Transportation	Independent in car if independent with transfer and wheelchair loading/ unloading; independent in driving modified van from captain's seat	Modified vehicle Transfer board			
Homemaking	Independent light meal preparation and homemaking; some to total assist for complex meal preparation and heavy housecleaning	Adaptive devices as indicated			
Assist required	Personal care: 6 hr/day Homecare: 2 hr/day		8*	12*	2-24*

*Hours per day.

Continued

Table 27-1 Expected Functional Outcomes—cont'd

Expected Functional Outcome		Equipment	FIM/ASSISTANCE DATA Exp	Med	IR
Level T1-9					
Functionally relevant muscles innervated: intrinsics of the hand including thumbs; internal and external intercostals; erector spinae; lumbricals; flexor/extensor/abductor pollicis					
Movement possible: upper extremities fully intact; limited upper trunk stability; endurance increased secondary to innervation of intercostals					
Patterns of weakness: lower trunk paralysis; total paralysis of lower extremities					
NSCISC sample size: FIM = 144/assist = 122					
Respiratory	Compromised vital capacity and endurance				
Bowel	Independent	Elevated padded toilet seat or padded tub bench with commode cutout	6-7	6	4-6
Bladder	Independent		6	6	5-6
Bed mobility	Independent	Full to king standard bed			
Bed/wheelchair transfers	Independent	May or may not require transfer board	6-7	6	6-7
Pressure relief/ positioning	Independent	Wheelchair pressure-relief cushion Postural support devices as indicated Pressure-relief mattress or overlay may be indicated			
Eating	Independent		7	7	7
Dressing	Independent		7	7	7
Grooming	Independent		7	7	7
Bathing	Independent	Padded tub transfer bench or shower/ commode chair Handheld shower	6-7	6	5-7
Wheelchair propulsion	Independent	Manual rigid or folding lightweight wheelchair	6	6	6
Standing/ ambulation	Standing: independent Ambulation: typically not functional	Standing frame			
Communication	Independent				
Transportation	Independent in car; including loading and unloading wheelchair	Hand controls			
Homemaking	Independent with complex meal preparation and light housecleaning; total to some assist with heavy housecleaning				
Assist required	Homemaking: 3 hr/day		2*	3*	0-15*
Level T10-L1					
Functionally relevant muscles innervated: fully intact intercostals; external obliques; rectus abdominis					
Movement possible: fair to good trunk stability					
Patterns of weakness: paralysis of lower extremities					
NSCISC sample size: FIM = 71/assist = 57					
Respiratory	Intact respiratory function				
Bowel	Independent	Padded standard or raised padded toilet seat	6-7	6	6
Bladder	Independent		6	6	6
Bed mobility	Independent	Full to king standard bed			
Bed/wheelchair transfers	Independent		7	7	6-7
Pressure relief/ positioning	Independent	Wheelchair pressure-relief cushion Postural support devices as indicated Pressure-relief mattress or overlay may be indicated			
Eating	Independent		7	7	7
Dressing	Independent		7	7	7

*Hours per day.

Table 27-1 Expected Functional Outcomes—cont'd

Expected Functional Outcome		Equipment	FIM/ASSISTANCE DATA		
			Exp	Med	IR
Grooming	Independent		7	7	7
Bathing	Independent	Padded tub transfer bench Handheld shower	6-7	6	6-7
Wheelchair propulsion	Independent all indoor and outdoor surfaces	Manual rigid or folding lightweight wheelchair	6	6	6
Standing/ ambulation	Standing: independent Ambulation: functional, some assist to independent	Standing frame Forearm crutches or walker Knee-ankle-foot orthosis (KAFO)			
Communication	Independent				
Transportation	Independent in car; including loading and unloading wheelchair	Hand controls			
Homemaking	Independent with complex meal preparation and light housecleaning; some assist with heavy housecleaning				
Assist required	Homemaking: 2 hr/day		2*	2*	0-8*
Level L2-S5					
Functionally relevant muscles innervated: fully intact abdominals and all other trunk muscles; depending on level, some degree of hip flexors, extensor, abductors; knee flexors, extensors; ankle dorsiflexors, plantar flexors					
Movement possible: good trunk stability; partial to full control of lower extremities					
Patterns of weakness: partial paralysis of lower extremities, hips, knees, ankle, foot					
NSCISC sample size: FIM = 20/assist = 16					
Respiratory	Intact function				
Bowel	Independent	Padded toilet seat	6-7	6	6-7
Bladder	Independent		6	6	6-7
Bed mobility	Independent	Full to king standard bed			
Bed/wheelchair transfers	Independent		7	7	7
Pressure relief/ positioning	Independent	Wheelchair pressure-relief cushion Postural support devices as indicated			
Eating	Independent		7	7	7
Dressing	Independent		7	7	7
Grooming	Independent		7	7	7
Bathing	Independent	Padded tub bench Handheld shower	7	7	6-7
Wheelchair propulsion	Independent all indoor and outdoor surfaces	Manual rigid or folding lightweight wheelchair	6	6	6
Standing/ ambulation	Standing: independent Ambulation: functional, some assist to independent	Standing frame Forearm crutches or cane as indicated Knee-ankle-foot orthosis (KAFO) or ankle-foot orthosis (AFO)			
Communication	Independent				
Transportation	Independent in car; including loading and unloading wheelchair	Hand controls			
Homemaking	Independent with complex meal preparation and light housecleaning; some assist with heavy housecleaning				
Assist required	Homemaking: 0-1 hr/day		0-1*	0*	0*

From Consortium for Spinal Cord Medicine, Paralyzed Veterans of America: *Outcomes following traumatic spinal cord injury: clinical practice guidelines for health-care professionals,* Washington, DC, 1999, the Consortium.

*Hours per day.

FIM/assistance data: *Exp,* expected *FIM* score; *Med,* NSCISC median; *IR,* NSCISC Interquartile Range.

FIM/assistance data: *Exp,* expected *FIM* score; *Med,* NSCISC median; *IR,* NSCISC Interquartile Range.

FIM/assistance data: *Exp,* expected *FIM* score; *Med,* NSCISC median; *IR,* NSCISC Interquartile Range.

FIM/assistance data: *Exp,* expected *FIM* score; *Med,* NSCISC median; *IR,* NSCISC Interquartile Range.

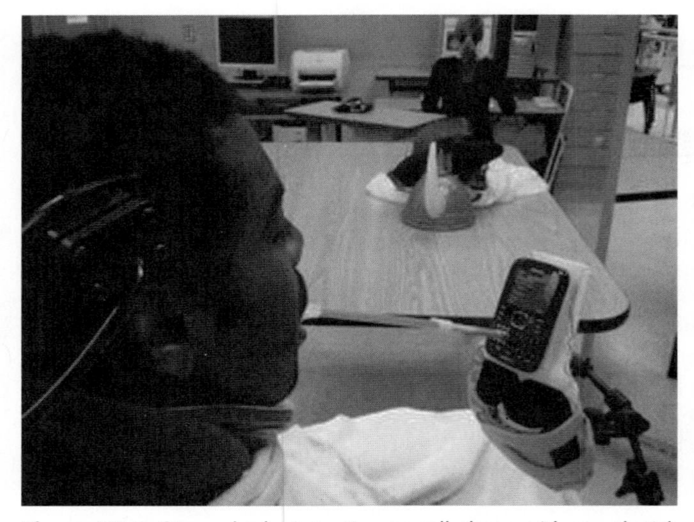

Figure 27-9 C4 quadriplegic texting on cell phone with mouthstick and custom-adapted wheelchair mount.

rehabilitation programs. The treatment and equipment needs of these individuals are unique and extremely specialized, ranging from mouthsticks and assistive technology to ventilators and sophisticated electric wheelchairs and drive systems (Table 27-1, levels C1-3 and C3-4). Commercially available assistive technology such as cell phones, electronic readers, and notebook computers have greatly enhanced the options available to high-level tetraplegics (Figure 27-9).

Consultation with experienced resources to identify appropriate short- and long-term goals and equipment needs enhances the quality and functional ability of an individual who otherwise would be quite dependent. Rehabilitation centers that specialize in the care of high-level quadriplegic patients have particular expertise in addressing all aspects of care.

When place of discharge is determined and the patient can tolerate leaving the hospital for a few hours, a home evaluation will be performed. The occupational therapist, patient, and family members can then view and attempt activities in the home in anticipation of return to a safe and accessible environment. The OTA must be knowledgeable about safety and accessibility options for a variety of environments and often must reinforce the necessity of having appropriate modifications completed before discharge. The OTA should be aware of accessibility requirements in the home, as well as those required in the workplace by the Americans with Disabilities Act of 1990 (ADA) (see Chapter 17).

Decreases in the time of inpatient rehabilitation have moved the extended phase of treatment to an outpatient basis or home therapy. Adaptive driving, home management, leisure activities, or workshop skill assessments using hand- or power-based tools are feasible and appropriate treatment modalities for evaluating and increasing UE strength, coordination, and trunk balance; however, they may not be a priority during inpatient hospitalization. Such activities can improve socialization skills and can also assess problem-solving skills and potential work habits.

OT practitioners may assist in the exploration of vocational potential of persons with SCI. By the sheer magnitude of the physical disability, vocational possibilities for individuals with high-level SCI are limited. Many patients must change their vocation or alter former vocational goals. Decreased motivation, loss of health benefits, and lack of perseverance on the part of many patients make vocational rehabilitation challenging for the therapist.

The OTA can assist in observing the patient's level of motivation, functional aptitudes, attitudes, interests, and personal vocational aspirations throughout the treatment program, particularly in ADL, mobility, and work simulation activities. The OTA can observe the patient's attention span, concentration, manual ability with splints and devices, accuracy, speed, perseverance, work habits, and work tolerance level. The OTA can offer valuable information from observations during activities. When suitable vocational objectives have been selected, they may be pursued in an educational setting or in a work setting, usually out of the realm of OT.

Aging with Spinal Cord Injury

After survival of acute SCI, the primary goal of rehabilitation is independence. Independence as the measure of quality of life for people with disabilities is an idea accepted and often perpetuated by survivors and health care professionals alike.[16]

All clinicians treating patients with SCI have considerable responsibility in influencing the level of independence, whether in the acute setting, during active rehabilitation, or in follow-up care throughout the life of a spinal cord–injured individual. Understanding the aging process in both able-bodied and disabled individuals is necessary for providing appropriate options and fostering attitudes that prevent further injury and enhance the quality of the patient's life at any age.

Physical aging is a natural, nonpreventable process that all humans encounter. The signs of aging can occur at varying rates for each individual, affecting most systems of the body. In individuals with SCI, aging is often accelerated by secondary effects of the disability such as muscle imbalance, infections (urinary and respiratory), deconditioning, pain, and joint degeneration secondary to overuse.[12] Urinary problems brought on by years of catheterization, bladder infections, and urinary retention are common. Other aging-related problems for SCI survivors include osteoporosis, arthritis and joint degeneration, constipation, weakening of already precarious skin, substance abuse, and the need for increased personal care over time.

Twenty years after injury is the typical point at which the aging problems begin to increase. Because at least one of four SCI survivors in the United States has survived more than 20 years after the injury,[13] a significant portion of SCI survivors are prematurely experiencing the problems of aging. Individuals with SCI onset in their later years have different patterns of functional outcomes, program needs, and financial resources than do those with onset in their earlier years. For someone who acquired quadriplegia in his or her 20s (the age when the majority of SCIs occur) the degenerating conditions of normal aging become evident prematurely, usually before the 40s.[5] Thus someone who was independent in transfers at home and loading a wheelchair in and out of the car may by age 40 require assistance getting in and out of bed; this person may have to trade the car for a van, requiring costly modifications because his or her shoulders have given out.

Likewise, someone at a level that usually permits functional independence (e.g., T10 paraplegia) may, in fact, need personal care assistance and consider a power wheelchair because of aging. The occupational therapist/OTA team can help prevent fixed trunk and pelvic deformities such as kyphosis and scoliosis, which can lead to considerable skin problems and uncorrectable cosmetic deformities years later, by making good trunk alignment and seating a priority from the outset. Although use of a manual wheelchair provides the advantage of cardiopulmonary conditioning, the weight of the wheelchair combined with the distance from shoulder to push rim during propulsion can damage a weak or imbalanced shoulder complex.

When SCI is compounded by the increased fatigue and weakness often associated with normal aging, the functional status of the individual affected with SCI may decline. The OTA may note these status changes during the course of therapy. Many considerations must be weighed to make appropriate short- and long-term decisions, and it is the responsibility of the team to be aware of how aging affects this population.

Table 27-1 presents expectations of functional performance of SCI at 1 year after injury and at each of eight levels of injury (C1-3, C4, C5, C6, C7-8, T1-9, T10-L1, L2-S5). The outcomes reflect a level of independence that can be expected of a person with motor-complete SCI, given optimal circumstances. The OTA should have a good understanding of aspects of each level in order to accurately communicate with other members of the interdisciplinary team regarding the patient's clinical and treatment status.

The categories presented reflect expected functional outcomes in the areas of mobility, ADL, instrumental activities of daily living (IADL), and communication skills. The guidelines are based on consensus of clinical experts, available literature on functional outcomes, and data compiled from Uniform Data Systems (UDS) and the National Spinal Cord Injury Statistical Center (NSCISC).

Within the functional outcomes for people with SCI listed in Table 27-1, a series of essential daily functions and activities, as well as the attendant care likely to be needed to support the predicted level of independence at 1 year after injury, have been identified. These outcome areas include the following:

- *Respiratory, bowel, and bladder function.* The neurological effects of SCI may result in deficits in the ability of the individual to perform basic body functions. Respiratory function includes the ability to breathe with or without mechanical assistance and to adequately clear secretions. Bowel and bladder function includes the ability to manage elimination, maintain perineal hygiene, and adjust clothing before and after elimination. Adapted or facilitated methods of managing these bodily functions may be required to attain expected functional outcomes.
- *Bed mobility, bed/wheelchair transfers, wheelchair propulsion, and positioning/pressure relief.* The neurological effects of SCI may result in deficits in the ability of the individual to perform the activities required for mobility, locomotion, and safety. Adapted or facilitated methods of managing these activities may be required to attain expected functional outcomes in standing and ambulation.
- *Standing and ambulation.* SCI may result in deficits in the ability to stand for exercise or psychological benefit or to ambulate for functional activities. Adapted or facilitated methods of management may be outcomes in standing and ambulation.
- *Eating, grooming, dressing, and bathing.* The neurological effects of SCI may result in deficits in the ability of the individual to perform these ADL. Adapted or facilitated methods of managing ADL may be necessary to attain expected functional outcomes.
- *Communication* (keyboard use, handwriting, and telephone use). The neurological effects of SCI may result in deficits in the ability of the individual to communicate. Adapted or facilitated methods of communication may be required to attain expected functional outcomes.
- *Transportation* (driving, attendant-operated vehicle, and public transportation). Transportation activities are critical for individuals with SCI to become maximally independent in their community. Adaptations may be required to help the individual meet the expected functional outcomes.
- *Homemaking* (meal planning and preparations and home management). Adapted or facilitated methods of managing homemaking tasks may be required to attain expected functional outcomes. Individuals with complete SCI at any level will require some level of assistance with some homemaking activities. The hours of assistance with homemaking activities are presented in Table 27-1.
- *Assistance required.* Table 27-1 lists the number of hours that may be required from a caregiver to assist with personal care and homemaking activities in the home. Personal care includes hands-on delivery of all aspects of self-care and mobility, as well as safety interventions.
- *Homemaking assistance* is also included in the recommendation for hours of assistance and includes activities previously presented. The number of hours presented in both the panel recommendations and the self-reported CHART data is representative of skilled and unskilled and paid and unpaid hours of assistance. The 24-hour-a-day requirement noted for the C1-3 and C4 levels includes the expected need for unpaid attendant care to provide safety monitoring. Adequate assistance is required to ensure that the individual with an SCI can achieve the outcomes set forth in Table 27-1. The hours of assistance recommended do not reflect changes in assistance required over time as reported by long-term survivors of SCI,[4] nor do they take into account the wide range of individual variables mentioned throughout this chapter that may affect the number of required hours of assistance. The Functional Independence Measure (FIM) estimates are widely variable in several of the categories. Whether the representative individuals with SCI in the individual categories attained the expected functional outcomes for their specific level of

injury is unclear. Also unclear is whether there were mitigating circumstances such as age, obesity, or concomitant injuries that would account for variability in assistance reported. An individualized assessment of needs is required in all cases.

- *Equipment requirements.* Minimum recommendations for DME and adaptive devices are identified in each of the functional categories. The most commonly used equipment is listed, with the understanding that variations exist among SCI rehabilitation programs and that use of such equipment may be necessary to achieve the identified functional outcomes. Additional equipment and devices that are not critical for most individuals at a specific level of injury may be required for some individuals. The equipment descriptions are generic so as to allow for varying program philosophies and financial resources. Rapid changes and advances in equipment and technology occur and therefore must be considered. Health care professionals should remember that the recommendations set forth in Table 27-1 are not intended to be prescriptive but rather to serve as a guideline. The importance of individual functional assessment of people with SCI before making equipment recommendations cannot be overemphasized. All DME and adaptive devices must be thoroughly assessed and tested to determine medical necessity, to prevent medical complications (e.g., postural deviations, skin breakdown, pain), and to foster optimal functional performance. Environmental control units and telephone modifications may be necessary for safety and maximal independence, and each person must be individually evaluated for the need for this equipment. Recommendations for disposable medical products are not included in this table.
- *FIM.* Evidence for the specific levels of independence provided in Table 27-1 relies on both expert consensus and data from FIM in large-scale, prospective, and longitudinal research conducted by the NSCISC. FIM is the most widely used disability measure in rehabilitation medicine, and although it may not incorporate all of the characteristics of disability in individuals recovering from SCI, it captures many basic disability areas. FIM consists of 13 motor and 5 cognitive items that are individually scored from 1 to 7. A score of 1 indicates complete dependence, and a score of 7 indicates complete independence (see Table 27-1). The sum of the 13 FIM motor score items can range from 13, indicating complete dependence for all items, to 91, indicating complete independence for all items. FIM is a measure usually completed by health care professionals; other observers (including the patient, family members, and caregivers) can contribute information to the ratings. Each of these observers may represent a different type of potential bias.
- Although the sample sizes of FIM data for certain neurological-level groups are quite small, the consistency of the data adds confidence to the interpretation. Other pertinent data regarding functional independence must be factored into outcome analyses including medical information, patient factors, social role participation, quality of life, and environmental factors and supports.
- In Table 27-1, FIM data, when available, are reported in three areas. First, the expected FIM outcomes are documented based on expert clinical consensus. The second number reported is the median FIM score, as compiled by the NSCISC. The interquartile range for NSCISC FIM data is the third set of numbers. In total, the FIM data represent 1-year postinjury FIM assessments of 405 survivors with complete SCI and a median age of 27 years. The NSCISC sample size for FIM and Assistance Data is provided for each level of injury. Different outcome expectations clearly should apply to different patient subgroups and populations. Some populations are likely to be significantly older than the referenced one. Functional abilities may be limited by advancing age.[14,19]
- *Home modifications.* To provide the best opportunity for individuals with SCI to achieve the identified functional outcomes, a safe and architecturally accessible environment is necessary. An accessible environment must take into consideration, but not be limited to, entrance and egress, mobility in the home, and adequate setup to perform personal care and homemaking tasks.

Research

Research in clinical settings and scientific laboratories around the world focuses on understanding the nature of SCI and defining the nervous system's response to this injury. The scientific community seems increasingly optimistic that it will be possible someday to restore function after SCI. This optimism is based on the combined research efforts of scientists in many different disciplines. It is important for all clinicians treating SCI to be aware of the scientific and technological advances so as to better educate patients while providing them with realistic and comprehensive rehabilitation interventions for their immediate and long-term needs.

Summary

SCI can result in substantial paralysis of the limbs and trunk. The degree of residual motor and sensory dysfunction depends on the level of the lesion, whether the lesion was complete or incomplete, and the area of the spinal cord that was damaged.

After an SCI, bony realignment and stabilization are established surgically, via an external immobilization device, or through a combination of both methods. The many possible complications of SCI include skin breakdown, rapid loss of bone density, and spasticity.

OT is concerned with facilitating the patient's achievement of optimal independence and functioning. Areas of focus are physical restoration of available musculature, self-care, independent living skills, short- and long-term equipment needs, environmental accessibility, and educational, work, and leisure activities. The psychosocial adjustment of the patient is important, and the occupational therapist and OTA offer emotional support toward this end in every phase of the rehabilitation program.

Selected Reading Guide Questions

1. Describe the functional and prognostic differences between complete and incomplete lesions.
2. When reference is made to C5 in quadriplegia, what is meant in terms of level of injury and functioning muscle groups?
3. What are some medical complications common to patients with SCIs that can limit achievement of functional potential?
4. How does postural hypotension affect function, and how should a caregiver respond?
5. What are the signs of autonomic dysreflexia, and how should a caregiver respond?
6. What is the role of the OTA in the prevention of pressure sores?
7. What additional muscle power does the patient with C6 quadriplegia have over the patient with C5 quadriplegia? What is the major functional advantage of this additional muscle power?
8. What is the first spinal cord lesion level that has full innervation of the UE musculature?
9. List five goals of OT for the patient with an SCI.
10. What are some of the first self-care activities that the patient with a C6 SCI should be expected to accomplish?
11. List four assistive devices commonly used by persons with quadriplegia, and tell the purpose of each.
12. Why would a person with paraplegia require homemaking assistance if he or she is independent in all self-care and mobility?

References

1. Amador MJ, Lynne CM, Brackett NL: Contemporary information regarding male infertility following spinal cord injury, *SCI Nursing* 15(3):61–65, 1998.
2. American Spinal Injury Association (ASIA): *Standards for neurological and functional classification of spinal cord injury*, Chicago, 1992, the Association.
3. Bromley I: *Tetraplegia and paraplegia: a guide for physiotherapists*, ed 5, New York, 1998, Churchill Livingstone.
4. Consortium for Spinal Cord Medicine, Paralyzed Veterans of America: *Outcomes following traumatic spinal cord injury: clinical practice guidelines for health-care professionals*, Washington, DC, 1999, the Consortium.
5. Freed MM: Traumatic and congenital lesions of the spinal cord. In Kottke FJ, Lehmann JF, editors: *Krusen's handbook of physical medicine and rehabilitation*, Philadelphia, 1990, WB Saunders.
6. Hanak M, Scott A: *Spinal cord injury: an illustrated guide for health care professionals*, New York, 1983, Springer-Verlag.
7. Heinemann AW, Magiera-Planey R, Schiro-Geist C, et al: Mobility for persons with spinal cord injury: an evaluation of two systems, *Arch Phys Med Rehabil* 68(2):90–93, 1987.
8. Hill JP, editor: *Spinal cord injury: a guide to functional outcomes in occupational therapy*, Rockville, Md, 1987, Aspen.
9. Institute for Medical Research, Santa Clara Valley Medical Center: *Severe head trauma, a comprehensive medical approach*, Project 13-9-59156/9, Nov 1982, report to National Institute for Handicapped Research.
10. Lammertse MD: Why some injured people get better and others don't. In Maddox S, editor: *Spinal network*, Boulder, 1987, Colo.
11. Malick MH, Meyer CMH: *Dynamic hand orthoses: manual on the management of the quadriplegic upper extremity*, Pittsburgh, 1978, Harmarville Rehabilitation Center.
12. Paulson S, editor: *Santa Clara Valley Medical Center spinal cord injury home care manual*, ed 3, San Jose, Calif, 1994, Santa Clara Valley Medical Center.
13. Pierce DS, Nickel VH: *The total care of spinal cord injuries*, Boston, 1977, Little, Brown.
14. Penrod LE, Hegde SK, Ditunno JF Jr: Age effect on prognosis for functional recovery in acute, traumatic central cord syndrome, *Arch Phys Med Rehabil* 71(12):963–968, 1990.
15. Spencer EA: Functional restoration. In Hopkins HL, Smith HD, editors: *Willard and Spackman's occupational therapy*, ed 8, Philadelphia, 1993, JB Lippincott.
16. Whiteneck GG, Charlifue SW, editors: *Aging with spinal cord injury*, New York, 1993, Demos Medical Publications.
17. Wilson DJ, McKenzie MW, Barber LM: *Spinal cord injury: a treatment guide for occupational therapists*, Thorofare, NJ, 1984, Slack.
18. Yarkony GM: *Spinal cord injury: medical management and rehabilitation*, Gaithersburg, Md, 1994, Aspen.
19. Yarkony GM, Roth EJ, Heinemann AW, et al: Spinal cord injury rehabilitation outcome: the impact of age, *J Clin Epidemiol* 41(2):173–177, 1988.

Suggested Readings

Adler C: Equipment considerations. In Whiteneck GG, et al, editors: *Treatment of high quadriplegia*, New York, 1988, Demos Publications.

Baer, Robert W: Is Fred Dead? A Manual on Sexuality for Men with Spinal Cord Injuries.

Bergen A, Presperin J, Tallman T: *Positioning for function*, Valhalla, NY, 1990, Valhalla Rehabilitation Publications.

Field-Fote, Edelle: Spinal Cord Injury Rehabilitation (Contemporary Perspectives in Rehabilitation), Philadelphia, FA Davis, 2009.

Ford JR, Duckworth B: *Physical management for the quadriplegic patient*, Philadelphia, 1974, FA Davis.

Gerhart KA, Koziol-McLain J, Lowenstein SR, et al: Quality of life following spinal cord injury: knowledge and attitudes of emergency care providers, *Ann Emerg Med* 23(4):807–812, 1994.

Hill JP, editor: *Spinal cord injury: a guide to functional outcomes in occupational therapy*, Rockville, Md, 1986, Aspen.

Klein SD, Karp G: *From There to Here: Stories of Adjustment to Spinal Cord Injury,* No Limits Communication, 2004.

Mayo Clinic: Guide to Living with a Spinal Cord Injury: Moving Ahead with Your Life.

Palmer S, Kriegsman K, Palmer J, Harris Kriegman K: *Spinal Cord Injury: A Guide for Living*, Baltimore, Md, 2000, Johns Hopkins University Press.

Paralyzed Veterans of America: *Outcomes following traumatic spinal cord injury: clinical practice guidelines for health-care professionals, Consortium for Spinal Cord Medicine*, Washington, DC, 1999, Paralyzed Veterans of America.

Paralyzed Veterans of America: *Preservation of upper limb function following spinal cord injury: a clinical practice guideline for health-care professionals, Consortium for Spinal Cord Medicine*, Washington, DC, 2005, Paralyzed Veterans of America.

Sisto SA, Druin E, Macht Sliwinski M: *Spinal Cord Injuries, Management and Rehabilitation*, St Louis, 2008, Mosby.

Somer, Martha Freeman: *Spinal Cord Injury: Functional Rehabilitation (3rd Edition)*, Upper Saddle River, NJ, Prentice Hall, 2009.

Suggested Websites

www.pva.org—Consortium for Spinal Cord Injury

www.spinalcord.uab.edu—spinal cord injury information network

www.disaboom.com

www.sci-info-pages.com

www.aparalyzed.com

www.contemporaryforums, online library—spinal cord injuries

www.spinalinjury.net—Spinal Cord Injury Resource Center

www.christopherreeve.org—Christopher and Dana Reeve Association

CHAPTER 28 Neurogenic and Myopathic Dysfunction*

JENNIFER NYBLOD

Key Terms

Motor unit
Neurogenic
Myopathic
Lower motor neuron dysfunction
Poliomyelitis
Contractures
Postpolio syndrome
Guillain-Barré syndrome
Peripheral nerve injury
Atrophy
Regeneration
Pain syndromes
Myasthenia gravis
Muscular dystrophies

Chapter Objectives

After studying this chapter, the student or practitioner will be able to do the following:

1. Describe the causes of lesions that result in motor unit dysfunction.
2. Name the clinical conditions that are characterized as motor unit dysfunction.
3. Identify the clinical manifestations of motor unit dysfunction conditions.
4. Contrast the goals and methods of occupational therapy treatment programs for the various motor unit conditions.

The motor unit is the elementary functional unit in the motor system.[45] Its components are the motor neurons and the muscle fibers that it innervates.[37] Diseases of the motor unit generally cause muscle weakness and atrophy of skeletal muscle and may be neurogenic (originating in the nerves) or myopathic (originating in the muscle). Neurogenic disorders affect the nerve cell bodies or the peripheral nerves. Myopathic diseases affect the neuromuscular junction or the muscle itself.[45] These conditions are commonly seen in clinical practice, and the occupational therapy assistant (OTA) should be familiar with their symptoms, courses, and treatments.

Neurogenic Disorders: Lower Motor Neuron Dysfunction

A lesion to any of the neurologic structures of the lower motor neuron system will result in lower motor neuron dysfunction.[12,13,45] Lesions can result from (1) nerve root compression; (2) trauma—bone fractures and dislocations, lacerations, traction, penetrating wounds, and friction; (3) toxins—lead, phosphorus, alcohol, benzene, and sulfonamides; (4) infections—poliomyelitis, Guillain-Barré syndrome; (5) neoplasms—neuromas and multiple neurofibromatosis; (6) vascular disorders—arteriosclerosis, diabetes mellitus, peripheral vascular anomalies, and polyarteritis nodosa; (7) degenerative diseases of the central nervous system—amyotrophic lateral sclerosis; and (8) congenital malformations.[3,24,55,59]

Poliomyelitis

The active immunization program (using the Salk and Sabin vaccines) in the United States since the mid-1950s has essentially eradicated poliomyelitis in the Western hemisphere. New cases are rare.[55,61] The last polio cases reported in the United States were in 1999. They were vaccine-associated paralytic polio cases caused by live oral polio vaccine. In 2009 only 1579 confirmed cases of polio were reported globally.[10] Adults who had poliomyelitis in early life in the United States and those from countries that lacked the benefits of

*Guy L. McCormack, Lorraine Williams Pedretti, Regina M. Lehman, and Lynn Roulette contributed large portions of this chapter to the previous editions of this book.

immunization and rehabilitation are referred to occupational therapy (OT) for vocational evaluation or improvement of quality of life.[51,59]

Poliomyelitis is a contagious viral disease that affects the anterior horn cells of the gray matter of the spinal cord and the motor nuclei of the brainstem. It results in a flaccid paralysis that may be local or widespread. The lower extremities, accessory muscles of respiration, and muscles that promote swallowing are primarily affected, but upper extremity (UE) involvement may also occur. Marked atrophy may be seen in the involved extremities, and deep tendon reflexes may be absent. Because poliomyelitis destroys the anterior horn cells, sensory roots are spared and sensation is intact. Contractures (permanent shortening of the muscles, tendons, and ligaments) can occur early in the course of the disease. In cases of local paralysis, the asymmetry of muscles pulling on various joints may promote deformities such as subluxation, scoliosis, and contractures. In severe cases osteoporosis (bone atrophy) may weaken the long weight-bearing bones (tibia and femur), and pathologic fractures can occur.[31]

The medical treatment for poliomyelitis during the acute phase includes bed rest, positioning, and applications of warm packs to reduce pain and promote relaxation. Because no known cure for poliomyelitis exists, the disease must run its course. The medical aspects of rehabilitation may include reconstructive surgery such as tendon transfer, arthrodesis, and surgical release of fascia, muscles, and tendons. Other rehabilitation measures may include therapeutic stretching, casts, muscle reeducation, orthoses, and bracing for standing or stability.[25]

Occupational Therapy Intervention

The OTA will most likely provide treatment to persons whose status is postacute phase and who are in the rehabilitation stage. It is hypothesized that during the recovery process, in an effort to compensate for the loss of neurons, surviving motor neurons sprout new endings to restore function to muscles.[35] Rehabilitation includes instruction in range of motion (ROM), muscle reeducation and graded strengthening, precautions against fatigue, psychological support, and retraining in activities of daily living (ADL).

Movement for the patient who is recovering from acute poliomyelitis proceeds from passive ROM (PROM) to active ROM (AROM), depending on the patient's level of voluntary control. Muscle reeducation should be preceded by gentle stretching exercises. All active motions should be performed under careful supervision of the therapist or assistant. Compensatory movement should be avoided. A limited but correct movement is preferred to a larger but incorrect movement. Active movements should be done in front of a mirror so that the patient may observe and correct motions accordingly.[25,28,52]

Muscle reeducation is accomplished in a graded fashion. At first the patient should learn "muscle-setting" exercises—alternating contraction and relaxation of muscles without moving the joints. Isometric exercises and electromyographic (EMG) biofeedback may be beneficial. As the patient progresses, the clinician can apply light resistance manually before using resistance equipment. This allows the therapy practitioner to estimate directly the patient's physical strengths and weaknesses. Weakened muscles must be protected at all times. Muscles that cannot resist the force of gravity are supported during exercise and rest periods. As a rule, resistive exercises are not attempted until the muscle can carry out a complete ROM against gravity. Weakened or flaccid muscles can be splinted at night to counteract the force of gravity or the pull of the stronger antagonist muscles. During resistive exercises the clinician should stress correct body positioning, joint alignment, and energy conservation. Periods of rest should be included in the exercise program. Activities that incorporate the same movements and musculature as the exercises are encouraged.[19]

The goals for resistive exercises in the rehabilitation of a patient with poliomyelitis are (1) to strengthen undamaged muscles and (2) to reinforce the slightest contraction by integrating it into a larger movement that permits the performance of a given activity. After 8 months, if the muscle cannot contract completely against gravity, it is unlikely that additional muscle strength will return. At this point the emphasis should be on maintaining existing muscles and functional ADL.

Psychological support for both patient and family should be a part of the treatment program. The OT practitioner should anticipate and respect the patient's fears and anxieties about the disabling effects of the disease. The patient may need encouragement and positive experiences to develop an optimistic outlook during the rehabilitation process. The family may also need assistance in adjusting to the patient's disability and new limitations. The occupational therapist or OTA should address these psychosocial issues with both the patient and the family during treatment. Additional support may be secured through a referral to the psychology service in the rehabilitation facility.

As the rehabilitation process progresses, the precautions against physical and body fatigue continue. Assistive devices, splints, and mobile arm supports may be used to gain independence in ADL. After the acute medical problems have subsided, the recovery stage may last as long as 2 years.[11]

The occupational therapist or OTA should administer a self-care evaluation to determine a baseline of function. Dressing activities may include donning and removing orthoses. Assistive devices should be tailored to the needs of the patient.[43] It may also be advantageous to begin activities for prevocational and vocational exploration. Patients' quality of life can be improved if they are employed and productive. The prognosis for successful rehabilitation depends on the personality of the patient and the perseverance of the clinician.

Postpolio Syndrome

OT practitioners are seeing more patients with postpolio syndrome in rehabilitation centers. Patients who had polio earlier in life are experiencing additional weakness and other disabling symptoms years after the initial disease.[55,61] The numbers of such persons have increased, in part because of the influx of immigrants from Southeast Asia and Latin America who suffered the original infection in their native lands.[20] It is estimated that more than 440,000 polio survivors are living in the United States. Of those, some 25% to 60% may be experiencing symptoms of postpolio syndrome.[35] Postpolio syndrome causes health and functional problems, and patients who are affected are likely to be referred for OT services.[61]

Postpolio syndrome is a combination of impairments occurring in individuals who have experienced poliomyelitis many years ago and have functioned quite satisfactorily in the interim. It is primarily characterized by increased weakness of muscles that were previously affected by the polio infection. This is considered to be due possibly to chronic strain of weakened musculature and ligaments or dysfunction in reinnervated motor units.[42] Symptoms include fatigue, slowly progressing muscle weakness and, at times, muscular atrophy. Joint pain and increasing skeletal deformities such as scoliosis are also common. The severity of the postpolio syndrome depends on the degree of residual weakness and disability after the original polio attack. Persons with only mild polio generally experience more mild postpolio symptoms. Those who experienced more severe polio with greater weakness may develop greater loss of function with postpolio syndrome.[35] One hypothesis about postpolio syndrome is that it occurs when motor neurons with excessive sprouting can no longer maintain the metabolic demands. Thus, slow deterioration of individual terminals results.[35]

Fatigue is the most debilitating symptom because it limits activity yet is not apparent to others. The fatigue may be severe and out of proportion to the apparent physical demands of the activity and can be overwhelming.[20,61] An increase in difficulties with ADL accompanies the symptoms. Problems with ambulation, transfers, using stairs, home management, driving, dressing, eating and swallowing, and bladder and bowel control may occur.[61]

Effective remedies aim to prevent muscle fatigue, improve body mechanics, and conserve energy. In general, it has been observed that patients who adjust their lifestyles experience improvement of symptoms and stabilization of function.[20]

Occupational Therapy Intervention

When a diagnosis of postpolio syndrome has been made, the affected person may be referred for rehabilitation services. Physical therapists assess strength, ROM, and endurance. Occupational therapists assess these factors separately for how they affect ADL, occupational performance, and psychosocial status. Gait and orthotic needs should be evaluated as well.[20] The OTA may participate in this assessment process in specific areas where proficiency and competence have been demonstrated.

The OT practitioner should begin by interviewing the patient to ascertain valued occupational roles and obtain an activity profile of daily life. The clinician should ask the patient which activities cause pain or fatigue; which activities have been curtailed or eliminated because of symptoms; when symptoms are most likely to occur (time, circumstances); and what kinds of aids, equipment, and human assistance are presently used. Manual muscle testing of the UEs may be indicated if there is weakness. It should be noted that due to being easily fatigued, postpolio muscles may actually function at levels of strength lower than estimated from scores on the manual muscle test and that UE strength varies markedly throughout the ROM.[61] Joint ROM measurements are important if contractures and muscle imbalances are present.

An assessment of psychosocial status is necessary to select the best approach for the patient to facilitate rehabilitation efforts and to adjust to new limitations. Changes in physical capacities and curtailment of valued life skills confront the individual with psychological issues of coping, adjustment, and adaptation. These may be as traumatic as they were at the time of the original illness. Reactions such as denial, anger, frustration, and hopelessness must be recognized, addressed, and processed.

As a group, persons who originally had polio assumed that the disease was over, that disability was in the past, and that any residual weakness would not worsen. They worked hard to overcome the effects of the initial paralysis and often performed well, achieved high levels of personal fulfillment, became well integrated into society, and so "disappeared" as a disabled group. The onset of new symptoms disrupts the performance and lifestyle achieved through years of hard work. Old remedies are ineffective in ameliorating the new limitations. The person often struggles to accept the reality of the circumstances. As a result, the clinician should introduce change gradually. Small changes may be more easily accepted than major ones, even if the latter are obviously necessary.[20]

The patient is confronted, for a second time, years after the disability was thought to be stabilized, with the notion of being "disabled" and with limited function and diminished participation in valued life activities. A supportive and realistic approach and patient education are key to lifestyle modification.[61]

Exercise may not be consistently beneficial because it may aggravate pain. Overwork of muscles that have a decreased number of motor units may be damaging. However, muscles weakened by disuse may benefit from a nonfatiguing trial of gentle exercises for purposes of strengthening and improving activity tolerance.[42] Strength may be maintained by performance of ADL. Muscles used for ADL should not be stressed further.[61] Patients should be encouraged to be active within limits of their comfort and safety. A regular routine of activity or nonfatiguing exercise is important and affords the patient the feeling of doing something positive. Exercise programs must be carefully supervised. Long-term strengthening or maintenance exercises are recommended only for muscles that show no EMG evidence of prior polio involvement. Further weakness, discomfort, pain, muscle spasm, or chronic fatigue resulting from exercise are signs of excessive activity.[20,61]

Pain can be managed or alleviated by improving body mechanics, supporting weakened muscles, and promoting lifestyle modification. The OTA can teach correct body mechanics in daily living tasks such as work and home management, ambulation, and transfers. Orthoses may be used to support weakened muscles and prevent deformity with muscle imbalance. Activities and lifestyle should be modified to reduce fatigue, stress, and overuse of muscles. Weight reduction is necessary for some patients.[16]

Perhaps the most important contribution of the OT practitioner is guiding and facilitating lifestyle modifications. Patients must avoid overuse of muscles. Evaluation and retraining in all aspects of ADL are important. Assistive devices for self-care and home management may be indicated. Home and workplace modifications can help prevent muscle overuse and decrease fatigue and potential deformity. Energy conservation and work simplification techniques should be taught. The patient and clinician should set priorities for occupational role performance. Energy conservation for the most valued activities may mean sacrificing less valued ones to be done by others or to be done with the assistance of equipment such as orthoses, assistive devices, or ambulation aids.[42,61] Adaptive devices are sometimes viewed by the person with postpolio syndrome as devices used by "disabled" and are therefore rejected by the person or by his or her family. Often, the device is more easily accepted when it is introduced as a tool to get a job done.

Guillain-Barré Syndrome

Guillain-Barré syndrome (also known as *acute idiopathic neuropathy, infectious polyneuritis,* and *Landry's syndrome*) is an acute inflammatory condition involving the spinal nerve roots, peripheral nerves, and—in some cases—selected cranial nerves. Guillain-Barré syndrome often follows a viral illness, immunization, or surgery and may affect both sexes at any age.[6,11,24,42,46,51,52,55,59]

Guillain-Barré syndrome has a rapid onset. Initially no fever presents, but pain and tenderness of muscles, weakness, and decreased deep tendon reflexes occur. As the disease progresses, it produces motor weakness or paralysis of the limbs, sensory loss, and muscle atrophy. Fatigue is also experienced and in many cases can be quite debilitating.[14] The prognosis in Guillain-Barré syndrome is varied. In severe cases cranial nerves 7, 9, and 10 may be involved, and the patient may have difficulty speaking, swallowing, and breathing. If vital centers in the medulla are affected, the patient may experience respiratory failure and require tracheostomy or assisted ventilation. In the majority of the cases, the patient completely recovers within a few weeks to a few months with relatively few residual effects.[24,55]

Occupational Therapy Intervention

Once the patient is medically stabilized, rehabilitation can be initiated. Comprehensive rehabilitation goals should be coordinated with the physician, nurse, physical therapist, and other members of the team. The patient may be referred to OT while still totally paralyzed. This initial phase of evaluation and treatment focuses on PROM, positioning, and splinting to prevent contracture and deformity, as well as to protect weak muscles. Passive activities such as watching television and light social activities such as visits from friends are encouraged. As improvement occurs and more active motion is possible, OT interventions include gentle, nonresistive activities and light ADL to alleviate joint stiffness and muscle atrophy and to prevent contractures.[42] The occupational therapist or assistant should grade the activity program to the patient's physical tolerance level. Fatigue should be avoided, and psychological support should be provided.[51]

The OT evaluation should include a test of strength, ROM measurement, and functioning in occupational performance areas. Sensory testing should also be conducted because the sensory pathways are often affected. In most cases this formal testing is performed by the occupational therapist. During the early stages of recovery the evaluation process itself may be fatiguing. It is often best to spread the evaluation over a few days.[42]

PROM should begin with gentle movement of the proximal joints and should proceed only to the point of pain. As the patient's tolerance increases, active assisted ROM (AAROM), AROM, and light exercises may be introduced. The program should stress joint protection, and the clinician should look for muscle imbalance and substitution patterns. Progressive resistive exercises should be used conservatively. Throughout the course of recovery the clinician should guard against fatigue and irritation of the inflamed nerves.

As the patient's strength and tolerance increase, resistance can be gradually and moderately increased and upgrades can be made to daily tasks. The clinician may introduce sedentary or tabletop activities during the early stages of recovery. As the patient's strength increases, activities promoting more resistance such as leather work, textiles, and ceramics can be added. Grooming, self-care, and other ADL should be included as soon as the patient is capable of some independence. These should be graded to include more activities as strength and endurance improve. Slings and mobile arm supports may be used to alleviate muscle fatigue and promote independence. Activities should be varied between gross and fine and resistive and nonresistive to prevent undue fatigue. Ongoing assessment of ADL status is important to determine which activities the patient can perform, where assistive or adaptive equipment is necessary, when energy conservation techniques are necessary, and where independence can be maximized.[22] Typically, as physical function improves the occupational therapist or OTA can recommend discontinuing the use of adaptive equipment or techniques to enable a return to normalcy.

Psychological support is important throughout the treatment program. The clinician should try to facilitate a feeling of self-worth, convey a positive attitude, and provide encouragement throughout the therapeutic process. Because the prognosis for recovery is good, the activities should be mentally stimulating and purposeful to the patient. The clinician should also respect the patient's level of pain tolerance during stretching and ROM exercises[57]

CASE STUDY

Holly

Holly is a 36-year-old who developed lower extremity (LE) pain, weakness, and numbness in all four extremities, severe fatigue, and facial droop after experiencing a minor respiratory illness. Holly was hospitalized and diagnosed with Guillain Barré syndrome. She quickly transitioned to the inpatient rehabilitation unit of the hospital. Holly was referred to physical therapy to address her LE weakness and mobility impairments, as well as to speech therapy for her facial droop and assessment of swallow function. On initial OT evaluation Holly required moderate to maximal assist with all basic ADL and moderate assist with functional transfers. She was unable to ambulate. Holly had full shoulder, elbow, wrist, and digit AROM but on testing she only had 3/5 strength in all major muscle groups and fatigued quickly. Holly's OT treatment plan was established and included adaptive device training for lower body (LB) dressing, toileting, and showering. Functional transfer training included use of adaptive devices and techniques, as well as instruction in safety strategies. She was instructed in energy-conservation techniques during all functional tasks to prevent overfatigue and maximize her independence. Holly participated in low-resistance and aerobic exercises to gradually improve her functional strength and activity tolerance. Because Holly had never heard of her diagnosis, education regarding the course of the disease and appropriate precautions was also a part of her treatment. As her strength returned, Holly's OT plan was upgraded to include a reduction in energy-conservation techniques and adaptive equipment, participation in functional tasks at a standing level instead of sitting, and training in higher-level tasks such as instrumental ADL. After a 4-week course of treatment, Holly returned home with her husband independent in all basic ADL, light meal prep, functional transfers, and ambulation within household distances. She required assist from her husband for grocery shopping and cleaning and was unable to yet return to work. She was referred to outpatient physical and occupational therapy to continue to address strength deficits, as well as to improve job-related skills so that she could return to work as a soda distribution plant manager.

Peripheral Nerve Injuries

General Characteristics

Regardless of the origin of the injury, peripheral nerve lesions produce similar clinical manifestations. The most obvious manifestation of peripheral nerve injury is muscle weakness or flaccid paralysis, depending on the extent of the nerve damage. Because of the loss of muscle innervation, atrophy will follow and deep tendon reflexes will be absent or depressed.

Sensation along the cutaneous distribution of the nerve will also be lost. Trophic changes such as dry skin, hair loss, cyanosis, brittle fingernails, painless skin ulcerations, and slow wound healing in the area of involvement may also be present. Occasionally, minute muscle contractions called *fasciculations* may be seen on the surface of the skin overlying the denervated muscle belly. As a result of disturbances of sympathetic fibers of the autonomic nervous system, the ability to sweat above the denervated skin surfaces will be lost.

The patient may experience paresthesias—that is, sensations such as tingling, numbness, and burning or pain (causalgia), particularly at night. Moreover, if the nerve damage was caused by trauma, edema will be a prominent clinical manifestation. EMG examinations may reveal extremely small muscle contractions called *fibrillations*.[3,4,11,12,13,18,26]

Extensive peripheral nerve damage may produce deformity if contractures, joint stiffness, and poor positioning are allowed to develop. Disfigurement of the hands is particularly noticeable and may produce some psychological complications. Other complications may include osteoporosis of bone and epidermal fibrosis of the joints.

The medical-surgical management of peripheral nerve lesions depends on the type of injury that has occurred and may include microsurgery, nerve grafts or transplants, and injections of alcohol, vitamin B_{12}, and phenol.

Peripheral nerve regeneration begins about 1 month after the injury. The rate of regeneration depends on the nature of the nerve lesion. If the nerve root has been cleanly severed and surgically repaired, the rate of regeneration will vary from ½ inch (1.3 cm) to 1 inch (2.6 cm) per month. Peripheral nerve injuries caused by burns, sepsis, or crushing will present other complications to the healing process. Age is another factor; children usually have a faster rate of regeneration than do adults.[39] In addition, proximal lesions regenerate faster than distal lesions and injuries to mixed nerves are slower to recover than single nerves.[5,36] Early medical treatment may require suturing the nerve and immobilizing the involved extremity to ensure good apposition of the severed nerves. In the past, full recovery of muscles was not probable because regenerated fibers lose about 20% of their original diameter and conduct impulses at a slower rate.[12,13,37] Microsurgery has resulted in an improved regenerative process in recent years.

Because peripheral nerves can regenerate, the course of recovery can be somewhat predictable. Although the clinical signs of regeneration do not always follow a specific sequence, the following clinical signs of nerve regeneration can be expected:

- *Skin appearance:* As the edema subsides and collateral blood vessels develop, the circulatory system should become more normalized. The skin should improve in its color and texture.
- *Primitive protective sensations:* The first signs of cutaneous sensation will usually be the gross recognition of crude pain, temperature, pressure, and touch.

- *Paresthesias:* Tingling or paresthesias ("pins and needles") distal to the presumed site of the lesion may indicate that regeneration is occurring.
- *Scattered points of sweating:* As the parasympathetic fibers of the autonomic nervous system regenerate, the sweat glands will recover their functions.
- *Discriminative sensations:* The more refined sensations such as the ability to identify and localize touch, joint position (proprioception), recognition of objects in the three-dimensional form (stereognosis), movement (kinesthesia), and two-point discrimination should be returning at this point.
- *Muscle tone:* Flaccidity will decrease, and muscle tone will increase. An important principle is that paralyzed muscles must first sense pressure before tone and movement can be realized.
- *Voluntary muscle function:* The patient will be able to move the extremity first with gravity eliminated and then proceed to full ROM as strength increases. At this point graded exercises can begin.

Specific Peripheral Nerve Injuries

Brachial Plexus Injury

The nerve roots that innervate the UE originate in the anterior rami between the C4 and T1 vertebrae. This network of lower anterior cervical and upper dorsal spinal nerves is collectively called the *brachial plexus.* This important nerve complex can be palpated just behind the posterior border of the sternocleidomastoid as the head and neck are tilted to the opposite side.[6,11,25,50]

Lesions to the brachial plexus usually result from a variety of traumatic injuries. Most brachial plexus injuries in children are caused by birth trauma. Such injuries are called *Erb's palsy* and *Klumpke's paralysis.* Erb's palsy is indicative of lesions to the fifth and sixth brachial plexus roots. Paralysis and atrophy occur in the deltoid, brachialis, biceps, and brachioradialis muscles. Clinically the arm hangs limp, the hand rotates inward, and functional movement is extremely limited.

Klumpke's paralysis affects the more distal aspect of the UE. The disorder results from injury to the eighth cervical and first thoracic brachial plexus roots. Consequently, there will be paralysis to the distal musculature of the wrist flexors and the intrinsic muscles of the hand.[6,11]

Long Thoracic Nerve Injury

The long thoracic nerve (C5 to C7) innervates the serratus anterior muscle, which anchors the apex of the scapula to the posterior of the rib cage. Although injury to this nerve is not common, it can be injured by carrying heavy weights on the shoulder, by neck blows, and by axillary wounds. The resulting clinical picture is winging of the scapula, difficulty flexing the outstretched arm above shoulder level, and difficulty protracting the shoulder or performing scapular abduction and adduction.

The treatment for injuries involving the long thoracic nerve usually involves stabilizing the shoulder girdle to limit scapula motion. The clinician must avoid activities that promote shoulder movements. If nerve regeneration is incomplete, surgery may be indicated to relieve the excessive mobility of the scapula. After medical treatment the occupational therapist or assistant encourages maximal functional independence and teaches the patient to use long-handled devices to compensate for shoulder limitations.

Axillary Nerve Injury

The axillary nerve arises from the C5 and C6 spinal nerves and is derived from the posterior region of the brachial plexus. The motor branches of the axillary nerve innervate the superior aspect of the deltoid muscle and the teres minor muscle. Although the axillary nerve is rarely damaged by itself, it is often damaged along with traumatic lesions to the brachial plexus. As a result, the patient will experience weakness or paralysis of the deltoid muscle, which causes limitations in horizontal abduction and hyperesthesia (extreme sensitivity to pain or touch) on the lateral aspect of the shoulder. In addition to the loss of muscle power, atrophy of the deltoid muscle produces asymmetry of the shoulders. If the nerve damage is permanent, a muscle transplantation may be required to provide some abduction of the arm.[6,11,47]

The OT practitioner should maintain ROM to prevent deformity and improve circulation. Passive abduction of the shoulder should be done daily. The teres minor and deltoid muscles should be protected from stretch during the manual ROM activities. The patient may be taught to use long-handled assistive devices to compensate for the abduction deficit. If a surgical transplant is performed, the clinician should be familiar with the surgical procedure to assist in muscle reeducation. An EMG biofeedback machine can be beneficial in providing the patient with visual and auditory incentives during muscle reeducation sessions. The clinician may also assist the patient in dressing activities. If the asymmetry of the shoulders presents a cosmetic problem when wearing shirts or jackets, a foam rubber or thermoplastic pad can be fabricated to fill in the space that was once occupied by the deltoid muscle. The patient should be encouraged to learn self-ranging techniques and to implement an exercise program to maintain the integrity of the unimpaired muscles of the involved extremity.

Lesions of the radial, median, and ulnar nerves and cumulative trauma disorders that affect the hand are discussed in Chapter 30.

Volkmann's Contracture

A fracture of the lower end of the humerus (in the supracondylar region) may result in a diminished supply of well-oxygenated blood to the muscles of the forearm. This phenomenon can occur when the fracture has been tightly cast and bandaged. Edema sets in near the site of the injury and shuts down the blood supply to the muscle bellies because the cast will not allow the tissue to swell outward. Ischemia deprives tissues of oxygen and nourishment. The muscle can become necrotic, causing atrophy and contractures of the wrist, fingers, and forearm. The flexor digitorum profundus and flexor pollicis longus muscles are severely affected. The median nerve is often more impaired than the ulnar nerve.[11,25]

Shortly after a fracture of the humerus has been immobilized, the patient may have a cold distal extremity with a smooth, glossy, or dusky appearance of the skin. If the clinician observes these symptoms and cannot detect a radial pulse, the physician should be informed immediately and the cast should be removed. Early detection and prevention of this problem can eliminate or minimize what would otherwise become a severe deformity. If, for example, the ischemia lasts 6 hours, some contracture will follow. Ischemia that lasts 48 hours or more will result in a permanent deformity of the forearm. If mild ischemia has occurred, the physician may prescribe vigorous, active exercises to increase circulation, activate musculature, and prevent joint stiffness.[6]

Occupational Therapy Intervention

Peripheral nerves convey sensory information from the environment to the central nervous system and then control the motor response of the muscles and glands to this sensory input.[37] Peripheral nerve injury results most commonly from trauma to the shoulder complex, UE, or hand. Management of peripheral nerve injury may involve surgery, orthopedic stabilization or immobilization, OT, and physical therapy.

The aim of treatment for peripheral nerve injuries is to assist the patient in regaining the maximum level of motor function and independence in performance areas. Treatment is directed to the stage of recovery and focuses on remediation and compensation for sensory, motor, and performance deficits. The rate of return and the residual impairments depend largely on the severity of the lesion and the quality of care during the rehabilitation process. Table 28-1 offers a useful summary of the major nerve roots and clinical manifestation of their lesions.

The OT practitioner may be involved during the acute and rehabilitation phases of treatment. During the acute phase (immediately after surgery), treatment aims to prevent deformity. Initially, immobilization splints are used to stabilize the extremity and protect the site of injury.[52,56] See Chapter 30 for more information on postoperative management of peripheral nerve repair.

Reduction of edema is important and is achieved by elevating the extremity above the level of the heart. This will decrease the hydrostatic pressure in the blood vessels and promote venous and lymphatic drainage. Manual massage with the extremity elevated may also reduce edema. The massage should consist of centripetal (small, circular) strokes to gently force the excess fluids toward the proximal aspects of the body. Care must be taken not to disturb the healing process of the site of injury. External elastic support can also be used to alleviate edema. PROM will assist in the prevention of edema by promoting venous return.[58]

As the patient's muscle function returns, an appropriate exercise program can be established. Resistive activities such as cooking, woodworking, ceramics, leather work, and copper tooling may be used in conjunction with isometric and isotonic exercises when muscle function is adequate. The clinician should not overtax the musculature where nerve regeneration and motor return are apparent and should protect the weaker muscle groups from stretch and fatigue. The clinician may fabricate splints or slings to protect weakened musculature from overstretching and to maintain functional position.

ADL assessment is necessary to identify difficulties with essential performance tasks. One-handed methods of dressing, eating, and hygiene activities may be necessary temporarily or

Table 28-1 Clinical Manifestations of Peripheral Nerve Lesions

Spinal Nerves	Nerve Roots	Motor Distribution	Clinical Manifestations
Brachial Plexus			
C5-C7	Long thoracic	Shoulder girdle, serratus anterior	Winged scapula
C5, C6	Dorsal scapular	Rhomboid major and minor, levator scapulae	Loss of scapular adduction and elevation
C7, C8	Thoracodorsal	Latissimus dorsi	Loss of arm adduction and extension
C5, C6	Suprascapular	Supraspinatus, infraspinatus	Weakened lateral rotation of humerus
C5, C6	Subscapular	Subscapularis, teres major	Weakened medial rotation of humerus
C6-C8, T1	Radial	All extensors of forearm, triceps	Wrist drop, extensor paralysis
C5, C6	Axillary	Deltoid, teres minor	Loss of arm abduction, weakened lateral rotation of humerus
C5, C6	Musculocutaneous	Biceps brachii, brachialis, coracobrachialis	Loss of forearm flexion and supination
C6-C8, T1	Median	Flexors of hand and digits, opponens pollicis	Ape-hand deformity, weakened grip, thenar atrophy, unopposed thumb
C8, T1	Ulnar	Flexor of hand and digits, opponens pollicis	Claw-hand deformity, interosseus atrophy, loss of thumb adduction
Lumbosacral Plexus			
L2-L4	Femoral	Iliopsoas, quadriceps femoris	Loss of thigh flexion, leg extension
L2-L4	Obturator	Adductors of thigh	Weakened or loss of thigh adduction
L4, L5, S1-S3	Sciatic	Hamstrings, all musculature below the knee	Loss of leg flexion, paralysis of all muscles of leg and foot
L4, L5, S1, S2	Common peroneal	Dorsiflexors of foot	Foot drop, steppage gait, loss of eversion
L4, L5, S1-S3	Tibial	Gastrocnemius, soleus, deep plantar flexors of foot	Loss of plantar flexion and inversion of foot

permanently. Assistive devices such as long-handled reaching aids and one-handed kitchen tools can be beneficial to increase independence in self-care ADL and instrumental ADL (IADL) tasks.

Sensory reeducation is used to assist the patient in establishing appropriate responses to sensory stimuli. Sensory reeducation for peripheral nerve injuries is discussed in Chapters 22 and 30.

Peripheral Nerve Pain Syndromes

Pain is a common complication in peripheral nerve injuries.[7,38] For some patients the pain itself becomes an overwhelming disability. Two pain syndromes associated with peripheral nerve injuries are causalgia and neuroma pain.[38,47,53] Causalgia is pain of great intensity. It commonly results from injury to the brachial plexus, median, and ulnar nerves.[5]

In the UE, causalgia is described as an intense burning sensation so excruciating that the patient holds the affected limb immobile for fear of stimulating the pain. The affected limb becomes extremely sensitive to temperature change, wind, and even noise.[17,36] Causalgia is also exacerbated by emotional stress.

Neuromas are incompletely regenerated nerve endings and fibers at the site where the peripheral nerve was damaged. Neuromas are particularly problematic in nerve endings serving the fingers and in amputated limbs. Phantom limb pain is often the result of neuroma formation.

Occupational Therapy Intervention

Research on pain management has revealed that certain activities and noninvasive techniques can modulate pain perception.[27,53,54] A better understanding of pain control mechanisms has provided therapists with new techniques for patients with peripheral nerve pain.[1,7,27,40,49]

The OT practitioner can modulate pain perception in several ways. The occupational therapist interviews the patient to evaluate the intensity, quality, and location of pain. The patient is asked to mark the point of pain on an anatomic drawing and then estimate pain intensity on a numeric scale. The patient is told to describe the personal experience of the pain with terms such as sharp, dull, aching, throbbing, sore, or burning. Factors that seem to contribute to pain are explored during the interview. For example, these factors might include specific foods and drinks, positions, and activities.[27]

Several intervention techniques can alter pain messages. Peripheral pain emitting from neuromas is managed with intervention from both the occupational therapist and the OTA. The occupational therapist may provide graded sensory input such as tapping or vibration over the neuroma, transcutaneous electrical nerve stimulation (TENS), or localized stimulation to acupressure points and trigger points.[1,8,23,29,30,48,49,53] Thermal modalities such as heat or cryotherapy may be used to minimize pain as well.[8] The OTA may instruct the patient to obtain pain relief by protecting the tender regions of the body during daily activities and by using protective devices fabricated from splinting materials.

Involving the patient in successful and purposeful activities may help manage pain by providing cognitive diversion from the pain experience. Engagement in purposeful activities can influence moods and emotions, an effect that in turn will alter the perception of pain intensity in chronic pain and causalgia and can ultimately modify the pain threshold.[15,21,27,36,53] The clinician can also use background music or music with earphones as a therapeutic modality. While the patient is engaged in activities, the volume of the music can be increased or decreased as a diversion to accommodate the pain intensity.[27]

Causalgia is related to tension and stress. To decrease these factors, the clinician can also instruct the patient in relaxation techniques[7,17] such as deep breathing, progressive relaxation, and visualization.[27,36,53] When the relaxation response is elicited, the patient's muscles relax; the heart rate and respiration rate slow; and the patient experiences a sense of well-being. Learning relaxation techniques allows the patient to exert some control over emotional tension and depression, both of which contribute to causalgia and the perception of pain[27]

CASE STUDY

Garrett

Garrett is a 45-year-old construction worker with a severe, traumatic brachial plexus injury to his right UE following a motorcycle accident. After surgical repair he was referred to outpatient OT to maximize functional use of his UE and to return to independence with all ADLs. On initial evaluation Garrett presented with severe pain throughout his right UE and had no active movement. His PROM was limited to 70 degrees of shoulder flexion and 60 degrees of abduction. His elbow also had extremely limited PROM due to pain and stiffness. Garrett was developing moderate to severe tightness in his wrist and digit flexors. He required minimal assist upper body (UB) dressing, LB dressing, grooming, and showering. A treatment plan that consisted of physical agent modalities (such as hot packs before exercise to decrease joint stiffness and increase soft tissue elasticity and TENS to decrease pain) was established. It also included ADL training using one-handed techniques for basic ADL. Garrett also participated in aggressive PROM and stretching to improve joint mobility and was given a home exercise program to supplement his therapy services. A resting hand splint was fabricated for support and stability of his wrist and hand, as well as to prevent contractures. Garrett progressed well with his functional independence and was able to independently perform BADL using one-handed techniques after two sessions of OT. With pain management, splinting, and exercise he was able to return to full PROM in his UE after 1 month. As his peripheral nerves regenerated, his OT treatment plan was upgraded to include AROM and neuromuscular facilitation techniques to obtain functional use of his UE. Due to Garrett's motivation and compliance with therapy techniques including strict adherence to all recommendations and exercises, Garrett now has full AROM in his hand, wrist, and elbow and 120 degrees of shoulder flexion and abduction. He is able to independently use his right UE for all self-care tasks but continues to require bilateral assist for heavier household and work-related duties due to continued strength impairments.

Disease of the Neuromuscular Junction

Some motor unit disorders originate in diseases of the junction between the motor nerve and the muscle it innervates.

Myasthenia Gravis

Myasthenia gravis is a disease of chemical transmission at the nerve-muscle synapse or neuromuscular junction. It results in weakness of skeletal muscle.[44] It occurs at all ages but primarily affects younger women and older men.[24,55] Medical management of these patients varies and may include removal of the thymus gland (thymectomy), treatment with pharmacologic agents, or plasmapheresis (blood filtering).[2,23,24,44,55,60]

Myasthenia gravis is characterized by abnormal fatigue of voluntary muscle.[19] The disease can affect any of the striated skeletal muscles of the body but in particular targets the muscles of the eyelids and eyes and oropharyngeal muscles. Therefore the muscles most often affected are those that move the eyes, eyelids, tongue, jaw, and throat. The limb muscles may also be affected. The muscles that are used most often fatigue sooner.[19,44,60] Therefore the patient may have double vision, drooping of the eyelids, and difficulty with speech or swallowing as muscles fatigue.

Patients with myasthenia gravis may experience life-threatening respiratory crises that require hospitalization and the use of a ventilator. The incidence of these crises has declined significantly in recent years, probably because of increased use of thymectomy.[44,60] The intensity of the disease fluctuates, and its course is unpredictable.[60] Spontaneous remissions occur frequently, but relapse is usual.[11] Remissions or decrease in symptoms and improvement in strength and function can last for years. However, there may be exacerbations of unpredictable severity induced by exertion, infection, or childbirth.[46] The prognosis for myasthenia gravis varies with each individual, but for most it is a progressively disabling disease; the patient may ultimately become bedridden with severe permanent paralysis. Death usually results from respiratory complications.[11,51,55]

Occupational Therapy Intervention

The primary role of the OT practitioner is to help the patient regain muscle power and build activity tolerance or endurance. It is important that the therapeutic program not cause fatigue. The clinician should monitor the patient's muscle strength on a regular basis, taking into account factors that would contribute to fatigue and the effects of medications. A running record noting any significant changes in muscle strength should be kept. The clinician should report any changes in the patient's physical appearance (such as ptosis of the eyelids, drooping facial muscles, or alterations of breathing or swallowing) to the physician.

The clinician should provide gentle, nonresistive activities that are intellectually and psychologically stimulating. The activities should be graded so that they do not fatigue the patient. Overexertion must be avoided and respiratory problems prevented. The treatment plan should include energy conservation, work simplification, and necessary adaptive and assistive devices to reduce effort during daily activities. If appropriate, electronic communication devices can be installed in the patient's home so that contact with social supports and community agencies can be maintained. In addition, the clinician may assist with home planning to determine architectural barriers, bathroom adaptations, and furniture rearrangements. Mobile arm supports and splints may be used to protect weakened musculature from overstretching and to aid in positioning for function.[42,46]

The clinician should assist in educating the patient about the disease. The patient should avoid emotional stress, overexertion, fatigue, and excessive heat or cold because these factors can exacerbate the symptoms of the disease. All clinicians should follow infection control procedures because minor infections can also exacerbate the symptoms.

Myopathic Disorders

Another group of motor unit disorders is caused by disease of the muscles.

Muscular Dystrophies

The muscular dystrophies are a group of nine genetic, degenerative diseases primarily affecting voluntary muscles.[32] The four major types of muscular dystrophy (MD)[45,60] have in common the progressive degeneration of muscle fibers while the neuronal innervation for motor action and sensation remain intact. As the number of muscle fibers declines, each axon innervates fewer and fewer of them, thus resulting in progressive weakness.[41]

Duchenne's and Becker's Muscular Dystrophy

Duchenne's MD affects males only. It is inherited as an X-linked recessive trait. The disease begins at birth and is usually diagnosed between the ages of 18 and 36 months. It begins in the muscles of the pelvic girdle and legs and then spreads to the shoulder girdle. The child has difficulty walking, has a waddling gait, and usually must use a wheelchair by age 12. Ultimately the child becomes bedridden, and death usually occurs by the age of 30.[42,45,51,60] Becker's MD is a much milder form of Duchenne's MD with a later onset, slower course, and far less predictability. Though Duchenne's MD and Becker's MD affect boys almost exclusively, in rare cases Becker's MD can affect girls.[33]

Facioscapulohumeral Muscular Dystrophy

This form of MD has its onset in adolescence and primarily affects the muscles of the face and shoulder girdle, hence its descriptive name. It progresses slowly, and its victims have a normal life expectancy.[60] It is inherited through an autosomal dominant gene and equally affects males and females.[45]

Myotonic Muscular Dystrophy

This type of MD not only causes weakness but also has another component, myotonia (tonic spasm of muscles), that makes relaxation of muscle contraction difficult. It is inherited through an autosomal dominant gene and affects males and females. In addition to the myotonia, its unique features are that it involves the cranial muscles and shows a pattern of limb weakness that is distal rather than proximal.[45,60] Other symptoms involve the gastrointestinal system, vision, heart, or respiration. Learning disabilities occur in some cases. The more severe congenital form begins at birth. The more common form may begin in teen or adult years.[32]

Limb-Girdle Dystrophy

Limb-girdle dystrophies are a group of disorders that present with weakness and wasting first affecting the muscles around the shoulders and hips (limb girdles). These problems usually progress slowly, and cardiopulmonary complications sometimes occur in the later stages of the disease. Some types of dystrophies are autosomal dominant; others are recessive.[34]

Occupational Therapy Intervention

Because this group of diseases is degenerative, decline of muscle function cannot be prevented. Medical management is largely supportive, and rehabilitation measures are vital to delaying deformity and achieving maximal function within the limits of the disease and its debilitating effects. The primary goal of OT is assisting the patient in attaining and maintaining maximal independence in ADL and other occupational performance areas for as long as possible.

Gentle passive stretch should be taught to the family with emphasis on maintaining good body alignment and joint integrity. Instruction in bed positioning is provided to prevent further trunk, hip, and extremity contractures. Self-care activities, assistive devices for independence, and leisure activities are key elements of the treatment program. Wheelchair prescription and mobility training may be included, and power wheelchairs are necessary in some instances.[9,42]

The wheelchair may require a special seating system or supports to minimize scoliosis and to prevent or reduce hip and knee flexion contractures and ankle plantar flexion deformity. A wheelchair lap board, suspension slings, or mobile arm supports are indicated to optimize self-feeding, writing, reading, use of a computer, and tabletop leisure activities when there is significant shoulder girdle and upper limb weakness. Built-up utensils may be helpful when grip strength declines.[51] Home and workplace modification may be necessary for some patients.[16]

Active exercises, especially low-impact aerobic exercise, may be helpful, but overexertion and fatigue should be avoided.[9] For patients with respiratory involvement, exercises for breathing control may be administered by the physical therapist.[51]

Psychosocial problems and educational and vocational requirements also need attention from the OT practitioner. Deficits in cognitive function and verbal intelligence have been reported in some types of MD. Depression and personality disorders may be concomitant problems.[16] Patient and family education is an important part of the OT program. A supportive approach to the patient and family is helpful as function changes and as new mobility aids, assistive devices, and community resources become necessary.[51]

Summary

The motor unit consists of the lower motor neuron, neuromuscular junction, and muscle. Some motor unit disease conditions are reversible, and others are degenerative. The occupational therapist and the OTA both play vital roles in the management of patients with motor unit dysfunction. The occupational therapist coordinates formal assessment of functional capabilities in all areas of occupation and related performance skills. Either the occupational therapist or OTA can implement specific interventions. Provision of positioning, exercise, pain management techniques, and orthoses is necessary in the treatment of these patients. ADL skills including self-care, home management, mobility, and work-related tasks are central to recovery of function. Compensatory measures such as energy conservation, work simplification, and joint protection techniques are important elements of the OT intervention program. Assistive devices, communication aids, and mobility equipment, as well as training in their use, may be necessary. Psychosocial considerations and patient and family education are important aspects of the OT program.

Selected Reading Guide Questions

1. Name three causes of lesions that will result in motor unit dysfunction.
2. Describe the differences in the OT treatment programs for patients with poliomyelitis and postpolio syndrome.
3. Describe the symptoms of postpolio syndrome.
4. What are the elements of the OT program for the patient with postpolio syndrome?
5. Describe the OT intervention for Guillain-Barré syndrome.
6. List at least six clinical manifestations of peripheral nerve injury.
7. Describe the sequential signs of recovery after peripheral nerve injury.
8. Describe some treatment strategies for peripheral nerve injuries.
9. Describe four noninvasive methods for modulating pain perception.
10. Discuss the clinical signs of myasthenia gravis.
11. Describe the role of OT for patients who have myasthenia gravis.
12. What is the primary treatment precaution in myasthenia gravis?
13. Name and differentiate four types of MD. Which one primarily affects children?
14. What are the OT treatment goals for MD?

References

1. Adler M: Endorphins, enkephalins and neurotransmitters, *Med Times* 110:32, 1982.
2. Barone D: Steroid treatment for experimental autoimmune myasthenia gravis, *Arch Neurol* 37(10):663–666, 1980.
3. Barr ML: *The human nervous system*, ed 2, New York, 1974, Harper & Row.

4. Bateman J: *Trauma to nerves in limbs*, Philadelphia, 1962, WB Saunders.
5. Birch R, Grant C: Peripheral nerve injuries—clinical. In Downie P, editor: *Cash's textbook of neurology for physiotherapists*, ed 4, Philadelphia, 1986, JB Lippincott.
6. Brashear RH, Raney RB: *Shand's handbook of orthopaedic surgery*, ed 9, St. Louis, 1978, Mosby.
7. Brena SF, editor: *Chronic pain: America's hidden epidemic*, New York, 1978, Atheneum.
8. Bracciano AG: *Physical agent modalities: theory and application for the occupational therapist*, ed 2, Thorofare, NJ, 2008, Slack.
9. Carter GT: *Rehabilitation management of neuromuscular disease*, http://emedicine.medscape.com/article/321397 Retrieved 09-21-10.
10. Centers for Disease Control and Prevention: *Poliomyelitis*. http://www.cdc.gov/vaccines/pubs/pinkbook/downloads/ polio.pdf Retrieved 11/18/11.
11. Chusid JG: *Correlative neuroanatomy and functional neurology*, ed 19, Los Altos, Calif, 1985, Lange.
12. Clark RG: *Clinical neuroanatomy and neurophysiology*, ed 5, Philadelphia, 1975, FA Davis.
13. deGroot J: *Correlative neuroanatomy*, ed 21, Norwalk, Conn, 1991, Appleton & Lange.
14. deVries JM, Hagemans MLC, Bussmann JBJ, Van der Ploeg AT, van Doorn PA: Fatigue in neuromuscular disorders: focus on Guillain-Barré syndrome and Pompe disease, *Cell Mol Life Sci* 67(5):701–713.
15. Fisher GS, Emerson L, Firpo C, Ptak J: Chronic pain and occupation: an exploration of the lived experience, *Am J Occup Ther* 61(3):290–302.
16. Fowler WF, Goodgold J: Rehabilitation management of neuromuscular diseases. In Goodgold J, editor: *Rehabilitation medicine*, St. Louis, 1988, Mosby.
17. Gandhavadi B: Autonomic pain: features and methods of assessments, *Postgrad Med* 71(1):85–90, 1982.
18. Gardner E: *Fundamentals of neurology*, ed 6, Philadelphia, 1975, WB Saunders.
19. Gilroy J, Meyer J: *Medical neurology*, ed 3, New York, 1979, Macmillan.
20. Halstead LS: Late complications of poliomyelitis. In Goodgold J, editor: *Rehabilitation medicine*, St. Louis, 1988, Mosby.
21. Heck SA: The effect of purposeful activity on pain tolerance, *Am J Occup Ther* 42(9):577–581, 1988.
22. Khan F: Rehabilitation in Guillain Barré syndrome, *Aust Fam Physician* 33(12):1013–1017, 2004.
23. Kornfeld P: Plasmapheresis in refractory generalized myasthenia gravis, *Arch Neurol* 38:478, 1981.
24. Krupp MA, Chatton MJ: *Current medical diagnosis and treatment, 1984*, Los Altos, Calif, 1984, Lange.
25. Larson CB, Gould M: *Orthopedic nursing*, ed 9, St. Louis, 1978, Mosby.
26. Laurence TN, Pugel AV: Peripheral nerve involvement in spinal cord injury: an electromyographic study, *Arch Phys Med Rehabil* 59(7):309–313, 1978.
27. McCormack GL: Pain management by occupational therapists, *Am J Occup Ther* 42(9):582–590, 1988.
28. Melville ID: Clinical problems in motor neurone disease. In Obeham P, Rose FC, editors: *Progress in neurological research*, London, 1979, Pitman.
29. Melzack R: Prolonged relief from pain by brief, intense transcutaneous somatic stimulation, *Pain* 1(4):357–373, 1975.
30. Melzack R, Wall PD: Psychophysiology of pain, *Int Anesthesiol Clin* 8:3–34, 1970.
31. Morrison D, Pathier P, Horr K: *Sensory motor dysfunction and therapy in infancy and early childhood*, Springfield, Ill, 1955, Charles C Thomas.
32. Muscular Dystrophy Association: *Facts about Duchenne and Becker muscular dystrophies*, updated December 2009. http://www.mda.org/publications/fa-dmdbmd-what.html. Retrieved 09-30-10.
33. Muscular Dystrophy Association: *Facts about myotonic muscular dystrophy*. http://www.mda.org/publications/fa-mmd-qa.html updated December 2009. Retrieved 09-30-10.
34. Muscular Dystrophy Association: *Facts about limb girdle muscular dystrophy*, updated December. http://www.mda.org/publications/fa-lgmd-qa.html2009 Retrieved 09-30-10.
35. National Institute of Neurological Disorders and Stroke: *NINDS post-polio syndrome fact sheet*, updated 05-06-10. http://www.ninds.nih.gov/disorders/post_polio/detail_post_polio.htm Retrieved 09-20-10.
36. Newburger PE, Sallan SE: Chronic pain: principles of management, *J Pediatr* 98(2):180–189, 1981.
37. Noback CR, Demares RJ: *The nervous system: introduction and review*, ed 2, New York, 1977, McGraw-Hill.
38. Parry CB, Withrington RH: Painful disorders of peripheral nerves, *Postgrad Med J* 60(710):869–875, 1984.
39. Phelps PE, Walker E: Comparison of the finger wrinkling test results to establish sensory tests in peripheral nerve injury, *Am J Occup Ther* 31(9):565–572, 1977.
40. Piercey MF, Folkers K: Sensory and motor functions of spinal cord substance P, *Science* 214:1361–1363, 1981.
41. Portney L: Electromyography and nerve conduction velocity tests. In O'Sullivan SB, Shmitz TJ, editors: *Physical rehabilitation: assessment and treatment*, ed 2, Philadelphia, 1988, FA Davis.
42. Reed KL: *Quick reference to occupational therapy*, ed 2, Gaithersburg, Md, 2001, Aspen.
43. Robinault I: *Functional aids for the multiply handicapped*, New York, 1973, Harper & Row.
44. Rowland LP: Diseases of chemical transmission at the nerve-muscle synapse: myasthenia gravis. In Kandel ER, Schwartz JH, Jessell TM, editors: *Principles of neural science*, New York, 1991, Elsevier.
45. Rowland LP: Diseases of the motor unit. In Kandel ER, Schwartz JH, Jessell TM, editors: *Principles of neural science*, New York, 1991, Elsevier.
46. Schumacher B, Allen HA: *Medical aspects of disabilities*, Chicago, 1976, Rehabilitation Institute.
47. Seddon HJ: *Surgical disorders of the peripheral nerves*, ed 2, Edinburgh, 1975, Churchill Livingstone.
48. Shealy CN: Transcutaneous electrical nerve stimulation for control of pain, *Clin Neurosurg* 21:269–277, 1974.
49. Sjolund BH, Eriksson M: Electro-acupuncture and endogenous morphines, *Lancet* 2(7994):1085, 1976.
50. Smith B: *Differential diagnosis in neurology*, New York, 1979, Arco Publishing.
51. Spencer EA: Functional restoration, section 2. In Hopkins HL, Smith HD, editors: *Willard and Spackman's occupational therapy*, ed 8, Philadelphia, 1993, JB Lippincott.
52. Spencer EA: Functional restoration, specific diagnoses. In Hopkins HL, Smith HD, editors: *Willard and Spackman's occupational therapy*, ed 6, Philadelphia, 1983, JB Lippincott.
53. Swerdlow M: *The therapy of pain*, Philadelphia, 1981, JB Lippincott.
54. Tappan FM: *Healing massage techniques: a study of eastern and western methods*, Reston, Va, 1978, Reston.

55. Tierney LM, McPhee SJ, Papadakis MA: *Current medical diagnosis and treatment*, ed 33, Norwalk, Conn, 1994, Appleton & Lange.
56. Trombly CA, Scott AD: *Occupational therapy for physical dysfunction*, Baltimore, 1977, Williams & Wilkins.
57. Van Dam A: Guillain-Barré syndrome: a unique perspective, *Occup Ther Forum* 2:6, 1987.
58. Vasudevan S, Melvin JL: Upper extremity edema control: rationale of the techniques, *Am J Occup Ther* 33(8):520–523, 1979.
59. Walter JB: *An introduction to the principles of disease*, Philadelphia, 1977, WB Saunders.
60. Walter JB: *An introduction to the principles of disease*, ed 3, Philadelphia, 1992, WB Saunders.
61. Young GR: Occupational therapy and the postpolio syndrome, *Am J Occup Ther* 43(2):97–103, 1989.

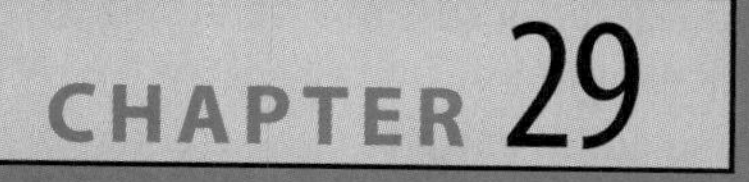

Arthritic Diseases*

PAMELA HARRELL

Key Terms

Connective tissues
Inflammation
Chronic
Systemic
Autoimmune
Synovitis
Tophi
Crepitation
Osteophytes
Joint laxity

Chapter Objectives

After studying this chapter, the student or practitioner will be able to do the following:

1. Identify common signs and symptoms and differences among rheumatoid arthritis, osteoarthritis, and gout.
2. Identify common joint and hand deformities seen in arthritis.
3. Recognize medications commonly used in the treatment of arthritis and identify the side effects of these medications.
4. Recognize surgical interventions commonly performed on persons with arthritis.
5. Discuss the psychological impact of arthritis.
6. Identify important areas for the occupational therapist to evaluate in patients with arthritis.
7. Identify treatment objectives of occupational therapy intervention for persons with arthritis.
8. Identify appropriate treatment methods for persons with arthritis based on diagnosis, stage of disease, functional limitations, type of deformity, and lifestyle.
9. Identify resources helpful to persons with arthritis.
10. Identify treatment precautions for arthritic conditions.

Although arthritis literally means *joint inflammation,* it is used to describe many different conditions that cause aching and pain in joints and connective tissues throughout the body. Some of these diseases such as osteoarthritis (OA) do not involve inflammation. Three of the more common forms of arthritis are rheumatoid arthritis (RA), osteoarthritis, and gout.[4,19]

Description of Major Arthritic Diseases

Rheumatoid Arthritis

RA is a chronic, systemic, autoimmune disorder. It is long lasting and involves multiple body systems. In RA the immune system of the body attacks itself. The course of the disease is different for each person. Some may have a single episode of joint inflammation and a long-lasting remission. The majority of persons with RA will experience inflammation of the joints over long periods of time. The disease process may progress continuously or may progress as a series of flare-ups or exacerbations and complete or incomplete remissions. Remissions provide a period of pain relief; however, the condition has not been cured. It may flare up again. In addition, any damage done during an active stage remains. The patient's functional skills may vary depending on the course of the disease and the severity of the symptoms.[2,7,19]

The systemic symptoms characteristic of RA include fatigue, loss of appetite, fever, overall achiness or stiffness, and weight loss. Morning stiffness, an overall stiffness that occurs on awakening, also indicates systemic involvement. The severity of the systemic symptoms usually matches the severity of joint involvement. As in many chronic diseases, a resulting depression or lack of motivation may also occur. In a small percentage of persons, the blood vessels, heart, lungs, or eyes may be involved.[2,7,19]

RA is an inflammatory arthritis and is considered to be an autoimmune disease. It occurs most commonly between the ages of 30 and 40, and women are three times more commonly affected than men.[2,7,17] Its outstanding clinical feature is synovitis, or inflammation of the synovial tissue lining the inside of the joints. The function of the synovial tissue is to produce fluid

*Wendy Buckner contributed large portions of this chapter to the first edition of this book.

to lubricate the joint. Joint swelling results from an abundance of synovial fluid, enlargement of the synovium, and thickening of the joint capsule. These changes weaken the joint capsule, tendons, and ligaments. Inflamed joints are warm, swollen, tender, often red, and difficult or painful to move. Range of motion (ROM), strength, and endurance usually diminish. As the inflammation continues, it invades the cartilage, bone, and tendons and secretes enzymes that damage them. If the inflammation is not controlled, the cartilage, bone, tendons, and ligaments surrounding the involved joint(s) can be damaged. Scar tissue can form between the bone ends, and the joint can become fused, permanently rigid, and immovable.[2,3,7,19]

Joint involvement is commonly bilateral and symmetrical.[3] If one hand is involved, the other is also involved. However, the disease progression may be different on the two sides. One side may be more involved than the other and may have different deformities. The joints most affected by RA are the small joints of the wrist, thumb, and hand. RA is most commonly seen in the proximal interphalangeal (PIP) and metacarpophalangeal (MCP or MP) joints, whereas the distal interphalangeal (DIP) joints are usually spared from the inflammatory process. The elbows, shoulders, neck, jaw, hips, knees, ankles, and feet may also be involved. The thoracic and lumbar spine are usually not directly affected.[2,3,19]

Osteoarthritis (Degenerative Joint Disease)

OA is a disease that causes the breakdown of cartilage in joints, leading to joint pain and stiffness. Unlike RA, OA is not inflammatory or systemic but limits its attack to individual joints. It is often referred to as the *wear-and-tear* disease because the involved joints wear down with age, overuse, or injury. Up to the age of 45 years, OA is more common in men; beyond age 54, it is more common in women.[2]

In OA the breakdown of joint tissue occurs in several stages. First, the smooth cartilage softens and loses its elasticity. This allows it to be more easily damaged. Eventually, large sections of the cartilage wear away completely and permit the bones to rub together, thus causing pain. The joint may lose its normal shape. As the ends of the bone hypertrophy (thicken), spurs (bony growths) are formed where the ligaments and capsule attach to the bone (Figure 29-1). These spurs are also referred to as *osteophytes.* Fluid-filled cysts may form in the bone near the joint or around the joint itself. Bits of bone or cartilage may float loosely in the joint space. The joint becomes stiff or unstable. Joint motion becomes restricted and painful. Occasionally, the process of osteoarthritis causes irritation of the joint and local inflammation may occur.[1,19]

OA can affect any joint but is seen most commonly in the weight-bearing joints of the hips, knees, and spine, as well as the metatarsophalangeal (MTP) joint of the big toe, where it produces bunions.[1,3] In the hand the DIP joints, the PIP joints, and the carpometacarpal (CMC) joint at the base of the thumb are most commonly affected. Hip and knee involvement causes the most severe disability and may require surgery for joint replacement.

The symptoms of OA usually begin slowly and may appear as a minor ache or soreness with movement. Pain is felt most often in the affected joint(s) after overuse or long periods of inactivity. The joint becomes stiff, although movement is possible. If the joint is not moved, surrounding musculature becomes weak. Coordination and posture may also be impaired.[1,3]

Degenerative joint disease (DJD) occurs in some degree among many people older than age 60. Although it is most common in the elderly, other factors such as obesity, heredity, injury, and overuse of joints can contribute to the disease process.[1,3,19]

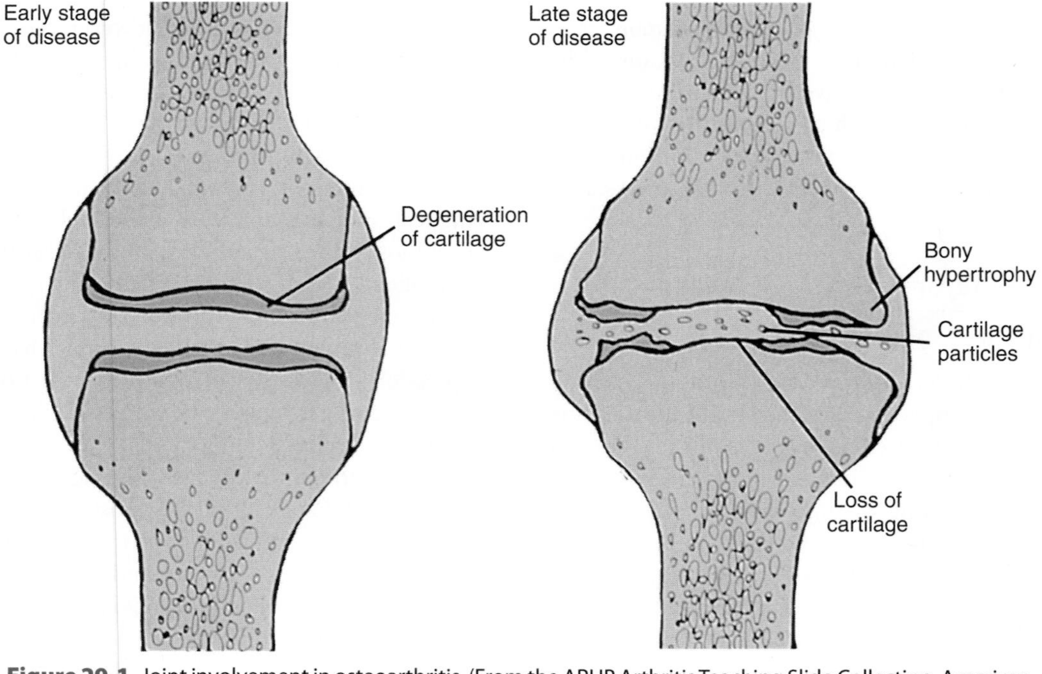

Figure 29-1 Joint involvement in osteoarthritis. (From the ARHP Arthritis Teaching Slide Collection, American College of Rheumatology.)

Gout

Gout occurs when there is an excess of uric acid in the body. These uric acid crystals may become deposited in the joints, causing a sudden onset of severe joint inflammation. It occurs most often in middle-aged men (40 to 50 years old). It rarely occurs in women until after menopause.[3,5,19]

The exact cause of gout is unknown. It appears to be the result of a genetic defect in body chemistry that causes uric acid, a normal body substance, to be either overproduced or produced faster than the kidneys can dispose of it. The increased concentration of uric acid may lead to the formation of tophi (needlelike crystals of sodium urate) in bones, joints, or tissues.[3,5,19]

Gout follows an intermittent course and often leaves patients free of symptoms for months or years between attacks. The acute onset is rapid. The inflamed joint displays extreme heat, pain, redness, and swelling within several hours. Gout is an extremely painful arthritis; it usually affects one joint, although multiple joints can become involved. The most common site of involvement is in the big toe. The MTP joint of the big toe becomes inflamed first (podagra); then the instep, ankle, heel, knee, or wrist joints follow (Figure 29-2). With treatment, the prognosis is good. Appropriate medication can limit the initial attack to a few days and prevent further attacks.[3,5,19]

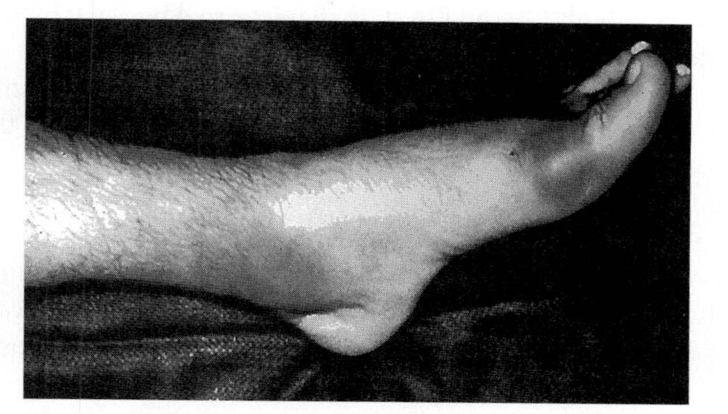

Figure 29-2 Podagra—gout. (From the ARHP Arthritis Teaching Slide Collection, American College of Rheumatology.)

Without proper medication, recurrent episodes may affect more than one joint. Severe attacks may persist for days or weeks. The accumulation of urate crystals can erode into the joints, cartilage, synovial membranes, tendons, and soft tissue, with resulting joint deformity. Other conditions related to gout may include kidney stones, hypertension, and impaired kidney function.[3,5,19] Occupational therapy (OT) is seldom necessary for an acute attack of gout, unless resting splints are required. Referral to OT may be for decreased hand function as a result of tophi or loss of joint mobility. Adapted equipment and assistive techniques may be beneficial for the patient's functioning.[3,5,19]

Description of Common Upper Extremity Joint and Hand Deformities

The destructive processes seen in arthritis can result in tendon, muscle, and nerve dysfunction and many joint deformities. A brief explanation of some of the most common deformities follows.

Crepitation is seen in both RA and OA and occurs as the joints degenerate. It is characterized by a grating, crunching, or popping sensation (and/or sound) that occurs during joint or tendon motion. When the presence of crepitus is documented, the location and/or motion that caused the sensation should be noted.[1,19]

Osteoarthritis

In osteoarthritis, osteophytes, or bone spurs, may form in the fingers or at the base of the thumb.[1,3,19] This excess bone formation indicates cartilage damage. Osteophytes are hard to the touch and may or may not be painful or tender. They are most commonly seen at the DIP joint and are called *Heberden's nodes* (Figure 29-3, *B*). If seen at the PIP joint they are called *Bouchard's nodes* (see Figure 29-3, *A*). Heberden's and Bouchard's nodes can both lead to a loss of motion in the fingers, which can limit grasping and hand dexterity.

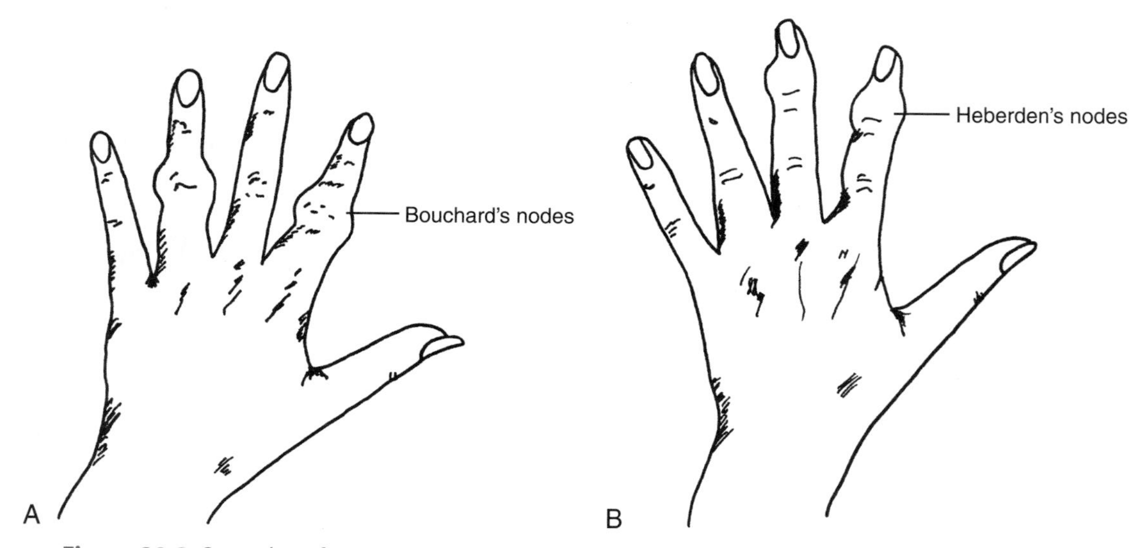

Figure 29-3 Osteophyte formation in the **(A)** proximal interphalangeal joints (Bouchard's nodes) and **(B)** distal interphalangeal joints (Heberden's nodes) is characteristic of osteoarthritis.

Osteoarthritis may also involve the CMC joint at the base of the thumb. This joint is highly mobile and is subject to a large amount of stress during pinch activities. The most common symptom is pain with pinching and gripping. Patients may be limited in many activities because the thumb accounts for 45% of hand function.[19] As the disease progresses, osteophytes may form. In this case the joint can sublux, creating a squared appearance (Figure 29-4).[6]

Rheumatoid Arthritis

The hands are the sites most severely affected by RA.[2,3,19] A typical sign of RA is the fusiform (spindle-shaped) swelling in the PIP joints (Figure 29-5). Swan-neck, boutonnière, and MCP ulnar deviation deformities may also result from the inflammatory process, which weakens supportive structures around the joints. Muscle and tendon contractures and imbalances also contribute to these deformities. The swan-neck deformity involves hyperextension of the PIP joint and flexion of the DIP joint (Figure 29-6). It may also involve a flexion deformity of the MCP joint. Patients who have a swan-neck deformity may have difficulty with or be unable to make a fist or to flex the PIP joint to hold small objects. The boutonnière deformity may look worse than a swan-neck deformity, but it usually does not impair function as much. It is a combination of PIP flexion and DIP hyperextension (Figure 29-7). Its cause is the detachment of the central slip of the extensor tendon, which renders the patient unable to extend the PIP joint.[2,3,19]

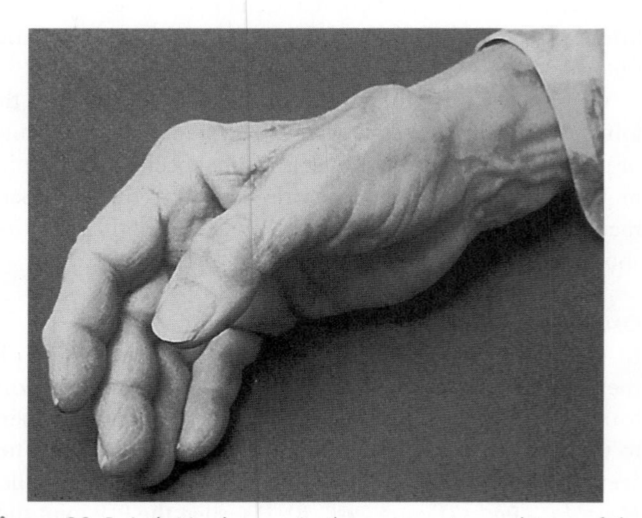

Figure 29-4 Arthritic changes in the carpometacarpal joint of the thumb result in a squared appearance. (From the ARHP Arthritis Teaching Slide Collection, American College of Rheumatology.)

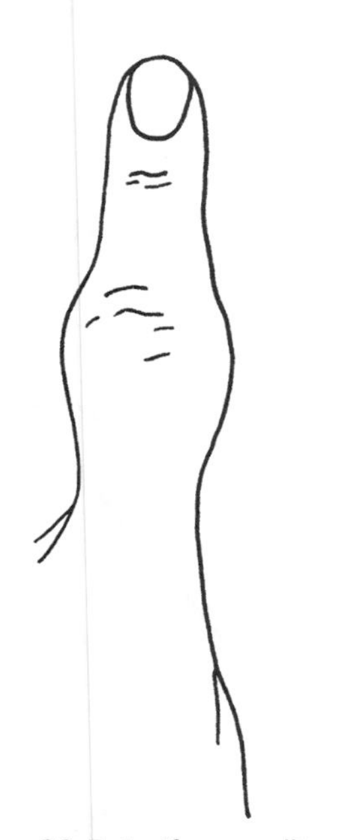

Figure 29-5 Fusiform swelling.

Trigger finger is caused by a nodule or thickening of the flexor tendon at the entrance of the tendon sheath and pulley. The tendon's gliding motion through its sheath and pulley is hindered, thus snapping or catching the finger during active flexion or extension (Figure 29-8). Persistent triggering may result in lost ROM or tendon rupture.[3,19]

The MCP and CMC joints are the most common sites of inflammation in the thumb[2,5] (Figure 29-9). The boutonnière-type deformity of the thumb is the thumb deformity most commonly seen in RA. It begins with chronic synovitis of the MCP joint, leading to stretching of the joint capsule and flexion of the MCP joint with hyperextension of the interphalangeal (IP) joint. The swan-neck–type thumb deformity is seen in both RA and OA. It is characterized by MCP hyperextension and flexion of the IP joint.[7,19]

Joint laxity is a term that describes ligamentous instability and can be a major cause for loss of hand function. In the fingers and thumb, the collateral ligaments support the joint capsule on either side. Chronic synovitis can result in stretching or lengthening of the ligaments and abnormal lateral or anterior-posterior movement of the joint. When the thumb MCP or IP joint becomes unstable, the thumb joints can easily be moved laterally by the therapist and the patient loses

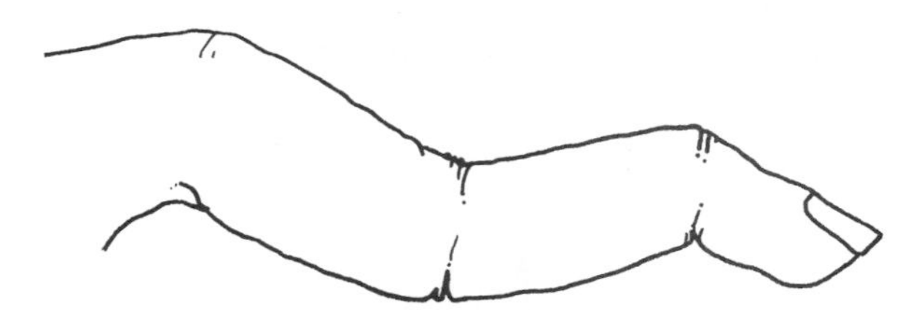

Figure 29-6 Swan-neck deformity results in PIP hyperextension and DIP flexion.

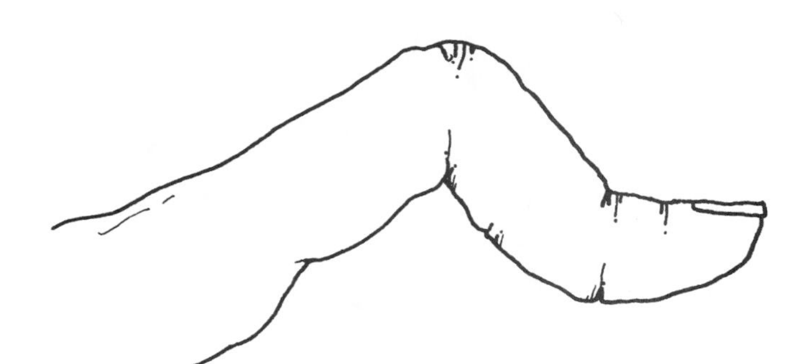

Figure 29-7 Boutonnière deformity results in DIP hyperextension and PIP flexion.

stability of the thumb to pinch and manipulate small objects (Figure 29-10). Joints may also become subluxed or dislocated (Figure 29-11) because of weakened ligaments. The most common sites of subluxation are in the wrist and MCP joints.[3,7,19]

A characteristic sign of RA is ulnar drift or deviation of the MCP joint (Figure 29-12). MCP ulnar deviation is often seen in combination with palmar or volar subluxation of the joint and is caused by several factors including synovitis of the joint, which leads to weakness or destruction of the ligaments supporting the joint. Normal muscle force of the long finger flexors is in an ulnar direction, and when the MCP joints are unstable, gripping forces can pull the joint toward the little finger. Forced contractions and especially forceful hand grip increase this tendency.[3,19,28] Other contributing factors to the development of MCP ulnar drift are displacement of the extensor tendons of the fingers onto the ulnar side of the joint and radial deviation of the wrist.

Loss of elbow and shoulder motion attributable to weakness, pain, and contractures is also a common occurrence in RA. Secondary conditions such as tendonitis and bursitis are common causes of pain. Frozen shoulder is a complication

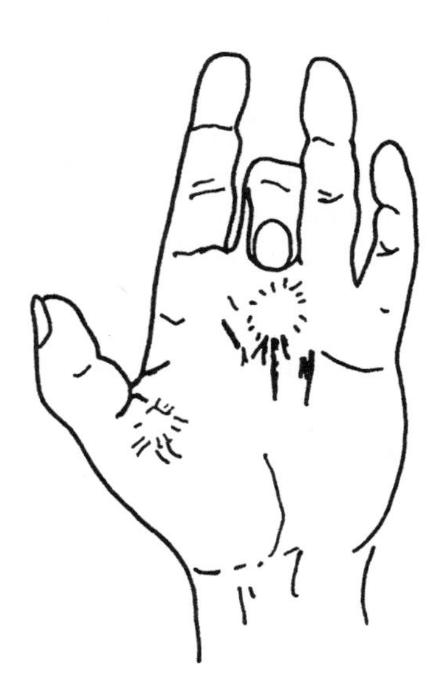

Figure 29-8 Trigger finger. (From Melvin JL: *Rheumatic disease in the adult and child: occupational therapy and rehabilitation,* ed 3, Philadelphia, 1989, FA Davis.)

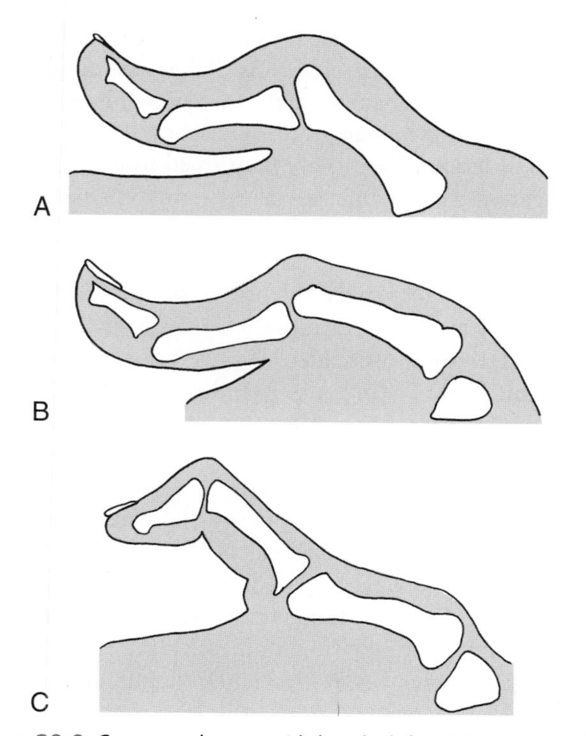

Figure 29-9 Common rheumatoid thumb deformities. **A,** Interphalangeal (IP) hyperextension, metacarpophalangeal (MCP) flexion. **B,** IP flexion, MCP hyperextension, carpometacarpal subluxation. **A** is most commonly seen in rheumatoid arthritis (RA). **B** is seen in RA and osteoarthritis of the carpometacarpal joint. (From Melvin JL: *Rheumatic disease in the adult and child: occupational therapy and rehabilitation,* ed 3, Philadelphia, 1989, FA Davis.)

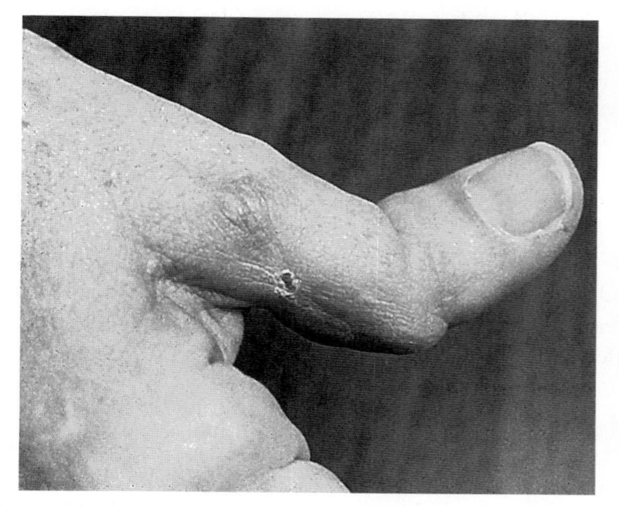

Figure 29-10 Joint laxity (instability). (From the ARHP Arthritis Teaching Slide Collection, American College of Rheumatology.)

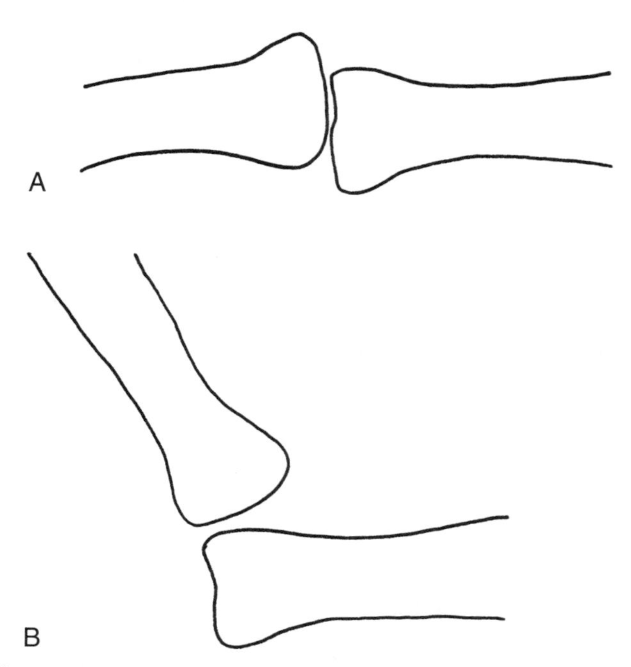

Figure 29-11 **A,** Subluxation. **B,** Dislocation. (From Melvin JL: *Rheumatic disease in the adult and child: occupational therapy and rehabilitation,* ed 3, Philadelphia, 1989, FA Davis.)

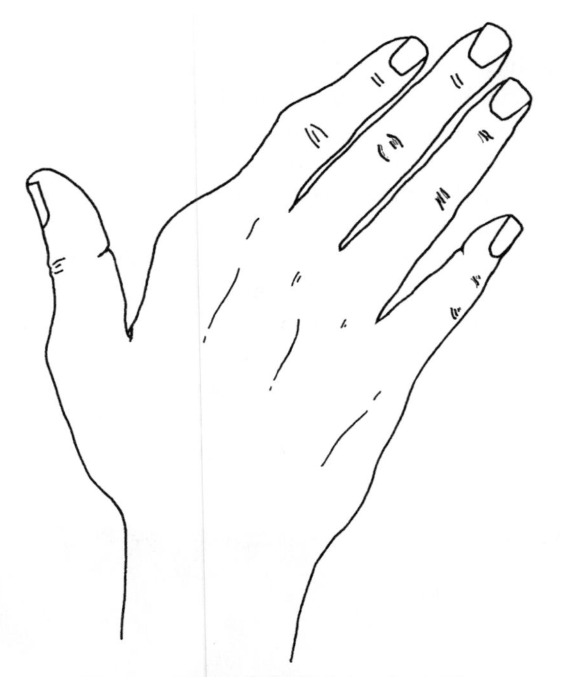

Figure 29-12 MP (MCP) joint ulnar drift.

of shoulder synovitis and is characterized by restricted ROM.[19] In addition, patients with RA may develop muscle weakness as a result of disuse, inflammation, and drug side effects.[15]

Medical Management

No cure for arthritis is yet available. Treatment is geared toward reducing inflammation, pain, and joint damage while maintaining functional abilities. Treatment methods include medication, exercise, use of heat and cold, joint protection techniques, weight control, surgery (when necessary), and coping strategies.[2,3,5,19] When making treatment decisions, both the benefits and risks (or costs) of one form of treatment over another must be considered.

Drug Therapy

Many drugs are used in treating arthritis. Drug therapy is constantly changing, and no single method is recommended over other methods.[19] Patients' needs and reactions change, and each physician develops his or her own philosophy and regimen. Allied health professionals need to be aware of the medical protocols used in their facilities and of the specific medications taken by their patients, as well as their side effects.

Several categories of medications are used to treat arthritis, and patients may be on combinations of medications. Many of these medications help to relieve pain and inflammation. Some are specifically designed to reduce the chances of joint damage and to slow progression of the arthritis.

Nonsteroidal antiinflammatory drugs (NSAIDs) are used to reduce inflammation and pain in both OA and RA. Examples of NSAIDs include ibuprofen, naproxen, and aspirin. Common side effects include stomach pain, diarrhea, dizziness, headache, and nausea.[2,7,19]

Disease-modifying antirheumatic drugs (DMARDs) and biologic response modifiers (BRMs) are used alone or in combination in inflammatory types of arthritis including RA to slow joint damage by suppressing the immune system. Examples of these drugs include methotrexate, gold salts, hydroxychloroquine, etanercept, and infliximab. Some of these medications may be effective within a week or two, whereas others may require 2 to 3 full months of therapy before their full benefit is seen. These drugs may have serious side effects and require careful monitoring. Side effects may include diarrhea, nausea, skin rashes, mouth ulcers, and bone marrow suppression (bruising, bleeding, fever, fatigue). Any of these symptoms should be promptly reported to the physician.

Analgesic medications relieve the pain associated with arthritis. They have no effect on the inflammatory process or in prevention of joint damage. Analgesics taken orally include acetaminophen and prescription pain medications. Topical analgesics are applied directly to the joint or painful area and may include agents such as antiinflammatory medications, camphor, salicylates, or capsaicin.

Steroids may be used either orally or by injection into the joint to reduce joint inflammation and pain. Serious side effects may occur with long-term use and include bone loss, diabetes, weight gain, and hypertension. Steroids are usually prescribed for a short period if the disease is not adequately controlled by other medications alone.[2,19]

Surgical Intervention

Treatment of the patient with long-term RA may include operative procedures to repair soft tissue or replace joints destroyed by the rheumatoid process.[4,19] Several surgical procedures may benefit patients with RA. Synovectomy (removal of the diseased synovium) and tenosynovectomy (removal of diseased tendon sheath) are performed to prevent further complications. These surgeries relieve symptoms and slow the process of joint destruction or tendon rupture and help preserve vascular supply to the joint. The removal of the excessive tissue does not prevent the progression of the disease. A synovectomy may be performed on the ankle, knee, hip, MCP joint, wrist, elbow, or shoulder.[4,19]

Tendon surgery (including tendon relocation, tendon repair, tendon transfer, and tendon release) is considered a corrective strategy for specific hand impairments. Tendon surgery is most often performed on the extensor tendons of the hand and wrist.[4,19] Arthroplasty (joint reconstruction) and arthrodesis (joint fusion) may be done when joint restoration is not possible. Both types of surgery may be performed to relieve pain, improve function, provide stability, and correct deformity. Common sites for these surgeries are the knee, hip, first CMC joint, MCP, PIP and DIP joints, and wrist.[4,19]

Psychological Factors

Any person with a chronic illness must develop coping strategies to deal with the daily challenges they face. The effects of arthritis on a patient's function and lifestyle can cause an adjustment process similar to the grief process after a death. Because the disease is both painful and unpredictable, reactions such as depression, denial, and anxiety are common. Psychological stressors may also contribute to an exacerbation of the disease.[24]

Family relationships and culture will influence the patient's response to the disability.[16] OT practitioners need to understand their patients' responses and work to facilitate their adjustment to the disease (see Chapter 2 for information on psychosocial adjustment to physical disability). Patients and their families must learn all they can about the disease and have opportunities to share their concerns.[3,19] The arthritis support groups available through the Arthritis Foundation will be helpful for many (see Resources list at the end of the chapter).

Occupational Therapy Intervention

Evaluation of Functional Abilities and Activities of Daily Living

The functional abilities of the patient with arthritis must be the first consideration in evaluation. Deformity and decreased function do not necessarily go hand in hand. For example, impaired ROM and joint deformities may be seen in the patient who functions well independently. Such a patient may use substitute or compensatory motions to complete tasks. In contrast, the patient with no apparent deformities may be severely disabled for routine tasks because of pain, edema, or joint laxity.[3,19] It is also important to consider the effect of medication and levels of fatigue on performance.[19]

The initial interview should consider such factors as the medical history, joints involved, presence of pain, medication, functional abilities, and the current symptoms the patient is experiencing.[19] It is also important to find out how much the patient already knows about arthritis and to learn whether any exercise or splinting program is being followed. If the patient reports pain, it is important to ask "where is it?," "when does it occur?," and "how does it limit your abilities?" The patient should be asked to complete a numeric pain rating on a scale of 0 (no pain) to 10 (greatest pain) at different times of the day or with different activities. The patient should be asked whether morning stiffness is experienced and, if so, what is the duration of the stiffness? Morning stiffness that lasts a half hour or less would be more characteristic of OA. With RA, the stiffness may last for longer than an hour and may affect the patient's ability to perform normal morning activities of daily living (ADL). The interview should address present abilities and the potential for independence in self-care. The patient's tolerance for activity should be noted. This type of interview may be conducted by either the occupational therapist or OTA with a structured format such as the Arthritis Evaluation Checklist (Figure 29-13).

The patient should be observed for signs of acute inflammation such as pain, heat, swelling, and/or redness.[2,19] When observing the patient's movements, the OT or OTA should look for signs of pain, loss of ROM, decreased muscle strength, and the presence of joint deformities. Strength of the lower extremities (LEs) can be observed in the patient's gait pattern and when the patient rises from a chair. If the patient must use arms and hands to push off, this indicates weakness of the lower extremities. The patient's use of joint protection techniques can be observed during functional activities.[3,19]

The occupational therapist determines whether objective measurements of ROM, strength, gross and fine motor coordination, sensation, and cognition should be taken (see Chapters 6, 7, 8, and 9). The actual testing may be done by the occupational therapist or by an OTA who has met service competencies in the specific areas. When completing these measurements, the OT practitioner should be careful not to stress the joints. For this reason, grip and pinch strength may be tested with an adapted blood pressure cuff and measured in mm Hg.[3,19] Manual muscle testing may be difficult because of joint instability and alterations in the line of muscle pull. Touch, pain, temperature, and proprioceptive sensations may be impaired as a result of nerve compression or damage. Depression may cause deficits in attention span, short-term memory, and problem-solving skills.[7]

The evaluation of ADL for patients with arthritis is similar to ADL evaluations for other physical disabilities (see Chapter 13). However, the evaluation should consider such factors as morning stiffness, medication schedule, activity tolerance, degree of difficulty with activities, and proper positioning.[16,19] Patients with arthritis may report both "good days" and "bad days." It is important to find out the relative percentage of each and how the patient's functional abilities differ on good and bad days. Such information may help the patient learn how to prevent pain and stress to the joints and to increase functional independence.[16,19]

Evaluations for ADL, work, and leisure activities should consider both psychological and social factors. What is the patient's attitude toward the disability? What specific goals does the patient have? What strategies are used to deal with pain and fear? The patient's abilities may be determined in part by interview. The actual performance should be observed at the normal time each activity is performed because the patient's abilities may change at different times of the day. Ideally, a home evaluation should be done in the patient's home. On site or simulated experiences may be used to assess job performance. In all areas of ADL, it is essential to determine whether the patient is using energy conservation and joint protection techniques.[3,16,19]

Treatment Objectives

Treatment of the patient with arthritis must consider the chronic and progressive nature of the disease.[16] An overall goal of treatment is to decrease pain and inflammation. According to Hittle and colleagues,[16] the general objectives of treatment in OT therapy are the following: (1) maintain or increase joint mobility and strength; (2) increase physical endurance; (3) prevent, correct, or minimize the effect of deformities; (4) maintain or increase ability to perform ADL; (5) increase knowledge about the disease and the best methods of dealing with the physical, psychological, and functional effects; and (6) assist with stress management and adjustment to physical disability.

The treatment plan should be designed for the individual patient and be based on the severity of the symptoms, as well as the general health status, lifestyle, and personal goals of

ARTHRITIS EVALUATION CHECKLIST

Name: ______________________ Diagnosis: ______________________

Referral: ______________________

Initial Interview:

Which joints bother you the most? ______________________

Pain: (0–10 scale) at rest _____ on movement _____ constant _____ Description ______________________

Do you experience morning stiffness? _____ Duration? ______________________

Which medications are you presently taking? ______________________

Since taking the medication, have you noticed any of the following? (circle)

headaches nausea itching rash ringing in ears other ____________

Surgeries? ______________________

Exercise program? ______________________

Splints? ______________________

What do you know about arthritis? ______________________

What are your goals? ______________________

UPPER EXTREMITY ROM:

		RIGHT		LEFT		COMMENTS
		Active	Passive	Active	Passive	
Shoulder	Extension/flexion					
	Adduction/abduction					
	Internal rotation					
	External rotation					
Elbow	Extension/flexion					
Forearm	Supination					
	Pronation					
Wrist	Flexion					
	Extension					
	Ulnar/radial deviation					

Limitations:

HAND PLACEMENT EVALUATION:

Key: 0—Easily 2—With moderate difficulty
1—With minimal difficulty 3—Unable

	RIGHT	LEFT	COMMENTS
Reach overhead			
Touch top of head			
Touch mouth			
Touch back of neck			
Touch behind back			

Figure 29-13 Arthritis evaluation checklist.

the patient. The patient should be an active participant in the treatment process. Both the patient and significant others need to understand the disease process and treatment methods. Rehabilitation intervention will most likely be intermittent so that the patient's ability to follow through with the treatment methods between visits will greatly influence the success of the treatment.[3,19]

Treatment Methods

A number of treatment strategies are used in OT for the management of arthritis. Traditional methods include rest, positioning, physical agent modalities (PAMs), exercise, therapeutic activity, splinting, ADL training, and patient education. The choice of methods will depend on the patient's condition and reaction to the various procedures.

HAND	RIGHT	LEFT
9 hole peg (seconds)		
Grip strength		
Pinch: lateral, 3-jaw		
Opposition		

COMMENTS

Sensation:
Soft tissue and hand deformities noted: (including flexion contractures, swan neck, boutonnière, ulnar deviation, subluxation, edema, redness, warmth)

____

____

FUNCTIONAL ABILITIES: Key: 0—Easily; 1—With minimal difficulty; 2—With moderate difficulty; 3—Unable

	COMMENTS
Grasp spoon or fork	
Carry to mouth	
Cut meat	
Drink from glass/cup	
Bilateral activities	
Button	
Manipulate coins	
Turn key in lock	
Write name	
Turn pages	
Use telephone	
Open doors	
Open jars	

Endurance: ______________________________

Marital status: ________ Family members/supportive persons at home: ______________________________

Household responsibilities: ______________________________

Do you have difficulty in ADL? ______________________________

Architecture: ______________________________

Vocational responsibilities: ______________________________

RECOMMENDATIONS: Adaptive equipment (circle): key extension feeding device writing device telephone device car door opener dressing stick buttonhook other ______________________________

Splints: ______________________________

Joint protection: ______________________________

Home program: ______________________________

Evaluation completed by: ______________________________ Date: ______________

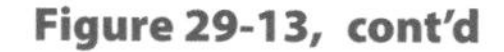

Figure 29-13, cont'd

Rest

Rest is an important part of treatment and should be considered an effective way of reducing inflammation and increasing energy levels. Rest can take several forms. The required amount of systemic rest varies with individuals, depending on disease activity—from complete bed rest during severe flare-ups to short naps during the day. Localized rest to individual joints might include wearing a splint to support the involved joint during activity or lying in non-weight-bearing positions to prevent joint stress. Psychological rest may be experienced with a short diversion from routine activities or a refocusing of attention on enjoyable instead of stressful events.[7,9,15]

Positioning

Positioning against the patterns of deformity is recommended to prevent contractures and joint deformities. To prevent flexion contractures, persons with arthritis should *not* sleep with a pillow under the knees and should use only a small pillow under the neck. Prone lying is recommended for periods of time for both the hip and knee joints to maintain full extension of these joints.

Maintaining good postural alignment when standing and sitting will discourage the development of deformities and prevent undue stress to the muscles and joints. Patients may benefit from using chairs with high seats and armrests because these features will make it easier to facilitate rising from a seated to a standing position and can also reduce stress on involved joints of the upper extremities.[16,19]

> ***Black Box Warning***
>
> Patients with MCP ulnar drift should NOT exercise into composite fist (full fist) or use putty to do this because contraction of long finger flexors promotes ulnar drift. Instead, direct the patient to keep MPs (same as MCPs) extended while working on finger flexion.

Physical Agent Modalities

PAM such as heat, cold, transcutaneous electrical nerve stimulation (TENS), and biofeedback are helpful for relieving pain.[7,19] Local applications of heat including paraffin wax treatments and moist or dry heat packs help to reduce stiffness and increase mobility. At home, patients may enjoy the benefits of heat by taking a warm bath or shower. The application of heat should be limited to 20 minutes because longer periods of warmth can increase inflammation and edema.[7,19,20] Ice packs are used both for pain relief and to decrease inflammation and edema. Occupational therapists and OTAs must be aware of their state licensure requirements and be trained in the use of PAM if they plan to use these treatments as an adjunct to the treatment plan for patients with arthritis.

Therapeutic Activity and Exercise

Therapeutic activities and exercise are used to promote joint function, muscle strength, and endurance. Any functional program needs to be coordinated with the physical therapy program to avoid overworking any group of muscles. The specific types of activity that might be prescribed will depend primarily on the stage of disease the patient is experiencing, as well as his or her level of pain and fatigue. The stages of the inflammatory process have been described as acute, subacute, chronic active, and chronic inactive.[10,19]

Clinical symptoms seen in the acute stage include limited movement; pain and tenderness at rest that increases with movement; overall stiffness; weakness; hot, red, swollen joints; and possible symptoms of nerve entrapment including numbness and tingling. In the subacute stage, limited movement and stiffness remain. A decrease in pain and tenderness indicates that inflammation is subsiding. Stiffness is limited to morning stiffness, and the joints appear pink and warm. The chronic-active stage is characterized by reduced pain and tenderness and increased activity tolerance, although endurance remains low. Minimal signs of inflammation are present in the chronic-inactive stage. The patient's low endurance, pain, and stiffness at this stage are due to disuse. Overall functioning may be decreased because of fear of pain and limited ROM, muscle atrophy, and contractures.[16,19,27,29]

Any treatment program should begin slowly and gradually increase in intensity, duration, and frequency of the various activities.[3] Splints, braces, and positioning devices may be used throughout the stages to provide joint rest and stability. The patient may perform self-care activities as tolerated while incorporating the principles of joint protection. During the acute stage, active assistive exercises and exercises with gravity eliminated may be performed within the limits of pain tolerance. As the patient's abilities improve, the activities will progress to include active and resistive exercises. The exercises should be done at the best time of the day for the patient—that is, when the patient feels more limber and has the least pain (such as after a warm shower or a short time after receiving pain medication).[3,19]

In the acute stage, gentle passive and active ROM exercises to the point of pain (without stretch) should be done twice daily. As few as one to two repetitions of complete joint range are necessary to prevent loss of ROM.[16,19] However, several attempts at movement may be necessary before full range is achieved. The patient may complete self-ranging exercises of the neck, elbows, and hands, but the therapy practitioner should passively range the shoulder to promote muscle relaxation.[19] Some believe that isometric exercises without resistance may be attempted to preserve strength. One to three contractions per muscle group per day is the recommended number.[16,19] Resistive exercises and stretching at the end range should be avoided during the acute phase.[16,19]

> **CLINICAL PEARL**
>
> Exercises for RA tend to focus on antideformity positions:
> - For MCP involvement, work on MP (MCP) extension and radial deviation because the position of deformity is MP flexion and ulnar deviation.
> - For boutonnière deformity, work on PIP extension and DIP flexion because the position of deformity is loss of PIP extension with DIP hyperextension.
> - For swan-neck deformity, focus exercise on PIP flexion and DIP extension because the position of deformity is PIP hyperextension and DIP flexion.

Active and passive ROM exercises that may include a gentle passive stretch may be started in the subacute stage. Isotonic exercises and graded isometric exercises may be performed provided there is minimal stress to the joints.[16,19]

In the chronic-active and chronic-inactive stages, stretch at the end of the range may be included during ROM. Resistive isotonic and isometric exercises are permissible if they do not overstress the joints.[3,16,19]

The level of pain the patient experiences with exercises and activities should be a guiding factor in determining the correct type and amount to perform. Isotonic resistive exercise is sometimes considered controversial for patients with arthritis.[16,19] The occupational therapist must determine whether stable inactive joints will benefit from a strengthening program, without jeopardizing other joints. If pain resulting from exercise lasts longer than 1 hour, the vigor of the exercise should be reduced.[16,19]

Whether choosing therapeutic activities or exercise, the occupational therapist and OTA should apply the principles of joint protection to treatment.[19] Activities should not overstress the joints but should offer enough repetition of movement to help improve ROM and strength. The activities should be nonresistive and avoid patterns of deformity. In general, resistive squeezing of the hand should be avoided because it can promote ulnar deviation, MP subluxation, and extensor tendon displacement.[11,19] When choosing an activity, one must consider how it will affect all joints. Although sanding a board on an inclined plane may be helpful for increasing shoulder and elbow range, it could be harmful for the hand to grip a piece of sandpaper. This problem could be remedied by using a standard sanding block or one with a dorsal strap or other special adaptation.

It is recommended that patients with arthritis avoid activities that require the use of the hand in prolonged static contractions. However, sometimes the psychological benefits of doing activities one enjoys may outweigh the risks involved, especially if the risks can be minimized. According to Melvin,[19] activities such as knitting and crocheting are contraindicated only in cases of active MP synovitis, developing swan-neck deformity, or thumb CMC joint involvement. Wearing a hand or thumb splint while performing the activity may prevent these problems. In addition, regular rest breaks and stretching exercises for the intrinsic muscles may help to prevent complications.[7,19]

Other leisure activities may be introduced to patients as a means of helping them cope with their disabilities. An interest survey completed by the patient can be analyzed to determine appropriate activities. The patient may need help modifying or substituting similar activities.

> ***Black Box Warning***
>
> Be sure to assess the symptoms of the patient at each session and adjust activity accordingly. For example, a patient may arrive for therapy with a prescription for active exercise and strengthening but be in the midst of a symptom flare with inflamed joints. In such cases, treatment should be modified to include resting splints, pain relief modalities, and energy conservation for resting principles. The OTA must notify the OT of the need to change the plan and obtain approval but should not proceed with aggressive exercise while the patient is having acute symptoms.

Splinting

The goals of splinting are to support the joint in an optimal position for function and to reduce inflammation by providing rest or support to the joint.[16,19] Splints may also be used to correct deformity. Splints can be useful for the wrists, fingers, thumbs, neck, elbows, knees, and ankles. The occupational therapist should determine the need for splinting based on a thorough evaluation and consultation with the patient's physician. Inappropriate use of splints can be harmful.[12,25] The splinting of one joint may put added stress on the surrounding joints (e.g., increased stress on the MCP joints when splinting the wrist).[19] Splints worn for too long may cause unnecessary stiffness of a joint or weakness of muscles surrounding the joint. Patients should receive proper instruction in the purpose and wearing schedule of the splint.

Some of the more commonly used splints in the treatment of the arthritic hand include the resting hand splint, wrist immobilization splint, wrist cock-up splint with MCP support, ulnar drift positioning splint, thumb spica splint, and individual finger splints such as a figure-8 splint or a Silver Ring Splint. Specific directions for splints may be found in several sources.[19,32] In addition, several splints designed for the arthritic hand such as the Silver Ring Splint are commercially available.

The resting hand splint (see Chapter 20) is useful for treating acute synovitis of the wrist, fingers, and thumb. It properly aligns MCPs, thus protecting them from ulnar drift, and maintains the thumb web space. Its primary use is to provide rest for the involved joints, but it may also help to prevent multiple joint contractures. Because it restricts movement, it is usually worn during sleep. If the patient requires resting splints for both hands, each splint may be worn on alternate nights so that the patient has one free hand.[19,32]

A wrist immobilization splint (Figure 29-14) is used to immobilize a painful wrist while allowing the hand to remain functional. Wrist immobilizations splints have been shown to be highly effective in reducing wrist pain during functional activities.[30] The wrist is supported in slight extension; this also relieves symptoms of nerve compression in the carpal tunnel.[19,32] If the MPs are involved, a wrist cock-up splint with MCP support may be necessary (Figure 29-15). This splint places the MCP joints in normal alignment, allowing them 0 to 25 degrees of MP flexion.

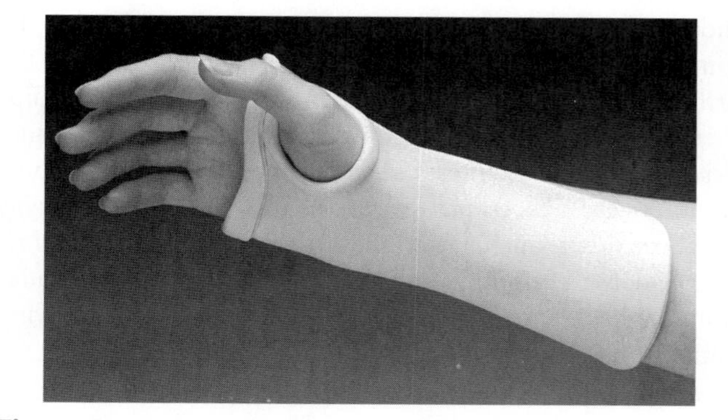

Figure 29-14 Wrist immobilization splint. (From North Coast Medical, Inc., San Jose, Calif.)

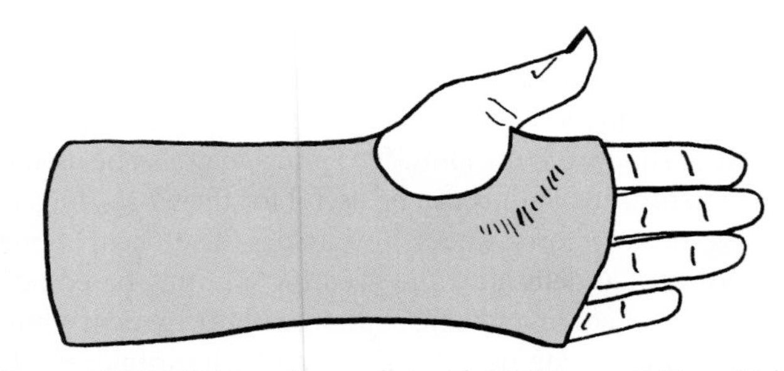

Figure 29-15 Wrist cock-up splint with MCP support. (From Melvin JL: *Rheumatic disease in the adult and child: occupational therapy and rehabilitation,* ed 3, Philadelphia, 1989, FA Davis.)

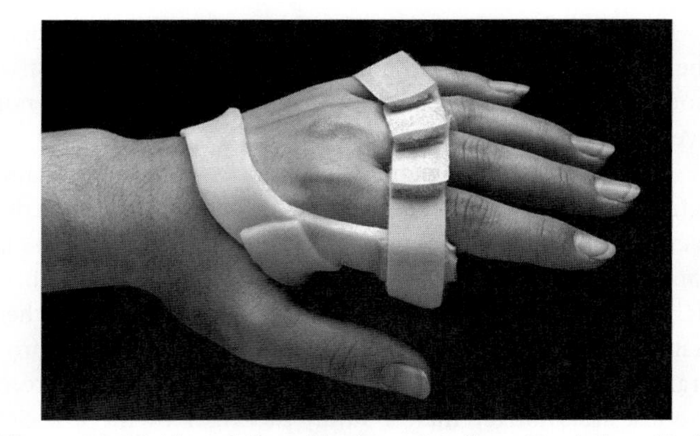

Figure 29-16 Ulnar drift positioning splint. (From North Coast Medical, Inc., San Jose, Calif.)

During pinch and grasp activities, an ulnar drift positioning splint (Figure 29-16) may be used to align the MCPs properly in order to avoid ulnar deviating forces. Individual finger splints such as Silver Ring Splints (Figure 29-17) may be used to support unstable or misaligned fingers during functional activities. In order to prevent stiffness from occurring, removing splints and other orthoses on a regular basis is important. This practice allows ROM exercises to the involved joints.[19,32] Table 29-1 describes specific splinting and treatment strategies for upper extremity (UE) deformities previously described.[16]

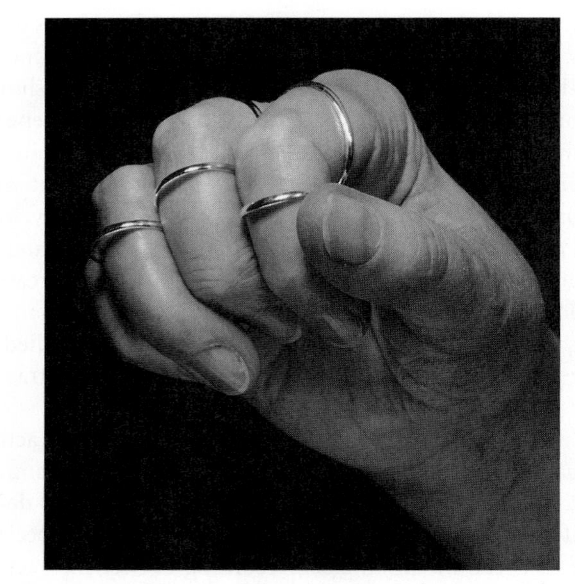

Figure 29-17 Silver Ring Splint. (Courtesy Silver Ring Splint Company, Charlottesville, Va.)

CLINICAL PEARL

Every encounter with the patient provides an opportunity for education about the arthritis disease process and management. Teach patients to recognize signs of inflammation and to change their use of splints and home-based PAM (hot and cold packs) depending on how they are feeling and how their disease is presenting.

Occupational Performance

An effective method of minimizing the effects of disuse and bed rest is to have patients perform ADL to their tolerance.[3,7,16,19] When the patient's condition is acute, activities may be limited to feeding and facial hygiene. As the patient's condition improves, ADL should be resumed to help maintain muscular tone and improve endurance. Adaptive equipment and joint protection methods may be used with bathing, dressing, feeding, work/home management, and leisure activities to promote independence and to prevent pain and further injury to the joints. Occupational therapists and OTAs who work with the arthritic population should be familiar with adaptive equipment and joint protection and work simplification techniques described in this chapter and in Chapter 11. Two additional resources are *The Arthritis Helpbook* and *Tips for Good Living with Arthritis,* available from the Arthritis Foundation. *Arthritis Today* is a bimonthly publication of the Arthritis Foundation that has current articles regarding various topics of living with arthritis (see Resources list at end of chapter).

An important but often neglected aspect of self-care training is sexual counseling (see Chapter 16). Patients may approach any member of the health care team with questions related to sexual concerns. In addition to open discussion of sexual problems, patients and their partners are often helped by illustrations of more comfortable positions for intercourse. Several excellent treatments of this subject are available.[8,23,26]

Energy Conservation

Because patients with arthritis have decreased energy and may require more energy to do things, they can benefit from using energy conservation techniques (Figure 29-18).[15,16,19] OT practitioners can teach the techniques to their patients and help the patients to apply the principles to daily activities. Patients may have difficulty fitting the principles into their lifestyle because doing so often requires a change in lifelong habits. Practice in using the techniques during hospitalization will help with carryover after discharge.

Assistive Devices

Assistive devices should be used only when necessary and must be selected with the patient's needs in mind.[3,16,18,19] Patients are less likely to use expensive or cumbersome equipment. Assistive devices can be used as tools of joint protection to reduce stress on joints during ADL. Patients may need to be taught

Table 29-1 Treatment for Specific Deformities

Deformity	Possible Medical Care	Treatment Methods	Splinting	Methods to Avoid
Swan-neck deformity	Synovectomy in the early stages	Daily ROM to each finger joint and gentle stretches for the PIP joints and intrinsics	Three-point finger splint for the PIP joint to prevent hyperextension	Isotonic, isometric, and resistive exercise
Boutonnière deformity	Synovectomy and tendon repair	Daily ROM to each finger joint, gentle assisted and active extension of the PIP joints, and active DIP flexion with the PIP extended	Extension mobilization or resting splints for the PIP joints	Isotonic, isometric, and resistive exercise
Trigger finger	Steroid injections	Tendon protection techniques—heat/ice for inflammation, avoidance of repetitive gripping activities	Trigger finger splint	Gripping exercises or activities
MP ulnar drift	Synovectomy Tendon realignment Joint replacement	Daily ROM to MP joints with emphasis on MP extension and radial deviation; joint protection techniques	Soft ulnar deviation splints during the day; immobilization splints with the MP joints in neutral deviation and 30 degrees of flexion at night	Isotonic, isometric, and resistive exercise Positions of deformity
MP volar palmar subluxation-dislocation	Joint replacement or repair	AROM of the MP joints emphasizing extension; joint protection techniques	Resting splints at night	Positions of deformity
Wrist subluxation	Arthroplasty or arthrodesis	—	Wrist support during the day and immobilization splint at night	—
Elbow synovitis	Steroid injections; synovectomy and resection of the radial head; arthroplasty	Rest for acute synovitis; use of cold; daily AROM and PROM exercise; isotonic or isometric exercise	Resting splint or splint for stabilization	Overuse
Shoulder synovitis	Steroid injections; applicable surgery	AROM and isotonic exercises preceded by hot packs	—	Slings

AROM, Active range of motion; *DIP,* distal interphalangeal; *MP or MCP,* metacarpophalangeal; *PIP,* proximal interphalangeal; *PROM,* passive range of motion; ROM, range of motion.

to use some of the assistive devices (such as those that compensate for loss of ROM) when they are experiencing a flare-up. When the inflammation has subsided, patients should be encouraged to begin using their own ROM and muscle power to maintain their strength and mobility and, if possible, to rely less on assistive devices. Table 29-2 describes the principles used in selecting devices and examples for each.[3,16,19]

CLINICAL PEARL

Effective use of assistive devices depends on proper body mechanics. The OTA should observe the patient carefully during the return demonstration of how the device is used and counsel the patient to correct any errors, redemonstrating as needed. Be sure that the patient understands the joint protection reason for using the device and the principles behind it including optimum alignment. This helps with carryover to other situations. Practice and feedback will help ensure better outcomes and safer use of devices.

Joint Protection

Joints affected by arthritis have an increased potential for developing further damage. Joint protection techniques are taught to patients to reduce deforming forces on joints and to minimize risk of injury during daily activities. These techniques are especially helpful for patients with RA or with OA involving the hands.[7,9,16,28]

1. *Respect pain.* Pain is one way the body signals that something is wrong and is an indicator that there may be too much stress on the joint. Many patients with arthritis may feel that they can "tough it out," but ignoring pain will often lead to more pain. As a rule of thumb, pain that lasts for more than 1 or 2 hours after completing a task indicates that the activity was too stressful and that it should be changed. This might include breaking the task into steps, using less effort or a different joint position, or possibly using an assistive device to complete the task. Activities that put strain on an already painful joint should be avoided.[7,9,16,28]
2. *Maintain muscle strength and joint ROM.* This may be accomplished by using each joint to its maximal available ROM and strength during daily activities. When ironing, sweeping, or mopping, the patient should use long, flowing strokes, straightening and bending the arms as much as possible (Figure 29-19). Light items such as cereal or noodles can be stored in high cabinets so that full shoulder ROM will be used when reaching.[7,9,16,28]

Attitudes and Emotions
- Remove yourself from stressful situations.
- Avoid concentrating on things that make you tense.
- Close your eyes and visualize pleasant places and thoughts.

Body Mechanics
- When lifting something that is close to the floor, bend your knees and lift by straightening your legs. Try to keep your back straight.
- Avoid reaching (or use reachers). Avoid stretching, bending, carrying, and climbing. If you have to bend, keep your back straight.
- Incorporate good posture into your activities.
- Sit while working whenever possible.
- To get up from a chair, slide forward to the edge of the chair. With your feet flat on the floor, lean forward and push with your palms on the arms or seat of the chair. Stand by straightening your legs.
- Before you get tired, stop and rest.

Work Pace
- Plan on getting 10 to 12 hours of rest daily (through naps and sleeping at night).
- Work at your own pace.
- Spread tedious tasks throughout the week.
- Do the tasks that require the most energy at the times you have the most energy.
- Alternate easy and difficult activities, and take a 10- to 15-minute rest break each hour.

Leisure Time
- Devote a portion of your day to an activity that you enjoy and find relaxing.
- Check out what activities are available in the community.

Work Methods
- Keep items within easy reach.
- Provide good light, proper ventilation, and a comfortable room temperature.
- Use joint protection techniques.
- Make sure work surfaces are at the correct height.

Organization
- Plan ahead—do not rush or push yourself.
- Decide which jobs are absolutely necessary.
- Share your work load with family and friends.

Figure 29-18 Principles of energy conservation.

3. *Avoid positions that put stress on involved joints.* The "normal way" of doing things may need to be changed so that joints are used in their most stable position. Activities involving a tight grip can be avoided by using items with enlarged handles.[7,9,16,28]

Holding a knife in the traditional manner puts too much direct pressure on the fingers. Instead, the patient should use the knife as if it were a dagger or use a pizza cutter. A vegetable peeler should be held parallel to MP joints and not diagonally across the palm. A butter knife can be used to open milk cartons. The palm of the hand (not just the fingers) should be used when pushing from a chair to stand up.[7,9,16,28]

Other hand positions to avoid are those that involve tight pinching, squeezing, or twisting motions. Instead, patients should be encouraged to use the hand in an open position with the fingers held straight and pressure on the palm. A dusting mitt will help to keep the fingers extended while dusting. Sponges or rags may be wrung out by spreading the hand flat over them or by squeezing them between the palms. Several methods may be used to open a screw-top jar. The person can lean on the jar with the palm of the hand and turn the lid with shoulder motion (Figure 29-20) or hold the jar in a drawer as the cap is twisted.[7,9,16,28] A variety of assistive devices are also available for opening jars.

To discourage the development of ulnar drift deformities, patients are taught to turn their hands toward the thumb when turning doorknobs. The right hand is used to open a jar and the left hand to close it. To stir, a person moves the

How to Begin

- Plan ahead by charting your daily routine.
- Make a list of tasks and spread them out in your schedule.
- Include daily rest periods and rest breaks during energy-consuming times.

Weekly Schedule

TIME	Sunday	Monday	Tuesday	Wednesday	Thursday	Friday	Saturday
7:00 AM							
8:00							
9:00							
10:00							
11:00							
12:00 PM							
1:00							
2:00							
3:00							
4:00							
5:00							
6:00							
7:00							
8:00							
9:00							
10:00							

Check your schedule for the following:

- Is one day longer than another?
- Are heavier tasks distributed through the week?
- Is there a long task that could be done in several steps?
- Will your plan allow flexibility?
- Have you devoted part of your day to a relaxing activity?
- Does your plan use the principles of energy conservation?

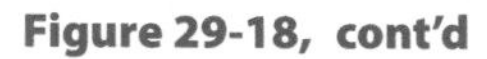

Figure 29-18, cont'd

spoon counterclockwise (right hand) or clockwise (left hand) (Figure 29-21). Patients should be discouraged from leaning their chins on the hands or fingers and from using their fingers to pick up a mug because pressure on the thumb side of the fingers may promote ulnar deviation.[7,9,16,28]

The following are some useful guidelines:

1. *Avoid staying in one position for a long time.* Staying in one position can cause excess fatigue and stiffness. Instead of holding a book with the fingers in a flexed position, use a book stand to hold a book. When stirring, place the bowl in a partially opened drawer or on a rubber mat to eliminate holding. Never begin an activity that cannot be stopped immediately if pain or fatigue sets in.[7,9,16,28]
2. *Use the strongest joints and muscles available.* The use of the larger joints reduces the stress on the smaller joints. One example is carrying a purse on the shoulder instead of in the hands. (Backpacks and fanny packs are also helpful.) The weight should be either balanced between both shoulders or frequently alternated between the two sides. Other examples include pushing doors open with the side of the arm or the whole body instead of the hand, adding cloth loops to drawer pulls so that they can be opened with the

Table 29-2 Assistive Devices

Problem	Principle	Examples
Decreased range of motion	Lengthen the handle on objects Organize objects within easy reach	Reachers, long-handled shoe horn, extended mop handle, long-handled bath sponge Revolving space saver, pegboards
Impaired grasp	Enlarge the circumference of handles	Built-up soft handles, large pens, universal cuffs
Instability	Stabilize objects and provide support for safety	Nonskid mats, suction brushes, handrails, grab bars
Decreased energy	Facilitate performance, energy-conservation techniques	Lightweight tools, electrical tools, Zim jar opener, sit with proper posture while working, pacing of activities, balancing of rest and activity
Potential for joint deformities	Increase leverage Prevent static or prolonged holding	Extended faucet handles, enlarged handles, adapted key holder, vegetable peeler held at MPs, lever-type doorknobs Book stand, bowl holder
Decreased strength	Modify work heights Raise the height of beds and chairs to make standing easier	Raised toilet seats, shower seats

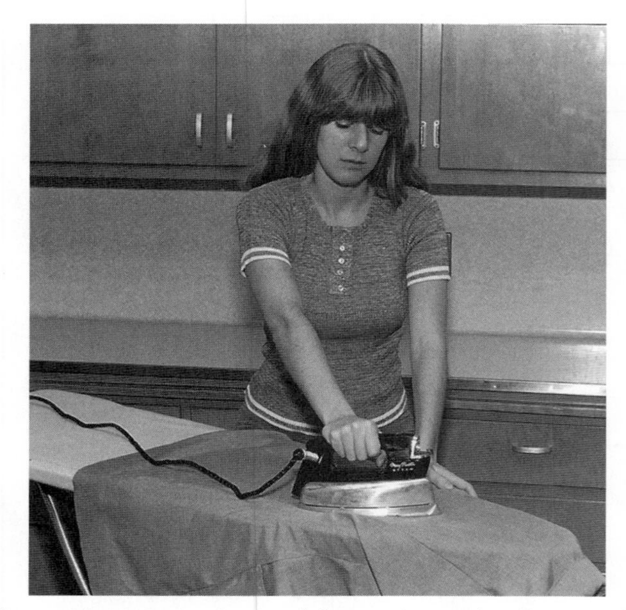

Figure 29-19 During ironing, full extension at the elbow can be practiced.

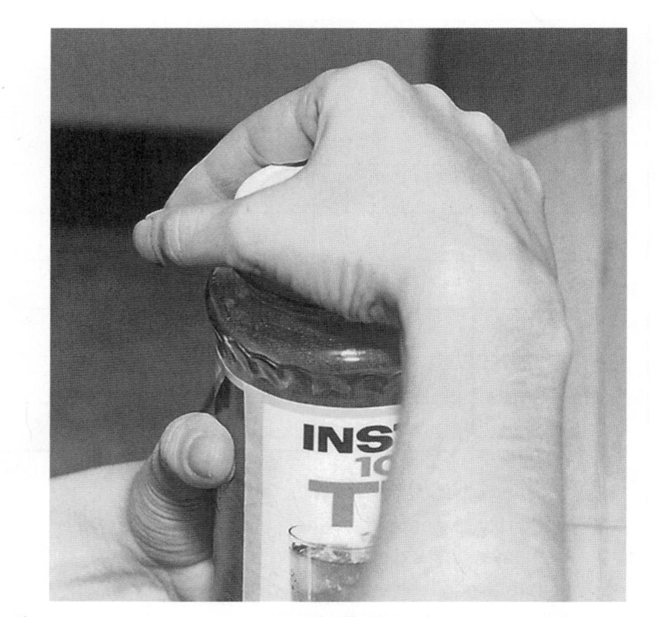

Figure 29-20 Jar cap is twisted off with palm of right hand, or with left hand and opened with right hand, to prevent ulnar drift.

forearm, using palms with the fingers straight instead of bent fingers to pick up a coffee mug, and using the stronger leg first to go up the stairs and last to go down the stairs. It is also important to keep weight under control to avoid stress on the weight-bearing joints.[7,9,16,28]

3. *Distribute the workload over several joints.* For example, use the palms of both hands to lift and hold cups, plates, pots, and pans instead of grasping them with the fingers. Use oven mitts to carry hot dishes. Carry heavy loads close to the body in the arms instead of holding them with the hands. Slide objects along the counter instead of carrying them. If necessary, lift objects by scooping them up with forearms and both palms turned upward. Stress and pain may also be reduced by wearing a wrist splint during functional activities.[7,9,16,28]

Discharge Planning

Discharge planning begins as soon as the patient is referred to OT. Patients who are encouraged to be active participants throughout their treatment program are more likely to follow through with treatment once discharged.[7,26] Patient education will help patients to use the many appropriate resources available to them.

Education of the patient and family should provide information about the disease process including signs of inflammation, potential disability, and realistic treatment options.[7] It is important for families to understand the patient's abilities and to know when they should help (or not help) the patient do things.[21,22] They must be cautioned against medical quackery that promotes worthless arthritis remedies. Because more

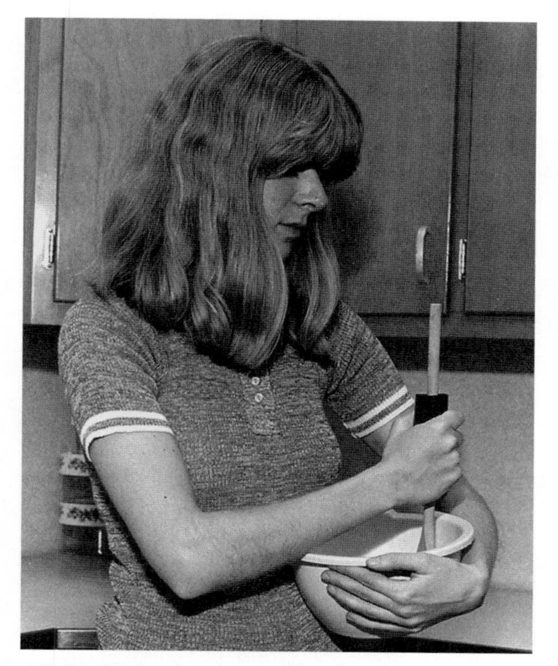

Figure 29-21 Mixing bowl is stabilized with forearm. Spoon with soft, built-up handle is held so that pressure is toward radial side of the hand.

than 40 million Americans suffer from arthritis, health fraud in this area is a lucrative business.[1]

When providing patient education, the OT practitioner should pay particular attention to the patient's questions. Information should be reviewed even if the patient may have heard it before.[3] Repetition and reinforcement are the keys to education. Approach the topics in a variety of ways. Use examples that relate directly to the patient's interest and experiences.[3]

Group treatment (e.g., movement or exercise classes, water exercise classes, home management classes, or arthritis education classes) can use the process of the group for mutual support and problem solving. Seeing others with similar problems may serve as a powerful motivational tool.[3,13,16,19] OT practitioners may lead or participate with other members of the rehabilitation team in such activity groups.

One group program, designed by an occupational therapist, is the ROM Dance Program.[14] Based on the principles of *tai chi chuan,* it promotes involvement in daily exercise and rest. Components include the ROM dance itself, relaxation techniques, group sharing, and health education. Information on the ROM Dance Program and other arthritis exercise programs can be obtained from the address listed at the end of the chapter.

Both the occupational therapist and the OTA should develop a home program and train the patient in its use. A variety of topics including energy conservation, joint protection, and appropriate activities and exercises might be included. An example of a home exercise program can be found in Figure 29-22. Verbal and written directions with pictures should be geared to the patient's level of education and understanding. The patient should be made aware of the resources available from the local or national chapter of the Arthritis Foundation. The Foundation supports research and offers literature and classes designed to improve the quality of life for patients with arthritis (see Resources list at end of chapter).

Treatment Precautions

The following is a list of treatment precautions to be followed when working with patients with arthritis.[16] More specific information on each can be found in the appropriate sections in this chapter.

- Avoid fatigue.
- Respect pain.
- Avoid static, stressful, or resistive activities.
- Limit the application of heat to 20 minutes.
- Use resistive exercises with caution and never with unstable joints.[31]
- Be aware of sensory impairments.

ARTHRITIS RANGE OF MOTION EXERCISES

The following exercises will help you to maintain your mobility. Do only those checked by the therapist.

INSTRUCTIONS

1. Start doing five of each exercise two times per day.
2. Progress to ten of each, two times per day.
3. Do all exercises *slowly* while sitting.
4. If having an active flare-up, cut down or eliminate exercises. After symptoms subside, start at the beginning to build up tolerance.

Shoulder

___ Hold your hands on your shoulders and make small to large circles with your elbows. Go clockwise and then counterclockwise.

___ With your hands on your shoulders, bring your elbows together in front of you and then spread your elbows apart to the side and as far back as you can reach.

Elbow

___ Hold your hands on your shoulders. Bring them out straight in front of you with your palms up.

___ With your elbows bent at your side, turn your palms up and down.

___ Roll up a newspaper and hold onto the ends of it with each hand facing down. Rest the paper on your knees. Bend your elbows to bring the paper to your right shoulder and back to your knees. Bend your elbows to your left shoulder and back to your knees.

Wrist

___ Hold your hand facing down. Make a fist as you bend your wrist up. Open your fingers as you bend your wrist down.

___ Hold your hands together in a praying position. Keeping your hands together and moving only your wrist, point your fingertips away from and toward you.

Hands

___ Touch your thumb to each finger.

___ Make a fist and stretch your fingers open and out.

Please call if you have any questions.

Figure 29-22 Arthritis range of motion exercises.

SAMPLE TREATMENT PLAN

The following treatment plan[16] is not comprehensive because it deals with only four of the eight problems identified and two stages of the disease process. The reader is encouraged to add objectives and methods to the plan to make it more complete.

Case Study

Mrs. B. is a 36-year-old woman with a diagnosis of RA. The onset was 3 years ago. She is a wife and the mother of an 8-year-old girl. She lives with her husband and daughter in a three-bedroom, single-level home. Mrs. B.'s primary role is that of homemaker. However, she has held a part-time job at a florist shop designing and constructing wreaths and arranging flowers. She enjoys this work and sees her salary as a necessary adjunct to the family income.

Mrs. B. experiences intermittent acute disease episodes that have primarily involved the elbows, wrists, MP joints, and PIP joints bilaterally. Slight losses of ROM and strength exist in all involved joints.

To date there is no permanent deformity, but ulnar deviation, MP subluxation, boutonnière deformity, wrist subluxation, and further limitation of ROM at all involved joints are possible deformities.

Medical management has been through rest and medication. Medical precautions include no strenuous activity, no resistive exercise or activity, and prevention of fatigue.

Mrs. B. was referred to OT during the acute phase of her most recent episode for prevention of deformity and loss of ROM and maintenance of maximal function. She continued with OT services during the subacute period with the same goals.

Personal Data

Name: Mrs. B.
Age: 36
Diagnosis: Rheumatoid arthritis
Disability: Limited ROM, decreased strength, potential deformity of elbows, wrists, MP and PIP joints bilaterally
Treatment aims stated in the referral: Prevent deformity, prevent loss of ROM, maintain maximal function.

Other Services

Physician: Supervise medical management and rehabilitation therapies.
Physical therapy: Use if needed for specific exercise program.
Social services: Provide patient and family counseling if needed, and explore financial arrangements if appropriate.
Vocational counseling: Explore feasibility of return to same or modified occupation in floral work.

Treatment Approach

Biomechanical and rehabilitation approaches

OT Evaluation

Active and passive ROM: test
Muscle strength: observe, test
Hand deformities: observe, test MP stability
Ulnar drift (measure if present): wrist subluxation, MP subluxation, boutonnière deformity, swan-neck deformity, thumb deformities
Hand function: test
Endurance: observe, interview
Sensation: test
Pain level: assess with numeric scale with various ADL at different times of the day

Cognitive Functioning

Memory: observe, interview
Functional language skills: observe, interview comprehension of written/spoken language
Occupational role performance: observe, interview
Adjustment to disability: observe, interview
Coping and time management skills: observe
Family and community support: interview

Occupational Performance

ADL: observe, interview
Home management: observe, interview
Work: observe, interview
Leisure: observe, interview

Evaluation Summary

Mrs. B. reports that she tires easily but desires to continue her job as a floral designer. She admits that working at her job exacerbates her pain at times. She says her family is helpful with housework and that she can let them help her. Mrs. B. expresses frustration that she cannot do more and is annoyed with herself for being short-tempered and impatient when she is in pain.

In the physical examination, weakness is noted particularly in wrist and finger extensors (F) and to a lesser degree in flexor groups (G). Mild ROM limitations are present in elbows, wrists, and fingers with some MP instability noted (10-degree ulnar drift). No subluxation or other deformities are noted. Hand function testing revealed difficulty with fingertip prehension. Pinch and grip are good but not normal in strength. Forceful use of the thumb in opposition enhances ulnar drift and produces MP discomfort.

Sensation is intact. Pain is rated at 3/10 at rest and increases to 5/10 with household and work activities. Cognitive state is within normal limits. The patient's family has noted that the patient demonstrates withdrawal from social situations during flares and has limited patience when she is fatigued and in pain. Her family appears to be supportive, and her daughter helps with household tasks. During inactive disease periods the patient is independent for light housekeeping, self-care, and work. She fatigues after 2 hours of light to moderate activity and requires a 20-minute rest period. During flares she is severely limited in ADL, leaves home management tasks to her family, and cannot work. She manages to do only light self-care activities independently.

Observation of the job by another worker and Mrs. B. in simulated tasks revealed that some aspects of her job would contribute to development of deformity. Cutting and twisting floral wire, forcing stems and stem supports into floral foam, and binding wreaths were thought to be likely to enhance ulnar drift and MP subluxation because of the resistance and direction of joint forces. However, wreath design and layout and fresh flower arrangement are possible alternatives. Mrs. B.'s employer is willing to retain her on a part-time basis to perform these duties.

Assets

No LE involvement
Good preservation of function
Supportive and intact family unit
Potential job skills, flexible employer
Intelligence, motivation

Continued

SAMPLE TREATMENT PLAN—cont'd

Problem List

1. Muscle weakness
2. Limited ROM
3. Potential deformity
4. Pain at rest and increased with activities
5. Fluctuating vocational role
6. Limited ADL independence
7. Fluctuating role as wife and mother
8. Tendency to social withdrawal
9. Limited endurance

Acute Stage—Problem 1

Muscle weakness

Objective

Maintenance of muscle strength to enable return to work and maximum participation in ADL

Method

Isometric exercise without added resistance to elbow and wrist flexors and extensors, one to three repetitions once a day; active ROM exercise to elbows and wrists, two to three repetitions once a day; self-care to tolerance

Gradation

Increased number of exercise sessions or repetitions as synovitis and pain subside

Acute Stage—Problem 2

Limited ROM

Objective

Maintenance of ROM of affected joints to enable return to work and maximum participation in ADL

Method

Active or active-assisted ROM exercises to elbow, MP and PIP flexion and extension, wrist flexion and extension, radial and ulnar deviation; may carry out active ROM exercises in a warm bath or shower or immediately after bathing

Gradation

Graded to active exercises and addition of gentle active and passive stretching during subacute stage

Acute Stage—Problems 3 and 5

Potential deformity

Limited ADL independence

Pain increases with household and work activities

Objective

With adaptive equipment and use of joint protection techniques, performance of self-care activities independently without increased pain and without causing stress to involved joints

Method

Instruction from OT practitioner in joint protection techniques and specific recommendations for modifications to existing equipment (building up handles on toothbrush, hairbrush, eating utensils, tools used at work, etc.); provision of necessary adaptive equipment (button hook, washing mitt, etc.) and instruction in their use; treatment sessions within the clinic that include household and work tasks to facilitate problem solving and permit patient to demonstrate competence with adaptive equipment and joint protection techniques

Gradation

As synovitis subsides, gradual tapering off from the use of adaptive equipment and increase in activity level

Subacute Stage—Problem 1

Muscle weakness

Objective

Increase in strength of weakened muscles by a half grade as compared with the initial evaluation, to enable return to work and maximum participation in ADL

Method

Light housekeeping activities (ironing, dust mopping, dish washing) to increase home activity level; isometric exercise with resistance to elbow and wrist flexor and extensors, MP and PIP extensors, 3 to 10 repetitions 3 times daily

Subacute Stage—Problem 2

Limited ROM

Objective

Increase in or maintenance of ROM of affected joints to enable return to work and maximum participation in ADL

Method

Active ROM exercises to elbow, wrist, MP and PIP joints; gentle passive stretching to elbow flexion; stretching to PIP extension; active DIP flexion with PIP extended; instructions to use full ROM for light resistance ADL such as dust mopping, folding linens, and ironing

Gradation

Increased resistance for stretching exercise, as tolerated

Summary

Three of the more common forms of arthritis are RA, OA, and gout. Although their causes and symptoms differ, methods for treating the joint involvement are similar. Potential for further joint damage can be reduced with proper medication, exercise, surgery, and a balance between rest and activity. In OT, patients learn how to protect their joints while performing day-to-day tasks at work and at home. Successful treatment depends on patient education, early intervention, and ongoing care and reassessment.

Selected Reading Guide Questions

1. What is the outstanding clinical feature that causes joint damage in RA?
2. What are the major differences between OA and RA?
3. When is OT indicated for the treatment of patients with gout?
4. What are three systemic signs of RA?
5. What are the clinical signs of joint inflammation?
6. When is resistive exercise appropriate for persons with RA?
7. Why are activities such as crocheting and knitting controversial for patients with RA?
8. What adaptive equipment would be useful for patients with arthritis?
9. Why is it important to know the type and schedule of medication the patient is taking?
10. Why should patients with RA avoid opening doors in the usual method?
11. What areas are evaluated in patients with arthritis?
12. Why is grip strength measured with an adapted blood pressure cuff for patients with RA?
13. Why is rest an important part of treatment for patients with arthritis?
14. Identify five principles of joint protection.
15. Describe how energy conservation techniques can be applied to daily activities.
16. Identify five assistive devices and describe why they are useful for patients with arthritis.

References

1. The Arthritis Foundation: *Osteoarthritis: the basics about the disease that affects 27 million Americans.* Retrieved March 21, 2011 from, http://www.arthritis.org/osteoarthritis.php.
2. The Arthritis Foundation: *Rheumatoid arthritis: the basics about the disease that affects 1.3 million Americans.* Retrieved March 21, 2011 from, http://www.arthritis.org/rheumatoid-arthritis.php.
3. Arthritis Health Professions Selection Task Force: *Arthritis teaching slide collection for teachers of allied health professionals,* New York, 1980, The Arthritis Foundation.
4. The Arthritis Foundation: *American Academy of Orthopaedic Surgeons Fact Sheets.* Retrieved March 21, 2011 from, http://www.arthritis.org/aaos-fact-sheets.php.
5. *Arthritis: the basic facts,* Atlanta, 1974, The Arthritis Foundation.
6. Banwell B: Physical therapy in arthritis management. In Ehrlich G, editor: *Rehabilitation management of rheumatic conditions,* ed 2, Baltimore, 1986, Williams & Wilkins.
7. Batts C: Rheumatoid arthritis. In Hansen RA, Atchison B, editors: *Conditions in occupational therapy: effect on occupational performance,* Baltimore, 1993, Williams & Wilkins.
8. Comfort A: *Sexual consequences of disability,* Philadelphia, 1978, George F. Stickley.
9. Cordery JC: Joint protection: a responsibility of the occupational therapist, *Am J Occup Ther* 19:285, 1965.
10. Engleman E, Shearn M: Arthritis and allied rheumatic disorders. In Krupp M, Chatton M, editors: *Current medical diagnosis and treatment,* Los Altos, Calif, 1980, Lange Medical Publications.
11. Fries JF: *Arthritis: a comprehensive guide to understanding your arthritis,* Reading, Mass, 1986, Addison-Wesley.
12. Hanten DW: The splinting controversy in rheumatoid arthritis, *Phys Disabil Spec Interest Newsl* 5:4, 1982.
13. Harcom TM, Lampman RM, Banwell BF, Castor CW: Therapeutic value of graded aerobic exercise training in rheumatoid arthritis, *Arthritis Rheum* 28:32, 1985.
14. Harlowe D: The ROM dance program, *Phys Disabil Spec Interest Newsl* 5:4, 1982.
15. Harris E: Rheumatic arthritis: the clinical spectrum. In Kelley WH, editor: *Textbook of rheumatology,* Philadelphia, 1981, WB Saunders.
16. Hittle JM, Pedretti LW, Katch MC: Rheumatoid arthritis. In Pedretti LW, Zoltan B, editors: *Occupational therapy practice skills for physical dysfunction,* St. Louis, 1995, Mosby.
17. Lipsky P: Rheumatoid arthritis. In Harrison TR, Braunwald E, editors: *Principles of internal medicine,* ed 11, New York, 1987, McGraw-Hill.
18. Mann WC, Hurren D, Tomita M: Assistive devices used by home-based elderly persons with arthritis, *Am J Occup Ther* 49(8):810, 1995.
19. Melvin JL: *Rheumatic disease in the adult and child: occupational therapy and rehabilitation,* ed 3, Philadelphia, 1989, FA Davis.
20. Michlovitz SL: *Thermal agents in rehabilitation,* ed 2, Philadelphia, 1990, FA Davis.
21. Navarro A: Rheumatic conditions causing hip pain. In Rigg G, Galle E, editors: *Rheumatic diseases: rehabilitation and management,* Boston, 1984, Butterworth.
22. Potts MG: *Psychosocial aspects of rheumatic diseases: rehabilitation and management,* Boston, 1984, Butterworth.
23. Richards JS: Sex and arthritis, *Sex Disabil* 3:97, 1980.
24. Rudolph M: The psychosocial effects of rheumatoid arthritis, *OT Forum* 2:24, 1987.
25. Seeger M: Splints, braces and casts. In Riggs G, Gall E, editors: *Rheumatic diseases: rehabilitation and management,* Boston, 1984, Butterworth.
26. Sidman JM: Sexual functioning and the physically disabled adult, *Am J Occup Ther* 31:81, 1977.
27. Sliwa J: Occupational therapy assessment and management. In Ehrlich G, editor: *Rehabilitation management of rheumatic conditions,* ed 2, Baltimore, 1986, Williams & Wilkins.
28. Slonaker D: *Arthritis information: using your joints wisely,* Atlanta, 1992, The Arthritis Foundation.
29. Talbott JH: *Clinical rheumatology,* ed 2, New York, 1981, Elsevier.
30. Veehof MM: Efficacy of wrist working splints in patients with rheumatoid arthritis: a randomized controlled study, *Arthritis Care Res* 59:12, 2008.
31. Wickersham B: The exercise program. In Riggs G, Gall E, editors: *Rheumatic diseases: rehabilitation and management,* Boston, 1984, Butterworth Publishers.
32. Ziegler EM: *Current concepts in orthotics: a diagnosis-related approach to splinting,* Chicago, 1984, Rolyan Medical Products.

Recommended Reading

Association of Rheumatology Health Professionals: *Clinical care in the rheumatic diseases,* ed 3, Atlanta, 2006, American College of Rheumatology.

Lorig K, Fries J: *The arthritis help book,* ed 6, Reading, MA, 2006, Da Cappo Press.

Marx H: *Arthritis: best use of the hands,* Phoenix, 1988, Video Education Specialist (videotape).

Melvin JL: *Rheumatic disease in the adult and child: occupational therapy and rehabilitation,* ed 3, Philadelphia, 1989, FA Davis.

Resources

Arthritis Foundation
PO Box 7669
Atlanta, GA 30357-0669
www.arthritis.org
(800) 283-7800

Association of Rheumatology Health Professionals
2200 Lake Boulevard NE
Atlanta, GA 30319
www.rheumatology.org

The ROM Dance Program
Tai Chi Health
P.O. Box 756
Taos, NM 87571
www.taichihealth.com
(575) 776-3470

CHAPTER 30 Acute Hand Injuries

SALLY E. POOLE

Key Terms

Observation
Range of motion (ROM)
Total active ROM (TAM)
Total passive ROM (TPM)
Edema
Grip strength
Pinch strength
Joint assessment
Sensibility
Sympathetic function
Sensory reeducation
Evaluation of hand function
Coban
Sensory desensitization
BTE Technologies
Weight well
Theraband
Immobilization approach
Early passive motion
Early active short arc program
Peripheral nerve injuries
Contracture
Fracture
Complex Regional Pain Syndrome, Types I and II
Cumulative trauma disorders (CTDs)

Chapter Objectives

After studying this chapter, the student or practitioner will be able to do the following:

1. Differentiate the roles of the occupational therapist and the occupational therapy assistant in the evaluation and treatment of the patient with an injured hand.
2. Explain the general principles for conducting assessments of range of motion, strength, sensibility, edema, soft tissue, and function.
3. Explain the treatment principles for selected acute hand injuries.
4. Practice specific assessments and treatment techniques under supervision.
5. Explain the impact of a hand injury on physical, cognitive, psychological, and contextual performance areas.

Work-Related Musculoskeletal Disorders

Three days before his wedding, while removing construction debris from a home he is building, a 32-year-old police officer and avid tennis player falls down a short flight of stairs. As he attempts to break his fall, his right dominant arm goes through the window pane of the door at the bottom of the steps, resulting in a deep laceration at the level of the midforearm. All the flexor tendons to the wrist and hand, as well as the median nerve, are severed. He is referred to occupational therapy (OT) for splinting and treatment 2 days after the accident, 24 hours after the surgical repair of all damaged structures. Will this patient make it to his wedding? Will he ever return to work? Will he be able to finish building his new home? Will he be able to play tennis again? What will the OT team do?

The case illustrated is not at all unusual for an occupational therapist and occupational therapy assistant (OTA) working in a facility where people with acute hand injuries are treated. It demonstrates the challenge of working with this population: how to balance the necessary focus on impairment-directed treatment with the "application of an intervention process that facilitates engagement in occupation to support participation in life."[1] With OT's renewed focus on helping people reengage in activity and occupations that are meaningful and interesting to them, therapists must consider more than the specific structures that have been injured.

Treatment of the upper extremity (UE) is important to all OT practitioners who work in the physical disability practice area. UE injuries account for approximately one third of all injuries.[59] Hands and fingers are the most commonly injured body parts in the work environment, leading to more than 1 million visits to the emergency department.[89] Most of those injured are between the ages of 25 and 44 years old; approximately three times more men than women are injured, but all are considered to be in the prime of their lives.[89] Manufacturing, construction, and the retail trade produce the highest number of work-related hand injuries.[90] But hand injuries may also occur in the home, during sports, and while driving a car. Other causes of UE dysfunction include disease such as arthritis and congenital anomalies. Estimates suggest that only 15% of those with severe cerebrovascular accidents ever recover hand function.[59] These injuries and other causes of hand disability can cost our society as much as $19 billion dollars in direct and indirect costs.[59]

The hand is vital to human function and appearance. It flexes, extends, opposes, and grasps thousands of times daily, facilitating necessary daily activities. Sensibility of the hand allows feeling without looking and provides protection from injury. The hand touches, gives comfort, and expresses emotions. Hands, like the face, are exposed for all to see and often have great cosmetic importance. Therefore loss of hand function through injury or disease affects more than the mechanical tasks that the hand performs. Hand injuries may, at the very least, affect every daily activity but also, depending on the severity of the injury, may jeopardize the family's livelihood and compromise a person's self-esteem. Hand injury has a psychological impact and often changes subsequent life roles.[69,86] Effects of a hand injury can interfere with the person's ability to participate fully in meaningful roles, occupations, and activities. The occupational therapist with training in physical and psychological assessment, prosthetic evaluation, fabrication of orthoses, and assessment and training in activities of daily living (ADL) and functional restoration is uniquely qualified to treat UE disorders. The OTA with the desire and motivation to acquire and build knowledge and skills in this area can be a valuable member of the hand rehabilitation team.

Hand rehabilitation, or hand therapy, has grown as a specialty area of both occupational and physical therapy. Hand therapy is defined, in part, as "the art and science of rehabilitation of the upper quarter of the human body. Hand therapy is the merging of occupational therapy and physical therapy theory and practice that combines comprehensive knowledge of the upper quarter, body function, and activity."[49] Treatment techniques have evolved from both professions. The purpose of this chapter is to provide a fundamental knowledge base for treating hand-injured patients. It is assumed that treatments will be provided by the therapist best trained to provide them. Hand rehabilitation requires advanced and specialized training for the OTA or physical therapy assistant. The OTA or physical therapy assistant, with close supervision of the therapist, may assist in providing care for hand-injured patients. The present chapter provides a broad scope of information to serve as a base for the OTA who is interested in developing skills in this area, ideally with the mentorship of an occupational therapist who has advanced service competencies in hand rehabilitation, and with much additional study and experience on the part of the OTA. Detailed information on assessments and results is provided, but it is understood that the OT manages the evaluation process and delegates to the OTA only those portions for which the OTA has attained service competency. The American Occupational Therapy Association's position is that physical agent modalities (PAMs) may be used in preparation for or as an adjunct to purposeful activity.[2] This chapter discusses PAMs within this context.

Successful treatment of the injured hand requires timing and judgment. After trauma or surgery, the body must repair all the damaged tissue including bone. A series of complex overlapping cellular-level events occurs. These events begin at the time of injury and may continue for many months. The healing process is divided into three phases: inflammatory, proliferative, and remodeling.[46,91] Occupational therapy treatment guidelines differ depending on the phase of wound healing, and although sample timetables are often available, the therapist should always coordinate the application of any treatment with the referring physician. Surgical techniques may vary, and inappropriate treatment of the hand patient can jeopardize the results of a surgical procedure. Communication among a surgeon, therapist, and patient is critical. Without the patient's cooperation, gains will be limited. The psychological loss suffered by the patient with a hand injury must be recognized and addressed. A comfortable environment in which group interaction is possible may increase patient motivation and cooperation.

Hand therapy is provided in treatment settings ranging from private therapy offices, outpatient rehabilitation clinics, and hospitals. Reimbursement for services may come directly from the patient or through private medical insurance, worker's compensation insurance, or automobile insurance, all of which may use managed care entities. The number of authorized visits may therefore be limited. Therapists will be asked for documentation that supports the need for continued services. Documented patient improvement is required for ongoing occupational therapy visits to be authorized by the managed care entity and subsequently reimbursed by the insurance company. With fewer authorized visits, the therapy team must be more adept at instructing the patient in self-management of his or her condition. OT practitioners must understand the greater need to justify treatment as the national trend to control medical costs continues. Certified assistants, aides, and other support personnel will be used increasingly, but service must continue to meet all professional and ethical standards.

Information Gathering and Observation

Information Gathering

The OTA must clarify the diagnosis either by reading the medical chart or operative report or by communicating with other health professionals—that is, the physician or therapist. Only then can the OTA accurately understand and implement the treatment. Looking at the x-rays or other test results may help the therapy practitioner understand more fully the patient's condition. The OTA should also make note of any plans for further surgery or conservative treatment.

The OTA may be asked to gather demographic information about the patient such as age, hand dominance, general medical conditions, occupation, living situation, avocational interests, and the patient's goals for therapy. This information will assist the therapist in setting appropriate goals and in selecting appropriate treatment activities with the patient.

When working with a hand-injured patient, one must understand not only the medical condition but also the patient's concerns regarding present and future ability or inability to participate in meaningful occupations. It is important learn how the habits, routines, and roles of the patient have been affected by the hand injury. The Canadian Occupational Performance Measurle (COPM)[68] is an excellent tool that can be employed by the service-competent occupational therapy practitioner to gather the patient's perspective on his or her occupational performance.

Observation

Observation of the patient by the clinician takes two forms. First, if possible, the patient is observed entering the clinic or office. Is the patient alone and able to negotiate contact with office personnel? Or does the patient enter the office with an entourage of family and friends who negotiate the system for him or her? How does the patient hold the injured hand? Is it carefully guarded and overprotected, or is it ignored? Is the hand wrapped in a silk scarf? Observe the patient's posture; is the shoulder hiked and upper arm kept close to the body? Is ambulation impaired? Or is the patient attempting to use the hand within the confines of the injury? The position of the hand and arm at rest, as well as the carrying posture, can yield valuable information about the dysfunction and the patient's response to it.

Second, the hand and arm must be carefully observed and inspected. The skin condition should be noted. Are there lacerations, sutures, or evidence of recent surgery? Is the skin dry or moist? Are there scales or crusts? Does the hand appear swollen? Does the hand have an odor? Palmar skin is normally less mobile than dorsal skin. The degree of mobility, elasticity, and adherence of scars is determined. Trophic changes (dryness, thinning, decreased sweating) in the skin should be observed. The vascular system is assessed by observing the skin color and temperature of the hand and evaluating for the presence of edema. Are there contractures of the web spaces? The therapist will observe the relationship between the hand and arm function as the patient moves about and performs test items or tasks.

The therapist may ask the patient to perform some simple bilateral ADL tasks such as buttoning a button, putting on a shirt, opening a jar, and threading a needle and will observe the amount of spontaneous movement and use of the affected hand and arm.

Physical Evaluation of Body Functions

The effect of trauma or dysfunction on anatomic structures is the first consideration in evaluating hand function. To administer a thorough evaluation of the hand-injured patient, each of the following areas must be investigated: joints, ligaments, tendons, muscles, and peripheral nerves. Usually, the occupational therapist performs the formal initial evaluation and subsequent interim evaluations.

The joints must be assessed for active and passive mobility, fixed deformities, and any tendency to assume a position of deformity. The ligaments must be evaluated for laxity or contracture and their ability to maintain joint stability. Tendons must be examined for integrity, contracture, or overstretching; muscles are tested for strength and function. Peripheral nerves are evaluated indirectly via the sensibility and muscle strength assessments.

The results of these individual assessments will be crucial in determining the patient's overall function in the areas of ADL, instrumental activities of daily living (IADL), education, work, play, leisure, and social participation.

Range of Motion Assessment

When indicated, goniometric measurements are an essential part of an initial evaluation. Measuring joint **range of motion (ROM)** with a goniometer is expected but may be clinically impossible at times because of surgical pins, the patient's position, or edema. In the hand, goniometric measurements give information about the joint, the soft tissue surrounding the joint, and the long finger flexors and extensors.

Unless it is medically contraindicated, active ROM (AROM) is usually measured first, to assess the available ROM at the joints when they are moved volitionally.[23] Passive ROM (PROM) need not be measured when full AROM is present. A specific method of recording finger ROM known as **total active ROM (TAM)** and **total passive ROM (TPM)** requires additional clinical training but considers the dynamics of tendon excursion and joint mobility (Figure 30-1). In addition to goniometric measures, a gross measurement of finger flexion can be obtained by measuring, in centimeters, the distance between the finger pulp and the distal palmar crease (Figure 30-2).

Edema Assessment

A normal consequence of an acute hand injury is localized **edema,** defined by Brand as "the collection of water and electrolytes in the tissues. Tissue fluid may accumulate in the hand because of dependency or diminished muscle action."[18] Hand volume is measured to assess the presence of edema and to determine the effect of treatment and activities. By measuring the volume at different times of the day, the effects of rest versus activity and of splinting or treatment techniques designed to reduce edema may be determined.

A commercially available volumeter[29] may be used to assess hand edema (Figure 30-3). The volumeter has been shown to be accurate to 10 ml[106] when used in the prescribed manner. Variables that have been shown to decrease the accuracy of the volumeter include (1) the use of a faucet or hose that introduces air into the tank during filling; (2) movement of the arm within the tank; (3) inconsistent pressure on the stop rod; and (4) the use of a volumeter in a variety of places. The same level surface should always be used.[53] The edema assessment is performed as described in Box 30-1.

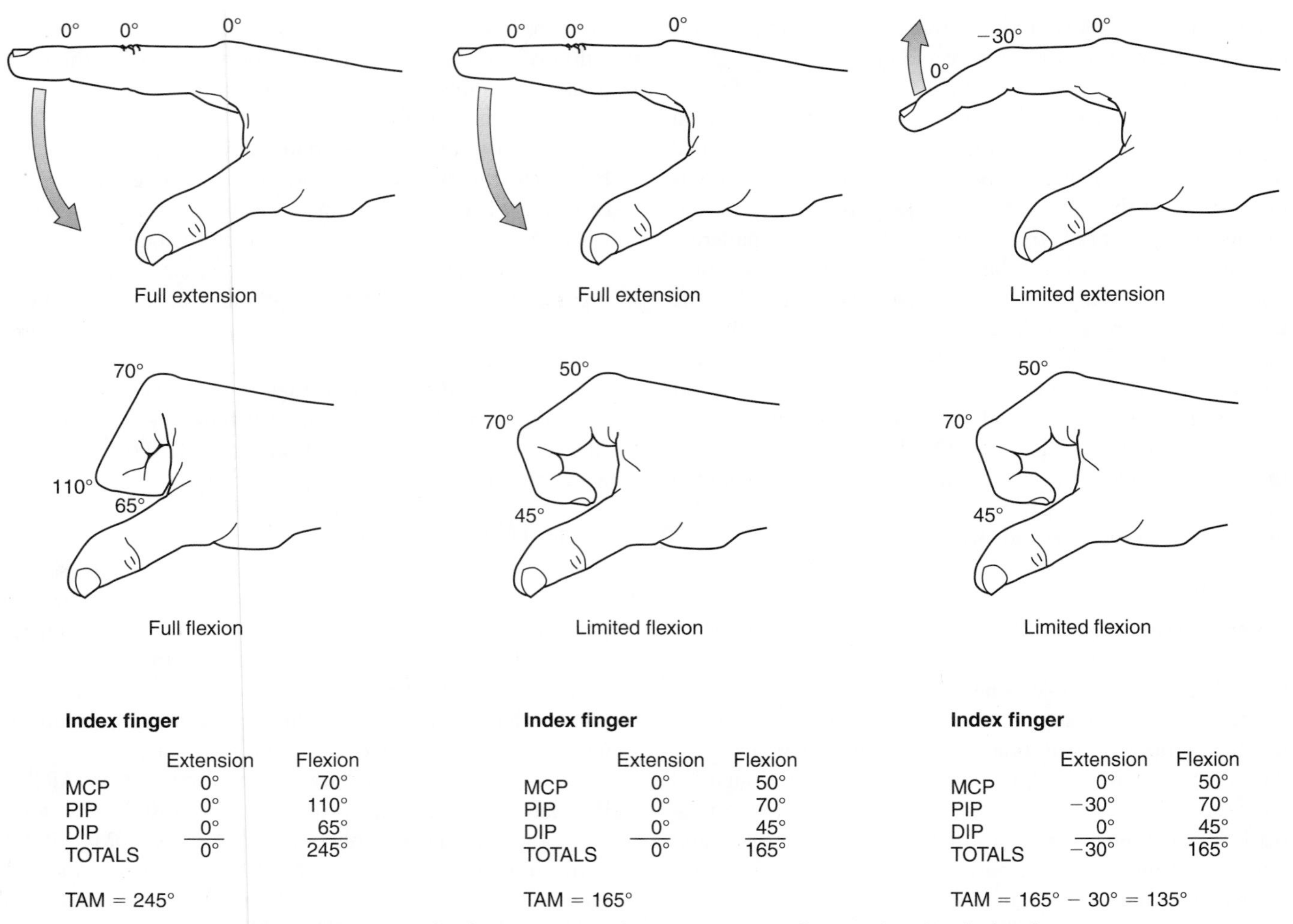

Figure 30-1 Example of measurement of total active range of motion (TAM) in the hand.

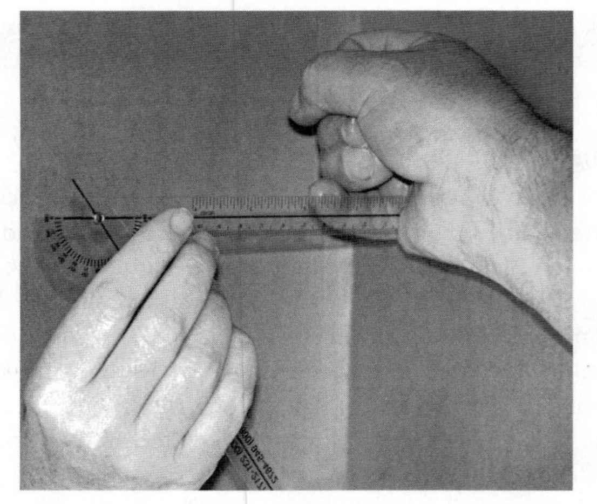

Figure 30-2 Measuring distance between finger pulp and distal palmar crease.

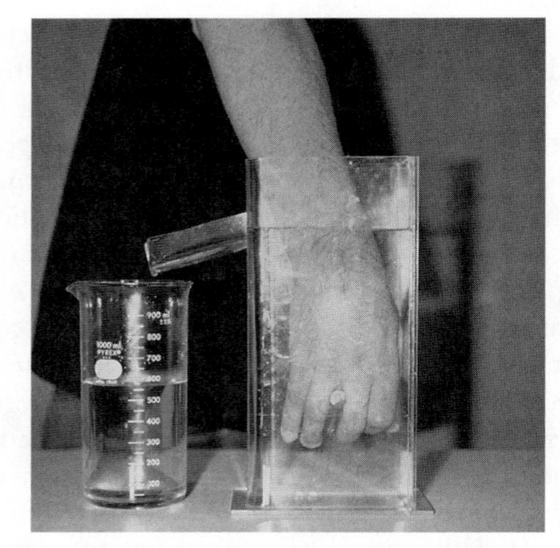

Figure 30-3 Volumeter used to measure volume of both hands for comparison. Increased volume indicates edema.

Not all patients are candidates for the volumeter. Patients who have open wounds, sutures, staples, or pins in place or any questionable skin condition should not use the volumeter. A tape measure can be used to measure parts of the hand or forearm. Common measuring sites are around the distal palmar crease, around the ulnar styloid of the wrist, or over the joints or phalanges. When using a tape measure for the hand, one must note the exact site and time of day of the measurements so that meaningful comparison can be made in repeat assessments.

To assess an individual finger (or when a volumeter is contraindicated), a tape measure or jeweler's ring-size standards

Box 30-1

Volumeter Assessment of Edema

1. Fill the plastic volumeter until the water reaches spout level. Allow excess water to drip out of the spout. Empty and dry the beaker thoroughly.
2. Instruct the patient to slowly immerse his or her hand into the plastic volumeter, being careful to keep the hand in the midposition, until the web space between the middle and ring fingers rests gently on the dowel rod. The hand must not press onto the rod.
3. Keep the hand still and in position until no more water drips into the beaker.
4. Pour the water from the beaker into a graduated cylinder.
5. Place the cylinder on a level surface, and read the amount of water displaced.

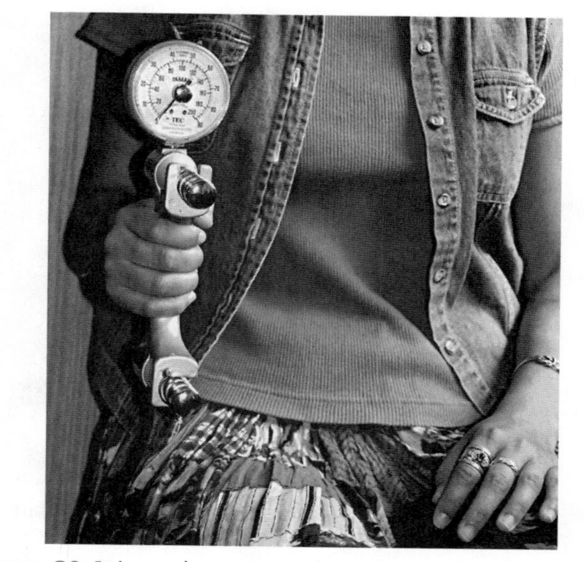

Figure 30-4 Jamar dynamometer is used to measure grip strength.

can be used. Measurements should be taken before and after treatment, especially after the application of thermal modalities or splinting. When patients report a range of subjective complaints relating to swelling, objective data of circumference or volume help the therapist assess the response of the tissues to treatment and activity. Edema control techniques are discussed later in this chapter.

Strength Assessment

UE strength assessment should be performed well after the inflammatory phase of healing. Strength testing is not performed after recent trauma or surgery and should be deferred until the patient has been cleared for full-resistive activities, usually 8 to 12 weeks after injury. Strength in the hand is measured in several ways: grip strength, pinch strength, and manual muscle testing.

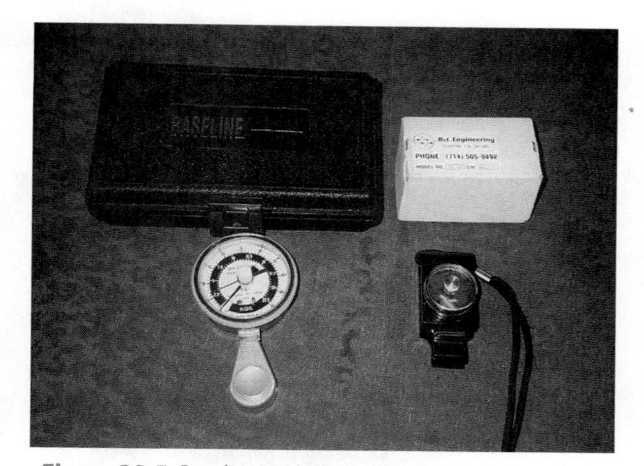

Figure 30-5 Baseline and B&L Engineering pinch gauges.

Grip Strength

The dynamometer is recommended for assessing **grip strength** (Figure 30-4). The recommended patient position[75] is seated with the shoulder adducted and neutrally rotated, the elbow flexed at 90 degrees, the forearm in the neutral position, and the wrist between 0 and 15 degrees of ulnar deviation. The patient is asked to squeeze using his or her maximal effort. Three trials of each hand are taken with the dynamometer handle set at the second position.[76] The dynamometer can be held lightly by the examiner to avoid the patient's dropping the instrument. A mean of the three trials should be reported. The noninjured hand is measured for comparison. Normative data may be used to compare strength scores.[58,74] Variables such as age will affect the strength measurements.

Pinch Strength

Pinch strength is tested with either of the commercially available pinch gauges (Figure 30-5). Two-point pinch (thumb tip to index fingertip), lateral or key pinch (thumb pulp to lateral aspect of the middle phalanx of the index finger), and three-point pinch (thumb tip to tips of index and long fingers) are measured. The patient position is the same as for grip testing and the patient is asked to give his or her maximal effort (Figure 30-7). Three successive trials are obtained and compared bilaterally.[58]

Manual Muscle Testing

Manual muscle testing is also used to evaluate UE strength. Accurate assessment is especially important when the patient is to undergo tendon transfers or other reconstructive surgery because it individuates each intrinsic and extrinsic muscle of the hand. A manual muscle test is not customary during a routine hand evaluation, except when a specific diagnosis (e.g., peripheral nerve injury or neuromuscular disease) warrants a detailed investigation. Kendall[60] is an excellent text reference for assessing individual muscle strength.

Maximum voluntary effort during grip, pinch, or muscle testing will be affected by pain in the hand or extremity. Therefore subjective complaints should be noted if the patient's ability to exert true force is limited. Localization of the pain or symptoms and consistency of pain complaints will help the therapist to determine the role that pain is playing in the recovery from injury.

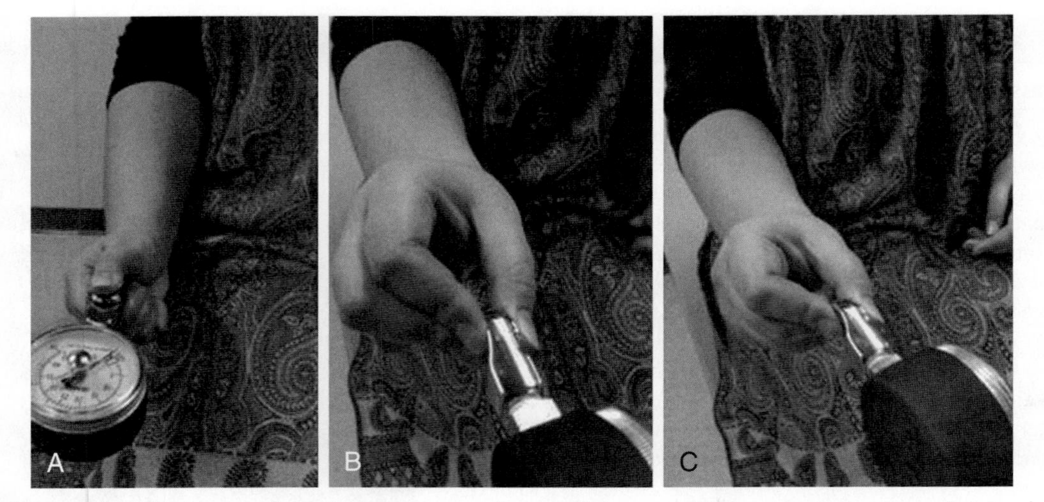

Figure 30-6 Pinch gauge is used to measure pinch strength in a variety of prehension patterns. **A,** Lateral pinch. **B,** 3-jaw chuck. **C,** 2-point pinch.

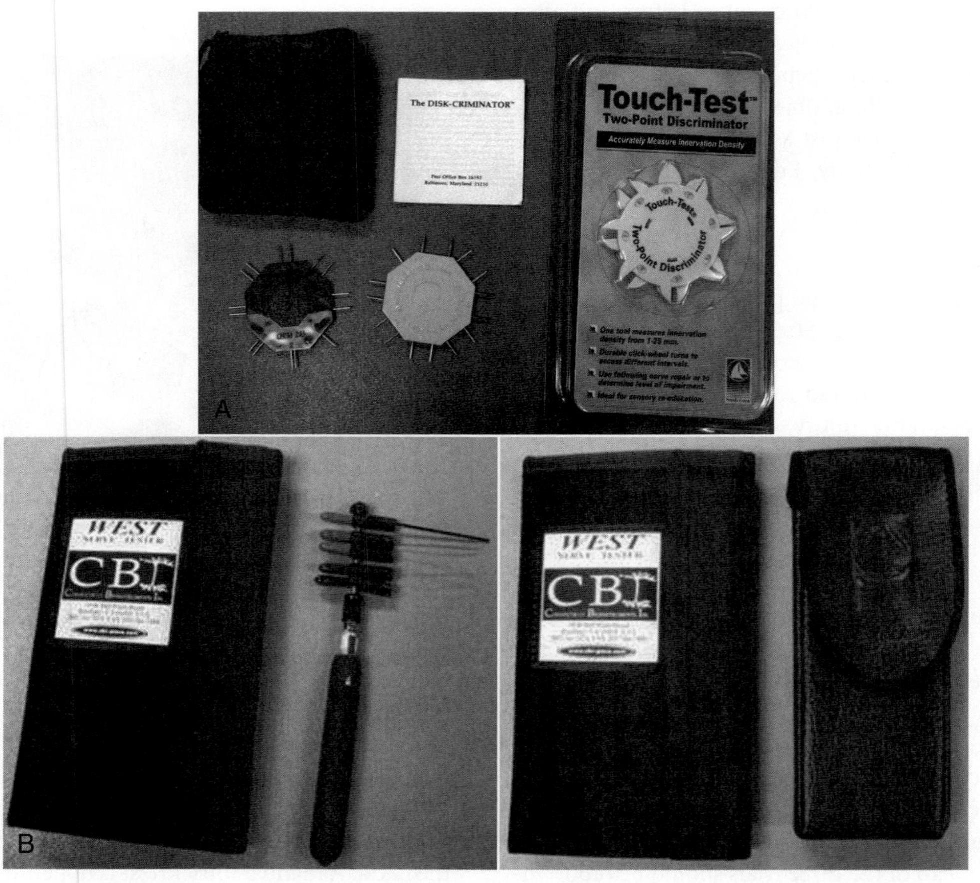

Figure 30-7 **A,** Pocket sized monofilament touch tests available from West and North Coast Medical. **B,** The Disk Criminator and the Touch Test (TM) Two-Point Discriminator can be used to assess static or moving two-point discrimination.

Soft Tissue Assessment

Joint Assessment

Joints may develop dysfunction after trauma, immobilization, or disuse. Decreased AROM is one way this dysfunction can be seen. Limited ROM is often caused by tightness in the ligaments and other soft tissue that surround a joint. For a joint to have full AROM, small passive involuntary movements must occur inside the joint at the joint surfaces. These movements are called *joint play,*[78,110] or *accessory* or *component motions.*[81] These movements must be present for a joint to express normal ROM.[78] Because these motions are passive and not under voluntary control, they cannot be produced at will and can be facilitated only by someone other than the patient.[61]

The technique to assess or help to restore these motions is called *joint mobilization.*[84] An example is joint distraction, in which the occupational therapist firmly but gently applies a traction (pulling) force at the joint, thereby stretching the ligaments surrounding that joint. It may be helpful to restore joint play with this technique before attempting PROM or AROM.[39,55,110] Guidelines must be followed for applying joint mobilization techniques, which should not be attempted by the untrained or inexperienced practitioner. Continuing education courses are offered in joint mobilization of the extremities, and the therapist must be familiar with the arthrokinematics (movements of joint surfaces) of each joint, as well as with the techniques used.

Extrinsic and Intrinsic Assessment

Tightness of the extrinsic muscles/tendons (origins outside of the hand proper) or intrinsic muscles/tendons (origins and insertions inside the hand proper) may also limit joint motion. Various injuries may cause adhesions or shortening (tightness) of the intrinsic hand muscles. In order to determine whether the joint limitation is a result of shortening of the tissues surrounding the joint, or shortening of muscles and/or tendons, the occupational therapist passively places these joints—metacarpophalangeals (MCPs), proximal interphalangeals (PIPs), and distal interphalangeals (DIPs)—in a series of recommended positions.[3]

Sensibility Assessment

Any patient who has sustained a direct injury to a peripheral nerve or who is suspected of having a condition that may compress a peripheral nerve needs to be fully assessed in the area of **sensibility.** The ability of the hand to function, explore, and interact with the environment depends on sensibility.[5] Therefore the OTA must be familiar with all sensibility tests and how their results affect treatment and function. However, the occupational therapist performs the assessment.

Mapping

Sensibility testing can begin with sensory mapping of the entire volar surface of the hand.[22] The areas are carefully marked and transferred to a permanent record, usually a diagram of the hand. Mapping should be repeated at monthly intervals during nerve regeneration.

Categories of Tests

A variety of tests may be required to adequately assess sensibility. These tests can be divided into four categories: (1) *threshold* tests for pain, vibration, temperature, and touch pressure; (2) *functional* tests to assess the quality of sensibility or what Moberg described as "tactile gnosis," such as stationary and moving two-point discrimination and the Moberg Pick-up Test; (3) *objective* tests that do not require active participation by the patient including the O'Riain wrinkle test, the triketohydrindene hydrate (Ninhydrin) sweat test, and nerve conduction studies[79]; and (4) *provocative* or *stress* tests that either attempt to reproduce the patient's complaints of pain or determine if a peripheral nerve is regenerating at the appropriate rate. To reproduce symptoms, the patient or part of the upper limb is placed in certain positions or postures that will provoke or elicit the symptoms. Tapping over a peripheral nerve can help determine whether the nerve is regenerating appropriately or whether the nerve is being entrapped by other body tissue.[22]

Sympathetic Function

Recovery of the **sympathetic function** (sweating, pain, and temperature discrimination) may occur early but does not correlate with functional recovery.[31] O'Riain[84] observed that denervated skin does not wrinkle. Therefore nerve function may be tested by immersing the hand in water for 5 minutes and noting the presence or absence of skin wrinkling. This test may be especially helpful in diagnosing a nerve lesion in young children or cognitively impaired adults. The ability to sweat is also lost in a nerve lesion. A Ninhydrin test[22,84] evaluates sweating of the finger.

The wrinkle test and the Ninhydrin test are objective tests of sympathetic function. Recovery of sweating has not been shown to correlate with the recovery of sensation, but the absence of sweating correlates with the lack of discriminatory sensation. Other signs of sympathetic dysfunction are smooth, shiny skin; nail changes; and "pencil pointing," or tapering of the fingers.[105]

Nerve Compression and Nerve Regeneration

Sensibility testing is done (1) to assess the recovery of a nerve after laceration and repair; (2) to determine the presence of a nerve compression syndrome and the return of nerve function after surgical decompression; and (3) to determine the efficacy of conservative treatment to reduce compression. Therefore vibratory tests and other relative assessments may be interpreted differently depending on the mechanism of nerve dysfunction.

Tinel's Sign and Phalen's Test

Although the Tinel's sign and Phalen's tests are not considered tests of sensibility, they are used to assess the rate of nerve recovery (Tinel's) and are considered "provocative" tests in nerve compression syndromes because they aim to elicit a pathologic response of the nerve. During the first 2 to 4 months after nerve repair, axons regenerate and travel through the hand at a rate of about 1 mm per day or 1 inch per month (2.54 cm). Tinel's sign may be used to follow this regeneration.[70] The test is performed by tapping gently along the course of the nerve, starting distally and moving toward the nerve repair site to elicit a tingling sensation in the fingertip. The point at which tapping begins to elicit a tingling sensation is noted and indicates the extent of sensory axon growth. As regeneration occurs, hypesthesias will develop. Although this hypersensitivity may be uncomfortable to the patient, it is a positive sign of nerve growth. A treatment program for desensitization of hypersensitive areas can be initiated as soon as the skin is healed and can tolerate gentle rubbing and immersion in textures. Desensitization is discussed further in the treatment section of this chapter.

The examiner may attempt to elicit a Tinel's sign in nerve compression disorders such as carpal tunnel syndrome. The therapist taps the median nerve at the level of the wrist.[22,78] The Tinel's sign is considered positive if the patient reports tingling along the course of the nerve distally when tapped. The Phalen's test will also produce the nerve paresthesias present in compression of the median nerve. The patient is asked to hold the wrist in a fully flexed position for 60 seconds. The test is considered positive if tingling occurs within this time.[22,78]

Vibration

Tuning forks of 30 and 256 cps (cycles per second) are used for assessing the return of vibratory sensation after nerve repair as regeneration occurs and as a guideline for initiating a **sensory reeducation** program.[31,32] Commercially available vibrometers may also be used to detect abnormal sensation.

Vibration and the Semmes-Weinstein monofilament tests[15] are more sensitive in picking up a gradual decrease in nerve function in the presence of nerve compression where the nerve circuitry is intact. Therefore vibration, Semmes-Weinstein, and electrical testing are reliable and sensitive tests for early detection of carpal tunnel syndrome and other nerve compression syndromes. Vibration and Semmes-Weinstein tests can be performed in the clinic with no discomfort to the patient and are excellent screening tools when nerve compression is suspected.[15,47]

CLINICAL PEARL

To determine if pain sensibility has returned, use the 30 CPS tuning fork rather than a pin to avoid risk of injury and/or infection.

Touch Pressure

Moving touch is tested with the eraser end of a pencil. The eraser is placed in an area of normal sensibility and, with light pressure, is moved to the distal fingertip. The patient notes when the perception of the stimulus changes. Light and heavy stimuli may be applied and noted.[31] Constant touch is tested by pressing with the eraser end of the pencil, first in an area with normal sensibility and then moving distally. The patient responds when the stimulus is altered; again, light and heavy stimuli may be applied.[31] The Semmes-Weinstein monofilaments test provides the most accurate instrument for assessing cutaneous pressure thresholds.[15] The test employs 20 nylon monofilaments, of increasing thickness, housed in plastic handheld rods. Markings on the probes range from 1.65 to 6.65. Normal fingertip sensibility has been found to correspond to the 2.44 and 2.83 probes.

The monofilaments must be applied perpendicular to the skin and are applied until the monofilament just begins to bend. Results can be graded from normal light touch (probes 2.83 and above) to loss of protective sensation (probes 4.56 and below). There are commercially available pocket-size monofilament touch tests containing five monofilaments that are easy to use and are in protective cases (Figure 30-7, *A*).

Static Two-Point and Moving Two-Point Discrimination

Discrimination requires the patient to distinguish between two direct stimuli. These tests elicit information about the patient's potential for function. To assess static two-point discrimination, a variety of commercially available devices such as the Disk-Criminator[73] or Touch-Test Two-Point Discriminator (Figure 30-7, *B*) are used. The Disk-Criminator is a small tool with parallel prongs of variable distances apart. It has blunted ends that will not hurt the patient and should produce replicable results. The patient is touched with the device and asked to indicate whether he or she perceives one or two points (Box 30-2).

Moving two-point discrimination is slightly more sensitive than stationary two-point discrimination,[71] and it provides information about the patient's potential to manipulate objects in the hand. Two-point values increase with age in both sexes (as the skin becomes less discriminating), with the smallest values occurring between the ages of 10 and 30. Women tend to have smaller values than men have, and no significant differences exist between dominant and nondominant hands.[71]

Modified Moberg Pick-Up Test

Recognition of common objects is the final level of sensory function. Moberg used the phrase "tactile gnosis" to describe the ability of the hand to perform complex function by feel. Moberg described the Pick-Up Test in 1958,[79] which Dellon[31] later modified. This test is used with either a median nerve injury or a combined injury of median and ulnar nerves. Clinically, it takes twice as long to perform the tests with vision occluded than with vision not occluded. The therapist performs the test as described in Box 30-3.

Functional Evaluation

Evaluation of hand function or performance is important because the physical evaluation does not measure the patient's

Box 30-2

Interpretation of Static Two-Point Testing

Norms	
Normal	5 mm or less apart
Fair	6 - 10 mm apart
Poor	11 - 15 mm apart
Protective	Only 1 point is perceived
Anesthetic	No point is perceived

From American Society for Surgery of the Hand: *The hand, examination and diagnosis*, ed 3, New York, 1990, Churchill Livingstone.

Box 30-3

Modified Moberg Pick-Up Test

1. Place 9 or 10 small objects (coins, paper clips, etc.) on a table.
2. Ask the patient to place them one at a time in a small container as quickly as possible while looking at them. Time the patient.
3. Repeat the test for the opposite hand with vision.
4. Repeat the test for each hand with the vision occluded.
5. Ask the patient to identify each object, one at a time, with and then without vision.
6. Observe substitution patterns that may be used when the patient cannot see the objects.

ingenuity and ability to compensate for the loss of strength, ROM, and sensation, or for the presence of deformities. The results of the physical evaluation will, however, increase the therapist's understanding of functional impairment and of why patients function the way they do.[77]

The occupational therapist should observe the effect of dysfunction on use of the hand during ADL. In addition, a standardized performance evaluation such as the Jebsen Test of Hand Function[54] can be administered. With service competency, delegated administration of some of these tests may be within the scope of the OTA.

Jebsen Hand Function Test

This test was developed to provide objective measurements of standardized tasks with norms for patient comparison. It is a short, inexpensive test that is easily assembled by the administrator. The test consists of seven subtests: (1) writing a short sentence; (2) turning over 5-inch cards three times; (3) picking up small objects and placing them in a container; (4) stacking checkers; (5) eating (simulated); (6) moving large empty cans; and (7) moving large weighted cans. Norms are provided for dominant and nondominant hands for each subtest and are also divided by sex and age. The authors provide instructions for assembling the test and specific instructions for administering it.[54] It has been found to be a good test for overall hand function.

Dexterity Tests

Dexterity is the ability to manipulate small objects with the fingers with speed and accuracy.[6] An evaluation of the hand is not complete without a dexterity measurement. One of the most commonly used dexterity tests is the commercially available Nine-Hole Peg Test.[48] It has normative data and is quick and easy to administer; again, once service competency is assured, the OTA could administer this test.

Other tests that have been found to be useful in the evaluation of hand dexterity are the Crawford Small Parts Dexterity Test,[28] the Bennett Hand Tool Dexterity Test,[17] the Purdue Pegboard Test,[98] and the Minnesota Manual Dexterity Test.[44] The Valpar Corporation has developed a number of standardized tests that measure an individual's ability to perform work-related tasks. They provide information about the test taker's results in comparison to industry performance standards. All of these tests include comparison with normal subjects working in a variety of industrial settings. This information can be used in predicting the likelihood of successful return to a specific job. These tests are especially useful when administering a work capacity evaluation. Tests may be purchased and come with standardized norms and instructions for administration and scoring.[77]

CLINICAL PEARL

Do not use the tools of any assessment (such as Nine-Hole Peg Test or any other test for dexterity) for treatment activities. The retest would not be valid because there would be a learning effect for the patient.

Outcome Measures

Initial hand evaluations are beginning to include outcome measures to determine a patient's health status, functional status, and overall satisfaction level. Outcome measure tools are primarily by self-report (i.e., the patient determines the answers to specific questions). A therapist does not observe function or behavior. There are three categories[101] of outcomes measures: *generic* measures, which compare overall health conditions; *regional* measures, which look at specific body systems or areas; and *disease-specific* measures (see Box 30-4 for a partial list of outcomes measures by category). The DASH (Disability, Arm, Shoulder, and Hand) and the Michigan Hand Questionnaire are often selected for use in a hand therapy clinic because these tools direct their questions to the outcomes related to the UE.[72] The Barthel ADL Index is widely used to assess lifestyle task performance, and a newer tool, the MAMS (Manual Ability Measure), is being developed to look at hand function across diagnostic categories.[26] Many clinics use the generic Sickness Impact Profile (SIP) to assess overall health status; however, in facilities where hand-injured patients are treated, the SF-36 Health Survey is favored.[103]

Goal-Directed Treatment Techniques

Edema Reduction

Edema is a normal consequence of trauma but must be quickly and aggressively treated to prevent permanent stiffness and disability. Within hours of trauma, vasodilation and local edema occur.

Early control of edema is ideally achieved through elevation, massage, compression, and AROM. The patient is instructed at the time of injury to keep the hand elevated, and a compressive dressing is applied to reduce early swelling. Pitting edema is present early and can be recognized as a bloated swelling that "pits" when pressed by the examiner's finger. This may be more pronounced on the dorsal surface where the skin is looser and where venous and lymphatic systems provide

Box 30-4

Categories of Functional Outcome Measures*

Generic Measures:
- Canadian Occupational Performance Measure (COPM)
- Short Form 36 (SF36)
- Short Musculoskeletal Functional Assessment (SMFA)

Regional Measures:
- Disabilities of the Arm, Shoulder, and Hand (DASH)
- Michigan Hand Questionnaire (MHQ)
- Patient-Rated Wrist/Hand Evaluation (PRWHE)

Disease-Specific Measures:
- Arthritis Impact Measurement Scales (AIMS2-SF)
- Australian/Canadian Osteoarthritis Hand Index (AUSCAN)
- Rotator Cuff Quality of Life (RC-QOL)

*This does not represent a fully comprehensive list.
From Von Der Heyde R: Assessment of functional outcomes. In Cooper C (ed): *Fundamentals of hand therapy,* St. Louis, 2007, Mosby Elsevier, pp 98-111.

return of fluid to the heart. Active motion is especially important to produce retrograde venous and lymphatic flow; AROM moves this fluid back into the general circulatory system.

If swelling continues, a serofibrinous exudate (a fluid that contains both serum and fibrin) invades the area. Fibrin is deposited in the spaces surrounding the joints, tendons, and ligaments, resulting in reduced mobility, flattening of the arches of the hand, tissue atrophy, and further disuse.[100] Normal gliding of the tissues is reduced, and stiffness and pain in the hand often result. Scar adhesions are likely to form and further limit tissue mobility. If untreated, these losses may become permanent.

Early recognition of persistent edema through volume and circumference measurement is important. Several of the suggested edema control techniques may be necessary.

Elevation

Early elevation with the hand above the heart is essential. Slings should be avoided if possible because they tend to reduce blood flow because of the flexed elbow posture and may lead to shoulder stiffness as well. Resting the hand on pillows while seated or lying down is effective. Resting the hand on top of the head or using devices that elevate the hand with the elbow in extension have been suggested. Suspension slings may be purchased or fabricated.

The patient should use the injured hand for ADL within the limitations of resistance prescribed by the physician. Light ADL that can be accomplished while the hand is in the dressing are permitted because these facilitate gentle active ROM.

Contrast Baths

Contrast baths, immersing the hand alternately in warm water and then cold water, have traditionally been used by many therapists to help reduce edema and facilitate ROM in hand-injured patients. The alternating of warm and cool water will cause vasodilation and vasoconstriction, resulting in a pumping action on the edema. Many patients report that they like contrast baths. Although the technique is described in textbooks, little research has been done on its effectiveness. A recent systematic review[92] on the effectiveness of contrast baths concludes that although contrast baths may increase skin temperature and superficial blood flow, there is little evidence that they affect edema and even less evidence that ROM or function is improved. Practitioners are urged to study the literature and make an informed decision before using this treatment strategy; the OTA should consult with the supervising OT.

Retrograde Massage

The practitioner may perform retrograde massage, which can also be taught to the patient (and caregiver or family member) so that it can be done frequently throughout the day. The massage assists in blood and lymph flow. Start the massage distally and stroke smoothly and lightly in a proximal direction with the extremity in elevation.[30] Active motion should follow the massage if possible, but avoid muscle fatigue.

In more severe cases, when the hand and forearm are involved, retrograde massage is a two-stage procedure. First, it begins proximally (i.e., midforearm) to empty the proximal body part. Next, the hand, or distal part, is massaged so that this fluid may be emptied into an available space.

Manual Edema Mobilization

In 1997 Artzberger[8] described a massage technique she developed based on manual lymphatic treatment (MLT), a treatment technique used for people with lymphedema. She modified MLT and coined the term Manual Edema Mobilization (MEM) for this new technique and began to use it on subacute hand patients with some success. MEM is used in cases where the impairment of the lymph system is temporary (edema) rather than caused by damage to the lymphatic system (lymphedema). This technique is grounded in a thorough understanding of the anatomy and physiology of the lymphatic system, as well as research data.[8] Although the technique is described in the literature,[9] therapy practitioners are encouraged to study and take hands-on continuing education courses to become skilled in this massage technique. Although MEM can be helpful in reducing edema, it must be used selectively with appropriate patients to avoid medical complications. Again, the OTA must be service competent and follow OT direction.

Pressure Wraps

Light compression may be applied throughout the day with a light **Coban** wrap, an Isotoner glove, or a custom-made garment by Bioconcepts or Jobst (Figure 30-8). Wrapping with Coban elastic[36] may be used to reduce edema (Figure 30-9). Starting distally, the finger is wrapped snugly with Coban. Care must be taken not to pull the Coban too tightly because it can restrict circulation. Each involved finger should be wrapped distal to proximal until the wrap is proximal to the edema. The wrap remains in place for 5 minutes and then is removed. Active exercise may be done while the finger is wrapped or immediately after. Measurements should be taken before and after treatment to document an increase in ROM and a decrease in edema. The wrapping may be repeated three times a day.

Any method of compression should not be constricting and must be discontinued if ischemia results. Elastic Ace bandages may be used for larger areas. An elastic bandage of 3 or 4 inches in width may be used when the entire hand and forearm require a gentle pressure wrap. A variety of pressure wraps are used by hand centers. Tubular gauze and Digisleeves[3] provide compression to a specific finger. No single method is superior to the other. A combination of techniques used at different stages of healing and according to patient comfort may be most effective.

CLINICAL PEARL

Instead of Coban Wrap, consider purchasing Vet Wrap at a veterinary or equestrian supply source. It is cheaper, comes in colors (to match the jockey's silks), and is wider; therefore you or the patient will need fewer rolls.

Physical Agent Modalities

Two modalities are particularly helpful in the reduction of edema: neuromuscular electrical stimulation (NMES) and high-voltage pulsed current stimulation (HVPC). Both modalities are applied in such a way as to facilitate a muscle contraction, thereby improving the muscle's ability to pump. Improved pumping action will boost lymphatic return, which will reduce edema.[64] In OT treatment, these modalities must be used in conjunction with purposeful activity and may be used only by an occupational therapist with documented competency.

Active Range of Motion

Normal blood flow depends on muscle activity. Active motion does not mean wiggling the fingers but rather maximum available ROM done firmly and with purpose. Casts and splints must allow mobility of uninjured parts while protecting newly injured structures. The shoulder and elbow should be moved several times a day. The importance of AROM for edema control, tendon gliding, and tissue nutrition cannot be overemphasized.

Range of Motion Improvement

To improve ROM, the practitioner must answer the following questions:

- What is the available PROM?
- Is muscle strength available?
- Can the tendons glide?

PROM gives information about noncontractile structures such as ligaments surrounding the joint. PROM is assessed by the therapist moving the joint throughout its available range. AROM gives information about the contractile units moving the joint. When PROM is greater than AROM, there is a problem with the contracting unit (i.e., muscle weakness or tendon adherence). If PROM is limited, the therapist must address the specific cause of the limitation and choose treatment strategies to improve AROM.

To improve PROM, the occupational therapist may use a combination of the following: modalities to improve tissue elasticity, joint mobilization techniques to restore joint play, PROM to the involved joint, and dynamic or static progressive splinting. The OTA may supplement these PROM treatment strategies with specific exercises or activities that target the involved structures. The clinician must be sensitive to the patient's age and interest when selecting activities. As with any rehabilitation program, the patient should be provided with a specific home exercise program that will supplement and reinforce therapy.

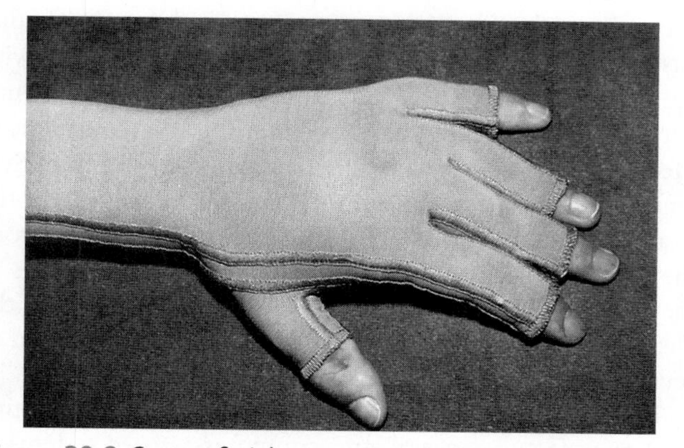

Figure 30-8 Custom-fit Jobst garment may be used to reduce edema and to reduce or prevent hypertrophic scar formation after burns or trauma.

Soft Tissue Mobility Improvement

Many hand therapy patients have experienced an invasive event to the hand, whether through trauma or surgical intervention. Therefore the OTA must be familiar with wound-healing theory to assist the occupational therapist in managing the acute hand injury or surgery. All wounds lead to formation of scars, which are necessary for healing. It is the therapist's responsibility to select and use techniques that will modify and remodel the scar to preserve soft tissue mobility.

Tissues that have restored gliding have different scar architecture from those that do not develop the ability to glide. With gliding, the scar resembles the state of the tissues before injury, whereas the nongliding scar remains fixed on or adherent to the surrounding structures. Controlled tension on a scar has been shown to facilitate remodeling. Scar formation is also influenced by the patient's age and the quantity of scar deposited.[100]

Pressure

A hypertrophic scar, or a scar that is randomly laid down and thickened, cannot glide properly and therefore may restrict AROM, contribute to deformity, or be cosmetically unacceptable. The principal technique used to modify a scar is the application of pressure, similar to the techniques used in burn rehabilitation.

Several types of commercially available products, when used in combination, enable the clinician to manage scars effectively. For example, the following products can be used as the contact medium with the skin: Otoform, Silastic Elastomer, and Prosthetic Foam. These products are generally held in place with pressure devices such as Coban wrap, Isotoner gloves, Ace bandages, or pressure elastic garments. Pressure should be applied for most of the 24-hour period and removed for bathing and exercise. As the scar changes in response to pressure, the contact medium needs to be replaced. For patients with burns, a custom-measured pressure garment is worn 23 hours per day and may need to be worn for 6 months to 18 months, depending on the severity of the burn.

Massage

Gentle to firm massage of the scarred area with a thick ointment such as lanolin, Deep Prep, or Aliprep Deep Tissue massage cream will rapidly soften scar tissue and should be followed immediately with active hand use so that tendons will glide against the softened scar.[30] Vibration to the area with a small, low-intensity vibrator will have a similar effect.[56] Active exercise with facilitation techniques, exercise against resistance, or functional activity should follow vibration. Massage and vibration may be started 4 weeks after the injury.

Thermal heat in the form of a paraffin bath, hot packs, or fluidotherapy immediately followed by stretching while the tissue cools will provide stretch to scar tissue. Gently wrapping the scarred or stiff digit into flexion with Coban during the application of heat will often increase mobility in the area. Heat should not be used with insensate areas or if swelling persists.[57] Scar reduction techniques can be carried out by the OTA under close supervision of a therapist.

Active Range of Motion and Physical Agent Modalities

AROM provides an internal stretch against a resistant scar, and its value cannot be overstated. When the patient cannot achieve active range because of scar adhesions or weakness, an occupational therapist may use NMES to assist the motion.[51,64] High-voltage, direct-current ultrasound and a continuous passive motion machine may also be judiciously used by the therapist. These modalities help increase motor activity and help remodel the scar. The use of any modality requires a prescription from a physician and must be administered by a service-competent clinician.

Normalization of Sensation

As an injury to the hand resolves, the hand or a portion of it may be either hypersensitive or hyposensitive, having either too much or too little sensation. For example, after trauma to a peripheral or digital nerve, sensibility can be expected to return in a certain order.[33] To facilitate the return of function to the peripheral or digital nerve, a program of sensory *reeducation* may be used. Alternatively, a patient may have a hypersensitive area, one that is excessively sensitive to even the lightest touch, making it almost impossible for that person to manipulate ordinary items. In this case, a program of sensory *desensitization* is indicated.

Sensory Reeducation

Evaluation of sensibility has been described earlier in this chapter. The occupational therapist would use this information to prepare a program of sensory reeducation after nerve repair.

When a nerve is repaired, regeneration is not perfect, resulting in fewer and smaller nerve fibers and receptors distal to the repair. The goal of sensory reeducation is to maximize the functional level of sensation. All programs emphasize a variety of stimuli used in a repetitive manner to bombard the sensory receptors. A sequence of eyes-closed, eyes-open, eyes-closed is used to provide feedback during the training process. Sessions are limited in length to avoid fatigue and frustration. To avoid further trauma, objects must not be potentially harmful to insensate areas. A home program should be provided to reinforce learning that occurs in the clinical setting.

Several authors[22,31,105] have found that sensory reeducation can result in improved functional sensibility in motivated patients. Objective measurement of sensation after reeducation must be performed and then compared with initial testing to accurately assess the success of the program. A program of sensory reeducation does not begin until the patient has at least protective sensibility.

Sensory Desensitization

Sensory desensitization techniques are based on the theory that nerve fibers that carry pain sensation can be positively influenced through the use of pressure, rubbing, vibration, transcutaneous electrical nerve stimulation (TENS), percussion, and active motion. Hypersensitivity is sometimes the result of a lacerated nerve, but a too tight cast or splint may also cause nerve irritation requiring a program of sensory desensitization.[80]

Yerxa and colleagues[109] have described a desensitization program that "employs short periods of contact with three sensory modalities: dowel textures, immersion or contact particles, and vibration." This program allows the patient to rank 10 dowel textures and 10 immersion textures on the degree of irritation produced by the stimulus. Treatment begins with a stimulus that is irritating but tolerable. The stimulus is applied for 10 minutes three or four times a day. The vibration hierarchy is predetermined and is based on cycles per second (cps) of vibration, the placement of the vibrator, and the duration of the treatment. The Downey Hand Center hand sensitivity test can be used to establish a desensitization treatment program and to measure progress in decreasing hypersensitivity.[109]

Strength Improvement

Acute care is followed by a gradual return of motion, sensibility, and preparation to return to normal ADL. Strengthening of the injured and neglected extremity usually begins in the clinic, but because visits to therapy are often limited by insurance carriers, the therapist must also provide a written home program. It is also critical to educate the patient as to what are and are not appropriate strengthening techniques to allay any fears they may have of further injury or pain. Because every hand clinic has its own armamentarium of strengthening exercises and media, only a few suggestions are provided here.

Computerized Evaluation and Exercise Equipment

Cedaron Medical, Inc. manufactures Dexter ImpairmentCare, which is a computerized evaluation system (www.cedaron.com). The system allows therapists to complete an upper extremity evaluation, using some of the tools previously discussed in this chapter. A printed report is then generated with the evaluation data. The system can also calculate the patient's Permanent Impairment Level as established by the American Medical Association. The Dexter Evaluation and Therapy System can be used to evaluate the patient, record and report the results of evaluation, establish an exercise program, record the results of each therapy session, and compare changes in the individual's strength or ROM. Any clinician using the Dexter system is encouraged to get sufficient training and to review the published validity studies.[16,19]

BTE Technologies, Inc. (formerly Baltimore Therapeutic Co.) manufactures several large computer-assisted systems to meet the evaluation and rehabilitation needs of occupational and physical therapists.[20] The Simulator II (Figure 30-10)

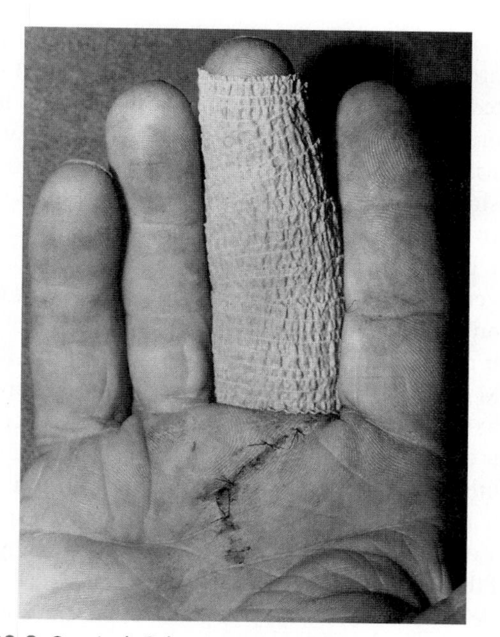

Figure 30-9 One-inch Coban is wrapped with minimal pressure from distal to proximal.

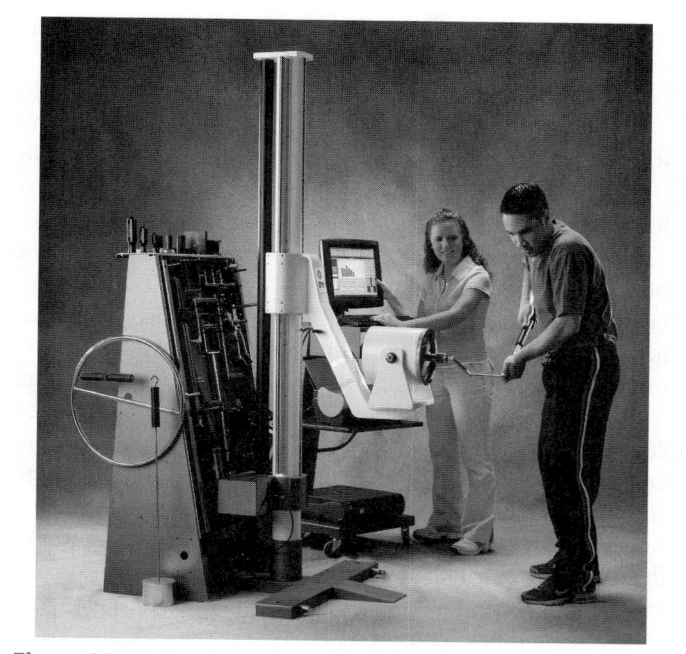

Figure 30-10 Simulator II from BTE Technologies for upper extremity rehabilitation.

system is primarily used for upper extremity rehabilitation. A variety of handles and tools can be attached to the system to serve three functions: (1) provide upper extremity strengthening exercise such as shoulder flexion and extension, (2) simulate upper extremity industrial tasks such as climbing a ladder or auto repair, and (3) simulate ADL tasks such as ironing or putting on shoes. When using the Simulator II for strength training, set the resistance low and gradually increase the resistance with concurrent increases in the length of exercise.

Resistive Pulley Weights

The **weight well**[11] (Figure 30-11) is one type of resistive pulley system that is commercially available. A variety of handle shapes are attached to rods with suspended weights. The rods are turned against resistance throughout the ROM to encourage wrist flexion and wrist extension, pinch, pronation and supination patterns, and full grasp and release of the injured hand. The weight well can be graded for resistance and repetitions and is an excellent tool for progressive resistive exercise. Pulley systems can have single or double handles, and can be mounted on walls and/or ceilings for shoulder and general upper extremity resistive exercise. Not all systems will include an attachment for the hand and wrist.

Theraband

Theraband is a 6-inch-wide (15.2-cm) rubber sheet available by the yard and color-coded by degrees of resistance. It can be cut into any length and is used for resistive exercise for the UE. Use of the Theraband is limited only by the therapist's imagination; it can be adapted to diagonal patterns of motion, wrist exercises, follow-up treatment of tennis elbow, and other uses. The Theraband can be combined with dowel rods and other equipment to provide resistance throughout the ROM. It is inexpensive and easy to incorporate into a home treatment program.

Hand-Strengthening Equipment

Hand grips of graded resistance are available from rehabilitation supply companies and sporting goods stores. They can be purchased with various resistance levels and used for progressive resistive hand exercises. The practitioner is cautioned against using overly resistive spring-loaded grippers such as those sold in sporting goods stores. These devices may be beneficial to the seasoned athlete but are usually too resistive for the recently injured. Therapy putty can be purchased in bulk and in grades of resistance. It is color-coded to allow easy progression of the patient as strength improves. It can be adapted to most finger motions and is easily used as part of a home program; the amount given to the patient is adjusted to hand size and strength.

Household items such as spring-type clothespins have been used to increase strength of grasp and pinch. Imaginative use of common objects may originate with the clinician or the patient and is highly beneficial and motivating.

Functional Improvement in Activities of Daily Living

Functional Activities

Functional activities are an integral part of rehabilitation of the hand. By engaging in occupation-based activities early, the patient will, in most cases, be able to achieve long-term goals in desired performance areas.[4] Functional activities may include crafts, games, dexterity activities, ADL, and work samples. Many of the treatment techniques described to this point are used to condition and prepare the hand for normal use.

Activities should be started as soon as possible at whatever level the patient can perform them, with adaptations to compensate for limited ROM and strength. Activities should be used in conjunction with other treatments. The occupational therapist must continually assess the patient's functional capacities and initiate changes in the treatment program to introduce a graded program of activities as soon as possible in the restorative phase of healing.

Vocational and avocational interests and goals should be noted at the time of initial evaluation and taken into account when planning treatment so that the patient can eventually resume meaningful life roles. The needs of a brick mason are likely to be quite different from those of a mother with small children—the environmental needs of the patient must not be neglected. Crafts should be graded from light to heavy resistance and from gross to fine dexterity. Crafts that have been found to work extremely well with hand injuries include macramé, Turkish knot weaving, clay, leather, and woodworking.

All of these crafts can be adapted and graded to the patient's capabilities and have been found to have a high level of patient acceptance. When integrated into a program of total hand rehabilitation, they provide another milestone of achievement rather than a diversion to fill up empty hours. For example, the pride of accomplishment felt by a patient who sustained a Volkmann's contracture caused by ischemia and then completed the first project in nearly 4 years is evidence that crafts belong in hand rehabilitation.

Activities that do not have an end product but provide practice in dexterity and ADL skills also fit into the category of functional activities. Developmental games and activities that require pinch or grasp and release may be graded and timed to increase difficulty. ADL boards that have a variety of opening and closing devices provide practice for use of the hand at home and increase self-confidence. String and finger games are challenging and entertaining coordination activities that can be done in pairs. Many times a hobby can be adapted for use in the clinic. Fly-tying (making lures for trout from string and feathers) is a difficult dexterity activity but one that will be enjoyed by avid fishermen. Golf clubs and fishing poles can be adapted in the clinic to allow early return to a favorite form of relaxation. Humor and interaction with the therapists and other patients provide vital but intangible benefits. Treatment should be planned to promote both.

Specific Interventions for Selected Hand Injuries

Amputations

A common injury among people using machinery such as saws and snow blowers is a traumatically amputated fingertip or partial finger amputation. Chapter 33 provides information on UE amputations; the discussion here is concerned solely with partial finger and fingertip amputations.

The surgeon's goal is to ensure good skin coverage of the amputated part when replantation is not an option. This goal may be achieved by a variety of surgical methods. The goals of OT, however, remain essentially the same: wound care, edema reduction, restoring ROM, scar management, desensitization if necessary, and restoring full function. Edema reduction is a concern that must be addressed immediately. Elevation, massage, and gentle wraps can be initiated early postoperatively, possibly before ROM therapy is begun. However, all uninvolved joints must be ranged immediately.

Very often, patients with a partial finger or fingertip amputation are left with a hypersensitive residual fingertip. If left untreated, a patient would be unable to use that finger to touch or pick up most common objects. Once the wound is closed with satisfactory coverage (i.e., skin thick enough to act as a cushion to the underlying bone yet not so thin that skin breakdown is a constant concern), a program of desensitization can begin. Traditionally, this includes tapping on or near the fingertip, sensory stimulation with a variety of textures, vibration, and submerging the finger in a container of raw rice or other materials.[31]

ROM of the affected digit and adjacent fingers may be limited as a result of the patient's decreased pain tolerance, edema, and fear of moving. This problem must be addressed immediately with an appropriate program in the clinic and followed up with a home exercise program. Occasionally, a splint may be indicated to improve ROM in a stiff joint, generally the PIP joint of the involved finger.

While these concerns are being addressed, the patient can be encouraged to use his or her hand in as many functional activities as possible such as dressing, feeding, and other light activities. If the patient has a sedentary job, an early return to work is advised. People whose work demands heavy bimanual activity may have to increase strength and endurance before returning to work. With appropriate rehabilitation, a single partial finger or fingertip amputation should have limited impact on a person's ability to return to full employment.

CLINICAL PEARL

Suggest that patients with fingertip amputations purchase a Dr. Scholl's toe guard, which is lined with silicone to help reduce scar, shape tip, and help cushion against vibration.

Introduction to Tendon Injuries

Historically, one of the most difficult treatment problems for surgeons and therapists has been the return of normal function to the finger or hand in which a tendon has been injured.[63] In order to better understand the management of tendon injuries, the International Federation of Societies for Surgery of the Hand agreed on anatomic nomenclature that divided the hand, both flexor (palmar) and extensor (dorsal) surfaces, into tendon zones[63] (Figure 30-12). The tendon zones illustrated were adopted in 1980 and are still in use today. The purpose of the zone designation was to help the surgeon—and subsequently the therapist—better understand the treatment of a specific tendon injury. Surgical and rehabilitation protocols are often determined by the level, or zone, of injury.

When a tendon moves, it is said to "glide." When a person makes a fist, for example, the flexor digitorum superficialis and flexor digitorum profundis muscle bellies contract and the tendon portion of the muscle slides or glides proximally. At the same time, the extensor digitorum communis muscle must relax, allowing its tendon to glide distally and releasing to allow the fingers to fully flex in a fist position. An injury to a tendon that involves excessive scarring may cause a tendon to become adherent or stuck to other tissues or bone, preventing

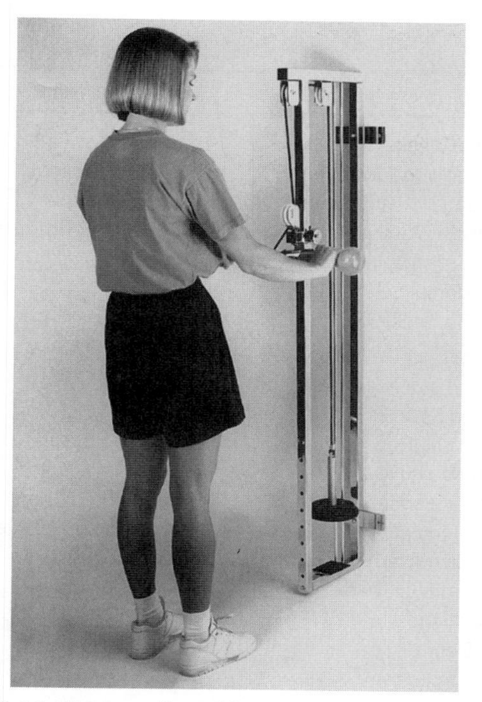

Figure 30-11 Weight well used for upper extremity and pinch and grip strengthening. (Courtesy Karen Schultz Johnson.)

this necessary gliding. A properly gliding tendon is like a skater's blade on ice. A tendon trying to glide in scar is like trying to walk through wet concrete.

Sometimes the tendon alone is injured, but more typically, other structures are injured as well. For example, when a person suffers a crush injury or fracture of bone, the tendons are often affected. The treatment protocols discussed in this chapter must be modified when other structures are injured in conjunction with the tendon. An understanding of tendon and hand anatomy and of the type of surgical repair is critical to rehabilitation of a patient with any tendon injury, as is good communication with the surgeon.

Flexor Tendon Injuries

The goal of flexor tendon surgery and rehabilitation is a strong repair that allows the tendon to glide freely.[94] Because of the complicated anatomy and mechanical considerations, treatment protocols have been developed for almost every level or zone of injury. A flexor tendon that has been injured between the distal palmar crease and the insertion of the flexor digitorum superficialis (Zone II) is considered the most difficult to treat because the tendons lie in their sheaths in this area beneath the fibrous pulley system, and any scarring will cause adhesions. This area is often called *no man's land.* The treatment strategies discussed in this chapter are primarily for tendons injured in Zones II and III.

Primary repair of the flexor tendons within these zones is attempted most often after a clean laceration. Several methods of postoperative management have been proposed with the common goal of promoting tendon glide and minimizing the formation of scar adhesions. Three methods of postoperative flexor tendon management are (1) immobilization, (2) controlled passive mobilization, and (3) early active mobilization (Table 30-1). *Note:* in each of the three rehabilitation methods, the patient is placed in a dorsal blocking splint to prevent wrist and finger extension. The wrist is positioned in 10 to 30 degrees of flexion with the MCP joints at 40 to 60 degrees of flexion and the PIPs and DIPs in full extension.

Immobilization Technique

This treatment strategy completely immobilizes the tendon for 3½ weeks after tendon repair. Immobilization may not result in consistently good results because it often leads to scar adherence and may lead to a greater incidence of tendon rupture. However, in the presence of other injuries (e.g., a fractured phalanx that cannot be moved), this technique may be necessary. Also, if a patient appears unable to participate fully in treatment (as might be the case for a child or a person with cognitive impairments), this method may be selected.

Controlled Passive Motion

Duran and Houser[38] suggested the use of controlled passive motion, which allows 3 to 5 mm of tendon excursion, to achieve optimal results after primary tendon repair. They found this practice sufficient to prevent adherence of the repaired tendons. On the third postoperative day, the patient begins a twice-daily exercise regimen of passive flexion and extension of 6 to 8 motions for each tendon. Care is taken to keep the wrist flexed and the MCPs in 70 degrees of flexion during passive exercise. After 4½ weeks the protective dorsal splint is removed and the rubber band traction is attached to a wristband (Figure 30-13). Active extension and passive flexion are done for 1 additional week and gradually increased over the next several weeks.

Early Active Motion

Dr. Harold Kleinert, a pioneer of flexor tendon surgery, was an early advocate of rubber band traction after repair of flexor tendons. This technique is often called the *Kleinert technique.* After surgical repair, rubber bands are attached to the nails of the involved fingers with a suture through the nail or with a hook held in place with cyanoacrylate glue. A dorsal blocking splint is fabricated from low-temperature thermoplastic material with the MCP joints held in about 60 degrees of flexion and the PIPs in gentle flexion. The patient must be able to fully extend the interphalangeal (IP) joints actively within the splint; otherwise, joint contractures will develop (Figure 30-13). Kleinert's original protocol has been modified but remains the basis for most of the early active motion protocols described in the literature and described briefly in Table 30-1. His protocol and the Washington approach use early active extension but passive flexion. The Indiana and MAMTT (minimal active muscle-tendon tension) protocols allow for early gentle supervised active flexion of the injured tendon. There is some evidence[99] that early active motion such as "place-and-hold" exercises do result in greater finger motion after a Zone II tendon injury.

In the Kleinert and Washington protocols the patient wears the splint 24 hours a day for 3 weeks and is instructed to actively extend the fingers several times a day in the splint, allowing the rubber bands to pull the fingers into flexion.

Table 30-1 Flexor Tendon Rehabilitation Protocol*

Treatment Protocol	Indications/ Discussion	Early Treatment Phase	Middle Treatment Phase	Late Treatment Phase
Immobilization	Patient under 10 years old Cognitively impaired When movement would adversely affect other healing structures Usually leads to adherent scar	0 to 3 Weeks *Positioning Splint* Postoperative cast or dorsal blocking splint Wrist 10-30° flexion MCP 40-60° flexion IP full extension *Exercise:* AROM uninvolved shoulder, elbow	3 to 6 Weeks *Positioning Splint* Change wrist to neutral *Exercise*: Passive finger flexion with wrist in 10° extension Tendon glide exercise (Figure 30-13)	4 to 6 weeks *Positioning Splint* Discontinue splint May need nighttime static extension splint *Exercise:* Blocking Light resistance Light ADL
Early passive mobilization protocols 1. Kleinert 2. Duran and Houser 3. Modified Duran	Early passive motion Facilitates tendon glide and decreases adherent scar formation	0 to 4.5 Weeks (Duran & Houser) *Positioning Splint* Wrist 20° flexion MCP relaxed flexion IP extension *Exercise:* Passive PIP and DIP flexion/extension in protected position Modified Duran *Positioning Splint* Wrist varies from 20° flexion to 20° extension MCP 40-50° flexion Strap finger in extension at night and when not exercising *Exercise:* PROM as above Active extension of PIPs and DIPs with MCPs held in maximum flexion In OT clinic only: protected tenodesis	4.5 to 8 Weeks (Duran & Houser) *Positioning Splint* Replace splint with wrist band with rubber band traction applied to finger *Exercise:* Active extension Blocking FDS glide Fisting	8 Weeks (Duran & Houser) *Positioning Splint* Discontinued *Exercise:* Begin gentle graded resistance
Early active motion protocols 1. Washington 2. Indiana Protocol 3. Minimal Active Muscle Tendon Tension (MAMTT)	Generally favored protocols Places gentle active tension on the repaired tendon Therapist and MD must agree on protocol Patient must be able to comply fully with treatment regimen	0 to 4 Weeks (Washington) *Positioning Splint* Wrist 30-45° flexion MCP 40-70° flexion IP full extension Rubber band traction with palmar bar pulley *Exercise:* Active IP extension to splint Passive flexion MCP, PIP, and DIP Composite passive flexion to distal palmar crease	4 to 6 Weeks (Washington) *Positioning Splint* Week 5 begin nighttime splinting only, wrist changed to 15° flexion May apply wrist cuff with rubber band traction *Exercise:* Active tendon glides or "place & hold" exercise, cleared by MD Blocking flexion of PIP and DIP, cleared by MD Composite extension to neutral	6 to 8 Weeks (Washington) *Positioning Splint* Discontinue protective splint but may begin dynamic PIP extension if indicated *Exercise:* Blocking to PIP and DIP Passive wrist, finger extension Light putty with MD approval Light ADL At 8 weeks can begin graded resistance

Data from Cifaldi CD, Schwarze L: Early progressive resistance following immobilization of flexor tendon repairs, *J Hand Ther* 4:111, 1991; Duran RJ et al: Management of flexor tendon lacerations in zone 2 using controlled passive motion postoperatively. In Hunter JM, Mackin E, Callahan A et al, editors: *Rehabilitation of the hand*, ed 3, St. Louis, 1990, Mosby; Evans RB, Thompson DE: The application of force to the healing tendon, *J Hand Ther* 6(4):266-284, 1993; Halikis MN, Manske PR, Kubota H et al: Effect of immobilization, immediate mobilization, and delayed mobilization on the resistance to digital flexion using a tendon injury model, *J Hand Surg* 22(3):464-472, 1997; Schenck RR, Lenhart DE: Results of zone II flexor tendon laceration in civilians treated by the Washington regime, *J Hand Surg* 21(6):984-987, 1996; Stewart Pettengill KM, van Strein G: Postoperative management of flexor tendon injuries. In Mackin EJ, Callahan AD, Osterman AL et al, editors: *Rehabilitation of the Hand and Upper Extremity*, ed 5, Vol I, St. Louis, 2002, Mosby.

*This table is meant only as a basic outline of the variety of rehabilitation protocols for a flexor tendon injury. Not all protocols have been listed or described under each category. It is the responsibility of the therapist to consult the appropriate and complete sources. It is expected that the occupational therapist will study the original complete protocols and be in contact with the surgeon before beginning tendon rehabilitation. The OTA must also have knowledge of tendon anatomy and the protocols to assist the occupational therapist in treatment.

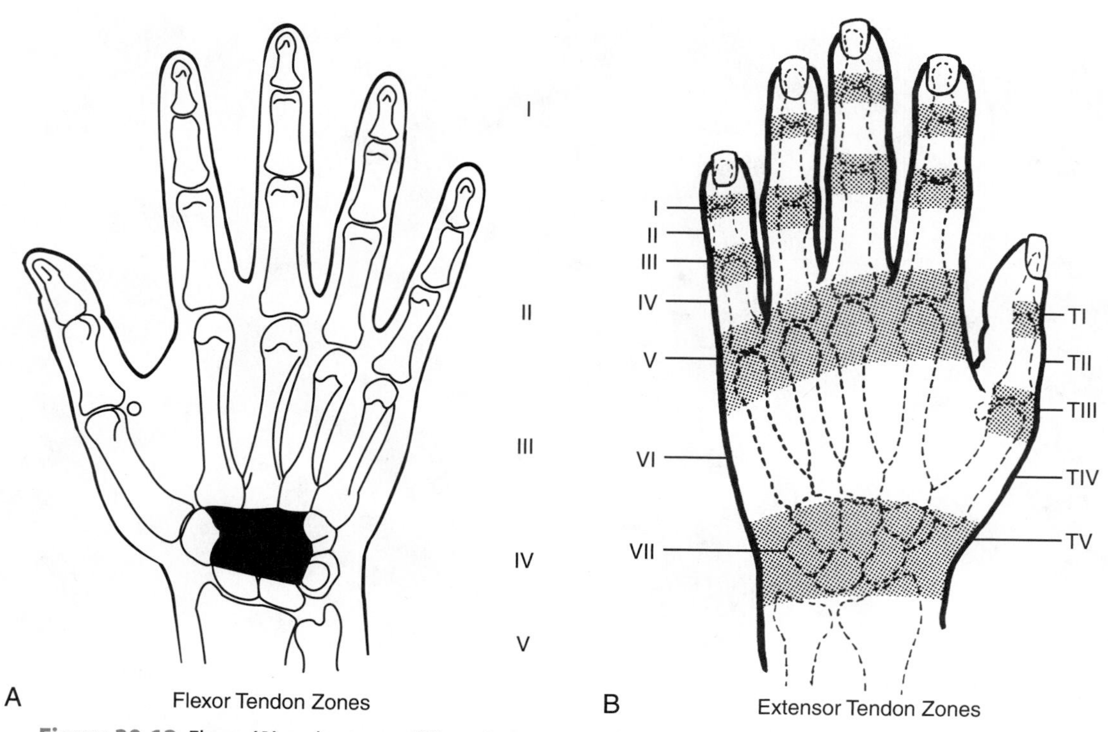

Figure 30-12 Flexor **(A)** and extensor **(B)** tendon zones as determined by the First Congress of the International Federation of Societies for Surgery of the Hand, 1980. (From Kleinert HE, Sibrand S, Gill T: Flexor tendon injuries, *Surg Clin North Am* 61(2):268-269, 1981.)

The movement of the tendon through the tendon sheath and pulley system minimizes scar adhesions while enhancing tendon nutrition and blood flow. The dorsal blocking splint is removed at 3 weeks, and the rubber band is attached to a wristband, which is worn for 1 to 5 additional weeks, depending on the surgeon's judgment.

To be successful, all of the early mobilization techniques require a motivated patient who thoroughly understands the program. Some early active mobilization protocols currently allow early active extension and flexion of the repaired tendons, as well as other changes.[24,94] Only the most experienced occupational therapist who has good communication with the surgeon should attempt these treatment approaches.

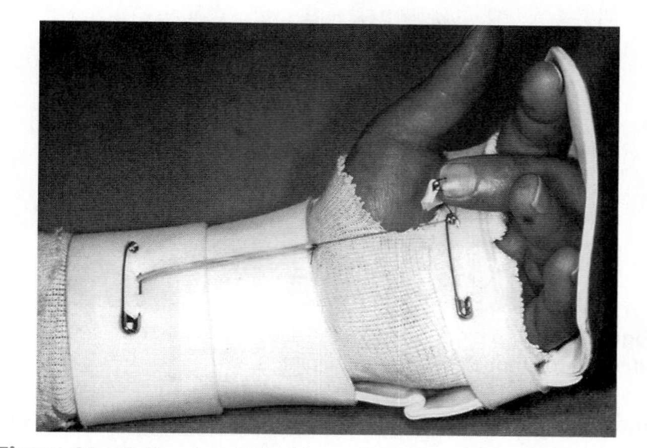

Figure 30-13 The dorsal blocking splint allows for passive flexion of the digit(s) and full active extension at the PIP and DIP joints.

Postacute Flexor Tendon Rehabilitation

Although each protocol has a specific, and sometimes slightly different time line, when active flexion is begun out of the splint after any of the postoperative management techniques described previously, the patient should be instructed in exercises to facilitate differential tendon gliding.[107,108] Wehbe[107] recommends three positions—hook fist, straight fist, and composite fist—to maximize isolated gliding of the flexor digitorum superficialis and the flexor digitorum profundus tendons, as well as stretching of the intrinsic musculature and gliding of the extensor mechanism. These tendon glide exercises (Figure 30-14) should be repeated 10 times in each position, two to three times daily. Isolated exercises to assist tendon gliding may also be performed with a blocking splint[40] (Figure 30-15) or by using the opposite hand (Figure 30-16). The MCP joint is held in extension during blocking, so the intrinsic muscles that act on it cannot overcome the power of the repaired flexor tendons. Care should be taken not to hyperextend the PIP joint because this would overstretch the repaired tendons.

After 6 to 8 weeks, passive extension may be started and a volar finger splint may be necessary to correct a flexion contracture at a PIP joint. Alternately, the therapist may fabricate a cylindrical plaster splint to apply constant static pressure on the contracture[14] (Figure 30-17).

After approximately 8 weeks, the patient may begin light resistive exercises, light ADL, and other activities. The patient must avoid lifting with or applying excessive resistance to the affected hand. Sports activities should be discouraged. However, activities such as working with soft clay, woodworking,

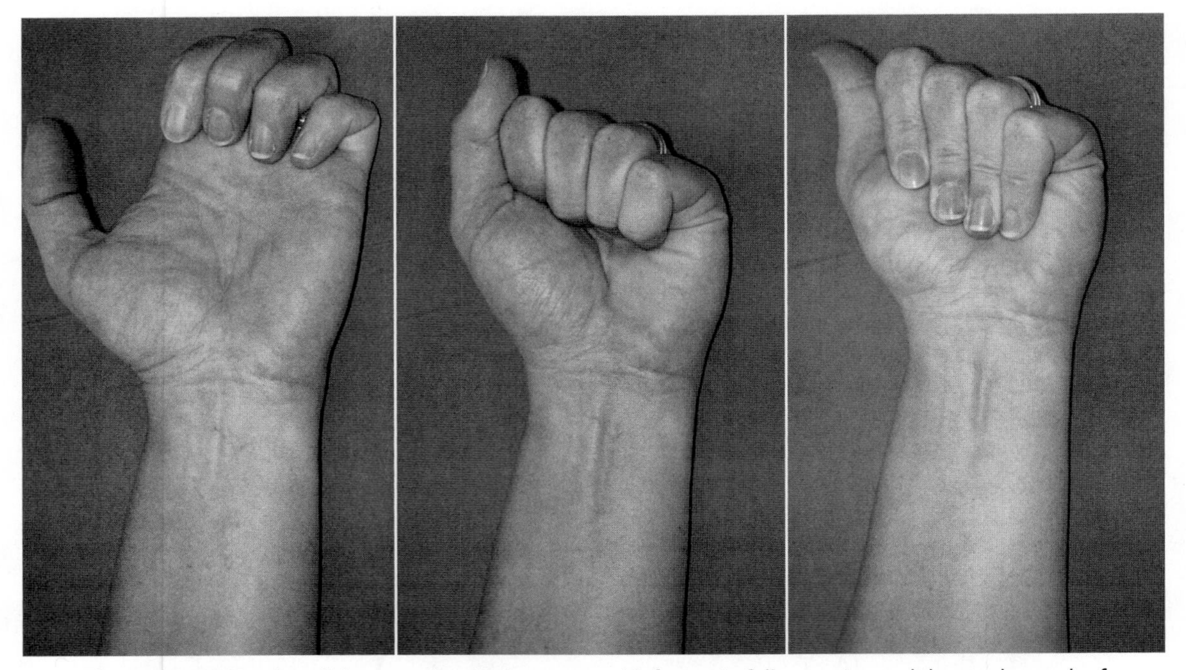

Figure 30-14 Tendon gliding exercises. Patient starts with fingers in full extension and then makes each of these fist positions.

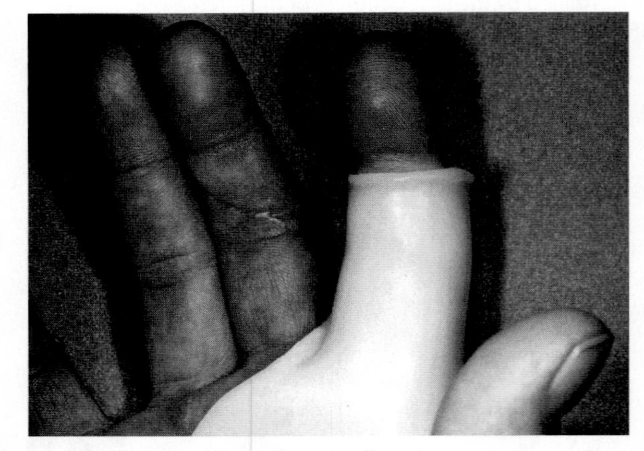

Figure 30-15 A blocking splint can allow the patient to perform isolated tendon motion at a specified joint.

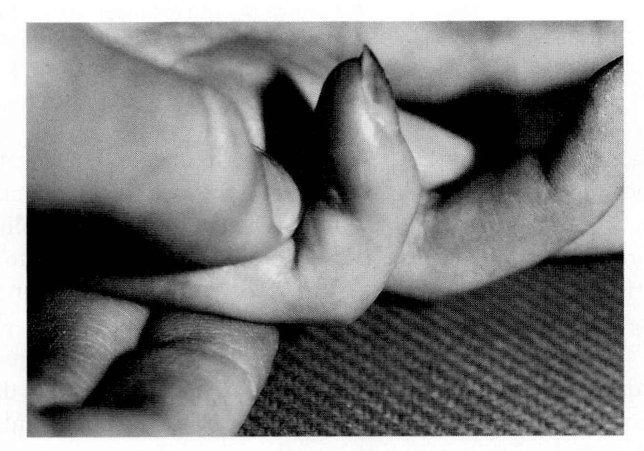

Figure 30-16 Manual blocking of the MCP during active flexion of the PIP joint.

and macramé are excellent. Full resistance and normal work activities may resume at 3 months after surgery.

Although performance of ADL is generally not a problem, therapy providers should ask patients about any problems they may have or anticipate. Disuse and neglect of a finger, especially the index finger, are common and should be prevented.

Gains in finger flexion and extension may continue to be recorded for 6 months postoperatively. A finger with limber joints and minimal scarring preoperatively will function better after repair than one that is stiff and scarred or that has trophic skin changes.[25] A "functional" to "excellent" result is obtained when there is minimal extension lag at the PIP and DIP joints and the finger(s) can flex to the palm.

Extensor Tendon Injuries

Traditionally, extensor tendons have been treated via immobilization protocols. However, because of their anatomy (they are broad, thin, and structurally flat), they easily become adherent to the tissue above (skin) and below (fascia, bone) after injury. They can rupture more easily than flexor tendons. Scar adherence limits extensor tendon gliding and can impair not only extension of the digits but also flexion. Incomplete extension is known as *extensor lag.* Because of the frequency and ease with which the extensor tendons can become scarred and adherent, new treatment philosophies have developed during the past 20 years.[41] Three current treatment approaches to extensor tendon rehabilitation are (1) immobilization, (2) early controlled passive mobilization, and (3) early active motion. Extensor tendons are divided into zones (see Figure 30-12), and rehabilitation depends on the zone of injury regardless of which of the three treatment methods is used. As with flexor tendon injuries, the therapist who works with patients with extensor tendon injuries must understand tendon anatomy and biomechanics and facilitate communication with the surgeon. A study of the literature[41-43,52] before one works with patients with extensor tendon injuries is essential.

The **immobilization approach** keeps the tendons in a shortened position through splinting or casting. Tendons are immobilized for 3 weeks; in week 4, gentle active motion of the repaired tendons is introduced. Extensor tendons injured proximal to the MCP joints often become adherent to the structures above and below them. This problem will require the occupational therapist to begin a splinting program. A removable volar splint is used between exercise periods to protect the tendon for 2 additional weeks. Dynamic flexion splinting may be started 6 weeks after surgery to regain flexion if needed.

Extensor tendons injured proximal to the MCP joint may be immobilized for 3 weeks. After this, the finger may be placed in a removable volar splint that is worn between exercise periods for an additional 2 weeks. Progressive ROM is begun after 3 weeks, and if full flexion is not regained rapidly, dynamic flexion may be started after 6 weeks.

Extensor tendon injuries that occur distal to the MCP joint require a longer period of immobilization (usually 6 weeks). A progressive exercise program is then initiated with dynamic splinting during the day and static splinting at night to maintain extension.

The **early passive motion** approach reverses what was done for the flexor tendons. The extensor tendons are held in extension by dynamic, gentle rubber band traction, and the patient is allowed to actively flex the fingers, thereby passively moving the repaired extensor tendons. These splints must have a dorsal component to provide a block to flexion so as not to move the tendons too much, which could lead to overstretching or rupture of the extensor tendon.[41,43] This method facilitates tendon strength and can prevent the scarring that ultimately limits motion and function.

The early active short arc program, developed by Evans,[41,42] allows the tendon (except a Zone I injury) to actively move 3 days after surgery. The therapist must take care to ensure that the stress applied by **early active motion** does not overpower the strength of the surgical repair. The splinting program is quite complex and specific and requires a skilled occupational therapist.[41,42,52,97]

Peripheral Nerve Injuries

In 1943 Seddon[13] devised the following three categories of **peripheral nerve injuries:**

1. *Neurapraxia* is contusion or bruise of the nerve. The nerve recovers function without treatment within a few days or weeks.
2. *Axonotmesis* is an injury in which nerve fibers distal to the site of the injury degenerate, but the internal organization of the nerve remains intact. No surgical treatment is necessary, and recovery usually occurs within 6 months. The length of time may vary depending on the level of injury.
3. *Neurotmesis* is a complete laceration of the nerve. Microsurgical repair is required.

The mechanisms by which peripheral nerve injuries occur are numerous.[88] The peripheral nerve can be injured by one of the following mechanisms: (1) compression from within by a tumor or fracture (which can also lacerate a peripheral nerve); (2) compression from without such as a hand or finger crushed in a machine or car door; (3) laceration by a fractured bone, knife, or lid of a can; (4) stretching, which deranges the internal structure of the nerve beyond its ability to function, as may occur in a motor vehicle accident when the arm and therefore brachial plexus may be stretched by the force of the accident; (5) inadvertent injection into a peripheral nerve; (6) radiation such as may be administered to the axillary lymph node area because of breast cancer; and (7) electricity (consider the child who puts his or her finger into an electrical outlet). Peripheral nerves have both motor and sensory functions. Symptoms of peripheral nerve injuries include muscle weakness or paralysis and sensory loss in the area innervated by the injured peripheral nerve. The therapist who assesses the patient for nerve loss must be familiar with the muscles and areas that are innervated by the three major forearm nerves. A summary of UE peripheral neuropathies can be found in Table 30-2.

Peripheral Neuropathy

Occupational therapists may administer several quick clinical tests of the motor function of the individual peripheral nerves to detect impairment. The ulnar nerve may be tested by asking the patient to pinch a piece of paper between his or her thumb and index finger while the therapist tries to pull the paper way. This is called the Froment's sign (Figure 30-18). The therapist may also palpate the first dorsal interosseous muscle. The radial nerve may be tested by asking the patient to extend the wrist and fingers together (Figure 30-19). Median nerve function is tested by asking the patient to oppose the thumb to the fingers[27] (Figure 30-20). Early signs of median nerve compression are commonly sensory in nature and may be tested by performing provocative tests such as the Phalen's test and percussing over the median nerve at the wrist to elicit a Tinel's sign, as described earlier in this chapter.

Patients may also develop compression syndromes of the ulnar and radial nerves that will be indicated by paresthesias along the course of those nerves.

Radial Nerve

The radial nerve innervates the extensor and supinator group of muscles of the forearm. The sensory distribution of the radial nerve is a strip of the posterior upper arm and the forearm, the dorsum of the thumb, and the index and middle fingers and radial half of the ring finger to the PIP joints. Sensory loss of the radial nerve does not usually result in dysfunction or have serious functional ramifications.

A dorsal splint that provides wrist extension, MCP extension, and thumb extension is provided to protect the extensor tendons from overstretching during the healing phase and to position the hand for functional use (Figure 30-21).

Median Nerve

The median nerve innervates the flexors of the forearm and hand and is often called the *eyes* of the hands because of its importance in sensory innervation of the volar surface of the hands. Median nerve loss may result from lacerations, as well as from compression syndromes of the wrist such as carpal tunnel syndrome.

Table 30-2 Nerve Injuries of the Upper Extremity

Nerve	Location	Affected	Test
Radial nerve (posterior cord; fibers from C5, C6, C7, C8)	Upper arm	Triceps and all distal motors; sensory to SRN	MMT, sensory test
Radial nerve	Above elbow	Brachioradialis and all distal motors, sensory to SRN	MMT, sensory
Radial nerve	At elbow	Supinator, ECRL, ECRB, and all distal motors; sensory to SRN	MMT, sensory
Posterior interosseous nerve	Forearm	ECU, ED, EDM, APL, EPL, EPB, EIP; no sensory loss	Wrist extension—if present indicates PIN rather than high radial nerve
Radial nerve at ECRB, radial artery, arcade of Froshe, origin of supinator	Radial tunnel syndrome	Weakness of muscles innervated by PIN, no sensory loss	Palpation for pain over extensor mass; pain with wrist flexion and pronation; pain with wrist extension and supination; pain with resisted middle finger extension
Median nerve (lateral cord from C5, C6, C7; medial cord from C8, T1)	High lesions (elbow and above)	Paralysis/weakness of FCR, PL, all FDS, FDP, I and II; FPL, pronator teres, and quadratus, opponens pollicis, APB, FPB (radial head), lumbricals I and II; sensory cutaneous branch of median nerve	MMT, sensory
Median nerve	Low (at wrist)	Weakness of thenars only	Inability to flex thumb tip and index fingertip to palm; inability to oppose thumb, poor dexterity
Median nerve under fibrous band in PT, beneath heads of pronator, arch of FDS, origin of FCR	Pronator syndrome	Weakness in thenars but *not* muscles innervated by AIN; sensory in median nerve distribution in hand	Provocative tests to isolate compression site
Median nerve under origin of PT, FDS to middle	Anterior interosseous nerve syndrome	Pure motor, no sensory; forearm pain preceding paralysis; weakness of FPL, FDP I and II, PQ	Inability to flex IP joint of thumb and DIP of index; increased pain with resisted pronation; pain with forearm pressure
Median nerve at wrist	Carpal tunnel syndrome	Weakness of median innervated intrinsics, sensory	Provocative tests, Tinel's, sensory
Ulnar nerve at elbow (branch of medial cord from C7, C8, T1)	Cubital tunnel syndrome	Weakness/paralysis of FCU, FDP III and IV, ulnar intrinsics; numbness in palmar cutaneous and dorsal cutaneous distribution; loss of grip and pinch strength	Pain with elbow flexion/extension
Ulnar nerve at wrist	Compression at Guyon's canal	Weakness and pain in ulnar intrinsics	Reproduced by pressure at site

SRN, Superficial radial nerve; *MMT*, manual muscle test; *ECRL*, extensor carpi radialis longus; *ECRB*, extensor carpi radialis brevis; *ECU*, extensor carpi ulnaris; *ED*, extensor digitorum; *EDM*, extensor digiti minimi; *APL*, abductor pollicis longus; *EPL*, extensor pollicis longus; *EPB*, extensor pollicis brevis, *EIP*, extensor indicis proprius; *PIN*, posterior interosseous nerve; *FCR*, flexor carpi radialis; *PL*, palmaris longus; *FDS*, flexor digitorum superficialis; *FDP*, flexor digitorum profundus; *FPL*, flexor pollicis longus; *APB*, abductor pollicis brevis; *FPB*, flexor pollicis brevis; *AIN*, anterior interosseous nerve; *PT*, pronator teres; *FCR*, flexor carpi radialis; *PQ*, pronator quadratus; *IP*, interphalangeal; *DIP*, distal interphalangeal; *FCU*, flexor carpi ulnaris.

Motor distribution of the median nerve is listed in Table 30-2. Sensory distribution of the median nerve includes the volar surface of the thumb, index, and middle fingers; the radial half of the ring finger and dorsal surface of the index and middle fingers; and the radial half of the ring finger distal to the PIP joints. The sensory loss associated with median nerve injury is particularly disabling because sensory innervation is lacking in the fingers that perform all pinch patterns. The patient is unable to judge the amount of pressure or force needed to accomplish a pinch task and so the task becomes almost impossible to do. When vision is occluded, the patient will substitute pinch to the ring and small fingers to compensate for this loss.

Splints that position the thumb in palmar abduction and slight opposition will increase functional use of the hand (Figure 30-22). If clawing of the index and long fingers is present, a splint should be fabricated to prevent hyperextension of the MCP joints. Patients report that they avoid use of the hand with a median nerve injury because of lack of sensation rather than because of muscle paralysis. Despite this, the weakened or paralyzed muscles should be protected.

Ulnar Nerve

The ulnar nerve in the forearm innervates only the flexor carpi ulnaris, the median half of the flexor digitorum profundus, and the intrinsic muscles of the hand (see Table 30-2). The

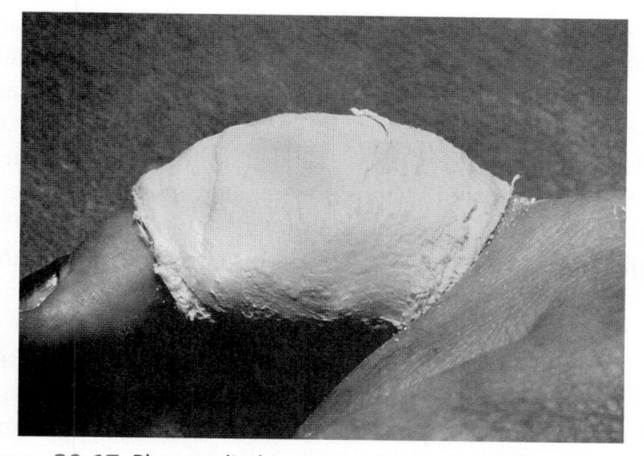

Figure 30-17 Plaster cylindric cast used to apply gentle static stretch to PIP joint.

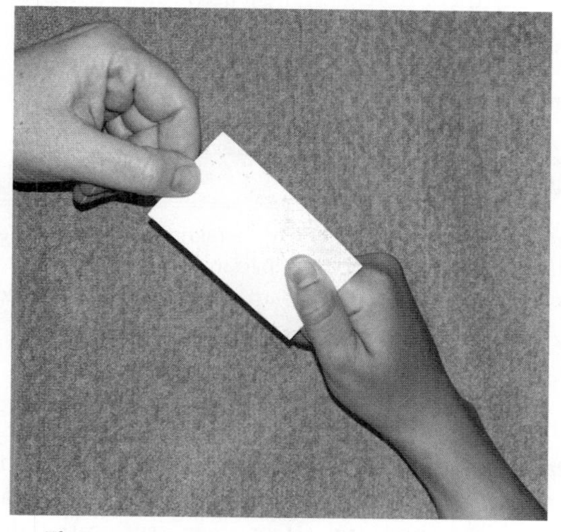

Figure 30-18 Quick ulnar nerve function test.

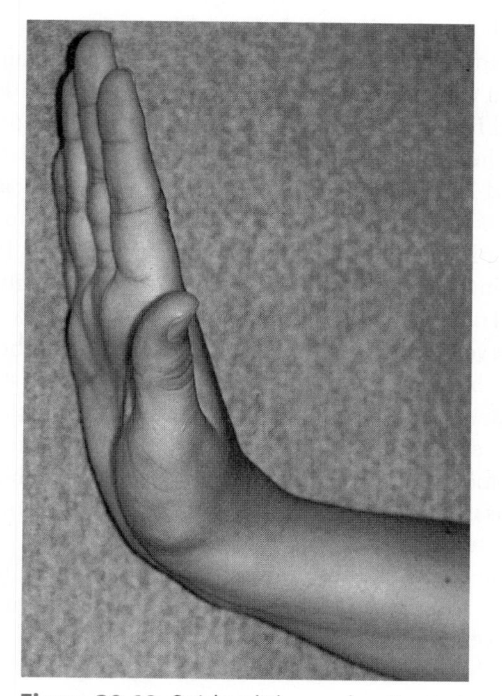

Figure 30-19 Quick radial nerve function test.

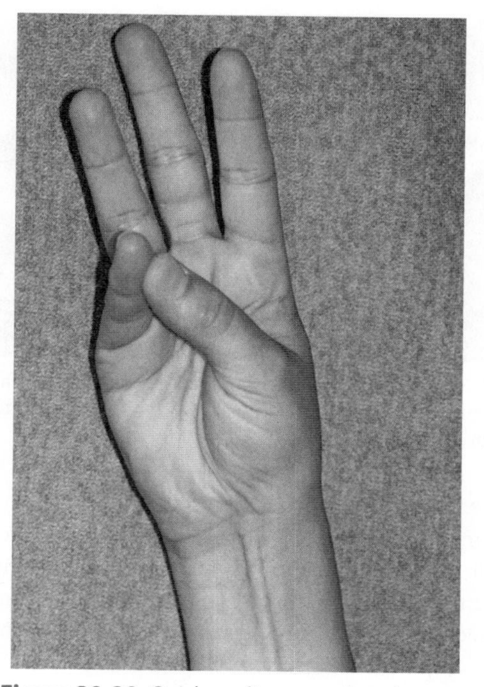

Figure 30-20 Quick median nerve function test.

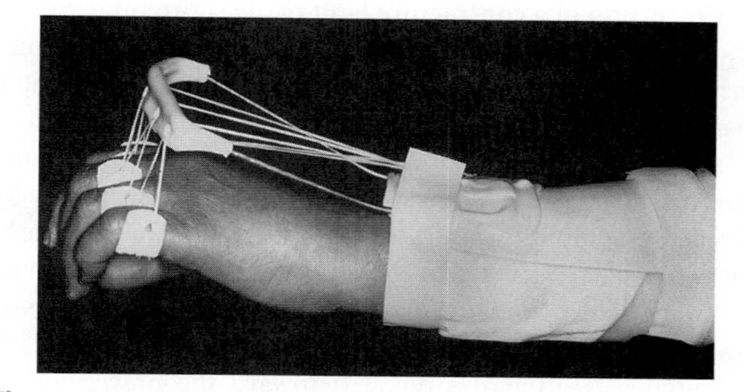

Figure 30-21 Low-profile radial nerve splint is carefully balanced to pull MCP joints into extension when wrist is flexed and allows the MCP joints to fall into slight flexion when wrist is extended, preserving normal balance between two joints and preventing joint contracture. (Courtesy Judy C. Colditz.)

sensory distribution of the ulnar nerve includes the dorsal and volar surfaces of the little finger and the ulnar half of the dorsal and volar surface of the ring finger. An ulnar nerve injury results in hyperextension of the MCP joints of the ring and small fingers *(clawing)* caused by action of the extensor digitorum communis that is not held in check by the third and fourth lumbricals.[83]

Splints should block hyperextension of the MCP joints (Figure 30-23). The IP joints of the ring and small fingers will not demonstrate a great flexion deformity because of the paralysis of the flexor digitorum profundus. The hypothenar muscles and interossei will be absent. The wrist will assume a position of radial extension caused by the loss of the flexor carpi ulnaris.

Sensory loss of the ulnar nerve results in frequent injury (especially burns) to the ulnar side of the hand and small finger. Patients must be instructed in visual protection of the anesthetic area.

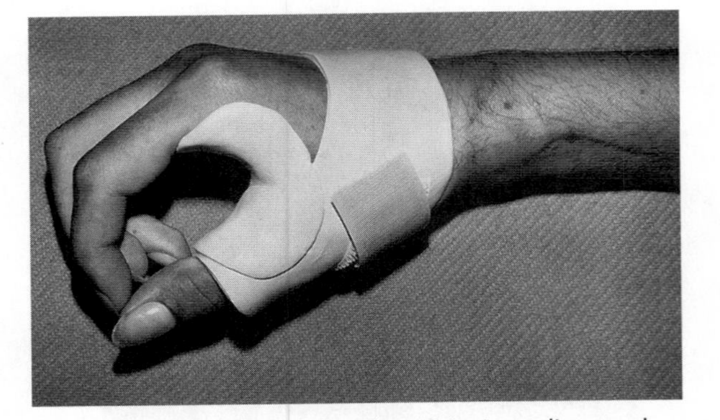

Figure 30-22 A hand-based thumb-positioning splint may be used with median nerve injury to preserve the web space and to position thumb for function.

Postoperative Management after Nerve Repair

After surgical nerve repair the hand is placed in a position that will minimize tension on the nerve. For example, after the repair of the median nerve the wrist will be immobilized in a flexed position. Immobilization usually lasts 2 to 3 weeks, after which protective gentle motion of the joints may begin. The clinician must exercise great care not to put excessive traction on the newly repaired nerve.

Correction of a **contracture** (soft tissue shortening around a joint) may take 4 to 6 weeks. Active exercise is the preferred method of gaining full wrist extension, although a light dynamic splint may be applied with the surgeon's supervision. Splinting to assist or substitute for weakened musculature may be necessary for an extended period during nerve regeneration. Splints should be removed as soon as possible to allow for active exercise of the weakened muscles. However, instructing the patient in correct patterns of motion is important so that substitution is minimized.

Initially, treatment is directed toward the prevention of deformity and correction of poor positioning during the acute and regenerative stages. PROM is an essential component of the clinic and the home exercise programs so that as the muscle begins to work, it does not have to move a tight or contracted joint. Patients must be instructed in visual protection of the anesthetic area. The patient's ADL status should be evaluated in case alternative methods or devices are needed for functional independence. Use of the hand in the patient's work should be evaluated, and the patient should be returned to employment with any necessary job modifications or adaptations of equipment as soon as possible.

Careful muscle, sensory, and functional testing is performed frequently. As the nerve regenerates, splints may be changed or eliminated. Exercises and activities are revised to reflect the patient's new gains, and adaptive equipment should be discarded as soon as possible.

As motor function begins to return to the paralyzed muscles, a careful program of specific active and active-assistive exercises is devised to facilitate the return. The occupational therapist may use NMES (neuromuscular electrical stimulation)[37] to provide an external stimulus to help strengthen the newly innervated muscle. When the muscle grade receives a good rating, functional activities are used to complete the return to normal strength.

An intact peripheral nerve gives sensory feedback and stimulates a motor response. A sensory disturbance may take two forms; first, the area of innervation may be hypersensitive. This commonly occurs in fingertip injuries. Consider a carpenter who might have to reach into a pocket to retrieve nuts, screws, and bolts with a finger that cannot tolerate even a light touch. The task would be difficult, if not impossible. This patient would require a program of sensory desensitization, as described earlier in this chapter, with the goal of reducing hypersensitivity.

The second sensory disturbance problem involves insufficient protective sensibility. Without intact sensation the carpenter could become injured on a sharp object. Sensory reeducation attempts to help the patient learn to recognize and interpret normal sensory impulses. Sensory reeducation is not begun until the patient has protective sensibility. In both treatment strategies, the patient must understand the treatment objectives, be willing and able to carry out the prescribed program at home, and consciously incorporate his or her hand into daily tasks.[66]

CLINICAL PEARL

Patients with upper extremity peripheral nerve injury often experience intolerance to cold. The clinician may suggest a mitten or glove lined with Thinsulate to guard against pain experienced in a cold environment.

Fractures

In treating a hand or wrist **fracture** (broken bone), the surgeon attempts to achieve good anatomic position through either a closed (nonsurgical) or open (surgical) reduction. Closed reductions are usually immobilized with a cast or, in some cases, a splint. Open reductions are immobilized with internal fixation devices such as Kirschner wires, metallic plates, and screws so that the desired position is maintained. External fixation may be used alone or in combination with internal fixation. Whenever the injury allows, the position in which the hand is immobilized is wrist extension, MCP flexion, and PIP and DIP extension.[51] This position is called the *safe position*[45] or *intrinsic plus position*[51] because it maintains the length of the collateral ligaments of the MCP, PIP, and DIP joints, thereby preserving the eventual mobility of the hand. Trauma to bone may also involve trauma to tendons and nerves in the adjacent area. Treatment must be geared toward the recovery of all injured structures. In fact, it is often joint contracture and tendon adherence that present the most difficult challenges for postfracture hand rehabilitation.[51]

OT may be initiated during the period of immobilization, which is usually 3 to 5 weeks. Goals of OT intervention during this phase include the following:

- Edema reduction via elevation of the limb
- Skin care, especially in the presence of an external fixation device
- AROM of the noninvolved joints, especially the elbow and shoulder

If possible, the patient should be encouraged to use the involved hand as an ADL assist (with light activities only) so that he or she does not become completely one-handed during the immobilization period.

As soon as bone stability is sufficient, the surgeon will remove the immobilization apparatus (internal plates, screws, and pins are not usually removed) and allow mobilization of the injured part. The surgeon will provide guidelines for the amount of resistance or force that may be applied to the fracture site. Activities that correct poor motor patterns and encourage use of the injured hand are started as soon as the hand is pain free. Many patients believe that they will be fine once the cast or hardware has been removed and may be upset at the prospect of a protracted period of rehabilitation. Therefore a careful assessment of the patient's emotional status will be helpful to the therapists working with the patient. Early motion will prevent the adherence of tendons and reduce edema through stimulation of the lymphatic and blood vessels.

When the brace or cast is removed, the patient's hand must be assessed. If edema is present, edema control techniques can be initiated with techniques described earlier in this chapter. A baseline ROM should be established, and the application of appropriate splints may begin. A splint may be used to correct a deformity that has resulted from immobilization or may be used to protect the hand or finger from additional trauma to the fracture site. An example of this type of splinting is the Velcro "buddy" splint (Figure 30-24). A dorsal blocking splint that limits full extension of the finger may be used after a fracture or dislocation of the PIP joint. A dynamic splint may be used to achieve full ROM or prevent the development of further deformity at 6 to 8 weeks after fracture.

Intraarticular (inside the joint) fractures may result in injury to the cartilage of the joint, resulting in additional pain and stiffness. An xray will indicate whether damage to the joint surface might limit the treatment of the joint. Joint pain and stiffness after fracture without the presence of joint damage should be alleviated by a combination of thermal modalities, restoration of joint play (joint mobilization), and corrective and dynamic splinting, followed by active use. Resistive exercises can be started when bony healing has been achieved.

Wrist fractures of the distal radius are common and may present special problems for the surgeon and therapist. There are several categories of distal radius fractures,[67] but the Colles fracture of the distal radius is the most common injury to the wrist[96] and may result in limitations in wrist flexion and extension, as well as forearm pronation and supination, resulting from the involvement of the distal radioulnar joint. Treatment objectives from the medical and therapeutic perspectives are to establish joint alignment through anatomic reduction and to restore pain-free hand and wrist function with full ROM of the proximal joints.[67] Use of splints, active motion that emphasizes wrist movement, and joint mobilization may be beneficial. The weight well (see Figure 30-11) may be used to provide resistance to wrist motions.

The scaphoid is the second most commonly injured bone in the wrist[96] and is often fractured when the hand is dorsiflexed at the time of injury. Fractures to the proximal portion of the scaphoid may result in nonunion because of poor blood supply to this area. Scaphoid fractures will require a prolonged period of immobilization, sometimes up to several months in a cast, with resulting stiffness and pain. Care should be taken to mobilize noninvolved joints early.

Stiffness and pain are common complications of fractures, but the control of edema coupled with early motion and good patient instruction and support will minimize these complications.

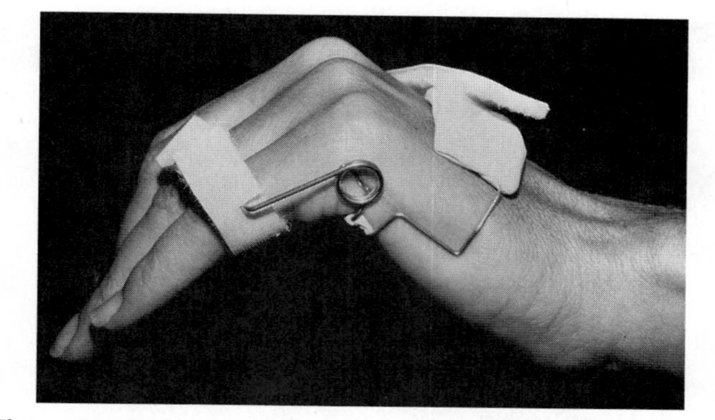

Figure 30-23 A dynamic ulnar nerve splint blocks hyperextension of the MCP joints, thus allowing extension of the PIP joints. (Splint courtesy Mary Dimick, University of California—San Diego Hand Rehabilitation Center, Calif.)

CLINICAL PEARL

For distal radial fractures: use a wrist cock-up splint to maintain wrist extension at night to allow the tissue to rest at a proper position.

CLINICAL PEARL

For all distal fractures: Both passive and active range of motion of the noninvolved joints is critical for preventing stiffness of shoulder and elbow. When the patient cannot use his or her hand and is not reaching overhead, around, etc., the proximal joints can easily become stiff.

Complex Regional Pain Syndrome

Complex regional pain syndrome (**CRPS**) is a relatively new term for a condition that has been documented since the American Civil War.[50] It is a painful disorder that can occur in the upper or lower extremity after injury or immobilization; it is characterized by pain, irregular blood flow, edema, changes in skin temperature and color, and often limitations of movement.[34,35] Reflex sympathetic dystrophy (RSD) had been the term used to identify this condition but was changed at a conference of the International Association for the Study of Pain in 1993 because of the confusion as to what was and was not RSD, as well as because the designation was being used indiscriminately.[93] Rather than the name implying the cause of the condition, the new name describes the "clinical features, location, and specifics of the injury."[65]

Box 30-5

Diagnostic Criteria for Complex Regional Pain Syndrome

1. Pain that is out of proportion to initial event or injury
2. One symptom in each of the four categories:
   a. Sensory: acutely sensitive to touch
   b. Vasomotor:
      1) Changes in skin temperature, limb may be cooler or warmer than noninvolved side
      2) Changes in skin color—may be red, blue, pale, blotchy
   c. Sudomotor/Edema: limb may be swollen, sweaty, or dry
   d. Motor/Trophic:
      1) Decreased ROM
      2) Changes in nails, hair and skin
3. One sign in two of the categories
   a. Sensory: aversion to pinprick or light touch
   b. Vasomotor: asymmetric skin color or temperature
   c. Sudomotor/Edema: edema, sweating irregularities
   d. Motor/Trophic: decreased ROM, weakness, tremors, changes in nails, hair or skin
4. Another diagnosis cannot explain signs and symptoms

From Harden RN, Bruehl SP: Diagnosis of complex regional pain syndrome: signs, symptoms, and new empirically derived diagnostic criteria. *Clin J Pain* 22:415-419, 2006.

There are two subsets of CRPS: CRPS Type I, which refers to the classic RSD, and CRPS Type II, which presents with similar signs and symptoms but can be attributed to a diagnosed nerve injury (see Box 30-5 for diagnostic criteria). The degree of trauma in both types may not correlate with the severity of the pain and may occur after any injury, even a seemingly minor one. The syndrome appears to be triggered by a cycle of vasospasm and vasodilation after an injury. Abnormal edema and constrictive dressings or casts may be a factor in initiating the vasospasm. A vasospasm can decrease the blood supply to tissue; edema and pain result and contribute to the abnormal cycle of pain.[85] When circulation is decreased, the extremity becomes cool and pale. Fibrosis after tissue anoxia and the production of protein-rich exudates results in joint stiffness. The patient may cradle the hand and prefer to keep it wrapped. There may be an exaggerated reaction to touch, especially light touch. Osteoporosis may be apparent on x-ray films by 8 weeks after trauma. Burning pain associated with CRPS Type II is a symptom that may be alleviated by surgical interruption of the sympathetic nerve pathways. Millions of people in the United States may be affected with CRPS[95]; women are affected more frequently than men, the upper extremity is more often involved than the lower extremity, and fractures are the most common initiating event.[34] CRPS Types I and II can present a real challenge to the treating physician and therapist. CRPS can be extremely disabling and is potentially a long-term condition that can prevent the patient from fully participating in life activities that are valuable to him or her.

The broad goals of occupational therapy are to control the symptoms of pain and edema, help normalize sensation, improve joint ROM and thereby functional abilities, and facilitate independence in activities of daily living with compensation strategies and/or assistive devices if necessary.[82] It is imperative to begin treatment as early as possible to prevent long-term consequences and complete dysfunction of the limb. The OT treatment program must avoid stressful interventions that aggravate pain or cause inflammation.

To control pain, the OT may consider thermal modalities (hot packs, fluidotherapy), TENS, splinting, and gentle AROM. Edema is controlled by elevation, gentle massage (with a very light touch so as not to compress the lymphatic system), active exercise, and gentle compression. Edema control techniques should be started immediately. A desensitization program, massage, gentle handling of the patient's hand, and acupressure may help alleviate hypersensitivity. To decrease joint stiffness and improve ROM, biofeedback with active exercise and activities may be helpful. Biofeedback may be used to improve general relaxation and reduce anxiety as well. Only if the patient can tolerate dynamic or static progressive splinting to reduce joint contracture should it be employed. Weight bearing (stress loading[104]) on the extremity and low-impact aerobic activity to improve blood flow will also help these patients in later stages of the condition.[10] A stress-loading program has been used effectively to reduce symptoms[104] and can easily be adapted for home use. At all times these patients must be treated by the most qualified OT team member. Frequent communication with the physician may be necessary, and caution must be used to avoid causing an increase in pain.

The physician uses medication and sometimes regional anesthesia techniques[10] to control the symptoms of CRPS. Medication regimens and surgical options are complicated and numerous.[10,65,102]

CRPS may trigger shoulder pain and stiffness, resulting in shoulder-hand syndrome or a "frozen" shoulder. Therefore early in the treatment program, AROM and functional activities should include the entire upper quadrant. Skateboard exercises are helpful in the early stages for active-assistive exercise of the shoulder. Splints that reduce joint stiffness should be used as tolerated. A tendency to develop a CRPS should be suspected in any patient who seems to complain excessively about pain, appears anxious, and complains of profuse sweating and temperature changes in the hand. Patients will tend to overprotect the hand. Early intervention with a structured therapy program of functional activities, group interaction, psychological support, and exercises that include all joints from the hand to the shoulder may prevent the occurrence of a fully developed pain syndrome. This problem is best recognized early and treated with tempered aggressiveness and empathy. The OTA who suspects a patient may be developing CPRS must report this immediately to the supervising occupational therapist.

Cumulative Trauma Disorder

Work-Related Musculoskeletal Disorder

A number of terms have described the conditions that occur when the musculoskeletal system is subjected to repeated stress: overuse syndromes, cervicobrachial disorders, repetitive stress or strain injuries (RSIs), repetitive motion injuries, and **cumulative trauma disorders (CTDs)**. In the United States the term CTD is most commonly used. Cumulative disorders are thought to be work related and are often referred to as work-related musculoskeletal disorders (MSDs). Musculoskeletal disorders are defined as "injuries or disorders of muscles, nerves, tendons, joints, cartilage, or spinal disks associated with risk factors at the workplace."[62] Between 1981 and 1992, reported CTDs increased from 18% to 62% of all workers' compensation claims filed,[59] although there has been a decline since then. In 2007 the number of reported cases of work-related MSDs was 335,900[12]; the indirect and directs costs to the economy are thought to be $54 billion annually.[62]

The term *cumulative trauma disorder* or *work-related musculoskeletal disorder* should be considered descriptive; it describes the mechanism of injury but is not a diagnosis. Today, many workers are required to perform the same repetitive motor task 6 or more hours a day. For example, a worker who is required to stand on an assembly line doing the same task repeatedly or type on a computer all day long is at risk for MSD. Work-related high-risk factors for CTD are repetition, high force, awkward joint posture, direct pressure, vibration, and prolonged static positioning.[7] The human body was not made to work this way, even though today's technology and productivity may encourage this behavior. In addition, many people have second jobs or pursue rigorous leisure activities. It is important to recognize that CTD may take many weeks, months, or years to develop and may take just as long to resolve.

Cumulative trauma occurs when force is repeatedly applied to the same muscle or muscle group, causing an inflammatory response in the tendon, muscle, or nerve.[85] Muscle fatigue is an important aspect of cumulative trauma and can be relieved by rest. However, chronic fatigue, the usual condition of these patients, cannot be relieved by rest alone. In these circumstances, it is important to examine the patient's job requirements, as well as home and leisure activities.

Diagnoses associated with cumulative trauma usually fall within the following three categories: tendonitis, nerve compression or entrapment syndromes, and myofascial pain. Common examples of CTD involving the tendons are lateral epicondylitis (tennis elbow) and de Quervain's disease.

Patients can also demonstrate nerve pain associated with CTDs. Peripheral nerves become entrapped in scar tissue or irritated by low levels of edema in the surrounding tissue. Like tendons, nerves have to slide or glide as the extremity moves. When a nerve is entrapped or caught in scar, "friction can develop along the nerve tract, most likely at the vulnerable tunnel sites."[21] Thus the patient often reports vague symptoms of pain in the extremity. A well-known nerve compression syndrome is carpal tunnel disease, which is a compression of the median nerve at the level of the wrist. However, the peripheral nerve can also be entrapped along its entire pathway. A skilled therapist may perform a neural tension or neurodynamic test of the peripheral nerve.[87] Tests (Figure 30-25), which lengthen the peripheral nerve path, are

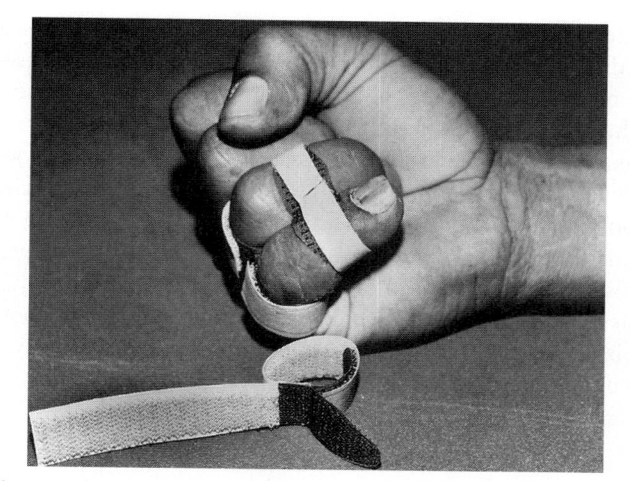

Figure 30-24 Velcro "buddy" splint/strap may be used to protect a finger after a fracture or to encourage movement of a stiff finger.

provocative; they can reproduce the patient's symptoms. The OT would advise the patient that he or she may experience an increase in pain symptoms after the test.

Poor posture and positioning of the body out of normal alignment are often the cause of myofascial pain. This diagnosis is difficult to make because the pain is often referred to a distal area. An accurate diagnosis of any of these conditions is difficult and should be done by a skilled physician, often with input from an experienced occupational therapist.

When supervised, the OTA may assist in the treatment of these patients. In the acute phase, when muscle or tendon involvement exists, treatment aims to reduce inflammation through rest. Splints are used for immobilization, often in combination with physician-prescribed antiinflammatory medication. In this phase the patient may be placed on an active therapy program consisting of modalities to reduce pain and stretching of the affected musculature to prevent joint stiffness. The patient should be instructed not to engage in activities that cause pain.

As the acute symptoms decrease, the patient begins the exercise phase of treatment. Resistive exercise can be added, but only after the muscle has been warmed by slow stretching and the physiological muscle length has been fully restored. Resistance should be increased slowly and should not result in increased pain. Patients are instructed to stretch at home, especially before activity, three times daily for an indefinite period of time.

When the source of the problem is nerve related, the treatment goal is to decrease pain by decreasing tension on the nerve tissue and to decrease any muscle imbalance that might be impinging on the nerve tissue. To achieve these goals, the OT, with the assistance of the OTA, may perform soft tissue massage, nerve gliding exercises, and strengthening when appropriate. Active release technique may be beneficial with these patients. Education related to postural awareness and ergonomic problem solving with the patient are critical to complete recovery.

To control symptoms in the long term, patients must become aware of what triggers their symptoms and learn early intervention strategies if symptoms reappear. Modalities to reduce pain—splints, stretching, and modified activities—combined with proper body mechanics are usually effective. The key is that patients learn self-management techniques and take an active role in their treatment. When the patient's job demands have caused the CTD, an evaluation of the job site, tools used, and body mechanics during work activities may be indicated. The OT undertakes the job site evaluation with permission from the patient and employer. The OTA may assist the therapist in gathering information from the patient about job requirements to help determine whether a job site analysis is indicated.

CLINICAL PEARL

Begin your occupational therapy program with postural training exercises such as "chin tuck" exercises and "scapular pinching" that will lengthen anterior body muscles.

CLINICAL PEARL

Teach diaphragmatic breathing to take the stress off the intercostals and upper trapezius, which are accessory breathing muscles.

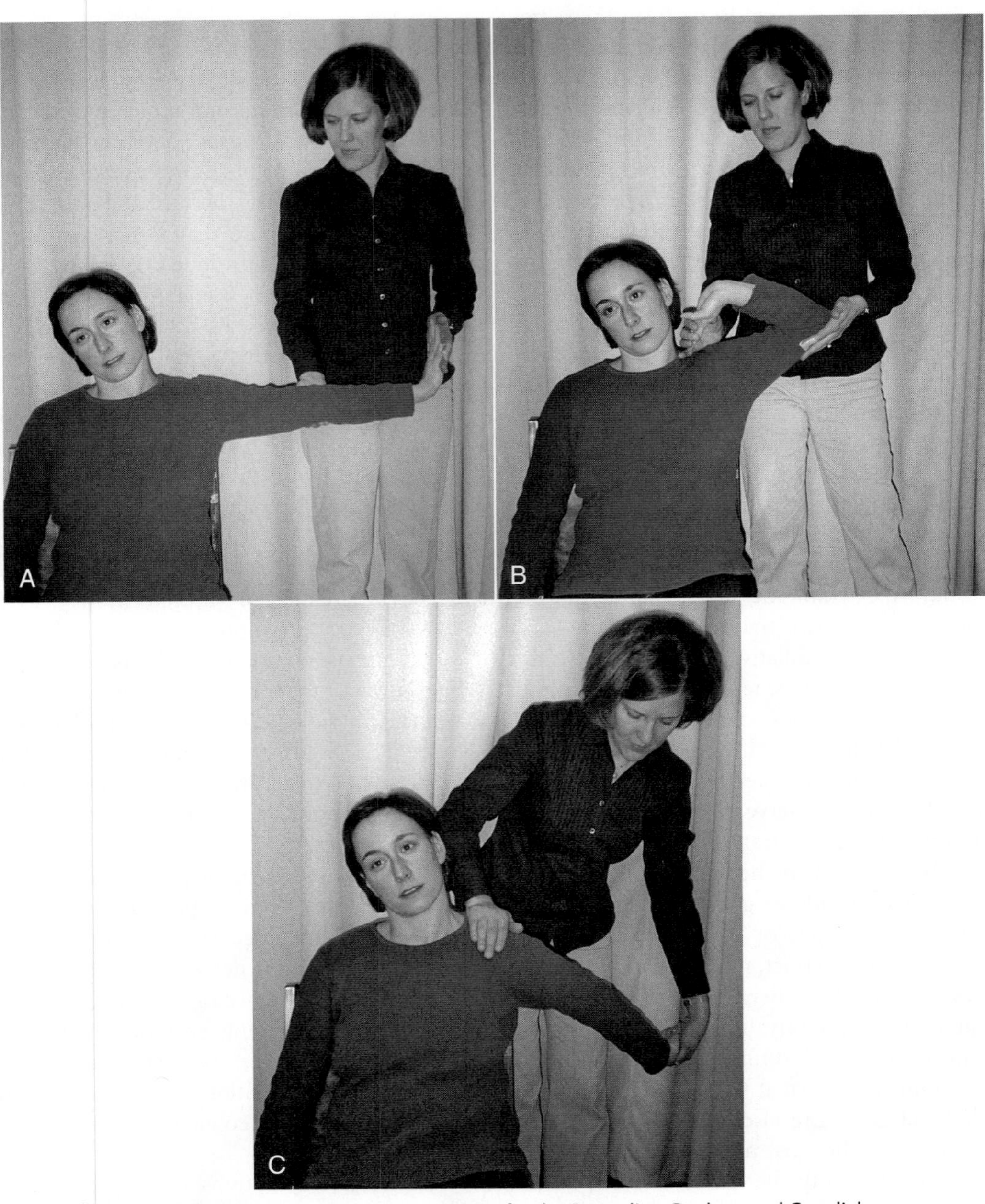

Figure 30-25 Neurodynamic testing positions for the **A,** median, **B,** ulnar, and **C,** radial nerves.

CASE STUDY

JC

JC is typical of a patient with an acute hand injury seen in an OT hand clinic. He is a 65-year-old retired police officer who injured his left, nondominant, hand in a home accident with a circular saw. He suffered subtotal amputation of the tips of the index and middle fingers, which were successfully replanted. The ring finger, which could not be replanted, was amputated at the level of the DIP joint. The accident and surgery occurred on December 3; he is seen for the first time in OT on January 10. Pictured is the patient's hand at rest in comparison with the noninjured side (Figure 30-26) and the patient attempting to make a fist (Figure 30-27).

For results of JC's initial evaluation in OT, refer to Figure 30-28. Consider the following questions:

1. Determine a problem list for JC and list problems in priority order. What rationale guides this order?
2. For each problem that you have described, discuss the intervention strategy you would use. What is your rationale for the strategy?
3. For each treatment strategy, describe exactly what the therapy practitioner would do including patient position and therapist action.
4. Discuss the ADL areas in which the patient may have difficulty. What are the best recommendations for these possible limitations?

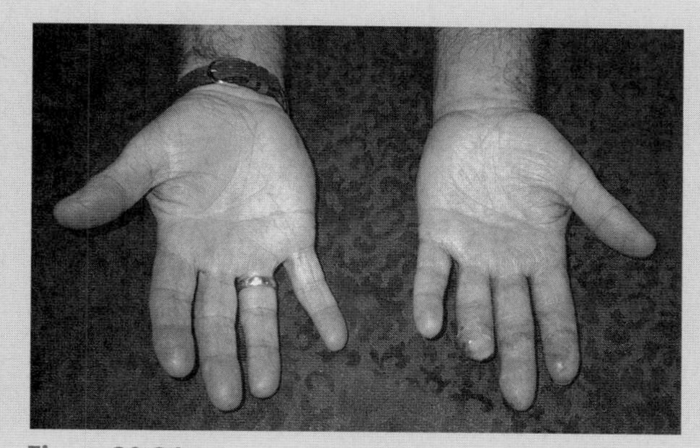

Figure 30-26 Palmar surface, injured and noninjured hands.

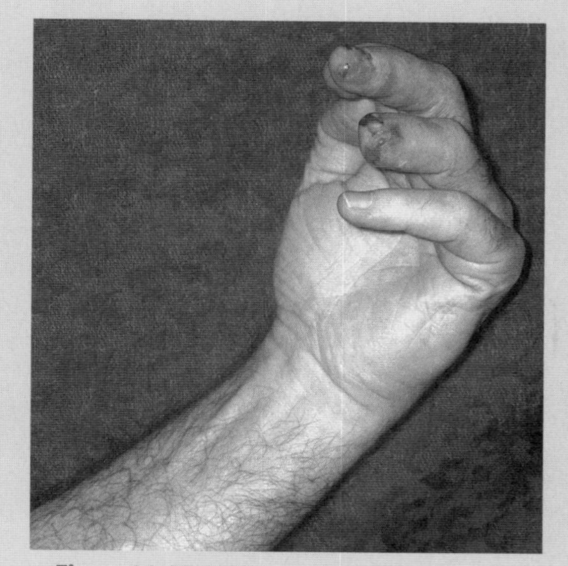

Figure 30-27 Patient attempting to make a fist.

OCCUPATIONAL THERAPY INITIAL EVALUATION RESULTS

Patient: JC

History: Left carpal tunnel release 1991, no other relevant PMH

Wound appearance: Well-healed scars volar surface of index and middle fingers; amputation of ring finger at DIP joint

Edema: Moderate

Circumference	Right	Left
Wrist	6.75 inches	6.75 inches
Midpalmar (DPC)	8.50 inches	8.25 inches
PIP joint ring fingers	2.50 inches	2.75 inches

Pain: 4 out of 10 (intermittent, not constant, patient bothered by numbness more than pain)

Hand active ROM Right noninjured

Finger	MCP joint	PIP joint	DIP joint	TAM
Index	0/85	0/100	0/60	245
Middle	0/90	0/100	0/65	255
Ring	0/80	0/90	0/55	225
Small	0/80	0/85	0/60	225
Thumb	0/40	−/60		100

Hand active ROM Left injured

Finger	MCP joint	PIP joint	DIP joint	TAM
Index	0/70	0/45	0/30	145
Middle	0/70	0/45	0/10	125
Ring	0/60	0/30	Amp	0/40
Small	0/70	0/50	0/10	130
Thumb	0/40	0/60		100

Finger tip to distal palmar crease

Finger	Right	Left injured
Index	0 cm	6 cm
Middle	0 cm	7 cm
Ring	0 cm	6 cm
Small	0 cm	5.5 cm

Strength (recorded in pounds)

Test	Right	Left injured
Gross grasp	105	20
2 point pinch	18	4
3 jaw chuck	22	8
Lateral	26	10

Dexterity

9-hole peg test Right = 15 seconds Left = 27 seconds

Sensibility

Semmes-Weinstein monofilament test

Finger tip	Radial side	Ulnar side
Thumb	3.61	3.61
Index	3.61	3.61
Middle	3.61	4.31
Ring (amp at DIP)	3.61	3.61
Small	3.61	3.61

Figure 30-28 Case study: occupational therapy initial evaluation results.

Summary

The occupational therapist usually assesses the hand-injured patient with assistance from the OTA. The occupational therapist establishes the intervention strategy for each patient. The OTA may assist in certain defined areas and in some areas may carry out the treatment independently. However, OTAs who work with this population must be familiar with assessment and intervention concepts. OTAs who elect to work in this specialty area are encouraged to further develop service competency by participating in continuing education and on-site supervision.

Selected Reading Guide Questions

1. Describe the various sensory tests and their appropriate uses.
2. What are two tools used to measure edema? Discuss the rationale for each.
3. Name two objective tests of sympathetic function.
4. What is the only technique that is always appropriate for acute hand injury?
5. Name the components of a hand evaluation.
6. What are the benefits of using the Jebsen Test of Hand Function?

7. If no goniometer is available, describe another method of evaluating gross finger flexion.
8. What are the goals of OT with a patient who has had a fingertip amputation?
9. Name the three types of pinch that are routinely assessed for strength. Name two functional activities for each of these pinch types.
10. Name the three levels of peripheral nerve injury.
11. Why is the median nerve sometimes referred to as the "eyes of the hand?"
12. Why does "clawing" occur in the small and ring fingers after ulnar nerve injury?
13. What splint position is indicated after a low-level median nerve injury that has resulted in paralysis?
14. Once a patient has been cleared for strengthening, name two clinic activities and two craft activities that will achieve this goal.
15. Describe two treatment strategies to reduce fingertip hypersensitivity.
16. Describe the appropriate splint immediately after flexor tendon repair. What is the rationale of the Kleinert protocol?
17. What is Complex Regional Pain Syndrome? What is the difference between CRPS Type I and CRPS Type II? What is a key caution when working with patients with CRPS?
18. Discuss the risk factors for work-related musculoskeletal or cumulative trauma at the workplace. What body tissues are affected by work-related musculoskeletal disorders? What is the goal of OT during the acute rehabilitation phase when working with a patient with this disorder?

References

1. American Occupational Therapy Association: Occupational therapy practice framework: domain and process, ed 2, *Am J Occup Ther* 56(6):609–639, 2002.
2. American Occupational Therapy Association: Physical agent modalities position paper, *Am J Occup Ther* 51(10):870–871, 1997.
3. American Society for Surgery of the Hand: *The hand, examination and diagnosis*, ed 3, New York, 1990, Churchill Livingstone.
4. Amini DA: Renaissance in occupational therapy and occupation-based hand therapy, OT Practice, vol 9, No. 32004.
5. Anthony MS: Sensory evaluation. In Clark G, Shaw-Wilgis EF, Aiello B, et al: *Hand rehabilitation: a practical guide*, New York, 1993, Churchill Livingstone.
6. Apfel ER, Carronza J: *Dexterity. In the American Society of Hand Therapists, Clinical assessment recommendations*, ed 2, Chicago, 1992, AHST.
7. Armstrong TJ: Cumulative trauma disorders of the upper limb and identification of work-related factors. In Millender LH, Louis DS, Simmons BP, editors: *Occupational disorders of the upper extremity*, New York, 1992, Churchill Livingstone.
8. Artzberger SM: Edema control: new perspectives, *Phys Disabil Special Interest Section Q*, vol 20, 1997. No 1.
9. Artzberger SM: Manual edema mobilization: treatment for edema in the subacute hand. In Mackin EJ, Callahan AD, Osterman AL, et al, editors: ed 5, *Rehabilitation of the hand and upper extremity*, vol I, St. Louis, 2002, Mosby.
10. Astifidis RP: Pain related syndromes: Complex regional pain syndrome and fibromyalgia. In Cooper C, editor: *Fundamentals of hand therapy*, St. Louis, 2007, Mosby Elsevier, pp 376–387.
11. Barber LM: Occupational therapy for the treatment of reflex sympathetic dystrophy and post-traumatic hypersensitivity of the injured hand. In Fredericks S, Brody GS, editors: *Symposium on the neurologic aspects of plastic surgery*, St. Louis, 1978, Mosby.
12. Barr AE: Approach to management of work-related musculoskeletal disorders. In T. Skirven TM, Osterman AL, et al, editors: *Rehabilitation of the hand and upper extremity*, ed 6, vol 2, Philadelphia, 2011, Elsevier.
13. Batha M, Gupta R: Basic science of peripheral nerve injury and repair. In T. Skirven TM, Osterman AL, et al: *Rehabilitation of the hand and upper extremity*, ed 6, vol 2, Philadelphia, 2011, Elsevier.
14. Bell-Krotoski JA: Tissue remodelling and contracture correction using serial plaster casting and orthotic positioning. In Skirven TM, Osterman AL, Fedorczyk J, Amadio P, editors: *Rehabilitation of the hand and upper extremity*, ed 6, vol 2, Philadelphia, 2011, Elsevier.
15. Bell-Krotoski JA: Sensibility testing with the Semmes-Weinstein monofilaments. In Mackin EJ, Callahan AD, Osterman AL, et al, editors: *Rehabilitation of the hand and upper extremity*, ed 5, vol I, St. Louis, 2002, Mosby.
16. Bellace JV, Healy D, Besser MP, et al: Validity of the Dexter Evaluation System's Jamar dynamometer attachment for assessment of hand grip strength in a normal population, *J Hand Ther* 13(1):46–51, 2000.
17. Bennett GK: *Hand-tool dexterity test*, New York, 1981, Harcourt, Brace, Jovanovich.
18. Brand PW, Hollister A: *Clinical mechanics of the hand*, ed 3, St. Louis, 1999, Mosby.
19. Brown A, Cramer LD, Eckhaus D, et al: Validity and reliability of the Dexter hand evaluation and therapy system in hand-injured patients, *J Hand Ther* 13(1):37–45, 2000.
20. BTE Technologies: *Smart physical therapy and physiotherapy equipment, occupational therapy equipment, & athletic training equipment*, 2011, . Retrieved from http://www.btetech.com/eval_rehab_systems.htm.
21. Butler DS: *Mobilisation of the nervous system*, Edinburgh, 1991, Churchill Livingstone.
22. Callahan AD: Sensibility assessment for nerve lesions-in-continuity and nerve lacerations. In Mackin EJ, Callahan AD, Osterman AL, et al: editors *Rehabilitation of the hand and upper extremity*, ed 5, vol I, St. Louis, 2002, Mosby.
23. Cambridge CA: Range of motion measurement of the hand. In Mackin EJ, Callahan AD, Osterman AL, et al; editors: *Rehabilitation of the hand and upper extremity*, ed 5, vol I, St. Louis, 2002, Mosby.
24. Cannon NM: Post flexor tendon repair motion protocol, *Indiana Hand Center Newsl* 1:13–17, 1993.
25. Cannon NM, Foltz RW, Koepfer JM, et al: Control of immediate postoperative pain following tenolysis and capsulectomies of the hand with TENS, *J Hand Surg* 8:626, 1983.
26. Chen C, Granger CV, Peimer CA, et al: Manual ability measure (MAM-16): a preliminary report on a new patient-centered and task-oriented outcome measure on hand function, *J Hand Surg* 30(2):207–216, 2005.

27. Chusid JG: *Correlative neuroanatomy and functional neurology*, ed 19, Los Altos, Calif, 1985, Lange.
28. Crawford JE, Crawford DM: *Crawford small parts dexterity test manual*, New York, 1981, Harcourt.
29. Creelman G: *Volumeters unlimited*, Idyllwild, Calif.
30. Cyriax JH: Clinical application of message. In Basmajian JV, editor: *Manipulation, traction, and massage*, ed 3, Baltimore, 1985, Williams & Wilkins.
31. Dellon AL: *Evaluation of sensibility and reeducation of sensation in the hand*, Baltimore, 1981, Williams & Wilkins.
32. Dellon AL: The vibrometer, *Plast Reconstr Surg* 71(3):427–431, 1983.
33. Dellon AL, Curtis RM, Edgerton MT: Reeducation of sensation in the hand after nerve injury and repair, *Plast Reconstr Surg* 53(3):297–305, 1974.
34. deMos M, deBruijn AGJ, Huygen FJ, et al: The incidence of complex regional pain syndrome: a population based study, *J Int Assoc Study Pain* 129(1):12–20, 2007.
35. Dommerholt J: Complex regional pain syndrome-1: History, diagnostic criteria and etiology, *J Bodywork Movement Ther* 8:167–177, 2004.
36. Donatelli R, Owens-Burkhart H: Effects of immobilization on the extensibility of periarticular connective tissue, *J Orth Sports Phys Ther* 3:67–72, 1981.
37. Duff SV, Estilow T: Therapist's management of peripheral nerve injury. In Skirven TM, Osterman AL, et al, editors: *Rehabilitation of the hand and upper extremity*, ed 6, vol I, Philadelphia, 2011, Elsevier.
38. Duran RJ, et al: Management of flexor tendon lacerations in zone 2 using controlled passive motion postoperatively. In Hunter JM, Mackin E, Callahan A, et al, editors: *Rehabilitation of the hand*, ed 3, St. Louis, 1990, Mosby.
39. Edmond SL: *Manipulation mobilization extremity & spinal techniques*, St. Louis, 1993, Mosby.
40. English CB, Rehm RA, Petzoldt RL: Blocking splints to assist finger exercise, *Am J Occup Ther* 36(4):259–262, 1982.
41. Evans RB: Clinical management of extensor tendon injuries: The therapist's perspective. In Skirven TM, Osterman AL, et al, editors: *Rehabilitation of the hand and upper extremity*, ed 6, vol 2, Philadelphia, 2011, Elsevier.
42. Evans RB: Immediate active short arc motion following extensor tendon repair, *Hand Clin* 11(3):483–512, 1995.
43. Evans RB, Burkhalter WE: A study of dynamic anatomy of extensor tendons and implications for treatment, *J Hand Surg* 11(5):774–779, 1986.
44. Fess EE: Documentation: essential elements of an upper extremity assessment battery. In Mackin EJ, Callahan AD, Osterman AL, et al, editors: *Rehabilitation of the hand and upper extremity*, ed 5, vol I, St. Louis, 2002, Mosby.
45. Fess EE: *Hand and upper extremity splinting principles & methods*, ed 3, St. Louis, 2003, Mosby.
46. Fishman TD: Phases of wound healing, http://medicaledu.com/phases.htm, copyright 1995-2010, retrieved 12/2/11.
47. Gelberman RH, Szabor M, Williamson RV, et al: Sensibility testing in peripheral nerve compression syndromes: an experimental study in humans, *J Bone Joint Surg Am* 65(5):632–638, 1983.
48. Grice KO, Vogel KI, Le V, et al: A brief report—adult norms for a commercially available nine hole peg test for finger dexterity, *Am J Occup Ther* 57(5):570–573, 2003.
49. *Hand Therapy Certification Committee*: www.htcc.org/about/index.cfm. Accessed February 1, 2005.
50. Harden RN, Bruehl SP: Diagnosis of complex regional pain syndrome: signs, symptoms, and new empirically derived diagnostic criteria, *Clin J Pain* 22(5):415–419, 2006.
51. Hardy MA, Freeland AE: Hand fracture fixation and healing: skeletal stability and digital mobility. In Skirven TM, Osterman AL, et al, editors: *Rehabilitation of the hand and upper extremity*, ed 6, vol I, Philadelphia, 2011, Elsevier.
52. Hung LK, Chan A, Chang J, et al: Early controlled active mobilization with dynamic splintage for treatment of extensor tendon injuries, *J Hand Surg* 15(2):251–257, 1990.
53. Jaffe R, Farney-Mokris S: *Clinical assessment recommendations*, ed 2, Chicago, 1992, American Society of Hand Therapists.
54. Jebsen RH, Taylor N, Trieschmann RB, et al: An objective and standardized test of hand function, *Arch Phys Med Rehabil* 50(6):311–319, 1969.
55. Kaltenborn FM, Evjenth O: *Manual mobilization of the extremity joints*, ed 4, Oslo, 1989, Olaf Norlis Bokhandel.
56. Kamentz HL: Mechanical devices of massage. In Basmajian JV, editor: *Manipulation, traction and massage*, ed 3, Baltimore, 1985, Williams & Wilkins.
57. Kasch MC: Clinical management of scar tissue, *OT Health Care* 4(3):37–52, 1988.
58. Kellor M, Kondrasuk R, Iversen I, et al: *Technical manual of hand strength and dexterity test*, Minneapolis, 1971, Sister Kenny Rehabilitation Institute.
59. Kelsey JL, McEwing G: *Upper extremity disorders: frequency, impact, and cost in the United States*, New York, 1997, Churchill Livingstone.
60. Kendall FP, McCreary EK, Provance PG, et al: *Muscles: testing and function*, ed 5, Baltimore, 2005, Williams & Wilkins.
61. Kessler RM, Hertling D: Joint mobilization techniques. In Kessler RM, Hertling D, editors: *Management of common musculoskeletal disorders*, New York, 1983, Harper & Row.
62. Kietrys DM, Barr AE, Barbe M: Pathophysiology of work-related musculoskeletal disorders. In T. Skirven TM, Osterman AL, et al,editors: *Rehabilitation of the hand and upper extremity*, ed 6, vol 2, Philadelphia, 2011, Elsevier, p 1769.
63. Kleinert HE, Schepel S, Gill T: Flexor tendon injuries, *Surg Clin North Am* 61(2):267–286, 1981.
64. Knight KL, Draper DO: *Therapeutic modalities: the art and science*, Baltimore, 2008, Lippincott, Williams & Wilkins.
65. Koman LA, Li Z, Smith BP, Smith TL: Complex regional pain syndrome: types I and II. In Skirven TM, Osterman AL, Fedorczyk J, et al, editors: *Rehabilitation of the hand and upper extremity*, ed 6, vol I, Philadelphia, 2011, 2011 Elsevier.
66. Larson RN: Desensitization and reeducation. In Burke SL, Higgins JR, McClinton MA, et al: *Hand and upper extremity rehabilitation*, St. Louis, 2006, Elsevier, pp 151–165.
67. Laseter GF, Carter PR: Management of distal radius fractures, *J Hand Ther* 9(2):114–128, 1996.
68. Law M, Baptiste S, Carswell A, et al: *Canadian occupational performance measure*, ed 3, Ottawa, Canada, 1998, CAOT Publications ACE.
69. Bear-Lehman J, Poole SE: The presence and impact of stress reactions on disability among patients with hand injury. *J Hand Ther* 24:89–93, April-June 2011.
70. Lister GL: *The hand: diagnosis and indications*, ed 3, New York, 1993, Churchill Livingstone.
71. Louis DS, Greene TL, Jacobson KE, et al: Evaluation of normal values for stationary and moving two-point discrimination in the hand, *J Hand Surg* 9(4):552–555, 1984.

72. MacDermid JC: Outcome measurement in the upper extremity. In Mackin EJ, Callahan AD, Osterman KL, et al, editors: *Rehabilitation of the hand and upper extremity*, ed 5, vol I, St. Louis, 2002, Mosby.
73. Mackinnon SE, Dellon AL: Two-point discrimination tester, *J Hand Surg* 10(6):906–907, 1985.
74. Mathiowetz V, Kashman N, Vollard G, et al: Grip and pinch strength: normative data for adults, *Arch Phys Rehabil* 66(2): 69–74, 1985.
75. Mathiowetz V, Remmells C, Donoghue L: Effects of elbow position on grip and key pinch strengths, *J Hand Surg* 10(5): 694–697, 1985.
76. Mathiowetz V, Weber K, Vollard G, et al: Reliability and validity of grip and pinch strength evaluations, *J Hand Surg* 9(2): 222–226, 1984.
77. Melvin JL: *Rheumatic disease occupational therapy and rehabilitation*, ed 3, Philadelphia, 1989, FA Davis.
78. Mennell JM: *Joint pain*, Boston, 1964, Little, Brown.
79. Moberg E: Objective methods for determining the functional value of sensibility in the hand, *J Bone Joint Surg Br* 40-B(3): 454–476, 1958.
80. Moscony AMB: Common nerve problems. In Cooper C, editor: *Fundamentals of hand therapy*, St. Louis, 2007, Mosby Elsevier, pp 201–250.
81. Oatis CA: *Kinesiology: the mechanics and pathomechanics of human movement*, Philadelphia, 2004, Lippincott Williams & Wilkins.
82. Oerlemans HM, Oostendorp RAB, deBoo T, et al: Adjunctive physical therapy versus occupational therapy in patients with reflex sympathetic dystrophy/complex regional pain syndrome type I, *Arch Phys Med Rehabil* 81:49–56, 2000.
83. Omer GE Jr: Tendon transfers for traumatic nerve injuries, *J Am Soc Surg Hand* 4(3):214–226, 2004.
84. O'Riain S: New and simple test of nerve function in the hand, *Br Med J* 3:615–616, 1973.
85. Rempel DM: Work-related cumulative trauma disorders of the upper extremity, *JAMA* 267(6):838–842, 1992.
86. Schier JS, Chan J: Changes in life roles after hand injury, *J Hand Ther* 20(1):57–68, 2007.
87. Shacklock M: *Clinical neurodynamics: a new system of musculoskeletal treatment*, Sydney, 2005, Butterworth Heinemann.
88. Smith K: Nerve response to injury and repair. In Skirven TM, Osterman AL, Fedorczyk J, et al, editors: *Rehabilitation of the hand and upper extremity*, ed 6, vol I, Philadelphia, 2011, Elsevier.
89. Sorock GS, Lombardi DS, Hauser RB, et al: Acute traumatic occupational hand injuries: Type, location, and severity, *J Occup Environ Med* 44:4, 2002. 345–3351.
90. Sorock GS, Lombardi DS, Courtney TK, et al: Epidemiology of occupational acute traumatic hand injuries: a literature review, *Safety Sci* 38:241–256, 2001.
91. Staino MJ: Common elbow diagnoses. In Cooper C, editor: *Fundamentals of hand therapy*, St. Louis, 2007, Mosby Elsevier, pp 183–200.
92. Stanton DB, Lazaro R, MacDermid JC: A systematic review of the effectiveness of contrast baths, *J Hand Ther* 22(1):57–69, 2009.
93. Stanton-Hicks M, Janig W, Hassenbusch S, et al: Reflex sympathetic dystrophy: changing concepts and taxonomy, *Pain* 63: 127–133, 1995.
94. Stewart Pettengill KM, vanStrein G: Postoperative management of flexor tendon injuries. In Skirven TM, Osterman AL, et al, editors: *Rehabilitation of the hand and upper extremity*, ed 6, vol I, Philadelphia, 2011, Elsevier.
95. Stralka SW: Reflex sympathetic dystrophy. In Brotzman SB, editor: *Clinical orthopaedic rehabilitation*, St. Louis, 1996, Mosby.
96. Taleisnik J: *The wrist*, New York, 1985, Churchill Livingstone.
97. Thomas D, Moutet F, Guinard D: Postoperative management of extensor tendon repairs in zones V, VI, VII, *J Hand Ther* 9(4):309–314, 1996.
98. Tiffin J: *Purdue pegboard examiner manual*, Chicago, 1968, Science Research Associates.
99. Trumble TE, Vedder NB, Seiler JG, et al: Zone II flexor tendon repair: a randomized prospective trial of active place-and-hold therapy compared with passive motion therapy, *Am J Bone Joint Surg* 92:1381–1389, 2010.
100. Villeco JP, Mackin E, Hunter J, et al: Edema: therapist's management. In Mackin EJ, Callahan AD, Osterman AL, editors: *Rehabilitation of the hand and upper extremity*, ed 5, vol I, St. Louis, 2002, Mosby.
101. Von Der Heyde R: Assessment of functional outcomes. In Cooper C, editor: *Fundamentals of hand therapy*, St. Louis, 2007, Mosby Elsevier, pp 98–111.
102. Walsh MT: Therapist's management of complex regional pain syndrome. In T. Skirven TM, Osterman AL, et al, editors: *Rehabilitation of the hand and upper extremity*, ed 6, vol 2, Philadelphia, 2011, Elsevier.
103. Ware JJ, Sherbourne CD, The MOS: 36-item short-form health survey (SF-36), part I: conceptual framework and item selection, *Med Care* 30:473–483, 1992.
104. Watson HK, Carlson L: Treatment of reflex sympathetic dystrophy of the hand with an active "stress loading" program, *J Hand Surg* 12(5):779–785, 1987.
105. Waylett-Rendall J: Sensibility evaluation and rehabilitation, *In Orthopedic Clin North Am* vol 19(1):43–56, 1988.
106. Wayletl-Rendell J, Seibly D: A study of the accuracy of a commercially available volumeter, *J Hand Ther* 4(1):10–13, 1991.
107. Wehbé MA: Tendon gliding exercises, *Am J Occup Ther* 41(3):164–167, 1987.
108. Wehbé MA, Hunter JM: Flexor tendon gliding in the hand, part II: differential gliding, *J Hand Surg* 10(4):575–579, 1985.
109. Yerxa EJ, Barber LM, Diaz O, et al: Development of hand sensitivity test for the hypersensitive hand, *Am J Occup Ther* 37(3):176–181, 1983.
110. Zohn DA: *Musculoskeletal pain*, Boston, 1988, Little Brown & Company.

CHAPTER 31

Hip Fractures and Lower Extremity Joint Replacement

SONIA LAWSON AND LYNNE MURPHY

Key Terms

Open reduction and internal fixation (ORIF)
Weight-bearing restrictions
Osteoarthritis
Degenerative joint disease
Avascular necrosis
Arthroplasty
Hip precautions
Knee immobilizer
Leg lifter
Commode chairs
Abduction wedges
Minimally invasive technique

Chapter Objectives

After studying this chapter, the student or practitioner will be able to do the following:

1. Outline the etiology of hip fractures and lower extremity joint replacements and how these conditions limit participation in daily activities and meaningful occupations.
2. Outline the medical management and precautions for these conditions.
3. Describe occupational therapy interventions that address all areas of occupation affected by lower extremity joint replacement or hip fracture.
4. Analyze and apply appropriate adaptive equipment and environmental modifications for these conditions.
5. Distinguish areas of intervention for the occupational therapist and the occupational therapy assistant.

CASE STUDY

Ms. Johnson, Part 1

Ms. Johnson is a 50-year-old single parent of a 12-year-old daughter. Ms. Johnson was a strong long-distance runner when she was in high school until a knee injury curtailed her running. Currently, she runs only occasionally due to involvement with church activities and her daughter's Girl Scout troop. Over the years, she progressively gained weight, aggravating the pain not just in the injured knee but the other as well. She works as an administrative assistant and recently participated in a weight loss program, losing 50 of the 100 lb she expected to lose. She was diagnosed with degenerative joint disease in both knees.

Because of increased knee pain, she has limited her participation in many activities with her daughter and in her church. She is most upset at not being able to ride a bike or do more active kinds of things with her daughter. She wants to set a good example for health and exercise but is limited by her bilateral knee pain. Ms. Johnson states, "Getting in and out of the car is excruciating!" She uses a cane for walking and feels "really old." She decided to go ahead with bilateral total knee replacement (surgeries spaced 1 week) apart. Her goals are to relieve pain and become more active, to be able to enjoy being a mom and church member, and to improve her self-esteem through exercise and weight loss.

The incidence of hip fractures and lower extremity (LE) joint replacements has increased in the past decade for several reasons: the elderly population is at risk for falls[17] and likely to sustain fractures due to aging joints; active middle-aged adults place increased amounts of stress on joints through participation in sporting or other strenuous activities; and medical advances in the management of orthopedic conditions have made joint replacement widely available.

Replacement is considered a reasonable option when a large weight-bearing joint (i.e., hip or knee) has become unstable or painful, thus limiting an individual's participation in meaningful daily occupations.

The elderly population is at greatest risk for hip fractures because of diminished abilities due to the aging process and the prevalence of osteoporosis. Osteoporosis is reduced bone density that causes bones to be more brittle and susceptible to fracture. Elderly women are more likely to develop osteoporosis than men and thus are more likely to fracture a hip when they fall.[6,17]

Adults with a history of arthritis or other joint disease are primary candidates for LE joint replacement. These individuals have lived with increasing pain in their joints for many years and have become limited in performance of daily activities and occupations. They hope that having the painful joint(s) replaced will enable them to return to a more active and satisfying lifestyle.

The occupational therapist and occupational therapy assistant (OTA) play key roles in assessing and remediating functional problems and returning the patient to optimal performance of safe, independent, and meaningful occupations.

This chapter discusses the medical management of hip fractures and LE joint replacements, the psychological implications of hospitalization and disability, the role of occupational therapy (OT) for individuals with these conditions, types of OT interventions, and the health care team approach in acute hospital and rehabilitation settings.

Hip Fractures

The OTA who works with orthopedic patients must understand the site, type, and cause of the fracture before starting treatment. A basic understanding of fracture healing and medical management is also necessary to appreciate risks, precautions, and complications involved, as well as to effectively communicate the related therapeutic techniques to the patients. The OTA is advised to consult an orthopedic manual for specific information with respect to the fracture healing process. A good blood supply is necessary for proper healing. The fracture site is protected during the healing process by pins, plates, and wires. In some cases in which extra protection is necessary, a brace may be used to stabilize the hip. The brace extends around the pelvis and down the thigh of the fractured hip, often with an adjustable hinge at the level of the hip joint. Other types of casts or immobilization devices may be used for fractures at other parts of the LE. Several months may be required for a bone fracture to heal completely. The time required varies with the age and health of the patient, site and configuration of the fracture, initial displacement of the bone, and blood supply to the fragments.[5]

Etiology

Trauma is the major etiology or cause of fractures. In most cases the trauma occurs from falling. Poor lighting, throw rugs, and unmarked steps can increase the risk for a fall. Fracture is more likely when the person has osteoporosis, a condition of decreasing bone density. Osteoporosis involves mostly the vertebral bodies and the neck of the femur, humerus, and distal end of the radius. Because the bone becomes porous and therefore fragile, the affected bones are prone to fracture. A pathological fracture, where there has been no obvious trauma, can occur in a bone weakened by tumor or disease such as osteomyelitis and cancers that have metastasized to the bone.[4]

Medical Management

Fracture interventions aim to relieve pain, maintain optimal positioning of the fracture site, facilitate fracture healing, and restore optimal function to the patient.[4] Reduction of a fracture refers to restoring the fragments to normal alignment.[4] This restoration can be achieved by a closed reduction (manipulation) or by an open procedure (surgery). A closed reduction is performed by the physician applying a force to the displaced bone opposite to the force that produced the fracture. Depending on the nature of the fracture, the reduction is maintained in a cast, brace, traction, or skeletal fixation.

With open reduction, the fracture site is exposed surgically so that the fragments can be aligned. The fragments are held in place with internal fixation consisting of pins, screws, a plate, nails, or a rod. Further immobilization by a cast or a brace may be necessary. Usually an open reduction and internal fixation (ORIF) must be protected from excessive forces after surgery; therefore weight bearing is usually restricted.[4]

Several levels of weight-bearing restrictions exist. The physician will indicate the level and will reduce restrictions as the fracture site heals and becomes stronger. The levels of weight-bearing restrictions are listed in Box 31-1.[7]

Box 31-1

Weight-Bearing Restrictions

NWB (non–weight bearing) indicates that no weight at all can be placed on the extremity involved.

TTWB (toe-touch weight bearing) indicates that only the toe can be placed on the ground to provide some balance while standing—90% of the weight is still on the unaffected leg. In toe touch weight bearing, the patient is instructed to imagine that an egg is under his or her foot.

PWB (partial weight bearing) indicates that only 50% of the person's body weight can be placed on the affected leg.

WBAT (weight bearing at tolerance) indicates that patients are allowed to judge how much weight they can put on the affected leg without causing too much pain.

FWB (full weight bearing) indicates that patients should be able to put 100% of their weight on the affected leg without causing damage to the fracture site.

Hip Fractures: Types of Hip Fractures and Medical Management

Knowledge of hip anatomy helps the OTA understand the medical management of hip fractures. An anatomy and physiology reference should be consulted for details. Figure 31-1 illustrates the normal hip joint.

The typical levels of fracture lines are shown in Figure 31-2. The names of the fractures generally reflect the site and severity of injury and may suggest the appropriate medical intervention. For example, a femoral neck fracture will be treated with femoral neck stabilization.[9]

Femoral Neck Fractures

Femoral neck fractures (subcapital, transcervical, and basilar fractures) are common in adults older than 60 years of age and are more common among women. Even slight trauma or rotational force causes fracture in osteoporotic bone.[6]

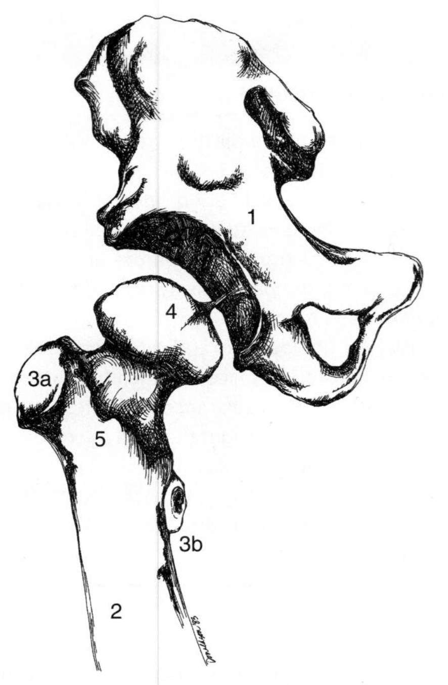

Figure 31-1 Normal hip anatomy. *1,* Acetabulum; *2,* femur; *3a,* greater trochanter; *3b,* lesser trochanter; *4,* ligamentum teres; *5,* intertrochanteric crest. (Modified from Crouch JE: *Functional human anatomy,* ed 3, Philadelphia, 1978, Lea & Febiger and Grant LC: *Grant's atlas of anatomy,* ed 6, Baltimore, 1972, Williams & Wilkins.)

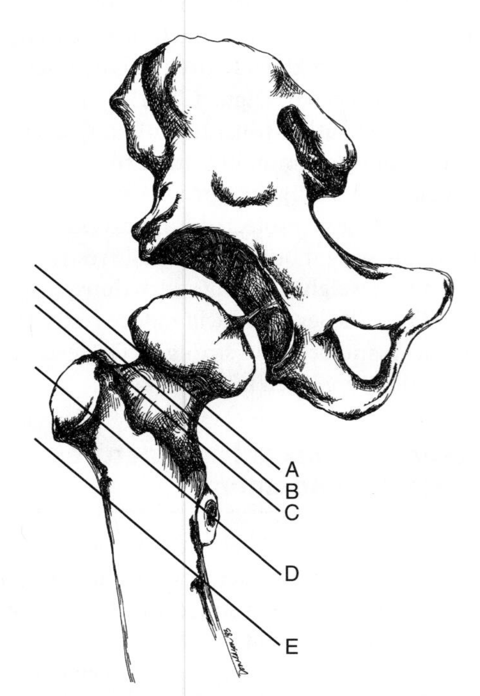

Figure 31-2 Levels of femoral fracture. *A,* Subcapital; *B,* transcervical; *C,* basilar; *D,* intertrochanteric; *E,* subtrochanteric. (Modified from Crow I: Fracture of the hip: a self study, *ONA J* 5:12, 1978.)

The age and health of the patient affect the surgeon's choice of surgical procedure. Generally, hip pinning or application of a compression screw and plate is used when displacement is minimal to moderate and blood supply is intact. With physician approval, the patient usually can begin out-of-bed activities 1 to 3 days after surgery. Per physician orders, weight-bearing restrictions may need to be observed with the aid of a walker or crutches for at least 6 to 8 weeks while the fracture heals. Weight-bearing restrictions may extend beyond this time if precautions are not observed or if a delayed union occurs.[13]

Box 31-2

Hip Precautions

Posterior Approaches

- No hip flexion greater than 90 degrees
- No internal rotation
- No adduction (crossing legs or feet)

Anterior Approaches

- No external rotation
- No adduction (crossing legs or feet)
- No extension

With severe displacement or poor blood supply (avascular condition), the femoral head and acetabulum are surgically removed and replaced by an endoprosthesis. This process is called *bipolar arthroplasty*[9,13] and may also be referred to as a *total hip replacement* (THR). If only the femoral neck and head are replaced, the surgical procedure is called a hemiarthroplasty. Several types of metal prostheses can be used; each has its own shape and advantages. Weight-bearing restrictions are sometimes indicated. Precautions for positioning the hip must be observed to avoid dislocation following the surgical procedure. The precautions will vary according to the surgical approach but are the same as for total hip replacement, which is discussed later in this chapter (Box 31-2). Patients who have had a prosthesis implanted can usually begin out-of-bed activity, with physician approval, about 1 to 3 days after surgery.[9,13] Ambulatory devices or aids may also be indicated to ensure patient safety during functional mobility and are determined with other members of the rehabilitation team.

Intertrochanteric Fractures

Intertrochanteric fractures between the greater and lesser trochanter are extracapsular (or outside the articular capsule of the hip joint), and the blood supply is not affected. Like femoral neck fractures, intertrochanteric fractures occur most commonly in older women. The fracture typically results from direct trauma or force over the greater trochanter, as can occur in a fall. ORIF is the preferred medical intervention. A nail or compression screw with a side plate is used. Weight-bearing restrictions must be observed, sometimes for as long as 4 to 6 months, when a patient is ambulating. Again, the patient is allowed out of bed 1 to 3 days after surgery, pending physician approval,[11] with an appropriate ambulatory device.

Subtrochanteric Fractures

Subtrochanteric fractures (1 to 2 inches below the lesser trochanter) usually occur because of direct trauma, which may result from falls, motor vehicle accidents, or any direct blow to the hip area. These fractures occur most often in persons younger than 60 years of age. Skeletal traction and an ORIF is the usual surgical intervention. A nail with a long side plate or an intramedullary rod is used. The rod is inserted through the central shaft of the bone to help maintain proper alignment for bone healing.[4] In all types of hip fractures, the OTA should be aware of the coexisting conditions of soft tissue trauma, edema, and bruising that occur around the fracture site.[4,9,13] These conditions can greatly affect the amount of pain and discomfort a patient may experience.

Lower Extremity Joint Replacement

Etiology

Restoration of joint motion and management of pain by arthroplasty (insertion of a prosthesis), or total hip or knee replacement, is sometimes indicated for persons with osteoarthritis, rheumatoid arthritis, or other conditions such as dysplasia (congenital malformation of joints). Osteoarthritis or degenerative joint disease (DJD) may develop in middle age and progress with the normal aging process. It also may result from trauma, congenital deformity, or disease that damages articular cartilage. Weight-bearing joints such as the hip, knee, and lumbar spine are usually affected. In the hip, cartilage is lost centrally on the joint surface, and osteophytes (bone spurs) form on the periphery of the acetabulum. Pain arises from the bone, synovial membrane, and fibrous capsule, and from muscle spasm. When hip movement causes pain, movement becomes restricted and muscles shorten from disuse. The osteoarthritic hip may assume a flexed, adducted, and internally rotated position that also causes a painful limp.[11] In the knee, cartilage is also lost on the joint surfaces. This condition also causes pain and limping during ambulation and difficulty bending the knee for daily activities. Other disease processes (such as lupus and cancer) and some medications (e.g., corticosteroids such as prednisone) can compromise the blood flow to the hip joint and lead to avascular necrosis (AVN), a condition in which bone cells die because of poor blood supply, or to osteoporosis; both conditions may lead to hip pain.[11]

Total Hip Replacement: Medical Management

Total joint replacement or arthroplasty is designed to alleviate pain and restore joint motion. There are two components to a total hip replacement or bipolar arthroplasty. A high-density polyethylene socket is fitted into the acetabulum, and a metallic prosthesis replaces the femoral head and neck (Figure 31-3). Methylmethacrylate or acrylic cement fixes the components to the bone. Various surgical approaches are used according to the surgical skill or technique of the orthopedist, severity of the joint involvement, and history of past surgery to the hip. With an anterior or anterolateral approach, the patient will be unstable in external rotation, adduction, and extension of the operated hip and usually must observe precautions to prevent these movements for 6 to 12 weeks. With a posterior or posterolateral approach, the patient must be cautioned not to move the operated hip in specific ranges of flexion (usually 60 to 90 degrees) and not to internally rotate or adduct the leg. Failure to maintain hip precautions during muscle and soft tissue healing may result in hip dislocation (see Box 31-2).

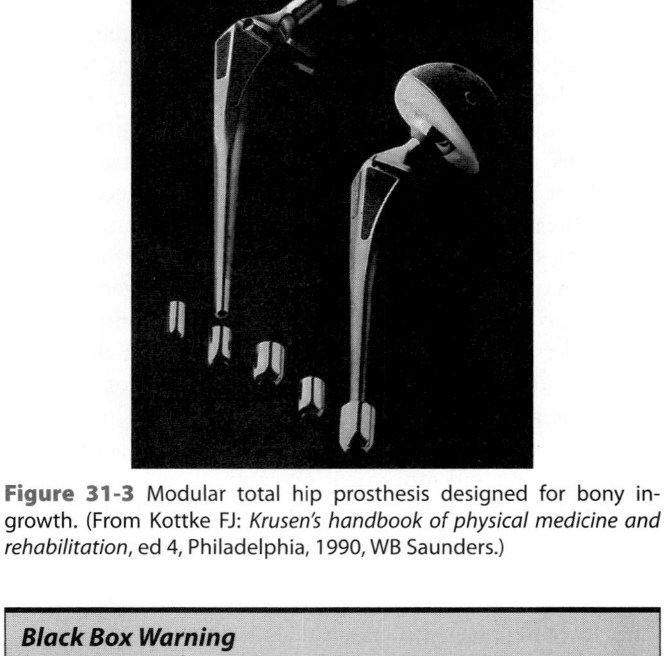

Figure 31-3 Modular total hip prosthesis designed for bony ingrowth. (From Kottke FJ: *Krusen's handbook of physical medicine and rehabilitation*, ed 4, Philadelphia, 1990, WB Saunders.)

> ***Black Box Warning***
>
> Patients may have difficulty understanding and following hip precautions. It is best to use lay language and real life examples of how hip precautions can be broken during everyday tasks. Rather than say, "Don't bend at the waist past 90 degrees," it is better to say, "Don't bend over to pick up the newspaper" or "Don't lift your foot to put on your socks." Rather than say, "Don't internally rotate the hip," say "Don't turn around to reach for items behind you while you are standing." In other words, replace the medical language with real-life examples pertinent to the patient.

Orthopedic surgeons now use a minimally invasive technique whenever possible to perform the anterior, anterolateral, and posterolateral approaches, thus reducing trauma to the tissues and allowing for faster recovery. The older traditional surgical technique requires that a long incision be made (about 10 inches) and muscles detached to get to the hip joint. In the minimally invasive technique, two incisions of approximately 2 inches each are necessary, and no detachment of muscles is required. Because no muscles are detached, the hip is more likely to remain in a stable position while healing. This technique is not appropriate for all people undergoing total hip arthroplasties. Persons with severe damage to the hip joint will require the traditional surgical method. The minimally invasive technique is more appropriate for persons without complicating medical conditions and who present with easier access for physicians to the hip joint. Hip precautions that are identified for the anterior, anterolateral, and posterolateral approaches are indicated for persons receiving the minimally invasive technique.[12,15]

Hip resurfacing, which is used less often than other procedures, is a variation of the total hip replacement.[11,18] The surface of the head of the femur is capped by a metallic shell, and the acetabular cavity receives a plastic or metal cup. Both are held in place by methylmethacrylate. This technique preserves the femoral head and neck. This technique has no weight-bearing or movement restrictions and is used primarily for younger, more active patients.[11]

The majority of patients with total hip replacements are permitted to place as much weight on the leg as tolerated (weight bearing at tolerance [WBAT]); however, the OTA must always check physician orders to ensure the patient maintains the prescribed weight-bearing restriction. An ambulatory aid, usually a walker or crutches, is necessary for at least the first month while the hip is healing and muscles are becoming stronger. Patients with total hip replacements usually begin out-of-bed activity 1 to 3 days after surgery.[9]

Therapy practitioners must recognize complications and understand special surgical procedures, and they must inquire about additional precautions and risks. For example, infections around the implanted prosthesis can occur and may result in the removal of the prosthesis. In this case, new weight-bearing and movement precautions will be imposed. Another special procedure involves using an abduction brace to immobilize the hip joint for individuals who are at high risk for a dislocation.[4]

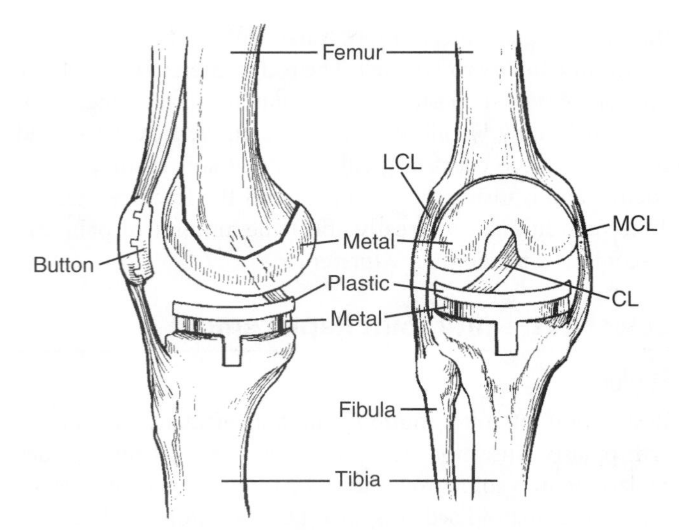

Figure 31-4 Total knee replacement prosthesis. The metal aspects of the prosthesis cover the distal portion of the femur and the end of the tibia. There is a polyethylene plastic-bearing surface *(plastic)* between the metallic aspects of the two surfaces. The patella is replaced by a polyethylene button. The medial collateral ligament *(MCL),* lateral collateral ligament *(LCL),* and cruciate ligaments *(CL)* are retained. (Modified from Calliet R: *Knee pain and disability,* ed 3, Philadelphia, 1992, FA Davis.)

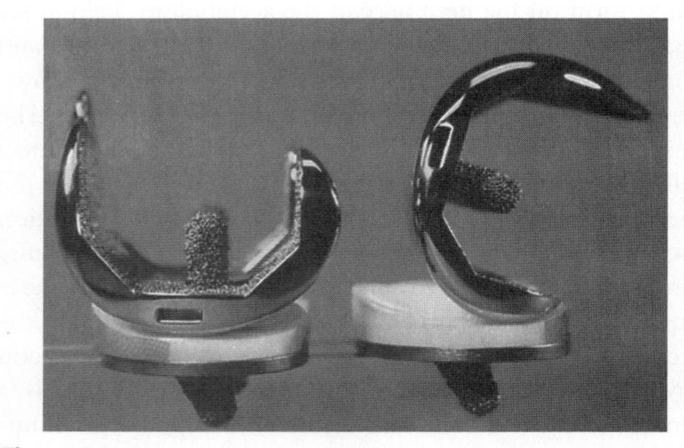

Figure 31-5 Porous-coated total knee prosthesis. Note resurfacing features of components and beaded surfaces for biologic fixation. (From Kottke FJ: *Krusen's handbook of physical medicine and rehabilitation,* ed 4, Philadelphia, 1990, WB Saunders.)

Total Knee Replacement: Medical Management

Total knee replacement or arthroplasty (TKA) is designed to alleviate pain, restore motion, and maintain alignment and stability of the knee joint. The process involves cutting away the damaged bone (as little bone as possible) and attaching a prosthesis for the new joint. The type of prosthesis used depends on the severity of joint damage (Figures 31-4 and 31-5). The prosthesis may be cemented to the bone. In a cemented prosthesis, patients usually can bear weight as tolerated on the operated leg. In a noncemented prosthesis, the patient is initially placed on weight-bearing precautions. Patients may start out-of-bed activities 1 to 3 days after surgery, pending the physician's approval.[3,8,9,13,14] Patients may use a knee immobilizer (Figure 31-6) to provide support to the knee when moving in and out of the bed and ambulating. The patient should avoid any rotation at the knee up to 12 weeks after surgery.[3,9,13] Postsurgical knee pain should be addressed by the entire treatment team. During occupational therapy, the occupational therapist or OTA may assist the patient in managing pain by positioning the knee in positions of comfort, using superficial cold modalities, and providing support to the lower extremity during transfers and movement transitions.[2]

As with hip replacement, a minimally invasive technique has been developed for knee replacements. Proponents of this technique report that patients can achieve greater knee flexion (up to 90 degrees) a couple of days after surgery. In addition, because fewer ligaments are cut, increased lateral and medial stability is obtained immediately, thus eliminating the need for a knee immobilizer.[5,19] The OTA needs to be aware of the surgical technique to know whether to reinforce the use of a knee immobilizer and to encourage an appropriate amount of knee flexion.

Emphasis in rehabilitation is on maintaining or regaining joint motion, slowly increasing the strength of surrounding musculature, decreasing swelling, and increasing independence in activities of daily living (ADL) and instrumental ADL (IADL). The role of occupational therapy in this process is primarily to educate the knee replacement patient in adaptive techniques for ADL and IADL.

Individuals with joint changes that result in increasing pain may have multiple joint involvement (i.e., both knees or hips). Some individuals opt to have both joints replaced during the same hospitalization, either at the same time or up to 1 week apart. Replacing both joints can complicate the rehabilitation process because the patient will not have a stronger leg to rely on for ambulation and performing daily activities.[10]

In Ms. Johnson's case, a traditional surgical technique rather than a minimally invasive technique was used because

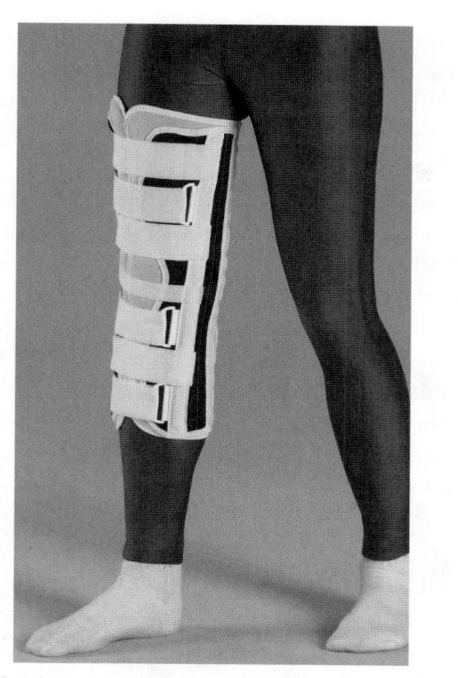

Figure 31-6 A knee immobilizer is used to support and stabilize the knee joint during mobility. (Courtesy DeRoyal, Powell, Tenn.)

of her weight and the extent of joint degeneration in her knees. She had the knee replacements 1 week apart and was placed on WBAT precautions after each knee surgery.

Psychological Factors

Psychological issues affect the overall intervention and prognosis for the orthopedic patient. A large number of such patients are faced with a chronic disability (e.g., rheumatoid arthritis), a life-threatening disease (e.g., cancer), chronic or postsurgical pain, or the aging process. Loss or potential loss of mobility and physical ability that limits participation in necessary and pleasurable activities is a major concern. Adjusting to loss is stressful and requires an enormous amount of physical and emotional energy.[6,16] Awareness of these issues and sensitivity toward the orthopedic patient are critical to the delivery of optimal patient care.

The OT practitioner must realize that each patient's experience of loss varies based on person factors (e.g., personality, physical diseases, specific changes, body image); contextual factors (e.g., family dynamics, home environment); and the types of occupations in which the patient typically engages.[6]

Patients with a chronic orthopedic disability often experience one or all of the following: a disease of a body part, fear, anxiety, change in body image, decreased functional ability, loss of roles, deformity, and pain. These events may occur at a relatively young age and then progress in rapid succession. When treating a patient with a chronic orthopedic disability, one must address these issues and provide the support needed for the mourning and grieving process. Without an opportunity to confront these issues, the patient may become depressed, filled with guilt and anxiety, and paralyzed with fear. These emotions inhibit progress and further damage self-image. Practitioners can help patients acknowledge and experience some of these feelings and ultimately enhance the rehabilitation process.

CLINICAL PEARL

It is always good to encourage patients to put on their own clothes if they are past the stage of their recovery where bandages need changing often. This helps them feel "more like themselves" and a change in affect is immediately evident!

An important issue experienced by the elderly disabled individual is the change to a more dependent status. With the onset of a disability late in life, the patient may be forced to let go of years of independence and self-sufficiency.[6] For some, this can be a devastating experience that requires prolonged grieving before adjustment. Others may use dependency for secondary gain, remaining in the hospital for extra attention or manipulating their support systems to avoid taking responsibility for themselves and others.

Another psychological phenomenon experienced by the hospitalized older adult is relocation trauma. Older people, when removed from their familiar environment, may decompensate cognitively and may experience confusion, emotional lability, and disorientation. Therefore it is important that any new environment be made as familiar as possible. Decorating it with familiar objects from their home and providing a calendar and current newspapers and magazines are often helpful in reducing this traumatic effect.

Learning to cope and adjust to the changes resulting from chronic disability or the aging process is a critical aspect of recovery. Practitioners must realize that a great deal of a patient's functional independence has been relinquished to the disease or disability. The psychological issues resulting from this loss must be addressed while focusing on increasing the patient's functional level of independence.[6,16]

An important area of ADL that is often overlooked is sexual activity. Persons with a hip fracture or LE joint replacement will have difficulty performing sexual activities in their usual manner. (See Chapter 16 for a further discussion of sexuality.) It is recommended that persons not engage in sexual activity for 6 weeks after surgery so that they maintain the movement precautions applicable to their condition.[9] Patients of all ages and both genders may have questions regarding the level of permissible sexual activity. The occupational therapy practitioner will need to create an environment in which the patient feels he or she has permission to ask personal questions. The therapist and assistant can do this by being open-minded and realizing that sexual activity is an important and meaningful occupation. The therapist and assistant can suggest ways for the patient to position the operated leg during sexual activity to maintain precautions. Side-lying on the nonoperated side is one option. Abduction precautions can be maintained via pillows between the knees. To prevent excessive external rotation at the hips while in the supine position, the patient can place pillows under the knees. Patients with knee replacements or weight-bearing precautions should avoid kneeling.[9] Written information with diagrams can be helpful when addressing such a personal issue. The patient can read it privately or with his or her partner at another time.

Rehabilitation Measures

Good communication and clear role delineation among members of the health care team are essential for an efficient and smooth therapy program. The health care team usually consists of a primary physician, nursing staff, an occupational therapist or OTA, a physical therapist or physical therapy assistant, a nutritionist or dietician, a pharmacist, and a case coordinator. Regular team meetings to discuss each patient's ongoing progress and discharge plans are necessary to coordinate interventions. Members from each service usually participate in the team meetings to provide information and consultation.

The role of the physician is to inform the team of the patient's medical status, medical history, diagnosis of the present problem, and a complete account of the surgical procedure performed. This report would include the type of appliance inserted, the anatomic approach, and any movement or weight-bearing precautions that are necessary to ensure patient safety. The physician is also responsible for ordering specific medications and therapies. The physician should approve any change or progression in therapy or changes in the patient's medication regimen.

The nursing staff is responsible for the actual physical care of the patient during hospitalization. Responsibilities of the nurse include administering medications, assisting the patient with bathing and hygiene, and monitoring vital signs and physical status. The orthopedic nurse must understand thoroughly the surgical procedures and movement precautions for each patient. The nurse ensures proper positioning with pillows and wedges, especially in the first few days after surgery. As the therapy program progresses, the patient can start to take more responsibility for proper positioning and physical care. The nursing staff works closely with the occupational therapy practitioners and physical therapy practitioners to carry through self-care and mobility skills that the patient has already learned in therapy.

The physical therapist is responsible for evaluation and intervention in the areas of musculoskeletal status, sensation, pain, skin integrity, and mobility (especially gait). In many cases involving total joint replacements and surgical repair of hip fractures, physical therapy is initiated on the first day after surgery. The physical therapist obtains baseline information including range of motion (ROM), strength of all the extremities, muscle tone, and mobility and adheres to the prescribed precautions. An intervention program that includes therapeutic exercises, ROM activities, transfer training, and progressive gait activities is established. The physical therapist is responsible for recommending the appropriate assistive device for ambulation. As the patient's ambulation status advances, instruction in stair climbing, managing curbs, and outside ambulation is given.[9]

The nutritionist or dietician consults with each patient to ensure that adequate and appropriate nutrition is received to aid the healing process. The pharmacist monitors the patient's drug therapy and provides information and assistance with pain management.

The case coordinator (usually a registered nurse or social worker) ensures that each patient is discharged to the appropriate living situation or facility with the appropriate equipment. With input from the health care team, the case coordinator arranges for ongoing therapy after hospitalization, admission to a rehabilitation facility for further intensive therapy, or nursing home care and assists in obtaining durable medical equipment.

CASE STUDY

Ms. Johnson, Part 2

Ms. Johnson was initially seen by OT when she had her first knee replacement on the right knee. Her first wish was to "go to the bathroom by myself."

The occupational therapist and OTA reviewed the chart, obtained an occupational profile, and assessed body functions and occupational performance. The initial goals for rehabilitation were set by the occupational therapist, keeping in mind that a second surgery was to come. The evaluation revealed that Ms. Johnson had difficulty bending at both the waist and the knees to perform ADL, had limited endurance for physical activity (3 minutes), and felt discouraged about not being the mother she wanted to be for her daughter.

Factors that could support therapy included her ranch-style home with only a few steps to navigate, a sister in the area who could help her if necessary, a daughter who was old enough to manage most of her own self-care activities, and a host of church members to provide support (both physical and spiritual) as needed. Unsupportive factors were her excess weight and the short time available for recovery (she only had 6 weeks of sick/vacation time available). She valued being a mother, a professional, and a church member and enjoyed performing all the routines associated with those roles.

In addition to degenerative joint disease in the knees, Ms. Johnson also experienced some right shoulder pain at times, which limited her participation occasionally. Before the surgery, Ms. Johnson was independent in all areas of occupational performance despite the pain. Ms. Johnson currently needed assistance with mobility, ADL, and IADL because of the knee replacement. She would be even more limited once she had the second knee replaced.

Role of Occupational Therapy

After a total joint replacement or surgical repair of a fractured hip, OT usually begins when the patient is ready to start getting out of bed, about 1 to 3 days after surgery. The actual time varies depending on age, general health, and surgical events or medical complications. Before any physical assessment, the

OT practitioner must review medical information, introduce and explain the role of OT, establish rapport, and complete an occupational profile. The profile includes gathering information about the patient's occupational history, prior functional status in ADL and IADL, performance contexts (e.g., home environment, social support), and personal goals. The goal of OT is for the patient to return home, independently performing daily activities and observing all movement precautions. It is the role of the occupational therapist and assistant to teach the patient ways and means of performing daily occupations safely.[9]

The role of the occupational therapist and OTA can be clearly distinguished in the cases of total joint replacement and hip fractures. The occupational therapist performs any assessments needed for the evaluation including obtaining an occupational profile and assessing body functions and performance skills. A baseline assessment of body functions is necessary to determine whether any physical limitations not related to surgery might prevent functional independence. Upper extremity ROM, muscle strength, sensation, and coordination are assessed before a functional evaluation is made. An assessment of mental functions by the occupational therapist is also necessary because many elderly patients may experience some mental status change after surgery due to relocation trauma, residual effects of anesthesia, and medications. The OTA participates in the assessment of performance skills, ADL, and IADL and can gather data to contribute to the occupational profile. During the evaluation process, the occupational therapist and OTA must observe any signs of pain and fear at rest and/or during movement.

OT intervention involves a program of functional activities that gradually enable a person to regain abilities and skills needed for greater participation in identified areas of occupation. This intervention plan is implemented with consideration of any required movement precautions. The OTA plays a major role in intervention planning and implementation by training patients in the use of assistive devices, proper transfer techniques, and adaptive techniques while maintaining movement precautions during purposeful and occupation-based activities. Both the occupational therapist and the OTA are involved in collaborative intervention planning, documentation, and discharge planning (including recommending equipment and home exercise programs). The patient's personal occupational goals are paramount to this collaborative process.

Total joint replacements for degenerative or chronic conditions are usually preplanned and scheduled for a specific date. The OTA can play a role along with the occupational therapist in providing education classes (e.g., a series on fall prevention, introduction of appropriate use of assistive devices). The OTA can coordinate and facilitate this type of group. Topics can include home modifications (e.g., removing throw rugs, telephone cords, clutter), safe transfer techniques, use of public transportation, and community mobility tips. The person who is having an elective total joint replacement can benefit from a class offered before surgery to explain the procedures and describe the therapy process.

CASE STUDY

Ms. Johnson, Part 3

After discussion with the occupational therapist, the OTA initiated mobility training to help Ms. Johnson reach her first goal of getting to the bathroom independently. This provided an opportunity to introduce bed mobility and dressing. The OTA took safety measures to ensure that the wheels of the bed were locked to prevent any shifting of the bed during the mobility and dressing training. Ms. Johnson put on the knee immobilizer, her robe, and her slippers. With instruction and assistance from the OTA, Ms. Johnson sat up and moved her right leg to the edge of the bed. After ensuring that Ms. Johnson was not dizzy or too fatigued and after applying a safety belt around her waist, the OTA assisted Ms. Johnson to stand and then hold onto the walker to ambulate to the bathroom. Ms. Johnson had already initiated walking short distances with the physical therapist before this OT intervention session. When they reached the bathroom, the OTA carefully assisted Ms. Johnson onto the raised commode seat, reminding Ms. Johnson to avoid rotating her body with her right leg planted on the floor, and ensuring safe transfer procedures.

Guidelines for Training in Adaptive Techniques

Some common assistive devices are useful for many people with hip fractures or joint replacements (Figure 31-7). The OT clinic should have samples of these and should be able to issue them to patients for use during the training process. Helpful assistive devices or adaptive aids include a dressing stick, a sock aid, a long-handled sponge, a long-handled shoe horn, a reacher, elastic shoelaces, an elevated toilet or commode seat, a leg lifter, and a shower chair or bench. These devices optimize safety and assist patients in reaching items when they are limited by movement precautions or decreased flexibility. Walker bags are helpful for people who are using walkers and need to carry small items from one place to another.

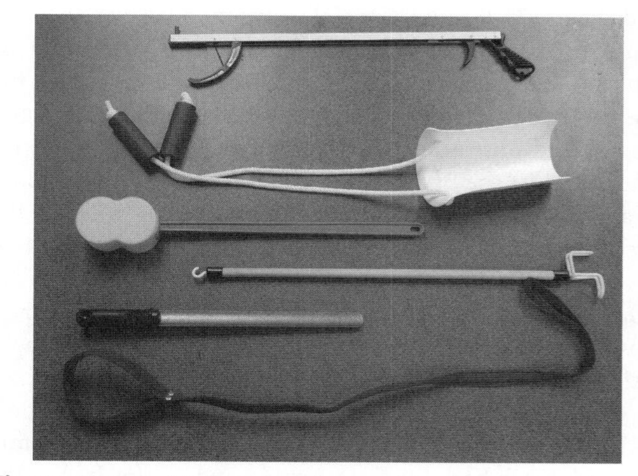

Figure 31-7 Assistive devices for activities, from top to bottom: reacher, sock aid, long-handled sponge, dressing stick, long-handled shoe horn, and leg lifter.

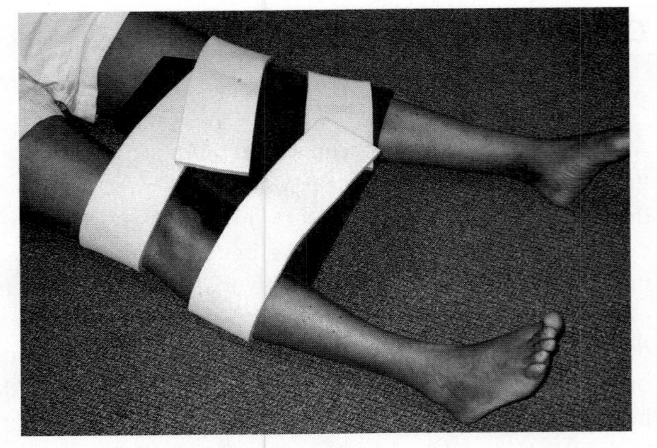

Figure 31-8 Patient is positioned with an abduction wedge to maintain hip precautions.

Hip Joint Replacement Procedures

Procedures for training (outlined as follows) apply to all types of hip joint replacement unless otherwise noted. It is important to remember the positions of hip instability for surgical procedures that generally fall more anterior or more posterior. For the posterior approaches, positions of instability include hip adduction, internal rotation, and flexion greater than precautions. For the anterior approaches, positions of instability include hip adduction, external rotation, and excessive hyperextension.

Bed Mobility

The supine sleeping position with an abduction wedge or pillow in place is recommended (Figure 31-8). If patients sleep on their sides, sleeping on the operated side is recommended if tolerable. When the patient is sleeping on the nonoperated side, the legs must be abducted with the wedge or large pillows and the operated leg must be supported to prevent rotation and adduction. The patient is instructed on getting out of bed on both sides, although initially it may be easier to maintain precautions by moving toward the nonoperated leg. The patient may support the upper body by extending the arms and leaning slightly back, then gradually turning the entire body as a unit toward the side of the bed (Figure 31-9, *A-C*). Careful instruction is given to avoid hip adduction past midline. It is important to determine the type and height of the patient's bed at home and adjust the hospital bed as needed for more realistic practice. When getting in and out of bed, the patient may initially use a leg lifter to assist the operated leg in moving from one surface to another; however, as the leg becomes stronger, use of the leg lifter should be discontinued.

Transfers

It is always helpful for the patient to first observe the proper technique for transfers before attempting the movement.

- *Chair:* A firmly based chair with armrests is recommended. The patient is instructed to extend the operated leg forward, reach back for the armrests, and sit slowly. For the person with a posterior approach, care should be taken to not lean forward when sitting down (Figure 31-10). To stand, the patient extends the knee of the operated leg and pushes off from the armrests and supports the body weight with the nonoperated leg. This procedure should also be followed for a commode transfer (Figure 31-11). Because of the hip flexion precaution for the posterior approach, the patient should sit on the front part of the chair and lean back (see Figure 31-10, *C*). Firm cushions or blankets can be used to increase the height of chairs and may be necessary, especially if the patient is tall. Low, soft, reclining, and rocking chairs should be avoided.[1]
- *Commode chair:* Three-in-one commode chairs with armrests are to be used in the hospital and at home (see Figure 31-11, *A*). For the person with a posterior approach, the height and angle can be adjusted so that the front legs are one notch lower than the back legs; thus with the patient seated, hip flexion will not exceed 90 degrees. A person with an anterior approach may have enough hip mobility to use a standard toilet seat safely at discharge. All patients should complete toileting hygiene by wiping between the legs in a sitting position or from behind in a standing position with caution to avoid rotation of the hip. The patient is to stand up and step to turn to face the toilet and flush rather than rotate the trunk and hip.[1]
- *Shower stall:* Generally, patients are advised to have another person in the home when they attempt to shower in case assistance is needed. Nonskid strips or stickers are recommended in all shower stalls and tubs. When the patient enters, the walker or crutches go first. The operated leg is next and is followed by the nonoperated leg. A shower chair with adjustable legs or a stool and grab bars should be installed if balance is a problem or if weight-bearing precautions are necessary.
- *Tub shower (without shower doors):* Sitting in the bottom of the tub for a bath is prohibited until the joint is fully healed. To preserve hip precautions, it is recommended that a tub bench be considered to facilitate a safe transfer. The patient sits on the edge of the bench as if sitting in a chair and then carefully swings the legs over the tub while observing flexion precautions, using a leg lifter if necessary. Sponge bathing at the sink is an alternative activity.[1]
- *Car:* Bucket seats in small cars should be avoided. Bench-type seats are recommended. The patient is instructed to back up to the passenger seat, hold onto a stable part of the car, place the operated leg forward of the nonoperated leg, and slowly sit in the car. Remembering to lean back, the patient then slides the buttocks toward the driver's seat. The upper body and LEs then carefully move as one unit to turn to face the forward direction. It is helpful to have the seat pushed back and reclined to accommodate the hip flexion precaution. Pillows in the seat may be necessary to increase the height of the seat. Prolonged sitting in the car should be avoided.

Lower Body Dressing

The patient is instructed to sit in a chair with arms or on the edge of the bed for dressing activities. The patient is instructed

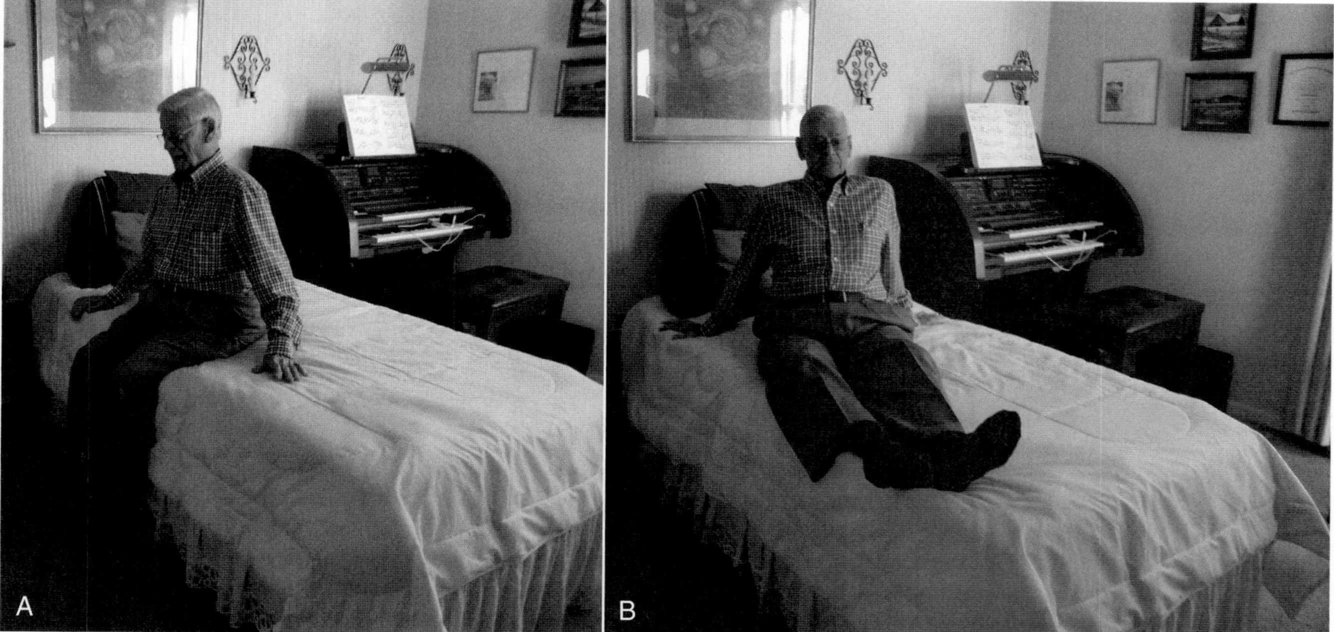

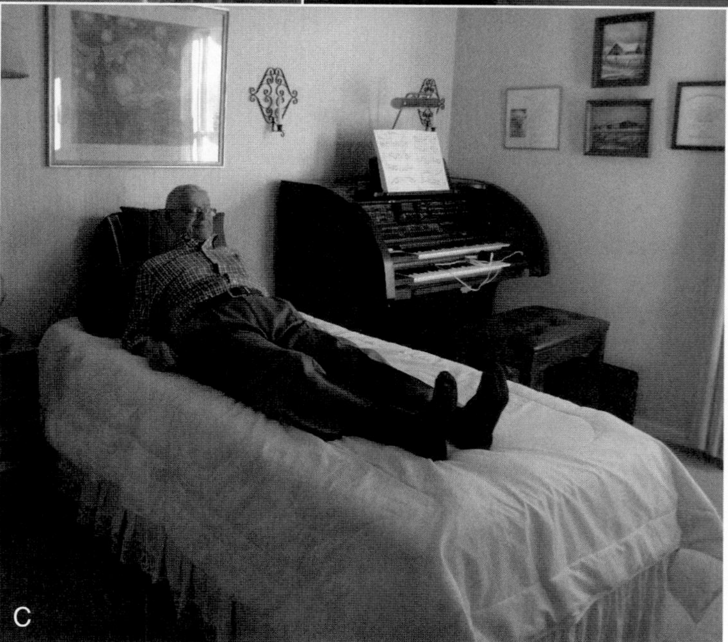

Figure 31-9 These three pictures show the technique for getting into a bed following a total hip replacement. **A,** Patient is directed to sit on the edge of the bed within total hip replacement precautions. **B,** To lift the lower extremities onto the bed within the hip precautions, patient is instructed to lean back onto the upper extremities. **C,** Ending position of sit to supine mobility.

to avoid hip adduction and rotation or crossing the legs to dress. Crossing the operated extremity over the nonoperated extremity at either the ankles or knees is to be avoided. Leaning the trunk forward or flexing the hips more than 90 degrees should also be avoided. Assistive devices may be necessary to observe precautions (see Figure 31-7). To follow hip precautions, the patient uses a reacher or dressing stick for donning and removing pants and shoes. When donning pants, the operated leg is dressed first by using the reacher or dressing stick to bring the pants over the foot and up to the knee. A sock aid is used to don socks or knee-high nylons, and a reacher or dressing stick is used to remove them. A reacher, elastic shoelaces, and a long-handled shoe horn can also be provided to limit hip flexion motion.[1] Clothes should be chosen that are loose fitting enough to allow ease of dressing. Slip-on shoes with soles that provide appropriate traction should also be used to prevent falls.

CLINICAL PEARL

The OTA is advised to practice LE dressing techniques in order to demonstrate the procedures properly before any interventions. Often, the patient must be shown how easy it is to use the devices. Otherwise, he or she may not be willing to try.

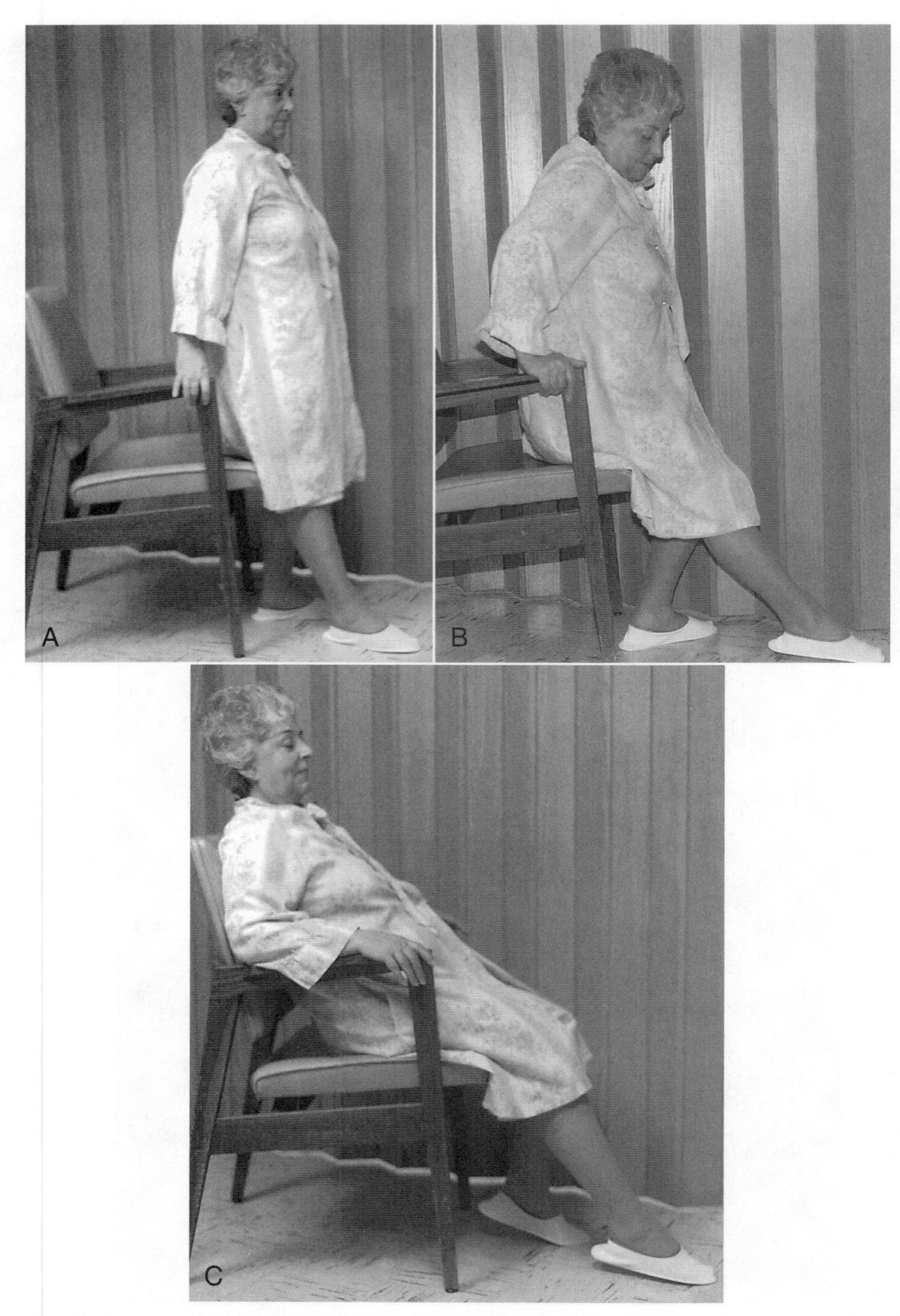

Figure 31-10 Chair transfer technique. **A,** Patient extends operated leg and reaches for arm rests. **B** and **C,** Bearing some weight on arms, patient sits down slowly while maintaining some extension of operated leg.

Lower Body Bathing

Refer to transfer section for method to get in/out of shower or tub. Sponge bathing at the sink is indicated until the physician permits the patient to shower. Patients are instructed to sit to wash their legs. A long-handled bath sponge or back brush is used to reach the lower legs and feet safely; "soap on a rope" is used to prevent the soap from dropping; and a towel is wrapped on a reacher to dry the lower legs.[1]

Hair Shampoo

Until patients can shower, they are instructed to obtain assistance for shampooing their hair. If the patient has no assistance, he or she may shampoo hair while standing or sitting on a stool at the kitchen or bathroom sink, observing hip precautions at all times.

Homemaking

Heavy housework such as vacuuming, lifting, and bed making should be avoided until the joint is fully healed. Commonly used items for kitchen activities should be kept at countertop level. Items can be moved by using an apron with large pockets, sliding items along the countertop, using a utility cart, attaching a small basket or bag to a walker, or wearing a pouch ("fanny pack") around the waist. Reachers

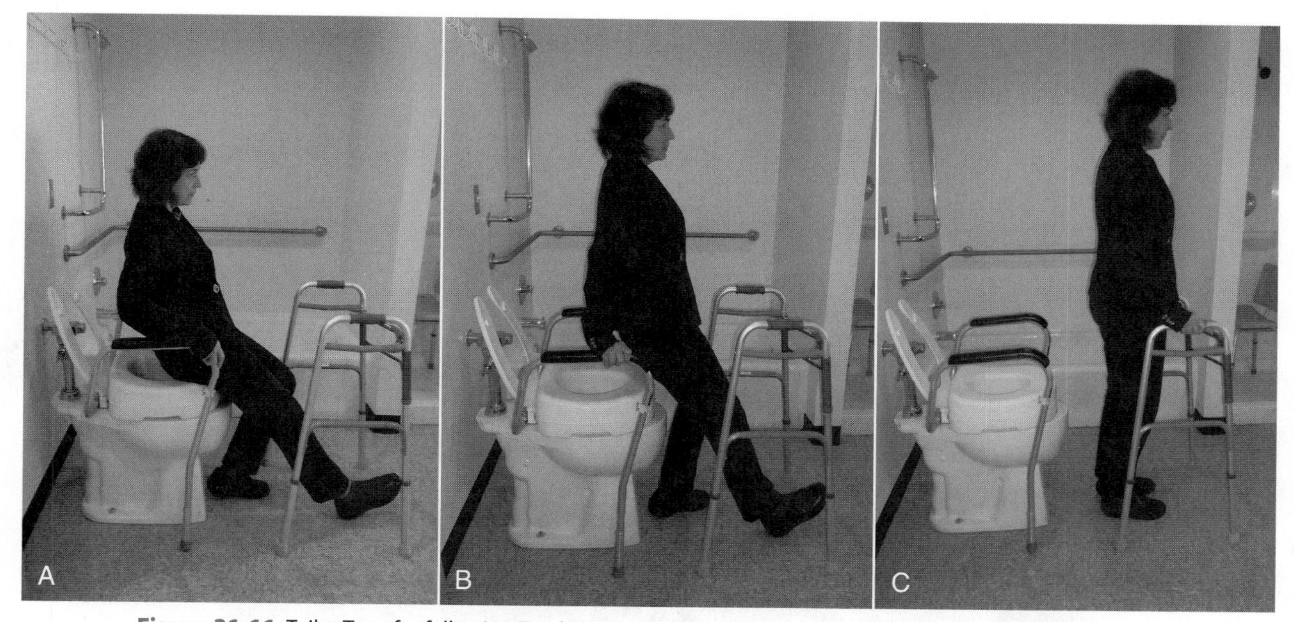

Figure 31-11 Toilet Transfer following Total Hip Replacement Precautions. **A,** Patient is instructed to place operated leg forward, to prevent hip flexion greater than 90°. **B,** Patient stands by placing weight through upper extremities and non-operated leg. **C,** Once standing, the patient can utilize the walker for balance and stability.

are used to grasp items in low cabinets or to pick them up from the floor. Light meal preparation should be done at the stovetop or with appliances such as a microwave oven or toaster oven within easy reach. Use of a standard oven should be avoided. Problem solving for pet care or other homemaking tasks must ensure adherence to hip precautions (Figure 31-12).

CLINICAL PEARL

Many times, patients will say that they have thought through how they will manage at home and do not need to actually practice certain skills. It is helpful to say "Well, let's see how your plan might actually work out by going to our simulated car (bathroom, kitchen) and you can show me." Many times, this brings up new questions or helps patients develop a better plan to ensure they observe hip precautions.

Caregiver Training

A family member, friend, or caregiver should be present for at least one OT treatment session so that any questions may be answered and the caregiver can appreciate the patient's current abilities and limitations. Appropriate supervision recommendations and instruction regarding activity precautions are given at this time. Instructional booklets on hip fractures and total hip and knee surgery can be purchased from the American Occupational Therapy Association[1] or other sources to supplement training.

Total Knee Replacement Procedures

The following are procedures for ADL and IADL training for persons with total knee replacement. Many of the techniques used with a hip replacement can be used for a patient with a knee replacement, even though in this case the hip can be flexed freely without precautions. Positions of knee instability include internal and external rotation of the hip with concurrent torque (twisting) at the knee joint and knee flexion greater than ROM permits.

Bed Mobility

Supine position is recommended with the leg slightly elevated via balanced suspension or pillows with or without a knee immobilizer. This position will help to reduce edema and prevent knee flexion contractures. Sleeping on the operated side is not recommended. As in hip replacement, a pillow or wedge can be placed in between the legs if this is necessary for side-lying and the person lies on the nonoperated side. Rolling is permitted to reach the side of the bed, and movement from side-lying may ease the transition from supine to sitting on the side of the bed.

Transfers

In general, patients can bend at the hip during transfers without restriction. Because of decreased knee flexion, the patient may need to use the same techniques as described for hip replacements for commode and car transfers. Grab bars and a shower chair or bench are recommended, especially for transferring to the shower over the tub, as well as for the individual with decreased standing endurance or inability to bend the knee enough to sit on the bottom of the tub. As an alternative to using the shower chair or transfer bench, the patient may stand parallel to the tub facing the shower fixtures. For extra stability, the patient may put the hands on the wall for support or use grab bars to assist in a side-step technique over the side of the tub. Patients are warned not to turn their bodies with

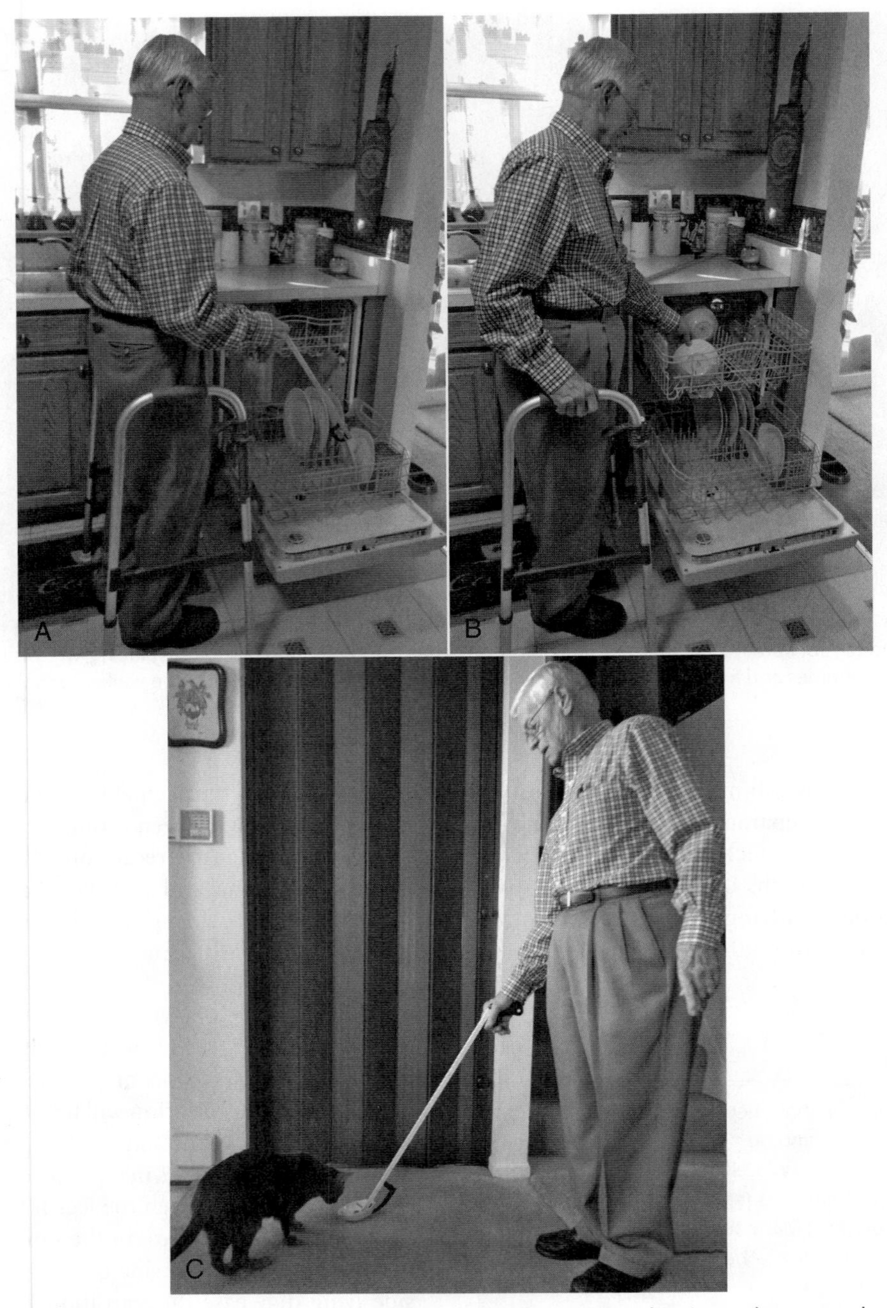

Figure 31-12 Homemaking procedures using hip precautions. **A,** Reacher is used to grasp low items. **B,** Where possible, use upper rack of dishwasher and maintain contact with walker handle with other hand. **C,** Present treats to pets using long-handled device, rather than bending over at hip.

their operated leg planted on the floor to prevent torque at the knee joint (Figure 31-13).

Lower Body Dressing

Lower body dressing presents a problem only if patients cannot reach their toes. In such a case, techniques described for hip replacement can be used. The patient should practice donning and removing the knee immobilizer. In addition, patients need to avoid donning shoes in a way that causes torque at the knee (e.g., by wiggling the foot into shoes while weight bearing).

The techniques for homemaking and caregiver training are the same as those used for hip replacement.

General Considerations for Occupational Therapy Intervention

In addition to the ADL and IADL specified earlier, the OTA should address all areas of occupation that the patient may find difficult and those that may pose a safety risk. Occupations such as care of a pet, navigating through a cafeteria for meals, traveling in vehicles other than cars, and attending religious activities that require transfer to a church pew all may be part of a patient's typical performance pattern and should be addressed in OT. The OTA can assist the patient in approaching meaningful occupations safely, observing any movement precautions that are required and promoting

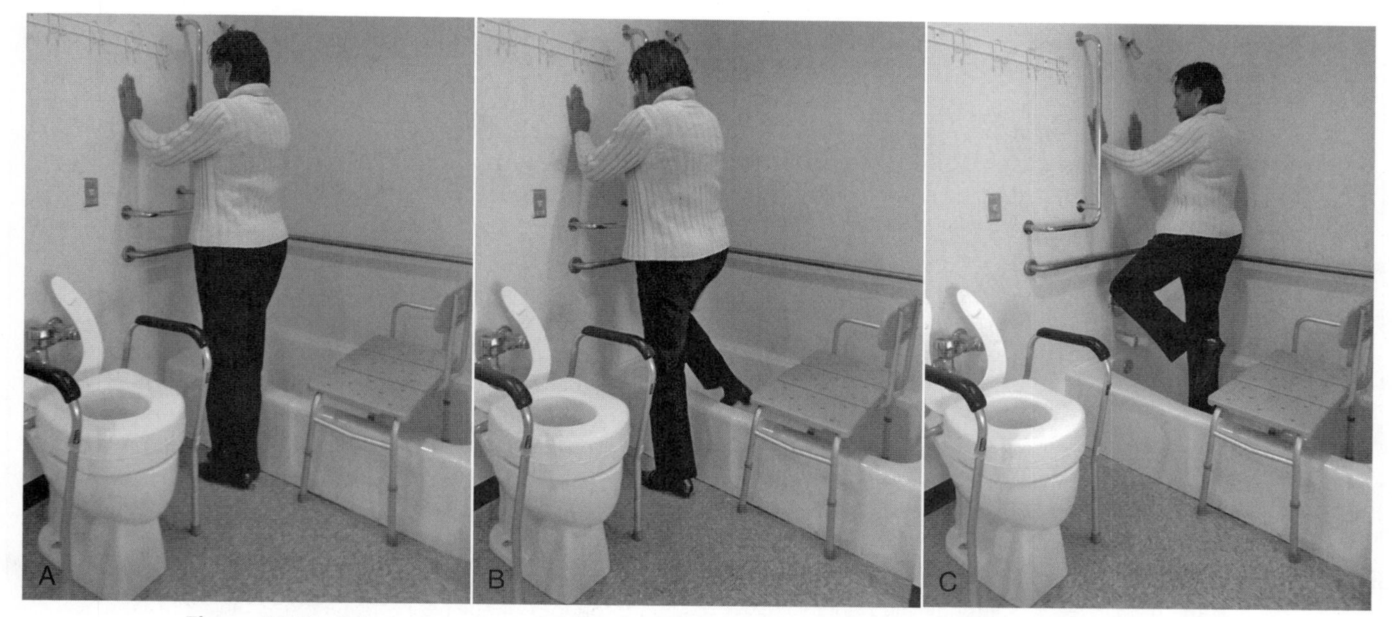

Figure 31-13 **A,** Patient stands parallel to tub, facing shower fixtures. **B** and **C,** Patient uses wall and/or grab bars for support when entering and exiting tub and steps deliberately, avoiding turning the body while the knee is planted on the floor.

alternative methods and/or use of assistive devices through patient education and demonstrated performance.

> ***Quote Box***
>
> Excerpt taken from *Ordinary Miracles: True Stories About Overcoming Obstacles & Surviving Catastrophies* (Labovitz, 2003).
>
> Dr. P was in a skilled nursing facility for rehabilitation following a hip fracture. He initially refused occupational therapy but when he was unable to put on his socks, he soon found out the value of occupational therapy! " ... I spotted Dr. P walking down the hall ... and poking out of his shirt pocket ... was the top of a pair of black socks. I glanced at his bare feet inside his shoes as I smiled and commented, 'I notice though that your socks are in your pocket, do you need help getting them on?''Oh, I'll find a nursing assistant to help me after a while' he grinned sheepishly. I said, 'That's fine, but where are you going to find a nursing assistant when you go home?' I quipped. ... That afternoon he offered no objection as I demonstrated how to put the sock onto the [sock] aid and put it on his foot. ... Dr. P decided that the OT was a pretty good person to know. After his sock success, he requested more occupational therapy and I worked with him on other activities such as cooking, small household chores, and driving. ... Several months later, I saw Dr. P at the grocery store... [He said] 'You know I still use that sock thing everyday. I'm sure glad you were around since there are no nursing assistants at my house' he chuckled." (pp. 207-209)

Special Equipment

The OT practitioner should be familiar with the following equipment that is commonly used in the treatment of hip fracture and lower extremity joint replacement.

Hemovac

During surgery a plastic drainage tube is inserted at the surgical site to assist with postoperative drainage of blood. It has an area for collection of drainage and may be connected to a portable suction machine. The unit should *not* be disconnected for any activity because this may create a blockage in the system. The Hemovac is usually left in place for 2 days after surgery.

Abduction Wedge

Large and small triangular abduction wedges are used when the patient is supine; they maintain the LEs in the abducted position (see Figure 31-8).

Balanced Suspension

Balanced suspension is fabricated and set up by the physical therapist or cast-room technician and physician and is often used for about 3 days after surgery when indicated. Its purpose is to support the affected LE in the first few postoperative days. The patient's leg should *not* be taken out of the device for exercise unless the physician has given written permission.

Reclining Wheelchair

A wheelchair with an adjustable backrest that allows a reclining position is used for patients who have hip flexion precautions while sitting.

Commode Chairs

The use of a commode chair instead of the regular toilet aids in safe transfers and allows the patient to observe necessary hip flexion precautions. The two front legs of the commode chair may be adjusted slightly lower than the back legs to increase the patient's ability to observe hip flexion limitations and decrease the risk of dislocation.

Sequential Compression Devices

Sequential compression devices (SCDs) are used postoperatively to reduce the risk of deep vein thrombosis. They are inflatable,

CASE STUDY

Ms. Johnson, Part 4

Ms. Johnson's rehabilitation program focused on mobility and adaptive strategies for basic ADL (e.g., going to the bathroom, donning a robe or slippers, sponge bathing, grooming) during the first few days before she had the second surgery on the left knee. After the second surgery, Ms. Johnson was a bit disheartened at how much more difficult it was to get moving again. She still had some pain in her right knee from the surgery a week ago; now there was excruciating pain in the left knee. Despite Ms. Johnson's training in adaptive techniques for bed mobility and ADL, she needed considerable additional assistance because of the pain now in both legs.

A couple of days after her second surgery, Ms. Johnson was discharged to a subacute rehabilitation facility where she could really "get back on my feet." By now her pain was decreasing slowly and the right knee was stronger and able to assist with movement more. Her ROM in both knees was improving daily. Since moving to the subacute facility, a new evaluation of Ms. Johnson's abilities was conducted by a new team of occupational therapist and OTA. After the plan of care was established by the occupational therapist, the OTA began dressing training, initially by loaning Ms. Johnson a reacher for dressing and encouraging her to bend her knees as much as she could. This functional activity also helped Ms. Johnson increase her knee flexion. Eventually, Ms. Johnson did not need the reacher or other dressing aids. Ms. Johnson was now highly motivated to get home to her daughter, who had been staying with Ms. Johnson's sister. The OTA outlined several activities that she could perform on her own to increase her independence. The OTA suggested that Ms. Johnson not ask for help with dressing and that she take walks around the nursing floor and get items from the cabinet, closets, and drawers herself. These activities reinforced prior performance habits and routines. Together, Ms. Johnson and the OTA improved independence in car and shower transfers and home management activities such as cooking, making the bed, light housekeeping, and laundry. The OTA recommended that Ms. Johnson go home with an elevated toilet seat or three-in-one commode chair.

Ms. Johnson was encouraged by her progress and asked the OTA to help her determine activities in which she could participate with her daughter. The OTA recommended that she and her daughter go swimming together. This active occupation would present Ms. Johnson with less risk of injuring the newly replaced knees. In addition to doing more active kinds of occupations, like swimming and walking, with her daughter, Ms. Johnson would be helping her daughter develop the healthy habits with which she herself had struggled lately. The OTA also encouraged Ms. Johnson to continue her participation as Girl Scout troop leader. She could enlist the help of the girls in the troop when necessary. By getting back into her previous habits and routines, she would remain motivated and feel like she was moving toward full engagement in all of the activities and occupations she found meaningful.

At discharge from the subacute rehabilitation facility, Ms. Johnson was to continue with outpatient physical therapy—primarily to continue to increase her knee ROM and LE strength. She met her OT goals while at the subacute facility. Ms. Johnson felt that she had the skills necessary to be independent in her own care, as well as her daughter's care. Even though she did not plan to return to work for a few weeks, Ms. Johnson felt that she could manage at home with her sister's assistance for transportation until she could drive herself.

external leggings that provide intermittent pneumatic compression of the legs.[3] They are typically used when the patient is sedentary (i.e., in bed) and can be removed during activity.

Antiembolus Hosiery

Antiembolus hosiery is thigh-high hosiery that is worn 24 hours a day and removed only during bathing. Its purpose is to assist circulation, prevent edema, and reduce the risk of deep vein thrombosis.[4]

Patient-Controlled Administration of Intravenous Analgesia (Pain Medication)

The amount of pain medication is predetermined and programmed by the physician and nurse to allow the patient to self-administer the medication by pushing a button without the risk of overdose. The medication may also be administered into the epidural space of the spine (patient-controlled epidural analgesia [PCEA]).

Incentive Spirometer

An incentive spirometer is a portable breathing apparatus used to encourage deep breathing and exercise of the muscles that aid in inspiration and expiration, as well as reduce the risk for postoperative pneumonia. Its use should be encouraged by the OTA.

Continuous Passive Motion Machine

Following a total knee replacement, patients may use a continuous passive motion (CPM) machine that supports the lower extremity with a hinge parallel to the knee joint. The speed and range of motion can be adjusted to promote slow and comfortable motion for a few hours daily while the patient is resting supine in bed. Use of the CPM is designed to facilitate the return to normal knee ROM and to discourage edema.

Summary

Hip fractures and LE joint replacement are orthopedic conditions in which OT intervention may speed the patient's return to optimal participation in daily activities safely and comfortably. The protocol for OT is determined by the surgical procedure performed and by the precautions prescribed by the physician. Patients who have weight-bearing precautions must be trained to observe these during all ADL and IADL. A simulation of the home environment or a home assessment is helpful in preparing the patient for potential problems that may arise after discharge. Areas to assess include the entry, stairs, bathroom, bedroom, sitting surfaces, and kitchen. The occupational therapist will recommend removing throw rugs and slippery floor coverings and obstacles because the patient will most likely be going home using an assistive device for ambulation. A kitchen stool or utility cart may be indicated. The occupational therapist must assess and instruct the patient and caregiver in ADL and IADL with adaptive equipment and in observing any movement precautions. Home therapy may be indicated after a hospital stay to ensure safety and independence in daily occupations if these goals were not met during hospitalization.

Preoperative teaching programs are invaluable in aiding patient adjustment. The group class orients and familiarizes the patient with the hospital, nursing, OT, physical therapy, and discharge planning. Procedures and equipment, concerns regarding the hospitalization and discharge, and therapy are addressed. Participation in this type of class has been shown to relieve anxiety and fear, empower the patient during the hospitalization, and decrease the hospital length of stay.

Selected Reading Guide Questions

1. Why is it critical for the OTA to understand hip anatomy and treatment of hip fractures?
2. What information should the occupational therapist (with assistance of the OTA) obtain for the occupational profile?
3. Identify four factors that will influence fracture healing.
4. Define the levels of weight-bearing restrictions.
5. List areas of OT intervention for hip fractures and joint replacements.
6. Why must hip position precautions be observed during activity by patients with total hip replacements?
7. Briefly describe the positions of instability in both the anterior and posterior approaches to hip replacement arthroplasty.
8. Briefly describe an abduction wedge and a knee immobilizer and the indications for their use and application.
9. After initial postoperative assessment, which functional activities are generally assessed in planning the initial OT intervention?
10. Briefly describe the transfer method to a chair after total hip replacement with a posterolateral approach. What is the rationale applied here? What types of chairs should be avoided? Why?
11. Briefly describe a car transfer recommended for the patient with hip replacement arthroplasty with an anterolateral approach.
12. Describe techniques for completing home management tasks for someone with a total hip replacement.
13. Outline the psychological issues faced by the elderly person with a hip fracture or joint replacement.
14. How might a person's rehabilitation program be affected by bilateral joint replacements?
15. List the most common types of adaptive equipment used during rehabilitation of hip fractures and LE joint replacements, and describe their purposes.

Application Exercises for Students

In a laboratory setting, the following role-playing activities may assist the OTA student to prepare for providing intervention to patients with LE joint replacements.

1. Instruct a peer in getting in and out of bed using hip precautions or a leg lifter.
2. Instruct a peer to prepare a light meal such as cooking soup at the stovetop. He or she should use a walker and be assigned a weight-bearing status for the activity. The goal is for the simulated patient and OTA student to problem solve appropriate strategies to obtain and transport items to prepare the meal and ensure safe use of the stove.
3. Review transfer techniques and then instruct a peer who is simulating a patient with bilateral total knee replacements with knee flexion less than 90 degrees and some level of pain. Identify the appropriate transfer techniques for patient instruction and ensure safe body mechanics for the OTA student in facilitating a transfer from the bed to a commode chair.
4. Complete dressing techniques using assistive devices. Attempt this activity with a variety of types of clothing and evaluate ease of dressing and use of assistive devices within hip precautions.
5. Assess your own living space. Is it accessible for a person who must observe strict hip precautions? Where would this person most safely sit? Could he or she cook in your kitchen? Are all rooms and hallways free of fall risks? What would need to be modified?

References

1. American Occupational Therapy Association: *After your hip surgery: a guide to daily activities*, Rockville, Md, 2001, American Occupational Therapy Association.
2. American Occupational Therapy Association: *After your knee surgery: a guide to daily activities*, Rockville, Md, 2001, American Occupational Therapy Association.
3. Calliet R: *Knee pain and disability*, ed 3, Philadelphia, 1992, FA Davis.
4. Delisa J, Gans B: *Rehabilitation medicine: principles and practice*, ed 2, Philadelphia, 1993, JB Lippincott.
5. Hanusch B, Lou T, Warriner G, et al: Functional outcome of PFC Sigma fixed and rotating-platform total knee arthroplasty. A prospective randomised controlled trial, *Int Orthop* 34(3): 349–354, 2010.
6 Kane RL, Saleh KJ, Wilt, et al: *Total knee replacement. Evidence report/technology assessment No. 86, AHRQ Publication No. 04-E006-1*, Rockville, Md, 2003, Agency for Healthcare Research and Quality.
7. Larson K, Stevens-Ratchford RG, Pedretti L, Crabtree J: *Role of occupational therapy with the elderly*, Bethesda, Md, 1996, American Occupational Therapy Association.
8. Luo S, Zhao J, Su W: Advancement in total knee prosthesis selection, *Chinese J Repar Reconstruct Surg* 24(3):301–303, 2010.
9. Melvin J, Gall V: *Rheumatic rehabilitation series: surgical rehabilitation*, vol. 5, Bethesda, Md, 1999, American Occupational Therapy Association.
10. Noble J, Goodall JR, Noble DJ: Simultaneous bilateral knee replacement: a persistent controversy, *The Knee* 16:420–426, 2009.

11. Opitz J: Reconstructive surgery of the extremities. In Kottle F, Lehmann J, editors: *Krusen's handbook of physical medicine and rehabilitation*, ed 4, Philadelphia, 1990, WB Saunders.
12. Paillard P: Hip replacement by a minimal anterior approach, *Int Orthop* July, 27, 2007. Doi: 10.1007/s00264-007-0433-7.
13. Richardson JK, Iglarsh ZA: *Clinical orthopaedic physical therapy*, Philadelphia, 1994, WB Saunders.
14 Saccomanni B: Unicompartmental knee arthroplasty: a review of literature, *Clin Rheumatol* 29(4):339–346, 2010.
15. Sherry E, Egan M, Warnke PH, et al: Minimal invasive surgery for hip replacement: a new technique using the NILNAV hip system, *ANZ J Surg* 73:157–161, 2003.
16. Singh J, Sloan J, Johanson N: Challenges with health-related quality of life assessment in arthroplasty patients: problems and solutions, *J Am Acad Orthop Surg* 18(2):72–82, 2010.
17. Sirkka M, Branholm I: Consequences of a hip fracture in activity performance and life satisfaction in an elderly Swedish clientele, *Scand J Occup Ther* 10:34, 2003.
18. Treacy RC, McBryde W, Pynsent PB: Birmingham hip resurfacing arthroplasty: a minimum follow up of 5 years, *Br J Bone Joint Surg* 87B(2):167–170, 2005.
19. Tsai C, Chen C, Liu T: Lateral approach with ligament release in total knee arthroplasty: new concepts in the surgical technique, *Artif Organs* 25(8):638–643, 2001.

CHAPTER 32 Burns

ELIZABETH A. RIVERS

Key Terms

Skin
Epidermis
Dermis
Burn
Eschar
Extent of the burn
Percentage of the total body surface area (%TBSA)
Edema
Autograft
Split-thickness skin graft (STSG)
Full-thickness skin graft
Hypertrophic scar
Contracture
Wound maturation
Skin conditioning
External vascular supports or pressure garments

Chapter Objectives

After studying this chapter, the student or practitioner will be able to do the following:

1. List the functions of skin and identify changes caused by a burn injury.
2. List the treatment goals for the three phases of burn wound healing.
3. Discuss the value of elevated, antigravity positioning for the burn patient and give one example.
4. Discuss scar management and give one example of a technique used to prevent or minimize scarring.
5. Prioritize rehabilitation goals to achieve maximum recovery with the least cost to the patient.
6. List two ways the occupational therapy practitioner prevents infection transfer.
7. Prioritize adaptations for function and list two reasons why such adaptations are discontinued early for burned survivors.
8. Discuss the benefits and challenges of using video games and Wii to improve motivation for rehabilitation.
9. List two additional diagnoses that benefit from "burn"-style rehabilitation.

The annual incidence of burn-related injuries in the United States is decreasing. Current estimates suggest that 500,000 burn patients are treated annually in the United States. Of these, more than 45,000 require hospitalization. Thirty-five hundred (3500) deaths occur from residential fires, and 500 result from other causes such as motor vehicle and aircraft crashes, contact with electricity, chemicals or hot liquids and substances, and other sources of burn or freezing injury.[1] Improvements in comprehensive burn rehabilitation continue.[2,3,10] Recovery after a burn is a long and arduous process.[7,20,22] Severely burned survivors experience a myriad of continuing medical, functional, and psychosocial problems. Nonetheless, those who want to return to the level of function they had before their injuries can anticipate recovery near that capacity.[33,55]

Beyond ensuring their patients' survival, burn care professionals use advanced medical and surgical techniques and focus on minimizing pain and maximizing motion, functional recovery, and quality of life after a burn.

Although this chapter is concerned mainly with thermal burns, the reader is advised that burn style rehabilitation is also being applied to conditions such as *toxic epidermal necrolysis* (in which the skin dies after exposure to a toxin such as spider bite or infection) and *necrotizing fasciitis* (in which the deep fascia and connective tissue dies after toxic exposure).

Skin

The skin[12,18,23] is the largest organ of the body and serves primarily as an environmental barrier. Skin is waterproof, protects from infection, helps control body temperature, prevents fluid loss, provides vast sensory information, and contributes to identity.

Skin has two basic layers: the epidermis and the dermis[12,18,23] (Figure 32-1). The skin growth cells (germinal keratinocytes) are in the epidermis. The melanocytes (pigment or color-producing cells) are found at the dermo-epidermal junction.

The dermis[18] is composed of highly structured and organized collagen; wandering cells (white blood cells, macrophages, fibroblasts, endothelial cells); blood vessels; elastic fibers; and a gluelike substance of glycosaminoglycans (GAG),

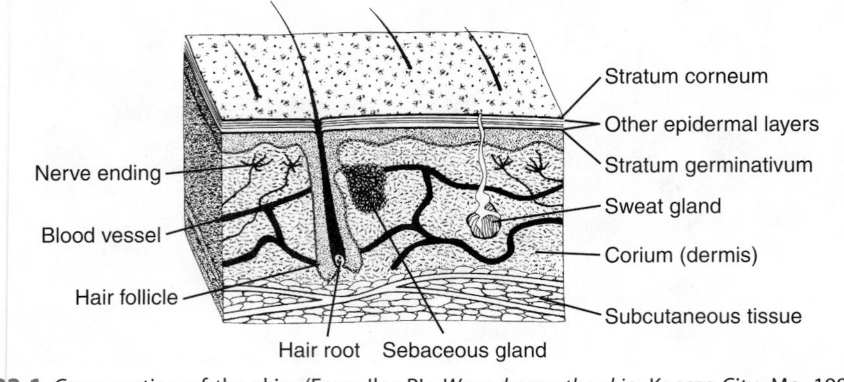

Figure 32-1 Cross-section of the skin. (From Iles RL: *Wound care: the skin,* Kansas City, Mo, 1988, Marion Laboratories.)

which is also known as "ground substance." The dermis does not regenerate and heals by scar formation.

A burn is a permanent destruction of tissue caused by release of energy from an external agent. Eschar, pronounced "es-kar," is the dead epidermis and necrotic dermis that remain attached to the wound bed. Most thermal burns are of varying depths (Table 32-1).

When the skin is damaged, innumerable systemic, physiological, and functional problems begin.[23,29,36,40,50] The basis for safe burn treatment is detailed knowledge and understanding of normal skin anatomy, physiology, wound healing, and infection control; this expertise requires continuing study and research by all team members. Detailed wound healing is beyond the scope of this chapter, but the recommended readings list at the end of this chapter suggests other helpful resources. With increasingly high levels of training in staff, hospital stay is reduced and outcomes improve in burn centers.[47,48,55]

Measures of Burn Injury Severity

Percentage of Total Body Surface Area Involved

The extent of the burn is classified as a percentage of the total body surface area (%TBSA) burned. Two methods used to estimate burn size are the "rule of nines" and the Lund and Browder chart.[32] The rule of nines, developed in the 1940s by Pulaski and Tennison and communicated by word of mouth, divides the body surface into areas of 9%, with the perineum making up 1%. Although simple, the rule of nines is relatively inaccurate, especially for children (Figure 32-2). The Lund and Browder chart[32] provides a more accurate estimate of %TBSA involved and is used in most burn centers.

Burn Depth

An accurate depth of burn is difficult to estimate. Assessment is based on experienced clinical observation of the appearance, sensitivity, and pliability of the wound.[11,12,16] The burn is described as a superficial-, partial-, or full-thickness injury (see Table 32-1). For treatment planning, the team should remember that the wound is constantly changing and must be reassessed frequently.[24,38]

Mechanism of Injury

Thermal injuries are caused by exposure to flames, steam, hot liquids, hot metals, electricity, radiation, toxic chemicals, or extreme cold. Heat injury accounts for most burns[1,55]; about 75% of these accidents are preventable.

Hospital Medical Management

Initial Care

Burn injury causes extensive shifts of body fluids.[26,28,57,60] Fluids and electrolytes are replaced intravenously to prevent shock and death. Edema (swelling) is the first problem that occupational therapy (OT) practitioners treat.

In circumferential full-thickness burns, the leathery eschar is inelastic, thus impairing normal circulation. The surgeon performs an escharotomy (incision through destroyed skin) to improve circulation.[2,10] The procedure is usually painless because the nerve endings are destroyed in a full-thickness burn (Figure 32-3).

Wound Care

A shower, shower cart hydrotherapy (SCH), submersion cleansing, or local cleansing of the wound and uninvolved areas is done on admission and, depending on dressings used, weekly or biweekly. Various topical agents are applied to reduce bacterial counts in the wounds. All staff observe universal infection control precautions according to the hospital's rules (see Chapter 3). The OT practitioner decontaminates all equipment, materials, and surfaces between patient contacts. All family, staff, and visitors wash hands frequently and consistently.

Skin Grafting

When the depth and extent of the wound will require 3 or more weeks for healing, surgery will decrease hospital length of stay, pain, and scar or contracture complications.[48] With the patient anesthetized, the surgeon excises (removes) the eschar, controls bleeding in the recipient area, and places an autograft. An autograft is a surgical transplantation of the person's own skin from an unburned area (donor site). The sheet or meshed (perforated evenly by machine) split-thickness skin graft (STSG) is applied to the clean excised

Table 32-1 Depth of Injury Correlated with Anticipated Healing Time and Treatment Interventions

Injury Depth	Healing Time	Wound Outcome	Therapy Treatment Modalities
Superficial epidermis (first-degree burn)	1-5 days for spontaneous healing	No problems after healing	Elevation decreases limb pain. Wash wound to prevent infection. On healed wound, aloe or other moisturizer reduces dry skin and itching. Therapist rarely consulted.
Superficial dermis (superficial partial-thickness burn or second-degree burn)	14 days for spontaneous healing	Possible pigment (color) changes	Above, plus more careful wound care. Active elevated exercise to preserve joint function and improve wound circulation, especially venous return. Protective garments. Sunscreen. Acknowledge patient's pain and inconvenience. Coordinate treatments with adequate analgesia.
Deep reticular dermis (deep partial-thickness burn or second-degree)	21 days* for spontaneous healing. (If grafted, see below)	Probable pigment changes Reduced skin durability Severe scarring Sensory changes Sweating changes Edema in dependent limbs, usually temporary	Above, plus: Therapists consulted by burn team. More frequent active elevated exercise. Elevated positioning or splints or both. Vascular support garments.† Healed areas may need inserts or silicone tapes to manage hypertrophic scars. Moisturization and lubrication to healed skin. Prolonged stretch to involved joints twice daily until contractures resolve. Daily living skills practice. Psychological therapy. Team collaboration to prevent stress disorder.
Subcutaneous tissue (full-thickness burn or third-degree burn)	Variable healing time Graft needed or if small area, approximated wound edges with primary closure Very large burn, cultured epithelial autograft (CEA)‡	Same as above Additional sweating loss Possible loss of involved finger or toe nails Possible additional sensory loss No hair over grafts	Same as above plus: Postoperative positioning or immobilization. Initiate exercise despite pain, very slow weaning from analgesics and medications for stress. Vibration for itching. Additional education for skin precautions. Wear support/pressure garments and inserts and overlays to manage concave areas. Participate in peer support group. Early return to recreation and work, school, family, and community responsibilities.
Muscle, tendon, bone (fourth-degree burn, historic term, rarely used)	Healing time variable Amputation or reconstructive surgery such as flaps needed.§	Variable	Same as above plus: Deep tendon massage to prevent tethered skin. Adapted equipment. Prosthetic fitting and training if indicated. Additional counseling for stress. Watsu (water shiatsu) therapy for posttraumatic stress. Memory retraining. Participate in peer support group. Work retraining if unable to return safely to preburn employment.

*If surgeon grafts burn by 14 days, scar formation is reduced with improved functional outcome, less pain, and shortened length of hospital stay.
†Gradient pressure progressively decreases the rate of pressure applied by an elastic bandage or cylindrical pressure sleeve, keeping the most pressure on the distal limb and the least pressure around the proximal area of the extremity.
‡Areas of cultured epithelial autograft (CEA) show permanent fragility; loss of temperature control; dry, blister-prone skin with permanently changed sensation.
§Early amputation with closure using noninjured tissue shortens length of hospital stay, decreases pain and wound breakdown, improves prosthesis fit, and simplifies prosthesis use. However, wounds are rarely of single depth, through skin and muscle.

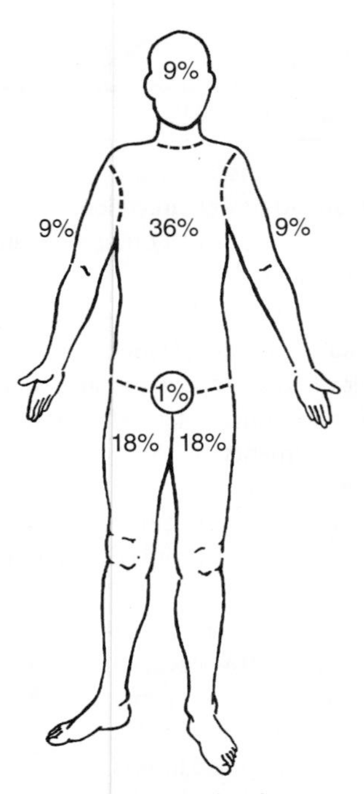

Figure 32-2 Rule of nines.

wound (graft recipient site). As the size of a survivable burn increases, available donor sites for autograft decrease. For this reason, alternatives to autografts such as the cultured epidermal autograft (CEA), other cultured skin substitutes, biological dressings/temporary graft, or synthetic coverings are being explored.[1,2,10] When the wound is limited in size but the defect is so deep that tendon survival or graft adherence is extremely doubtful, a plastic surgeon covers the area with a microvascular skin flap autograft. Because a full-thickness skin graft requires donor wound closure by an STSG or by edge-to-edge closure, it is usually reserved for reconstruction.

Pain

Pain[9,14,36] is defined as an unpleasant sensory and emotional response to a stimulus associated with actual or potential tissue damage.[36] Burn pain severity cannot be predicted; it is influenced by burn depth and location, patient age, gender, ethnicity, education, occupation, history of drug or alcohol abuse, and psychiatric illness. A burn medication protocol includes long-acting narcotics for background pain, short-acting drugs for procedural pain, and medications to decrease anxiety. Procedural pain occurs during activities such as wound cleansing, dressing changes, or therapy.[4,13,38] If possible, therapists schedule exercise sessions when pain medications are at peak effectiveness. As the wound heals, a patient gradually decreases the dosage and frequency of drugs and usually requires minimal pain medications after wound closure.

Scar Formation

A hypertrophic scar is a hard, red, collagenous bundle of connective tissue raised above the surface of the burn wound.[3,16,28,31] Initially, healed burn wounds usually appear red and flat. Hypertrophic scars commonly become visible

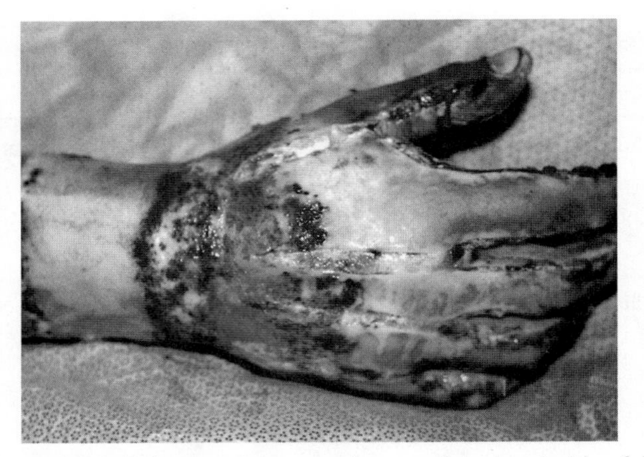
Figure 32-3 Escharotomies on the dorsum of the hand with a full-thickness burn injury.

6 to 8 weeks after wound closure. The functional or cosmetic significance of hypertrophic scars varies with the anatomical location of the wound. Race, age, and the location and depth of the burn wound have been reported to influence hypertrophic scarring.[28,31,45,56]

Contracture Development

Normal wound healing occurs by contraction.[2,45] In addition, the burned patient often chooses to lie in a flexed, adducted, "fetal" position, the position of withdrawal from pain. If the patient does not actively stretch the healing wound to its original length, the new collagen fibers in the wound shorten.[3,6,16,20] A contracture is limited joint motion caused by shortened soft tissue, tendons, ligaments, blood vessels, and nerves or by calcium deposits surrounding the involved joint.

Psychosocial Factors

During hospitalization, the patient experiences fear, isolation, dependency, and pain. Potential psychological reactions include posttraumatic stress disorder,[9] depression, withdrawal, reactions to disfigurement, regression, and anxiety and uncertainty about the ability to resume work, family, community, and leisure roles.[3,5,9,20] During each contact, the occupational therapy assistant (OTA) and occupational therapist provide emotional support and education to facilitate adjustment, coping, and self-direction, as well as managing exercise and/or splint fitting.

Burn Rehabilitation

Team

The burn care multidisciplinary team comprises the patient and family, physicians, nurses, physical therapists[49] and physical therapy assistants,[39] registered occupational therapists,[49] OTAs,[38] dietitians, social workers, respiratory therapists, art and play therapists, massage therapists, recreational therapists,[21] personal clergy, case managers, visiting caregivers, chaplains, and vocational counselors. Nationally, team members available to the burn patient vary widely.[4,5,16,39,40,46] Specific role delineation varies with state licensure or certification regulations and with hospital or facility policies.[4,5,11]

Phases of Recovery

Burn management can be divided into three overlapping phases: (1) acute care; (2) surgical and postoperative care; and (3) rehabilitation (inpatient and outpatient).[39]

The acute care phase occurs in the first 72 hours after a major burn injury. If the wound is superficial, a person experiences only this phase.

The surgical and postoperative phase follows the acute phase. Vulnerability to wound infection, sepsis, and septic shock predominate at this time.

The final phase is the postgrafting or wound maturation period when the patient is medically stable. Inpatient and outpatient treatments are provided during this phase, which the American Burn Association (ABA) calls *rehabilitation.*[40] Besides depth and %TBSA, other factors that affect outcome are the quality of wound healing, scar formation, and effectiveness of team collaboration. The final phase is the longest, most rigorous, and most challenging for the patients, family, and staff. The OTA provides treatments at this time, gradually increasing the patient's responsibility for exercise, return to hobbies, getting face masks revised, and resuming independent self-care.

Goals of Rehabilitation

Considering the functional, cosmetic, and psychosocial consequences of a severe burn injury, the team focuses on cost-effective, successful outcomes[7,33,34] (see Table 32-1).

Acute Care Phase

During the acute care phase, medical management and patient survival are the primary concerns. Occupational therapists, sometimes collaborating with an experienced OTA, assist with edema management and splints during this phase as ordered by the physician.

Surgical and Postoperative Phases

OT goals during the surgical and postoperative phases promote skin graft adherence while preserving or assisting function when possible. The graft recipient area is immobilized after surgery. The preferred position and length of immobilization vary by physician preference and burn center protocol; however, the range is from 1 to 7 days, usually in extension.[40,41]

Rehabilitation Phase

The overlapping third phase of recovery is the postgrafting, wound maturation period. It begins as wound closure occurs. The patient becomes medically stable, and external life support and monitoring tubes are discontinued. A wound is considered mature when it is soft, the proper color, flat, durable, and supple. Wound maturation time varies from less than a year to 2 years and in growing children up to 5 years.[42,43]

Care during the rehabilitation phase focuses on achieving independence while preventing deformity and contractures.[19] If a clear plastic face or neck splint is to be used to stretch facial contractures and soften scars, the fit is improved during this stage. The occupational therapist and OTA teach precautions to the patient and family.[15,25,31,34,41,43,54] The patient and family prepare for discharge, and the OTA recommends practical program modifications. Once the individual is home, therapists and physician follow-up, psychological support, and intervention are provided to restore motivation, self-confidence, social interaction, family participation, and return to work. Clinic visits include splint and custom garment evaluation, in addition to physician follow-up.

At discharge or soon after, the patient will do the following:

1. Direct skin conditioning and wound care, bathe, moisturize skin,[7] and perform self-care with minimal assistance; independently don and remove vascular supports; and preserve healed burn wounds, grafts, and donor areas while resuming preburn activity.
2. Recover at least 80% of preburn active range of motion (AROM), demonstrate prolonged stretching to decrease joint and skin contractures, and avoid joint deterioration while preserving full use of the extremities at work or school.
3. Recover 80% of preburn strength (in comparison to norms for age) to return to preburn functional activities in the home and community.
4. Develop endurance to tolerate 2 hours of work-equivalent activity and 8 hours of activities including safe homemaking or home chores, with the final goal of endurance for preburn level of activity.
5. Recover coordination sufficient for work and daily living skills with minimal adaptive equipment and at preburn flexibility and speed.
6. Control limb edema with vascular supports 23 hours a day combined with elevated positioning to prevent wound breakdown, decrease scar formation, and prevent cellulitis.
7. Demonstrate independent donning and removal of splints, inserts, and overlays to modify burn scars; remember to wear devices for the prescribed number of hours and explain the purpose of these devices.
8. Learn and use protective outdoor interventions such as flap hats or sunscreen clothing in the sun and layered winter clothing to avoid wound breakdown and hyperthermia or hypothermia.
9. Demonstrate successful use of interventions such as cutting nails, applying lotion, massage, vibrating, and desensitizing to control itching and avoid excoriation of wounds.
10. Participate in appropriate, coordinated planning for discharge from burn care.
11. Explore vocational issues with a vocational rehabilitation or school counselor to resume work or school and develop OT plan for skill practice if needed.
12. Explore and participate in recreational activities, leisure planning, and social and community reintegration while wearing external vascular supports and splints.
13. Hire and supervise appropriate attendant help if not consistently independent in hygiene, use of support garments, and homemaking.

14. Learn to cope constructively with stress symptoms, changed body appearance, intimacy issues, and adjustment to disability; seek assistance from psychologist, counselor, or family as needed.
15. Participate in a survey of home needs emphasizing independence and safety; use mobility aids and adaptive equipment in the home if necessary; determine the level of assistance required after discharge.

Role of Occupational Therapy

There is no substitute for early and consistent intervention by occupational therapists. When burn team disciplines work closely together and communicate accurately and frequently, patients benefit from the skills and viewpoints of all. Moreover, documentation and communication with third-party payers, home care facilities, and families are consistent and coordinated.

OT in burn care draws on specialized knowledge of environments, sexuality, cultural and family influences, anatomy, physiology, kinesiology, neurology, infection control, splint fabrication, activities of daily living (ADL), instrumental ADL (IADL), and psychosocial development. The occupational therapist's and the OTA's skills, therapeutic approaches, energy, and creativity become part of the strengths and resources available to the burned patient and his or her family.

Often an OTA is part of the team at a rehabilitation center to which grafted and medically stable burn patients are referred before returning as appropriate to previous participation in home, work, school, and community pursuits. After the patient is stable, an OTA—in collaboration with an occupational therapist—may provide inpatient and outpatient personal daily living skills practice and follow-up with exercise treatment such as BTE Technologies, Biodex, and adapted games.[17,21,35,59] The OTA can also make adaptations for support garments and clothing, remeasure patients for custom-fitted vascular support garments as assigned, and teach homemaking skills. Depending on local practice regulations, exclusion criteria for OTA treatment may include patients with more than 20% TBSA burn, more than one joint involved, exposed tendons, hand or toe burns, face grafts, or inhalation injuries, as well as those patients who are not yet medically stable. In some hospitals, a qualified and experienced OTA reports and documents patient change; recommends reevaluations; and collaborates with the patient and social worker to resolve transportation, shopping, and homemaking limitations. Massage therapy may be taught by an OTA. In centers where hard plastic splints are formed over plaster models of the face, neck, or other concave areas, the OTA provides the second set of hands to form the hot plastic over the model.

Assessment

If possible, the occupational therapist completes initial patient evaluation[2,27] within the first 24 to 48 hours, first obtaining data on burn etiology, medical history, any secondary diagnoses, and precautions from the medical chart. The occupational therapist looks at the wounds to determine the extent and depth of injury, notes critical areas involved, and interviews the patient to establish rapport and obtain specific information such as hand dominance, previous functional limitations, sensory limitations, daily activities before the injury, psychological status, and spiritual and cultural values.

When alert, the patient collaborates with the occupational therapist and OTA to develop the first week's care plan based on this information.

Acute Care Phase Treatments

Exercise

Acute care treatments[10,16,17,20] (see Tables 32-1 and 32-2) include range of motion (ROM), which is a primary component in every burn treatment plan. Active, active-assisted, or prolonged stretch exercises are selected based on the patient's condition. Exercise in acute care preserves ROM and functional strength and decreases edema.[26,28,57,60] Ambulation begins as soon as it is medically safe. The patient who has a lower extremity (LE) burn wears elastic wraps. These are applied in a figure-8 pattern from the metatarsal heads including the heel to the groin. During therapy, static standing or prolonged dangling of feet should be avoided to prevent edema formation and unnecessary discomfort. A walker improves safety when walking. If the arms are also involved, an overhead bar can be added since grasping this bar decreases upper extremity edema during ambulation.

Strength and endurance activities are introduced early. Research and experience have shown that graded progressive exercise is not deleterious in acute burn recovery.[8,20,22,29,53,56]

If comatose or on a ventilator, the patient depends on nursing for self-care. As soon as the patient is medically cleared to eat, the occupational therapist or experienced OTA assesses eating skills. Initially, self-feeding motions may be limited by dressings, edema, and pain, and adaptive equipment may be used for a short time. Temporary adaptive equipment includes built-up and extended-handle utensils and a plate guard. Depending on amputations and the burn site, early simple grooming, toileting, and phone management are encouraged. All professional staff convey the expectation of early, independent, patient-initiated ADL with normal movement patterns and at a normal speed. Therapy staff encourage IADL before discharge, beginning with independent telephone use, as soon as possible.

Edema Management

During acute care, elevated positioning limits edema formation.[26,28,57,60] The extremity or head is raised above heart level (Table 32-2, Figure 32-4). Positions should be varied to improve patient comfort and normal joint function. The occupational therapist or experienced OTA makes the daily positioning program and changes clearly visible to all team members including the patient, family, nurses, and doctors by posting the information prominently in the patient's room.

Table 32-2 Antideformity Positioning, Equipment, and Techniques

Body Area	Antideformity Position	Equipment/Technique
Mouth	Varied	Regular food (i.e., not cut into small pieces), straw for thick liquids, exercise, microstomia splint
Ears/face	Positions that prevent pressure	No pillows, ear protection headgear, cut-out cushions in airbed, head of bed elevated to decrease edema and risk of aspiration
Neck	Neutral/slight extension	No pillow (or neck extended by foam wedge), elevation and head cut-out airflow or bead bed, foam neck splint conformer, multiple rings of plastic tubing collar (sometimes called *watsu*), triple component neck splint
Chest/abdomen	Trunk extension, shoulder retraction	Head of bed lowered, towel roll beneath spine, clavicle straps
Axilla	Shoulder abduction 90-100 degrees	Arm boards, foam wedges, overhead traction slings, axillary total contact splint, clavicle straps, overhead wheeled walker
Elbow/forearm	10 degrees short of full elbow extension, forearm neutral	Foam wedge pillows, arm boards, conformer splints, dynamic splints
Wrist/hand	Wrist extension 30 degrees, thumb abducted and extended, MCP flexion 50-70 degrees, IP extension	Elevation above heart with pillows or foam wedges when lying down or sitting; suspension slings, deltoid aid, overhead bar on wheeled walker with overhead bar for walking
Hip/thigh	Neutral extension, hips abducted 10-15 degrees	Bed elevation changed for prone/side-lying positions, trochanter rolls, pillow between knees, wedges to abduct hips
Knee/lower leg	Knee extension for circumferential burn, slight flexion for anterior burn	Foot of bed positioned to elevate feet when sitting in bed, knee conformer, casts, dynamic splints, knee extension with feet elevated when sitting, normal gait when walking
Ankle/foot	Neutral or 0-5 degrees dorsiflexion	Cut-out heel cushions, airflow bed with foot cushion, custom splint, cast, AFO, pillow under calf to prevent pressure on heels, footstool elevation when sitting, heel-to-toe motion when walking, slow normal to large step gait during ambulation

Note: All positioning must be varied throughout 24 hours. Any position held for many days can result in contractures.
AFO, Ankle-foot orthosis; *IP*, interphalangeal; *MCP*, metacarpophalangeal.

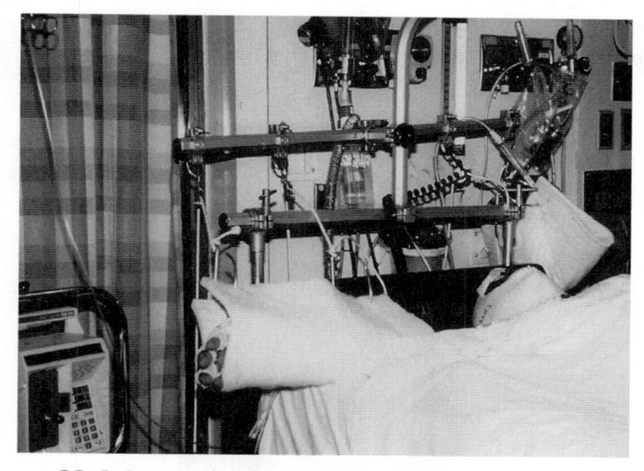

Figure 32-4 Supine shoulder positioning using overhead traction and felt slings.

Splinting

A splint used during the acute phase is usually applied during rest, with activity and exercise emphasized while the patient is awake. The volar burn hand splint is designed to provide approximately 30 degrees of wrist extension, 50 to 70 degrees of metacarpophalangeal (MCP) joint flexion, full interphalangeal (IP) extension, and the thumb abducted and extended (Figure 32-5). It is secured in place with a figure-8 wrap of gauze bandage. Straps are not used on acute burn splints because of the potential tourniquet effect and infection control concerns. Splints require daily assessment and alteration as edema and fit change.

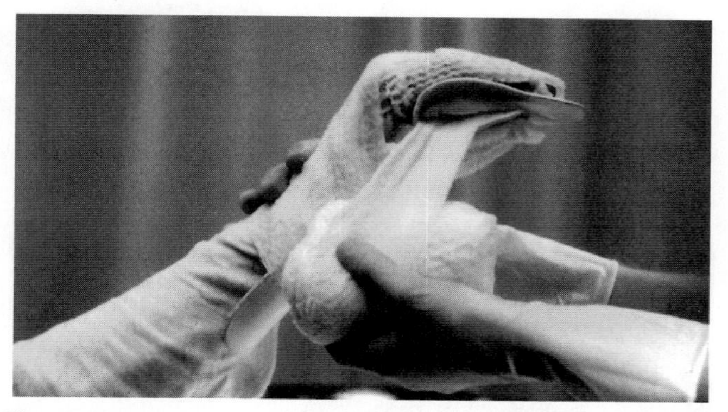

Figure 32-5 Postburn hand splint. Note wrapping approach for the thumb.

Surgical and Postoperative Phase Treatments

A period of postoperative immobilization assists graft adherence and vascularization. Bulky restrictive dressings with standard positioning equipment (see Figure 32-4) often are adequate. Splints may be ordered. Positioning procedures are checked by the team each day for graft and patient safety.

Exercises for adjacent body areas are discontinued until the physician indicates they may resume. The average immobilization is 3 to 5 days, with 7 to 10 days for cultured epidermal grafts. The physician, occupational therapist, and experienced OTA view the unbandaged graft and donor sites to determine graft integrity, exposed tendons, and bleeding areas before resuming exercises.

If permitted, temporary, simple equipment such as overhead mirrors, prism glasses for those supine in bed, or universal cuffs and extended-handle utensils for self-care are provided by the experienced OTA. These devices may help to preserve feelings of self-worth and orientation.

Rehabilitation Phase Treatments

Exercise is the most important treatment component in the rehabilitation phase (see Table 32-1 and Table 32-2, and Figures 32-6 to 32-10) and is not unique to burn injuries (see Figures 32-6 through 32-8). Depending on joints involved, every treatment during the intense rehabilitation phase overlaps with another treatment. For example, active exercise during ambulation includes stretching shoulders, elbows, and hands by grasping and releasing an overhead walker bar (see Figure 32-9) and increasing the number of laps the patient makes. Stair climbing and more vigorous patient-initiated exercises begin along with independent tub and car transfers. Rehabilitation equipment such as grippers, hand-manipulation boards, pipe trees, reciprocal pulleys, stationary bicycle, the BTE work simulator, Work Evaluation Systems Technology (WEST), the Valpar whole body exerciser (see Figure 32-8), musical or computer keyboards, Wii games,[21,35,38,58] homemaking work simulation activity, or weighted pulleys

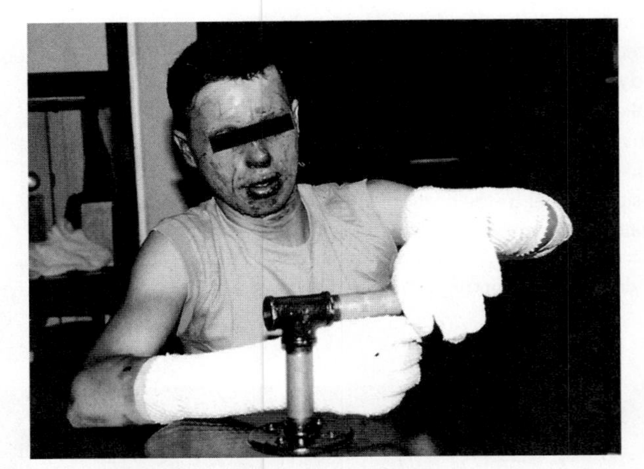

Figure 32-6 A commonly used pipe tree is a good activity for hand exercise after a burn injury.

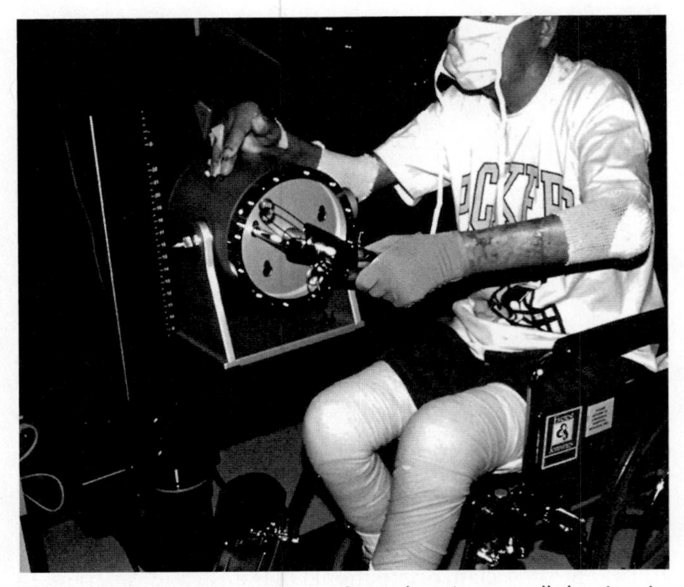

Figure 32-7 A presized intermediate glove is worn all the time including during exercise and activity to condition the skin and control edema. BTE Technologies (www.btetech.com) provides work simulation. Note elastic wraps to legs, toe to groin, bilaterally.

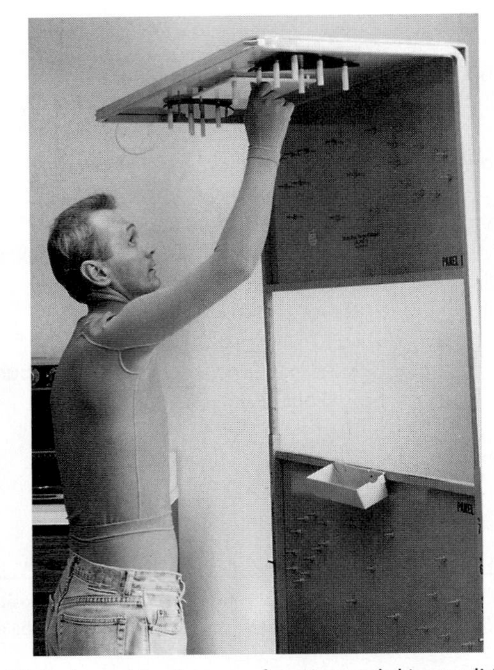

Figure 32-8 A combined range of motion and skin conditioning activity. Use of the Valpar whole body range of motion for upper extremity exercise while wearing compression garments.

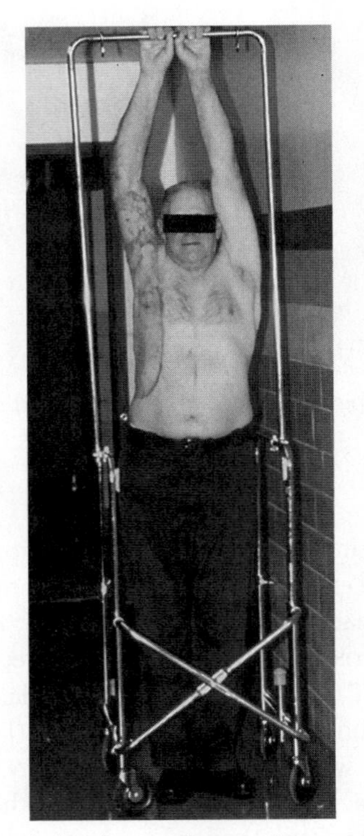

Figure 32-9 Wheeled walker equipped with an overhead bar helps patient stretch axillary contracture during ambulation.

may be used to increase range, strength, and endurance. Timers and written graph reminders give the person control of the duration and frequency of activity and provide objective documentation of improvement.

Stretching increases flexibility and fluidity of movement.[7,8,11] Patients perform a slow, sustained stretch in front of a full-length mirror to see and correct abnormal postures. The OT practitioner may ask the patient to combine activities and do composite stretches. An example is using plastic syringe cases as mouth cones (Figure 32-11) while lying prone to stretch hips, shoulders, and elbows. Other possibilities include (1) stretching shoulders and elbows while vibrating an itching back or combing hair; (2) reaching overhead to punch a balloon after every 10 repetitions of stationary bicycling; (3) cutting foods independently, drinking from a cup without a straw or using straw with thickened liquids only, or opening the mouth to eat regular raw fruits or vegetables; and (4) elevating arms while eating and tucking feet under a chair to stretch knee flexion and ankle dorsiflexion during a meal.

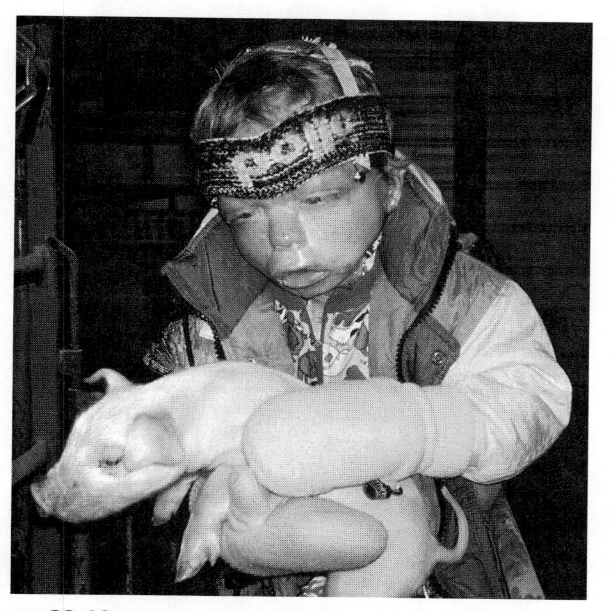

Figure 32-10 Mittens, layered clothing, and scarves protect child doing winter chores from frostbite.

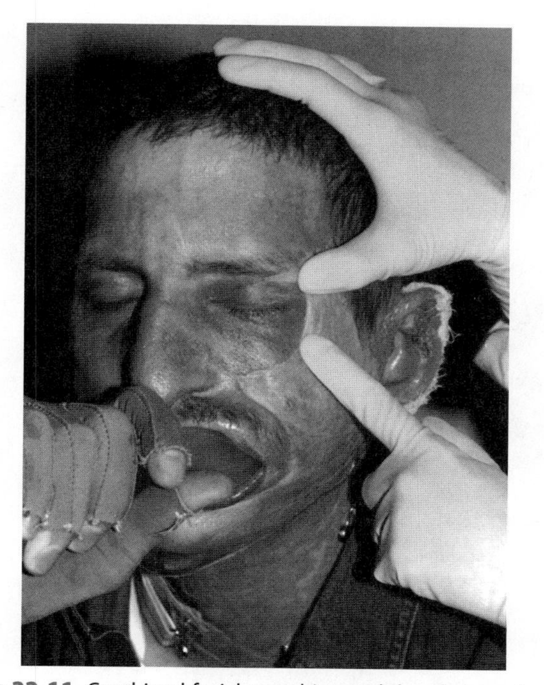

Figure 32-11 Combined facial stretching with hand strengthening. A patient wearing an Isotoner glove for hand edema uses a syringe case to stretch the left cheek pouch while an occupational therapy assistant stretches the facial contracture band. Note the neck splint.

It is important to control edema until swelling ceases.[26,28,57,60] In severe burns of the hand[7] that have healed, edema occurs because of decreased hand use, dependent positioning without adequate external support, and the tourniquet action of circumferential upper extremity (UE) scarring. When edema is present, motion is limited and painful, the skin is prone to damage from shearing forces, and fibrosis may result. Often an Isotoner glove adequately controls hand swelling (see Figure 32-7).

In addition to controlling edema, **external vascular supports or pressure garments** help to manage hypertrophic scars[26,28] but use must be supervised to avoid complications.[13,24,37,44,45] Custom-made support garments can be fitted once the patient's weight is stable, the healed skin does not stick to support, and the skin is durable. Motivated by anecdotal information, many surgeons recommend garments for all donor sites, graft sites, and burn wounds that take more than 2 to 3 weeks to heal. Inserts and/or overlay splints are needed to modify scars in areas where body contours such as finger webs and breast contours tent the garment (see Resources at end of chapter). The occupational therapist or experienced OTA often measures, orders, and checks the fit (Figure 32-12) of the custom-made garments (see Resources at end of chapter).

All custom-made garments need to be measured and ordered according to the special instructions of each company. To provide adequate scar compression, garments must be worn 23 hours a day; they are removed only for bathing, massage, or changing into a clean garment.

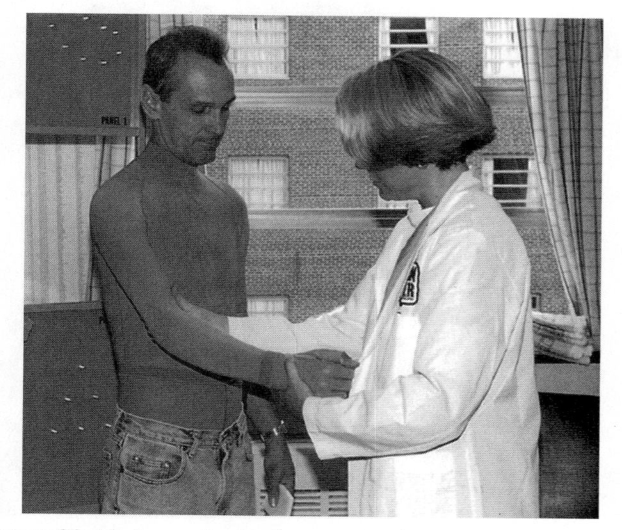

Figure 32-12 Assess the fit of custom-made compression garments frequently to ensure adequate compression for scar management.

Scar contracture is often the primary cause of dysfunction (Figure 32-13). Splints at this stage (1) limit or reverse potentially disabling or disfiguring contracture formations (Figures 32-14 and 32-15); (2) increase ROM; (3) distribute pressure over problem hypertrophic scar areas; or (4) assist function. Serial drop-out casts[30,37,51] (see Figure 32-15), which are used for progressive scar elongation, have the additional advantages of moisturizing and softening the scar, preventing orthotic slippage, and ensuring a consistent wearing schedule.

Before discharge, fears of heat sources such as hot water, the stove, or an iron are addressed during homemaking practice. The OTA teaches burn prevention techniques at this time and consults with the psychologist when behavioral desensitization procedures are indicated.

Assessment of physical tolerance and work skills should precede return to work. Vocational rehabilitation referrals are sometimes needed. Functional activities and work skills are assigned to improve work tolerance, strength, endurance, and flexibility. Lifting, stooping, pushing, pulling, handling, and manipulating are a few examples of common job activities that therapists incorporate. A job analysis interview will provide a basis for beginning work conditioning. Outpatient OT

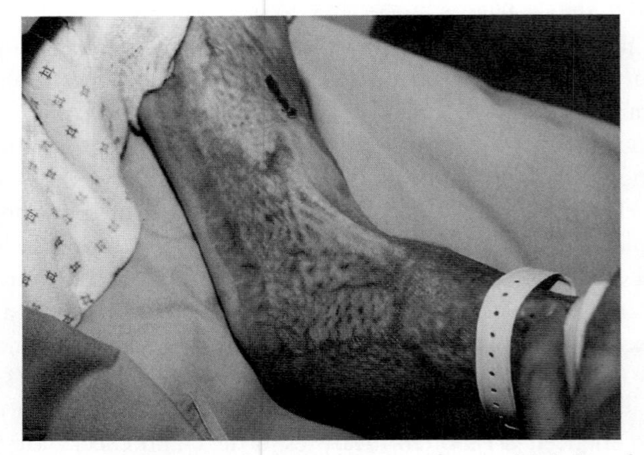

Figure 32-13 Example of scar contracture of antecubital skin of elbow. Note taut, shortened skin when elbow is extended.

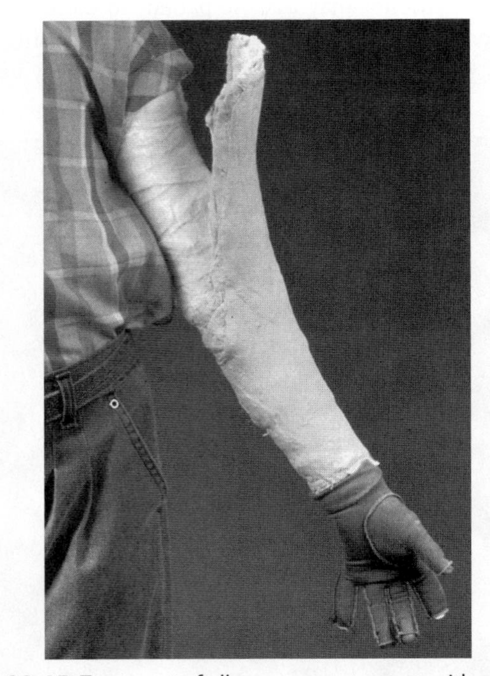

Figure 32-15 Treatment of elbow scar contracture with a serial fall-out elbow cast applied at maximum elbow extension at night blocks flexion and allows full, painless extension by morning when the cast is removed. After several weeks, contracture does not re-form and the cast is discontinued.

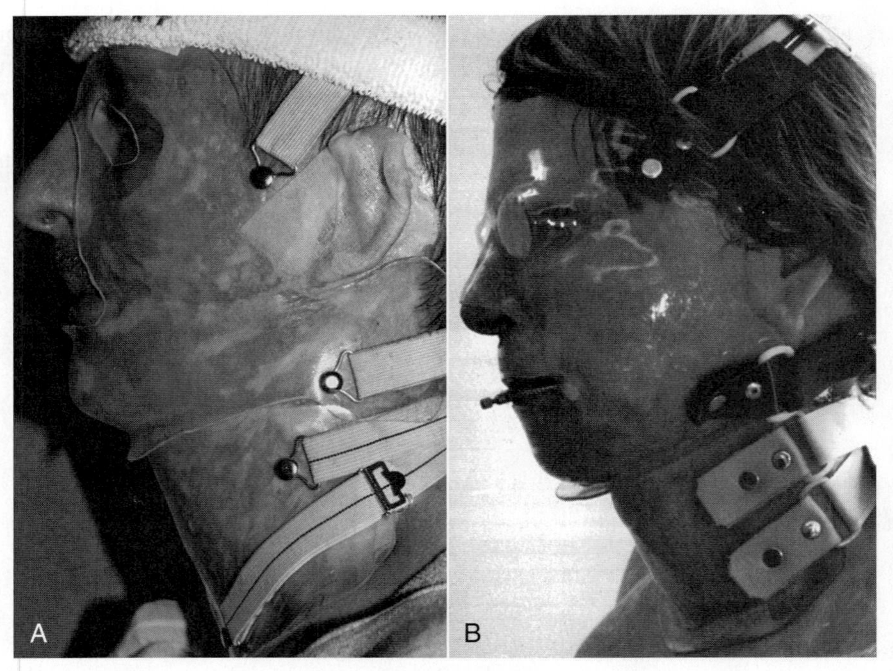

Figure 32-14 Transparent facial orthosis and neck orthosis. **A,** Day facial and neck orthoses fitted to blanch or turn raised scar tissue white. **B,** Night face and neck orthoses with humidity domes for eyes and microstomia prevention appliance for mouth stretch.

is replaced as soon as possible by participation in health clubs, swimming, gymnastic or sports programs, general home management, and work activity.

In the outdoor environment, special techniques are necessary to protect the patient. The OTA gives the following suggestions to avoid injuries from sun exposure: wear light-colored, lightweight, nonrestrictive clothing, sandal shoes, and a cool flap hat or wide-brimmed hat; use a battery fan and spray bottle to increase evaporative cooling; wear sunglasses; drink more fluids; avoid vasoconstricting drugs such as cigarettes; work in a shaded area; and apply sunscreen. Unprotected sun exposure results in blotchy, unpredictable tanning. If pigment is absent in the healed wound, severe tissue damage can result from sun exposure.

A healed wound has increased sensitivity to cold because of a changed ability to sweat and constrict or dilate capillaries in the scar tissue. If the patient lives in a cold climate, the OTA gives these general safety recommendations: keep vehicles well maintained; have a cell phone; keep blankets, extra mittens (not gloves), warm clothing/boots, candles, and snacks in the vehicle; wear insulated, waterproof boots; use safety shoes with fiberglass toe and shank if approved by employer; wear hats or an insulated hood and multiple-layer, nonrestrictive clothing made of wind-resistant fabric (see Figure 32-10); and avoid vasodilating drugs such as alcohol or vasoconstricting drugs such as cigarettes.

Many burn centers offer school reentry programs for children that educate teachers and students about burn injuries and explain the purpose of compression garments, splints, exercise, and care of the skin.[5] The program goals are to prevent unnecessary restrictions to the child's activities, decrease teasing and bullying, ensure splint and exercise assistance, remind schoolmates that the burned child is the same as before on the inside, and ease the transition back to school.[5]

Patient and family collaboration and motivation promote successful outcomes. For example, Lauren Manning survived a more than 82% burn from a fireball that escaped the elevator of One World Trade Center on September 11, 2001. Three months later she walked out of New York Presbyterian Hospital to begin a 3-month stay in Burke Rehabilitation Center. She then returned to life at home with her young son and husband. Her heroism is remarkable. She benefited from her own personal strength and committed family, community, and professional support. Her recovery is recorded in her husband's e-mails to their family.[33]

Olympic achievement and the support of Fidel Castro were incentives for the 1996 Cuban 800-meter silver medalist Ana Quirot to recover full function after a 40% TBSA full-thickness burn of the face, neck, and upper torso from a cooking fire. Cliff Meidl is an inspiring American example of the triumph of the human spirit over burn injury. Three heart attacks, two toe amputations, loss of the use of both knees, and a severe burn from a 30,000-volt electrical injury during construction work sidelined the former soccer player. His doctor reconstructed his legs with a muscle transplant. Then he said, "Now you do your 50%. Go for it and try to prove us wrong. Try to walk." This was something Meidl and the doctors thought he would never do. "Someone told me winners never quit and quitters never win, and that there's no such thing as an overachiever or underestimator," Meidl said. "I lived by that philosophy and used it a lot as a crutch because there's lots of dips and turns along the road." He was selected for the 1996 U.S. Olympic team in the four-man flatwater kayak 1000-meter event.

CASE STUDY

Sample Burn Treatment Plan, Mr. J.

Personal Data

Name: Mr. J.
Age: 36
Religion: Native American who uses healing stones
Diagnosis: Partial-thickness and full-thickness burn; 20% TBSA involving right arm and hand, right anterior axillary fold, chest, neck, and face
Mechanism of injury: Carburetor backfired while he was examining it and clothing caught fire
Marital status: Recently married, planning to have children
Employer: Northwest Airlines
Job duties: Computer design, drafting, onsite management of building construction
Education: College degree
Wife's employer: Hospital-laboratory technician
Insurance: Both covered by Mr. J.'s insurance
Financial status: Both incomes needed for mortgage payments and remodeling of new home
Recreational hobbies: Spectator sports, motorcycle riding and repair, home renovations
Dominant hand: Right
Length of stay: 21 days
Grafts: STSG meshed to right hand, sheet STSG to face
See the OT Evaluation Summary that follows for details of the evaluation and treatment plan. Based on the summary of the acute care and OT treatment plan, assess OT treatment changes in surgical and rehabilitative stages of care.

Follow-Up Care

Mr. and Mrs. J., the OTA, and the occupational therapist collaborate to update the treatment plan and revise the face mask fit every 2 weeks for a minimum of 2 months. If scar activity is stabilized and the patient independently evaluates scar control, therapy visits are reduced to once a month with the scheduled clinic time until the patient is discharged from all follow-up care.

Continued

CASE STUDY—cont'd

OT Evaluation Summary

Acute Care Phase	*Current Status*	*Short-Term (1-Week) Goals (Including Education)*
UE, LE, face, trunk function	ROM—eyelids do not close when asleep	Close eyelids tightly 3 to 5 times each hour from 6 AM to 11 PM to elongate contracting upper and lower lids, so he avoids corneal scratches or edema, keeps the ability to see, read and do vocational and avocational activities.
ROM	Mouth has increased from small to medium size microstomia prevention appliance (MPA)	Increase mouth stretches to 6 cc tube by next week so that he can eat normal foods and safely be intubated for general anesthesia.
Strength	Shoulder flexion and abduction limited to 0-150 degrees; elbow flexion limited to 10-90 degrees	Improve wound healing by keeping right UE flexible and participating more vigorously in active ROM in all joints burned within limits of pain, endotracheal tube, and intravenous lines to improve wound healing and assist return to work activities.
Sensation	Right wrist extension decreased—unable to extend wrist actively past neutral, approximately 20-degree wrist extension after 20 minutes of prolonged stretch	Four times daily, reach for bed traction bar above head with both hands, hold stretch, count to 15, exaggerate extension to prepare for self-feeding.
Mobility	Supination limited 20 degrees actively and 60 degrees passively bilaterally	As soon as vent discontinued, use BTE in rehabilitation clinic and soft foam gripper increasing to rubber band exerciser when IPs closed so that he can use hands for driving.
	Hand function—active ROM: MCPs 0-45 degrees, PIPs 15-30 degrees, DIP 0 degrees	
	Unwilling to do prolonged stretch independently because of pain and medication sleepiness	
	When cued, does relaxation breathing before exercise	
	Increased sensitivity to touch and co-contraction from pain in past week	Remember to use overhead walker for ambulating.
		Learn quad sets and ankle pumps to use when grafted.
	Distraction from pain, irritation from nasogastric feeding tube, coughing up secretions	Discuss pain and distraction with surgeon and psychologist, use recommendations, and share information with therapist.
	Needs cueing for each exercise	
	Since off ventilator, ambulates to chair independently and forgets tall walker	
	Good functional strength	
Positioning and edema management	Positioning—no head pillow because of face and neck burns, elevated head of bed; shoulders at 90 degrees forward flexion in chair, at 90-degree abduction in bed (using bedside table to support end of wedge); elbow extension; forearm in neutral; hands slightly elevated	Keep injured areas elevated. Use wedges or airplane bed attachment at all times.
Foam wedge		Change position every 2 hours when awake by elevating head of bed, flexing knees, turning, and when off vent dangling; sitting, standing, or walking.
Traction	Pillow behind neck when in chair to allow neck extension when sitting	Be able to state importance of using tall walker for edema control when ambulating.
		Beginning middle of week, when off vent, independently direct elevation and move furniture to achieve elevated positioning for arms and, if needed, legs.
		Review positioning with OTA each afternoon.
Orthotics	Wears large or extra-large MPA	Keep MPA in mouth all night and loosen (not remove) to avoid discomfort of insertion and removal. Change to wearing 5-30 minutes of each waking hour as soon as tolerated.
Splints	Uses Exudry pad or equivalent neck dressing to improve neck contours	
Casts		
Support garments	Wears wrist-hand-finger orthosis in IP extension, MP flexion, wrist 30-degree extension, thumb abduction/flexion secured with Kerlix coarse mesh gauze wrap at bedtime	Remember to ask for wrist-hand-finger orthosis at bedtime.
	Wears elastic wraps on legs during day	Remove leg elastic wraps at bedtime as soon as tolerated.

CASE STUDY—cont'd

Acute Care Phase	*Current Status*	*Short-Term (1-Week) Goals (Including Education)*
Daily living skills (evaluation done by OTA and occupational therapist)	Unable to pick up anything because of open fingertips Uses elastic wrap or tape on comb, toothbrush, fiber pen, spoon and fork for eating because of hand edema Needs assistance bathing Cannot apply lotion to dry lips before eating or moisturize healed areas yet Can remove elastic wraps with help Cannot don own clothing because of too much wound drainage, tube feeding supplements, and gas pains causing clothing to be temporarily too tight around waist	Operate nurse call button with foot or arm by middle of week. Independently eat, brush teeth, comb hair, sign forms, and clean glasses by end of week using gross grasp. Family will bring large jogging shorts and shirt. Slip on shoes after grafting.
Patient and family involvement with therapy	Given outpatient instruction book for education in anticipated course of wound, graft, and donor healing Home therapy program and education reviewed with wife and parents on several occasions Written exercise program being followed by patient-still needs maximum help from therapist at this point, facial and hand edema interfere, groggy from medications, and does not remember exercises from one session to the other Works with vigor and is cooperative during therapy sessions when analgesia effective Wears healing stones	Family will begin to learn active ROM exercise program for face, neck, UEs and follow through in the evening with patient. Work on memory, negotiation, and teamwork during therapy. Take responsibility to inform others of desires and wishes. Family will follow through with patient's independent exercises and therapy program. Change Velcro healing stone pocket as needed.
Equipment		Use foam wedge, overhead walker, foam tape, and large handles temporarily for utensils.

Summary

Advances in burn care continue to improve burn injury outcomes. Today, most patients recovering from a burn injury can expect to return to a near-normal life including early return to school or work. The American Burn Association[1] (ABA) Guidelines for the Operation of Burn Centers do not specify a particular patient-to-therapist ratio, only that there must be one full-time equivalent burn therapist (either an occupational or physical therapist) assigned to the burn center. The guidelines further specify that staffing must be based on patient activity but do not specify ratios or acuity considerations. Some burn centers have developed their own frequency of therapy guidelines.[4]

The occupational therapist and OTA provide exercise, ADL, IADL, skin-conditioning activities, positioning techniques, splints, casts,[1] patient education, vascular support, and compression garments. Reassessment of patient needs and function throughout recovery promotes effective and economical treatment progression.

Burn scars last forever, but they can be modified somewhat by plastic surgery or camouflage make-up. Three-fourths of burn injuries could have been prevented. Thoughtful OTAs incorporate burn prevention when they do therapy with the frail, the elderly,[52] the socioeconomically burdened, or risk-taking youth who have immature judgment. The American Burn Association and local fire fighting departments provide free prevention materials.

Selected Reading Guide Questions

1. What are the two layers of the skin?
2. Why may a patient need temporary adaptations for self-care during the acute care phase?
3. What is the primary objective for positioning during acute care?
4. Why are patients immobilized postoperatively?
5. How soon after grafting can gentle, active ROM be resumed?

6. How soon after grafting should an intermediate garment or support dressing be applied?
7. Why are skin-conditioning activities used in burn rehabilitation? Name two examples of skin-conditioning techniques.
8. When a splint is ordered in the acute phase, what is the preferred wearing schedule? Why?
9. What is the primary cause of dysfunction after a burn injury?
10. Which points should be covered in a home program?
11. What are possible causes of limitations in ADL during the rehabilitation phase?
12. How does a patient recover work skills?
13. Are splints always used during the rehabilitation care phase?
14. Name three interventions to prevent sunburn.
15. When should patient education about burn injury and rehabilitation begin?

References

1. American Burn Association: *Burn care resources in North America* (800):548–2876, 2007.
2. Atiyeh BS, Gunn SW, Hayek SN: State of the art in burn treatment, *World J Surg* 29:131–148, 2005.
3. Baker CP, Russell WJ, Meyer W 3rd, Blakeney P: Physical and psychologic rehabilitation outcomes for young adults burned as children, *Arch Phys Med Rehabil* 88:S57–S64, 2007.
4. Bailes AF, Reder R, Burch C: Development of guidelines for determining frequency of therapy services in a pediatric medical setting, *Pediatr Phys Ther* 20:194–198, 2008.
5. Blakeney P, Moore P, Meyer W III, et al: Efficacy of school reentry programs, *J Burn Care Rehabil* 16:469–472, 1995.
6. Celis MM, Suman OE, Huang TT, Yen P, Herndon DN: Effect of a supervised exercise and physiotherapy program on surgical interventions in children with thermal injury, *J Burn Care Rehabil* 24:57–61, 2003.
7. Chapman TT, Richard RL, Hedman TL, et al: Combat casualty hand burns: evaluating impairment and disability during recovery, *J Hand Ther* 21:150–158, 2008.
8. de Lateur BJ, Magyar-Russell G, Bresnick MG, et al: Augmented exercise in the treatment of deconditioning from major burn injury, *Arch Phys Med Rehabil* 88:S18–S23, 2007.
9. Ehde DM, Patterson DR, Wiechman SA, et al: Post-traumatic stress symptoms and distress 1 year after burn injury, *J Burn Care Rehabil* 21(2):105–111, 2000.
10. Esselman PC, Thombs BD, Magyar-Russell G, Fauerbach JA: Burn rehabilitation: state of the science, *Am J Phys Med Rehabil* 85:383–413, 2006.
11. Fakhry SM, Alexander J, Smith D, et al: Regional and institutional variation in burn care, *J Burn Care Rehabil* 16:86–90, 1995.
12. Falkel JE: Anatomy and physiology of the skin. In Richard RL, Staley MJ, editors: *Burn care and rehabilitation principles and practice*, Philadelphia, 1994, FA Davis.
13. Ferguson JS, Franco J, Pollack J, et al: Compression neuropathy: a late finding in the postburn population: a four-year institutional review, *J Burn Care Res* 31(3):458–461, 2010.
14. Field T, Peck M, Hernandez-Reif M, et al: Postburn itching, pain, and psychological symptoms are reduced with massage therapy, *J Burn Care Rehabil* 21(3):189–193, 2000.
15. Fricke N, Omnell M, Dutcher K, et al: Skeletal and dental disturbances in children after facial burns and pressure garment use: a 4-year follow-up, *J Burn Care Rehabil* 20(3):239–249, 1999.
16. Gibran NS: Practice guidelines for burn care, 2006, *J Burn Care Res* 27:437–438, 2006.
17. Glass TM, Bruns MM: *Exercises for pediatric burn therapy*, San Antonio, 2000, Therapy Skill Builders.
18. Harris S, Harris J: The skin, *Permachart Quick Reference Guide, Papertech, Inc*, 1999. (1-800-387-3626).
19. Helm PA: The status of burn rehabilitation services in the United States: results of a national survey, *J Burn Care Rehabil* 13(6):656–662, 1993.
20. Helm P, Herndon DN, Delateur B: Restoration of function, *J Burn Care Res* 28:611–614, 2007.
21. Hoffman HG, Doctor JN, Patterson DR, et al: Virtual reality as an adjunctive pain control during burn wound care in adolescent patients, *Pain* 85(1-2):305–309, 2000.
22. Holavanahalli R, Cromes G, Kowalske K, Helm P: Factors predicting satisfaction with life over time in patients following a major burn injury, *J Burn Care Rehabil* 21:S139, 2000.
23. Iles RL: *Wound care: the skin*, Kansas City, MO, 1988, Marion Laboratories.
24. Johnson C: Pathologic manifestations of burn injury. In Richard RL, Staley MJ, editors: *Burn care and rehabilitation principles and practice*, Philadelphia, 1994, FA Davis.
25. Kowalske K, Holavanahalli R, Serghiou M, et al: Contractures following burn injuries in children and adults - a multicenter report, *J Burn Care Rehabil* 24:S85, 2003.
26. Kramer G, Lund T, Beckum O: Pathophysiology of burn shock and burn edema. In Herndon D, editor: *Total burn care*, ed 2, London, 2007, WB Saunders, pp 93–118.
27. Kurtz L: Creating productivity standards, *OT Pract* 26–30, May 1999.
28. Laubenthal KN, Lewis RW, et al: Prospective randomized study of the effect of pressure garment therapy on pain and pruritus in the maturing burn wound, *Proc Am Burn Assoc* 28:161, 1996.
29. Leman CJ, et al: Exercise physiology in the acute burn patient: do we really know what we're doing? *Proc Am Burn Assoc* 24:91, 1992.
30. Leslie G, et al: Native Americans: a challenge for the pediatric burn team (poster), *Proc Am Burn Assoc* 28:147, 1996.
31. Leung KS, Cheng JC, Ma GF, et al: Complications of pressure therapy for post-burn hypertrophic scars: biochemical analysis based on 5 patients, *Burns* 10(6):434–438, 1984.
32. Lund C, Browder N: The estimation of area of burns, *Surg Gynecol Obstet* 79:352–355, 1944.
33. Manning G: *Love, Greg & Lauren*, New York, 2002, Bantam Books.
34. Nahieli O, et al: Oromaxillofacial skeletal deformities resulting from burn scar contractures of the face and neck, *Burns* 27(1):65–69, 1995.
35. Neugebauer CT, Serghiou M, Herndon D, Suman OE: Effects of a 12-week rehabilitation program with music and exercise groups on range of motion in young children with severe burns, *J Burn Care Res* 29:939–948, 2009.
36. Pain management of the burn patient, *J Burn Care Rehabil* 16(3):343–376, 1995.
37. Parry I, Doyle B, Mollineaux C, et al: Foot drop in children with burn injury, *J Burn Care Rehabil* 24:S100, 2003.
38. Reeves SU: Adaptive strategies after severe burns. In Christiansen CH, Matuska KM, editors: *Ways of living, adaptive strategies for special needs*, ed 3, Bethesda, Md, 2004, AOTA Press.

39. Richard R, et al: Algorithm to guide burn patient treatment by physical therapist assistants (PTAs), *Poster Proc Am Burn Assoc* 28:160, 1996.
40. Richard R, Baryza MJ, Carr JA, et al: Burn rehabilitation and research: proceedings of a consensus summit, *J Burn Care Res* 30(4):543–573, 2009.
41. Richard R, Ward RS: Splinting strategies and controversies, *J Burn Care Rehabil* 26:392–396, 2005.
42. Ricks N, Meager D: The benefits of plaster casting for lower extremity burns after grafting in children, *J Burn Care Rehabil* 13(4):465–468, 1992.
43. Robertson CF, Zuker R, Dabrowksi B, Levison H: Obstructive sleep apnea: a complication of burns to the head and neck in children, *J Burn Care Rehabil* 6(4):353–357, 1985.
44. Schneider JC, Holavanahalli R, Helm P, et al: Contractures in burn injury part 2: investigating joints of the hand, *J Burn Care Res* 29:606–613, 2008.
45. Schneider JC, Holavanahalli R, Helm P, et al: Contractures in burn injury: defining the problem, *J Burn Care Res* 27:508–514, 2006.
46. Serghiou M, Ott S, Farmer S, et al: Comprehensive rehabilitation of the burned patient. In Herndon D, editor: *Total burn care*, ed 3, Philadelphia, 2007, Elsevier, pp 620–651.
47. Sheridan R, Hinson MI, Liang MH, et al: Long-term outcome of children surviving massive burns, *JAMA* 283(1):69–73, 2000.
48. Sheridan R, Weber J, Prelack K, et al: Early burn center transfer shortens the length of hospitalization and reduces complications in children with serious burn injuries, *J Burn Care Rehabil* 20(5):347–350, 1999.
49. Simons M, King S, Edgar D: Occupational therapy and physiotherapy for the patient with burns: principles and management guidelines, *J Burn Care Rehabil* 24:323–335, 2003.
50. Sorenson W, Fisher S, Rivers E: Burn rehabilitation. In O'Young BJ, Yong MA, Steins SA, editors: *Physical medicine and rehabilitation secrets*, Philadelphia, 2001, Hanley & Belfus.
51. Staley M, Serghiou M: Casting guidelines, tips, and techniques: proceedings from the 1997 American Burn Association PT/OT Casting Workshop, *J Burn Care Rehabil* 19(3):254–260, 1998. discussion 253.
52. Still JM, Law EJ, Belcher K, et al: A regional medical center's experience with burns of the elderly, *J Burn Care Rehabil* 20(3):218–223, 1999.
53. Suman OE, Herndon DN: Effects of cessation of a structured and supervised exercise conditioning program on lean mass and muscle strength in severely burned children, *Arch Phys Med Rehabil* 88:S24–S29, 2007.
54. Sungur N, Ulusoy MG, Boyacgil S, et al: Kirschner-wire fixation for postburn flexion contracture deformity and consequences on articular surface, *Ann Plast Surg* 56:128–132, 2006.
55. Supple KG: Handle with care, *Adv Phys Ther Rehab Med* 16(23):60–63, 2010.
56. Tredget E, Anzarut A, Shankowsky H, Logsetty S: Outcome and quality of life of massive burn injury: the impact of modern burn care, *J Burn Care Rehabil* 23:S95, 2002.
57. Ward RS: Pressure therapy for the control of hypertrophic scar formation after burn injury: a history and review, *J Burn Care Rehabil* 12(3):257–262, 1991.
58. Wolfram D, Tzankov A, Pulzi P, Katzer H: Hypertrophic scars and keloids—a review of their pathophysiology, risk factors, and therapeutic management, *Am Soc Dermatol Surg* 35:171–181, 2009.
59. Yohannan SK, Schwabe E, et al: The Wii gaming system for rehabilitation of an adult with lower extremity burns: a case report. Proceedings from the 2009 American Burn Association, *J Burn Care Rehab* 43:S65, 2009.
60. Zuther J: *Compression bandages. Lymphedema management: the comprehensive guide for practitioners*, New York, 2005, Thieme Medical Publishers. pp 113–114.

Recommended Reading

Richard RL, Staley MJ, editors: *Burn care and rehabilitation principles and practice*, Philadelphia, 1994, FA Davis.
Herndon D, editor: *Total burn care*, ed 3, Philadelphia, 2007, Elsevier.
Richard R, Chapman T, Dougherty M, et al: *An atlas and compendium of burn splints*, San Antonio, 2005, Splint Atlas.

Resources for Custom-Made Garments

Barton Carey
P.O. Box 421
Perrysburg, OH 43552
(800) 421-0444

Bio-Concepts
2424 E. University Dr.
Phoenix, AZ 85034
(800) 421-5647

Resources for Overlay and Insert Materials

Liquid Silicone
any splint supply catalog

Silon Woundcare Products
Bio Med Sciences
7584 Morris Court, Suite 218
Allentown, PA 18106
(800) 257-4566

Internet Websites and Blogs

http://www.burntherapist.com/QuarterlySplints.htm

www.healthgamesresearch.org (Robert Wood Johnson Foundation, Pioneer Portfolio)

www.humanagames.com

www.games4rehab.com

http://www.wiihabilitation.org/

www.wiihabilitation.co.uk/resources.shtml

http://www.ipaconed.com/

CHAPTER 33

Amputation and Prosthetics

EUGENIA PAPDAPOULOS AND **BETH DEVERIX**

Key Terms

Transhumeral
Transradial (below-elbow) amputation (BE)
Phantom pain
Cosmesis
Mechanical prosthesis
Terminal devices (TDs)
Socket
Myoelectric prosthesis
Electrode
Early postoperative prosthesis
Transfemoral (above-knee) amputations (AKAs)
Transtibial (below-knee) amputations (BKAs)
Syme's amputation
Rigid removal dressing
SACH foot
Pylon
C-leg
Ischial weight-bearing prosthesis

Chapter Objectives

After studying this chapter, the student or practitioner will be able to do the following:

1. Appreciate the role of occupational therapy within the context of the rehabilitation team.
2. Understand the relationship between levels of amputation and the function of the amputee.
3. Appreciate the importance of maximizing the amputee's skill with prosthetics.
4. Understand why recovery can be slow and physically draining for the patient and family.
5. Teach new methods for basic and advanced activities of daily living with prosthetics.

The vast majority of people who undergo amputations do not know what to expect when they come to the medical center. This traumatic crisis will affect both the family and the patient. A successful rehabilitation program requires the coordinated efforts of the rehabilitation team. This chapter addresses teamwork, surgical management, psychological adjustment, levels of losses in upper and lower extremities (UEs and LEs), mechanical and myoelectric prostheses, and treatment planning.

The chapter also addresses the ongoing collaboration between the occupational therapist and occupational therapy assistant (OTA) in amputation and prosthetics programs.

Team Members

The rehabilitation of the individual with limb loss requires the skills of many health care professionals: general or vascular surgeon, orthopedic surgeon, plastic surgeon, physiatrist, prosthetist, occupational therapist and OTA, physical therapist, social worker, psychologist, pastoral counselor (spiritual guidance), and vocational counselor. Ideally these health care specialists function together as an integrated team.

Successful amputee rehabilitation programs focus on individual needs, development of new surgical techniques, improvements in technology, and a better understanding of the psychosocial implications of limb loss.

Congenital and Acquired Amputations

Incidence and Cause

The cause of limb loss and associated medical conditions varies. Loss of a limb is generally divided into two broad categories: congenital and acquired.[19]

Congenital amputation is the absence of a limb or part at birth, usually the result of a defect in development.[23] The loss of part or all of an extremity as the direct result of trauma or by surgery is known as an *acquired amputation.*[19] This chapter discusses and focuses only on acquired amputations sustained in adulthood and will consider both UEs and LEs.

Acquired amputations result from surgery and trauma.[35] Surgical amputations of both UEs and LEs are performed in cases of severe infections or gangrene, to remove cancerous tumors, and in cases of severe injury in which extremities are not salvageable.

In 2005, 1.6 million persons were living with the loss of a limb in the United States. Thirty-eight percent of these people had an amputation due to dysvascular (diabetes-related) disease with a comorbidity of diabetes mellitus. It is estimated that 3.6 million people will have undergone limb amputation by the year 2050. If, however, the incidence of dysvascular disease can be reduced by 10%, this number would be lowered by 225,000.[39] Projected annual hospital costs for an estimated 158,000 people who undergo amputations are $4 billion.[25] Traumatic amputations are often results of motor vehicle accidents (MVAs), work-related injuries, recreational injuries, tumors, burns, electrical injuries, and war injuries. Rates for trauma-related and cancer-related amputation declined by approximately 50% in the 20 years from 1984 to 2004.[22] In the LE, approximately 82% of all acquired amputations are related to diabetes or peripheral vascular disease, especially in the population aged 60 and older.[6a,7] The highest rates of dysvascular amputations occur in men and in African-Americans.[7]

Surgical amputation is a last resort after all conventional treatments have been tried. Conventional treatments include testing, medication adjustment, and therapy. When these treatments have not improved the medical situation, the physician will reassess the individual for intervention. If amputation is required, the physician will consult with the internist, neurologist, orthopedic and plastic surgeons, as necessary. The orthopedic surgeon will determine the level of the amputation by considering the potential for wound healing and optimal prosthetic fit and function. During the surgery, attention will be directed to the management of the various tissues involved, with an eye toward rehabilitation and prosthetic restoration. This process includes preserving length of the residual limb to improve prosthetic suspension and force transmission from the residual limb to the socket,[6a] beveling the ends of bones, sharp transaction of the nerves (which are allowed to retract into proximal soft tissues so that they do not adhere to the scar or remain in a location where they might be traumatized by a prosthesis), appropriate myofascial closure of muscle or myodesis to provide good control of the remaining bone in the residual limb, and appropriate placement of skin incision line(s) to avoid bony prominences and prevent adherence of skin to the underlying bone.[9] Such attention to detail results in a well-shaped residual limb that can be fitted with a prosthesis, thus permitting maximum prosthetic function. During and after medical and surgical interventions, the team members try to facilitate the psychosocial adjustment of the patient and family members.

Psychological Adjustment

Responses to UE and LE amputations have often been compared with the grieving process. The amputee experiences identifiable stages of denial, anger, depression, coping, and acceptance.[10] Some individuals will progress through these stages and ultimately adapt to the loss. The cause of the amputation may contribute significantly to the individual's response. Factors associated with positive psychosocial adjustment to the amputation are: the individual's disposition toward optimism, the individual's active coping mechanisms, the quality of the social support systems available, controllable pain levels, a good prosthetic fit, and the comprehensive care provided by the team.

It is common for a new amputee to experience depression and anxiety for up to two years post-amputation. Other psychosocial challenges experienced by the amputee are social discomfort (adjusting to the fact they appear different from other people) and body-image anxiety (adapting to a changed body image) resulting from activity restriction, depression, and anxiety.[12]

Postoperative Complications

The following conditions may occur in upper and lower limbs after amputation.

Neuromas

A neuroma is a bulbous benign tumor that may develop at the proximal end of a severed nerve. It is generally made up of nerve fibers and Schwann cells.

Phantom Sensation

Phantom sensation is present when the amputee feels sensations coming from the amputated limb. Phantom sensation is experienced by the majority of traumatic amputees and to a lesser degree in congenital amputees. Sensations that are felt in the amputated limb include numbness, tingling, temperature changes, pressure, itching, and muscle cramps. Some amputees feel as though the amputated limb moves on its own or as if they can control its movement. For new lower extremity amputees, the phantom sensation can feel so real that they may try to stand up and walk again. Phantom sensation endures differently for each individual. For some, it may last for a few months; for others, it may diminish in intensity, but may linger for many years.[8,36]

Phantom Limb Pain

Phantom limb pain is the unpleasant sensation of burning and shooting pain as well as a squeezing sensation in the part that was amputated. The medical community believes that phantom limb pain and phantom sensation result from abnormal sensory processing within the nervous system. Fortunately, phantom limb pain tends to improve with time.[8,36]

Contractures

A contracture is the shortening of ligaments and muscles which would otherwise allow for good motion of a joint. The joint above the amputation site typically develops a contracture if full range of motion is not initiated immediately after the amputation. Contractures frequently occur when the patient keeps the extremity in a flexed position for comfort. This is a significant complication that will interfere with prosthetic fitting and training, as significant joint stiffness and loss of range of motion occurs.

Weakness

Prolonged muscle inactivity leads to weakness. The individual is encouraged to get out of bed and move around as soon as possible. Generally the amputee will be up the day after surgery. The longer the amputee stays in bed, the longer it will take to recover, and more complications may ensue.

Skin Breakdown

This condition is mainly caused by excess pressure. Poor blood supply from lack of mobility might also cause breakdown; decreased sensation leading to poor awareness is another cause. Skin breakdown may be avoided by instructing the patient to frequently check his or her skin.

Upper Extremity Amputations

Role of the Occupational Therapy Assistant

UE amputee training is a specialized area of treatment. A program is usually directed by a skilled and experienced senior clinician. Under guidelines established by the American Occupational Therapy Association (AOTA), the occupational therapist would complete the evaluation and prosthetic checkout and establish the goals and treatment plan. Under close supervision the OTA may implement a program for the patient with an amputation. Close supervision is essential because of the complex problems and degree of change commonly seen, which may require a modified treatment approach or reevaluation by the occupational therapist. The OTA is responsible for keeping the supervising therapist informed of all changes in patient performance and any other pertinent facts. As treatment progresses and changes are noted, the assistant may contribute suggestions for program modifications or additions that will help the patient reach the established goals. Communication and feedback between occupational therapist and OTA are the keys to a successful program.

Levels of Amputation

Levels of amputations of the UE are illustrated in Figure 33-1. A new system of classification adopted by professional organizations including the International Society for Prosthetics and Orthotics replaces the previous system.[31] Some terms are retained. Figure 33-1 shows the current terminology and includes the deleted terms in parentheses (see Figure 33-14 for the equivalent terms for the LE). The reader may still encounter the terms "above elbow" and "below elbow"; however, these have been replaced by "transhumeral" and "transradial," indicating the bone transected by the surgery.

Level of amputation significantly affects function. The higher (more proximal) the level of amputation, the greater the functional loss and the more the amputee must depend on the prosthesis for function and cosmesis (appearance). The higher-level amputations require more complex and extensive prostheses and prosthetic training. More complex prostheses can be more difficult to operate and use effectively.[33]

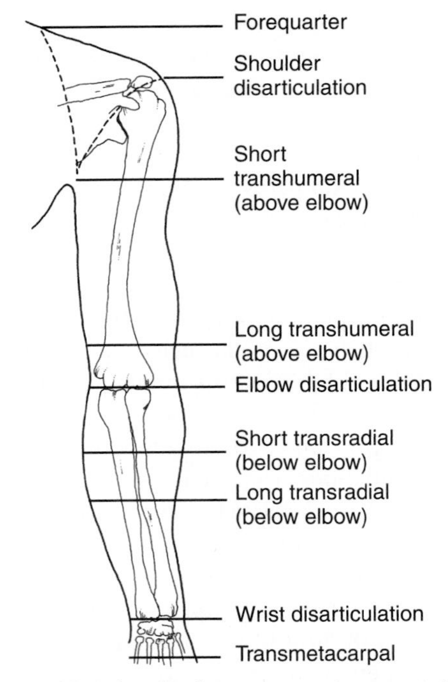

Figure 33-1 Levels of upper extremity amputation.

The shoulder forequarter and shoulder disarticulation (SD) amputations will result in the loss of all arm and hand functions. The short transhumeral amputation will result in the loss of all hand, wrist, and elbow functions and rotation of the shoulder. The long transhumeral and elbow disarticulation amputations will result in the loss of hand, wrist, and elbow functions, but good shoulder function will remain.

The short transradial amputation will result in loss of hand and wrist function, forearm pronation and supination, and reduction in the force of elbow flexion. Shoulder function will be intact and good. The long transradial amputation will result in loss of hand and wrist function and most forearm pronation and supination. Elbow function and force of elbow flexion will be good. The wrist disarticulation will result in complete loss of hand and wrist function; pronation and supination remain full.

Amputations across the metacarpal bones, are called transmetacarpal or partial hand amputations. Functions of all the unaffected joints of the arm are intact, and some hand function may be available, depending on whether the thumb was amputated or left intact.[5] Many types of prostheses are available for each level of amputation. Each prosthesis is individually prescribed according to the client's needs and lifestyle and is individually fitted and custom-made.[33]

Rehabilitation Philosophy

Current philosophy dictates that prosthetic fitting within the first 30 days of amputation is the most important element in achieving successful upper-limb amputation rehabilitation.[8,21] This 30-day period is termed "the golden period." At one time, the standard approach for providing a prosthetic device was to wait for complete wound healing and stump maturation, which might take 3 to 6 months. Waiting often resulted in late fitting of amputees and poor rehabilitation results. By the time amputees were fitted with a prosthetic device, they had become one-handed individuals who could see little use for an assistive prosthetic device. The multiple advantages to early prosthetic fit include the following:

- Decreased edema
- Decreased postoperative and phantom pain
- Accelerated wound healing
- Maintenance of two-handed function
- Decreased length of hospital stay
- Increased prosthetic use and acceptance
- Increased proprioceptive input through the residual limb
- Improved psychological adjustment
- Improved patient rehabilitation

Types of Prostheses

Prostheses are of two main types. Body-powered prostheses (mechanical) are cable-controlled, like the hook prosthesis. This type is most durable, requires gross limb movement, but is less cosmetically pleasing. The other option is the externally powered prosthesis. This type may be electrically powered, like the myoelectric prosthesis. External motor power may provide proximal function and greater grip strength. This type is more acceptable cosmetically, but can be heavy and expensive.

Component Parts of a Body-Powered/Mechanical Prosthesis (Proximal to Distal Components of the Prosthesis)

Stump Sock

A stump sock is worn over the residual limb. It absorbs perspiration and protects from discomfort or irritation that could result from direct contact of the skin with the socket of the prosthesis. It accommodates volume change in the stump and aids with fit and comfort of the stump in the socket.[33,38]

Harness

The purposes of the harness are to suspend the prosthesis and to anchor the control cables. The figure-eight harness is a common design, but others are available. Extra straps may be added to the figure-eight as needed. The higher the level of amputation, the more complex the harnessing system must be. Variations in available muscle power and ROM may necessitate variations in the harness design. A properly fitted harness is important for both comfort and function.

Cable and Components

The cable is made of stainless steel and is contained in a flexible stainless steel housing. It is fastened to the prosthesis by a retainer unit made of a base plate and a retainer butterfly or by a housing crossbar and a leather loop. A ball or ball swivel fitting at one end of the cable attaches it to the TD while a T-bar or hanger fittings at the other end attach it to the harness.[30,37]

Socket

The forearm socket for the transradial below-elbow (BE) amputee may be made of plastic resins or carbon graphite. The latter is lightweight, comfortable, and durable. The socket may have a single or double wall. The socket must be stable on the stump to allow the wearer full power and control of the prosthesis. The transradial stump socket may be constructed to allow any remaining pronation and supination to be used. The single wall socket is used when the outside diameter of the distal end of the stump is sufficient to permit tapering to the wrist unit. The double wall socket is used when the stump is too short or slender to achieve the desired contour or tapering. The inner wall conforms to the stump, and the outer wall gives the required length and contour for the forearm replacement. The socket must fit snugly and firmly but allow full ROM at the first available joint.

A recent technology considered experimental in the United States involves the use of osseo-integration. A suspension system connects the prosthesis directly to the bone via a titanium implant which is partially external. There is no need for a socket.[8]

Elbow Unit

The elbow unit on the transhumeral above-elbow (AE) prosthesis allows the maximal range of motion (ROM) possible and allows locking of the elbow in various degrees of motion as well as positioning of the prosthesis for arm rotation by a manual control friction turntable unit.

Wrist Unit

The wrist unit is usually selected for its ability to meet the needs of the amputee in daily living and vocational activities.[33] It orients the terminal device (TD) in the forearm socket and serves as a disconnecting unit so that TDs may be interchanged. Once positioned, the wrist unit is held in place by one of a number of lock options: friction lock, quick-disconnect, locking unit, or flexion unit.

- The friction lock slips on and is easy to position; however, this lock can easily slip off when heavy objects are carried.
- The quick-disconnect allows for easy changing of TDs that have specialized functions.
- A locking unit option is chosen when there is a need to prevent rotation during grasping and lifting.
- A wrist flexion unit allows for improved self-care functions in midline, such as shaving, buttoning, and perineal care. It is especially helpful for a bilateral UE amputee.

Terminal Devices

Current prosthetic devices cannot completely substitute for all of the functions of the hand, which is anatomically and physiologcially complex. All prostheses lack sensory feedback and provide only limited mobility and dexterity. Prosthetic hands provide three-jaw chuck pinch and hooks provide lateral pinch. Slip control is a recently-introduced technology that can improve prehension to prevent accidental dropping of objects.[8]

Two main categories of terminal devices (TDs) are available: passive, and active.

Passive TDs are designed primarily for cosmesis, do not have moveable parts, and do not have any function, other than to serve as a gross assist. The passive hand and mitt-shaped prostheses are examples of passive TDs. The passive hand is a cosmetically-pleasing and socially-acceptable hand that is positioned in a static grasp position. The mitt shape

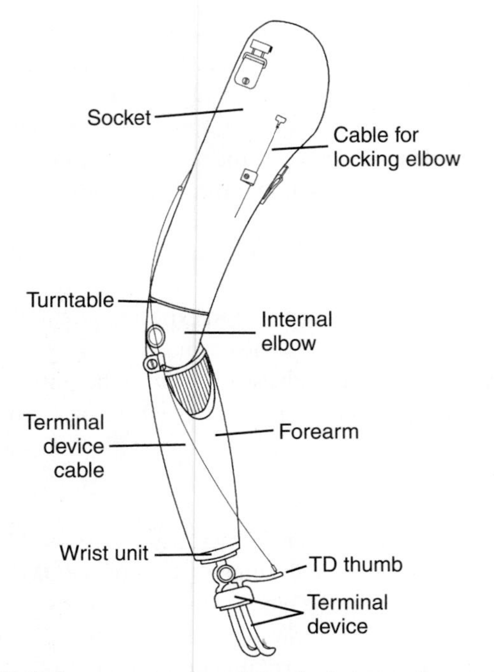

Figure 33-2 Component parts of standard above-elbow prosthesis. (Modified from Santschi W, editor: *Manual for upper extremity prosthetics,* ed 2, Los Angeles, 1958, University of California Press.)

is similar to a cupped hand and is recommended for infants. This TD may be used as a shock absorber in sports for younger children.

Active TDs are designed primarily for function and less so for cosmesis. The hook and the mechanical hand (Figure 33-2) are examples of active TDs. The hook TD may be made of aluminum or stainless steel alone or in combination with each other and with titanium. The hook may have canted or lyre-shaped fingers and usually has a neoprene or polyethylene gripping surface to protect grasped objects and prevent slippage. The hook is the most functional, durable, and most commonly prescribed and used TD. Several types of hooks are available to meet individual needs. The farmer's and carpenter's hooks make handling tools easier, and narrow-opening hooks may be used for handling fine objects.

On the hook TD, the number of rubber bands controls the amount of grasp pressure. Training usually begins with one rubber band, and the number increases to three to four rubber bands as training progresses. The mechanical hand is a functional hand that may be attached to the wrist unit and is activated by the same control cable that operates the hook. The fingers are controlled at the metacarpophalangeal (MCP) joints by the prosthesis control cable. The hand TD sacrifices grip force (2 lbs maximum) for improved cosmesis. A natural-looking plastic glove fits over the mechanical hand.[33]

Terminal devices are used to attempt to replicate 5 types of grip/prehension.

- Precision grip, which includes the pads of the thumb and index finger in opposition, providing the ability to pick up or pinch small objects.
- Tripod grip/3-jaw chuck pinch, in which the pad of the thumb is opposed to the index and middle finger
- Lateral grip/key pinch, in which the pad of the thumb is lateral to the index finger, which is employed in turning a key in a lock
- Hook power grip, where the distal and proximal interphalangeal joints are flexed, and the metacarpals are straight such as in holding a briefcase
- Spherical grip, in which the tips of all fingers are flexed, such as in opening a round doorknob.[8,17]

Materials and construction used in prosthetic components have greatly improved over the past several years. Recent developments include: lightweight socket fabrication materials (carbon graphite or high temperature flexible thermoplastics), custom-fitting techniques, suspension systems (such as osseo-integration), slip controls, power sources and electric controls.[8]

Component Parts of a Myoelectric Prosthesis

A myoelectric prosthesis is controlled by electrical signals from muscles. The first practical myoelectrically controlled prosthesis was demonstrated in 1948.[14] In the next several decades a considerable research effort followed; as a result, myoelectric prostheses have been improved so much that their clinical value is well established.[14] The concept of myoelectric control is simple: an electric signal from a muscle is used to control the flow of energy from a battery to a motor. The muscles in the residual limb produce the control signal by contracting through voluntary control. The motor is activated by the signal, and a prosthetic hand, wrist, or elbow is directed to move into action.

Socket/Suspension

Socket design is very important to the functional use of the myoelectric prosthesis. When the prosthetist is designing the socket for the patient, the following areas must be considered: (1) residual limb comfort; (2) overall cosmesis; (3) electrode contact; and (4) suspension style.

Residual limb comfort within the socket will often determine the wear and use pattern of the prosthesis. The socket must not compromise skin integrity by causing pressure points or pressing on sensitive areas of the residual limb. The amputee will not wear or use the device if it is not comfortable.

The same principle applies to the overall appearance of the prosthesis. To encourage the patient's acceptance, the prosthetic socket should be pleasing in skin tone, size, length, and muscle bulk. It is most essential that the socket design provide constant contact between the skin and the electrodes with very little movement of the arm within the socket. Without careful design and fit of electrode to muscle site contact, the operation of the prosthesis will be difficult (if not impossible), thus setting the patient up for failure.

Finally, the socket design determines the type of suspension to be used. For transradial (BE) amputees, self-suspension is always an option. This means the total elimination of a harness and its restriction of movement. In most cases the transhumeral (AE) amputee still requires a harness in addition to self-suspension to distribute the weight of the prosthesis. The type of suspension used should be determined by the length

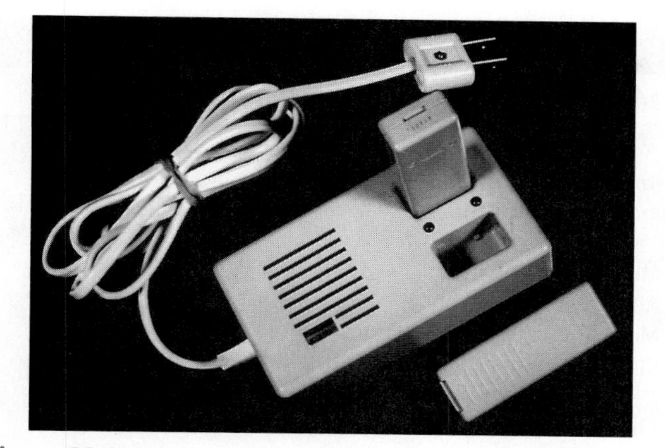

Figure 33-3 Battery of a myoelectric arm is inserted in a battery charger and charged overnight.

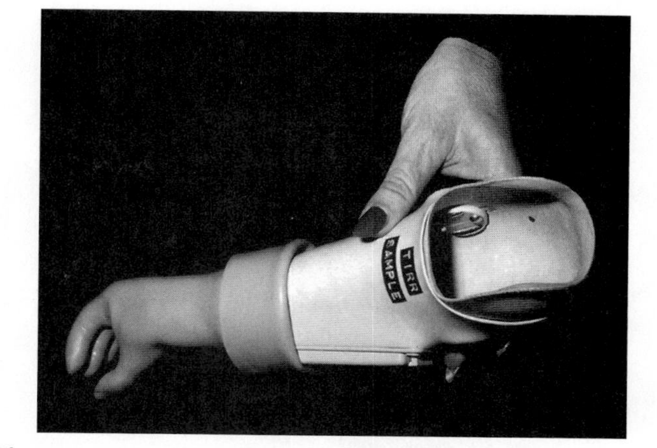

Figure 33-4 Surface electrodes recessed within the wall of a myoelectric socket detect muscle contractions.

of the residual limb, the patient's preference based on comfort and ease of prosthetic application and removal, and the prosthetic use pattern. The three types of suspension are the following: sleeve suspension, supracondylar suspension, and suprastyloid suspension.[4]

The prosthetist is the expert on the various socket suspensions available. However, the therapy practitioner must know the suspension options to assist the patient and the prosthetist in choosing one that will best meet the functional demands of the patient.

Battery

The battery (Figure 33-3) provides the energy from which the motor runs to operate the component parts of the prosthesis. A removable rechargeable 6-V lithium ion battery is used. The battery operates the prosthesis during the day and is recharged at night. The amputee may have several batteries to interchange as needed. The normal charge life of a battery varies from 6 hours to 24 hours of use, depending on the capacity and age of the battery. The capacity of these batteries to hold a charge will decrease in time, eventually requiring complete replacement of the battery approximately every 2 years, depending on the patient's use and on care patterns of the battery itself.[14] The battery is normally positioned at the surface of the prosthesis to allow for easy removal for charging. On the transradial prosthesis, the battery is located on the forearm; on the AE prosthesis, the battery is fitted at the elbow joint or is internal. The goal of the prosthetist in positioning the battery is two-fold–easy removal and good cosmetic appearance.

Electrodes

Surface electrodes (Figure 33-4) are mounted inside the socket at predetermined muscle sites that display strong myoelectric signals. Good electrical contact is the key to achieving a usable myoelectric prosthesis. The electrode reads the muscle activity and sends a message to the controller that moves the motor at the terminal device. For instance, for a transradial (BE) amputee, electrodes are placed on the wrist extensors and flexors. With normal movement, the flexors when activated would close the hand and the extensors would open the hand. In other words, when the electrodes read a signal from the flexors, the message would be sent to the motor. The hand would respond by closing. In the case of transhumeral (AE) amputation, the electrodes are placed on the triceps to open the hand and the biceps to close the hand. These sites are also used to send the signal to the elbow device, triggering elbow flexion from the biceps and elbow extension from the triceps.

Shoulder Unit

When a patient has a shoulder disarticulation or a forequarter amputation, a shoulder unit is used. It provides cosmesis for a symmetrical body appearance. Passive and friction components permit manual positioning of the shoulder but no active function.

Elbow Unit

Myoelectrically controlled elbow units are available for transhumeral (AE) amputees. The amputee with a high-level amputation requires an electric elbow because the force required to pull the mechanical prosthetic cable to operate a TD or mechanical elbow is too great for a short residual limb. Previously, prosthetic choices for these individuals were greatly limited. The development of the electric elbow has made it possible to restore upper-limb function to even the highest-level amputee. The motions of elbow flexion and extension are controlled by electrical signals from the muscle surface. When a muscle contracts, the muscle membrane generates an electric potential. The control unit senses, amplifies, and processes this potential. The same muscle sites used for hand control are used for elbow movement. Therefore no retraining of new muscle sites is needed. No large shoulder movements are required, only the natural contraction of the triceps and biceps. The elimination of awkward gross body movements allows more natural, smooth, body movements. The elbow has 21 available stopping positions within the range of 15 to 150 degrees of elbow flexion.[14] Currently, the elbow unit can perform only flexion and extension movement patterns through myoelectric control. A passive humeral rotation joint provides side-to-side positioning of the forearm. The elbow, when locked, can

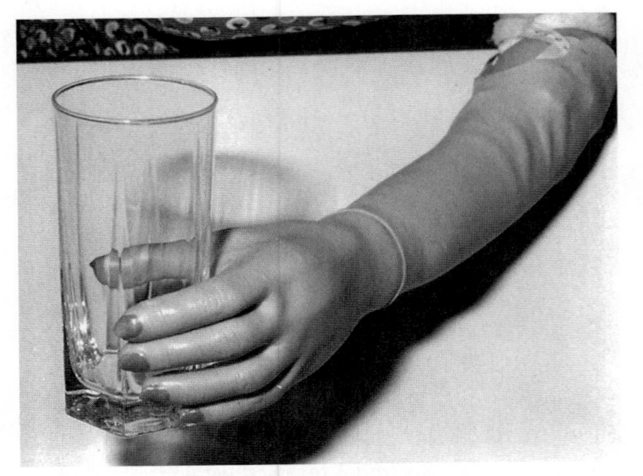

Figure 33-5 Myoelectric hand.

sustain a maximum load of 50 pounds and a live-lift of 2 pounds (when unit is not locked).[14] A common complaint about the electric elbow is its weight. The elbow unit itself adds 2 pounds of weight to the prosthesis, with an additional I pound for the electric hand. The finished product usually weighs a total of 3 to 4 pounds. However, the amputee who develops competence in operating the unit usually finds that its function more than compensates for the initial discomfort.

Wrist Unit

The following are the available wrist unit options: (1) passive friction wrist; (2) quick disconnect wrist; (3) flexion wrist; and (4) electric wrist rotator.

The quick disconnect wrist is the most commonly used wrist component in a myoelectric prosthesis. Several reasons for this are that (1) manually positioning the wrist is faster than waiting for a myoelectric signal to activate a motor to turn a component; (2) it eliminates an additional movement that would have to be incorporated into the amputee's repertoire for prosthetic movement; and (3) it provides for easy exchange of TDs.

Terminal Devices

Most myoelectric prostheses use an electric hand as a terminal device (Figure 33-5). They are available in various sizes to fit small children to adults. A latex glove covers the mechanism and is made to look as similar to the sound hand as possible, with skin tone choices and male or female features. The hand offers a simple open/close function. No individual finger movements are available, and there is no gradation of grip force. However, the hand opens at varying widths to provide for grasp of small objects such as a piece of paper or large objects such as a can of soda. The grip is strong (25 lbs of force). Adults who are active and perform heavy upper-body activities may use a Greiffer TD for heavy work in industry or farming; it provides quick handling and precise manipulation of small objects. Features of the Greiffer include a 38-lb grasp, parallel gripping surfaces, and a flexion joint for dorsal and volar wrist flexion.[29] Endless accessories are available for specific activities, such as sports, unusual work tasks, and leisure activities. The prosthetist is a good resource for these specialized TDs.

Box 33-1

Advantages and Disadvantages of Myoelectric Prostheses

Advantages

- Improved cosmesis
- Increased grip force (approximately 25 lb in an adult myoelectric hand)
- Minimal or no harnessing
- Ability to use overhead
- Minimal effort needed to control device
- Closely corresponds to human physiological control

Disadvantages

- Cost of prosthesis
- Frequency of maintenance and repair
- Fragile nature of glove and need for frequent replacements
- Absence of sensory feedback (some sense of proprioceptive feedback provided in a *body-powered* prosthesis)
- Slow response of electric hand
- Increased weight

Mechanical versus Myoelectric Prostheses

Many positive and negative aspects influence decisions concerning mechanical and myoelectric prostheses (Box 33-1). The best solution for an amputee is to have both prosthetic devices available to meet the changing demands of specific activities. An amputee may use the mechanical prosthesis when he is working on a car, but later that day he might wear the myoelectric prosthesis to go out with his friends to play pool. Different tools are used for different applications; both have value.

Progression of the Prosthesis

Assuming an amputee enters the prosthetic rehabilitation process at the time of surgery and has no complications, has good funding sources, has an optimal length of the residual limb, and is motivated for treatment, the progression would proceed as follows: (1) immediate/early postoperative prosthesis; (2) preparatory mechanical prosthesis; (3) preparatory myoelectric prosthesis; (4) definitive mechanical prosthesis; and (5) definitive myoelectric prosthesis. In many cases this progression is not practical or realistic. Many factors interfere with the preferred prosthetic progression. The progression differs from patient to patient, depending on variables such as stump length, funding sources, patient motivation, and time of entry into the rehabilitation process. A patient can start or stop at various points in the progression as a result of these factors.

Immediate/Early Postoperative Prosthesis

An immediate prosthesis and an early postoperative prosthesis are identical in fabrication. The name given varies with the time of fabrication. The immediate prosthesis is applied in surgery at the time of final closure. The early postoperative prosthesis is applied sometime after surgery but before suture removal. In both cases the socket is made from fiberglass casting tape wrapped around the residual limb. A thermoplastic frame is attached to the socket, and the terminal device and elbow unit are stabilized onto this frame.[4] If an elbow unit is required, a lightweight manual hinge elbow is placed on this prosthesis with eight set-locking points to position the elbow. A figure-8 harness with a simple cable to control the TD is used. Only one rubber band is provided for grip force at this stage. The prosthesis is used mainly as a gross stabilizer. The immediate/postoperative prosthesis introduces the patient to prosthetic use and wear and provides a rigid dressing for edema control and proprioceptive input.[4]

Preparatory Mechanical Prosthesis

The preparatory mechanical prosthesis is applied when full healing is complete and the sutures are removed, usually 10 to 14 days after surgery. The socket is fabricated from a plaster mold of the residual limb for a customized fit. The socket is made out of clear plastic to allow for monitoring of stump changes in volume and socket fit. The preparatory prosthesis is made from more durable materials than the postoperative prosthesis and can be used like a definitive (final) prosthesis. Its construction permits easy interchangeability of parts and components to evaluate which works best for this patient. The purposes of the preparatory mechanical prosthesis are the following:

- To continue edema control
- To condition tissues to accept forces exerted by the prosthetic socket
- To help the patient and clinic team determine which parts will functionally be the best
- To demonstrate the patient's level of motivation and compliance
- To give the patient a chance to see the value and limitations of a mechanical prosthesis[4]

The preparatory prosthesis allows the patient to develop skill and strength while determining which specifications work best. It is more cost-effective to make changes to this (temporary) prosthesis. Thus patients are free to evaluate their prosthetic needs.

Preparatory Myoelectric Prosthesis

Once the patient has demonstrated good muscle site control and funding is ensured for a myoelectric prosthesis, a preparatory myoelectric prosthesis is fabricated. A preparatory myoelectric prosthesis is a cost-effective way to analyze the patient's ability to use the prosthesis and to evaluate the components best suited to the patient's needs. The preparatory myoelectric prosthesis is fitted similarly to the definitive prosthesis, except that it has a transparent test socket to monitor electrode contact and evaluate socket stability. A fitting frame is attached to the socket to provide a surface for the electronic components to be attached. A standard protective outer glove is placed over the electronic hand for cosmesis and protection of the inner shell of the hand. Suspension, socket design, and electrode placement are all easily changeable to allow the patient to explore options. The purposes of the preparatory myoelectric prosthesis are the following:

- To determine a patient's motivation and commitment to get the maximum use out of the prosthesis
- To evaluate in a cost-effective way appropriate components and suspension systems
- To condition the tissues in a self-contained socket
- To determine the patient's use, skill, and wear patterns with myoelectric control[4]

Definitive Mechanical Prosthesis

Once the patient has determined the components needed, has established a full wear pattern with good prosthetic skill, and has reached full residual limb maturation, a definitive mechanical prosthesis is considered. The definitive prosthesis is designed around choices made by the patient in the preparatory stage. The definitive prosthesis is fabricated with durable parts and provides a good cosmetic appearance.

Definitive Myoelectric Prosthesis

The cost of a definitive myoelectric prosthesis in 2004 was approximately $45,000 for a transhumeral (AE) prosthesis and $20,000 for a transradial (BE) prosthesis. The preparatory myoelectric prosthesis is an essential step in determining whether myoelectric control is functional enough for the patient to incur this cost. The decision is based on the patient's wear, use, and skill patterns during the preparatory stage. The design incorporates the components that best suited the patient during the use of the preparatory myoelectric prosthesis.

Upper Extremity Prosthetic Training Program

Preoperative Care

Seventy-five percent of amputations result from trauma, and an opportunity to treat a patient before amputation is unusual. However, some amputations are the result of elective or needed surgery (after cancer or unsuccessful UE reattachment). Intervention before surgery emphasizes psychological support, education on prosthetic options available, training for the postoperative exercise program, and introduction to one-handed survival techniques for activities of daily living (ADL).

Postoperative Care

The usual patient length of stay in the hospital after an amputation is 3 to 4 days if no complications arise. Within these several days, patients are fitted with their prostheses, and the therapist or assistant makes the initial contact with them. The initial contact should focus on emotional and psychological support. Patients are typically overwhelmed with feelings of uncertainty and anxiety about the future. Answers to unspoken questions will begin to put them at ease about starting a rehabilitative process. During the postoperative period, patients may be counseled about accepting the amputation and about the prosthesis and its benefits. The clinician should be sensitive to what the amputation and the prosthesis may mean to the client. Grieving is a natural response to loss of a body part; the patient may imagine a total loss of the functions and occupations formerly controlled by that part.

A preprosthetic evaluation is completed by the occupational therapist, and the training program is introduced at this time. On the basis of this evaluation and with the patient's input, a treatment program is established that is designed to promote stump shrinkage, desensitize the stump, maintain ROM of proximal joints, and begin building prosthetic skill. Adjusting to the loss and achieving independence in self-care are other important aspects of the training program.[20] The following areas should be addressed in the postoperative training stage before the patient is discharged from the acute care hospital.

Stump Care/Skin Hygiene

The client is encouraged to move and use the stump as much as possible during the healing period. This movement will help give normal proprioceptive input to the brain and prevent muscle atrophy and contractures that result from guarding the residual limb at the side of the body. Instruction in proper residual limb hygiene is provided.

Stump Wrapping

Shrinking and shaping the residual limb is necessary to form a tapered-shaped limb that will tolerate a prosthesis. Compression aids in the shrinking and shaping process, with an elastic Ace bandage, a tubular bandage, or a shrinker sock applied to the residual limb. A figure-8 method is used when an elastic bandage is applied to the limb. Care must be taken to apply the bandage smoothly, evenly, and not too tightly from the distal to the proximal end of the residual limb. Circular wrapping, which may cause loss of circulation and further tissue loss, should not be used. The elastic bandage should be rewrapped several times a day to keep the correct tension. The patient is instructed to wrap the stump when he or she is not wearing the postoperative prosthesis.

Range of Motion Exercise

With medical approval, stump exercises may begin. These exercises are designed to encourage use of the stump, maintain ROM of joints proximal to the amputation site, and strengthen muscles of the arm and shoulder. Many of these muscles ultimately will be used to operate the prosthesis; therefore strength and endurance are the desired results of training.[27] A simple active ROM (AROM) routine without resistance is recommended for all the nonaffected muscles and available movements.

Desensitization

A program is established to normalize sensation in the residual limb, which is often hypersensitive after surgery, with extreme discomfort in response to normal tactile stimulation. Treatment aims to decrease hypersensitivity. Graded stimuli are introduced; materials are graded from soft to hard, and force of application is graded from light touch to rubbing to tapping to prolonged pressure. The patient should carry out a desensitization program so that tolerance is increased without pain.

Wear Schedule and Use Schedule

The patient is instructed to wear the postoperative prosthesis three times a day, beginning with 15-minute periods with 5 minutes of active use. The wear schedule is increased to 30 minutes of wear three times a day with 10 minutes of active use by the third day. Wear and active use progressively increase on an individual basis. The patient is instructed to check the residual limb after wear periods to identify pressure spots and any problems with healing. An activity list suggests ways to build skills. Examples of appropriate activities are picking up small objects such as paper clips, wrapping a present, and playing cards. The early use of a temporary prosthesis aids in psychological adjustment and will increase the likelihood of acceptance and use of the prosthesis by the amputee.

Prosthetic Skill Training

The patient will need instruction in the use of the early postoperative prosthesis. The mechanical training section in this chapter provides specifics of prosthetic use training. The postoperative prosthesis is basic in design, with a lightweight working hook TD that requires little exertion to operate. The TD has only 1 lb of grip force and therefore has limited practical use. The patient must be made aware of this limitation to prevent undue frustration. The patient should also be reassured that the next prosthetic device will be more functional. The patient is encouraged to incorporate the prosthesis in two-handed patterns and use it actively as much as possible. Most of the prosthetic skill training will occur on an outpatient basis, and only simple instructions are provided at first to avoid overwhelming the patient and to encourage use of the prosthetic device.

Components of Mechanical Prosthetic Training

A preparatory mechanical prosthesis is fabricated immediately after the sutures are removed. Once the patient has this device, training can begin full force with emphasis on prosthetic wear; skill; use; acceptance; grip-strength tolerance; a two-handed pattern; and a return to independence in ADL, work, and leisure activities. Other goals include retraining dominance if necessary, normalizing sensation in the residual limb, and strengthening the residual limb.

Training the Unilateral Transradial (BE) Amputee

- *Introduction to prosthetic parts:* The amputee should learn the names and functions of the parts of the prosthesis so that he or she can communicate with the therapist, physician, or prosthetist using common terminology. Knowledge of terms is especially important when the amputee is having difficulties with the prosthesis or if it is in need of repairs.
- *Donning and removing the prosthesis:* The amputee dons the stump sock with the sound arm. To apply the prosthesis, the amputee places it on a table or bed and pushes the stump between the control cable and Y-strap from the medial side into the socket (Figure 33-6, A). The sound arm is then slipped into the axilla loop. The amputee grasps the harness

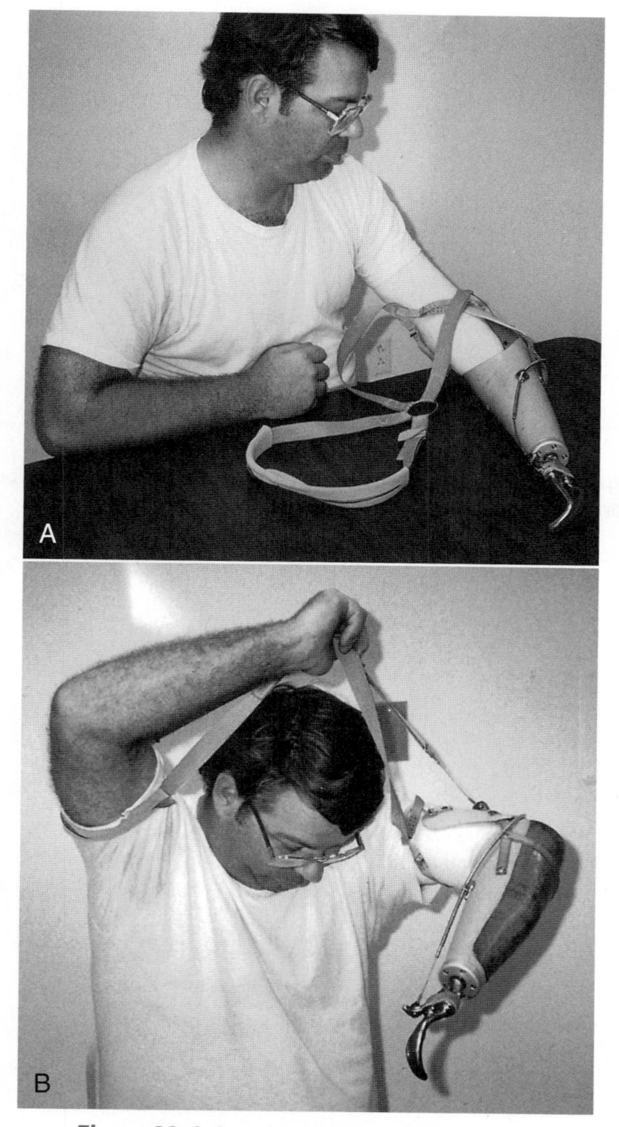

Figure 33-6 Donning a mechanical prosthesis.

and lifts it over the head so that it is positioned properly in back (Figure 33-6, B). The shoulders are shrugged to shift the harness forward and into the correct position. To remove the prosthesis, the amputee slips the axilla shoulder strap off on the sound side with the TD and then slips the shoulder strap off on the amputated side. The harness is slipped off like a coat.

- *TD control training:* Biscapular abduction and humeral flexion on the amputated side are the motions necessary to operate the TD. The clinician passively moves the patient through the motions (Figure 33-7). During this procedure the amputee watches the TD operate and gains a sense of the tension on the prosthesis control cable. The amputee then repeats the motions without assistance and verbalizes the actions that occurred during operation. The clinician instructs the amputee to repeat all of the motions in one continuous sequence in both sitting and standing positions until they are smooth and natural.[37] The amputee will then be instructed to open and close the TD in a variety of ranges of elbow and shoulder motion. TD opening and closing should be accomplished easily with the elbow extended, at 30 degrees, 45 degrees, 90 degrees, and with full elbow flexion, as well as with the arm overhead, down at the side, out to the side, and leaning over to floor level.[38]

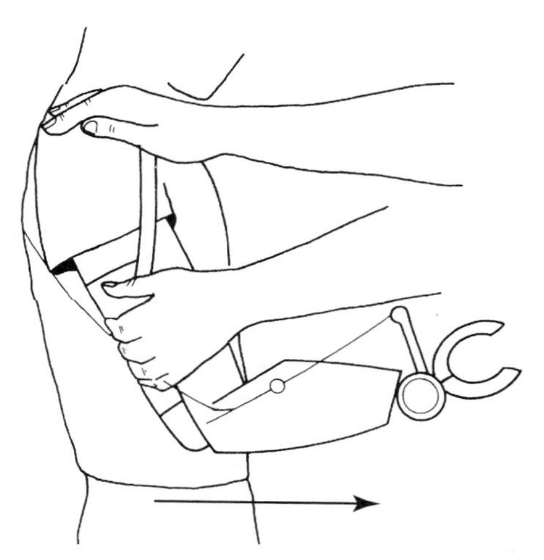

Figure 33-7 Therapist moves stump forward to attain cable tension and terminal device opening.

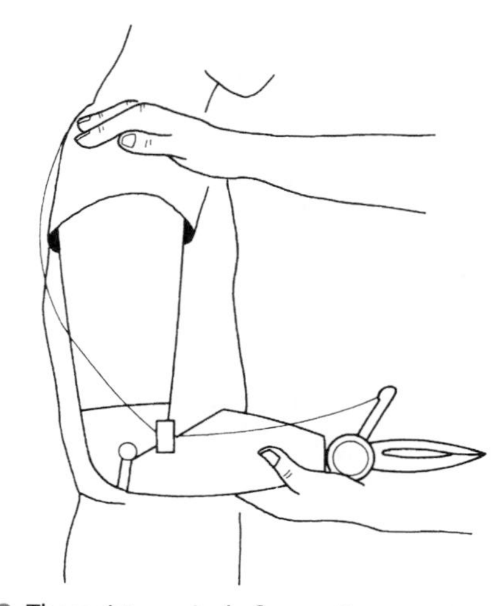

Figure 33-8 Therapist passively flexes elbow to cause slackening of control cable.

Training the Unilateral Transhumeral (AE) Amputee

- *Elbow control training:* Learning to flex the mechanical elbow is the first step in the training process. Once again, humeral flexion and scapular abduction are the control motions. The clinician passively flexes the prosthesis into full elbow flexion, noting that the control is slackened by this maneuver (Figure 33-8). The clinician then flexes the amputee's shoulder forward and asks the amputee to hold this position while the clinician lets go (Figure 33-9). The amputee gains a sense of the control cable tension across the scapula from this maneuver. The amputee is asked to relax the stump to the side of the body once again, slowly allowing the forearm to extend (Figure 33-10). The amputee is then asked to again flex the humerus and abduct the scapula to accomplish elbow flexion and relax the stump

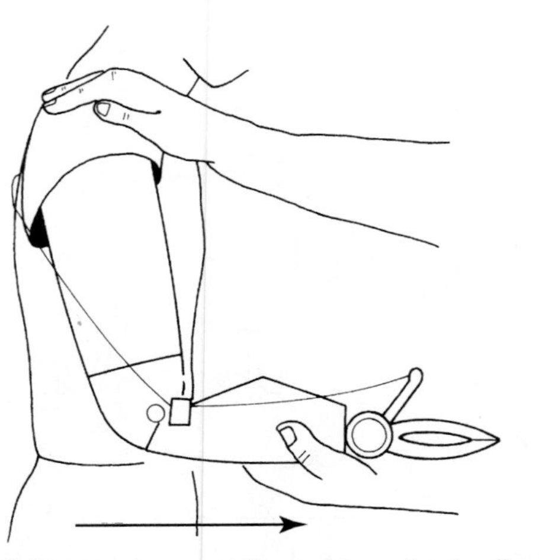

Figure 33-9 Forearm is moved forward to maintain elbow flexion, thus creating tension on control cable.

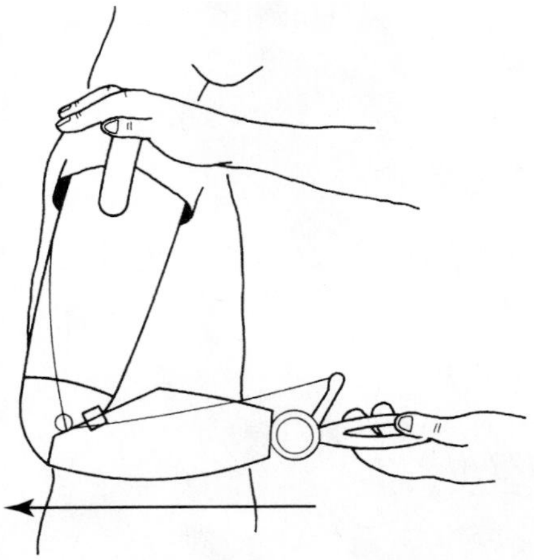

Figure 33-11 Therapist pushes humerus into hyperextension to lock elbow.

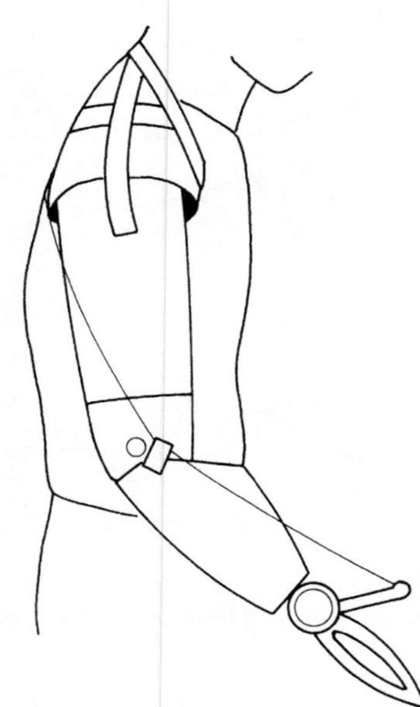

Figure 33-10 Amputee relaxes stump to allow controlled extension of forearm.

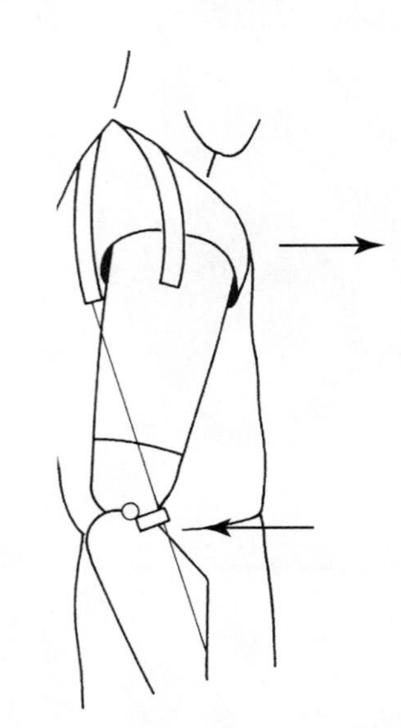

Figure 33-12 Shoulder is rolled forward, scapula abducted, and humerus hyperextended to lock or unlock elbow at various points in range of motion.

back slowly into shoulder extension to achieve elbow extension. This is repeated until the amputee gains enough control of cable tension to accomplish elbow flexion and extension smoothly and with ease.[38] The clinician then teaches elbow locking by passively pushing the humerus into hyperextension with the elbow flexed, thus locking the elbow (Figure 33-11).

- The clinician brings the arm back to the neutral position and then lets go, demonstrating that the elbow mechanism is locked. The clinician repeats this maneuver, demonstrating that the elbow is now unlocked. The amputee is then asked to lock the elbow by moving the humerus into hyperextension and rolling the shoulder forward, using scapular depression and abduction at the same time to lock the elbow. The amputee is then asked to practice locking and unlocking the elbow in various ranges of elbow flexion and extension until full flexion and extension are obtained (Figure 33-12).[38]
- *Use training:* Once the controls are mastered, use training begins. The first stage is prepositioning the TD. Prepositioning involves rotating the TD to the best position to grasp an object or perform a given activity. The goal of prepositioning the TD should be to allow amputees to approach an object or activity as they would with a normal hand and to avoid overreaching and similar awkward body movements that might be used to compensate for poor prepositioning. Along with prepositioning, prehension training should begin with large, hard objects such as blocks, cans, and jars and progress to soft and then crushable objects such as rubber balls, sponges, paper boxes, cones, and paper cups. These objects should be placed at various heights and positions that demand prepositioning and TD opening and closing, elbow flexion, and locking and unlocking, at various heights.

The amputee should be encouraged to use a problem-solving approach to these and other tasks to determine the best position for the TD, as well as appropriate use of the sound arm and the prosthesis in activities. Use training should progress to performance of necessary ADL. The amputee is encouraged to analyze and perform activities of personal hygiene and grooming, dressing, feeding, home management, communication and environmental hardware use, avocation, and vocation as independently as possible. The OTA may help the amputee achieve success by training with a special method or gadget or repetitious practice.[37]

Components of Myoelectric Prosthetic Training

Myoelectric prosthetic training takes place simultaneously with mechanical prosthetic training. Once the patient has developed good skill and use with the mechanical prosthesis and can tolerate learning another skill, muscle site testing and weight training are introduced. A typical treatment session at this point might focus on mechanical prosthetic functional use training for 15 minutes, muscle site training for 15 minutes, and weight training for the remaining 30 minutes. The therapist must thoroughly understand the myoelectric prosthesis and be able to differentiate patient errors from possible equipment malfunctions. The ability to pinpoint the source of the problem (whether it be equipment or operator error) is the key to successfully teaching and training the amputee about myoelectric control.

The goals of the myoelectric training program are the following:

- To operate the prosthesis automatically with minimal effort
- To care for the prosthesis
- To use the prosthesis smoothly and efficiently for commonly encountered tasks
- To analyze the best methods for unusual or new tasks[32]

Signal Training

Signal training is the process of learning to produce the muscle signals necessary to operate the myoelectric prosthesis.[32] Electrodes placed on the residual limb are connected to a feedback system that lets the patient know when the control muscles are contracting and at what level of intensity. Signal training helps the patient develop the ability to produce clear, strong contractions without wasting energy and to relax the control muscles even when the rest of the arm is actively moving.[24] Once the muscle sites are located by the occupational therapist, the OTA uses the same biofeedback device for training. Individuals with an amputation must receive adequate training and practice in initiating the desired muscle contractions before receiving the myoelectric prosthesis. The patients' success and effectiveness in using the prosthesis are closely related to the quality of the muscle site training process.

Weight Training

The occupational therapist designs a strengthening program to be carried out at home to strengthen the shoulder so that the added weight of a myoelectric prosthesis can be managed. The OTA may implement the weight-training program, providing instruction to ensure follow-through. A Theraband, free weights, or weight-training equipment all work equally well to accomplish this goal. The prosthetist often provides a socket with weights equaling the myoelectric prosthesis attached to it for the patient to wear several weeks before receiving the prosthesis to accustom him or her to the additional weight.

Care of Prosthesis

When patients are given the myoelectric preparatory prosthesis, they are instructed in the basic care of the prosthesis including how to charge the batteries, clean the prosthesis, and take care of the glove.

Donning/Removing

The method of application is determined by the type of suspension and socket design that the patient uses. Therefore no single method can be discussed. Regardless, donning the prosthesis should be done with the electronics in the "off" position.

Use Training

Training focuses on a combination of skill-building activities to learn prosthetic control and functional activities to encourage carryover of skills in daily tasks, thus culminating in an occupational task important to the patient.[1,2] Training must begin with learning to use the myoelectric hand in simple approach, grasp, and release activities. Classic therapeutic activities for hand control can be used, such as the pegboard or hook-and-loop fastening (Velcro) checkers. The patient should be able to judge the amount of hand opening or closing required to pick up an item. For instance, if the patient is trying to pick up a cotton swab, full hand opening would not be necessary and would demonstrate a lack of control. The clinician emphasizes good problem-solving skills for the patient to first position the TD in the optimum position for the specific activity. It is a common error for the amputee to "adjust" the body with compensatory large body motions rather than adjusting or prepositioning the hand first.

Another important aspect in training is mastery of the gripping force of the terminal device. This involves close visual attention to grade the muscle contraction to get a specific result in the calibration of the myoelectric hand. Too strong a grasp will result in crushing an object that is being held (Figure 33-13). Training with foam cups, sponges, and cotton balls will help develop the control needed to grasp and lift and move paper cups, eggs, potato chips, and sandwiches; ultimately, the patient can learn sufficient sensitivity to hold someone's hand. Eventually the movements will take less cognitive effort and become automatic. Each session should focus on both functional training and skill-building activities. Occupationally based two-handed tasks should include those the patient finds difficult and those that fit the patient's interests. The therapist should observe the patient closely when he or she is performing a functional task and ask the following questions: (1) Is the patient using the prosthesis spontaneously in the activity? (2) Is it being used as a gross stabilizer or in a nonactive pattern of use? (3) Does the patient use large compensatory body movements instead of prepositioning the components to

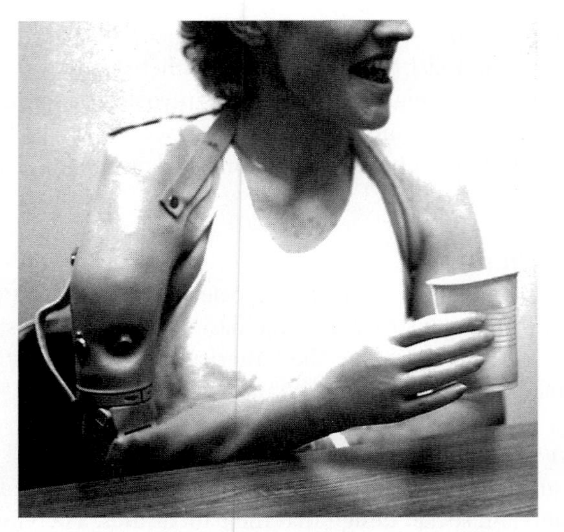

Figure 33-13 Above-elbow amputee demonstrates how too strong a grasp will crush the object being held.

the optimal position? (4) Is the patient overshooting the target? and (5) Is the patient using the proper grip force? Appropriate activities to focus on deficit areas can be selected on the basis of these answers.

Vocational and Leisure Activities

As training proceeds and the patient develops a sense of self-acceptance and comfort with the amputation, the clinician should broach the subject of return to work. If possible, job requirements can be discussed and then practiced in a simulated step-by-step process. Ideally, the clinician could make an on-site visit, and several requirements of the job could be practiced. If changes and adjustments to the work environment are necessary, the clinician could advise on these modifications (see Chapter 17).

Leisure and social participation contribute to significant physical and psychological well-being and are critically important. The terminal devices for recreational activities are not myoelectric but can be placed on the socket of a myoelectric prosthesis. Therapeutic Recreation Systems (TRS) has some excellent adaptation components.[27]

Expected Outcomes

At the completion of a training program, patients should be proficient in the use and care of both the mechanical and myoelectric prostheses and should demonstrate a full-day wear pattern. Patients should incorporate the use of a prosthesis into all occupational tasks, and they should demonstrate good spontaneous prosthetic use with skilled precision of movement. They should also have resolved psychological issues related to limb loss and have a realistic outlook on the usefulness of the prosthesis as a replacement arm.

Non-Use of Prosthetics

Approximately one-third of individuals using prostheses are dissatisfied with the comfort of the socket in addition to the suspension and control system; as a result they often do not use the prosthesis.[16,25,28]

Future Developments and Plans of Action

As a consequence of the wars of Operation Iraqi Freedom and Operation Enduring Freedom, several thousand military personnel have experienced polytrauma and multiple limb loss. Amputee healthcare for wounded military is the responsibility of the Department of Defense and the Veterans Administration (VA). In 2003, clinical scientists from the VA, Walter Reed Army Medical Center (WRAMC), academic institutions and the nonprofit sector met in Arlington, VA to brainstorm initiatives to address the need for innovative and functional prostheses as well as to advance medical management and post-prosthetic rehabilitation.

Discussions of critical importance included: upper-limb prostheses, platform technology, osseointegration, computer-aided design/computer-aided manufacturing (CAD/CAM), continuing education in amputee healthcare and prosthetic design, and post-prosthetic amputee rehabilitation. The group identified questions for investigation in upper-limb prosthetics and areas for research, including barriers to prosthetic use. Technologies discussed included tissue engineering, osseointegration, microstimulation, muscle actuation, and robotics. The VA and Department of Defense are designing research protocols to answer targeted questions as well as to develop shared outcome measures and databases, so as to provide a continuum of care between medical facilities and the VA. The hope is that this information will also be disseminated to the private sector to maximize comfort and function for the non-military amputees as well.[18]

Lower Extremity Amputations

OT for lower extremity (LE) amputees focuses on positioning, transfer training, strengthening of UE, ADL and instrumental activities of daily living (IADL), dynamic balance (with and without a prosthesis), strengthening the LE for the amputee to perform IADL (with and without a prosthesis), driving, prevocational and vocational activities, leisure education, and facilitating reintegration into the community. Critical to these aims are family education, a home visit, a home program, and provision of appropriate durable medical equipment (DME) for the home such as tub seats, tub benches, raised toilet seats, and grab bars. The OTA may assist the occupational therapist or assume responsibility for many of these areas once service competency with this population is achieved.

CASE STUDY

Cathy: Upper Extremity Amputee

Referral

Cathy is an 18-year-old right-hand-dominant Chinese-American girl who, at age 17, sustained a right transradial amputation in an automobile accident. She was fitted with a cable-driven harness with a hook TD. She now desires a cosmetic hand and training with a myoelectric prosthesis.

CASE STUDY—cont'd

Occupational History and Profile

Cathy is a high school senior. She has lived in the United States for the past three years, since her family (both parents, one other sibling) emigrated from Guangdong province in China. She plans to attend college next year and has been awarded a full scholarship. She spends her time studying and helping her parents with household chores. She occasionally works as a receptionist in her family's restaurant. She enjoys downloading music, taking photographs, and hanging out with her girlfriends.

Client Factors and Performance Skills

The occupational therapist assessed passive and active ROM, muscle strength, sensory function, and coordination of both UEs. The left UE was normal in all measures; the amputated right UE showed some distal sensory loss but good coordination, ROM, and strength across existing joints. Cathy performed all basic ADL including make-up application skillfully.

Cathy stated that she wanted the myoelectric hand for cosmetic reasons because she felt self-conscious going away to college wearing a hook. She also said she was afraid no one would want to go out with her.

Interventions

OT was provided on an outpatient basis in a rehabilitation hospital three times a week for 45- to 60-minute sessions. The occupational therapist and the prosthetist worked with Cathy to place the controls. The OTA trained Cathy in using the myoelectric device for BADL and IADL. Because of her strong motivation and family support, Cathy progressed rapidly in wearing time and skill in calibration and positioning of the device. She completed training in time for the fall semester.

Physical therapy assumes major responsibility for the preprosthetic preparation and prosthetic training of the LE amputee; however, an OT can incorporate the prosthetic training as part of the ADL routine beginning with stump care, which involves stump wrapping, inspection of the wound, and donning and doffing of stockings and prosthesis. Physical therapy manages the wound care and application of any physical modalities to minimize the pain and promote healing. Understanding the levels of an LE amputation is important for managing an LE amputee in OT.

Levels of Amputation and Functional Losses in the Lower Extremity

Levels of amputation, described with current terminology, are shown in Figure 33-14. The higher the level of amputation is, the greater the functional loss of the part and the more the amputee will depend on the prosthesis for function and cosmesis. The higher-level amputation requires more complex and extensive prostheses and prosthetic training. Hemipelvectomy and hip disarticulation amputation results in loss of the entire LE; thus hip, knee, ankle, and foot functions are lost.[23,24] Transfemoral (above-knee) amputations (AKAs) and knee disarticulation amputations result in loss of knee, ankle, and foot motion. The stump of the transfemoral amputated limb can vary in length from 10 to 12 inches (5.4 to 30.5 cm) below the greater trochanter.[23,24]

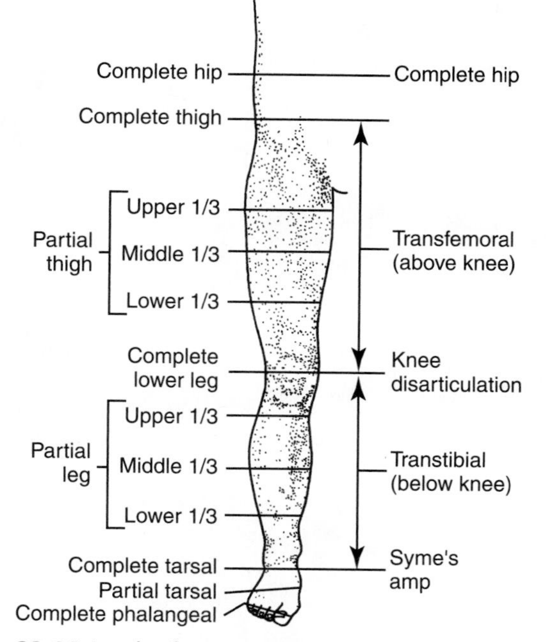

Figure 33-14 Levels of amputation and functional losses in lower extremity. (From O'Sullivan SB, Cullen K, Schmitz T: *Physical rehabilitation: evaluation and treatment procedures,* Philadelphia, 1981, FA Davis.)

Transtibial (below-knee) amputations (BKAs) result in a stump that is approximately 4 to 6 inches (10.1 to 15.2 cm) in length from the tibial plateau.[23,24] Other classification systems further delineate the amputations into thirds. *Upper, middle,* and *lower third* indicate the distance below the ischium for transfemorals. For the transtibials, these divisions indicate the distance below the tibial plateau.[23] The Syme's amputation is equivalent to an ankle disarticulation and results in loss of ankle and foot function.[3] In a transmetatarsal amputation, the foot is severed through the metatarsal bones and the ankle function remains intact.[3] Loss of the small toes does not result in functional impairment. Loss of the great toe, however, prevents toe-off during ambulation.[34]

Component Parts of the Lower Extremity Prosthesis

Rigid Removal Dressing

The major component parts in the immediate postoperative prosthesis for LE amputees can include the rigid removal dressing (i.e., cast or a stiff solid dressing of plaster of Paris or other material) that is applied just after surgery to ensure control of swelling, to apply firm pressure, and to contour the stump in preparation for the permanent prosthesis. The cast is changed approximately every 10 days or earlier if the cast becomes loose until the stump is healed and ready for a permanent artificial leg (Figure 33-15). The cast is held in position with a canvas band and secured with a Velcro strap. Alternatively, suspension straps can be used to overcome the weight of the cast.

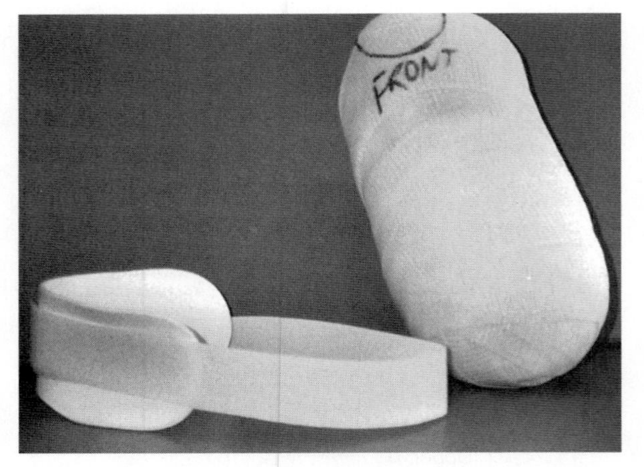

Figure 33-15 Rigid removal dressing with Velcro strap.

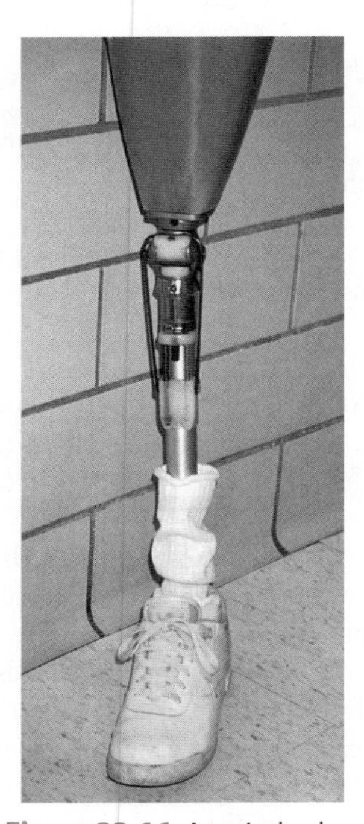

Figure 33-16 A typical pylon.

Suspension Straps

The suspension straps can go to the waist or shoulder belt to keep the cast in position. The end of the cast can be made to take a simple training prosthesis (usually called a *pylon*) so that training in standing and walking can be started immediately. A typical pylon is shown in Figure 33-16.

The casts are normally designed to take only 30 to 45 lb of the body weight. Too much weight on the cast may result in slow healing or even cause the wound to open. An adjustment quadrilateral socket attached to the upright of a bail suspension and a solid ankle cushion heel (SACH foot) are used for the foot.[24] An immediate postoperative prosthesis for the LE amputee allows greater independence early on in the rehabilitation program.

Types of Prostheses

The pylon is a temporary artificial leg. The pylon will serve as a working prosthesis to allow the amputee to use the stump and proximal musculature, maintain joint ROM, and provide a sense of pressure, motion, and weight that may be similar to that of the actual prosthesis.[34]

The computerized C-leg system from Otto Bock features a microprocessor-controlled knee-shin system. It is customizable and allows for increased comfort while ambulating a variety of surfaces and inclines. The amputee can safely and easily climb stairs and uneven terrain. Although it is expensive (approximately $60,000 in 2004), this device provides state-of-the-art function and versatility and is consistently used for wounded military personnel with transfemoral amputations (Figure 33-17).[13]

The Canadian-type disarticulation prosthesis meets the needs of the hemipelvectomy and hip disarticulation amputee (Figure 33-18). This prosthesis is suspended from the pelvis and equipped with hip and knee joints and a SACH foot. Pelvic movements provide energy for use of the limb.[34]

The Syme's amputee uses the Canadian-type Syme's prosthesis or a plastic Syme's (Figure 33-19). This prosthesis consists of a total contact plastic socket and SACH foot; there is no ankle joint.[34]

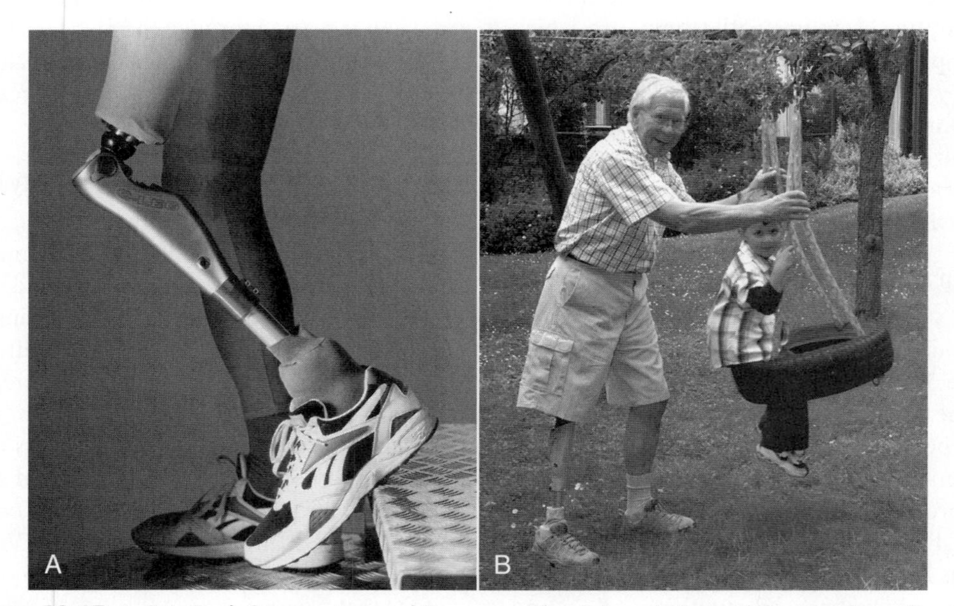

Figure 33-17 **A,** Otto Bock C-Leg system and **B,** a man with a C-Leg playing with his grandson. (Courtesy Otto Bock HealthCare, Minneapolis.)

Transmetatarsal and toe amputations do not require prostheses. These amputees need a shoe-toe-filler.[34] In the complete tarsal, the amputation is the same as in the Syme's. In the partial tarsal the instep is intact. In the complete phalangeal, all the toes are amputated.

Lower Extremity Preoperative Training

Preoperative care includes psychological support; keep in mind that individuals' cultural backgrounds and lifestyles will influence their abilities to cope with the loss of a limb. If amputations are viewed with aversion in individuals' cultures or lifestyles, they are likely to have the same feelings.[10] Support groups can help them express feelings. Group members are generally sensitive to others' needs and encourage constructive and creative thinking, which helps to motivate initiative and self-assurance. Visits by other amputees who have adjusted to the loss of a limb can also offer support.

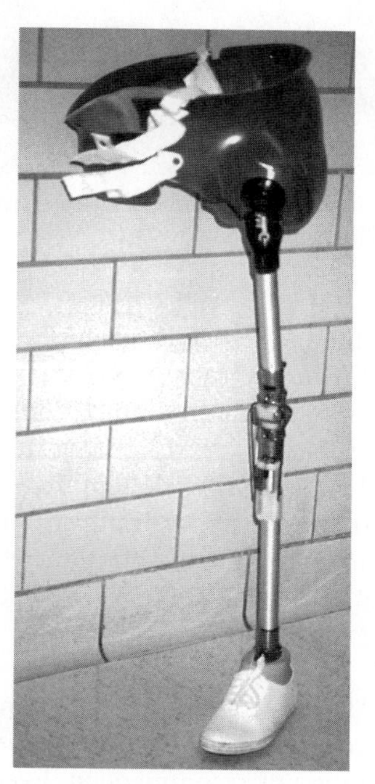

Figure 33-18 The Canadian prosthesis meets the needs of the hemipelvectomy and hip disarticulation amputee.

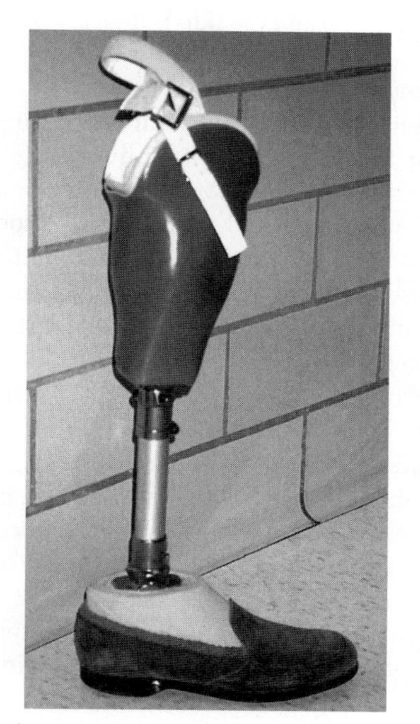

Figure 33-19 Plastic Syme's prosthesis.

Postoperatively, the therapy practitioner trains the individual in edema management, exercise, balance, and pain management. In most settings, physical therapy is responsible for this training. For transfemoral (AK) and transtibial (BK) with swelling (edema) at the stump site, the practitioner instructs the amputee on how to apply the elastic wrap(s) in a figure-8 pattern to prevent a tourniquet effect. The elastic wrap(s) should be placed around the stump site with firm pressure distally that decreases as the wrapping continues proximally. Bandages are reapplied three or four times a day.[26] If the amputee cannot wrap properly, a stump shrinker (an elastic stocking to control edema) is worn when the prosthesis is not being worn. Maintaining postoperative ROM in the involved extremity is necessary to maintain joint integrity and prevent contractures. Because balance can be affected by the loss of the LE, additional training will be required for ADL. Pain management is important. The aim is to decrease pain whenever possible.

Occupational Therapy Evaluation

The occupational therapist and OTA work in close partnership with *all* the rehabilitation team members to obtain information on the new amputee in the rehabilitation unit. The occupational therapist and OTA have important and distinct roles in the practice setting. The OTA's responsibilities in the initial evaluation process may include data collection from chart review, interviews with patient and family members, general observations, behavioral checklists, and administering standardized tests once competency is demonstrated (in accordance with the OTA's experience and the facility's regulations). The OTA and occupational therapist should both have the following knowledge of the patient's medical condition: (1) date and level of amputation (including complications during hospitalization); (2) reason for amputation; (3) exact site and level of amputation; (4) periods of dependent positioning allowed by physician; (5) wear schedule for the prosthesis; and (6) other medical conditions that might influence treatment (e.g., fractures, vascular involvement, medication, edema, infection, lab values, pertinent comorbidities).[20] The OT evaluation should cover the following areas: physical functions and skills, ADL, assessment of vocational interests/pursuits, home safety and accessibility, and architectural barriers within the community.

The OT plan of care requires assessment, reassessment, and ongoing communication between the OT and OTA in order to provide a truly individualized course of treatment to a person with an amputation. The assessment of the ROM, muscle strength, sensation, coordination, balance, vision, pain, and activity tolerance of the person with an amputation will be performed by the occupational therapist. A comprehensive and ongoing assessment of the person's prior level of function and occupational profile will provide guidance in determining discharge disposition. The occupational therapist prepares the intervention plan for any complex problem involving physical, emotional, or cognitive factors that arise throughout the course of treatment. The OTA implements the plan under the guidance and supervision of the occupational therapist. The OTA observes for any changes from the initial assessment and reports these to the occupational therapist; in collaboration with the OTA, the OT can change the plan of care as needed to ensure individualized treatment is provided on the basis of information gathered and reported by the OTA. The OTA provides training for the routine/structured techniques for ADL, bed mobility, wheelchair mobility, seating and positioning, transfers, toileting, hygiene, and dressing, with supervision from the occupational therapist as directed by the established plan of care.

An OTA can gather data regarding IADL, leisure, and social interests and pursuits and report such findings to the OT; however, it is the responsibility of the OT to integrate these findings into the plan of care in order for the OTA to provide intervention. The OTA can also provide training for IADL such as homemaking, meal preparation, laundry, shopping, and cleaning. The OTA can lead groups on home safety and accessibility, exercise, pacing and energy conservation, home modifications, discharge planning, work simplification, and joint protection and may document the individual's participation.

Home assessment for architectural barriers within the individual's home and community and while driving is performed by the occupational therapist or experienced service-competent OTA, in accordance with state practice acts and standards of practice. When indicated, the occupational therapist assesses cognition, psychological adjustment to amputation and its limitations, and visual/perceptual components.

The occupational therapist and OTA will formulate the OT discharge and follow-up plan, along with the interdisciplinary team, and report factual and objective data at time of discharge orally and in writing.[6] A partnership between the occupational therapist and OTA will accelerate the rehabilitation of the person with an amputation. The occupational therapist and OTA can also work effectively in another area of importance—sexual counseling—at the individual's request (see Chapter 16).[11]

Basic Activities of Daily Living

Positioning

Prevention of muscle contracture is an immediate postoperative concern.[20] Joint contracture is a common preprosthetic problem among LE amputees.[24] The transfemoral amputee typically develops a flexion, external rotation, and abduction contracture of the affected hip. The transtibial amputee develops an external rotation deformity of the hip and flexion of the knee.[24] Daily ROM exercise is encouraged. One should avoid placing pillows beneath the knee of a transtibial amputee and under the stump of a transfemoral amputee. Proper positioning reduces excessive edema in a limb when the individual is up in a wheelchair (Figure 33-20).[24] The OTA needs to consider the seating and positioning of the person with an amputation. Proper cushion selection can assist with obtaining neutral hip alignment and prevent pelvic obliquity, thereby reducing the risk of developing contractures. Appropriate cushions also address comfort and pain management and reduce the risk of decubitus ulcers.

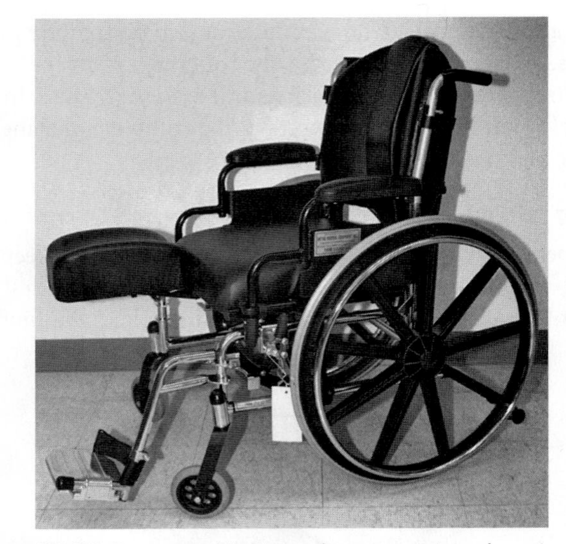

Figure 33-20 Proper positioning reduces excessive edema in a limb when individual is in a wheelchair.

Stump Hygiene

Once the wound is healed and sutures are removed, the stump should be washed with warm water and dried with a towel. Lotion or alcohol is not recommended. Evening care is recommended so that the stump is not softened immediately before prosthetic use.[19] As part of the ADL routine, the OTA should instruct the person on stump inspection with a long-handled mirror to ensure the skin is intact.

Dressing Training

Most LE amputees are independent in UE dressing but require assistance for LE dressing. Grade LE dressing from performing in bed, to sitting [bedside to sinkside], to standing.[24] Socks and shoes should be donned while sitting. A sock aid, long-handled shoe horn, long-handled reacher, and elastic shoelaces may ease donning and doffing for the individual with loss of flexibility, poor sitting balance, or impaired vision. A footstool may also be useful.

Bed Mobility

Individuals are taught bed mobility activities to promote independence without rails or an overhead trapeze bar. They are encouraged to roll from side to side, perform bridging activities with knee and hip flexion, and push the foot of the existing limb so that they can push up in bed and don LE clothing over the hips (Figure 33-21).[24] Bed mobility is an important aspect to master in preparation for bedside ADL and in preparation for transfers.

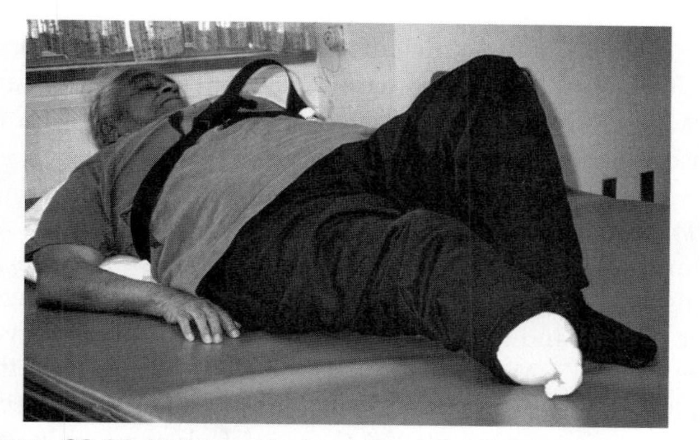

Figure 33-21 *Bridging,* a bed mobility skill called for pushing up in bed to don lower extremity.

Wheelchair Mobility and Parts Management

The wheelchair will be the main source of postoperative mobility for some persons with LE amputations and should be assessed by the OT (see Chapter 15 for information on wheelchair training).

Transfer Training

The unilateral LE amputee generally uses a standing pivot transfer (90-degree pivot), transferring toward the existing limb when possible. Having the individual practice transfers toward the amputated side or 180-degree pivots increases independence when he or she is transferring in more restrictive environments (e.g., a bathroom or bedroom).[24] The use of a pivot disc with crutches and/or a standard walker can assist with stand pivot transfers. Sliding board transfers may be taught to bilateral amputees and to those with a weak existing limb; however, UE and core strength should be assessed before attempting slide board transfers. Bilateral amputees may consider purchasing a wheelchair with a zippered or removable back to allow transfer by sliding backward to a surface and by sliding forward to return to the wheelchair (anterior/posterior).[20] Transfer training for a person with an amputation should be practiced for various surfaces and situations such as toilet transfers, tub/shower stall transfers with and without a seat or bench, bed transfers to and from a chair or wheelchair, and transfers from wheelchair to and from a chair.

Bathing

Bathing is a self-care activity that includes dressing and undressing, transferring to and from shower chair or tub transfer bench, and balancing while managing the water controls (faucets) and body parts. Adaptive devices (i.e., long-handled bath brush, flexible shower hose, grab bars and a tub-transfer bench/chair) can promote independence and safety.[24]

Balance Activities

The prerequisite to performing ADL and IADL is balance. The person with an amputation must have good dynamic sitting and standing balance while performing LE dressing activities and while bathing, transferring, reaching for objects in cupboards overhead, and retrieving objects from the floor. These tasks may be done from the wheelchair and while wearing an immediate postoperative prosthesis. The OT practitioner must provide graded functional activities to facilitate postural adjustment in all planes.[24] The OT practitioner must also address core strengthening and UE strengthening to assist with balance.

Pain Management

No specific protocol for the treatment of phantom sensation and pain exists. Medication, biofeedback, and other compensatory techniques can decrease the pain and sensation. The occupational therapist can instruct the person with an amputation on techniques such as applying pressure (to tolerance), rubbing, tapping, and other modalities such as heat or cold applications on the stump for relief.[20] An experienced OTA will observe the amputee's performance and collaborate with the occupational therapist when problems arise. Alternative treatment ideas to address pain management that can be addressed by the OTA include deep breathing, yoga, tai chi, visualization, and progressive muscular relaxation.

Energy Conservation and Work Simplification

The person with an amputation will expend more energy during ADL than a person of the same sex, age, and stature who has no amputations.[3] Energy expenditure increases with age and obesity.[24] The OTA should incorporate pacing in all activities to prevent fatigue and injury. The OTA should determine the person's activity tolerance through vital signs, rate of perceived exertion, and use of the BORG scale (see Chapter 34).

Home Management

Living alone will require independence and safety during homemaking tasks. Home management should be addressed near discharge but should be considered day one on initial evaluation and may involve a combination of individual and group sessions. Areas discussed and practiced are preparing simple and full meals, purchasing food, cooking, serving, cleaning, doing laundry (light and heavy), cleaning house, stripping and making beds (a hospital bed and double bed), and working at various levels (e.g., with a wheelchair, walker [standard or wheeled], cane, and crutches [axillary or loftstrand] with or without prosthesis).[24]

Driving

State laws regarding driving after LE amputation vary. The OT practitioner should know the law before recommending that the individual resume driving. When appropriate, the individual should be referred to a driver safety specialist for a driving assessment (see Chapter 15).

Prevocational and Vocational Activities

The evaluation will determine whether the person with an amputation can return to his or her previous job. The basic elements are psychological testing including interest and achievement; establishment of an initial vocational plan; vocational counseling; work evaluation including definition of functional skills and assessment of architectural barriers in the work environment; driver education and vehicle modification as needed; communication with state vocational rehabilitation agencies, insurance companies, and other sponsors; job analysis and modifications; and follow-up (see also Chapter 17).

Leisure and Social Participation

Recreation and the constructive use of leisure time enhance quality of life. Many individuals may view mobility limitations as obstacles to returning to premorbid leisure activities. Thus the overall program should include using community recreational resources, learning new leisure skills, making adaptations for previous leisure skills and interests, and refining of functional abilities related to specific leisure activities. Community skills groups feature both discussion and reentry trips to develop the skills necessary to take an active role in recreational opportunities.[15] Recreational LE prostheses are available for golf, swimming, and skiing[24] (see also Chapter 18).

Reintegration into Community

Ultimately, the individual must gain independence in and accessibility to the community. Here the person with an amputation attempts to manage curbs, inclines, steps, uneven surfaces, and elevators. The individual should be encouraged to problem solve specific architectural barriers.

Discharge Planning

Discharge planning includes educating the family, providing home exercise programs, and securing necessary DME. A home visit may be completed in anticipation of discharge.[29]

Family Education

During family education, the therapist (occupational therapist or OTA) demonstrates skills taught and encourages the patient and his or her family to practice with the recommended DME. The therapist observes closely how the family and individual perform the activities and corrects any unsafe practices. If the therapist feels the family will benefit from additional family education, this need should be discussed at that time. It is imperative that the therapist observe a return demonstration from the caregivers to assess their ability to care for the person with an amputation and to also determine a safe and reasonable discharge situation with appropriate social support. Exercise programs are reviewed with the family in clear and understandable language, and a written copy is provided. DME is discussed in great detail with the family, as are locations to purchase equipment in the community. To ensure accessibility in and out of the home and in tight spaces, a home visit is essential.

The occupational therapist and OTA work collaboratively as the case study situation illustrates.

CASE STUDY

Mrs. M.: Lower Extremity Amputation

Mrs. M. is a 76-year-old African-American woman. She had a surgical right transtibial amputation because of poor circulation. The stump is well healed, and there is good stump shrinkage. No significant medical issues are present, and there were no complications during hospitalization.

Referral

A referral was sent to OT to increase function in basic ADL, mobility, transfers, and IADL with a prosthesis and walker. The estimated length of stay is 14 days.

Mrs. M. was assigned to the amputee unit. The occupational therapist reviewed in conjunction with the OTA Mrs. M.'s medical chart to obtain data sent from the acute care facility.

Occupational History and Profile

Mrs. M. is a retired postal worker. She reported having completed 1 year of college. She enjoys the following leisure activities: playing cards, visiting friends, bowling, and traveling with her husband (Mr. M.) to Georgia to visit family members.

Mrs. M. lives with her husband in a single-family home. There are three steps to enter the front of the home with bilateral hand rails, as well as a ramp leading up to the side door. Her bedroom and a full bathroom are located on the first floor with a tub. Her husband is in poor health and is in a wheelchair. He cannot assist her physically; however, accommodations have been made to the home already: there is a hand-held shower with grab bars and a tub bench, as well as a raised toilet seat and grab bars near the toilet. Mrs. M. will need to be independent with adaptive equipment and devices for self-care skills and transfers with the ischial weight-bearing prosthesis and a standard walker. She will also need to be able to complete light meal preparation for both her husband and herself. Mrs. M. is also responsible for medication management for both her husband and herself, as well as financial management. Mrs. M.'s niece will perform the heavier home management activities such as laundry and housekeeping and other personal business in the community such as grocery shopping, driving, and obtaining medication from the pharmacy.

Client Factors and Performance Skills

The OTA's admissions interview included an introduction to the OT program. Mrs. M. was aware of her deficits and appeared motivated. The assessment began with UE passive ROM and active ROM, manual muscle test, and tests of

CASE STUDY—cont'd

sensory, coordination, pain, edema, skin, visual, and cognition performance by the occupational therapist. ADL performance, transfer status positioning and activity tolerance were assessed collaboratively by the occupational therapist and OTA. A treatment plan was developed after completion of all the assessments. Areas of deficits were identified. Short-term and long-term goals were identified with Mrs. M., who played an active part in setting goals.

Interventions

Mrs. M. was treated by the OTA in daily, 45- to 60-minute OT sessions. The OTA consulted daily with the occupational therapist.

Adaptive devices (i.e., long-handled bath brush, dressing stick, stocking aid, reacher) were issued to improve Mrs. M.'s self-care skills at bed or wheelchair levels. Transfers were initially performed with a sliding board to compensate for Mrs. M.'s decreased activity tolerance. At discharge, Mrs. M.'s mobility and transfers were independent at walker with walker basket level with prosthesis. She was able to complete light meal preparation in the kitchen such as obtaining a beverage from the refrigerator and making soup and sandwiches, as well as transporting items to the table. Mrs. M. was educated on energy-conservation techniques and was able to demonstrate 100% understanding and integration of these techniques during her OT sessions. Dressing the LE posed some problems initially, but Mrs. M. was independent with adaptive equipment at discharge. Mrs. M. was reassessed daily for areas that required more improvement. Family instruction was completed with her husband and niece present. A home evaluation was also completed by the OT and OTA to determine Mrs. M.'s ability to use current DME already in the home. Mrs. M. made significant progress in the rehabilitation program. She returned home with good family support and a UE home exercise program. Home therapy was recommended at discharge to ensure a safe transition into the home.

Three weeks after discharge, Mr. M. informed the staff that his wife had passed away. Mrs. M. will be remembered for her determination to regain her skills and return to the community.

Summary

Rehabilitation and prosthetic training of the UE amputee is a complex specialty practice area and is managed by an experienced occupational therapist in collaboration with the prosthetist and other rehabilitation team members. The OTA may assist, particularly in use training, donning and removing, and transfer of skills to ADL and work and leisure activities.

The rehabilitation of an individual with LE loss requires the skills of many health care specialists including OT practitioners. OT evaluation and training for the LE should focus on positioning, ADL training, and maintaining and improving the ROM and strength in the UE for training with the prosthesis in purposeful activities and occupations. The OT practitioner also assesses the feasibility of the amputee's returning to work and resuming or exploring leisure skills.

Facilitating psychological adjustment is another major role of the clinician working with the UE and LE amputees and their family members. The occupational therapist and OTA must collaborate to maximize the amputee's skills for reentry into the work force and community.

Selected Reading Guide Questions

1. What do the following abbreviations mean: AE, TD, BE?
2. Which arm functions are lost—and which functions are retained—in a long transradial amputation?
3. List the advantages and disadvantages of a myoelectric prosthesis.
4. Which motions accomplish TD opening with a mechanical prosthesis?
5. Which five questions should be asked when one is observing an amputee in an activity?
6. What is the recommended initial wearing period for the postoperative prosthesis?
7. What does "prepositioning the TD" mean?
8. Why is it important to wrap the stump?
9. What are the responsibilities of the OTA in initial evaluation of the LE amputee?
10. Which method can be used postoperatively to ensure control of stump swelling and to contour the stump for the permanent prosthesis?
11. Why is the LE amputee patient instructed *not* to place pillows under the hip and knee?
12. Amputees sometimes feel as if their missing limb is moving. What is this phenomenon called?
13. Which adaptive devices can ease donning of an LE prosthesis for an individual with loss of flexibility?
14. Which method can be used to teach the LE amputee to don pants in bed?
15. Which transfer approach is generally used by the LE amputee?
16. For which activities must the LE amputee have good dynamic balance?
17. For the LE amputee, which areas are assessed, discussed, and practiced in home management?
18. What will be reviewed by the occupational therapist or OTA during family education?
19. Describe what is included in discharge planning for the LE amputee.

References

1. American Occupational Therapy Association: Occupational therapy practice framework: domain and process, *Am J Occup Ther* 56(6):609–639, 2002.
2. American Occupational Therapy Association: *Occupational therapy practice framework: domain and process*, ed 2, Bethesda, MD, 2008, the Association.
3. Banerjee SJ: *Rehabilitation management of amputees*, Baltimore, 1982, Williams & Wilkins.
4. Brenner CD: *Atlas of limb prosthetics*, ed 2, St Louis, 1992, Mosby.
5. Bucchieri J, Poole BT, Schmidt CC, et al: Restoration of thumb function after partial or total amputation. In Mackin EJ, Callahan AD, Skirven TM, et al: *Rehabilitation of the hand and upper extremity*, ed 5, St Louis, 2002, Mosby.
6. DiDomenico R, editor: Lower limb amputation in the elderly: meeting the rehabilitation challenge, *Focus Geriatr Care Rehabil*, 4: 1–8, 1989pp .
7. Dillingham TR, Pezzin LE, MacKenzie EJ: Limb amputations and limb deficiency: epidemiology and recent trends in the United States, *Southern Med J* 95:875–883, 2002. Cited in National Limb Loss Information Center: Amputation statistics by cause: limb loss in the United States, 2004. Accessed July 25, 2005 from http://www.amputee-coalition.org/fact_sheets/amp_stats_cause.html.
8. Esquenazi A: Amputation rehabilitation and prosthetic restoration. From surgery to community reintegration, *Disability and Rehabilitation* 26(14/15):831–836, 2004.
9. Friedman LW: *The psychological rehabilitation of the amputee*, Springfield, Ill, 1978, Charles C Thomas.
10. Friedman LW: *The surgical rehabilitation of the amputee*, Springfield, Ill, 1978, Charles C Thomas.
11. Gurgold GD, Harden DH: Assessing the driving potential of the handicapped, *Am J Occup Ther* 32:41–46, 1978.
12. Horgan O, MacLachlan M: Psychosocial adjustment to lower-limb amputation: A review, *Disability and Rehabilitation* 26(14/15): 837–850, 2004.
13. Howard Col. WJ: Chief, Occupational Therapy Service, Walter Reed Army Medical Center, Washington DC. Personal communication, July 25, 2005.
14. Jacobsen S, Knutti DF, Johnson RT, Sears HH: Development of Utah Artificial Arm, *IEEE Trans Biomed Eng* 29(4):5, 1982.
15. Kegel B, Webster J, Burgress EM: Recreational activities of lower extremity amputees: survey, *Arch Phys Med Rehabil* 61:258, 1980.
16. Kejlaa GH: Consumer concerns and the functional value of prostheses to upper limb amputees, *Prosthet orthot int* 17(3):157–163, 1993 Dec.
17. Kelly BM, et al: *Upper limb prosthetics*, 2009, http://emedicine.medscape.com/article/317234-overview.
18. Kerkovich D: A report on the amputee healthcare and prosthetics workshop sponsored by Walter Reed Army Medical Center and the Department of Veterans Affairs (VA), *JRRD* 41(3B), May/June 2004.
19. Larson CB, Gould M: *Orthopedic nursing*, ed 8, St Louis, 1974, Mosby.
20. Lyons BG: The issue is: purposeful versus human activity, *Am J Occup Ther* 37:493, 1983.
21. Malone J, Fleming LL, Roberson J, et al: Immediate, early and late postsurgical management of upper limb amputation, *J Rehab Res Dev* 21, 1984.
22. National Limb Loss Information Center: *Amputation statistics by cause: limb loss in the United States*, 2004. Accessed July 25, 2005 from http://www.amputee-coalition.org/fact_sheets/amp_stats_cause.html.
23. O'Sullivan S, Cullen K, Schmitz T: *Physical rehabilitation: evaluation and treatment procedures*, Philadelphia, 1981, FA Davis.
24. Pedretti L, Pasquinelli S: Amputations and prosthetics. In Pedretti L, Zoltan B, editors: *Occupational therapy: practice skills for physical dysfunction*, ed 3, St Louis, 1990, Mosby.
25. Pezzin LE, Dillingham TR, MacKenzie EJ, et al: Use and satisfaction with prosthetic limb devices and related services, *Arch Phys Med Rehabil* 85:723–729, May 2004.
26. American Occupational Therapy Association: *Project to delineate the roles and functions of occupational therapy personnel*, Rockville, Md, 1972, the Association.
27. Rock L, Atkins A: Upper extremity amputations and prosthetics. In Pedretti L, Zoltan B, editors: *Occupational therapy: practice skills for physical dysfunction*, ed 4, St Louis, 1995, Mosby.
28. Roeschlein RA, Domholdt E: Factors related to successful upper extremity prosthetic use, *Prosthet Orthot Int* 13:14–18, 1989.
29. Rusk H, Taylor E: *Rehabilitation medicine: a textbook of physical medicine and rehabilitation*, ed 2, St Louis, 1964, Mosby.
30. Santschi WR, editor: *Manual of upper extremity prosthetics*, ed 2, Los Angeles, 1958, University of California Press.
31. Schuch CM, Pritham CH: International organization terminology: application to prosthetics and orthotics, *J Prosthet Orthot* 6(1):29–33, 1994.
32. Scott R, et al: Understanding and using your myoelectric prosthesis, *UNB Monogr Myoelectric Prostheses*, 1985.
33. Spencer E: Amputations. In Hopkins HL, Smith HD, editors: *Willard and Spackman's occupational therapy*, ed 5, New York, 1978, JB Lippincott.
34. Stoner EK: Management of the lower extremity amputee. In Kottke FJ, Stillwell GK, Lehmann JF, editors: *Krusen's handbook of physical medicine and rehabilitation*, ed 3, Philadelphia, 1982, WB Saunders.
35. United States Department of Health and Human Services: Vital and health statistics: prevalence of selected impairments, 1977, *Series* 10: 155-29, 1993.
36. Weeks SR, Anderson-Barnes VC, Tsao JW: Phantom limb pain, *The Neurologist* 16(5):277–286, Sept 2010.
37. Wellerson TL: *A manual for occupational therapists on the rehabilitation of upper extremity amputees*, Dubuque, Iowa, 1958, Brown.
38. Wright G: *Controls training for the upper extremity amputee*, San Jose, Calif, Instructional Resource Center, San Jose State University (film).
39. Ziegler-Graham K, MacKenzie EJ, Ephraim PL, et al: Estimating the prevalence of limb loss in the United States: 2005 to 2050, *Arch Phys Med Rehabil* 89, March 2008.

Recommended Reading

Atkins DJ, Alley RD: Upper-extremity prosthetics: an emerging specialization in a technologically advanced field, *OT Pract* 8(3):CE1–CE8, February 10, 2003.

Atkins DJ, Meier RH, editors: *Comprehensive management of the upper-limb amputee*, New York, 1989, Springer-Verlag.

Christian A: *Lower limb amputation: a guide to living a quality life*, New York, 2006, Demos Medical Publishing.

Crepeau EB, Cohn E, Schell B, editors: *Willard and Spackman's occupational therapy*, ed 10, Philadelphia, 2000, Lippincott Williams & Wilkins.

Klute GK, Kantor C, Darrouzet C, et al: Lower limb amputee needs assessment using multistakeholder focus group approach, *J Rehabil Res Dev* 46(3):293–304, 2009.

Pedretti LW, Early MB: *Occupational therapy: practice skills for physical dysfunction*, ed 5, St Louis, 2001, Mosby.
Reed KL: *Quick reference to occupational therapy*, ed 2, Gaithersburg, Md, 2000, Aspen.
Van der Linde H, Hofstad CJ, Geertzen JHB, et al: From satisfaction to expectation: the patient's perspective in lower limb prosthetic care, *Disabil Rehab* 29(3):1049–1055, July 2007.
Watt J: On the road to recovery at Brooke Army Medical Center, *OT Pract* 10(14):16–18, August 8, 2005.
Yeager A: Low-tech adaptive devices for upper-extremity amputations, *OT Pract* 9(8):12–16, April 19, 2004.

Resources

American Academy of Orthotics and Prosthetics
http://oandp.org/

Amputee Coalition of America
http://www.amputee-coalition.org/aca_about.html

Amputee Information Network
www.amp-info.net

Hosmer-Dorrance, manufacturer of components
http://hosmer.com/

Otto Bock, supplier of prosthetics
http://www.ottobockus.com/

Therapeutic Recreation Systems (TRS), Inc.
2450 Central Ave #D
Boulder, CO 80301-2844
(800) 279-1865
(303) 444-4720

CHAPTER 34

Cardiac Dysfunction and Chronic Obstructive Pulmonary Disease

MAUREEN MICHELE MATTHEWS

Key Terms

Myocardium
Ischemia
Myocardial infarction (MI)
Cardiac rehabilitation
Congestive heart failure (CHF)
Cardiac risk factors
Signs of cardiopulmonary distress
Heart rate
Blood pressure
Rate pressure product (RPP)
Chronic obstructive pulmonary disease (COPD)
Pulmonary rehabilitation
Dyspnea control postures
Pursed-lip breathing (PLB)
Diaphragmatic breathing
Cardiovascular responses to activity
Basal metabolic equivalents (MET)
Energy conservation

Chapter Objectives

After studying this chapter, the student or practitioner will be able to do the following:

1. Briefly describe the cardiovascular system and its function.
2. Identify the significance of ischemic heart disease and valvular diseases of the heart.
3. Identify major risk factors, modifiable risk factors, and contributing conditions for heart disease.
4. Identify signs and symptoms of cardiac distress.
5. Describe the course of action to take if signs and symptoms of cardiac distress are present.
6. List the psychosocial considerations for persons with cardiovascular or pulmonary disease.
7. Describe methods for taking heart rate and blood pressure.
8. Determine rate pressure product, given heart rate and blood pressure.
9. Give a brief overview of the respiratory system and identify its primary function.
10. Define chronic obstructive pulmonary disease.
11. Identify pulmonary risk factors and psychosocial considerations.
12. Describe dyspnea control postures, pursed-lip breathing, and diaphragmatic breathing.
13. Describe a relaxation technique and its purpose.
14. List interview questions that will help the clinician know what the patient understands about treatment.
15. Explain the significance of a basal metabolic equivalent chart in the progression of activity and describe how to use it.

Individuals with disorders of the cardiovascular or pulmonary system can be severely limited in endurance and performance of activities of daily living (ADL). Occupational therapy (OT) services can benefit such individuals. An understanding of the normal function of the cardiopulmonary system, the pathology of cardiopulmonary disease, common risk factors, clinical terminology, medical interventions, precautions, and standard treatment techniques will guide the occupational therapy assistant (OTA) in providing effective care and promoting recovery of function in persons with compromised cardiovascular or pulmonary systems.

Every cell of the body has three major requirements for life: (1) a constant supply of nutrients and oxygen; (2) continual removal of carbon dioxide and other waste products; and (3) a relatively constant temperature. The cardiovascular and pulmonary systems play key roles in these processes.

Cardiovascular System

Anatomy and Circulation

The heart and blood vessels work together to maintain a constant flow of blood throughout the body. The heart, located between the lungs, is pear shaped and about the size of a fist. It functions as a two-sided pump. The right side pumps blood from the body to the lungs; simultaneously the left side pumps blood from the lungs to the body. Each side of the heart has two chambers, an upper atrium, and a lower ventricle.

Blood flows to the heart from the venous system. It enters the right atrium, which contracts and squeezes the blood into the right ventricle. Next, the right ventricle contracts and ejects the blood into the lungs, where carbon dioxide is exchanged for oxygen. Oxygen-rich blood flows from the lungs to the left atrium. As the left atrium contracts, it forces

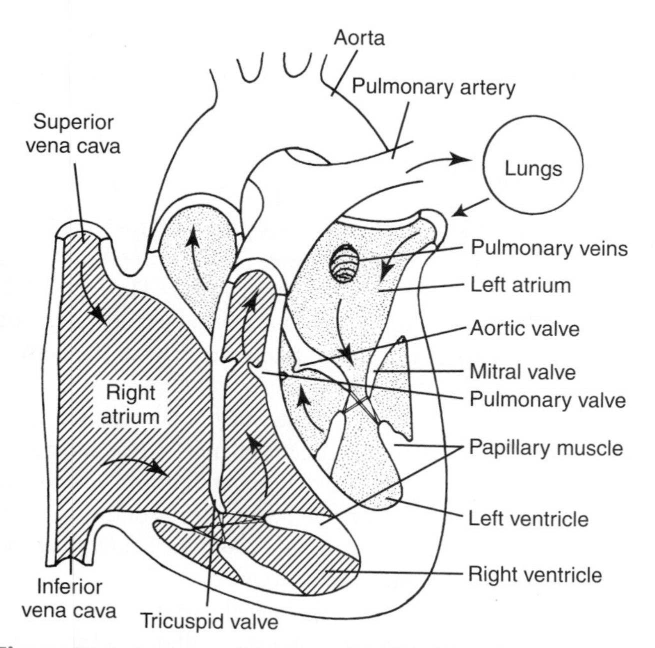

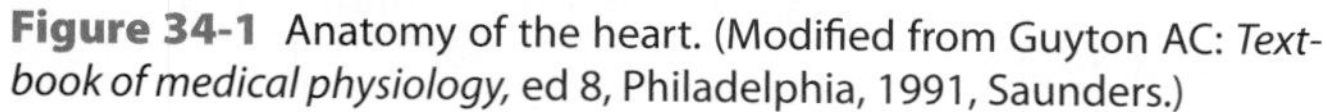

Figure 34-1 Anatomy of the heart. (Modified from Guyton AC: *Textbook of medical physiology,* ed 8, Philadelphia, 1991, Saunders.)

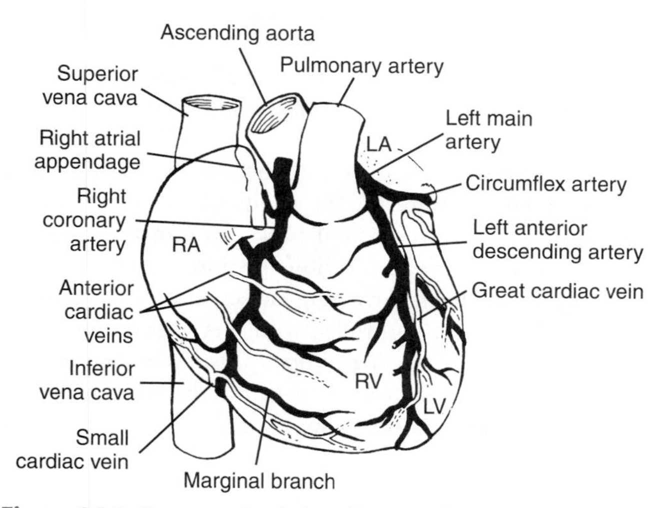

Figure 34-2 Coronary circulation. (From Underhill SL et al, editors: *Cardiac nursing,* Philadelphia, 1982, JB Lippincott.)

blood into the left ventricle, which then contracts and ejects its contents into the aorta for systemic circulation (Figure 34-1). Blood travels from the aorta to the arteries and through progressively smaller blood vessels to networks of tiny capillaries. In the capillaries, blood cells exchange their oxygen for carbon dioxide.

Each of the ventricles has two valves: an input valve and an output valve. The valves open and close as the heart muscle (**myocardium**) contracts and relaxes. These valves control the direction and flow of blood.

The heart is living tissue and requires a blood supply (arterial and venous system) of its own or it will die. Coronary arteries cross over the heart muscle to supply the myocardium with oxygen-rich blood. The coronary arteries are named for their location on the myocardium (Figure 34-2). Cardiologists refer to these arteries by abbreviations, such as *LAD* for left anterior descending. A blockage of the LAD will interrupt the blood supply to the left ventricle. Because the left ventricle supplies the body and brain with blood, a heart attack caused by LAD blockage can have serious consequences.[5,19,33] Look at Figure 34-2 and locate the LAD. This is the general area of Mr. F.'s heart attack.

CASE STUDY

Mr. F.

An occupational therapist has evaluated Mr. F., a 48-year-old realtor who experienced 10/10 substernal chest pain, nausea, and shortness of breath during closing of a large commercial transaction. In preparing for the closing, he had continued to work despite extreme fatigue, occasional chest pain, and shortness of breath. He was diagnosed with an acute anterolateral myocardial infarction (MI) complicated by acute congestive heart failure (CHF). After being stabilized in an acute hospital, he was discharged to a skilled nursing facility (SNF) for further therapy.

Mr. F. wants to return to his family and his real estate work. He is a married father of three children, ages 13, 11, and 7. His wife works full-time and cannot manage his care at home until he is self- sufficient. He was referred to OT for ADL evaluation and progression of activity.

Evaluation Summary

Medical history: unremarkable. Risk factors: age, sex, family history, and a sedentary lifestyle. Current clinical status: Normal sinus rhythm, enlarged left ventricle, and diffuse coronary artery disease. He performed a 2 basal metabolic equivalent (MET) seated sponge bath with minimal assistance. Vital signs were appropriate during the evaluation, except systolic blood pressure fell 20 mm Hg in recovery (3 minutes after completion of bathing), and patient became symptomatic (nausea and shortness of breath). Symptoms and vital signs stabilized after 5 minutes of rest. Mr. F. reports smoking 1 pack of cigarettes a day for the past 30 years. He states that he drinks socially, a few beers on weekends.

Mr. F. is anxious. He eats his meals in bed. He transfers independently and per physical therapy can safely walk to the bathroom. He expressed concern that he will die "before age 50, just like Dad." Before his MI, Mr. F. enjoyed playing catch with the kids and taking occasional walks with his wife. He describes himself as a "weekend warrior."

Problem List

1. Decreased functional capacity and endurance for self-care
2. Lack of ability to pace activity and monitor own signs and symptoms
3. Potential for alteration in sexual function
4. Positive risk factors of sedentary lifestyle and cigarette smoking
5. Anxiety amplified by family history of cardiac death

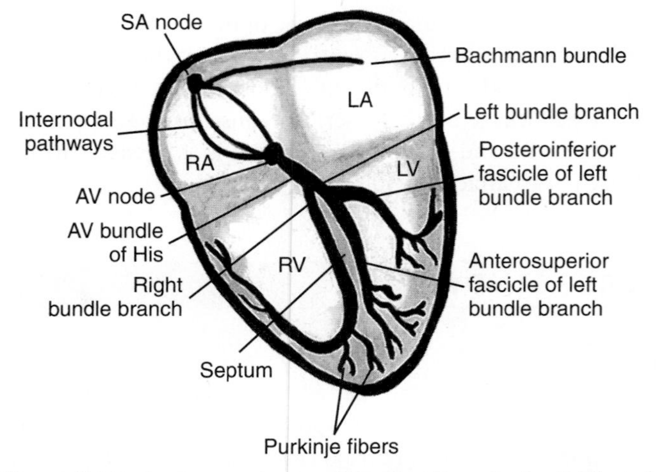

Figure 34-3 Cardiac conduction. (Modified from Andreoli KG et al: Comprehensive cardiac care: a text for nurses, physicians, and other health practitioners, St Louis, 1983, Mosby.)

Mechanism of Heart Contraction

The heart has an electrical conduction system that regulates contraction and relaxation of the myocardium (Figure 34-3). Electrical impulses usually originate in the right atrium at the sinoatrial (SA) node and travel along internodal pathways to the atrioventricular (AV) node, through the bundle of His, to the left and right bundle branches, and finally to the Purkinje fibers. Nerve impulses normally travel this pathway 60 to 100 times every minute, causing both atria to contract and then both ventricles. The SA node responds to vagal and sympathetic nervous system input.[5] Heart rate increases in response to exercise and anxiety and decreases in response to relaxation behaviors such as deep breathing and meditation.

Electrical impulses generated below the SA node cause the heart to contract abnormally. Some conduction irregularities can be life threatening. Impulses generated by the heart's conduction system can be studied by electrocardiography (ECG). ECG is used to assist in diagnosing cardiac disease.[5,17]

Pathology of Cardiac Disease

Ischemic Heart Disease

Cardiovascular disease (CVD) refers to diseases of the heart or blood vessels. *Atherosclerosis* is a CVD process that develops over a period of many years.[25] The walls of arteries can become injured by years of cigarette smoking or high blood pressure. Once the wall is damaged, it becomes irregular in shape and prone to collecting plaque (fatty deposits, like cholesterol). Platelets also gather along the arterial wall and clog the artery (which is called a *lesion*). The artery narrows and allows less blood to pass through it. Atherosclerosis may occur in any part of the body but is most dangerous when it affects arteries supplying the brain, heart, kidneys, or legs.[2] The leading cause of death for men and women in the United States is atherosclerotic CVD.[14] Coronary artery disease (CAD) refers to atherosclerosis of the arteries supplying the heart muscle.

If a coronary artery is partially or completely blocked, the heart may not get enough oxygen (a condition called ischemia). Persons with CAD may be free of symptoms at rest but develop angina, a type of chest pain, while eating or during exercise, exertion, or exposure to cold. Angina varies from individual to individual. Rest, medication, or both may relieve angina, usually without permanent heart damage. However, angina is a warning sign and should not be ignored.

Chest pain that is not relieved by rest or medication is indicative of a myocardial infarction (MI), or heart attack. A physician should evaluate the patient promptly. During an MI, part of the heart muscle dies. If a substantial part of the heart is damaged, the heart will stop (cardiac arrest) and the person may die.

For about 6 weeks after an MI, tissue damage can spread if the heart works too hard. A delicate balance of rest and activity must be maintained for cardiac rehabilitation so that the heart can heal without the patient becoming deconditioned. In about 6 weeks, scar tissue forms and the risk of extending the MI decreases. Scar tissue does not contract with each heartbeat, so the heart will not pump as well. Graded exercise can strengthen the healthy part of the myocardium and improve cardiac output.

Mr. F. has CAD and had ignored his symptoms (shortness of breath, fatigue, and chest pain). The CAD became significant enough to cause an MI. His heart muscle was damaged by loss of its blood supply. During his rehabilitation, Mr. F. must learn to listen to and respect the signs and symptoms that he previously disregarded.

Mr. F.'s recovery is also complicated by heart failure. Congestive heart failure (CHF) results when the heart cannot pump effectively and fluid backs up into the lungs or the body. Fluid overload is serious because it puts a greater workload on the heart. Straining causes further congestion. Usually, CHF can be controlled with diet, medications, and rest. Patients who experience difficulty resuming their former level of activity after acute CHF may limit their own recovery. Persons with acute CHF can attain optimal function through graded activity.

Valvular Disease

Heart valves may become damaged with disease or infection, resulting in CHF, ischemia, volume overload, or pressure overload. If the aortic valve fails to close properly (aortic insufficiency), CHF or ischemia may result. In another disorder of the aortic valve, aortic stenosis (calcification), *pressure overload* occurs. The left ventricle, which is working harder to open the sticky valve, enlarges, and cardiac output decreases. Ventricular arrhythmia, cerebral insufficiency, confusion, syncope (fainting), and sudden death may result. Surgery to correct valve problems may be recommended. *Volume overload* results when fluid accumulates in the lungs and causes shortness of breath. The overload increases the potential for irregular and ineffective contractions in both atria (atrial fibrillation). Consequently, blood flow through the heart slows, and blood clots (emboli) may develop in the ventricles. Many cerebrovascular accidents are caused by emboli ejected from the heart into the circulatory system of the brain.

Cardiac Risk Factors

The Framingham study[16] identified many factors that put people at risk for developing atherosclerosis. Cardiac risk factors fall into the following three major categories: (1) unchangeable factors—heredity, male gender, and age; (2) changeable factors—cholesterol levels, cigarette smoking, high blood pressure, and an inactive lifestyle; and (3) contributing factors—diabetes, stress, and obesity. The more risk factors a person has, the greater the risk of developing CAD. Four risk factors—smoking, diabetes, hypertension, and excessive weight—have been associated with left ventricular enlargement, which is a major cause of CHF.[3]

Reduction of risk factors is an important goal for the patient and requires support from the rehabilitation team. Prevention of cardiac disease is ultimately in the hands of the individual. Health care professionals, aware of the changes that persons with heart disease must make to reduce risk factors, can facilitate these changes via education, dialogue, and affirmation of the individual's responsibility. It takes years for most CVD to develop. Early prevention can avert or delay the onset. Which risk factors did Mr. F. have, and into what category might each be classified?

Medical Management

Emergency personnel will administer aspirin to persons who experience a heart attack if they have not taken any before the onset of symptoms. In the emergency department the patient is evaluated to determine whether reperfusion (opening blood flow) of the coronary blood vessels would be helpful. The patient may be given intravenous fibrinolytic therapy (clot-busting medication) or surgery to restore the blood flow. These emergency measures improve chance of survival and limit cardiac damage.[6]

Various surgical options can correct circulatory problems associated with CAD. Balloon angioplasty (or percutaneous transluminal coronary angioplasty, PTCA) and coronary artery bypass grafts (CABGs) are most common. In PTCA, a balloon catheter is guided through the circulatory system into the coronary arteries. The site of the lesion is pinpointed and the balloon inflated, pushing plaque against the arterial wall. When the balloon is deflated, improved circulation to the myocardium usually results. During a PTCA a wire mesh tube, called a *stent,* may be implanted into the coronary artery to keep the artery open.[15]

In CABG the surgeon opens the patient's chest by sawing through the sternum and spreading the ribs to expose the heart. Diseased sections of the coronary arteries are bypassed with healthy blood vessels from the saphenous veins or the internal mammary arteries. Improved coronary circulation results.

When the heart's pumping ability is severely reduced, a heart or heart lung transplantation may be performed. If the operation is successful, the patient may be rehabilitated to a level of function that is significantly higher than in the months before surgery.

Once hospitalized, heart attack survivors are managed in a coronary care unit, where they are closely observed for complications. Ninety percent of all persons who have had an MI will develop arrhythmia.[8] Close medical management is imperative.

Cardiac Medications

Knowledge of the purpose and side effects of cardiac medication provides a framework for understanding the patient's response to activity. Table 34-1 lists common cardiac medications. Cardiac medications are adjusted at frequent intervals until an optimal therapeutic response has been attained. Adverse signs and symptoms should be reported to the physician or nurse promptly. In most settings the nurse is responsible for contacting the physician.

Psychosocial Considerations

Individuals entering cardiac rehabilitation programs suffer from psychological distress that is related both to physical compromise and to psychological factors.[26] Individualized assessments that focus on social, psychological, and occupational status of patients can be helpful in tailoring therapeutic intervention for optimal functional outcomes.[31] Persons who have experienced an MI pass through a number of phases of adjustment to disability. Fear and anxiety are common initially as patients confront their mortality. Education and supportive communication will do much to reduce anxiety.[22] As patients begin to resume more normal activities, feelings of helplessness may begin to subside. Patients feel more secure when familiar coping mechanisms allow them to respond to the stress, but some former coping mechanisms (smoking, drinking, or consuming fatty foods) are harmful. These patients must learn new strategies.

Denial is common in patients with cardiac disease. Persons in denial must be closely monitored during the acute phase of recovery because they may not believe precautions are necessary and could further damage their cardiovascular system by not complying with them.

Depression occurs typically in the third to sixth day after an MI and can last many months.[8] Forced inactivity during the recovery phase can frustrate a person who previously used exercising to exhaustion as a way to deal with stress. Including the patient's family in the education will correct misconceptions and decrease anxieties.

Consider Mr. F. and his psychosocial response. Did he express any anxiety during his evaluation? What healthy coping mechanisms to decrease anxiety are available to Mr. F.? What aspects of his history would be of concern?

Cardiac Rehabilitation

Cardiac rehabilitation is a program aimed at educating persons with CVD to improve their cardiac condition, improve physical conditioning, reduce symptoms of cardiac distress, improve overall health, and prevent cardiac problems. Working with the health care team, individuals recovering from acute MI, CABG, and other cardiac procedures are instructed in guided exercise to improve their recovery. Through active engagement in the rehabilitation process, individuals learn to manage and improve their health.

Table 34-1 Common Cardiac Medications—Modified from Cardiac Medications at a Glance: American Heart Association, 2008

Category	Common Names	Purpose	Uses
Anticoagulants	Coumadin (warfarin) Enoxaparin (Lovenox) Heparin	Prevents blood clots	Helps to prevent harmful clots from forming. May prevent clots from becoming larger and causing more serious problems. Often prescribed to prevent stroke.
Antiplatelet agents	Aspirin Ticlopidine Clopidogrel Dipyridamole	Prevents blood clots by preventing platelets from sticking together	Helps prevent clotting in patients who have had a heart attack, unstable angina, and other forms of CVD. Usually prescribed preventively, when plaque buildup is present.
Angiotensin-converting enzyme (ACE) inhibitors	Benazepril (Lotensin) Captopril (Capoten) Enalapril (Vasotec) Fosinopril (Monopril)	Expands blood vessels and decreases resistance. Allows blood to flow more easily and makes the heart's work easier	Used to treat CVD including HTN and CHF.
Angiotensin II receptor blockers (or inhibitors) (ARBs)	Candesartan (Atacand) Eprosartan (Teveten) Irbesartan (Avapro)	ARBs prevent this chemical from having any effects on the heart and blood vessels. Dampens BP.	Used to treat or improve symptoms of cardiovascular conditions including HTN and CHF.
β-blockers	Nadolol (Corgard) Propranolol (Inderal) Atenolol (Tenormin) Other drugs ending in "olol"	Decreases the heart rate and cardiac output, which lowers BP and makes the heart beat more slowly and with less force.	Used to lower BP. Used with therapy for cardiac arrhythmias and in treating angina. Used to prevent repeated heart attacks.
Calcium channel blockers	Diltiazem (Cardizem) Verapamil (Isoptin, Calan)	Interrupts the movement of calcium into the cells of the heart and blood vessels.	Used to treat HTN, angina, and some arrhythmias.
Diuretics	Lasix (furosemide) Dyazide Hydrochlorothiazide (HCTZ)	Lowers BP, decreases edema through increased urination	Used to help decrease BP and excessive fluid buildup in tissues of the body.
Vasodilators	Isosorbide dinitrate (Isordil) Nesiritide (Natrecor) Hydralazine (Apresoline) Nitrates (NTG) Minoxidil	Relaxes blood vessels and increases the supply of blood and oxygen to the heart while reducing its workload.	Used to decrease angina.
Cardiac glycosides (digitalis preparations)	Digoxin Lanoxin	Increases the force of the heart's contractions, which can be beneficial in heart failure and for irregular heart beats.	Used to relieve heart failure symptoms
Statins	Atorvastatin (Lipitor) Simvastatin (Zocor)	Can lower blood cholesterol levels	Used to lower LDL ("bad") cholesterol, raise HDL ("good") cholesterol and lower triglyceride levels.

BP, blood pressure; *CHF*, congestive heart failure; *CVD*, cardiovascular disease; *HTN*, hypertension.

During the first 1 to 3 days after an MI, stabilization of the cardiac patient's medical condition is usually attained. This acute phase is followed by a period of early mobilization. Phase 1 of treatment (inpatient cardiac rehabilitation) focuses on monitored low-level physical activity including self-care; reinforcement of cardiac and postsurgical precautions; instruction in energy conservation and graded activity; and establishment of guidelines for appropriate activity levels at discharge. Via monitored activity, the ill effects of prolonged inactivity can be averted and medical problems, poor responses to medications, and atypical chest pain can be addressed.

Phase 2 of treatment, outpatient cardiac rehabilitation, usually begins at discharge. During this phase exercise can be advanced while the patient is closely monitored on an outpatient basis.

Community-based exercise programs follow in phase 3. Some individuals require treatment in their place of residence because they are not strong enough to tolerate outpatient therapy.

Table 34-2 Signs and Symptoms of Cardiac Distress

Sign/Symptom	What to Observe
Angina	Look for chest pain that may be squeezing, tight, aching, burning, or choking in nature. Pain is generally substernal and may radiate to the arms, jaw, neck, or back. More intense or longer-lasting pain forewarns of greater ischemia.
Dyspnea	Look for shortness of breath with activity or at rest. Note the activity that brought on the dyspnea and the amount of time that it takes to resolve. Dyspnea at rest, and with resting respiratory rate over 30 breaths per minute, is a sign of acute CHF. The patient may need emergency medical help.
Orthopnea	Look for dyspnea brought on by lying supine. Count the number of pillows the patient sleeps on to breathe comfortably (1, 2, 3, or 4 pillows of orthopnea).
Nausea/emesis	Look for vomiting or signs that the patient feels sick to the stomach.
Diaphoresis	Look for a cold, clammy sweat.
Fatigue	Look for a generalized feeling of exhaustion. The Borg Rate of Perceived Exertion (RPE) scale is a tool used to grade fatigue.
Cerebral signs	Ataxia, dizziness, confusion, and fainting (syncope) are all signs that the brain is not getting enough oxygen.
Orthostatic hypotension	Look for a drop in systolic blood pressure of greater than 10 mm Hg with change of position from supine to sitting or from sitting to standing.

When patients engage in a comprehensive cardiac rehabilitation program, health care costs can be significantly reduced and positive health effects can result.[28] Patients who acquire skills in relaxation and breathing control after an MI have been found to need fewer hospitalizations and have less expensive medical management even 5 years post MI.[34] Increased functional independence, prevention of disability, and a decreased need for custodial care have been attained in elderly cardiac rehabilitation patients.[21] Acute inpatient rehabilitation consists of monitored ADL and instruction in cardiac and postsurgical precautions, energy conservation, graded activity, and risk factor management. The patient is also instructed in guidelines for discharge activities. The ill effects of prolonged inactivity can be averted by means of monitored activity while medical problems, poor responses to medications, and atypical chest pain can be rooted out. Cardiac rehabilitation may continue in the home, community, or outpatient setting.

Prompt, accurate identification of the signs and symptoms of cardiac distress and immediate modification of treatment are imperative. If any signs of cardiac distress (Table 34-2) are observed during treatment, the proper response is to stop the activity, have the patient rest, seek emergency medical help if the symptoms do not resolve, report the symptoms to the team, and modify future activity to decrease the workload on the heart. Part of the OT intervention for Mr. F. should include identification of adverse response to activity. What signs and symptoms did Mr. F. ignore before his heart attack? Mr. F. would be unlikely to stop an activity when signs of cardiac distress occur if he could not recognize them in himself. During his evaluation, Mr. F.'s blood pressure dropped after assisted seated sponge bathing. He also experienced nausea and shortness of breath. What precautions should the OT practitioner review with Mr. F. before his next treatment session?

The Borg Rate of Perceived Exertion (RPE) scale measures perception of workload.[7] Patients are shown the scale (which ranges from 6 to 20) and instructed that a rating of 6 means no exertion at all and a 19 equals the most strenuous activity they have ever performed. After the activity, they are asked to appraise their feelings of exertion and rate the task.

Tools for Measuring the Patient's Response to Activity

Heart rate, blood pressure, rate pressure product, and ECG readings are other measures for evaluating the cardiovascular system's response to work.

Heart Rate

Heart rate (beats per minute) can be monitored by palpating the radial, brachial, or carotid pulse. The radial pulse is located on the volar surface of the wrist, just lateral to the radial head. The brachial pulse is slightly medial to the antecubital fossa. The carotid pulse, located lateral to the Adam's apple, should be palpated gently because overstimulation can cause the heart rate to fall. The OTA must establish service competency in palpating the carotid pulse before attempting palpation independently.

Heart rates can be regular (even) or irregular. Although an irregular heart rate is abnormal, many persons function quite well with one. To determine the heart rate, one applies the second and third fingers flat (not tips) to the pulse site. If the pulse is even (regular), count the beats for 10 seconds and multiply the finding by 6. When the heart rate is irregular, the number of beats should be counted for a full minute.

A sudden change in heart rate from regular to irregular should be reported to the physician. In addition, patients can be taught to take their own pulses and monitor their heart rates' responses to activity. As a general rule of thumb, the heart rate should rise in response to activity.

Blood Pressure

Blood pressure is the pressure that the blood exerts against the artery walls as the heart beats. A stethoscope and blood pressure cuff (sphygmomanometer) are used to determine blood pressure indirectly. Place the cuff snugly around the patient's upper arm just above the elbow, centering the bladder of the cuff above the brachial artery. Inflate the cuff while palpating the brachial artery to 20 mm Hg above the point at which a pulse is last felt. With the ear pieces of the stethoscope angled forward in the practitioner's ears, he or she places the dome of the stethoscope over the patient's brachial artery. The practitioner supports the patient's arm in extension with the brachial artery and the stethoscope gauge at the patient's heart level. The practitioner deflates the cuff at a rate of approximately 2 mm Hg per second. Listening carefully, the practitioner first hears two sounds that correspond to the systolic blood pressure. The practitioner listens for when pulse fades (diastolic blood pressure). This procedure should be practiced under immediate supervision until competency is established.

Rate Pressure Product

Heart rate and blood pressure will fluctuate in response to activity. Cardiac output is affected by both. Rate pressure product (RPP) measurement gives a more accurate indication of how well the heart is pumping. RPP is the product of heart rate and systolic blood pressure (RPP = HR × SBP). It is usually a five-digit number but is reported in three digits by dropping the last two digits (e.g., HR 100 × SBP 120 = 12000 = RPP 120). During any activity RPP should rise at peak and return to baseline in recovery.

ECG provides another objective measure of heart activity. It takes hours of instruction, study, and practice to become proficient in ECG reading and interpretation. The OTA is not qualified to read an ECG unless service competency is established under a qualified clinical instructor. See Dubin's *Rapid Interpretation of ECG*[17] as a resource on the subject.

Many similarities exist between the evaluation and treatment of persons with cardiac disease and those with pulmonary dysfunction. A review of the pulmonary system and chronic obstructive pulmonary disease follows.

Anatomy and Physiology of Respiration

While the heart provides oxygen-rich blood to the body and transports carbon dioxide and other waste products to the lungs, the respiratory system exchanges oxygen for carbon dioxide. The cardiac and pulmonary systems are interdependent. If no oxygen were delivered to the bloodstream, the heart would soon stop functioning for lack of oxygen; conversely, if the heart were to stop pumping, the lungs would cease functioning for lack of a blood supply.

The respiratory system supplies oxygen to the blood and removes waste products, primarily carbon dioxide, from the blood. Air enters the body through the nose and mouth and travels through the larynx or voice box to the pharynx. From there it continues downward into the lungs by way of the trachea or windpipe. If the trachea or pharynx becomes blocked, a small incision may be made into the trachea to allow air to freely pass into the lungs. This procedure is called a *tracheotomy.*

Two main bronchi branch off from the trachea, carrying air into the left and right lungs. The bronchi continue to branch off into smaller tubes called *bronchioles.* Bronchioles segment into smaller passages called the *alveolar ducts.* Each alveolar duct divides and leads into three or more alveolar sacs. The entire respiratory passageway from bronchi to alveolar ducts is often called the *pulmonary tree.*

Each alveolar sac contains more than 10 alveoli. A fine, semipermeable membrane separates the alveolus from the capillary network. Across this membrane, oxygen is transported and exchanged for carbon dioxide. Exhaled carbon dioxide travels upward through the pulmonary tree and out through the mouth and nose.

The muscle power for breathing air into the lungs, or inspiration, is provided primarily by the diaphragm. Originating from the sternum, the ribs and lumbar vertebrae, and the lumbocostal arches, the diaphragm forms the inferior border of the thorax. The muscle fibers of the diaphragm insert

CASE STUDY

Mrs. P.

Mrs. P. is a 64-year-old woman with a 3-year history of chronic obstructive pulmonary disease (COPD). She was released from the acute care hospital 3 days ago, having been stabilized after an acute exacerbation of COPD. She is widowed and lives alone in a small one-bedroom apartment. She has one daughter who is married, works full-time, and has one child. Mrs. P. was referred to OT for pulmonary rehabilitation. An occupational therapist evaluated her and established a treatment plan for the OTA to follow.

Evaluation Summary

Mrs. P. has been smoking cigarettes since age 20 and currently smokes one pack per day. She has had three prior exacerbations of COPD. She states that she cannot quit smoking because all of her friends smoke. Her apartment is on the first floor and is across the street from a grocery store. There is a first-floor laundry room in her building. Mrs. P.'s daughter lives three blocks away and checks on her daily. She empties the bedside commode and provides groceries and dinner. Mrs. P. wants to empty the commode herself. Mrs. P. is extremely anxious and demonstrates only minimal understanding of pursed lipped and diaphragmatic breathing. The home health aide provides total assistance with a bed bath. Mrs. P. experiences dyspnea on exertion and does not apply breathing techniques to activity. She gets herself a light breakfast and snack with a complaint of severe dyspnea on exertion. Mrs. P. does not use her prescribed oxygen during activity because it is too heavy to carry around. According to physical therapy, she was a limited community ambulator before her recent hospitalization.

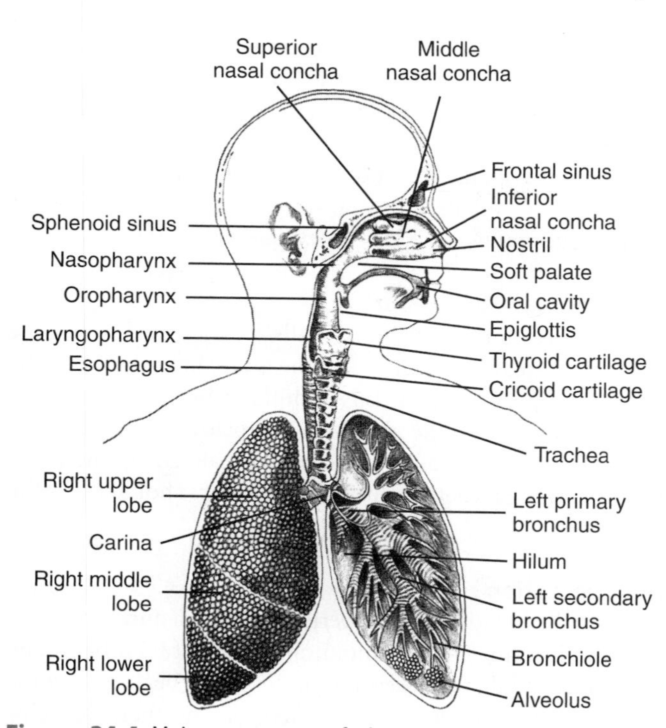

Figure 34-4 Major structures of the respiratory system. (From Springhouse Publishing Company Staff-Respiratory Support, Philadelphia, 1991, Lippincott Williams & Wilkins.)

into a central tendon. Innervated by the left and right phrenic nerves, the diaphragm domes downward as it contracts, enlarging the volume of the thorax and causing a drop in pressure in the lungs. Air then enters the lungs, equalizing lung and outside air pressures. Accessory muscles—the intercostals and scalene—are also active during inspiration. They maintain the alignment of the ribs and help elevate the rib cage, respectively.

At rest, expiration is primarily a passive relaxation of the inspiratory musculature. Forced expiration requires active contraction of the abdominal muscles to compress the viscera and squeeze the diaphragm upward in the thorax. Expiration can be further forced by flexing the torso forward and pressing with the arms on the chest or abdomen. As the volume of the thorax decreases, air is forced out of the lungs. Figure 34-4 shows the structure of the respiratory system.[9,33]

Innervation of the Respiratory System

Breathing is mostly involuntary. A person does not have to think to take a breath. The autonomic nervous system controls breathing. With anxiety and increased activity, the sympathetic nervous system will automatically increase the depth and rate of inspiration. Parts of the brain provide the central control for breathing; they adjust their response to input from receptors in the lungs, the aorta, and the carotid body.

Although the act of breathing is primarily involuntary, there is also a volitional component that allows for measured and deliberate mediation of the outflow of breath during activities requiring controlled breathing such as swimming or playing the harmonica.[9,33]

Chronic Obstructive Pulmonary Disease

Common chronic disorders of the lungs for which pulmonary rehabilitation is ordered include chronic obstructive pulmonary disease (COPD) and asthma.[9] COPD (actually a group of diseases) is characterized by "damage to the alveolar wall and inflammation of the conducting airways"[4] and includes emphysema, peripheral airway disease, and chronic bronchitis. More than 15 million Americans have been diagnosed with COPD.

The most common signs of COPD are daily coughing, shortness of breath, and increasing fatigue with exercise.[37] In COPD the onset of physical disability is typically gradual, with dyspnea on exertion representing the initial phase of disability. The disease evolves toward shortness of breath at rest. Uncoordinated, ineffective breathing patterns contribute to shortness of breath.[11]

Asthma is characterized by irritability of the bronchotracheal tree and is typically episodic in its onset. Individuals with asthma may be free of symptoms for periods of time between the episodes of wheezing and dyspnea.[20] A genetic predisposition seems to influence development of asthma in some individuals. Allergic causes of asthma may include pollens and respiratory irritants such as perfume, dust, pollen, and cleaning agents. If left untreated, a severe asthmatic episode may result in death.[4,9]

Pulmonary Risk Factors

Smoking is the primary cause of COPD. The best method for preventing COPD or for controlling it is to not smoke.[37] Because cigarette smoke is a pulmonary irritant, it may also be a causative agent in asthmatic episodes. Other environmental irritants such as air pollution and chemical exposure are contributory risk factors in the development of COPD and asthma.[4,9]

Medical Management

COPD is a progressive, chronic disease process. The onset of the disease process is gradual. Medications prescribed for pulmonary disease include antiinflammatory agents (e.g., steroids, cromolyn sodium); bronchodilators (e.g., albuterol, theophylline) that help to open the airways; and expectorants (e.g., iodides, guaifenesin) that help loosen and clear mucus. Oxygen therapy, at a specific liter flow, may also be prescribed. Some persons on oxygen therapy may be tempted to increase the liter-per-minute flow, erroneously thinking that more is better. This practice can result in CO_2 retention and lead to right heart failure.

Persons with acute respiratory distress initially may be managed on a ventilator before being weaned to oxygen. Ventilators provide a mechanical assist to the process of inspiration. Ventilators will not slow down the end-stage disease process of COPD.

When a patient's endurance decreases enough to impair ADL performance, the physician may refer the patient to OT.[4,9]

Signs and Symptoms of Respiratory Distress

Dyspnea is the most obvious sign that an individual is having difficulty breathing. In its most severe form, the patient is short of breath at rest. Persons with this level of dyspnea will be unable to utter a short phrase without gasping for air. When reporting that a patient has dyspnea, the practitioner should note the precipitating factors (e.g., "Mr. S. becomes short of breath when washing his face while seated in front of the sink").

Other signs that the body is not getting enough oxygen include extreme fatigue, a nonproductive cough, confusion, impaired judgment, and cyanosis (a blue tinge to the skin).[4,9]

Psychosocial Considerations

COPD is a progressive and debilitating physical illness, and the psychosocial effects of the disease are considerable. Depression and anxiety are not uncommon; 96% of patients with COPD have reported disabling anxiety.[1] Others complain of faintness or difficulty concentrating.[18] Progressive muscle relaxation has been shown to be successful for controlling dyspnea and anxiety and for lowering heart rate.[35] Dyspnea-related anxiety (fear related to shortness of breath and inability to manage symptoms) leads to avoidance of physical exertion.[12] A spiral of functional decline can follow in which the individual stops participating in activities that cause symptoms, lowering one's physical capacity for activity. This leads to deconditioning in which the individual experiences shortness of breath in activities that are progressively less physically demanding. Controlling and reducing dyspnea-related anxiety is important; patients can be taught breathing techniques using guided mastery and can be made more aware of symptoms and their management.[12]

Pulmonary Rehabilitation

The goals of pulmonary rehabilitation are to stabilize or reverse the disease process and return the patient's function to its highest capacity. A multidisciplinary rehabilitation team working with the patient can design an individualized treatment program to meet this end. An accurate diagnosis, medical management, therapy, education, and emotional support are components of a pulmonary rehabilitation program. OT personnel are often part of the team that also includes the physician, nurse, and patient. Respiratory therapists, dietitians, physical therapists, social workers, and psychologists may also be team members. When OT is part of the pulmonary rehab team, the outcome for severely disabled COPD patients is improved.[29] Knowledge of specialized pulmonary treatment techniques is imperative to treating persons with pulmonary disease.

Treatment Techniques

Dyspnea Control Postures

Breathlessness can be reduced in patients with COPD by having them adopt dyspnea control postures. When sitting, the patient bends forward slightly at the waist while supporting the upper body by leaning the forearms on the table or thighs. When standing, leaning forward and propping the body on a counter or shopping cart may relieve the problem.

Pursed-Lip Breathing

Pursed-lip breathing (PLB) is thought to prevent tightness in the airway by providing resistance to expiration. This technique increases use of the diaphragm and decreases accessory muscle recruitment.[10] PLB is sometimes instinctively adapted by persons with COPD, whereas others may need to be instructed in the technique. Instructions for PLB are the following: (1) purse your lips as if you are going to whistle; (2) slowly exhale through pursed lips—you should feel some resistance; (3) inhale deeply through your nose; and (4) it should take you twice as long to exhale as it does to inhale.

Diaphragmatic Breathing

Another breathing pattern that calls for increased use of the diaphragm to improve chest volume is diaphragmatic breathing. Many persons learn this technique by placing a small paperback novel on the abdomen just below the thorax. The person lies supine and is instructed to inhale slowly and make the book rise. Exhalation through pursed lips should cause the book to fall.

Desensitization

As individuals with COPD experience dyspnea during activity, manage their anxiety, and monitor and adjust their breathing in a controlled therapeutic environment, they begin to become desensitized to dyspnea-related anxiety. The therapist reinforces dyspnea control postures, paced activity, and breathing techniques while ensuring safe performance of activity. Oxygen saturation monitors, when available, provide another measure of safety. When oxygen saturation drops below 90%, activity should be stopped.[32]

Relaxation

Progressive muscle relaxation in conjunction with breathing exercises can be effective in decreasing anxiety and in controlling shortness of breath. One technique involves tensing muscle groups while slowly inhaling and then following with relaxation of the muscle groups when exhaling twice as slowly through pursed lips. It is helpful to teach the patient a sequence of muscle groups to tense and relax. One common sequence involves tensing and relaxing the face; then the face and the neck; then the face, neck, and shoulders; and so on down the body to the toes. A calm, quiet, and comfortable environment is important for the novice in learning any relaxation technique. Biofeedback in conjunction with relaxation therapy promotes a more rapid mastery of relaxation skills.[23]

Management of Dyspnea Guidelines for Practice[32]

Migliore[32] developed guidelines for the treatment of individuals with COPD. Treatment focuses initially on control of respiration at rest. Initial patient competency is attained in PLB and diaphragmatic breathing with dyspnea control postures. Biofeedback (paced breathing, metronomes, and recording of the patient's breathing pattern) reinforces learning. Clients are then progressed to controlled breathing with activity. Management of dyspnea-related anxiety is attained by therapeutic discussions to improve the patient's understanding of how poor breathing patterns create false danger signals and signs or symptoms of true hypoxia. Using both individual and group treatment, Migliore's guidelines provide the clinician with an organized and meaningful approach to treatment.

Other Treatments and Considerations

Physical therapists may teach chest expansion exercises, a series of exercises intended to increase the flexibility of the chest. Percussion, postural drainage, and vibration are other techniques used to loosen secretions and assist with draining them from the lungs. Other team members usually teach these techniques.

Humidity, pollution, extremes of temperature, and lack of air movement have been reported to have a deleterious effect on persons with respiratory ailments. These factors should be taken into consideration when one is planning activities.

Occupational Therapy Evaluation and Treatment of Persons with Cardiopulmonary Dysfunction

OT intervention can promote improvements in performance of ADL for persons with limitations caused by chronic respiratory or cardiovascular limitations. The following information is to be used for both cardiac and pulmonary conditions, occurring separately or together.

Evaluation

Review of the Medical Record

A review of the medical record will identify the patient's medical history (diagnosis, severity, associated conditions, and secondary diagnoses); social history; test results; and precautions. Although the OTA may not perform the initial evaluation of the patient, familiarizing oneself with changes in the patient's condition as documented in the medical record should be standard practice.

Patient Interview

It is common courtesy and good medical practice to begin every patient encounter with an introduction and an explanation of the purpose of treatment. Good interview skills include asking the right questions, listening to the patient's response, and observing patients as they respond. Look for signs of anxiety, shortness of breath, confusion, difficulty comprehending, fatigue, posture, endurance, ability to move, and family dynamics. Interview questions should not only seek clarification of information that was not clear in the medical record but also clarify the patient's understanding of his or her condition and treatment.

Not uncommonly, a patient may have cardiac AND pulmonary conditions. Patients with a history of angina should be asked to describe their angina. If the patient has also had an MI, he or she should be asked if he or she can differentiate between angina and MI chest pain and pulmonary symptoms. Clarification of symptoms before treatment can prove invaluable should symptoms arise.

Asking patients to describe a typical day, identify activities that bring on shortness of breath or angina, and tell how their physical limitations interfere with the things they enjoy doing most in life will reveal problems that are relevant to the patient.

Clinical Assessment

The purpose of the clinical assessment is to establish the patient's present functional ability and limitations. The content of an occupational therapist's clinical assessment will vary from patient to patient and setting to setting. Persons with impairments of the cardiovascular system will be monitored for heart rate, blood pressure, and signs and symptoms of cardiac distress during an evaluation of tolerance to postural changes and a functional task. Table 34-3 summarizes appropriate and inappropriate cardiovascular responses to activity. Individuals with disorders of the respiratory system must be monitored for signs and symptoms of respiratory distress. Range of motion, strength, and sensation may be grossly assessed within the context of the ADL evaluation. The patient's cognitive and psychosocial status will become apparent to the skilled clinician through interview and observation.

After the evaluation, the occupational therapist has sufficient information to formulate a treatment plan. In consulting the patient about the treatment plan, the clinician informs the patient of the expected outcome of treatment and verifies that goals will be meaningful and relevant to the patient.

Treatment

Both Mr. F. and Mrs. P. have a decreased functional capacity for self-care. They share a similar goal of wanting to take a standing shower (3.5 basal metabolic equivalents [MET]) and tolerate being out of bed for most of the day. The clinical techniques and cueing provided by the therapist or assistant will be unique to the condition of each of them. In reading this treatment section and comparing Mr. F.'s cardiac condition to Mrs. P.'s compromised respiratory status, consider which interventions would be most appropriate for each individual.

Table 34-3 Cardiovascular Response to Activity

	Appropriate	Inappropriate
HR	Increases with activity, to no more than 20 beats/min above resting heart rate	HR more than 20 beats/min above RHR with activity, RHR ≥120, HR drops or does not rise with activity.
BP	SBP rises with activity	SBP ≥220 mm Hg, postural hypotension (≥10-20 mm Hg drop in SBP), decrease in SBP with activity
Signs and symptoms	Absence of adverse symptoms	Excessive shortness of breath, angina, nausea and vomiting, excessive sweating, extreme fatigue (RPE ≥15), cerebral symptoms

BP, blood pressure; *HR*, heart rate; *RPE*, rate of perceived exertion; *RHR*, resting heart rate; *SBP*, systolic blood pressure.

Progression of treatment for persons with cardiovascular impairment or respiratory impairment is guided by present clinical status, recent functional history, response to current activity, and prognosis. Persons with significant cardiac or pulmonary impairment, limited recent functional ability, inappropriate orthostats (cardiovascular responses to changes in position, e.g., sit to stand), or poor reaction to activity and a poor prognosis will progress slowly in comparison with individuals with little impairment of the heart or lungs, a recent history of normal functional ability, appropriate responses to orthostats and activity, and a good prognosis. The OTA should keep these factors in mind when treating persons with cardiopulmonary deficits.

In both case studies in this chapter, the patients might benefit from working on seated bathing during the next therapy session, but the focus of treatment will be different for each. Mr. F.'s session might focus on early recognition of symptoms, pacing his self-care, and exhaling on exertion. Mrs. P.'s treatment would include coordination of PLB and diaphragmatic breathing with activity and use of dyspnea control postures at rest. If tolerated, dyspnea control postures could be extended to a simple light hygiene task, like seated teeth care.

Energy costs of an activity and the factors that influence them can further guide the OTA in the safe progression of activity. Oxygen consumption suggests how hard the heart and lungs are working, providing an indication of the amount of energy required to complete a task. Resting quietly in bed requires the least amount of oxygen per kilogram of body weight, 1 MET, roughly 3.5 ml O_2 per kilogram of body weight. As activity increases, more oxygen is required to meet the demands of the task. For instance, dressing requires 2 MET, or roughly twice the amount of energy that lying in bed takes. Guided by a MET table (Table 34-4) and the patient's response to activity, the OTA can determine a logical treatment progression tailored to the patient's prognosis and goals. As a general rule, once patients tolerate an activity (i.e., seated sponge bathing) with appropriate responses, they can progress to the next higher MET level activity (i.e., standing sponge bath).

At all times during interactions with patients, therapy personnel focus on attaining the safest and highest level of function. With a cardiac rehabilitation patient in denial, the OTA might best focus on paced activity and teaching the patient to recognize and identify symptom exacerbation as a time to stop and rest. In pulmonary rehabilitation the focus shifts to performing compensatory breathing strategies and dyspnea control postures. Here patients are learning to push their limits safely; education focuses on improving patient understanding that increased work requires increased respiratory effort. By focusing on helping the patient learn appropriate activity responses, the OTA guides the patient toward improving independent function in a safe and sustainable manner.

The duration of any physical activity must also be taken into account when determining activity guidelines. Obviously, persons who have difficulty performing a 2 MET activity must still use a commode (3.5 MET) or bedpan (5 MET) for their bowel management. A person can perform at a higher than usual MET level for brief periods without adverse effects.

Sexual activity at 5 MET is often a grave concern to persons with impaired cardiovascular function and their partners. Sexual intercourse is intermittent in its peak demands for energy. Patients often can return to sexual intercourse once they can climb two flights of steps in 1 minute with appropriate cardiovascular responses.[38] Providing the patient with information as to when it is safe to resume sexual activity can reduce anxiety surrounding the resumption of sexual intercourse. Discussing sexual activity guidelines with the patient and partner may further decrease anxiety. The patient should be instructed to monitor heart rate and symptoms of cardiac distress before and after intercourse. In addition, the patient and partner should be informed that cardiac medications can affect the patient's libido. The patient should be encouraged to inform the physician of problems related to sexual activity. Medications can often be adjusted to alleviate these problems.

Energy Conservation

When patients learn to conserve their energy resources, they can perform at a higher functional level without expending more energy. The basic principles of energy conservation and work simplification, covered in Chapter 11 and other chapters,

Table 34-4 Basal Metabolic Equivalent Table of Areas of Occupation

MET Level	Activities of Daily Living	Instrumental Activities of Daily Living, Work, Play, and Leisure
1-2	Eating, seated[30]; transfers, bed to chair; washing face and hands; brushing hair[30]; walking 1 mph	Hand sewing,[13] machine sewing, sweeping floors,[13] driving automatic car, drawing, knitting[36]
2-3	Seated sponge bath,[36] standing sponge bath,[36] dressing and undressing,[27] seated warm shower,[36] walking 2-3 mph, wheelchair propulsion 1-2 mph	Dusting[30]; kneading dough[13]; hand washing small items[13]; vacuuming, electric[30]; preparing a meal[27]; washing dishes[36]; golf[36]
3-4	Standing shower, warm[27]; bowel movement on toilet[13]; climbing stairs at 24 ft/min[36]	Making a bed,[27] sweeping, mopping, gardening[36]
4-5	Hot shower,[27] bowel movement on bedpan,[27] sexual intercourse[36]	Changing bed linens,[30] gardening, raking, weeding, rollerskating,[24] swimming 20 yards/min[36]
5-6	Sexual intercourse,[36] walking up stairs at 30 feet/min[36]	Biking 10 mph level ground[36]
6-7	Walking with braces and crutches	Swimming breaststroke,[36] skiing, playing basketball, walking 5 mph, shoveling snow, spading soil[36]

should prove useful in teaching persons with cardiovascular or pulmonary compromise how to decrease energy demands on the body while promoting function.

Exhaling with exertion is an energy conservation strategy particularly helpful for persons with compromised cardiac or pulmonary function. This technique helps control the rate of increase of systolic blood pressure with activity. It is important for the patient to practice energy conservation skills during treatment. Therapeutic support is critical in learning. Both Mr. F. and Mrs. P. would benefit from this technique.

Patient and Family Education

OT personnel, as members of the health care team, share the responsibility for patient and family education. Cardiac and/or pulmonary anatomy, disease process, symptom management, risk factors, diet, exercise, and energy conservation must be taught and reinforced to patient and family members by the team. Including family members in an education program provides support indirectly to the patient through the family unit. Such support is critical when a patient depends on the help of a family member to accomplish everyday tasks.

In progressing treatment for Mr. F. and Mrs. P., their individual goals will evolve into the areas of instrumental ADL. For Mr. F., sexual activity guidelines, guidelines for resuming sporting activities with his youngsters, and return to work are all possible venues for further therapeutic intervention. Mrs. P. has expressed an interest in basic homemaking tasks (emptying her commode). Given the proximity of laundry facilities to her apartment, independence in personal laundry may be of interest to her. Smoking cessation is essential for optimal outcomes for Mrs. P.

Summary

Healthy individuals can meet the varying demands of their bodies for oxygen because their heart and respiratory rates adjust to meet oxygen demand. When the cardiovascular and/or pulmonary system is compromised, the ability to perform normal activity declines. This chapter is designed to guide the OTA in the treatment of persons with impairments of the heart or lungs.

Selected Reading Guide Questions

1. Describe the heart's size and explain the function of its right and left sides.
2. What do the heart valves control?
3. Explain the significance of the coronary arteries in heart disease and heart attacks.
4. Identify the symptoms of cardiac distress. Explain why modifying activity in response to them is important.
5. Explain the significance of left ventricular dysfunction.
6. Using the MET chart, identify a safe self-care task for a person who can function at 2.5 MET.
7. If the patient could perform a seated sponge bath but could not stand because of a secondary disability, which activity would you choose to promote progress in rehabilitation? Explain.
8. Describe the appropriate therapeutic response when a patient develops chest pain during activity.
9. What is COPD?
10. Name the breathing techniques used in pulmonary rehabilitation and their purposes.
11. Describe dyspnea control postures.
12. Explain how treatment concerns for activity tolerance vary and are similar for persons with cardiac compromise and those with respiratory conditions.
13. Using the cardiac medications chart, explain how cardiac medications might affect heart rate or blood pressure.
14. What are cerebral signs? What do they signify, and why is this important? What action would you take if a patient were to suddenly develop cerebral signs?

Exercises

1. Demonstrate dyspnea control postures in sitting and standing.
2. Teach your partner pursed-lip and diaphragmatic breathing.
3. Choose a cooking task. Explain how to modify the activity by using three energy conservation principles.
4. Determine your partner's heart rate and respiratory rate.
5. Have your partner run in place for 3 minutes. Immediately take your partner's blood pressure and heart rate. Calculate the RPP for before and immediately after activity. Was your partner's response appropriate?
6. Pretend that your partner is Mr. F. (case study) and that he is asking about when it will be safe for him and his wife to resume sexual activity. How will you respond?
7. Pretend your partner is Mrs. P. (case study). She has a resting respiratory rate of 33. While panting, she tells you to "Leave" (pant) "me" (pant) "alone" (pant). Demonstrate an appropriate response.

References

1. Agle DP, Baum GL: Psychological aspects of chronic obstructive pulmonary disease, *Med Clin North Am* 61(4):749–758, 1977.
2. American Heart Association, Inc. (2011) Atherosclerosis: Retrieved from: http://www.heart.org/HEARTORG/Conditions/Cholesterol/WhyCholesterolMatters/Atherosclerosis_UCM_305564_Article.jsp.
3. American Heart Association rapid access journal report (2009): *Four risk factors raise probability of developing precursor of heart failure; new 30-year risk estimates developed for serious cardiac events.* Dallas: Retrieved from: http://www.newsroom.heart.org/index.php?s=43&item=746.
4. American Thoracic Society: Definitions and classifications of chronic bronchitis, asthma, and pulmonary emphysema, *Am Rev Respir Dis* 85(8):762–768, 1962.
5. Andreoli KG, Fowkes VK, Zipes DP, et al: *Comprehensive cardiac care: a text for nurses, physicians and other health practitioners*, ed 5, St Louis, 1983, Mosby.
6. Antman EM, Ande DT, et al: ACC/AHA guidelines for the management of patients with ST-elevation myocardial infarction: a report of the America College of Cardiology/American Heart Association Task Force on Practice Guidelines (Committee to Revise the 1999 guidelines for Management of Patients with Acute Myocardial Infarction), *J Am Coll Cardiol* 4(3):671–719, 2004 Aug 4.

7. Borg GA: Psychosocial bases of perceived exertion, *Med Sci Sports Exerc* 14(5):377–381, 1982.
8. Bragg TL: Psychological response to myocardial infarction, *Nurs Forum* 14(4):383–395, 1975.
9. Brannon FJ, Foley MW, Starr JA, et al: *Cardiopulmonary rehabilitation: basic theory and application*, ed 3, Philadelphia, 1997, FA Davis Company.
10. Breslin EH: The pattern of respiratory muscle recruitment during pursed-lip breathing, *Chest* 101(1):75–78, 1992.
11. Collins EG, Langbein WE, Fehr L, Maloney C: Breathing pattern retraining and exercise in persons with chronic obstructive pulmonary disease, *AACN Clin Issues* 12:202–209, 2001.
12. Carrieri-Kohlman V, Douglas MD, Gormley JM, Stulbarg MS: Desensitization and guided mastery: treatment approaches for the management of dyspnea, *Heart Lung* 22:226–234, 1995.
13. Colorado Heart Association: *Exercise equivalent 1970 cardiac reconditioning & work evaluation unit*, Spaulding Rehabilitation Center.
14. D'Agostino RB, Russell MW, Huse DM, et al: Primary and subsequent coronary risk appraisal: new results from the Framingham Study, *Am Heart J* 139:272–281, 2000.
15. Dangas G, Kuepper F: Cardiology patient page, restenosis: repeat narrowing of a coronary artery: prevention and treatment, *Circulation* 105(22):2586–2587, 2002.
16. Dawber R: *The Framingham study: the epidemiology of atherosclerotic disease*, Cambridge, Mass, 1980, Harvard University Press.
17. Dubin D: *Rapid interpretation of EKGs*, ed 6, Tampa, 2000, Cover Publishing.
18. Dudley DL, Glaser EM, Jorgenson BN, et al: Psychosocial concomitants to rehabilitation in chronic obstructive pulmonary disease, part 2: psychosocial treatment, *Chest* 77(4):544–551, 1980.
19. Elliot MA, Anbe DT, Armstrong PW, et al: ACC/AHA guidelines for the management of patients with ST-elevation myocardial infarction, executive summary: a report of the American College of Cardiology/American Heart Association Task Force on Practice Guidelines (Writing committee to revise the 1999 guidelines for the management of patients with acute myocardial infarction), *Circulation* 110(5):588–636, 2004.
20. Farzan S: *A concise handbook of respiratory diseases*, ed 2, Reston, Va, 1985, Reston.
21. Ferrara N, Corbi G, Bosimini E, et al: Cardiac rehabilitation in the elderly: patient selection and outcomes, *Am J Geriatr Cardiol* 15(1):22–27, Jan-Feb 2006.
22. Gentry WD, Haney T: Emotional and behavioral reaction to acute myocardial infarction, *Heart Lung* 4(6):738–745, 1975.
23. Green E, Walters ED, Green AM, et al: Feedback technique for deep relaxation, *Psychophysiology* 6(3):371–377, 1969.
24. Goldman L, Hashimoto B, Cook EF, et al: Comparative reproducibility and validity of systems for assessing cardiovascular functional class: advantages of a new specific activity scale, *Circulation* 64(6):1227–1234, 1981.
25. Goldberger E: *Essentials of clinical cardiology*, Philadelphia, 1990, JB Lippincott.
26. Jette DU, Downing J: The relationship of cardiovascular and psychological impairments to the health status of patients enrolled in cardiac rehabilitation programs, *Phys Ther* 76(2):130–139, Feb 1996.
27. Kottke FJ: Common cardiovascular problems in rehabilitation. In Krusen FH, Kottke FJ, Elwood PM, editors: *Handbook of physical medicine and rehabilitation*, Philadelphia, 1971, WB Saunders.
28. Levin LA, Perk J, Hedback B: Cardiac rehabilitation: a cost analysis, *J Intern Med* 230(5):427–434, 1991.
29. Lorenzi CM, Cilione C, Rizzardo R, et al: Occupational therapy and pulmonary rehabilitation of disabled COPD patients, *Respiration* 71:246–251, 2004.
30. Maloney FP, Moss K: Energy requirements for selected activities, *Unpublished manuscript*, 1974.
31. McKenna K, Mass F, Tooth L: Predictions of quality of life after angioplasty, *Scand J Occup Ther* 5:173–179, 1998.
32. Migliore A: Management of dyspnea guidelines for practice for adults with chronic obstructive pulmonary disease, *Occup Ther Health Care* 18(3), 2004.
33. Mythos for SoftKey: *BodyWorks 4.0: human anatomy leaps to life*, Cambridge, Mass, 1993-95, SoftKey International.
34. Oldridge NB, Guyatt GH, Fischer ME, et al: Cardiac rehabilitation after myocardial infarction. Combined experience of randomized clinical trials, *JAMA* 260(7):945–950, 1988.
35. Renfroe KL: Effect of progressive relaxation on dyspnea and state anxiety in patients with chronic obstructive pulmonary disease, *Heart Lung* 17(4):408–413, 1988.
36. Santa Clara Valley Medical Center: *Graded activity sheets*, San Jose, Calif, 1994.
37. Santa Clara Valley Medical Center: *Chronic obstructive pulmonary disease (COPD)*, San Jose, Calif Mar 23, 2007.
38. Scalzi C, Burke L: Myocardial infarction: behavioral responses of patient and spouses. In Underhill SL, Woods ES, Sivarajan Froelicher ES, et al, editors: *Cardiac nursing*, Philadelphia, 1982, JB Lippincott.

CHAPTER 35 Oncology

ANN BURKHARDT

Key Terms

Neoplasm
Cancer
Carcinoma
Sarcoma
Lymphoma
Leukemia
Paraneoplastic syndrome
Chemotherapy
Blood levels
Radiation therapy
Palliative care
Hospice
Mastectomy
Radical neck dissection
Stomas
Colostomy
Urostomy

Chapter Objectives

After studying this chapter, the student or practitioner will be able to do the following:

1. Describe cancer and its diagnosis and medical-surgical treatments.
2. Identify strategies for helping patients cope with side effects of chemotherapy and radiation.
3. Describe the role of occupational therapy in the treatment of cancer patients.
4. Identify techniques to be used in addressing a variety of occupational therapy goals with cancer patients.

Cancer is a broad category of conditions found when a tumor, or neoplasm (new abnormal growth of cells), is present in the body. A cancer (carcinoma) is an abnormal tissue that grows and spreads or that may metastasize (move and start in new sites) throughout the body. Cancers may be low grade, with a natural history of slow development and spread, or may be high grade, with a tendency to grow quickly and spread rapidly. The cancer type is diagnosed by the tissue from which it first develops. For example, if a person has breast cancer that metastasizes to the lung, the biopsy of the lung lesion will contain breast cancer cells, not lung cancer cells. This condition would be labeled "breast cancer metastatic to the lung."

The cancer is further defined by the tissue in which it arises. For example, a carcinoma arises from epithelial tissue, a sarcoma from connective tissue, a lymphoma from the cellular components of lymph nodes, and leukemia from blood-forming organs such as the bone marrow. Many cancers are solid tumors or masses in the tissue of origin. Cancers arising in the bone marrow are often characterized by abnormal blood cell counts such as those associated with anemia. When cancers arise in endocrine tissues (glands), the cancer may produce a pseudohormone that mimics a hormone normally present in the bloodstream. In these instances, the free-circulating hormone level will be abnormally elevated. People occasionally show neurologic signs (e.g., seizures, cognitive changes) caused by the free circulation of the pseudohormones. This is an example of paraneoplastic syndrome, a group of symptoms indirectly caused by the presence of cancer elsewhere in the body. Because no solid tumor is present, the paraneoplastic syndrome is sometimes the first clinical sign of a cancer that is difficult to diagnose.

Medical Background Information

A variety of xrays and scans are used to assist in the diagnosis of cancer. A lung cancer, for instance, may be detected initially by chest xray. The xray is the initial screening test. It is crude and not clear in its definition but still sensitive enough to be used for cancer screening. Moreover, it is much less expensive than a computed tomography (CT) scan or magnetic resonance imaging (MRI) procedure. Mammograms—xrays of the breast tissue—are a form of xrays used to detect breast tumors.

CT scans may be done with or without the use of contrast dye. Contrast dye is radioactive and circulates in the bloodstream, outlining all vascular (blood vessel) structures. To receive the nutrients they need to grow, tumors usually develop vascular networks that are highlighted by dye during this test. CT with contrast dye is a fairly good tool to diagnose the presence of a solid tumor.

MRI is helpful in the diagnosis of soft tissue lesions. No radiation is used in an MRI, a scan that uses magnetic properties of biological tissues to form the basis of an image. Abnormal tissues respond to magnetic radio frequencies differently than do normal tissues and produce a different image in an MRI. The scan cannot differentiate, however, among blood clots, cancers, or demyelinating plaques (like those found in patients with multiple sclerosis). Gadolinium is a magnetically active material used with the MRI as a contrast dye. It enhances the image of the vascular system with magnetic properties of the dye. MRI is particularly helpful for diagnosing spinal disorders.[16]

Bone scans are tomographic scans (serial xrays that, when viewed in composite, produce a three-dimensional representation of the segment of the body scanned) of the skeletal system. Contrast dye is injected 2 hours before the scan is taken. Bone scans are helpful in diagnosing metastatic lesions to bone and some primary bone tumors. They are used to stage cancers that metastasize to bone such as breast cancer and prostate cancer. They are also used for regular, routine follow-up for persons with an initial diagnosis of these cancers to check for recurrence of the cancer.

A positron emission tomography (PET) scan is used to look at the structure and function of body tissues and is effective at spotting tumors in the body.[15]

Biopsies are surgical procedures in which a section or segment of tumor is removed so that a pathologist may examine it to determine a diagnosis. Biopsies can be done in a number of ways (e.g., scrape, smear, needle biopsy).

Regional lymph nodes may be suspected of involvement, either from a primary cancer such as lymphoma, or as a sign of regional spread of disease, as in breast cancer. Lymph nodes are dissected at the time of a surgery to detect regional spread of the cancer and to stage the cancer. Imaging with ultrasound is sometimes used instead of biopsy of lymph nodes for staging a cancer.

Staging the Disease

A few systems are in use for staging cancers, but most are based on the same underlying principles. At diagnosis, the cancer may be localized to one region. At this point, the cancer is usually an early stage and may be classified as stage I disease. Cancer that has spread to an adjacent local region of the body such as from the right breast to the right axilla is classified as stage II disease (a tumor and one metastasis). If the disease spreads to another organ such as from the breast to the lung, then stage III disease is evident. When multiple systems/organs are involved and the disease is widespread, stage IV is present.[7]

Another staging system commonly used is the tumor, node and metastasis (TNM) system. *Tumor* (T) represents the number of actual tumor sites, primary and metastatic. *Node* (N) refers to the number of positive or involved lymph nodes that have cancer present in a surgical pathology sample. *Metastasis* (M) may be regional or widespread.

Staging of the disease is helpful, along with other information concerning the specific cancer, in determining a treatment course and prognosis for the patient. The past few years have seen an improvement in the treatment of several forms of advanced stage (stage IV) cancer, thus resulting in higher rates of survival with improved quality of life. For example, hormone-mediated cancers such as breast cancer and prostate cancer are being managed by combining a drug that blocks formation of bony metastases with hormone site blockers or chemotherapy regimens. Some forms of cancer are now considered chronic diseases rather than immediate life-threatening conditions. The demand for rehabilitation and improvement in quality of life has increased.

Treatment

After a diagnosis and staging of cancer, choices concerning treatment are made. Most tumors with a solid mass are treated by surgery. The mass may be resected, and a margin of normal tissue may be taken from the surrounding area to remove the risk of local spread to normal tissues. When a tumor is encapsulated, tightly localized in its own capsule, sometimes a limited resection or lumpectomy is sufficient. If a tumor has invaded some of the local region or structures, a resection of the tumor and the involved structures as a whole mass may be done. If the surgery removes bone, sometimes reconstructive or joint replacement surgeries may be necessary to improve cosmetic appearance or function. When a tumor is aggressive but interferes with a normal body function, a surgical bypass procedure may be performed to prolong function or alleviate pain. If a tumor has invaded surrounding tissues and structures and the neurovascular bundle (nerves and their blood supply), sometimes an amputation is the surgery of choice.

Cancer is now viewed as a chronic illness. People who have been in remission for up to decades after their initial diagnosis and treatment may have exacerbations, or recurrence of disease.[22]

Medical Oncology and Chemotherapy

Tumors are composed of different types of tissue, so the same treatment will not work for all tumors. Some tumor cells are sensitive to chemotherapy agents. Chemotherapy is a means of affecting change with chemicals. Most chemotherapeutic agents are toxic to normal tissues, as well as cancer cells; therefore side effects are inevitable. The chemotherapy drug can interfere with the tumor cells' genetic material, so the tumor cells stop dividing, multiplying, and surviving. Tumor cells often have a higher metabolic rate than normal cells, so they take up the chemicals and die first before the normal tissue shows signs of destruction.

Other chemotherapies work by bonding with the surface of the cancer cells and blocking their interaction with other cells. Because many cells rely on interactions with other cells to travel through membranes and become biologically active, this mechanical blocking mechanism stops their ability to act.

Monoclonal antibodies, hormones, and some antitumor antibiotics act in this manner.[13]

Patients who accept the concept of chemotherapy typically dread the side effects. The drugs are poisonous to normal tissues and can affect almost any body organ. For instance, many chemotherapies deplete the bloodstream of platelets, cells that help to clot blood. A person whose platelet count is low bleeds easily.[23] Simple activities such as brushing teeth may provoke abnormal bleeding. Overuse of a joint can trigger bleeding into a joint space or a muscle compartment, which can abnormally raise the pressure in the enclosed area and cause the normal tissues to die. In extreme cases, a compartment syndrome may result. If this goes undetected and the tissues become necrotic, an amputation may be necessary to save the person's life. Therapy personnel need to stay informed about the person's blood cell counts, monitor the sensory and motor function, and inform the doctor of any changes involving a limb.

It is helpful to use blood levels, such as white blood cell and platelet counts and hematocrit, to guide treatment choices in therapy (Table 35-1). The crisis with platelets may last only a few days, when the chemotherapy is at the maximum level in the bloodstream. Once the platelets begin to recover, more normal and increasingly stressful activities may be graded to adjust to the change and restore normal function.

Neutropenia is a severe impairment of the immune response with decreased resistance to infection. A cold can cause severe illness in someone who is immunosuppressed. Neutropenic patients may be kept on protective isolation to limit the risk of cross-infection.[12]

Anemia reduces an individual's tolerance for treatment. The oxygen level in the system is depleted because of reduced hemoglobin. Fatigue should be respected, and activities must be paced and prioritized to encourage a sense of self-direction and to maximize functional ability. With overactivity, the person may require oxygen to recover from shortness of breath.

Peripheral neuropathy is a common side effect of neurotoxic chemotherapeutic agents. The person may have both motor and sensory involvement of the peripheral nerves, experiencing diminished (hypoesthesia) or heightened (hyperesthesia) sensory awareness, particularly in the hands and feet.[9] Diminished awareness can lead to a loss of protective sensation, and the person may be at risk for cutting, burning, or entrapping a limb, depending on which neurologic components are involved. Patients with heightened sensation may complain of pain and burning sensations so intense as to interfere with tolerance for even basic activities of daily living (ADL). Mild compression garments (toning gloves or tubular support bandages) may muffle the painful sensation and provide comfort and protection of the limb. In addition, sensory stimulation may decrease pain; examples include massage and exposure to graded textures (very soft to somewhat rough).

Table 35-1 Blood Values Reference Chart

Complication	Normal Range	Precaution
Neutropenia (white blood cell count)	47.6-76.8%	Avoid exposure to infection
Platelets (thrombocytopenia)	<130,000	Avoid resistive activities Avoid skin breakage
Hematocrit (anemia)	Men: 40-54% Women: 37-47%	Monitor vitals and respiratory rate

Another difficult side effect of some chemotherapies is *alopecia* (hair loss), which may also affect eyebrows, pubic hair, and extremity hair. Alopecia is one of the most obvious outward signs that identify a person who has a serious illness and may invoke the social stigma of cancer. Hair is also a significant element of individual identification. Hair usually grows back after completion of chemotherapy treatment, but the person may experience premature graying, other color shifts, and changes in texture and distribution of hair. Some people respond well to the suggestion to use wigs or hairpieces; others prefer to wear hats, scarves, or turbans; some prefer to go bald. It is a personal choice. Identifying the choices and providing community resources, names of stores, and access to catalogs is often helpful.

Some chemotherapies and radiation can detrimentally affect the reproductive organs. Patients should be informed of the effects of the cancer treatment on the ability to reproduce (have children by natural means). Men can have sperm frozen in a sperm bank for future use. Embryos can also be frozen for later use. Even adolescents who do not currently have a sexual partner may choose this option to keep future choices open. For those who do not save eggs or sperm, parenting is still possible through donors or adoption.

Radiation Therapy

Radiation therapy uses radioactive materials to kill or control the growth of cancer cells. Some (but not all) cancers are sensitive to radiation; therefore it is not always the treatment of choice. However, when a tumor is sensitive to its beams, radiation can be curative on its own or in combination with a chemotherapeutic agent.

The radioactive isotope may be placed in a machine that pinpoints the location of the tumor. A lead plate protects tissues from exposure until the person is correctly positioned and ready for treatment. External beam radiation directs the radiation over a set field, exposing the tumor and surrounding tissues to treatment. The beam can also be directed to a specific spot by placing a cone over the lens of the linear accelerator (radiation machine), thus concentrating the beam in one specific region. Exposure is given over a period of days, weeks, or months to deliver a total dose of radiation that could not be tolerated in one dose (because the radiation burns the tissues). Near the completion of treatment, the person may experience radiation burning. The radiologist will ask the patient to avoid using lotions, creams, perfumes, and soaps on the treatment zone because these products could increase the probability of a burn by changing the surface composition of the skin.[3]

Radiation can also be administered through implantation of radioactive seeds into the tumor bed or affected gland *(brachytherapy)*. The seeds are removed when treatment is completed. The treatment course for brachytherapy is usually a few days to a week. The radioactive seed is either implanted directly into the tissues or inserted through a flexible straw. Brachytherapy is used in the treatment of thyroid cancer, prostate cancer, some cancers of the genitourinary tract in women, and soft tissue carcinomas. While a patient is radioactive with the seed implanted, personnel must take special precautions. Lead aprons are often available for short-term direct contact with the patient. The chart usually states the maximum time allowed for exposure to health care providers, thus limiting the rads delivered to the caregiver. Lead chariots (shields) are often provided at the doorway of the patient's room. The caregiver is protected behind the chariot but can speak with the patient inside the room.

In addition to its curative effect, radiation can also be used to treat cancer pain. Radiation may reduce pain in two ways: (1) by decreasing the size of a mass that is pressing on structures or nerves; or (2) or by deadening the perception of the nerve. Radiation is particularly helpful with spinal tumors and bony metastases.[4]

The side effects of radiation may be seen immediately (as in the case of radiation burns), over time, or in conjunction with the healing process. Fibrosis is a form of scarring that may result from radiation. Some of the modalities used to treat burns have been found helpful in treating radiation fibrosis in its early stages. Silicone gel pads, for instance, keep the tissues soft, hydrated, and pliable.

Normal activity during the scar management phase may help to reverse the soft tissue contracture effect.[3] Soft tissues are soft in part because of their elastic properties and their relationship to fascia, the tissue layer beneath the skin. Fascia covers the muscle compartments and reduces the effect of friction that occurs with normal movement and work. When the soft tissues are irradiated, they are burned. On healing, the tissues stiffen and harden. Beneath the skin, the fascia may also lose its elasticity and resilience. The person who receives radiation therapy may report pulling, tightening, or stiffness associated with the fibrotic change. The patient may describe the body as feeling hard, even like wood.

Radiation to the region of the head and neck may contribute to the development of dysphagia, or swallowing disorders. Initially, the irradiated tissues are inflamed and swollen. Open sores can form in the oral cavity and oropharyngeal cavity, thus slowing the swallowing reflex and diminishing the function of the musculature supporting the swallowing mechanism. Food can spill into the airway and be aspirated (breathed into the lungs).[10]

Head and neck irradiation can also cause stiffening of the muscles of the jaw, mouth, neck, and shoulder. Scar management, range of motion, and movement activities are helpful in restoring normal function and preventing pain and discomfort.

Radiation may also cause neutropenia; therefore care should be taken to protect the neutropenic patient from cross-infection. If the caregiver has an infection, good handwashing technique and the use of masks is expected. If the patient participates in a group activity, avoiding proximity with a patient who has an infection is important.

Myelopathy (pathological loss of the myelin surrounding a nerve) and *neuropathy* (weakness or sensory loss) can also result in the short term or long term after radiation therapy. Permanent nerve damage usually results; therefore restoration of function is unrealistic. A patient with a *brachial plexopathy* (sensory or motor dysfunction of nerves arising at the proximal level of division of the peripheral nerves of the arm) can benefit from positioning and comfort measures, as well as adapted equipment to compensate for lost function. The nerves will not regenerate; therefore the goals will be the following: (1) to support the remaining function; (2) to prevent subluxation and pain; and (3) to compensate for loss of arm function. Chronic pain syndromes may accompany this condition. Restoration of function is often the primary goal, rather than total relief of pain. Treatments administered by the occupational therapist or physical therapist such as transcutaneous electrical nerve stimulation (TENS) can help to alleviate pain. The occupational therapy assistant (OTA) may provide stress reduction techniques such as relaxation breathing or guided imagery.

Cancer treatment and survival with a diagnosis of cancer typically interrupt and alter normal activities. The patient may experience change in expectations concerning future roles and may need to define new roles. The therapy practitioner can help by determining the activities that are most important to the individual and enabling participation in those that are realistic. Counseling patients may empower them to recognize their ability to strive for new goals and accept their inability to resume some activities.

Patients who receive radiation may experience alopecia. The response and management are the same in this instance as in the management of alopecia after chemotherapy.

New Therapies

Nanotechnology is being advanced for the use in the treatment of cancers. Nanoparticles are being used both to target specific malignant cells as direct transporters of chemotherapy to the malignancy, and in diagnostic scanning procedures to transport contrast materials directly to a malignancy so that spread of disease can be directly visualized and pinpointed. It is anticipated that nanotechnology will dramatically lessen side effects of chemotherapy and make targeting of malignant cells more exact and direct.[19]

Reasons for Referral to Occupational Therapy

The reasons for referral to occupational therapy (OT) may be described along a continuum of expected functional gain and prognosis of disease—prevention, restoration, support, and palliation.[6] Reference to this continuum is helpful in guiding treatment choices and determining realistic goals for the individual undergoing treatment (Box 35-1).

Prevention is an optimal goal in treatment because it supports normal living and avoids the development of conditions or complications that could otherwise arise from high-risk

Box 35-1

Key Concepts for Treatment Planning with Cancer Patients

Prevention—Treatment that can decrease a risk behavior for development of a disease
Restoration—Treatment that can restore function with little or no evidence that the dysfunction existed
Support—Treatment that uses substitution actions or equipment to optimize function
Palliation—Treatment that provides physical comfort or peace of mind by empowering patients to focus on goals of their choosing

behaviors. An example of prevention is a smoking cessation program to prevent lung cancer.[15] OT practitioners might work with healthy adolescents in a smoking-prevention program. An occupational therapist in a community-based practice could run a women's health group and train women to do breast self-examinations.

Restoration focuses on a return to normal functioning without the need for adaptive equipment or techniques. Restoration is appropriate for individuals who have mild sequelae after medical treatment but who are expected to recover completely. For example, women who are diagnosed with breast cancer in the early stages, receive medical treatment, and are declared in remission typically become physically deconditioned. They may not have had good exercise habits before treatment but now are invested in health-promoting behaviors and wellness.

Supportive goals become the focus of treatment when individuals cannot resume doing things normally without adaptations because of medical, surgical, or disease-specific sequelae. For example, a patient who has lost intrinsic hand function after surgical resection and radiation therapy for a soft tissue sarcoma in the forearm may become independent in activities of daily living (ADL) again. Function may be supported by a wrist support or tenodesis splint and adaptive devices to substitute for fine mobility loss in the affected hand.

Palliation is emphasized when the disease has metastasized widely and the patient may have only a limited time to live. OT intervention may provide the patient with control over the environment or may reduce pain to allow increased activity for part of the day. Palliative care focuses on empowering the patient to determine which activity is personally important. Palliative care can sustain realistic hope and interest, as well as ward off overwhelming depression and accompanying feelings of helplessness and hopelessness.

There is a differentiation between hospice care and palliative care. In the United States hospice care is tied to third-party reimbursement. For example, Medicare pays hospices a capitated dollar amount to provide care to the dying person. The case manager for the hospice prioritizes what service the hospice client will receive based on the need and financial availability of services. Some hospices have consulting occupational therapists who provide services. Palliative care, in contrast, gives control to the client and is not necessarily linked to traditional service delivery models. Funding is generally from grant funding, private sources, and philanthropy.[1]

Personal Meaning and a Diagnosis of Cancer

A diagnosis of cancer may cause the individual to reflect more deeply on the personal meaning of life, death, health, and illness. Creswell[5] described the psychological context for personal meaning as the following:

1. What an experience means for the person who has the experience
2. The description the person gives and from which are derived individual descriptions and general or universal meanings or interpretations of their experience
3. The examination of the essence of the structures of the experience

Liminality, the sense that one personally recognizes the finality of one's life, has been described by Little and colleagues.[12] The experience of liminality initially produces a feeling of loss of control and the need to seek sources of rational straightforward answers. Over time, awareness of one's liminality persists, but living with the reality becomes bearable.

Royeen and Duncan[20] have described meta-emotion as the cognitive awareness of one's emotion and how one uses emotion to experience life moment to moment. The process is an intertwining of emotion and meaning. According to Royeen and Duncan, emotion is a constituent part of occupation. Over time emotion cannot exist without occupation as a constituent part.

Padilla[19] described occupational meaning as the insider's perspective. Meaning is experienced as it is being lived. Features or items that a person perceives are meaningful can be analyzed with respect to their role as structural units of meaning. When a person is living with a diagnosis of cancer, his or her sense of personal meaning will be influenced by the severity and context of problems or challenges that emerge, in particular with regard to how these changes influence personal values and broaden or narrow participation in the process of living.[2] OT treatment planning and intervention are based on listening, problem solving, and enabling the person who is living the experience to participate in the occupations, life roles, activities, and tasks that are meaningful and important for them to do and that give them a sense of self-control and sustainability or active presence in their own continued process of living. The OT practitioner assists clients who are living with chronic, potentially life-threatening illness to do what they want and need to do to live day to day.

A qualitative research study was done to explore occupational engagement and its meaning to individuals following a life-threatening diagnosis.[24] Semistructured interviews were conducted with three women diagnosed with breast cancer. The primary theme that emerged from the study was "Doing = Living." This theme illustrates the connection between meaningful occupational engagement and one's self-perception as capable and healthy. The practice implication is that, in a period of personal crisis such as a life-threatening diagnosis, individuals may turn to those occupations that are meaningful to regain a sense of control and normalcy in their lives.

Specific Diagnoses of Cancer and the Role of the Occupational Therapy Assistant

Breast Cancer

During the early postoperative phase after breast cancer surgery, the arm on the side of surgery is at risk for loss of range of motion (ROM) because the surgical incision may extend under the arm and thus limit chest wall and myofascial (soft tissue) gliding. Within the first 2 to 3 weeks after surgery, the patient should move gently to protect the incision and promote healing. In the next phase, the patient should stretch to regain normal movement in the arm. Because inpatient hospitalization is short (2 days for a mastectomy [removal of a breast]; 1 day for lumpectomy), outpatient and community group programs to encourage movement are appropriate and needed. In addition, education about sensory changes perceived as discomfort or pain, which occur normally after breast surgery, is necessary. Education helps to encourage movement and allay fear as to the meaning of the pain.

Education concerning lymphedema (swelling of the arm on the side of surgery that can occur because lymph nodes were removed or damaged) is also crucial. Patients with lymphedema should follow arm and hand precautions, avoiding trauma (cuts, insect bites, burns, and repetitive strain injuries) to the arm on the surgical side.[20] Community agencies may provide support groups and exercise programs. Putting patients in touch with these programs can be beneficial. Examples of programs include the Reach to Recovery or Look Good … Feel Better program of the American Cancer Society, SHARE, or ENCORE. Patients appreciate information about resources available for breast prostheses (e.g., corsetieres), wigs, salons, and other camouflage (hats or turbans). OT practitioners may initiate, coordinate, and lead groups for a Look Good … Feel Better program if one does not exist in the area.[19]

During chemotherapy and radiation therapy treatment, patients can benefit from movement programs to restore normal motion to the arm on the side of treatment. Radiation therapy can cause adhesive capsulitis (a stiffening and hardening of the glenohumeral joint capsule resulting in a loss of rotation and mobility of the shoulder joint) that leads to frozen shoulder in the irradiated shoulder as radiation fibrosis develops. Continuation of stretching exercises, especially overhead and shoulder rotation movements, is important for prevention of reflex muscle spasm and pain syndromes.

Chemotherapy can cause peripheral neuropathy: lost or diminished sensation or motor function of the arms or legs. Patients may complain of nerve-related pain such as burning, tingling, or numbness. In some instances this pain can be intense enough to limit participation in ADL. Providing the patient with isotonic gloves or tubular support bandages can sometimes soothe this pain enough to allow resumption of more normal activity. Sensory reeducation with textures can be soothing (see Chapter 22). Adaptation of assistive devices with large handles and soft grips may support function until the person completes chemotherapy and the peripheral nerve function improves or returns to normal.

Table 35-2 Peripheral Neuropathy and Precautions in Activities of Daily Living

Clinical Sign	Functional Problem	Solution
Numbness	Loss of sharp and dull perception, at risk for cutting and burning limb	Use vision, cueing, and adapted equipment
Burning pain	Cannot tolerate anything touching hand or foot	Wear toning gloves, cloth gloves, soft padding, and socks Use relaxation techniques
Proprioceptive loss	Unaware of where arm and leg are in space	Teach cueing and position for safety

If protective sensation (perception of hot, cold, sharp, dull, and position sense) is lost, participation in activities that rely on these sensations may put the person at risk for injury. For example, cooking activities rely on the patient's ability to use sharps. Patients are taught to use vision to avoid cutting themselves and oven mitts to prevent burns. Tables 35-2 and 35-3 summarize side effects, precautions, and techniques.

The psychosocial adjustment aspect of care is too often overlooked with cancer patients. Most are in the process of role adjustment and redefining themselves during the treatment phase of their disease. Encouraging group interaction and discussion, as well as providing opportunities to develop new hobbies or interests, may be beneficial. Research has shown that women with breast cancer who attend support groups tend to have a better quality of life and extended longevity even if they are in the advanced stage of disease. From a research perspective, little is known about the healing power of prayer and spiritual development.

Improved perception of the value of complementary medicine is promoting research in several allopathic medical centers regarding techniques such as stress reduction, massage, and energy therapies (e.g., therapeutic touch, Reiki). This potential area of development and participation is useful for OT practitioners who use groups in treatment settings. Functionally based standardized tests can be used to demonstrate improved functional outcomes with the use of complementary techniques.

Moreover, some patients may have defined psychiatric diagnoses and may require OT intervention based on that diagnosis. For instance, adjustment disorder occurs in many patients who react emotionally to the diagnosis or to a change in their condition. It is not uncommon for patients who develop acute lymphedema to also experience anxiety with a tendency to overfocus on details. These patients may require some counseling and limit-setting in addition to drug therapy to moderate their anxiety. Depression may also be associated with a cancer diagnosis. Depression may be reactional and appropriate to the situation or organically based.[15] Using activities with successful outcomes can be helpful to foster the development of self-esteem. In addition, structured activity can limit distractions and redirect the focus of the individual

Table 35-3 Functional Impact and Management of Side Effects from Cancer Treatment

Treatment	Side Effect	Functional Impact	Rehabilitation Management
Radiation	Burn (acute)	Avoid touch	Active ROM
stretching	Burn (subacute)	Soft tissue contracture	Scar management, stretching
	Myelopathy	Plexopathy	Positioning, ADL compensatory strategies
Chemotherapy	Neutropenia	Immunocompromise, fatigue	Protective isolation, paced activity
	Thrombocytopenia (low platelet count)	Decreased activity tolerance	Avoidance of skin breaks, paced activity
	Anemia	Shortness of breath, decreased activity tolerance	Frequent rest periods
	Peripheral neuropathy	Decreased sensation	Safety education and activity modification
Surgery	Incision	Movement limitation	Time for incision to heal (≈10 days), stretching after healing
	Referred pain	Reluctance to move	Coordination of pain medications with treatment, education regarding actual risk
	Phantom pain	Sleep disturbance, decreased activity tolerance	Application of light pressure to the area, education regarding meaning and actual risk

ADL, Activities of daily living; *ROM,* range of motion.

from a feeling of being overwhelmed to one of tolerating and coping with life in the present. Successful completion of a structured activity may also provide hope because concrete evidence of a positive change results.

Family and caregiver training is also important for breast cancer patients who will be responsible for participating in a home exercise program. The caregiver who is educated about the home program can better appreciate its value and assist the patient with recall of specific exercises or activities. Compliance with self-treatment may improve if a caregiver reminds the person about the importance of the home program.

Lung Cancer

In the early postoperative phase, patients who have undergone surgery to remove a portion of the lung may depend on oxygen because of shortness of breath.[3] ADL should focus on energy conservation and work simplification. It is advisable to monitor the patient's vital signs including respiratory rate (the number of breaths per minute), pulse, and blood pressure. In inpatient rehabilitation settings, it may be possible to monitor activity tolerance with a pulse oximeter (a digital machine with a finger electrode that measures the percentage of oxygen consumed). The goal is for the patient to do as much activity as physical tolerance allows.

The surgery for lung cancer, thoracotomy, involves a wide excision from the center of the chest to under the arm, terminating laterally at the spine. After the initial healing of the incision, the patient may benefit from scar management. Patients may complain of burning paresthesias and stabbing sensations in the scar. Silicone gel pads worn on the scar 22 hours a day for 4 to 6 weeks may prevent adhesion and soften and flatten the scar tissues while the collagen beneath the scar remodels. The silicone may also provide neutral warmth, a relaxing or comforting sensation that occurs from absorption and reflection of body heat. Sensory reeducation with textures may also help to reduce scar-related discomfort.

Gentle general conditioning exercises (GCEs) may assist the patient with increasing activity and respiratory tolerance. A program of GCEs may be taught to the patient or caregiver for a self-treatment regimen to support the OT program. The caregiver and patient can also be instructed in a ROM and positioning program for the shoulder on the side of surgery.

Head and Neck Cancer

Cancers of the head and neck region require surgical resection, usually augmented by radiation therapy and in some cases chemotherapy. The procedures most commonly done with oropharyngeal cancer patients require removal of cervical and submaxillary lymph nodes. The procedures for which OT is consulted most often are neck dissections (radical or modified radical) and resections involving the oralpharyngus and tongue.

Radical neck dissection involves removing the lymph nodes and vessels from the border of the jaw, the strap muscles of the neck, and the trapezius muscle. The spinal accessory nerve is usually impaired after a radical dissection. When this nerve does not work, the scapula "wings," which results in instability of the arm in overhead planes of motion because the scapula is unsupported. Therefore patients who have this surgery can develop painful shoulders and lose shoulder movement above 90 degrees of flexion and abduction. After surgery, some scar tissue must be allowed to develop in the neck to substitute for the lost function of the sternocleidomastoid muscle, which aligns the head at midline. Some neck stiffness tends to result and is necessary. However, what is not necessary is hardening of the tissues that are radiated. Scar management through application of silicone gel pads, gentle active ROM, and positioning with cervical support pillows is helpful for restoring more normal skin quality and preventing pain and deformity of the neck.[3]

Head and neck cancer patients also are at risk for developing oral-motor dysphagia. The swallowing team may find the patient can eat only if the diet is limited in consistency, or food will be aspirated. Some of these patients will be unable to eat orally and may need to be tube-fed for some time. If the patient's diet is limited, liquids may have to be thickened with a thickening agent to guarantee the consistency of the bolus.

In addition, patients may require special positioning or timed sitting after eating so that they do not aspirate after meals. The swallowing specialist, usually the speech or occupational therapist, provides the instructions. The OTA may be responsible for following through on the feeding program, using guidelines from a supervisor.

Again, training of the caregiver and patient is important for follow-through on exercise and activity programs. It is essential with dysphagia because the ability to swallow and protect one's airway is a vital (life-supporting) function.

Bone Tumors and Soft Tissue Sarcomas

Bone tumors and soft tissue sarcomas are usually first seen in the extremities. The surgical management depends on numerous factors including the type of tumor, the aggressiveness of the tumor, the status of the circulatory supply to the limb, the age and general health of the patient, and the functional prognosis. Some of the bone tumors are primary in bone, but most are metastases from other cancers. Soft tissue tumors are usually primary in nature. Some develop from prenatal influences and are called *embryonic in origin.* Some of these tumors are highly malignant and difficult to treat effectively.

If a tumor is aggressive and the blood or nerve supply to the limb is impaired, the patient may require an amputation. If the tumor is present but the blood and nerve supply are intact, it may be possible to salvage the limb. In this instance, the distal portion of the limb is preserved, the portion of bone is removed with some healthy tissue (a margin), and a prosthesis is implanted and cemented into place.[14] Amputees from cancer are rehabilitated similarly to amputees from other causes. However, some cancer amputations remove the total hindquarter or forequarter.

OT focuses on positioning and ADL. The patient will require training in positioning with the fracture brace and the sling, as well as self-ROM (with precautions as prescribed by the surgeon) and activities to restore hand strength and function. Cosmetic shoulder pads are also helpful in restoring the illusion of bulk to the arm because there will be loss of muscle and soft tissue with surgery.[3]

Because many of these patients are children or adolescents, parent training is important. Compliance with the use of the fracture brace and sling is crucial to prevent fracture of the limb and dislocation of the indwelling prosthesis.

Colon and Bladder Cancers

Patients with colon or bladder cancer have **stomas**—openings from the surgically resected site to the outside of the body—after surgery. **Colostomy** stomas (which have an opening between the colon and body surface) and **urostomy** stomas (which have an opening between the body surface and the organs that produce and collect urine) are common. Patients may also undergo chemotherapy as part of their treatment. They may develop peripheral neuropathy and lose fine motor sensibility and function—the very type of feeling and movement they must rely on to independently remove and clean their colostomy and urostomy bags and sites.

The OT practitioner may be asked to work collaboratively with the enterostomal nurse and the patient to develop strategies to restore independent function in stoma care and hygiene. Changing a clamp or using a built-up tool and practicing this adapted technique is often the single skill needed for discharge of these patients to the community.

This group can also benefit from peer support group activities because the presence of the stomas and the side effects of the disease and treatment affect body image, self-perception, sexual functioning, and life roles. Table 35-4 summarizes cancer conditions commonly seen in OT settings.

Issues Concerning Death and Dying

People who confront life-threatening illnesses are forced to face their own mortality. Grief is a common reaction and a necessary part of the adjustment process and is preceded by a dynamic interplay of behaviors or stages described by Kübler-Ross[9] as denial, bargaining, anger, depression, hope, and acceptance. At any given point the patient may exhibit one or several of these behaviors. Usually one stage prevails at a given time over the others. Denial is characterized by thoughts like, "A mistake has been made. This cannot be happening to me." Bargaining is manifested by thoughts such as, "If I do this one thing, then it will be all right." Anger may be volatile at times and may also be outwardly directed at a number of objects including, at times, the therapist. When people are predominantly angry, they may not tolerate therapy.

Depression is manifested by feelings of helplessness and hopelessness. When people are depressed, motivation generally wanes. Hope implies that some change for the good is possible. This restores motivation and participation in therapeutic goals. Acceptance is rarely achieved.[2,20] Great faith or self-actualization must be possessed for a person to accept the inevitable. Once acceptance is reached, therapy may no longer be a goal, unless the person has personal goals or requires the intervention of the therapist for comfort measures.

It may be hard for the therapy staff to react normally around the dying patient. It is difficult for most people to feel comfortable around death because it forces each of us to face our own individual issues, beliefs, and fears. Knowing the right thing to do or say is part of the art of practice. For some people, it is enough for a caregiver to be accountable and present; the physical act of following up indicates caring and support.

Some patients may seek existential (religious and spiritual) meaning.[20] The response of the caregiver is individualized and depends on the individual caregiver's comfort and willingness to engage in the therapeutic use of self. If the caregiver is uncomfortable, the patient could be assisted in contacting a spiritual or religious advisor. In this case, the clinician should just say, "I am not comfortable discussing this with you" or "I don't feel comfortable speaking about this topic."

Providing or facilitating activities that help the person deal with issues concerning death can be helpful. Some examples are creating memory books for significant others who will be left behind and writing personal diaries with humorous or special events—the stories that define the dying individual's life roles and experiences. Patients may also wish to write letters to family members or friends to resolve issues or say goodbye.

Table 35-4 Cancer Conditions Commonly Treated in Rehabilitation Settings

Type of Cancer	Side Effect Causing Physical Disability*	Possible Rehabilitation Diagnoses
Brain	Mass effect of the tumor displacing brain tissue Postradiation necrosis	Hemiparesis, quadriparesis, cognitive impairment Visual impairment, sensory impairment, ADL impairment, dysphagia
Head and neck	Facial disfigurement, sensory and motor loss (surgery) Oropharyngeal loss	Decreased movement of face or neck, shoulder pain and instability Facial/regional disfigurement, dysphagia, ADL impairment
Spinal	Sensory and motor loss below the level of the tumor	Paraparesis, quadriparesis, bowel and bladder dysfunction, pain, ADL impairment
Leukemia and lymphoma	Blood cell count changes, neurological signs	Weakness, fatigue, deconditioning, neuropathy, dysphagia, ADL impairment
Bone	Amputation, limb-sparing postsurgical complications	Mobility impairment, ADL impairment, wounds and scars, pain
Soft tissue	Amputation, scar adhesions, radiation fibrosis	Mobility impairment, ADL impairment, wounds and scars, pain
Colon and bladder	Colostomy, urostomy	Peripheral neuropathy, impaired mobility, ADL changes—toileting, bathing, and dressing
Lung	Postsurgical oxygen dependence and thoracic surgical movement limitations	Shortness of breath, ADL impairment, decreased mobility
Breast	Myofascial and joint changes in chest wall and shoulder Sensorimotor compromise in arm (brachial plexopathy) Uncontrolled lymphedema in arm, ADL impairment	Decreased mobility in arm, pain, myofascial scarring Muscle imbalance, sensory changes
Metastatic	Multiple organ and system involvement	Pain, fatigue, deconditioning, pain, impaired mobility, sensorimotor changes Cognitive changes

ADL, Activities of daily living.
*There may be accompanying psychological sequelae: depression (situationally or organically based), anxiety (including adjustment disorders), and hallucinations (related to medications or organic/disease processes). In addition, people with diagnoses of cancer often face issues concerning role adjustment and adaptation.

Palliative care also has its physical aspects. Techniques of comfort care that could be used are positioning, massage, complementary medicine (e.g., guided imagery, stress management, aromatherapy, therapeutic touch), adaptive devices, and rearrangement of the physical environment to allow maximum access for the patient with limited mobility. The practitioner can help maintain the patient's dignity by helping with toileting activities and strategies.

Summary

Cancer is a cluster of diseases with unique and identifiable problems for the OT practitioner to evaluate and treat. Although at one time many people did not survive cancer, with advances in medical care diagnoses are being made earlier and patients are being successfully treated for many cancer conditions. Many cancers are now viewed as chronic illnesses.

The role of OT for the person with cancer is always changing. The OT practitioner must be a good detective to search out the clues in each instance that may guide treatment. Skillful intervention interweaves the principles of physical disability practice and of mental health practice.

The partnership of the occupational therapist and OTA is imperative in cancer treatment, perhaps even more than in other areas of practice, because the case management for these conditions is highly technical. The OTA may perform many of the same evaluations and treatments used with the general physically disabled and mental health populations.

Selected Reading Guide Questions

1. List three tests commonly used to diagnose cancer.
2. What is the purpose of dissecting lymph nodes during cancer surgeries?
3. Which blood values are important to monitor in a cancer patient who is undergoing chemotherapy treatment?
4. What safety concerns would you have with a patient who has a chemotherapy-induced neuropathy?
5. List and describe the common effects of chemotherapy.
6. List and describe the common effects of radiation therapy.
7. What skin precaution should be followed while helping a cancer patient who is undergoing radiation therapy to perform basic self-care tasks?
8. A patient who has head and neck cancer is referred to a feeding group. What feeding problems might this person be expected to have? Must any precautions be followed?

9. Should a cancer patient who has neutropenia participate in the leisure group with patients of mixed diagnostic categories? Explain.
10. Are the goals for a patient with brachial plexopathy as a complication of breast cancer restorative, preventative, or palliative? Explain.
11. Give an example of a complementary treatment technique that can be used to reduce stress.
12. What approach could be used in counseling a cancer patient who cannot return to previous life roles?
13. What is alopecia, and is it a permanent condition in cancer patients?
14. List one restorative goal for a cancer patient (any diagnosis).
15. List a palliative goal for a patient who is confined to bed and has a progressive disease.
16. What education could be provided to prevent lymphedema in a breast cancer patient?
17. Which concern regarding ability to move applies to a breast cancer patient who is receiving radiation to her breast and shoulder?
18. Which strategies might be used to manage anxiety in a cancer patient who is diagnosed with an adjustment disorder?
19. Which ADL problems might be observed in a person with a diagnosis of lung cancer who has had a thoracotomy to remove the tumor?
20. List three ADL that are difficult for the head and neck cancer patient to perform after a radical neck resection and spinal accessory nerve dysfunction.
21. A head and neck cancer patient has winging of the scapula on the side of the surgery. What movement will be difficult for this patient?
22. Describe an activity that could be helpful for a patient who is coping with issues of death and dying.
23. From an OT perspective, what are the common functional problems of patients with cancer?

References

1. American Occupational Therapy Association: The Role of Occupational Therapy in End-of-Life Care: *Am J Occup Ther* 65 (6 Suppl), from http://www.aota.org/Practitioners/PracticeAreas/Rehab/Highlights/End-of-Life-Care.aspx?FT=.pdf, Accessed 12/14/11.
2. Burkhardt A: *Cancer and personal meaning*, Washington, DC, 2003, Short course presented at the American Occupational Therapy Association annual conference.
3. Burkhardt A, Joachim L: *A therapist's guide to oncology: medical issues affecting management*, San Antonio, Tex, 1996, Harcourt Brace.
4. Cook A, Burkhardt A: The effect of cancer diagnosis and treatment on hand function,, *Am J Occup Ther* 48(9):836–839, 1994.
5. Creswell JW: *Qualitative inquiry and research design: choosing among five traditions*, Thousand Oaks, Calif, 1998, Sage.
6. Dietz JH: Rehabilitation of the cancer patient: its role in the scheme of comprehensive care, *Clin Bull* 4:104–107, 1974.
7. Grunberg SM, Groshen S: Concepts of cancer staging. In Calabrese P, Schein PS, editors: *Medical oncology*, ed 2, New York, 1993, McGraw-Hill.
8. Hall SJ, Brown SE, Porter GJR, et al: Axillary ultrasound in stagin breast cancer: diagnostic accuracy and effect on subsequent axillary surgery - the Plymouth experience, *Breast Cancer Research* 2009, 11(Suppl 2):P21, doi:10.1186/br2391, from http://breast-cancer-research.com/content/11/S2/P21, Accessed 12/14/11.
9. Jost L, Roila F: Management of cancer pain: ESMO clinical practice guidelines, *Ann Oncol* (Suppl 5) v257–v260, 2010.
10. Kübler-Ross K: *On death and dying*, New York, 1969, Macmillan.
11. Lemoignan J, Chasen M, Bhargava R: A retrospective study of the role of an occupational therapist in the cancer nutrition rehabilitation program, *Support Care Cancer* 18(12):1589–1596, 2010.
12. Little M, Jordens CF, Paul K, et al: Liminality: a major category of the experience of cancer illness, *Soc Sci Med* 47:1485–1494, 1998.
13. Lowitz B, Casciato D: Cancer chemotherapeutics. In Casciato D, Lowitz B: *Manual of clinical oncology*, Boston, 1991, Little, Brown.
14. Marcove R: En bloc upper humeral intrascapular resection: the Tikoff-Limberg procedure, *Clin Orthop* 124:219–228, 1977.
15. Margary CJ: Aspects of psychiatric management of breast cancer, *Med J Aust* 148(5):239–242, 1988.
16. Mayo Clinic: *Positron emission tomography (PET) scan*, 2009, Retrieved January 28, 2011 from http://www.mayoclinic.org/pet/?mc_id=comlinkpilot&placement=bottom.
17. Mehls J: Occupational therapy in the rehabilitation of cancer patients. In American Occupational Therapy Association: *Cancer information packet*, Rockville, Md, 1987, the Association.
18. Miller GM, Forbes GS, Onofrio BM: Magnetic resonance imaging of the spine, *Mayo Clin Proc* 64(8):986–1004, 1989.
19. Padilla R: Clara: a phenomenology of disability, *Am J Occup Ther* 57(4):413–423, 2003.
20. Royeen C, Duncan M: *Meta-emotion of occupation*, Presentation, Midwest Dean's Conference, Omaha, Neb, 2002, Creighton University.
21. Sajja H, East M, Hui M, et al: Development of multifunctional nanoparticles for targeted drug delivery and non-invasive imaging of therapeutic effect, *Current drug discovery technologies [serial online]* 6(1):43–51, March 2009. Available from: Academic Search Premier, Ipswich, Mass. Accessed January 28, 2011.
22. Samphao S, Eremin J, El-Sheemy M, Eremin O: Treatment of established breast cancer in post-menopausal women: role of aromatase inhibitors, *Surg Edinburgh Univ Press [serial online]* 7(1):42–55, 2009. Available from: Academic Search Premier, Ipswich, Mass. Accessed January 28, 2011.
23. Silver JK, Gilchrist LS: Cancer rehabilitation with a focus on evidence-based outpatient physical and occupational therapy interventions, *Am J Phys Med Rehabil* 90(Suppl):S5–S15, 2011.
24. Vrkljan B, Miller-Polgar J: Meaning of occupational engagement in life-threatening illness: a qualitative pilot project, *Can J Occup Ther* 68(4):237–246, 2001.

Recommended Reading

Burkhardt A, Weitz J: Oncological applications for the use of silicone gel-sheets in soft-tissue contractures, *Am J Occup Ther* 45(5):460–462, 1991.

Delbrück H: *Rehabilitation and palliation of cancer patients: patient care*, New York, 2007, Springer Healthcare, p 438.

Rankin J, Robb K, Murtaugh N, et al: *Rehabilitation in cancer care*, Hoboken, NJ, 2008, Wiley-Blackwell, p 360.

Stubblefield MD, O'Dell MW: *Cancer rehabilitation: principles and practice*, New York, 2009, Demos Medical, p 1093.

Williams V, Burkhardt A, Royce J: Helping you call it quits, *OT Week* 9(9):18, 1995.

CHAPTER 36 HIV Infection and AIDS

MICHAEL PIZZI

Key Terms

Human immunodeficiency virus (HIV)
Acquired immunodeficiency syndrome (AIDS)
Context
Occupational role
Wellness
Control
Occupational choices
Functional activity
Adaptation

Chapter Objectives

After studying this chapter, the student or practitioner will be able to do the following:

1. Discuss the physical, mental health, and environmental factors associated with HIV disease that impede and enable engagement in occupation.
2. Understand the impact of HIV on body structures and functions, life activity, and social participation.
3. Understand the occupational therapy process for adults with HIV disease.
4. Understand the stages of HIV disease and its impact on occupational performance and participation.
5. Develop wellness strategies (in collaboration with the occupational therapist) for adults with HIV disease.

In 1982 five gay men from New York and California were diagnosed with a rare form of cancer and pneumocystis pneumonia (PCP), diagnoses not commonly seen in younger men. Soon thereafter, people with hemophilia, women, intravenous (IV) drug users, and children were becoming infected at dramatic rates with the same unnamed disease. This mysterious illness claimed the lives of hundreds before it was discovered to be fast and insidious, transmitted sexually or through blood products, transmitted consistently from blood to blood, and highly infectious. The disease came to be known as the human immunodeficiency virus, or HIV, from which the term acquired immunodeficiency syndrome, or AIDS, arises.

HIV attacks a person's immune system, the body's system that wards off infections and calls on T cells and B cells to help out when it recognizes a foreign substance. The virus often goes unrecognized until it has already attacked the system that helps a person get well. According to the Centers for Disease Control (CDC),[2] more than one million people are living with HIV in the United States with one out of five (21%) of those people living with HIV being unaware of their infection. The virus can lie dormant in the body for many years with the person showing no symptoms but always being a carrier of the virus.

Consequently, in the 1990s, the emphasis shifted to "living well with your disease" and to the view that HIV disease is a chronic and *not* a terminal illness. Occupational therapy (OT) was founded on the belief that it can help people with chronic diseases lead productive, active, and participatory lives; thus OT has an important role to play with people with HIV disease and their significant others.

The gay population, initially impacted, was quick to identify prevention and health promotion strategies that have decreased the number of new cases of HIV among that population. However, infection rates among women, minorities, and heterosexual men have increased dramatically. Most recently, a new wave of the epidemic has arisen among adolescents.[2] The virus does not discriminate. The "worried well" fear they may be infected because of a past or current history of high-risk behavior (behavior that puts them at higher risk for being infected with HIV). The prominent high-risk behavior is unprotected sex, the cause of increased numbers of cases in adolescents, young adults, and men who have sex with other men (many of whom identify themselves as heterosexual). Another high-risk behavior is sharing needles and injectables with others (including sharing steroid needles with workout partners). In the United States, the demographics continue to change, with more heterosexual cases reported, primarily among IV drug users and women. The people who have unprotected sex with affected individuals are sometimes infected unknowingly. Male-to-male unprotected sexual contact as a means of transmission also remains high.

A person infected with HIV does not necessarily have AIDS. HIV disease has several stages culminating in AIDS. The stages can be rapidly experienced or drawn out over time. HIV often first presents as a mononucleosis-like syndrome with fatigue, high fever, and some lymphadenopathy (swollen lymph glands). This syndrome usually occurs within a few weeks of infection. A person may then be asymptomatic for years, later developing persistent generalized lymphadenopathy (PGL). Finally, the last stage is characterized by clinical medical symptoms leading to the diagnosis of full-blown AIDS. These medical problems can include opportunistic infections like Kaposi's sarcoma or *Pneumocystis carinii* pneumonia (PCP). The person can also have medical complications such as high fevers, chronic diarrhea, painful neuropathies (that can affect sensation), and severe weight loss. The World Health Organization (WHO) categories for the stages of infection and specific illnesses within those categories that affect body structures and function are listed in Box 36-1.

The occupational therapy assistant (OTA) may work with individuals at any one of these stages, helping the person attain the highest level of occupational performance possible. An emphasis on holism and mind-body-spirit is essential to help people attain an optimal level of occupational participation. The OT goals of mastery and independence celebrate wellness, life, and living—not illness, death, and dying. It is vital that practitioners value individuals for their unique worth and contribution to the world and examine each person within the context of their environment and culture.

Considerations for Persons with HIV Disease and AIDS

The following are the physical, mental health, and contextual factors that the OTA might note in working with people with HIV disease.

Physical Considerations

Although HIV is now deemed a chronic and manageable illness, a person with HIV may experience a variety of impairments to body structures and functions over time, which also influence occupational participation. Given that each person is uniquely affected by the disease, not all of the following individual factors may be noted:

- Fatigue
- Peripheral and central nervous system disorders
- Visual impairments

Box 36-1

WHO Clinical Staging of HIV/AIDS for Adults and Adolescents with Confirmed HIV Infection

Clinical Stage 1

Asymptomatic
Persistent generalized lymphadenopathy

Clinical Stage 2

Moderate unexplained weight loss
(<10% of presumed or measured body weight)*
Recurrent respiratory tract infections sinusitis, tonsillitis, otitis media, and pharyngitis)
Herpes zoster
Angular cheilitis
Recurrent oral ulceration
Papular pruritic eruptions
Seborrhoeic dermatitis
Fungal nail infections

Clinical Stage 3

Unexplained† severe weight loss (>10% of presumed or measured body weight)
Unexplained chronic diarrhea for longer than 1 month
Unexplained persistent fever (above 37.6° C intermittent or constant, for longer than 1 month)
Persistent oral candidiasis
Oral hairy leukoplakia
Pulmonary tuberculosis (current)
Severe bacterial infections (such as pneumonia, empyema, pyomyositis,
bone or joint infection, mening:tis or bacteremia)
Acute necrotizing ulcerative stomatitis, gingivitis, or periodontitis
Unexplained anemia (<8 g/dl), neutropenia (<0.5 × 109 per liter) or chronic thrombocytopenia (<50 × 109 per liter)

Clinical Stage 4‡

HIV wasting syndrome
Pneumocystis pneumonia
Recurrent severe bacterial pneumonia
Chronic herpes simplex infection (orolabial, genital, or anorectal of more than 1 month's duration or visceral at any site)
Esophageal candidiasis (or candidiasis of trachea, bronchi, or lungs)
Extrapulmonary tuberculosis
Kaposi's sarcoma
Cytomegalovirus infection (retinitis or infection of other organs)
Central nervous system toxoplasmosis
HIV encephalopathy
Extrapulmonary cryptococcosis including meningitis
Disseminated nontuberculous mycobacterial infection
Progressive multifocal leukoencephalopathy
Chronic cryptosporidiosis (with diarrhea)
Chronic isosporiasis
Disseminated mycosis (coccidiomycosis or histoplasmosis)
Recurrent nontyphoidal *Salmonella bacteremia*
Lymphoma (cerebral or B-cell non-Hodgkin) or other solid HIV-associated tumors
Invasive cervical carcinoma
Atypical disseminated leishmaniasis
Symptomatic HIV-associated nephropathy or symptomatic HIV-associated cardiomyopathy

*Assessment of body weight in pregnant woman needs to consider the expected weight gain of pregnancy.
Retrieved from http://www.who.int/hiv/pub/guidelines/HIVstaging150307.pdf, September 17, 2010.
†Unexplained refers to where the condition is not explained by other causes.
‡Some additional specific conditions can also be included in regional classifications (such as reactivation of American trypanosomiasis [meningoencephalitis and/or myocarditis]) in the WHO Region of the Americas and disseminated penicilliosis in Asia).

- Cardiac problems
- Pain
- Weakness (neuromuscular)
- Changes in posture, gait, range of motion (ROM), strength, coordination, balance
- Changes in cognition (particularly affecting safety in carrying out tasks)

These physical client factors can and often do lead to changes in all areas of occupation as outlined by the Occupational Therapy Performance Framework (OTPF-2E).[1] These include activities of daily living (ADL), instrumental activities of daily living (IADL), rest and sleep, education, work, play and leisure, and social participation. They also often lead to altered performance patterns in habits and routines (e.g., increased time needed to complete basic and instrumental activities of daily living [B/IADL]).

Psychosocial/Mental Health Considerations

Physical changes may impair psychosocial and mental health because of the continuous interplay between mind and body. Those without physical impairments may experience mental health imbalance such as not coping well with the diagnosis or feeling stressed over the potential current and future impact of the disease on occupational performance. A person can become immobilized in carrying out performance patterns such as occupational habits, routines, roles, or activities while "waiting for the next shoe to drop" (i.e., waiting for the next diagnosis, symptom, or blood test to come back). Persons with HIV often feel overwhelmed with the numbers of medical appointments and tests and can easily fall into the "sick role" of not being able to view life positively. The person's identity may become wrapped up in T-cell counts or how many red and white blood cells he or she has rather than being based on how he or she can function on a day-to-day basis. OT assists people with managing their daily lives while helping them cope with the many new challenges of living with HIV, no matter the stage of illness. Other psychosocial and mental health considerations can include the following:

- Anxiety (which is often manifested in physical symptoms)
- Depression
- Guilt over being infected or the possibility of having infected others
- Preoccupation with illness or death
- Lack of interventions, limited access to health care, lack of insurance
- Anger (at the disease, lack of interventions, lack of social support, etc.)
- Neuropsychiatric problems (forgetfulness, apathy, withdrawal, memory loss)
- Altered self-image because of cancer or severe weight loss
- Lack of control over environment
- Hopelessness and helplessness
- Lack of meaning in daily activity and sense that "life is meaningless"
- Altered goals, plans, dreams for the future
- Grief and bereavement issues
- Societal stigma

It seems that people who have high standards of performance (perfectionists) or those who have a rigid schedule or routine of activity do not fare well in coping with illness. They are less able to adapt to the many changes that occur, sometimes on a daily basis. OT can help them identify how to adapt more easily so that they can continue to engage in occupation within a variety of contexts.

Contextual Considerations

The context and environment of a person with HIV/AIDS includes not just the physical setting in which a person lives but also the social, personal, cultural, temporal, and virtual contexts and environments in which they experience transactional relationships with occupation and participation.[1] People with HIV can function much better when the OTA incorporates contextual observations and awareness into interventions and understands the constant interplay among a person, his or her environment, and occupational performance. These interplays are explored as follows.

Physical Context

People with symptomatic HIV (and associated physical impairments) might have, for example, difficulty negotiating steps, and visual-motor impairments affecting driving, shopping, and traveling into the community. Mobility could be decreased because of impaired vision, reduced strength, or fatigue. Sensory problems such as neuropathies can alter balance, and taking a few steps can be painful.

Social Context

Stigma and discrimination often cause people with HIV to be seen as social pariahs or outcasts. Many people with HIV have already been victims of discrimination—gay men, persons of color, women, and IV drug users. This prejudice is important for the assistant to note in interventions. Relationships with significant others, family members, and work associates may change because of an HIV diagnosis. Health care providers may discriminate, consciously or unconsciously, which can make going to the hospital a frightening prospect instead of one that is welcomed for care and relief. The OTA may be one of the first people to physically touch a person with HIV—through ADL, ROM, or some creative interventions. Tactile contact that is accepting and caring can be as important to the person with HIV as any medication. Most importantly, the clinician who is skilled in therapeutic use of self and who has the goal of developing a healthy and nondiscriminatory therapeutic relationship can enable a person with HIV to carry on despite the diagnosis and its impact on daily occupations.

Cultural Context

As with other diagnoses, the person with HIV may come from any population or group of people. Occupational therapy interventions that are culturally specific and uniquely defined enhance patient health and promote well-being. Such interventions symbolically demonstrate that the OTA cares about and is attentive to the particular needs of that one individual;

this helps to establish rapport. For example, in the African-American culture, the status of a gay or bisexual man is rarely discussed. For this population, the better way to discuss such sexual activities is "men having sex with men."

Other Contexts

The American Occupational Therapy Association (AOTA) OTPF-2E[1] identifies other contexts (see earlier). True client-centered and occupation-focused holistic care can begin when the OTA considers all of the contextual factors for individuals with HIV and AIDS.

CASE STUDY

Mr. J.

Mr. J., a 38-year-old white male, was admitted to the hospital 6 months after an initial diagnosis of AIDS and after his first incident of pneumocystis pneumonia. He was referred to OT because of neuropathy in both feet. Mr. J. is a well-educated and well-traveled bank executive of French descent who speaks five languages. He was Catholic but left formal religion years ago because of the conflict between his gay lifestyle and the church's position on homosexuality. He rarely communicates with members of his nuclear family, who live outside the United States, and he lives with his supportive partner of 5 years. Mr. J. was referred to OT on the day of his hospital discharge. Because of this acute care situation (i.e., referred to OT in the morning and discharged that afternoon), assessment consisted only of interview and role, ADL, and biomedical assessments.

Assessment revealed Mr. J. to be independent in all self-care, home maintenance, and mobility activities except for minor standing balance deficits. No cognitive or sensory deficits were noted other than mild lower extremity neuropathy. Strength, active ROM, and coordination were all functional for task performance. Mr. J. complained of diminished endurance, which affected his occupational habits and pursuits of interests including exercise, history, collecting, photography, movies, concerts, classical music, and swimming. He had narrowed leisure activities to listening to classical music when he "felt up to it." He felt out of control and believed that HIV had taken over. He openly discussed his prognosis and his religious beliefs, examining his unresolved relationship with God and the possibilities of an afterlife. The occupational therapist referred him to Dignity (a gay Catholic organization), the unit social workers, and the hospital chaplain.

Critical Thinking Questions

1. What goals can you identify that Mr. J might desire?
2. What interventions (in addition to those discussed earlier) would be appropriate?

Adapted and reprinted with permission from Pizzi M: The model of human occupation and adults with HIV infection and AIDS, *Am J Occup Ther* 44(3):42-49, 1990.

Occupational Therapy

When Adolph Meyer, one of the founders of OT, identified the essential nature of occupation, he recognized several aspects of human behavior that today can be applied to work with people with HIV disease. These tenets include the following:

- An individual's health is measured by involvement in life tasks in the social and physical environments.
- The focus must be on a person's *lifestyle.*
- A healthy balance among work, rest, sleep, and play is necessary to fully function.
- Occupation can restore function, maintain functioning, and prevent dysfunction.
- Occupation helps people make better use of time and reorganize time.[3]

These important and fundamental concepts, as well as the following considerations that guide interventions, help to create a healthier lifestyle for people with HIV disease.

Environment

People are influenced by and have an impact on the environment because there is a constant interplay between them. Under both the International classification of functioning, disability, and health (ICF)[8] and the OTPF-2E, environmental considerations are of the utmost importance when developing and implementing interventions. The physical, social, temporal, attitudinal, and cultural environments are key to understanding occupational performance and creating adaptations to promote health and well-being. Occupations provide the most meaning when they are developed within the context of a familiar environment. For example, facilitating a chef or a homemaker in a wheelchair to make a home-cooked meal for a family gathering can include all aspects of the environment and the task is meaningful for the individual.

Occupational Roles

Role functioning (mastery and progress toward developing an occupational role) should be incorporated in intervention goals and activities. For example, if a patient is a worker, interventions designed to restore work habits, routines, and task performance would be appropriate. If a patient has no occupational role, role development might be important if that patient has no habits, routines, or meaningful activity during the day.

Wellness

In the OTPF-2E and other literature, wellness and health promotion have been emphasized both as interventions and as outcomes.[1,6,7] The WHO recently noted that HIV infections worldwide have been reduced by 17% and stated the following:

> HIV prevention programmes are making a difference. "The good news is that we have evidence that the declines we are seeing are due, at least in part, to HIV prevention," said Michel Sidibé, Executive Director of UNAIDS. "However, the findings also show that prevention programming is often off the mark and that if we do a better job of getting resources and programmes to where they will make most impact, quicker progress can be made and more lives saved."[9]

Occupation that holds meaning and in which the person can engage successfully promotes wellness. Wellness programming, facilitated and led by the OTA, can be implemented with individuals, populations, and communities. The immune system is supported and thus wellness created when a person engages in productive occupations and in purposeful and occupation-based activities adapted by the OTA and occupational therapist. Stacking cones in a clinic is not a wellness-oriented, meaningful occupation for a weight lifter with HIV (unless cones were stacked for a living!). Instead, a strengthening program (in collaboration with the physical therapist) while engaging in favorite occupations, balanced with rest and periods of leisure and good nutrition, is more client centered and appropriate.

Temporal Rhythms

Time is often organized through activity, and activity is often organized through time. A person with HIV might perceive that life is short and that time cannot be wasted. The OTA can help the person to organize routines, prioritize goals, and make the best use of time by using different techniques such as a time log or activity log that corresponds to how the person uses time. This exploration can give the person with HIV insight into how time can be used wisely and not wasted daily. Therapists should also recognize that many persons with HIV have an immediate need to get on with life and living, so they need to offer practical, functional, and meaningful occupations to people with HIV throughout the therapy process.

Control

HIV disease, or even the diagnosis of HIV, can take control away from a person, simply by the sheer magnitude of the disease process. The health care system also takes control away, especially in most hospitals, because it dictates how a person will spend waking moments. From the start of OT interventions, control must be shared with the patient through occupational choices in every session. For example, the OTA can have a list of 5 to 10 tasks in which the person can engage to increase physical or mental health and well-being and can ask the person to choose three for that session. Client-centered care is of the utmost concern in interventions and will provide an experience of control and choice to clients. The client is the expert on who they are and how best they "do" their lives; OTAs are the facilitators of health through their care and compassion and knowledge of the power of occupation in people's lives.

Occupational Therapy Assessment and Evaluation

The occupational therapist can assess all of the aforementioned areas with a variety of tools, from physical assessment tools like goniometry, balance, strength, and ADL evaluations through psychosocial assessment including a neuropsychiatric battery and coping assessments. It is also important to examine assessments done by other disciplines. The Pizzi Assessment of Productive Living (PAPL) for adults with HIV disease (Figure 36-1) gives the assistant an overview of other areas that need to be assessed for people with HIV. It also suggests how those areas can be addressed in interventions. The assistant can contribute to the assessment process by performing parts of the occupational profile, and carrying out an observational and written ADL evaluation, and a caregiver interview to determine level of social support and type of home environment (if possible) to which the person with HIV may be discharged.

The OTA then works with the evaluation information and the plan of care and goals set up by the occupational therapist. He or she develops the intervention sessions in collaboration with the person with HIV. It can also be appropriate for the occupational therapist and OTA to assess together, but this is not necessary. It is always important to collaborate with persons with HIV on their goals, plans, and desired functional outcomes from interventions. Employing a client-centered approach will further enable and empower people with HIV and AIDS.

Before assessment, it is vital that the OTA be conscientious about infection control. Masks are necessary if the person with HIV has tuberculosis or other airborne infectious disease or when the assistant has a cough, cold, or other health problem that might infect the person with HIV. Gloves are necessary to wipe up blood or other body fluid spills but are not normally worn for traditional interventions or written assessments or interventions. However, gloves should always be readily available. The practitioner should always check with his or her department and facility policy on universal precautions (see Chapter 3).

Interventions

Goal and intervention planning and implementation must take on a positive and supportive spirit; this responsibility belongs to the individual therapist. OTAs help to create environments, opportunities for and approaches toward health, wellness, and positive living for people with HIV disease. "Persons with HIV are often devastated physically, psychologically, and spiritually and most likely have encountered prejudice and discrimination before and after diagnosis. We have an opportunity to support people with HIV through nonjudgmental, positive approaches to life and living and to use our power as a catalyst for transformation. We can provide hope and meaning to patients through adaptation and a positive spirit without providing false hope for a cure."[5] Restoring and maintaining function and preventing dysfunction in self-chosen occupations related to the person's life and lifestyle are the focus of clinical interventions. Generally, traditional clinical interventions used with other diagnoses are implemented, along with the guidelines set forth thus far in this chapter. Other considerations must also be noted during interventions. These considerations include the following:

1. Incorporating nutritional education in interventions. Good nutrition maintains the body in good emotional and physical shape and is important to the immune system. This education can be incorporated into adaptive homemaking skills and ADL.
2. Use of alternative medicine therapies to complement traditional care. These can include visualization, imagery, massage, meditation, herbs, therapeutic touch, and several

CASE STUDY

Mr. J., Part 2

OT recommendations for Mr. J. included adaptive equipment for safety during bathing. Physical activity was tailored to his interests, values, and occupational choices. A new routine of daily living included a balance of activity and rest to maintain productivity. Adaptations of the worker role from office to home were also suggested because Mr. J. highly valued his work role.

Mr. J. was admitted to the hospital 1 year later with his third episode of PCP and severe neuropathy in both feet. This caused considerable pain even at rest. Physical limitations resulted in increased dependence.

This time the OT assessment was performed with the primary nurse and Mr. J.'s partner, Mr. F., in attendance. Their participation gave a more comprehensive perspective and helped meet the needs and goals of both Mr. J. and his caregiver.

Assessment

Mr. J. had poor endurance and severe pain in both feet, which limited standing tolerance to less than 2 minutes. His active range of motion, strength, coordination, vision, and cognition were within functional limits. No neuropathy was noted in his hands, but he had a flexion contracture as a result of a painful tubercular nodule that caused difficulties with writing and holding utensils.

Mr. J.'s daily living routine was severely altered, and his occupational roles of worker, home maintainer, and hobbyist were affected. His partner related he did nothing with his day except lie in bed and watch television or listen to music. He would not come to the dining room table for meals but demanded that Mr. F. bring them to the bedroom. Mr. F. related that he felt obligated to help Mr. J. but guilty about supporting Mr. J.'s dependent state, knowing that he could "do more."

Mr. F. reported that Mr. J. seemed to have much unresolved anger and depression related to helplessness and hopelessness but refused to acknowledge this or see a mental health professional. He participated in no leisure activity, was apathetic, and felt hopeless regarding current and future occupational performance. He was manipulating people into supporting his maladaptive style of dependency. He would often perform tasks for the occupational therapist yet tell nurses he could not perform these tasks, creating a division among staff regarding his occupational performance.

Critical Thinking Questions

1. How do you feel about Mr. J.'s behavior?
2. About his physical decline?
3. What interventions do you think would be appropriate?

manual therapies. The OTA can ask people with HIV if they currently use any alternative or complementary techniques and, if so, learn from them while introducing other techniques. The OTA should acquire service competency before administering any techniques and should discuss these with the occupational therapist.

3. Providing control and choices at each session conveys a healthy respect for the person with HIV and helps to establish rapport. It also symbolizes caring at its best.
4. Helping the person to adapt a routine or habit of daily living can promote healthier living. Illness of any kind disrupts a routine of activity. A progressive and chronic disease constantly interrupts routine. The OTA should work with the person with HIV to determine the best and worst times of day for activity and energy output. Is the person a morning or evening person? What is the normal routine of the person's day? How can the health care provider help to adapt the routine to make it as comfortable as possible? This is an often overlooked but vital part of interventions and overall caring that the OTA can implement.
5. Generalized weakness and fatigue disrupt routines and activity performance. Incorporating energy conservation, work simplification, and other strategies and adaptive devices can help maintain task performance.
6. Positioning for the bedbound or frail patient can prevent decubitus ulcers and promote healthier sleep and rest patterns. Ergonomic and appropriate positioning for tasks will optimize comfort and engagement in favored occupations.
7. Learning the use of adaptive equipment is vital for any person with functional limitations. Reachers for wheelchair-bound persons; lap trays, feeding equipment, and writing implements for people with hand neuropathies; and dressing sticks and sock aids for lower extremity dressing are just some examples of commonly used equipment. The OTA must ensure that the person accepts the equipment and knows how to use it.
8. Factors contributing to psychosocial stress must be considered. These can include (1) absence of a cure for the disease; (2) disruption of routines by interventions and regimens that may include 30 pills three times a day; (3) constant doctor and clinical appointments; (4) real and perceived discrimination; and (5) work roles and relationships that are lost because of the diagnosis. These are real factors for some people living with HIV disease—factors that are not commonly seen with other diagnoses. Perhaps the most important is that the person may have lost many, many friends and perhaps significant relationships to the same disease. Unresolved grief and bereavement issues and anger may exacerbate anxiety and other psychosocial factors related to HIV. The OTA must always note this possibility during interventions.
9. Health promotion and wellness programming are essential. HIV has become a chronic illness managed well by medications and improved health care strategies. OTAs have an opportunity to establish positive, healthy community-based programming that helps people with HIV remain active, resilient, and strong.

Demographics
Name: Age: Sex:
Lives with (relationship)
Identified caregiver:
Race: Culture: Religion: —practicing:
Primary occupational roles:
Primary diagnosis:
Secondary diagnosis:
Stage of HIV:
Past medical history:
Medications:

Activities of Daily Living (using ADL performance assessment)
Are you doing these now?
Do you perform homemaking tasks?
For areas of difficulty: Would you like to be able to do these again like you did before? Which ones?

Work
Job: When last worked:
Type of activity at job:
Work environment:
If not working, would you like to be able to?
Do you miss being productive?

Play/Leisure
Types of leisure activities engaged in:

Are you doing these now?
If not, would you like to? Which ones?
Would you like to try other things as well?

Is it important to be independent in daily living activities?

Physical Function
Active and passive range of motion:
Strength:
Sensation:
Coordination (gross and fine motor/dexterity):
Visual/perceptual:
Hearing:
Balance (sit and stand):
Ambulation/transfers/mobility:
Activity tolerance and endurance:
Physical pain:
Location:
Does pain interfere with doing important activities?
Sexual function:

Cognition (attention span, problem solving, memory, orientation, judgment, reasoning, decision-making, safety awareness)

Time Organization
Former daily routine (prior to diagnosis):
Has this changed since diagnosis? If so, how?

Are there certain times of day that are better for you to carry out daily living tasks?

Do you consider yourself regimented in organizing time and activity or pretty flexible?

What would you change if anything in how your day is set up?

Figure 36-1 Pizzi Assessment of Productive Living (PAPL) for adults with HIV infection and AIDS. (Courtesy Michael Pizzi.)

Body Image and Self-Image
In the last six months, has there been a recent change in your physical body and how it looks? How do you feel about this?

Social Environment (Describe support available and utilized by patient)

Physical Environment (Describe environments in which patient performs daily tasks and level of support or impediment for function)

Stressors
What are some things, people, and situations that are or were stressful?
What are some current ways you manage stress?

Situational Coping
How do you feel you are dealing with:
a. Your diagnosis
b. Changes in the ability to do things important to you
c. Other psychosocial observations

Occupational Questions
What do you consider to be important to you right now?

Do you feel you can do things important to you now? In the future?

Do you deal well with change?

What are some of your hopes, dreams, aspirations? What are some of your goals?

Have these changed since you were diagnosed? How?

Do you feel in control of your life at this time?

What do you wish to accomplish with the rest of your life?

Plan:

Short-term goals:

Long-term goals:

Frequency:

Duration:

Therapist:

Figure 36-1 cont'd

CASE STUDY

Mr. J., Part 3

Discussion among team members led to development of a structured and consistent approach that focused on sharing control of timing and choice of activities with Mr. P. The program of care was adapted to his preferences and promoted wellness by making interventions more meaningful to Mr. J.

The physical environment of the hospital was adapted, and items from Mr. J.'s home were brought in to create a more familiar physical space. Throughout the rehabilitation process, the occupational therapist worked with Mr. J.'s partner in his caretaker role. Attention was given to restructuring Mr. F.'s other roles, routines, time management, and activities to diminish his stress level, validate his own caregiving abilities, and work through impending loss of a partner. Mr. F. found these interventions helpful. He also stated that he felt like withdrawing from Mr. J. because of guilty feelings and impending loss. OT helped him focus on positive aspects of life and living.

One month before Mr. J.'s death, his mother, father, and sister visited him. The occupational therapist discussed the rehabilitation program with them; interventions were expanded to meet their needs to assist Mr. J. with his personal care, passive ROM, and work and leisure tasks and to incorporate their support for Mr. J.

Despite Mr. J.'s ability and choice to eat independently, his mother was observed feeding him. In acknowledging her overwhelming need to resume the role of caregiver, a role soon to be

CASE STUDY—cont'd

relinquished, the interventions team continued to learn the lesson of asking, "Whose need is it? Whose need is greater?"

Interventions

Mr. J.'s interventions focused on OT and physical therapy including a balance among self-care, mobility, work, and leisure tasks. The program incorporated rest and his medical regimen including vital signs and IV medications. As much as possible, he was given the opportunity to organize his schedule, which helped him to normalize his routine and incorporate new activities. Mr. J. chose to follow a program of holistic activities that included massage and back rubs, imagery and visualization, therapeutic touch, exercise, balance and gait training, and personal and instrumental ADL. Important leisure and social activities such as listening to classical music, attending plays at the hospital, praying and meditating, reading, working, spending time with loved ones, resting, and sleeping were included. The intervention team included OT and physical therapy, a nurse, a chaplain, a physician, a social worker, a recreation therapist, and Mr. J.'s significant others.

In addition, the OT program included the following:

- Provision of and teaching in use of adaptive equipment (tub bench, handheld shower, built-up handles for utensils, writing adaptations)
- Joint self-ranging, exercise, and upper extremity-strengthening occupations
- Energy conservation
- Development of new leisure tasks and engagement in those formerly enjoyed
- Discussion and activities centered around role changes and adaptation of favored roles (e.g., setting up tasks at bedside to continue his work in banking)
- Family and partner education to develop competence and confidence and to reduce fear in caring for Mr. J.

At the beginning of Mr. J.'s second hospitalization, a home program was designed to give direction, focus, and purpose and to establish goals for his hospitalization. (This is realistic and does not provide false hope to people with HIV because HIV is a process with great variability.)

Although Mr. J. hoped he would be discharged home, he came to accept that it was not possible as his medical condition rapidly worsened. His OT program was adapted accordingly.

At his highest level of function during his 6 weeks of hospitalization, Mr. J. participated in daily exercise, walked to and from therapy, engaged in work-related tasks, and was independent in personal care. At his lowest level of functioning, Mr. J. was positioned for comfort, had classical music at his bedside, and participated in as much personal care as he chose, which occasionally consisted of finger feeding while in bed.

As the nuclear family slowly became involved in Mr. J.'s care, the benefits of an occupation-centered approach were evident. The family restored their own forsaken occupational roles (particularly that of caregiver) and participation in occupations once enjoyed by the entire family assisted in healing old wounds. Open communication and self-expression were facilitated by the restoration of these roles and occupations. Mutual love, forgiveness, and support were shared among all family members, which assisted Mr. J. in envisioning his life as complete. The nuclear family first met Mr. J.'s partner at the bedside, and they immediately supported each other, which eased the loss felt by everyone when Mr. J. died.

Critical Thinking Questions

When a patient's functional abilities vary from day to day and decline, the OT practitioner must modify interventions to match the person's abilities. Identify several instances of such modifications in the case of Mr. J.

Summary

As highlighted by the following case study, OTAs have an important role in intervention sessions and may develop activities to promote health and well-being for people with HIV. OTAs must remember the guidelines set forth in this chapter and implement them without judgment, stigma, or discrimination. Communication with the occupational therapist on a consistent basis including asking questions or voicing concerns about safety and universal precautions while continuing to be client and occupation centered should be continuous. Maintaining an occupation-centered and client-centered approach to care will enhance health and well-being and promote a positive way of coping with HIV. This will ultimately help people with HIV/AIDS improve their quality of life, transition better and live productively in the community, enable active occupational participation, and live longer, successful lives.

Selected Reading Guide Questions

1. Describe the stages of HIV disease relative to their impact on occupational performance.
2. Describe the physical, psychosocial, and environmental factors to consider when working with adults with HIV.
3. Discuss the contextual considerations when implementing interventions.
4. Describe and discuss several themes related to OT intervention when working with people with HIV.
5. Describe and explain various interventions used in OT when working with adults with HIV, using the OT practice framework to guide you.
6. Discuss and explain how wellness approaches in OT guide clinical interventions for adults with HIV. How might you develop a wellness and prevention program for this population?

References

1. American Occupational Therapy Association: *Occupational therapy practice framework: domain and process*, ed 2, Bethesda, Md: Author, 2008. Available to AOTA members via website. http://www.aota.org/.
2. Centers for Disease Control (CDC): *Fact sheets*, http://www.cdc.gov/hiv/resources/factsheets/us.htm. Retrieved from, September 17, 2010.
3. Meyer A: The philosophy of occupation therapy, *Arch Occup Ther* 1:1, 1922. (Also in *Am J Occup Ther* 31(10):639-642, 1977).
4. Pizzi M: Nationally speaking: the transformation of HIV infection and AIDS in occupational therapy: beginning the conversation, *Am J Occup Ther* 44(3):1–5, 1990.
5. Pizzi M: The model of human occupation and adults with HIV infection and AIDS, *Am J Occup Ther* 44(3):42–49, 1990.
6. Pizzi, M., Reitz, S.M. & Scaffa, M.E: Wellness and health promotion for people with physical disabilities. In Pedretti's *Occupational therapy for physical dysfunction*, ed 6, Pendleton and Schultz-Krohn (editors), St Louis, Elsevier, 2006.
7. Scaffa ME, Reitz SM, Pizzi MA: *Occupational therapy in the promotion of health and wellness*, Philadelphia, 2010, FA Davis.
8. World Health Organization: *International classification of functioning, disability, and health (ICF)* Geneva, 2001a, Author. Available on the webhttp://www.who.int/classifications/icf/en/2001a.
9. *World Health Organization (WHO)*:Retrieved September 17, 2010 from http://www.who.int/mediacentre/news/releases/2009/hiv_aids_20091124/en/index.html.

Recommended Reading

Barrett HR: Women, occupation and health in rural Africa: adaptation to a changing socioeconomic climate, *J Occup Sci Australia* 4:93–105, 1977.

Bedell G: Daily life for eight urban gay men with HIV/AIDS, *Am J Occup Ther* 54:197–206, 2000.

Braveman BH: Development of a community-based return to work program for people with AIDS, *Occup Ther Health Care* 13(3/4):113–131, 2001.

Galantino ML, Pizzi M: Occupational and physical therapy for persons with HIV disease and their caregivers, *J Home Health Care Practice* 3(3):46–57, 1991.

Kielhofner G, Braveman B, Finlayson M, et al: Outcomes of a vocational program for persons with AIDS, *Am J Occup Ther* 58(1):64–72, 2004.

Phillips I: Occupational therapy students explore an area for future practice in HIV/AIDS community wellness, *AIDS Patient Care STDS* 16:147–149, 2002.

Pizzi M, editor: Special issue of the *Am J Occup Ther HIV AIDS*, 44(3), 1990.

Pizzi M: *HIV infection and AIDS: a professional's guide to wellness, health and productive living*, Silver Spring, Md, 1996, Positive Images and Wellness.

Pizzi M: Women and AIDS, *Am J Occup Ther* 46(11):1021–1026, 1992.

Pizzi M: Occupational therapy: creating possibilities for adults with HIV infection, ARC, and AIDS, *AIDS Patient Care* 3:18–23, 1989.

Pizzi M: Adaptive human performance and HIV infection: considerations for therapists. In Galantino ML, editor: *Clinical assessment and interventions in HIV: rehabilitation of a chronic illness*, Thorofare, NJ, 1991, Slack.

Pizzi M, Hinds-Harris M: Infants and children with HIV infection: perspectives in occupational and physical therapy. In Pizzi M, Johnson J, editors: *Productive living strategies for people with AIDS*, New York, 1990, Haworth Press.

Pizzi M, et al: HIV infection and occupational therapy. In Mukand J, editor: *Rehabilitation for patients with HIV disease*, New York, 1991, McGraw-Hill.

Schindler V: Psychosocial occupational therapy intervention with AIDS patients, *Am J Occup Ther* 42:507–512, 1988.

Spence DW, et al: Progressive resistance exercise: effect on muscle function and anthropometry of a select AIDS population, *Arch Phys Med Rehabil* 71:644–648, 1990.

Solomon GF, et al: An intensive psychoimmunologic study of long surviving persons with AIDS, *Ann New York Acad Sci* 496:647–655, 1987.

Villarino ME, et al: AIDS, infection control and employee health: considerations in rehabilitation medicine. In Munkand J, editor: *Rehabilitation for patients with HIV disease*, New York, 1991, McGraw-Hill.

Websites

AIDS Education and Training Centers National Resource Center
http://www.aidsetc.org/aidsetc?page=home-00-00
Resources including PowerPoint slides, CDs, and educational handouts

Centers for Disease Control
http://www.cdc.gov/hiv/default.htm
Provides most updated information about HIV/AIDS and programming for the disease including prevention guides, brochures, and slides

World Health Organization (WHO)
http://www.who.int/hiv/en/
Provides updated information on HIV from an international perspective

Index

A

Page numbers followed by *f* indicate figures; *b,* boxes; *t,* tables.

C

D

E

F

G

N

T